CORONARY ARTERY
MEDICINE AND SURGERY

CORONARY ARTERY MEDICINE AND SURGERY
Concepts and Controversies

Editor:

John C. Norman, M.D.

Director, Cardiovascular Surgical Research Laboratories, Texas Heart Institute; Clinical Professor of Cardiothoracic Surgery, University of Texas (UTSA); Clinical Associate in Surgery, Texas Heart Institute of St. Luke's Episcopal and Texas Children's Hospitals, Houston, Texas

Assistant Editor:

Evelyn P. Lawrence, B.A.

Editorial Assistant to the Cardiovascular Surgical Research Laboratories, Texas Heart Institute of St. Luke's Episcopal and Texas Children's Hospitals, Houston, Texas

Foreword by

Theodore Cooper, M.D.

Deputy Assistant Secretary of Health; formerly Director, National Heart and Lung Institute, National Institutes of Health, Bethesda, Maryland

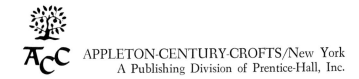

APPLETON-CENTURY-CROFTS/New York
A Publishing Division of Prentice-Hall, Inc.

LIBRARY OF CONGRESS CATALOGING IN PUBLICATION DATA
Main entry under title:

Coronary artery medicine and surgery.

     1. Coronary heart disease. 2. Aortocoronary
bypass. I. Norman, John C. [DNLM: 1. Coronary
disease—Congresses. 2. Coronary disease—Surgery—
Congresses. WG300 C821 1973]
RC685.C6C633   616.1'23   75-15891
ISBN 0-8385-1206-2

Prentice-Hall International, Inc., London
Prentice-Hall of Australia, Pty. Ltd., Sydney
Prentice-Hall of India Private Limited, New Delhi
Prentice-Hall of Japan, Inc., Tokyo
Prentice-Hall of Southeast Asia (Pte.) Ltd., Singapore

PRINTED IN THE UNITED STATES OF AMERICA

To Doris, Jill, Annemarie, sabrina, hither, and yonnie.

Contributors

WALTER H. ABLEMANN, M.D.
Professor of Medicine, Department of Medicine, Harvard Medical School, and Chief of Cardiology, Department of Cardiology, Beth Israel Hospital, Boston, Massachusetts

MAHDI S. AL-BASSAM, M.D.
Division of Cardiology, the Texas Heart Institute of St. Luke's Episcopal and Texas Children's Hospitals, and the Clayton Foundation Exercise and Non-invasive Laboratory, Houston, Texas

HAROLD ALDRIDGE, M.B.
Cardiovascular Unit, Toronto General Hospital, and Associate Professor of Medicine, Department of Medicine, the University of Toronto Faculty of Medicine, Toronto, Ontario, Canada

JAMES K. ALEXANDER, M.D.
Professor of Medicine, Baylor College of Medicine and Baylor Affiliated Hospitals, Houston, Texas

DAVID ALLEN, Ph.D.
Instructor of Pharmaceutical Sciences and Radiology, Division of Nuclear Medicine, Department of Medicine, Seattle Veterans Administration Hospital and the University of Washington School of Medicine, Seattle, Washington

FIROUZ AMIRPARVIZ, M.D.
Clinical Instructor, Department of Medicine, Loyola University of Chicago Stritch School of Medicine, Maywood, Illinois

KURT AMPLATZ, M.D.
Professor of Radiology, Department of Radiology, University of Minnesota Medical School and Affiliated Hospitals

EZRA A. AMSTERDAM, M.D.
Associate Professor of Medicine, Chief of Coronary Care Unit, Section of Cardiovascular Medicine, Department of Medicine, University of California at Davis, School of Medicine, Davis, California

RICHARD P. ANDERSON, M.D.
Associate Professor of Cardiopulmonary Surgery, Division of Cardiopulmonary Surgery, Department of Surgery, University of Oregon Medical School, Portland, Oregon

PAOLO ANGELINI, M.D.
Division of Cardiology, the Texas Heart Institute of St. Luke's Episcopal and Texas Children's Hospitals, Houston, Texas

WILLIAM W. ANGELL, M.D.
Chief of Cardiac Surgery, Cardiovascular Surgery Service, Palo Alto Veterans Administration Hospital, Palo Alto, California; Clinical Assistant Professor of Surgery, Department of Surgery, Stanford University School of Medicine, Stanford, California

CARL S. APSTEIN, M.D.
Assistant Professor of Medicine, Department of Medicine, Boston University School of Medicine; Director, Non-invasive Laboratories, Boston City Hospital, Boston, Massachusetts

DJAVAD ARANI, M.D.
Departments of General Surgery and Medicine, State University of New York at Buffalo School of Medicine and Buffalo General Hospital, Buffalo, New York

ROSTAM G. ARDEKANI, M.D.
Assistant Professor of Surgery, Division of Cardiovascular and Thoracic Surgery, the Abraham Lincoln School of Medicine, University of Illinois, and Cook County Hospital, Chicago, Illinois

RAYMOND G. ARMSTRONG, Col., USAF, MC
Thoracic Surgery Service, Wilford Hall United States Air Force Medical Center, Lackland Air Force Base, Texas

WILBERT S. ARONOW, M.D.
Adjunct Associate Professor, Department of Medicine, University of California at Irvine, Irvine, California, and Veterans Administration Hospital, Long Beach, California

STEPHEN M. AYRES, M.D.
Physician-in-Chief, St. Vincent Hospital, Worcester, Massachusetts; Professor of Medicine, University of Massachusetts Medical School, Worcester, Massachusetts

ROBERT C. BAHLER, M.D.
Assistant Professor of Medicine, Department of Medicine, Case Western Reserve University, and Cleveland Metropolitan General Hospital, Cleveland, Ohio

HENRY T. BAHNSON, M.D.
Professor and Chairman, Department of Surgery, the University of Pittsburgh School of Medicine, Pittsburgh, Pennsylvania

HAROLD A. BALTAXE, M.D.
Associate Professor in Radiology, Department of Radiology, the New York Hospital–Cornell Medical Center, New York, New York

BICHER BARMADA, M.D.
Arizona Heart Institute, St. Joseph's Hospital and Medical Center, Phoenix, Arizona

HENDRICK B. BARNER, M.D.
Professor of Surgery, Department of Surgery, St. Louis University, St. Louis, Missouri

F. R. BEGG, M.D.
Clinical Assistant Professor of Medicine, Department of Medicine, University of Pittsburgh School of Medicine and Allegheny General Hospital, Pittsburgh, Pennsylvania

LINDA A. BEGLEY, R.N., B.S.
Tufts University School of Medicine and Boston City Hospital, Boston, Massachusetts

ARTHUR R. BEIL, JR., M.D.
Associate Professor of Surgery, Department of Surgery, North Shore Hospital, Cornell University Medical Center, Manhasset, New York

SETH BEKOE, M.D.
Department of Thoracic Surgery, Allegheny General Hospital, Pittsburgh, Pennsylvania

RAYMOND BELANGER, M.D.
Department of Thoracic and Cardiovascular Surgery, Baylor University Medical Center, Dallas, Texas

PHILIP S. BERGER, M.S.E.E.
Division of Cardiothoracic Surgery, Department of Surgery, and the Biomedical Computer Laboratory, Washington University School of Medicine, St. Louis, Missouri

GEORGE E. BERK, M.D.
Division of Cardiology, North Shore Hospital and Cornell University Medical Center, Manhasset, New York

J. M. BHAYANA, M.D.
Veterans Administration Hospital, Oteen, North Carolina

WILLIAM C. BIRTWELL, B.S.
Associate Professor of Surgery (Electrical Engineering), Tufts University School of Medicine and Boston City Hospital, Boston, Massachusetts

JOE BISSETT, M.D.
Assistant Professor of Medicine, Department of Medicine, University of Arkansas School of Medicine and Veterans Administration Hospital, Little Rock, Arkansas

DAVID H. BLANKENHORN, M.D.
Professor and Chairman, Division of Cardiology, Department of Medicine, University of Southern California School of Medicine, Los Angeles, California; Rancho Los Amigos Hospital, Downey, California

ROBERT D. BLOODWELL, M.D.
Cardiovascular and Thoracic Surgery, Orlando and Winter Park, Florida

HOOSHANG BOLOOKI, M.D., F.R.C.S.(C)
Associate Professor of Surgery, Divisions of Thoracic and Cardiovascular Surgery, Department of Surgery, University of Miami School of Medicine, Miami, Florida

JOSEPH BONANNO, M.D.
Assistant Professor of Medicine, Section of Cardiology, Department of Medicine, University of California at Davis, School of Medicine, Davis, California

LAWRENCE I. BONCHEK, M.D.
Assistant Professor of Cardiopulmonary Surgery, Division of Cardiopulmonary Surgery, Department of Surgery, University of Oregon Medical School, Portland, Oregon

IRWIN B. BORUCHOW, M.D.
Assistant Director, St. Francis Hospital Cardiovascular Center, St. Francis Hospital, Miami Beach, Florida

FREDERICK O. BOWMAN, JR., M.D.
Associate Professor of Clinical Surgery, Department of Surgery, Columbia University College of Physicians and Surgeons, New York, New York

NORMAN BRACHFELD, M.D.
Associate Professor of Medicine, Department of Medicine, the New York Hospital–Cornell Medical Center, New York, New York

DAVID BREGMAN, M.D.
Assistant Professor of Surgery, Department of Surgery, Columbia University College of Physicians and Surgeons, Columbia-Presbyterian Medical Center, New York, New York

J. DAVID BRISTOW, M.D.
Professor and Chairman, Department of Medicine, University of Oregon Medical School, Portland, Oregon

WILLIAM R. BRODY, M.D., Ph.D.
National Heart and Lung Institute, Bethesda, Maryland

IVAN L. BUNNELL, M.D.
Associate Professor of Medicine, Department of Medicine, State University of New York at Buffalo and Buffalo General Hospital, Buffalo, New York

J. P. BYRNE, M.D.
Department of Surgery, University of Utah College of Medicine, Salt Lake City, Utah

ROBERT CAPONE, M.D.
Division of Cardio-Thoracic Surgery, Department of Surgery, Brown University and Rhode Island Hospital, Providence, Rhode Island

ROBERT G. CARLSON, M.D.
Assistant Professor of Surgery, Division of Thoracic and Cardiovascular Surgery, Department of Surgery, the New York Hospital–Cornell Medical Center, New York, New York

CRISTOPHER CAUDILL, M.D.
Section of Cardiology, Department of Medicine, University of California at Davis, School of Medicine, Davis, California

FRANK B. CERRA, M.D.
Clinical Assistant Instructor in Surgery, Department of Surgery, State University of New York at Buffalo and Buffalo General Hospital, Buffalo, New York

E. J. P. CHARRETTE, F.R.C.S.(C)
Associate Professor of Surgery, Division of Cardiovascular and Thoracic Surgery, Department of Surgery, Queen's University Faculty of Medicine, Kingston, Ontario, Canada

KANU CHATTERJEE, M.B., M.R.C.P. (London and Edinburgh), F.A.C.P.
Associate Professor of Medicine, Department of Cardiology, Cedars–Sinai Medical Center, Department of Medicine, UCLA School of Medicine, Los Angeles, California

SHEKHAR CHATTERJEE, M.D., M.Sc., F.R.C.S.(C)
Assistant Professor of Surgery, Mount Sinai Hospital and the University of Connecticut Health Center School of Medicine, Hartford, Connecticut

LUIGI CHIARIELLO, M.D.
Cardiovascular Surgical Fellow, Department of Surgery, Texas Heart Institute of St. Luke's Episcopal and Texas Children's Hospitals, Houston, Texas

H. P. CHIN, Ph.D.
Assistant Professor of Medicine, Cardiology Section, Department of Medicine, University of Southern California School of Medicine, Los Angeles, California; Rancho Los Amigos Hospital, Downey, California

RAY C. J. CHIU, M.D., Ph.D., F.R.C.S.(C), F.A.C.S.
Assistant Professor and Scholar of the MRC of Canada, Division of Cardiovascular and Thoracic Surgery, Department of Surgery, McGill University Faculty of Medicine, McIntyre Medical Sciences Center, Montreal, Quebec, Canada

JAMES CHRISTODOULOU, M.D.
Division of Cardiology, Department of Medicine, the New York Hospital–Cornell Medical Center, New York, New York

DAVID A. CLARK, M.D.
Western Heart Associates, Assistant Chief of Cardiology, Santa Clara Valley Medical Center, San Jose, California; Clinical Instructor, Department of Medicine, Stanford University School of Medicine, Stanford, California

DIANE K. CLARK, B.S., C.C.P.
Associate Director, School of Perfusion Technology, Perfusion Technology Section and Division of Surgery, Texas Heart Institute of St. Luke's Episcopal Hospital, Houston, Texas

RICHARD E. CLARK, M.D.
Associate Professor of Surgery, Division of Cardiothoracic Surgery, Department of Surgery; Biomedical Computer Laboratory, Washington University School of Medicine, St. Louis, Missouri

ROBERT E. CLINE, Lt. Col., USAF, MC
Thoracic Surgery Service, Wilford Hall United States Air Force Medical Center, Lackland Air Force Base, Texas

WILLIAM B. CLINE, B.A.
Department of Pathology, West Virginia University Medical Center, Morgantown, West Virginia

CHARLES T. CLOUTIER, Cmdr., USN, MC
Chief, Clinical Investigation Service, Naval Regional Medical Center, Philadelphia, Pennsylvania

JOSEPH D. COHN, M.D.
Chief, Physiology Service, Saint Barnabas Medical Center, Livingston, New Jersey; Clinical Professor of Surgery, Department of Surgery, College of Medicine and Dentistry at Newark, Newark, New Jersey

LAWRENCE H. COHN, M.D.
Assistant Professor of Surgery, Department of Surgery, Harvard Medical School; Division of Thoracic and Cardiovascular Surgery, Peter Bent Brigham Hospital, Boston, Massachusetts

JOHN J. COLLINS, JR., M.D.
Associate Professor of Surgery, Department of Surgery, Harvard Medical School, and Chief, Division of Thoracic and Cardiovascular Surgery, Peter Bent Brigham Hospital, Boston, Massachusetts

MARILYN A. COLOMBO
Department of Medicine, Boston University School of Medicine, Boston, Massachusetts

JOHN E. CONNOLLY, M.D.
Professor and Chairman, Department of Surgery, University of California at Irvine College of Medicine, Irvine, California; Veterans Administration Hospital, Long Beach, California

DENTON A. COOLEY, M.D.
Surgeon-in-Chief, Texas Heart Institute of St. Luke's Episcopal and Texas Children's Hospitals, Texas Medical Center, Houston, Texas

GEORGE N. COOPER, JR., M.D.
Assistant Professor of Surgery, Department of Surgery, Brown University Medical School, Providence, Rhode Island

ELIOT CORDAY, M.D.
Clinical Professor of Medicine, Department of Medicine, UCLA School of Medicine; Cedars–Sinai Medical Center, Cedars of Lebanon Hospital Division, Los Angeles, California

LUIS E. CORTES, M.D.
Clinical Instructor, Department of Surgery, New York University Medical Center School of Medicine, New York, New York

COSTANTINO COSTANTINI, M.D.
Research Fellow, Cedars–Sinai Medical Center, Cedars of Lebanon Hospital Division, Los Angeles, California

RICHARD S. CRAMPTON, M.D.
Associate Professor of Medicine, Department of Medicine, University of Virginia School of Medicine, Charlottesville, Virginia

GEORGE CURRY, M.D.
Associate Professor of Radiology, Department of Radiology, the University of Texas Health Science Center at Dallas, Southwestern Medical School, Dallas, Texas

BENEDICT D. T. DALY, M.D.
Sylvia R. Herring Scholar in Academic Thoracic and Cardiovascular Surgery, Cardiovascular Surgical Research Laboratories, Texas Heart Institute of St. Luke's Episcopal and Texas Children's Hospitals, Houston, Texas

JOHN T. DAWSON, M.D.
Division of Cardiology, Texas Heart Institute of St. Luke's Episcopal and Texas Children's Hospitals; the Clayton Foundation Exercise and Non-invasive Laboratory, Houston, Texas

DAVID G. DeCOCK, M.D.
Assistant Instructor in Surgery, Division of Thoracic-Cardiovascular Surgery, Department of Surgery, the Medical College of Wisconsin and Affiliated Hospitals, Milwaukee, Wisconsin

LOUIS R. M. DEL GUERCIO, M.D.
Director of Surgery, Saint Barnabas Medical Center, Livingston, New Jersey; Clinical Professor of Surgery, College of Medicine and Dentistry of New Jersey at Newark, Newark, New Jersey

HENRY DeMOTS, M.D.
Fellow in Cardiology, Division of Cardiology, Department of Medicine, University of Oregon Medical School, Portland, Oregon

KATHERINE M. DETRE, M.D., Ph.D.
Veterans Administration Cooperative Studies Center, West Haven, Connecticut; Department of Epidemiology, University of Pittsburgh, Pittsburgh, Pennsylvania

EDWARD B. DIETHRICH, M.D.
Director, Arizona Heart Institute, St. Joseph's Hospital and Medical Center, Phoenix, Arizona

MARGARET F. DiMODICA
Department of Medicine, Boston University School of Medicine, Boston Massachusetts

JAMES E. DOHERTY, M.D.
Professor and Chairman, Division of Cardiology, Department of Medicine, the University of Arkansas School of Medicine and Veterans Administration Hospital, Little Rock, Arkansas

ROBERT C. DUNCAN, Ph.D.
Associate Professor of Biometry, Cardiovascular Division, Department of Medicine, Medical University of South Carolina College of Medicine, Charleston, South Carolina

EDWARD F. DUNNE, M.D.
Divisions of Thoracic and Cardiovascular Surgery, Department of Surgery, the University of Southern California School of Medicine, Los Angeles, California

PAUL A. EBERT, M.D.
Professor and Chairman, Department of Surgery, the University of California at San Francisco, San Francisco, California

R. R. ECKER, M.D.
Division of Thoracic and Cardiovascular Surgery, Department of Surgery, and the Pauline and Adolph Weinberger Laboratory for Cardiac Research, the University of Texas Health Science Center at Dallas Southwestern Medical School, Dallas, Texas

RICHARD N. EDIE, M.D.
Assistant Professor, Department of Surgery, Columbia University College of Physicians and Surgeons and Surgical Service, Presbyterian Hospital, New York, New York

W. E. ELZINGA, Ph.D.
Associate Professor, Department of Mathematical Sciences, the Johns Hopkins University, Baltimore, Maryland

ROBERT ERLANDSON, Ph.D.
Department of Medicine, the New York Hospital–Cornell Medical Center, New York, New York

ROBERT G. EVANS, B.A.
Research Associate, Division of Cardiology, Department of Medicine, the St. Vincent Hospital, Worcester, Massachusetts

GORDON A. EWY, M.D.
Associate Professor of Internal Medicine, the University of Arizona College of Medicine, Tucson, Arizona

HENRY M. FARIS, JR., M.D.
Cardiovascular Division, Department of Medicine, Medical University of South Carolina College of Medicine, Charleston, South Carolina

HAROLD FEINBERG, Ph.D.
Department of Surgery, the Abraham Lincoln School of Medicine, and Department of Pharmacology, School of Basic Medical Sciences at the Medical Center, University of Illinois College of Medicine, Chicago, Illinois

THOMAS B. FERGUSON, M.D.
Clinical Professor of Surgery, Division of Cardiothoracic Surgery, Department of Surgery, Washington University School of Medicine, St. Louis, Missouri

J. FERNANDEZ, M.D.
The Deborah Heart and Lung Center, Browns Mills, New Jersey; Temple University Hospital of the Commonwealth System of Higher Education School of Medicine, Philadelphia, Pennsylvania

ROBERT J. FLEMMA, M.D.
Associate Clinical Professor of Thoracic and Cardiovascular Surgery, the Medical College of Wisconsin and Affiliated Hospitals, Milwaukee, Wisconsin

ATHANASIOS FLESSAS, M.D.
Physician in Charge, Hemodynamic Laboratory, University Hospital, and Assistant Professor of Medicine, Boston University School of Medicine, Boston, Massachusetts

JAMES S. FORRESTER, M.D.
Adjunct Assistant Professor of Medicine, Department of Medicine, UCLA School of Medicine; Department of Cardiology, Cedars–Sinai Medical Center, Cedars of Lebanon Hospital Division, Los Angeles, California

ARTHUR C. FOX, M.D.
Professor and Chairman, Department of Medicine, New York University Medical Center School of Medicine, New York, New York

STEPHEN L. FRANTZ, M.D.
Assistant Professor of Surgery, Department of Thoracic and Cardiovascular Surgery, Department of Surgery, North Shore Hospital, Manhasset, New York; Cornell University Medical College, New York, New York

ANDREW J. FRANZONE, M.D.
Lenox Hill Hospital, New York, New York

R.W.M. FRATER, M.D., F.R.C.S.
Professor and Chairman, Department of Surgery, Albert Einstein College of Medicine of Yeshiva University, Bronx, New York

ADRIANNE FRIED, R.N.
Division of Thoracic and Cardiovascular Surgery, Department of Surgery, and Cardiovascular Laboratories, Jackson Memorial Hospital, University of Miami School of Medicine, Miami, Florida

VINCENT E. FRIEDEWALD, M.D.
Department of Cardiology, Arizona Heart Institute, St. Joseph's Hospital and Medical Center, Phoenix, Arizona

JOHN FRIEDMAN, B.A.
Cedars-Sinai Medical Center, Cedars of Lebanon Hospital Division, UCLA School of Medicine, Los Angeles, California

WILLIAM H. FRISHMAN, M.D.
Division of Cardiology, Department of Medicine, the New York Hospital–Cornell Medical Center, New York, New York

JOEL E. FUTRAL, M.D.
Department of Cardiology, Arizona Heart Institute, St. Joseph's Hospital and Medical Center, Phoenix, Arizona

WILLIAM H. GAASCH, M.D.
Assistant Professor of Medicine and Director, Cardiology Non-invasive Laboratory, Tufts New England Medical Center Hospital, Boston, Massachusetts

ROGER GABRIEL, P.A.
Division of Thoracic-Cardiovascular Surgery, Department of Surgery, the Medical College of Wisconsin and Affiliated Hospitals, Milwaukee, Wisconsin

RAJ K. GANDHI, M.D.
Department of Surgery, North Shore Hospital, Manhasset, New York; Department of Surgery, Cornell University Medical College, New York, New York

EFRAIN GARCIA, M.D.
Director, Clayton Foundation Exercise and Non-invasive Laboratory, and Division of Cardiology, the Texas Heart Institute of St. Luke's Episcopal and Texas Children's Hospitals, Houston, Texas

ROBERT J. GARDNER, M.D.
Associate Professor of Surgery, Department of Surgery, West Virginia University, Morgantown, West Virginia

WILLIAM A. GAY, JR., M.D.
Assistant Professor of Surgery, Department of Surgery, the New York Hospital–Cornell Medical Center, New York, New York

PETER C. GAZES, M.D.
Professor of Medicine and Director, Cardiovascular Division, Department of Medicine, Medical University of South Carolina College of Medicine, Charleston, South Carolina

PETER W. GEIS, M.D.
Assistant Professor of Surgery and Chief, Section of Transplantation, Department of Surgery, Loyola University Stritch School of Medicine, Maywood, Illinois

ALI GHAHRAMANI, M.D.
Division of Thoracic and Cardiovascular Surgery, Department of Surgery; Cardiovascular Laboratories, Jackson Memorial Hospital, University of Miami School of Medicine, Miami, Florida

ISAAC GIELCHINSKY, M.D.
Assistant Director of Cardiac and Thoracic Surgery, Department of Surgery, Newark Beth Israel Medical Center, and Assistant Professor of Surgery, College of Medicine and Dentistry of New Jersey–New Jersey Medical School, Newark, New Jersey

LAWRENCE GILBERT, M.D.
Director of Cardiac and Thoracic Surgery, Department of Surgery, Newark Beth Israel Medical Center, and Associate Professor of Surgery, College of Medicine and Dentistry of New Jersey–New Jersey Medical School, Newark, New Jersey

EPHRAIM GLASSMAN, M.D.
Associate Professor of Medicine, Department of Medicine, New York University Medical Center School of Medicine, New York, New York

JAMES A. L. GLENN, M.D.
Cardiovascular Division, Department of Medicine, Medical University of South Carolina College of Medicine, Charleston, South Carolina

HERBERT GOLD, M.D.
Associate Clinical Professor of Medicine, Department of Medicine, UCLA School of Medicine, Los Angeles, California

DAVID GOLDFARB, M.D.
Department of Cardiovascular Surgery, Arizona Heart Institute, St. Joseph's Hospital and Medical Center, Phoenix, Arizona

BERNARD GOLDMAN, M.D.
Assistant Professor of Surgery, Cardiovascular Unit, Toronto General Hospital, the University of Toronto Faculty of Medicine, Toronto, Ontario, Canada

LANCE GOULD, M.D.
Assistant Professor of Medicine, Department of Medicine, University of Washington School of Medicine, and the Veteran's Administration Hospital, Seattle, Washington

YOUSEF GOUSSOUS, M.D.
The Clayton Foundation Exercise and Non-invasive Laboratory; Division of Cardiology, the Texas Heart Institute of St. Luke's Episcopal and Texas Children's Hospitals, Houston, Texas

DAVID G. GREENE, M.D.
Professor of Medicine and Associate Professor of Physiology, Department of Medicine, State University of New York at Buffalo and the Buffalo General Hospital, Buffalo, New York

HARVEY GREENFIELD, Ph.D.
Associate Research Professor of Computer Science, Division of Artificial Organs, Department of Surgery, University of Utah College of Medicine, Salt Lake City, Utah

S. R. GREENHALGH, B.S.
Division of Artificial Organs, Department of Surgery, University of Utah College of Medicine, Salt Lake City, Utah

STANLEY GROSS, M.D.
Director of Laboratories, North Shore Hospital, Manhasset, New York; Clinical Associate Professor of Pathology, Department of Pathology, Cornell University Medical College, New York, New York

BERTRON M. GROVES, M.D.
Assistant Professor of Medicine, Section of Cardiology, Department of Internal Medicine, University of Arizona College of Medicine, Tucson, Arizona

STEPHEN J. GULOTTA, M.D.
Division of Cardiology, Department of Medicine, North Shore Hospital, Manhasset, New York; Associate Professor of Medicine, Cornell University Medical College, New York, New York

ROLF M. GUNNAR, M.D.
Professor of Medicine and Chief, Section of Cardiology, Department of Medicine, Loyola University Stritch School of Medicine, Maywood, Illinois

EUGENE P. HADDOCK, M.D.
Department of Medicine, University of Pittsburgh School of Medicine, Pittsburgh, Pennsylvania

KENNETH G. HAGEN, M.S.
Thermo Electron Corporation Research and Development Center, Waltham, Massachusetts

RONALD W. HAGEN, M.S.E.E.
Biomedical Computer Laboratory, Washington University School of Medicine, St. Louis, Missouri

PETER HAIRSTON, M.D.
Associate Professor, Division of Thoracic Surgery, Department of Surgery, Medical University of South Carolina, Charleston, South Carolina

MILTON R. HALES, M.D.
Professor and Chairman, Department of Pathology, West Virginia University Medical Center, Morgantown, West Virginia

ROBERT J. HALL, M.D.
Director, Division of Cardiology, and Medical Director, Texas Heart Institute of St. Luke's Episcopal and Texas Children's Hospitals, Houston, Texas

GRADY L. HALLMAN, M.D.
Division of Surgery, Texas Heart Institute of St. Luke's Episcopal and Texas Children's Hospital, Houston, Texas

GLEN W. HAMILTON, M.D.
Chief, Nuclear Medicine, Veterans Administration Hospital, Seattle, Washington

KARL E. HAMMERMEISTER, M.D.
Assistant Chief of Cardiology, Veterans Administration Hospital, and Assistant Professor of Medicine, the University of Washington School of Medicine, Seattle, Washington

GRAEME L. HAMMOND, M.D.
Associate Professor of Surgery, Cardiothoracic Division, Department of Surgery, Yale University School of Medicine; Cardiothoracic Surgical Service, Yale–New Haven Hospital, New Haven, Connecticut

PAUL K. HANASHIRO, M.D.
Assistant Professor of Medicine, Cardiology Section, Department of Medicine, University of Southern California School of Medicine, Los Angeles, California; Rancho Los Amigos Hospital, Downey, California

E. LAWRENCE HANSON, M.D.
Department of Surgery, State University of New York Upstate Medical Center College of Medicine, Syracuse, New York

HAROLD HASTON, M.D.
Queen's Medical Center, University of Hawaii School of Medicine, Honolulu, Hawaii

W. CHARLES HELTON, M.D.
University of Minnesota Hospitals of the University of Minnesota Health Sciences Center, Minneapolis, Minnesota

E. J. HERSHGOLD, M.D.
Associate Professor of Medicine, Department of Internal Medicine, University of Utah College of Medicine Medical Center, Salt Lake City, Utah

GENERAL K. HILLIARD, M.D.
Assistant Clinical Professor, Section of Cardiology, Department of Medicine, University of California at Davis, School of Medicine, Davis, California

WILLIAM HOLLANDER, M.D.
Professor of Medicine, Department of Medicine, Boston University School of Medicine, Boston, Massachusetts

WILLIAM B. HOOD, JR., M.D.
Professor of Medicine, Department of Medicine, Boston University School of Medicine; Chief of Cardiology, Boston City Hospital, and Thorndike Memorial and Sears Surgical Laboratories, Boston, Massachusetts

JOHN HORNUNG, M.D.
University of Minnesota Hospitals of the University of Minnesota Health Sciences Center, Minneapolis, Minnesota

FRED N. HUFFMAN, Ph.D.
Project Manager, Thermo Electron Corporation Research and Development Center, Waltham, Massachusetts

DAVID A. HUGHES, M.D.
Mary A. Fraley Fellow in Cardiovascular Surgical Research, Cardiovascular Surgical Research Laboratories, Texas Heart Institute of St. Luke's Episcopal and Texas Children's Hospitals, Houston, Texas

HERBERT N. HULTGREN, M.D.
Chief of Cardiology Service, Veterans Administration Hospital, Palo Alto, California; Professor of Medicine, Department of Medicine, Stanford University School of Medicine, Stanford, California

G. BADGER HUMPHRIES, M.D.
Cardiovascular Division, Department of Medicine, Medical University of South Carolina, Charleston, South Carolina

EDWARD J. HURLEY, M.D.
Professor of Surgery and Chairman, Section of Thoracic Surgery, Department of Surgery, University of California at Davis, School of Medicine, Davis, California; Sacramento Medical Center of the University of California at Davis, Sacramento, California

ALBERT B. IBEN, M.D.
Associate Professor of Surgery, University of California at Davis, School of Medicine, Davis, California; Sacramento Medical Center of the University of California at Davis, Sacramento, California

STEPHEN R. IGO
Research Associate, Cardiovascular Surgical Research Laboratories, Texas Heart Institute of St. Luke's Episcopal and Texas Children's Hospitals, Houston, Texas

C. K. S. IYENGAR, F.R.C.P.(C)
Division of Cardiovascular and Thoracic Surgery, Department of Surgery, Queen's University Faculty of Medicine, Kingston, Ontario, Canada

RAMANUJA IYENGAR, M.D.
Director, Cardiac Catheterization Laboratory, St. Francis Hospital Cardiovascular Center, St. Francis Hospital, Miami Beach, Florida

S.R.K. IYENGAR, F.R.C.S.(C)
Assistant Professor of Surgery, Division of Cardiovascular and Thoracic Surgery, Department of Surgery, Queen's University Faculty of Medicine, Kingston, Ontario, Canada

DOV JARON, Ph.D.
Associate Professor, Department of Electrical Engineering, University of Rhode Island, Providence, Rhode Island

FREDERICK W. JOHNSON, M.D.
University of Minnesota Hospitals of the University of Minnesota Health Sciences Center, Minneapolis, Minnesota

CLAUDE R. JOYNER, M.D.
Chief of Medicine, Division of Cardiovascular Disease, Department of Medicine, Allegheny General Hospital, and Clinical Professor of Medicine, Department of Medicine, University of Pittsburgh School of Medicine, Pittsburgh, Pennsylvania

JAMES R. JUDE, M.D.
Director, St. Francis Hospital Cardiovascular Center, St. Francis Hospital, Miami Beach, Florida; Clinical Professor of Surgery, University of Miami School of Medicine, Miami, Florida

A. H. KAHN, M.D.
Assistant Clinical Professor of Medicine, Cardiology Section, Department of Medicine, University of Southern California School of Medicine, Los Angeles, California

JAMES KANE, M.D.
Veterans Administration Hospital and the University of Arkansas School of Medicine, Little Rock, Arkansas

MARTIN J. KAPLITT, M.D.
Chief, Cardiac Surgery, Department of Surgery, North Shore Hospital, Manhasset, New York; Assistant Professor of Surgery, Cornell University Medical College, New York, New York

KARL E. KARLSON, M.D., Ph.D.
Professor of Biomedical Science, Brown University Medical School; Surgeon-in-Chief, Division of Cardio-Thoracic Surgery, Rhode Island Hospital, Providence, Rhode Island

V. S. KAUSHIK, M.D.
Department of Cardiology, Cedars-Sinai Medical Center and Department of Medicine, University of California School of Medicine, Los Angeles, California

JEROME HAROLD KAY, M.D.
Associate Professor of Surgery and Chairman, Division of Thoracic Surgery, Department of Surgery, St. Vincent's Hospital and the University of Southern California School of Medicine, Los Angeles, California

J. S. KEATES, M.D.
Electrochemistry and Biophysics Research Laboratories, Vascular Surgical Services, Department of Surgery, State University of New York Downstate Medical Center, College of Medicine, Brooklyn, New York

ARTHUR S. KEATS, M.D.
Chief, Division of Cardiovascular Anesthesia, Texas Heart Institute of St. Luke's Episcopal and Texas Children's Hospitals, and Clinical Professor of Anesthesiology, Baylor College of Medicine, Houston, Texas

ROBERT M. KEENAN, B.S.
Perfusion Technology Sections and Division of Surgery, Texas Heart Institute; Department of Anesthesiology, Baylor College of Medicine, Houston, Texas

NADYA KELLER, Ph.D.
Assistant Professor of Biochemistry in Medicine, Department of Medicine, Cornell University Medical College, New York, New York

J. W. KENNEDY, M.D.
Chief, Cardiology, Veterans Administration Hospital, Seattle, and Associate Professor of Medicine, University of Washington School of Medicine, Seattle, Washington

THOMAS KILLIP, M.D.
Professor and Chairman, Division of Cardiology, Department of Medicine, the New York Hospital–Cornell Medical Center, New York, New York

SAMUEL A. KINARD, M.D.
Chief, Department of Cardiology, Arizona Heart Institute, St. Joseph's Hospital and Medical Center, Phoenix, Arizona

TOMAS KLIMA, M.D.
Department of Pathology, St. Luke's Episcopal and Texas Heart Institute, Houston, Texas

SUSAN A. KLINE, M.D.
Assistant Professor of Medicine, Department of Medicine, the New York Hospital–Cornell Medical Center, New York, New York

WILLEM J. KOLFF, M.D., Ph.D.
Professor of Surgery, Division of Artificial Organs, Department of Surgery, and Director, Institute for Biomedical Engineering, College of Engineering and College of Medicine, the University of Utah, Salt Lake City, Utah

YOSHIAKI KOMOTO, M.D.
Department of Surgery, State University of New York Downstate Medical Center, Brooklyn, New York

JON C. KOSEK, M.D.
Professor of Clinical Pathology, Department of Pathology, Veterans Administration Hospital, Palo Alto, California; Stanford University School of Medicine, Stanford, California

DIETER M. KRAMSCH, M.D.
Assistant Professor of Medicine, Department of Medicine, Boston University School of Medicine, Boston, Massachusetts

RAJ KUMAR, M.D.
Department of Medicine, Harvard Medical School; Medical Service, Boston City Hospital; and the Thorndike Memorial Laboratories, Boston, Massachusetts

THOMAS Z. LAJOS, M.D., F.R.C.S.
Assistant Professor of Surgery, Department of Surgery, State University of New York at Buffalo School of Medicine and Buffalo General Hospital, Buffalo, New York

HILLEL LAKS, M.D.
Department of Surgery, Harvard Medical School, and Division of Thoracic and Cardiac Surgery, Peter Bent Brigham Hospital, Boston, Massachusetts

TZU-WANG LANG, M.D.
Senior Research Scientist, Cedars–Sinai Medical Center, Cedars of Lebanon Hospital Division, Los Angeles, California

EUGENE LAPIN, M.D.
Divisions of Nuclear Medicine and Cardiology, Department of Medicine, Veterans Administration Hospital, Seattle, and University of Washington School of Medicine, Seattle, Washington

JOHN H. LAWSON, Ph.D.
Division of Artificial Organs, Department of Surgery, University of Utah College of Medicine, Salt Lake City, Utah

ROBERT D. LEACHMAN, M.D.
Professor of Medicine, Department of Medicine, Baylor College of Medicine, and Department of Cardiology, Texas Heart Institute of St. Luke's Episcopal and Texas Children's Hospitals, Houston, Texas

ARTHUR B. LEE, JR., M.D.
Assistant Professor of Surgery, Department of Surgery, State University of New York at Buffalo School of Medicine and Buffalo General Hospital, Buffalo, New York

WILLIAM H. LEE, JR., M.D.
Professor and Chairman, Division of Thoracic Surgery, Department of Surgery, Medical University of South Carolina, Charleston, South Carolina

ARMAND A. LEFEMINE, M.D.
Director, Cardiac Surgery, St. Elizabeth's Hospital; Associate Professor of Surgery, Tufts University School of Medicine, Boston, Massachusetts

G. M. LeMOLE, M.D.
The Deborah Heart and Lung Center, Browns Mills, New Jersey; Temple University Hospital, Philadelphia, Pennsylvania

DONALD F. LEON, M.D.
Associate Professor of Medicine, Division of Cardiology, Department of Medicine, University of Pittsburgh School of Medicine, Pittsburgh, Pennsylvania

DERWARD LEPLEY, M.D.
Clinical Professor of Surgery, Division of Thoracic-Cardiovascular Surgery, Department of Surgery, the Medical College of Wisconsin and Affiliated Hospitals, Milwaukee, Wisconsin

STEPHEN J. LESHIN, M.D.
Division of Thoracic and Cardiovascular Surgery, Department of Surgery, and the Pauline and Adolph Weinberger Laboratory for Cardiac Research, the University of Texas Health Science Center at Dallas, Southwestern Medical School, Dallas, Texas

DAVID C. LEVIN, M.D.
Assistant Professor of Radiology, Department of Radiology, the New York Hospital–Cornell Medical Center, New York, New York

SIDNEY LEVITSKY, M.D.
Associate Professor of Surgery, Division of Cardiovascular and Thoracic Surgery, Department of Surgery, the Abraham Lincoln School of Medicine, University of Illinois College of Medicine, Chicago, Illinois

JOSEPH LEWIS, M.D.
Department of Surgery, Yale University School of Medicine, Yale University, New Haven, Connecticut

G. A. LIEBLER, M.D.
Department of Thoracic Surgery, Allegheny General Hospital, and Clinical Instructor in Surgery, University of Pittsburgh School of Medicine, Pittsburgh, Pennsylvania

JAMES LIES, M.D.
Section of Cardiovascular Medicine, Departments of Medicine and Physiology, University of California at Davis, School of Medicine, Davis, California

C. WALTON LILLEHEI, M.D.
Professor of Surgery, Department of Surgery, Cornell University Medical College, New York, New York

KIRK LIPSCOMB, M.D.
Department of Medicine, University of Washington School of Medicine and Veterans Administration Hospital, Seattle, Washington

MARTIN M. LIPTON, M.D.
Cardiology Service, Veterans Administration Hospital, Palo Alto, California; Stanford University School of Medicine, Stanford, California

ROBERT H. LISS, Ph.D.
Director, Cytology Laboratories, Life Sciences, Arthur D. Little, Inc., Cambridge, Massachusetts; Visiting Scientist, Texas Heart Institute, Houston, Texas; Associate in Surgery, Harvard Medical School, Boston, Massachusetts

STEPHEN P. LONDE, M.D.
Assistant Professor of Surgery, Division of Thoracic and Cardiovascular Surgery, Department of Surgery of the Pauline and Adolph Weinberger Laboratory for Cardiac Research, the University of Texas Health Science Center at Dallas Southwestern Medical School, Dallas, Texas

ROBERTO LUFSCHANOWSKI, M.D.
Department of Cardiology, Texas Heart Institute of St. Luke's Episcopal and Texas Children's Hospitals, and Clinical Assistant Professor of Medicine, Department of Medicine, Baylor College of Medicine, Houston, Texas

ARTHUR J. LURIE, M.D.
Assistant Professor of Surgery, Section of Cardiovascular Medicine and Surgery, Department of Surgery, University of California at Davis, School of Medicine, Davis, California; the Sacramento Medical Center of the University of California at Davis, Sacramento, California

R. BEVERLY LYNN, F.R.C.S.
Professor of Surgery, Department of Surgery, Queen's University Faculty of Medicine, Kingston, Ontario, Canada

JOHN H. McANULTY, M.D.
Assistant Professor of Medicine, Division of Cardiology, Department of Medicine, University of Oregon Medical School, Portland, Oregon

PETER McCART, M.D.
Department of Surgery, University of California at Irvine, College of Medicine, Irvine, California; Veterans Administration Hospital, Long Beach, California

RITA McCONN, Ph.D.
Assistant Professor, Department of Surgery, Albert Einstein College of Medicine of Yeshiva University, Bronx, New York

PETER McLAUGHLIN, M.D.
Cardiovascular Unit, Toronto General Hospital and the University of Toronto Faculty of Medicine, Toronto, Ontario, Canada

J. JUDSON McNAMARA, M.D.
Professor of Surgery, Department of Surgery, University of Hawaii School of Medicine, Queen's Medical Center, Honolulu, Hawaii

IRVING M. MADOFF, M.D.
Associate Clinical Professor of Surgery, Department of Surgery, Boston University School of Medicine, Boston, Massachusetts

GEORGE J. MAGOVERN, M.D.
Clinical Associate Professor of Surgery, University of Pittsburgh School of Medicine, and Department of Thoracic Surgery, Allegheny General Hospital, Pittsburgh, Pennsylvania

JASBIR S. MAKAR, M.D.
Division of Cardiovascular Diseases, Department of Medicine, Allegheny General Hospital, and Department of Medicine, the University of Pittsburgh School of Medicine, Pittsburgh, Pennsylvania

JAMES R. MALM, M.D.
Professor of Clinical Surgery, Department of Surgery, Columbia University College of Physicians and Surgeons, and Department of Surgery, Columbia–Presbyterian Medical Center, New York, New York

PETER B. MANSFIELD, M.D.
Director, Reconstructive Cardiovascular Research Center, Providence Medical Center; Clinical Instructor, Department of Surgery, University of Washington School of Medicine, Seattle, Washington

FRANK I. MARCUS, M.D.
Professor of Internal Medicine, Department of Internal Medicine, University of Arizona College of Medicine, Tucson, Arizona

HAROLD S. MARCUS, M.D.
Department of Cardiology, Cedars–Sinai Medical Center, Cedars of Lebanon Hospital Division, and Adjunct Assistant Professor of Medicine, Department of Medicine, UCLA School of Medicine, Los Angeles, California

CLEMENT L. MARKERT, Ph.D.
Department of Surgery, Yale University School of Medicine, New Haven, Connecticut

DEAN T. MASON, M.D.
Professor of Medicine, Professor of Physiology, and Chief, Section of Cardiovascular Medicine, University of California at Davis, School of Medicine, Davis, California; the Sacramento Medical Center of the University of California at Davis, Sacramento, California

HUGOE R. MATHEWS, F.R.C.S.
Department of Surgery and Division of Biological Sciences, the University of Chicago, Chicago, Illinois

JACK M. MATLOFF, M.D.
Assistant Clinical Professor of Surgery, Department of Surgery, UCLA School of Medicine, and Cedars–Sinai Medical Center, Cedars of Lebanon Hospital Division, Los Angeles, California

JAMES E. MAY, M.D.
Assistant Professor of Surgery, Division of Thoracic Surgery, Department of Surgery, Medical University of South Carolina College of Medicine, Charleston, South Carolina

SAMUEL MEERBAUM, Ph.D.
Senior Research Scientist, Cedars–Sinai Medical Center, Cedars of Lebanon Hospital Division, UCLA School of Medicine, Los Angeles, California

MEENA M. MEHTA, M.D., F.R.C.S. (Edinburgh)
Saint Barnabas Medical Center, Livingston, New Jersey

A. MICHAEL MENDEZ, M.D.
Department of Thoracic and Cardiovascular Surgery, St. Vincent's Hospital and the University of Southern California at Los Angeles, Los Angeles, California

FREDERICK J. MERCHANT, M.D.
Macy Foundation Faculty Fellow, Departments of Surgery and Pharmacology, the Abraham Lincoln School of Medicine, and School of Basic Medical Sciences at Urbana-Champaign, University of Illinois College of Medicine, Chicago, Illinois

ARTHUR J. MERRILL, Maj., USAF, MC
Cardiovascular Diseases, Wilford Hall United States Air Force Medical Center, Lackland Air Force Base, Texas

JOSEPH V. MESSER, M.D.
Director of Cardiology, Rush–Presbyterian–St. Luke's Medical Center, and Professor of Medicine, Department of Medicine, Rush Medical College, Boston, Massachusetts

JOSEPH MEYER, M.D.
Division of Surgery, Texas Heart Institute of St. Luke's Episcopal and Texas Children's Hospitals, Houston, Texas

JOSEPH J. MIGLIORE, M.D.
Research Associate, Cardiovascular Surgical Research Laboratories, Texas Heart Institute of St. Luke's Episcopal and Texas Children's Hospitals, Houston, Texas

JOHN D. MILAM, M.D.
Associate Director, Department of Pathology, Texas Heart Institute of St. Luke's Episcopal Hospital; Associate Clinical Professor of Pathology, Baylor Medical School and University of Texas Medical School at Houston, Texas

ALAN B. MILLER, M.D.
Chief, Division of Cardiology, Department of Medicine, University Hospital of Jacksonville, Jacksonville, Florida

RICHARD B. MILLER, M.D.
Assistant Professor of Medicine, Section of Cardiovascular Medicine, Department of Internal Medicine, University of California at Davis, School of Medicine, Davis, California; the Sacramento Medical Center of the University of California at Davis, Sacramento, California

NOEL MILLS, M.D.
Clinical Assistant Professor of Surgery, Department of Surgery, Tulane University School of Medicine, and Oschsner Clinic and Oschsner Foundation, New Orleans, Louisiana

ALFONSO M. MIYAMOTO, M.D.
Department of Thoracic and Cardiovascular Surgery, City of Hope National Medical Center, Duarte, California

E. MIMS MOBLEY, JR., M.D.
Cardiovascular Division, Department of Medicine, Medical University of South Carolina College of Medicine, Charleston, South Carolina

MARIO MONTES, M.D.
Clinical Associate Professor of Pathology, Department of Pathology, State University of New York at Buffalo School of Medicine and Buffalo General Hospital, Buffalo, New York

HYUNG S. MOON, M.D.
Associate in Surgery, St. Elizabeth's Hospital, Boston, Massachusetts

JOHN F. MORAN, M.D.
Assistant Professor, Department of Medicine, Loyola University of Chicago Stritch School of Medicine, Maywood, Illinois

JOHN E. MORCH, M.D.
Associate Professor of Medicine, Department of Medicine, Cardiovascular Unit, Toronto General Hospital and the University of Toronto Faculty of Medicine, Toronto, Ontario, Canada

TOHRU MORI, M.D.
Department of Thoracic and Cardiovascular Surgery, the St. Vincent's Hospital and the Los Angeles County–University of Southern California Medical Center, Los Angeles, California

GEORGE C. MORRIS, JR., M.D.
Professor of Surgery, the Cora and Webb Mading Department of Surgery, Baylor College of Medicine, Houston, Texas

JOHN B. MORRISON, M.D.
Assistant Professor of Medicine, Division of Cardiology, Department of Medicine, North Shore Hospital, Manhasset, New York; Cornell University Medical College, New York, New York

DRYDEN P. MORSE, M.D.
The Deborah Heart and Lung Center, Browns Mills, New Jersey; Temple University Hospital, Philadelphia, Pennsylvania

BRIAN C. MORTON, M.D.
Cardiovascular Unit, Toronto General Hospital and the University of Toronto Faculty of Medicine, Toronto, Ontario, Canada

HILTRUD S. MUELLER, M.D.
Director of Cardiology, St. Vincent Hospital, and Associate Professor of Medicine, University of Massachusetts Medical School, Worcester, Massachusetts

MARVIN MURPHY, M.D.
Associate Professor of Medicine, Department of Medicine, the University of Arkansas School of Medicine and Veterans Administration Hospital, Little Rock, Arkansas

JOHN A. MURRAY, M.D.
Associate Professor of Medicine, Department of Medicine, the University of Washington School of Medicine and Veterans Administration Hospital, Seattle, Washington

BERNARDO NADAL-GINARD, M.D.
Department of Surgery, Yale University School of Medicine, Yale University, New Haven, Connecticut

ARNOLD NAGLER, Ph.D.
Assistant Professor of Surgery, Department of Surgery, Albert Einstein College of Medicine of Yeshiva University, Bronx, New York

ANTOINE NASRALLAH, M.D.
The Clayton Foundation Exercise and Non-invasive Laboratory and Division of Cardiology, Texas Heart Institute of St. Luke's Episcopal and Texas Children's Hospitals, Houston, Texas

RIMGAUDAS NEMICKAS, M.S.
Loyola University of Chicago Stritch School of Medicine, Maywood, Illinois

JOHN F. NEVILLE, JR., M.D.
Associate Professor of Surgery, Department of Surgery, State University of New York College of Medicine, Upstate Medical Center, Syracuse, New York

FREDRIC NEWMAN, M.D.
Division of Thoracic and Cardiovascular Surgery, Department of Surgery, North Shore Hospital, Manhasset, New York; Cornell University Medical College, New York, New York

DEMETRE M. NICOLOFF, M.D.
Associate Professor of Surgery, Department of Surgery, the University of Minnesota Health Sciences Center and Affiliated Hospitals, Minneapolis, Minnesota

EDWARD L. NIRDLINGER II, M.D., Ph.D.
Departments of Surgery and Pharmacology, the Abraham Lincoln School of Medicine, and School of Basic Medical Sciences at Urbana-Champaign, University of Illinois College of Medicine, Chicago Illinois

JOHN C. NORMAN, M.D.
Director, Cardiovascular Surgical Research Laboratories, Texas Heart Institute; Clinical Professor of Cardiothoracic Surgery, University of Texas (UTSA); and Clinical Associate in Surgery, Texas Heart Institute of St. Luke's Episcopal and Texas Children's Hospitals, Houston, Texas

ROBERT L. NORTON, M.D.
Tufts University School of Medicine and Boston City Hospital, Boston, Massachusetts

JOHN OCHSNER, M.D.
Clinical Professor of Surgery, Department of Surgery, Tulane University School of Medicine, and Ochsner Clinic and Ochsner Foundation, New Orleans, Louisiana

JOHN A. OGDEN, M.D.
Assistant Professor of Surgery, Department of Surgery and the Human Growth and Development Study Unit, Yale University School of Medicine, Yale University, New Haven, Connecticut

M. OKA, M.D.
Assistant Professor of Pathology, Department of Pathology, and Assistant Attending Pathologist, Department of Laboratories, North Shore Hospital, Manhasset, New York; Department of Pathology, Cornell University Medical College, New York, New York

YASU OKA, M.D.
Department of Surgery, Albert Einstein College of Medicine of Yeshiva University, Bronx, New York

CLAUDE OLIVER, M.D.
Department of Surgery, University of California at Irvine, California College of Medicine, Irvine, California; Veterans Administration Hospital, Long Beach, California

DONALD B. OLSEN, D.V.M.
Division of Artificial Organs, Department of Surgery, University of Utah College of Medicine Medical Center, Salt Lake City, Utah

JULES OSHER, B.A.
Cedars–Sinai Medical Center, Cedars of Lebanon Hospital Division, UCLA School of Medicine, Los Angeles, California

HARTMUT OSTER, M.D., Ph.D.
Division of Artificial Organs and Department of Anesthesiology, University of Utah, College of Medicine, Salt Lake City, Utah

JORGE OTERO, M.D.
Section of Cardiology, Department of Medicine, University of California at Davis, School of Medicine, Davis and Sacramento, California

VELLORE T. PADMANABHAN, M.D.
Assistant Professor of Medicine, Division of Cardiology, Department of Medicine, North Shore Hospital, Manhasset, New York; Cornell University Medical College, New York, New York

GEORGE PAPPAS, M.D.
Associate Professor of Surgery, Department of Surgery, University of Colorado School of Medicine, and Veterans Administration Hospital, Denver, Colorado

S. B. PARK, M.D.
Department of Thoracic Surgery, Allegheny General Hospital, Pittsburgh, Pennsylvania

FREDERICK B. PARKER, JR., M.D.
Assistant Professor, Department of Surgery, State University of New York School of Medicine, Upstate Medical Center, Syracuse, New York

WILLIAM W. PARMLEY, M.D.
Associate Professor of Medicine, and Chief, Division of Cardiology, Department of Medicine, University of California at San Francisco, School of Medicine, San Francisco, California

EDUARDO N. PARODI, M.D.
Department of Surgery, Columbia University College of Physicians and Surgeons, Columbia–Presbyterian Medical Center, New York, New York

VICTOR PARSONNET, M.D.
Director of Surgery, Department of Surgery, Newark Beth Israel Medical Center, and Clinical Professor of Surgery, College of Medicine and Dentistry of New Jersey–New Jersey Medical School, Newark, New Jersey

BRUCE C. PATON, M.D.
Professor of Surgery, Department of Surgery, the University of Colorado School of Medicine and Veterans Administration Hospital, Denver, Colorado

ROBERT M. PAYNE, M.D.
Department of Cardiology, Arizona Heart Institute, St. Joseph's Hospital and Medical Center, Phoenix, Arizona

JEFFREY L. PETERS, Ph.D.
Assistant Research Professor of Surgery, Division of Artificial Organs, Department of Surgery, University of Utah College of Medicine Medical Center, Salt Lake City, Utah

JAMES F. PFEIFER, M.D.
Instructor in Department of Medicine, Cardiology Service, Veterans Administration Hospital, Palo Alto, California; Stanford University School of Medicine, Stanford, California

BRENDAN P. PHIBBS, M.D.
Associate Professor of Medicine, Section of Cardiology, Department of Internal Medicine, University of Arizona College of Medicine, Tucson, Arizona

PETER A. PHILIPS, M.D.
Department of Thoracic and Cardiovascular Surgery, City of Hope National Medical Center, Duarte, California

ROQUE PIFARRE, M.D.
Clinical Professor of Surgery, Department of Surgery, Loyola University of Chicago Stritch School of Medicine, Maywood, Illinois

DAVID PITTMAN, M.D.
Division of Cardiovascular Diseases, Department of Medicine, Allegheny General Hospital, and Assistant Clinical Professor of Medicine, Department of Medicine, University of Pittsburgh School of Medicine, Pittsburgh, Pennsylvania

MELVIN R. PLATT, M.D.
Assistant Professor, Division of Thoracic Surgery and the Pauline and Adolph Weinberger Laboratory for Cardiac Research, the University of Texas Health Science Center at Dallas Southwestern Medical School, Dallas, Texas

CHARLES D. PRICE, M.D.
Department of Cardiology, Rhode Island Hospital, Providence, Rhode Island

R. BRADFORD PYLE, M.D.
University of Minnesota Hospitals of the University of Minnesota Health Sciences Center, Minneapolis, Minnesota

MIGUEL A. QUINONES, M.D.
Assistant Professor of Medicine, Department of Medicine, Baylor College of Medicine and Baylor Affiliated Hospitals, Houston, Texas

ROBERT A. QUINT, M.D.
Western Heart Associates, Assistant Chief of Cardiology, Santa Clara Valley Medical Center, San Jose, California; Clinical Instructor in Medicine, Stanford University School of Medicine, Stanford, California

SHAHBUDIN H. RAHIMTOOLA, M.D., F.R.C.P.
Professor of Medicine, Division of Cardiology, Department of Medicine, University of Oregon Medical School, Portland, Oregon

N. RAMASAMY, M.D.
Electrochemistry and Biophysics Research Laboratories, Vascular Surgical Services, Department of Surgery, State University of New York Downstate Medical Center, Brooklyn, New York

K. RAMASWAMY, M.D.
Assistant Professor, Tufts University School of Medicine; Director, Cardiac Catheterization Laboratories, St. Elizabeth's Hospital, Boston, Massachusetts

MARUF A. RAZZUK, M.D.
Department of Thoracic and Cardiovascular Surgery, the University of Texas Health Science Center at Dallas Southwestern Medical School, Dallas, Texas

RAYMOND C. READ, M.D.
Professor of Surgery, Department of Surgery, the University of Arkansas School of Medicine, Little Rock, Arkansas

PESARA S. REDDY, M.D.
Assistant Professor of Medicine, Division of Cardiology, Department of Medicine, University of Pittsburgh School of Medicine, Pittsburgh, Pennsylvania

CHARLES C. REED, B.S.
Director, Perfusion Technology Section, Texas Heart Institute of St. Luke's Episcopal and Texas Children's Hospitals, Houston, Texas

GEORGE E. REED, M.D.
Professor of Surgery, Departments of Medicine and Surgery, New York University Medical Center School of Medicine, New York, New York

KEITH REEMTSMA, M.D.
Professor and Chairman, Department of Surgery, College of Physicians and Surgeons, Columbia–Presbyterian Medical Center, New York, New York

ANNA RELIGA, M.D., Ph.D.
Director of the Metabolic Unit, St. Vincent Hospital, Worcester, Massachusetts; Adjunkt in the Department of Physiology, Medical School of Warsaw, Warsaw, Poland

ROBERT S. RENEMAN, M.D.
Formerly of the Cardiovascular Department, Janssen Research Foundation, Beerse, Belgium; presently Department of Physiology Biomedical Center, Medical Faculty Maastricht, Maastricht, The Netherlands

GEORGE J. REUL, JR., M.D.
Division of Surgery, Texas Heart Institute of St. Luke's Episcopal and Texas Children's Hospitals, Houston, Texas

JAMES L. RITCHIE, M.D.
Acting Instructor in Medicine, Department of Medicine, Veterans Administration Hospital and University of Washington School of Medicine, Seattle, Washington

ALEXANDER ROMAGNOLI, M.D.
Department of Anesthesiology, Texas Heart Institute of St. Luke's Episcopal and Texas Children's Hospitals, and Clinical Anesthesiologist, Baylor College of Medicine, Houston, Texas

JOSEPH RÖSCH, M.D.
Professor of Radiology, Department of Radiology, University of Oregon Medical School, Portland, Oregon

MICKI A. ROSENBLOOM
Saint Barnabas Medical Center, Livingston, New Jersey

JACOB ROSENSWEIG, M.D., Ph.D., F.R.C.S.(C)
Chief of Surgery, Department of Surgery, Mount Sinai Hospital and the University of Connecticut Health Center School of Medicine, Hartford, Connecticut

STEPHEN J. ROSSITER, M.D.
Department of Surgery, Veterans Administration Hospital, Palo Alto, California; Stanford University School of Medicine, Stanford, California

HENRY I. RUSSEK, M.D.
Research Professor in Cardiovascular Disease, Clinical Professor of Medicine, New York Medical College, New York, New York

THOMAS J. RYAN, M.D.
Head, Section of Clinical Cardiology, University Hospital, and Professor of Medicine, Boston University School of Medicine, Boston, Massachusetts

PHIROZE B. SABAWALA, M.D.
Department of Anesthesiology, Texas Heart Institute of St. Luke's Episcopal and Texas Children's Hospitals, and Clinical Anesthesiologist, Baylor College of Medicine, Houston, Texas

FRANK M. SANDIFORD, M.D.
Associate Surgeon, Division of Surgery, Texas Heart Institute of St. Luke's Episcopal and Texas Children's Hospitals, Houston, Texas

MIGUEL E. SANMARCO, M.D.
Assistant Professor of Medicine, University of Southern California School of Medicine, Los Angeles, California; Rancho Los Amigos Hospital, Downey, California

LESTER R. SAUVAGE, M.D.
Clinical Associate Professor of Surgery, Department of Surgery, University of Washington School of Medicine, Seattle, Washington

PHILIP N. SAWYER, M.D.
Director, Electrochemistry and Biophysics Research Laboratories, Vascular Surgical Services, and Professor of Surgery, Department of Surgery, State University of New York Downstate Medical Center, Brooklyn, New York

PATRICK J. SCANLON, M.D.
Director, Cardiopulmonary Laboratory, and Associate Professor of Medicine, Department of Medicine, Loyola University of Chicago Stritch School of Medicine, Maywood, Illinois

GEORGE SCHIMERT, M.D.
Associate Professor of Surgery, Department of Surgery, State University of New York at Buffalo School of Medicine, and the Buffalo General Hospital, Buffalo, New York

JOEL P. SCHRANK, M.D.
Assistant Professor of Medicine, Department of Medicine, University of Virginia School of Medicine, Charlottesville, Virginia

MEREDITH L. SCOTT, M.D.
Cardiovascular and Thoracic Surgeon, Orlando, Florida

STEWART M. SCOTT, M.D.
Chief, Division of Cardiovascular and Thoracic Surgery, Veterans Administration Hospital, Ashville, North Carolina; Assistant Clinical Professor of Surgery, Department of Surgery, Duke University School of Medicine, Durham, North Carolina

RONALD H. SELVESTER, M.D.
Professor of Medicine, Department of Medicine, University of Southern California School of Medicine, Los Angeles, California; Rancho Los Amigos Hospital, Downey, California

GULSHAN K. SETHI, M.D.
Assistant Chief, Division of Cardiovascular and Thoracic Surgery, Veterans Administration Hospital, Ashville, North Carolina; Assistant Clinical Professor of Surgery, Department of Surgery, Duke University School of Medicine, Durham, North Carolina

WILLIAM H. SEWELL, M.D.
Robert Packer Hospital, Guthrie Clinic, Ltd., Sayre, Pennsylvania

JAMES A. SHAVER, M.D.
Associate Professor of Medicine, Division of Cardiology, Department of Medicine, University of Pittsburgh School of Medicine, Pittsburgh, Pennsylvania

R. SHETTIGAR, M.D.
Cardiovascular Disease Service, Veterans Administration Hospital, Palo Alto, California; Stanford University Medical School, Stanford, California

JOHN H. SIEGEL, M.D.
Professor of Surgery, Department of Surgery, State University of New York at Buffalo School of Medicine and Buffalo General Hospital, Buffalo, New York

MALCOLM D. SILVER, M.D.
Cardiovascular Diseases, Toronto General Hospital and the University of Toronto Faculty of Medicine, Toronto, Ontario, Canada

SAMUEL M. SIMS, B.S.
Queen's Medical Center, University of Hawaii School of Medicine, Honolulu, Hawaii

ARUN K. SINGH, M.D.
Division of Cardio-Thoracic Surgery, Rhode Island Hospital, Providence, Rhode Island

HARJEET M. SINGH, M.D.
Department of Thoracic-Cardiovascular Surgery, Medical College of Wisconsin and Affiliated Hospitals, Milwaukee, Wisconsin

DAVID B. SKINNER, M.D.
Professor and Chairman, Department of Surgery, the University of Chicago Division of Biological Sciences and the Pritzker School of Medicine, Chicago, Illinois

ROBERT SLOAN, M.D.
Department of Thoracic and Cardiovascular Surgery, the University of Texas Health Science Center at Dallas Southwestern Medical School, Dallas, Texas

GREGORY T. SMITH, B.S.
Queen's Medical Center, University of Hawaii School of Medicine, Honolulu, Hawaii

JAMES C. SMITH, M.D.
Director of Experimental Surgery, Reconstructive Cardiovascular Research Center; Attending Staff, Providence Medical Center; and Children's Orthopedic Hospital, Seattle, Washington

CHARLES SMITHEN, M.D.
Assistant Professor of Medicine, Division of Cardiology, Department of Medicine, the New York Hospital–Cornell Medical Center, New York, New York

JOHN R. SOETER, M.D.
Assistant Professor of Surgery, Department of Surgery, University of Hawaii School of Medicine, Queen's Medical Center, Honolulu, Hawaii

HARRY S. SOROFF, M.D.
Professor and Chairman, Department of Surgery, State University of New York at Stony Brook Health Sciences Center, Stony Brook, New York

MERRILL P. SPENCER, M.D.
Clinical Associate Professor of Medicine, Department of Clinical Physiology, Providence Hospital, Medical Center, Seattle, Washington

RICHARD I. STAIMAN, M.D.
Department of Surgery, Yale University School of Medicine, and Cardiothoracic Surgical Service, Yale–New Haven Hospital, New Haven, Connecticut

B. STANCZEWSKI, M.D.
Electrochemistry and Biophysics Research Laboratories, Vascular Surgical Services, Department of Surgery, State University of New York Downstate Medical Center, Brooklyn, New York

WILLIAM STANFORD, Col., USAF, MC
Chief, Thoracic Surgery Service, Wilford Hall United States Air Force Medical Center, Lackland Air Force Base, Texas

THEODORE H. STANLEY, M.D.
Assistant Professor of Anesthesiology and Surgery, Institute for Biomedical Engineering and College of Medicine, University of Utah, Salt Lake City, Utah

H. C. STANSEL, JR., M.D.
Associate Professor of Surgery, Department of Surgery and the Human Growth and Development Study Unit, Yale University School of Medicine, New Haven, Connecticut

ALBERT STARR, M.D.
Professor and Chief of Cardiopulmonary Surgery, Department of Surgery, University of Oregon Medical School, Portland, Oregon

PETER P. STEELE, M.D.
Assistant Professor of Medicine, Department of Medicine, the University of Colorado School of Medicine; Section of Cardiovascular Diseases, Veterans Administration Hospital, Denver, Colorado

HARRY L. STEIN, M.D.
Department of Radiology, North Shore Hospital, Manhasset, New York; Cornell University Medical College, New York, New York

EDWARD A. STEMMER, M.D.
Associate Professor, Department of Surgery, University of California at Irvine, College of Medicine, Irvine, California; Veterans Administration Hospital, Long Beach, California

SIMON H. STERTZER, M.D.
Lenox Hill Hospital, New York, New York

KARL STRAUB, M.D.
Assistant Professor of Medicine, Department of Medicine, the University of Arkansas School of Medicine and Veterans Administration Hospital, Little Rock, Arkansas

WINFRED L. SUGG, M.D.
Chairman, Division of Thoracic and Cardiovascular Surgery, Department of Surgery, and the Pauline and Adolph Weinberger Laboratory for Cardiac Research, the University of Texas Health Science Center at Dallas Southwestern Medical School, Dallas, Texas

C. GERALD SUNDHAL, M.D.
Division of Cardiology, Department of Medicine, the University of Pittsburgh School of Medicine, Pittsburgh, Pennsylvania

HECTOR SUSTAITA, M.D.
Associate Surgeon, Department of Thoracic, Cardiac, and Vascular Surgery, Cedars–Sinai Medical Center, Cedars of Lebanon Hospital Division, Los Angeles, California

H. J. C. SWAN, M.D., Ph.D.
Professor of Medicine, Division of Cardiology, Department of Medicine, UCLA School of Medicine, and Cedars of Lebanon Hospital Division, Los Angeles, California

TIMOTHY TAKARO, M.D.
Chief, Surgical Service, Veterans Administration Hospital, Ashville, North Carolina; Associate Clinical Professor of Surgery, Department of Surgery, Duke University School of Medicine, Durham, North Carolina

JAMES V. TALANO, M.D.
Assistant Professor of Medicine, Department of Medicine, Loyola University of Chicago Stritch School of Medicine, Maywood, Illinois

RAVINDER TANDON, M.D.
Clinical Instructor in Medicine, Department of Medicine, State University of New York at Buffalo School of Medicine and Buffalo General Hospital, Buffalo, New York

CONSTANTINE J. TATOOLES, M.D., M.S.
Associate Professor of Surgery and Director, Division of Cardiovascular and Thoracic Surgery, Department of Surgery, the Abraham Lincoln School of Medicine, University of Illinois and Cook County Hospital, Chicago, Illinois

ALFRED J. TECTOR, M.D.
Associate Clinical Professor of Thoracic and Cardiovascular Surgery, Department of Surgery, the Medical College of Wisconsin and Affiliated Hospitals, Milwaukee, Wisconsin

U. F. TESLER, M.D.
Instructor in Surgery, Department of Surgery, Temple University School of Medicine, Philadelphia, Pennsylvania; the Deborah Heart and Lung Center, Browns Mills, New Jersey

CHARLES N. THOMAS, Col., USAF, MC
Cardiology Service, Wilford Hall United States Air Force Medical Center, Lackland Air Force Base, Texas

MARK E. THOMPSON, M.D.
Professor of Medicine, Division of Cardiology, Department of Medicine, University of Pittsburgh School of Medicine, Pittsburgh, Pennsylvania

JOHN R. TOBIN, JR., M.D., M.S.
Professor and Chairman, Department of Medicine, Loyola University of Chicago Stritch School of Medicine, Medical Center, Maywood, Illinois

ANTHONY J. TORTOLANI, M.D.
Division of Thoracic and Cardiovascular Surgery, Department of Surgery, North Shore Hospital, Manhasset, New York, and Cornell University Medical College, New York, New York

ROGELIO TRESPICIO, M.D.
Department of Anesthesiology, Saint Barnabas Medical Center, Livingston, New Jersey

ALAN S. TRIMBLE, M.D., F.R.C.S.
Assistant Professor of Surgery, Department of Surgery, Cardiovascular Unit, Toronto General Hospital and the University of Toronto Faculty of Medicine, Toronto, Ontario, Canada

YOUNG TSO LIN, M.D.
Divisions of Thoracic and Cardiovascular Surgery, Department of Surgery, St. Vincent's Hospital and the University of Southern California School of Medicine, Los Angeles, California

NAIP TUNA, M.D.
Associate Professor of Medicine, Department of Medicine, University of Minnesota Health Sciences Center and Affiliated Hospitals, Minneapolis, Minnesota

HATSUZO UCHIDA, M.D.
Department of Surgery, State University of New York Downstate Medical Center, Brooklyn, New York

HAROLD C. URSCHEL, M.D.
Clinical Associate Professor, Department of Thoracic and Cardiovascular Surgery, the University of Texas Health Science Center at Dallas Southwestern Medical School, Dallas, Texas

ABELARDO VARGAS, M.D.
Assistant Professor of Thoracic-Cardiovascular Surgery, Department of Surgery, University of Miami School of Medicine, and Cardiovascular Laboratories, Jackson Memorial Hospital, Miami, Florida

BERNARDO VIDNE, M.D.
Division of Cardiovascular Diseases, State University of New York at Buffalo School of Medicine and Buffalo General Hospital, Buffalo, New York

JAY VOLDER, M.D.
Division of Artificial Organs, Division of Surgery, University of Utah College of Medicine Medical Center, Salt Lake City, Utah

EUGENE WALLSH, M.D.
Chief, Cardiovascular Surgery, Department of Surgery, and Assistant Professor, New York University Medical Center School of Medicine, New York, New York; Lenox Hill Hospital, New York, New York

HERBERT E. WARDEN, M.D.
Professor and Assistant Chairman of Surgery, Department of Surgery, West Virginia University School of Medicine, Morgantown, West Virginia

JOHN T. WATSON, Ph.D.
Division of Thoracic and Cardiovascular Surgery, Department of Surgery, and the Pauline and Adolph Weinberger Laboratory for Cardiac Research, the University of Texas Health Science Center at Dallas Southwestern Medical School, Dallas, Texas

WATTS R. WEBB, M.D.
Professor and Chairman, Department of Surgery, State University of New York Upstate Medical Center College of Medicine, Syracuse, New York

GERALD WEINSTEIN, M.D.
Lenox Hill Hospital, New York, New York

BABETTE WEKSLER, M.D.
Assistant Professor of Medicine, Division of Cardiology, Department of Medicine, the New York Hospital–Cornell Medical Center, New York, New York

CLARENCE S. WELDON, M.D.
Chairman, Division of Cardiothoracic Surgery, Department of Surgery, and Biomedical Computer Laboratory, Washington University School of Medicine, St. Louis, Missouri

HARRY A. WELLONS, JR., M.D.
Assistant Professor of Surgery, Department of Surgery, University of Virginia School of Medicine, Charlottesville, Virginia

S. ADAM WESOLOWSKI, M.D.
Clinical Professor of Surgery, State University of New York Downstate Medical Center, Brooklyn, New York; Director, Cardiovascular Research Laboratory, Mercy Hospital, Rockville Centre, New York

JAMES T. WILLERSON, M.D.
Associate Professor of Medicine, Department of Medicine, the University of Texas Health Science Center at Dallas Southwestern Medical School, Dallas, Texas

DAVID O. WILLIAMS, M.D.
Assistant Professor in Residence, Section of Cardiovascular Medicine, Departments of Medical Sciences and Human Physiology, University of California at Davis, School of Medicine, Davis and Sacramento, California

G. DOYNE WILLIAMS, M.D.
Associate Professor of Surgery, Department of Surgery, University of Arkansas School of Medicine, Little Rock, Arkansas

WILLIAM G. WILLIAMS, M.D.
Lecturer, Division of Cardiovascular Surgery, Department of Surgery, Toronto General Hospital and the University of Toronto Faculty of Medicine, Toronto, Ontario, Canada

W. STAN WILSON, M.D.
Director, Cardiovascular Diagnostic Laboratory, St. Patrick Hospital and the Western Montana Clinic Foundation, Missoula, Montana

RICHARD E. WOOD, M.D.
Division of Thoracic and Cardiovascular Surgery, Department of Surgery, the University of Texas Health Science Center at Dallas Southwestern Medical School, Dallas, Texas

ROBERT D. WUERFLEIN, M.D.
Western Heart Associate, Santa Clara Valley Medical Center, San Jose, California

DON C. WUKASCH, M.D.
Division of Surgery, Texas Heart Institute of St. Luke's Episcopal and Texas Children's Hospitals, Houston, Texas

E. YELLIN, Ph.D., M.E.
Assistant Professor, Department of Surgery, Albert Einstein College of Medicine of Yeshiva University, Bronx, New York

LLOYD A. YOUNGBLOOD, M.D.
Research Assistant, Cardiovascular Surgical Research Laboratories, Texas Heart Institute of St. Luke's Episcopal and Texas Children's Hospitals, Houston, Texas

ROBERT ZELIS, M.D.
Associate Professor, Section of Cardiology, Department of Medicine, University of California at Davis, School of Medicine, Davis, California; Sacramento Medical Center of the University of California at Davis, Sacramento, California

PABLO ZUBIATE, M.D.
Associate Professor of Medicine and Associate Professor of Physiology, Department of Surgery, University of Southern California School of Medicine and St. Vincent's Hospital, Los Angeles, California

CONTENTS

Section III: DIAGNOSTIC TECHNIQUES AND FACILITIES

xxx   Contents

Section XIII: RESEARCH AREAS IN CORONARY ARTERY DISEASE

PREFACE

This edition of *Coronary Medicine and Surgery: Concepts and Controversies* was conceived in Houston, Boston, and Washington during meetings of the Presidential Advisory Committee on Heart Disease. The need for a reference source in this relatively new and currently burgeoning area of reparable ischemic heart disease was discussed with members of the committee. As a consequence of these discussions, 700 researchers, cardiologists, and surgeons gathered at the Texas Heart Institute in Houston a year later to discuss and debate an extended series of accepted, evolving, and controversial issues regarding the etiology, prevention, diagnosis, treatment, and prognosis of ischemic heart disease.

This text is a result of those discussions. Editing has been kept to a minimum in an effort to preserve the diversity of logic, approach, technique, and style of individual contributors. The careful reader will note degrees of redundancy, areas of unevenness, and perhaps even diametrically opposing opinions and conclusions. These, nonetheless, are the essentials of the presentations and discussions: cautious but firm, retrospective and preliminary, prospective and final. The result is a valid cross-sectional sampling of contemporary thought in coronory artery medicine and surgery.

We would like to acknowledge the continuing advice of Dr. Denton A. Cooley, Surgeon-in-Chief of the Texas Heart Institute, Houston; Robert R. Herring, Chairman of the Board of Trustees of the Texas Heart Institute; Newell E. France, Executive Director of St. Luke's Episcopal Hospital, the Texas Children's Hospital and the Texas Heart Institute; Dr. William V. McDermott, David Williams Cheever Professor of Surgery, Harvard Medical School; and Dr. M. Judah Folkman, Julia Dyckman Andrus Professor of Pediatric Surgery, Harvard Medical School.

Sincere appreciation must be expressed to Drs. William B. Hood, Martin J. Kaplitt, Jack M. Matloff, Joseph V. Messer, Joseph J. Migliore, William W. Parmley, and Edmond H. Sonnenblick for their help in planning and reviewing manuscripts in their areas of interest.

Special notes of appreciation are due Kathy Atkinson, Eugenia H. Campbell, Carolyn T. Cox, Dr. Benedict D. T. Daly, Patricia M. Devers, Charles H. Edmonds, Virginia D. Fairchild, John M. Fuqua, Dr. David A. Hughes, Stephen R. Igo, Liz Ann Johnson, Mark D. Johnson, John G. Kitsopoulos, Peter R. Maddeaux, James E. Martin, Alice G. Migliore, Susan Meixner, Dr. Ronald B. Ponn, Everett R. Price, William J. Robinson, Dr. William C. Scott, Mary J. Shyvers, and Nelly J. Stephan of the Cardiovascular Surgical Research Laboratories of the Texas Heart Institute; the Cardiovascular Division, Sears Surgical Research Laboratories, Harvard Medical School; the Countway Library of Harvard Medical School; the Board of Trustees of Texas Heart Institute and the Administration of St. Luke's Episcopal Hospital, Houston, Texas, for help with correspondence and manuscripts.

To the contributors, without whose time, effort, and expertise our text would not exist, again, a special note of appreciation. And, finally, we are most appreciative of the continued assistance, cooperation and encouragement of our publisher.

Houston and Boston   JOHN C. NORMAN, M.D.
                                                      EVELYN P. LAWRENCE

FOREWORD

Coronary artery disease in the United States is an awesome problem. It is awesome in the number of lives it takes each year, in the amount of suffering it causes, in the social dislocation it produces, and in financial costs. It is an important and extremely difficult scientific problem.

Each year in the United States more than one million people die of heart disease. As many as 75 percent of these have coronary artery disease as a primary or secondary cause of death. Of the one million cardiac deaths each year some 260,000 occur in patients who are under the age of 65.

Life is more than *not dying*, and disease is more than *just a cause of death*. One million Americans sustain their first heart attacks each year, and despite our best efforts, at least a third die within one month. In addition to those who suffer a symptomatic myocardial infarction, there are many who have no signs or symptoms at all. Yet a portion of their ventricular myocardium or interventricular septum becomes ischemic and subsequently fibrotic or aneurysmal or both. Theirs is a silent attack. Unfortunately, *silence* is not synonymous with *slight*. Not only does a silent, like a symptomatic, first myocardial infarction increase the risk of another attack, it also increases the probability that a subsequent infarction will result in a 40-percent or greater loss of viable functioning myocardium. It does not seem to matter whether this loss takes the form of scattered scars or one contiguous area. When the loss reaches the critical 40-percent level, cardiogenic shock and left ventricular power failure occur, and death is imminent and inexorable. Cardiogenic shock is an extremely ominous clinical condition with an 80- to 90-percent mortality.

The social costs of coronary artery disease need to be seen concurrently from the point of view of the patient and from the point of view of society. Looking first at the patient, it is all too clear that after recovery many victims of heart attacks have difficulty in getting back their former jobs or in obtaining new jobs. This may seem incredible, yet it is true, despite the outstanding example of one of Texas' most illustrious sons. Most people know that Lyndon Johnson had a heart attack while he was in the Senate. Certainly, they know that he went on to hold, for some six years, what has to be one of the world's most arduous jobs. Yet either they do not realize how severe his attack was or, like those who will not employ a heart-attack victim, they are unable to place themselves in the victim's position. In any case, patients are often rehabilitated physically but not socially or financially. This may be due in part to a lack of complete psychological rehabilitation. The patient must understand that he can, and must believe that he will, be able to do virtually everything that he did before his attack. Number are hard to come by in this area, but this must be true for *at least* half of those who survive a first heart attack, for whom complete rehabilitation is possible. Unfortunately, it is not true for all.

Thus, coronary artery disease, by virtue of its incidence and natural history, is almost as important to society as a whole as it is to the patient as an individual. For all ages and both sexes it is the primary factor limiting activities, the principal diagnosis on most hospital discharge sheets, the largest single cause of days spent in the hopital, and the primary reason for patients seeking advice from their physicians. Indeed, in 1971 heart disease accounted for some 22 million visits to physicians, or 18 percent of all visits to physicians for chronic conditions.

Coronary artery disease costs money as well. Clearly it is impossible to project individual lost earnings. However, if all the people who die of myocardial infarctions under the age of 65 in any one calendar year could be spared their diseases and their premature deaths, they would contribute during their remaining productive lifetimes some $2.6 billion to our gross national product.*

Given the complexity of the welfare structure throughout the country, it is not possible to determine with any reasonable degree of confidence the amount of money that society must expend to maintain the families of household heads who have died or been disabled and thereby removed from the work force by virtue of their coronary artery disease. We do know that heart disease accounts for $1.1 billion in disability allowances each year.

It is currently fashionable to decry the escalating costs of medical care. Some of the apparent increase in costs is due to more realistic accounting. Some of it is due to better wages being paid to nonprofessional service personnel in hospitals and clinics, and part of it is due to the improvements in medical therapy that, while costly in themselves, lead to shorter hospital stays and more complete recoveries. It certainly is true that treatment for patients with coronary heart disease does require, in one form or another, some subsidy by society. It is also true that a serious, life-threatening illness can be a financial catastrophe for any one individual or his family and that its repercussions may be crippling if, for example, it means that education of the children must be terminated or postponed. Similarly, if the patient is an independent employer, his illness may adversely affect many employees and their families.

By and large, when one hears about the magnitude of the health problem, it is usually in the context of these items, i.e., mortality, morbidity, social and psychological, and financial. By the same token, when one hears about the advances that have been made in the "war on heart disease," one hears about "scientific breakthroughs" and "technological advances." This dichotomy has some of the attributes of "riding one's horse while looking for him." Certainly, it contributes to a sense of dissatisfaction, discordance, and disunity between those who are attempting to solve the disease problems and those who control the federal purse strings, and between the physician and the patient. At a time when some medicine and a good deal of medical research requires federal support this is a most unfortunate state of affairs.

It may not be easy, but it is not impossible, to explain the scientific magnitude of the problem of coronary heart disease and the relationship between these scientific problems and their resolution to the morbidity, mortality, social, and financial problems of these same diseases. No one would quarrel with the statement that the scientific and medical problems of coronary artery disease are many and difficult.

Why, for example, does arteriosclerosis develop in coronary arteries in one patient, in cerebral arteries in another, yet remain confined to the aorta in a third? What is it that accounts for the marked variability within the coronary arteries of atherosclerotic plaques? Why is it that some transplanted hearts appear to be subject to an almost malignant progression of atherosclerosis, while others appear to be immune to this process? Turning to more immediate therapeutic problems, what is the best way to prevent the spread of ischemia secondary to coronary obstruction, and what is the easiest and best measure of the techniques being tried? In pathophysio-

---

* This is correct of coronary heart disease deaths. All cardiovascular diseases under the age of 65 cost $4.9 billion. All cardiovascular disease deaths for all ages cost $6.8 billion.

logical terms, how does a bypass relieve cardiac pain? Is it, in fact, through the production of a controlled infarction, or does the reversed saphenous vein graft manage to nourish the previously ischemic portion of the myocardium in a fashion yet to be discovered?

There seems to be general agreement between patients and physicians that patients with severe angina do receive relief from their pain after those procedures. How important is it then to determine whether the operation actually lengthens life? Is not the relief of pain in itself sufficient to justify the operation? Or is the operation so extensive in terms of trained people and special equipment that it must succeed simultaneously on all three fronts of the "magnitude of the problem?" Must it advance our scientific knowledge, relieve the patient's distress, and prolong his life in good health to be worthwhile? If so, how can we cost account new knowledge and/or pain?

There are, of course, many other questions that await answers. Possibly the most intriguing of these relate to the necessity for patency of the bypass. If, in fact, our goal is to produce a controlled infarction and to stimulate the development of collateral vessels, is it really necessary for the bypass to remain patent for more than a relatively short period of time? This is far from an academic question, since there are some who would judge the "success" of this procedure on the persistence of the patency of the graft without regard to the reduction in perceived pain (a soft end point) or the decrease in mortality (a hard end point).

Cynics will always be with us. Recognition of this fact, however, does not supply an answer to the contention that the fact that nothing else will help a patient is not a justification for surgery. Obviously, everything depends on the definition of the word "help." It is essential to keep in mind that, both from the public's point of view and from the patient's, the magnitude of the problem of coronary heart disease is the risk of getting the disease and the amount of suffering involved if one does get it.

If we suggest or imply that all new knowledge and every new technique is going to reduce the toll of coronary heart disease and forestall death, then it will not be long before it will be all too clear to everyone that at best we may have misled the patients and perhaps ourselves, and that at worst we have so exaggerated our claims that in essense we have told untruths.

Contrary to the claims of "miracle drugs," science and miracles have rarely kept company together. And most people know that if miracles happen at all, they happen only rarely and almost always to the other fellow. Patients are not looking for miracles from science or medicine in the realm of coronary artery disease; they are looking for progress, for more certain prevention, and more definitive care. And we can show them that we have made and are continuing to make progress in prevention and, especially, in therapy.

We should not belittle the magnitude of either the social or the scientific problem; nor should we claim or promise more than we have achieved or really expect to deliver. But to keep these in balance and perspective we need to know the nature and size of the problems and the amount of progress that is being made.

It is fitting and appropriate that Dr. John C. Norman has presented this book on coronary artery medicine and surgery. Speaking for all of us privileged to participate in its preparation, we offer him our congratulations and appreciation for an arduous task well done, and the readers our felicitations in having this summary available.

Washington, D.C.   THEODORE COOPER, M.D.

CORONARY ARTERY
MEDICINE AND SURGERY

1

SAPHENOUS VEIN AORTOCORONARY BYPASS
State of the Art

W. Stan Wilson

The emergence of the aorta-to-coronary artery bypass operation has made a major impact on the therapeutic approach to coronary artery disease. New information and concepts are accumulating rapidly and continued reassessment is essential. What, in fact, does the procedure accomplish? What are the risks and uncertainties? Is survival likely to be improved? To whom should surgery be recommended and for what indications? Many specific areas will be covered in more detail elsewhere in this volume. It is the purpose of this chapter to bring up to date previous reviews (Wilson, 1973; 1974) and provide an overview of the recent literature as well as a bibliographic basis for further study.

VEIN BYPASS FUNCTION: ENHANCED FLOW

The rationale of the saphenous vein bypass procedure centers on the assumption that increased quantities of oxygenated blood will reach the ischemic recipient distal vascular bed. Mean flow in bypass grafts measured immediately following insertion has consistently approximated normal coronary flow in many large series (Wilson, 1973) and contrasts strikingly with the very low flow rates observed in internal mammary artery implants, even after sufficient time for collateral development (Dart et al, 1970). Vein bypass flow is dependent on the relative lumenal diameters of vein and bypassed coronary artery (Furuse et al, 1972), the degree of stenosis in the bypassed artery (Urschel et al, 1972; Kakos et al, 1972; Furuse et al, 1972; Kirk et al, 1973), and the size

of the recipient vessel and its runoff (Segal et al, 1973). The influence of runoff bed size is demonstrated in the high flows noted when a single vein serves several runoff beds by means of side-to-side anastomoses, (Johnson, 1972a; Bartley et al, 1972; Johnson et al, 1972), in contrast to the limited flow that occurs through a vein graft serving a single small or diseased distal arterial system (Johnson, 1972a; Grondin et al, 1972; Lesperance et al, 1972a).

The bypass graft, unlike a significantly narrowed coronary artery, contributes little to total resistance to flow. The high fixed resistance of a critical proximal occlusive lesion is eliminated. Vascular tone in the peripheral vascular bed, previously near minimal in the setting of chronic hypoxia, returns to normal levels. The functioning graft thus reestablishes a more nearly normal situation whereby demand-dictated alterations in peripheral coronary vascular resistance distal to the bypass insertion can effect appropriate changes in coronary blood flow (Fig. 1). Flow sufficient to meet resting needs can increase when circumstances demand. Marked increases in flow are noted with the hypoxic hyperemia that follows release of graft occlusion or following injection of papaverine, isuprel, or nitroglycerin into the graft (Wilson, 1974). Appropriate increases in vein graft flow also have been noted postoperatively during exercise (Lichtlen et al, 1972) or with inhalation of amyl nitrite (Benchimol and Desser, 1973).

Collaterals participate in the distribution of flow as demonstrated by small increases in flow in one graft when a second graft to an adjacent coronary bed is clamped (Urschel et al, 1972; Mitchel et al, 1970; Webb et al, 1974). Flow

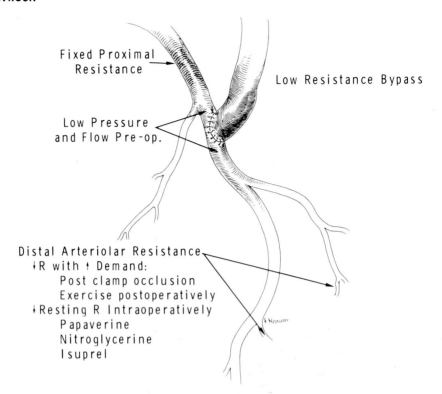

Fixed Proximal
Resistance

Low Resistance Bypass

Low Pressure
and Flow Pre-op.

Distal Arteriolar Resistance
↓R with ↑ Demand:
    Post clamp occlusion
    Exercise postoperatively
↓Resting R Intraoperatively
    Papaverine
    Nitroglycerine
    Isuprel

FIG. 1. Altered status of pressure, flow, and resistance after bypass (see text).

from a single graft distributes blood to a substantial mass of myocardium (Lichten et al, 1972; Hamilton et al, 1973; Greene et al, 1972).

Persisting substantial levels of flow have been measured a year or more after graft insertion by means of videodensitometry (Smith et al, 1972b), potassium-45 scanning (Bennett et al, 1973), xenon washout curves (Lichtlen et al, 1972; 1973), and flow meter measurement at reoperation (Diethrich, 1972). The presence of a widely patent graft at postoperative study is almost certain evidence that adequate flow is taking place (Lichtlen et al, 1972); grafts with low flow rates occlude early. This is in contrast to internal mammary artery implants where very low flow rates are present despite patency (Dart et al, 1970).

It must be noted that the presence of high rates of flow in a vein graft does not allow the conclusion that inadequate flow was present prior to graft insertion. Relative flow in two parallel conduits is determined by their relative diameters. Substantial flow occurs through a vein graft to a totally normal coronary artery due to the large relative size of the vein (Furuse et al, 1972). Attempts to demonstrate reduction in coronary blood flow among patients with coronary artery disease

have been largely unsuccessful (Rowe et al, 1969; Schwartz et al, 1973; Conti et al, 1970). These observations raise the question of whether graft flow really indicates increase in flow to the distal coronary bed or merely redistribution of flow through a preferred route of low resistance. Highly sophisticated studies of regional flow have suggested decrease in myocardial perfusion distal to occlusive lesions (Cannon et al, 1972; Dwyer et al, 1973), particularly during induced hyperemia (Gould et al, 1974). Careful observations at the time of vein bypass surgery demonstrate marked reductions in both pressure and flow in coronary arteries beyond areas of significant (70 to 80 percent or more) narrowing, even in the presence of collaterals (Urschel et al, 1972; Smith et al, 1972b; Webb et al, 1973; Webb et al, 1974; Parker et al, 1973; Johnson et al, 1970b; Kirk et al, 1973; Scherer et al, 1973; Leatherman et al, 1972). Release of clamp occlusion of a bypass graft to an adjacent collateralized bed does little to increase the low pressure in an ischemic bed whose graft is also clamped (Johnson et al, 1970b). Vein bypass grafts therefore not only achieve pressures and flows comparable to normal, they do so in areas where perfusion was seriously compromised.

1972; Bartel et al, 1973b; Lapin et al, 1972; Bowyer, 1973; Maurer et al, 1973; Helton et al, 1974; Trimble et al, 1974).

VEIN BYPASS FUNCTION: ENHANCED O₂ DELIVERY

Saphenous vein bypass grafting achieves a high rate of success in the relief of angina pectoris. In some patients, intraoperative myocardial infarction or the profound psychological impact of a thoracotomy may be responsible; such factors must be proposed for the improvement noted in some patients with totally occluded grafts (Griffith et al, 1973; Dodek et al, 1973). A number of widely confirmed observations, however, suggest that in most patients oxygen delivery is enhanced. Postoperative exercise capability is greatly improved in the absence of pain and with reduction of ST-T changes of ischemia noted preoperatively (Kaiser et al, 1972; Ross et al, 1972; Guiney et al, 1973; Dodek et al, 1973; Miller et al, 1972; Garcia et al, 1972; Bartel et al, 1973a; Bartel et al, 1973b; Matloff et al, 1973; Bowyer, 1973; Hammermeister and Kennedy, 1974; Hammermeister et al, 1974; Cline et al, 1974; Helton et al, 1974; Najmi et al, 1974; McDonough et al, 1974; Amsterdam et al, 1970a; Knobel et al, 1971). Reversal of ischemic ST changes has similarly been demonstrated with intraoperative release of clamp occlusion of the graft during rapid atrial pacing (Diethrich et al, 1973). Improved lactate metabolism during exercise suggests improved postoperative oxygen availability (Carlson et al, 1972, 1974; Smullens et al, 1972; Piccone et al, 1973; Kremkau et al, 1971; Hammond, 1970). Direct measurement of myocardial oxygen tension shows improvement after bypass insertion (Gardner et al, 1971). The observation that graft flow greatly increases following release of clamp occlusion at surgery (Wilson, 1974) or during postoperative exercise (Lichtlen et al, 1972; 1973) suggests autoregulatory function in the now-oxygenated distal coronary bed remains intact and that flow meeting resting demands is capable of increasing when demands increase. Coronary collaterals, presumably formed under the stimulus of poor perfusion, disappear after successful bypass and reappear after graft occlusion (Glassman et al, 1973; Solignac et al, 1973). Further evidence that improvement in symptoms reflects enhanced myocardial oxygen delivery is found in the high degree of correlation between improvement and graft patency; failure to improve or a return of symptoms similarly correlates with graft occlusion (Hammond and Poirier, 1973a; Alderman et al, 1973; Matloff et al, 1973; Manley et al, 1972; Ross et al,

VEIN BYPASS FUNCTION: IMPROVEMENT IN LEFT VENTRICULAR FUNCTION

The impact of saphenous vein bypass surgery on left ventricular function remains a subject of some controversy. Numerous studies appear to document improvement in at least some patients (Wilson, 1974). Perhaps the most convincing studies are those demonstrating marked reduction in ventricular function when the bypass graft is clamp occluded before sternotomy closure, with return to baseline values after release of the clamp (Emight et al, 1972; Anderson, 1972; Moran et al, 1973; Hairston et al, 1973; Wechsler et al, 1972; Bolooki et al, 1971; Rickards et al, 1974). Strain gauge measurements during such a sequence further demonstrate that improvement in left ventricular contractility is specific for the area of myocardium perfused by the graft (Moran et al, 1973; Hairston et al, 1973). Dramatic improvement is sometimes seen when moderate or marked left ventricular dysfunction accompanies rest pain (Sustaita et al, 1972; Fischl et al, 1973; Chatterjee et al, 1972b, 1973; Cheanvechai et al, 1973; Bolooki et al, 1973b, 1974b; Apstein et al, 1974; Hamby et al, 1974).

In many studies, improvement in ventricular function at rest has not been documented (Wilson, 1974; Hammermeister et al, 1974). Patients with chronic and more severe degrees of left ventricular dysfunction are least likely to improve, particularly if significant angina is absent (Wilson, 1974). Some studies showing enhanced function, furthermore, were performed in the early postoperative period when stress-induced increases in the contractile state may have been present (Rowe et al, 1969; Hammermeister et al, 1974). There is wide agreement that graft occlusion is well correlated with failure of left ventricular function to improve or, frequently, with deterioration in parameters of function (Wilson, 1973; 1974).

It is no surprise that noncontractile scar is not made functional by revascularization and that the chronically dysfunctional ventricle is most often unimproved after surgery. Profound degrees of dysfunction may occur in viable muscle in association with profound ischemia, however, and optimism is warranted when preoperative dysfunction accompanies rest or stress-induced pain. The distinction between scar and ischemic dysfunction, however, despite its central importance, is often difficult. A number of new approaches appear promising. A segmental area of hypokinesia is more likely to improve with revascularization than an area of akinesia (Campeau et al, 1973; Jacob et al, 1973; Hamby et al, 1974). Improvement in ventricular wall motion following nitroglycerin appears to correlate with improvement after revascularization (Pine et al, 1973; Reddy et al, 1974). Dysfunction appearing only with the stress of exercise or atrial pacing may be more frequently reversible (Hammermeister et al, 1974). Segmental contractile abnormalities involving areas distal to lesions of the anterior descending coronary artery are more likely to improve than are those of posterior or inferior walls (Banka et al, 1974; Saltiel et al, 1970; Chatterjee et al, 1972a). Segmental areas supplied by demonstrable collaterals may be more likely to demonstrate reversibility than those lacking collaterals (Banka et al, 1974). Electrocardiographic evidence of old infarction correlates with the presence of scar tissue and irreversible dysfunction (Jacob et al, 1973; Chatterjee et al, 1974; Banka et al, 1974; Hamby, et al, 1974), although islands of viable myocardium often exist in areas represented by Q waves on ECG (Dwyer et al, 1973). Differences in myocardial perfusion scanning (Gander et al, 1973; Dwyer et al, 1973; Jansen et al, 1973; Nener et al, 1973; McGowan et al, 1974), particularly after induced hyperemia (Ritchie et al, 1974), may offer clues as to the presence of scar or viable ischemic muscle. Refinement of these and other techniques may allow better selection of patients whose ventricular function is likely to improve following bypass graft surgery.

OPERATIVE MORTALITY AND MORBIDITY

Mortality within 30 days of vein bypass surgery is widely reported to be from 1 to 10 percent. Virtually all centers now experience surgical mortality of 5 percent or less for patients with stable angina and normal left ventricular function. Factors correlating with increased mortality include left ventricular dysfunction, increased severity of disease (particularly in the presence of a lesion of the left main), performance of less than "complete" revascularization, and recent myocardial infarction (Wilson, 1974). Increasing recognition of the importance of these factors has contributed to the decreasing mortality now reported. Diabetes mellitus and advanced age, independent of ana-

tomic considerations, do not greatly increase surgical risk (Verska et al, 1974; Hamby et al, 1973). Nonfatal intraoperative myocardial infarction occurs in 5 to 20 percent of patients and is a relatively uncommon mechanism in the relief of anginal pain (Wilson, 1974).

PATENCY OF THE BYPASS GRAFT: EARLY OCCLUSION BY THROMBUS

Patency is demonstrated at postoperative study in 65 to 90 percent of grafts in a large number of series (Wilson, 1973, 1974). Two institutions with wide experience report 90 percent patency at two years or longer following surgery (Urschel et al, 1972; Favaloro, 1973; Effler et al, 1971). Patency rates are based on angiographic series and may be overestimates in that nonsurvivors, many of whom have occluded grafts, are excluded.

Continued patency in the first few weeks after surgery may now be correlated with a number of factors, most of which relate to the amount of flow occurring in the graft. *Vein graft flow rates* of less than 20–40 cc's per minute (Davidson et al, 1973; Kaiser et al, 1972; Kaiser, 1972; Urschel et al, 1972; Urschel et al, 1974; Siderys et al, 1972; Girodin et al, 1971; Moran et al, 1971; Johnson, 1972b; Grondin et al, 1972) or lack of the usual post clamp occlusion hyperemic response (van der Mark et al, 1972) is associated with a high incidence of postoperative occlusion. Low graft flow is considered an indication for additional endarterectomy in some institutions (Urschel et al, 1972, 1974; Groves et al, 1972). Others propose high flow single grafts to multiple distal beds as a means of insuring patency (Johnson, 1972a; Bartley et al, 1972), although observed patency rates in such grafts are no higher (Bartley et al, 1972). A reliable prediction of the quantity of flow to be expected in a subsequent graft may be made from the preoperative angiogram. *Recipient artery diameter* of 1.5 to 2.0 mm or greater noted on preoperative coronary angiography (Lesperance et al, 1972a; Levin et al, 1972) or at surgery (Kaiser et al, 1972; Johnson, 1972a; Grondin et al, 1972, Lesperance et al, 1972a) predicts high flow and is associated with a high likelihood of postoperative patency. Although the arteriogram may occasionally underestimate distal arteries, particularly when they are filled by collaterals beyond major obstructions (Lesperance et al, 1972a; Levin et al, 1972; Rosch et al, 1972; Kay et al, 1974), distal segments not visualized by antegrade or retrograde collateral flow of contrast material are usually too small to sustain a patent graft (Levin et al, 1972). The presence of a large *distal runoff bed* free of arteriosclerotic disease correlates with much-improved postoperative patency (Lesperance et al, 1972a; Grondin et al, 1974). Similarly, the need for more distal placement of the graft is associated with increased risk of graft occlusion (Lesperance et al, 1972a). While *diabetes mellitus* often is associated with more distal disease (Chychrota et al, 1973), glucose intolerance in the presence of arteriographically favorable anatomy is not associated with an increased risk of graft occlusion (Chychrota et al, 1973; Barner et al, 1972). Decreased rates of patency have been noted in patients with poor *left ventricular function* (Apstein et al, 1974), perhaps reflecting decreased graft flow consequent to distal disease or increased wall tension.

One might expect *increased severity of arterial narrowing proximal to the graft* to be associated with increased graft patency in that experimental graft flow increases with increasing severity of acute proximal arterial obstruction (Kakos et al, 1972; Furuse et al, 1972). Such a relationship to patency has not been observed clinically (Johnson, 1972a; Alderman et al, 1973). The question may be asked as to whether a graft should ever be placed to an artery with less than a 70 percent obstructive lesion. Measurements in the dog with acute occlusion (Kakos et al, 1972; Furuse et al, 1972) and in the man at the time of operation (Urschel et al, 1972; Lichtlen et al, 1972; Smith et al, 1972b; Webb et al, 1973) suggest that perfusion is not compromised in such patients, at least at rest. Furthermore, flow in the graft (and hence patency prognosis) may be lessened. Such grafts have been proposed prophylactically to avoid reoperation as coronary disease progresses (Johnson et al, 1972). Consideration of graft patency and proximal graft-induced changes in the intrinsic circulation (*vide infra*) raise questions with regard to this policy.

The coronary artery bypassed is not an important factor with respect to early patency; equal patency rates are noted for bypass grafts to all three coronary divisions (Kaiser et al, 1972; Effler et al, 1971; Lesperance et al, 1972a; Flemma et al, 1972; Hammond and Poirier, 1973b; Grondin et al, 1974).

Experimental observations would suggest that decreased *diameter of the vein used for the graft* might enhance subsequent patency. Velocity of flow increases markedly as vein diameter decreases to approach that of the recipient artery (Urschel et al, 1972; Furuse et al, 1972). This increase in velocity occurs despite a lesser decrease in total flow. The increased sheer stress at the vessel wall consequent to increased velocity should discourage thrombus formation. The importance of this factor in early graft occlusion remains to be confirmed clinically. Many surgeons, nonetheless, are now using smaller saphenous veins taken below the knee despite the modest increase in technical difficulty of the anastomoses. *Technical factors* related to the aorta and coronary artery anastomoses may be incriminated in some early occlusions (Parsonnet et al, 1974; Urschel et al, 1974; Griffith et al, 1974). Use of single aortic anastomosis "Y" grafts is associated with higher rates of occlusion and to be avoided (Urschel et al, 1974; Walker et al, 1972).

Experimental observations suggest that *too many vein grafts* to adjacent areas connected by collaterals might reduce patency by competitive decrease in flow (Urschel et al, 1972). This too, remains to be observed clinically (Leatherman et al, 1972; Sewell, 1972). Despite the need for complete revascularization when possible, it is a rare heart in which more than three vein bypass grafts are indicated.

Postoperative mediastinal hemorrhage or infection carries a high risk of graft occlusion and must be carefully avoided and vigorously treated (Urschel et al, 1972; Adam et al, 1972). Fibrosis resulting from the inflammation of the postcardiotomy syndrome presents a similar threat, justifying the use of steroids when it occurs (Urschel et al, 1972).

PATENCY OF THE BYPASS GRAFT: LATE OCCLUSION BY PROLIFERATIVE CHANGE

Late occlusion does occur in a significant number of grafts that remain patent through the early postoperative period. Several studies in which series angiography has been performed suggest that as many as 12 to 19 percent of grafts patent in the early postoperative period have become occluded at restudy one year later (Sheldon et al, 1973; Lesperance et al, 1972a; Flemma et al, 1972; Sewell, 1972; Bourassa et al, 1973b).

Although numbers are as yet small, subsequent occlusion of grafts patent at 12 to 18 months would appear to occur rarely, and then only in graft segments where severe stenosis was noted on the earlier study (Manley and Johnson, 1972; Flemma et al, 1972; Lesperance et al, 1973; Grondin et al, 1974; Itscoitz et al, 1974). Excellent patency rates have been reported two years or more after operation (Urschel et al, 1972; Favaloro, 1973; Bruschke et al, 1973). Patency of one graft at seven years (Garrett et al, 1973) and another at six years (Itscoitz et al, 1974) after operation has been noted. It remains to be seen whether long-term patency will match the 65 percent patency rates noted at seven to ten years in femoral-popliteal grafts (Darling et al, 1967).

Late occlusion does not appear to correlate significantly with factors responsible for early graft occlusion (Lesperance et al, 1972a; 1972b), suggesting a differing mechanism. Atherosclerosis has been found in grafts of hyperlipidemic dogs (Brody et al, 1974), but has not yet been observed to play a role in late occlusion in man. Early occlusion results from thrombosis, often promoted by stasis; late occlusion usually results from venous subintimal hyperplasia. Initial observations of this proliferative process (Johnson et al, 1970a; Grondin et al, 1971; Vladover and Edwards, 1971) now have been confirmed by a large number of investigators (Wilson, 1974). A high percentage of late operative failures studied at reoperation or autopsy demonstrate this change (Adam et al, 1972; Vladover and Edwards, 1971; Kern et al, 1972). It is difficult to assess the frequency of subintimal hyperplasia among the majority of late postoperative survivors who are doing well. Only mild changes associated with wide patency have been noted following death from other causes as long as three years after insertion (Flemma et al, 1972). Two recent autopsy series of long-term survivors suggest that obstruction by this process is relatively uncommon (Staiman and Hammond, 1974; Klima and Milam, 1974). Angiography in long-term survivors suggests that a mild form of the process occurs in most grafts, with a mean reduction in vein diameter of approximately 30 percent developing between early and one-year postoperative study (Smith et al, 1972a; Lesperance et al, 1972b; Lesperance et al, 1973; Buis et al, 1973; Grondin et al, 1974). This reduction in vein diameter usually occurs diffusely along the length of the vein, but segmental narrowing of at least mild degree has been noted with a frequency as great as 35 percent (Lesperance et al, 1972b; 1973). No further reduction in vein diameter has been noted after one year (Lesperance et al, 1973; Grondin et al, 1974).

The etiology of subintimal hyperplasia is poorly understood and most likely is multifactorial. Incrimination of low flow or poor runoff (Vladover and Edwards, 1971) has not been confirmed (Lesperance et al, 1972a; 1972b). Furthermore, occluded grafts demonstrating this process have been

replaced by identically positioned new grafts that have then remained patent for at least one year (Johnson et al, 1972). The often segmental nature of the process suggests local trauma associated with manipulation. The frequent occurrence of the focal process in the proximal portion of grafts has suggested that turbulence may be important (Lesperance et al, 1972b). The fact that one graft may totally occlude by this process while others remain widely patent would appear to exclude systemic factors. Infrequently the process may be present in the vein prior to insertion as a result of venous disease (Urschel et al, 1972; Flemma et al, 1972). Of considerable interest is the fact that diffuse narrowing occurs to a greater extent in larger veins, resulting in an equalization of vein size to that approximating the 3–4 mm size of a major coronary artery (Lesperance et al, 1972b). This observation might suggest that decreasing diameter takes place to normalize increased wall tension and stress. Observations in the dog have suggested that interruption of the vasa vasorum and subjection of the vein to arterial pressure each makes an independent contribution to proliferative changes in the vein wall (Brody et al, 1972a; 1972b).

Care in dissection and manipulation, avoidance of exposure of the vein to nonphysiologic solutions, and an attempt to avoid dissection of the adventitia may decrease the incidence of late graft occlusion. Long-term aspirin therapy apparently has reduced long-term mortality following surgery in a single study (Al-Bassam et al, 1974; Mahdi et al, 1974). Whether this observation is correlated with vein graft patency is unknown. Steroids may retard development of the proliferative changes in the dog (Kaplitt et al, 1974). Additional study of avoidable factors in late proliferative occlusion is of high priority.

Reoperation may be considered in patients with good operative graft flow and subsequent late occlusion associated with the return of symptoms. Late occlusion may result from technical factors and, unlike most early occlusions, appears unrelated to local factors of inadequate runoff. A similarly placed second graft, then, need not meet the fate of the first. Results from reoperation in a limited number of patients have been reported by a number of groups (Reul et al, 1972; Cannom et al, 1973; Johnson et al, 1972; Hamaker et al, 1972; Favaloro, 1972). The surgery is more difficult, with longer operative and pump perfusion times required. Surgical mortality is in the range of 10 to 14 percent. Symptomatic results are generally good and patent grafts in sites of previous graft occlusions one year after reoperation have been reported (Johnson et al, 1972). The possibility of future reoperation for late graft occlusion adds practical importance to the careful documentation of graft flow rates at initial operation.

Very high rates of early and late postoperative patency are achieved with the increasingly popular internal mammary direct anastomosis. This procedure may be the operation of choice for lesions of the anterior descending coronary artery, particularly when distal vessel size or runoff is marginal and subsequent vein bypass graft patency questionable (Wilson, 1974).

CHANGES INDUCED BY THE BYPASS IN THE RECIPIENT CORONARY ARTERY

Aldridge and Trimble (1971) first observed the progression to total occlusion of proximal coronary artery lesions following bypass grafting (Fig. 2). This phenomenon subsequently has been observed by most investigators who have included visualization of the intrinsic coronary anatomy in postoperative evaluation, with incidence rates of 20 to 75 percent recorded (Griffith et al, 1973; Alderman et al, 1973; Ross et al, 1972; Segal et al, 1973; Johnson et al, 1972; Lichtlen et al, 1972; Malinow et al, 1972; Malinow et al, 1973; Bousvaros et al, 1972b; Adam et al, 1972; Green, 1972; Christie et al, 1973; Glassman et al, 1973;

Langston et al, 1973; Maurer et al, 1973; Zeft et al, 1974). Proximal artery occlusion is particularly common in patients with early graft occlusion (Griffith et al, 1973; Bourassa et al, 1973a; Ross et al, 1972). Proximal obstruction must be the result of the graft; nonbypassed arteries do not suffer this rate of progression in serial studies (Griffith et al, 1973; Bourassa et al, 1973a; Bemis et al, 1973; Kimbiris et al, 1972; Christie et al, 1973; Glassman et al, 1973).

Proximal narrowing proceeds to total occlusion after bypass presumably because high flow and high pressure introduced by the bypass into the recipient artery abolish the gradient across the proximal stenosis and reduce flow in the proximal coronary artery. Almost total cessation of flow across a narrowed proximal segment has been demonstrated in the dog following release of a clamp occluding a distal graft (Urschel et al, 1972; Furuse et al, 1972; Kakos et al, 1972). Occlusion then results from stasis-induced thrombosis. As might be expected, occlusion occurs at the previous site of narrowing and, particularly in the absence of large branches, may extend to the site of graft insertion. In some instances, failure of contrast material to proceed beyond an area of narrowing may reflect low levels of flow rather than true obstruction (Bourassa et al, 1973a; Bousvaros et al, 1972a; Tristani et al, 1973). Additional failure to visualize the proximal segment in retrograde fashion following vein graft injec-

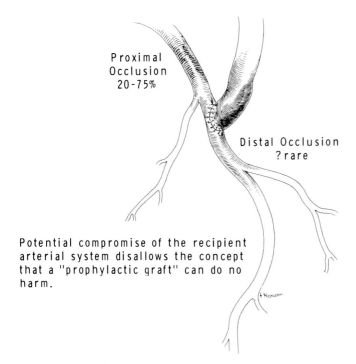

Proximal
Occlusion
20-75%

Distal Occlusion
?rare

Potential compromise of the recipient arterial system disallows the concept that a "prophylactic graft" can do no harm.

FIG. 2. Changes induced by the bypass in the recipient coronary artery (see text).

tion, included in most of the studies cited, is presumptive evidence of proximal artery occlusion. Progression of proximal arterial disease is not limited to use of the saphenous vein, for it has been observed following internal mammary anastomosis (Green, 1972).

Even when the graft remains patent, progression to occlusion of a proximal lesion may be clinically important. Simultaneous occlusion of branches between the sites of narrowing and anastomosis may result in infarction or return of angina (Bousvaros et al, 1972b). Preliminary information indicates, however, no increased incidence of infarction when the graft has remained patent (Malinow et al, 1972; Zeft et al, 1974). At least one remarkable patient remains alive and nearly asymptomatic seven years after bypass to the anterior descending coronary artery despite progression to total occlusion of a lesion in the left main coronary artery (Garrett et al, 1973). Progression to occlusion of a proximal lesion with the added insult of graft occlusion would be expected to have more grave consequences. Infarction and death attributed to this sequence of events have been noted (Alderman et al, 1973; Najmi et al, 1974).

Obstruction in the recipient coronary artery distal to the anastomosis site also has been reported (Griffith et al, 1973; Bourassa et al, 1973a; Arbogast et al, 1973; Grondin et al, 1974). Griffith et al (1973) noted a 10 percent incidence of distal obstruction at six months in association with a patent graft and a 26 percent incidence when the vein graft has been occluded. Most occlusions were bounded proximally by the anastomosis site in an area previously free of detectable disease. A 16 percent incidence of occlusion occurred in arteries not bypassed in the same patients, usually at a site of previous narrowing. Bourassa and coworkers (1973a) noted progression of disease (not necessarily to obstruction) distal to a patent graft in only 8 percent of recipient arteries in one year, a figure comparable to the 13 percent incidence of progression in arteries not bypassed. Glassman et al (1973) report new distal occlusion to be rare, irrespective of the patency status of the vein. Other reports of proximal arterial occlusion fail to mention the occurrence of distal occlusion. Such changes apparently are uncommon in the presence of a functioning bypass graft but may accompany graft occlusion. Extension of subendothelial proliferation from a vein graft into the wall of a coronary artery distal to the point of anastomosis has been observed in the dog (Jones et al, 1973).

Such changes have yet to be reported in man but could explain distal occlusion accompanying graft occlusion. Alternative explanations may be proposed. Thrombus may extend from a vein graft into a low flow recipient artery. Pressure distention of normal portions of a distal artery in some instances may create the illusion of increased severity of fixed diameter constricting lesions. Finally, the increase in pressure, turbulence, and flow may hasten the progression of arteriosclerotic disease in the distal vessel. Additional studies with regard to these important observations are needed.

These changes in recipient coronary arteries both proximal and distal to sites of graft anastomosis demand reappraisal of indications for bypass grafting. They disallow the romantic concept that a vein graft or an additional "prophylactic" graft *will do no harm.* Since occlusion in recipient arteries frequently accompanies early occlusion in vein grafts, an additional argument is made against insertion of a vein graft into an area where the recipient artery and runoff bed are small. The vein is unlikely to remain open, and its occlusion may be accompanied by further obstruction to the recipient artery.

IMPACT OF BYPASS SURGERY ON LONG-TERM SURVIVAL IN STABLE ANGINA

There is little doubt that vein bypass usually relieves angina. Coronary flow in previously compromised areas is increased, oxygen delivery is enhanced, and left ventricular function sometimes is improved. The quality of life is enhanced. A critical element in the decision to advise surgery to an individual patient, however, must remain the impact the operation may be predicted to have on his subsequent survival. On such information alone rests the decision for surgical intervention in the patient with few or no limiting symptoms. Large-scale controlled studies are now under way, but it may be some time before answers are available.

A single preliminary report of a prospective randomized series recently has appeared (Mathur and Guinn, 1973). Medical and surgical groups of 36 patients each have been followed slightly more than one year. Medical mortality has been 14 percent as compared to a total surgical mortality of 8 percent. Additional nonfatal infarctions have occurred in 8 percent and 3 percent, respectively. Quality of life and exercise capacity are better in the surgical group.

While additional reports encompassing more patients are awaited, tentative conclusions may be reached from examination of similar but unmatched postoperative patients and patients treated medically after angiographic documentation. Table 1 contains late mortality data from surgical series with reasonable followup. Of the patients in most of these series 70 to 80 percent had disease involving more than one artery and received multiple vein grafts. Surgical (30-day) mortality is excluded. Late attrition rates of 0.6 to 4.8 percent per year are noted. Of particular interest is the large series from the Cleveland Clinic (Sheldon et al, 1972; 1973) in which yearly attrition rates appear to decrease over the second and third years following surgery, perhaps in part reflecting a decreased tendency to late graft occlusion after one year.

The yardstick by which these data must be judged is the mortality observed with nonoperative management following angiographic definition. Such studies are largely retrospective, reporting subsequent follow-up of patients whose angiograms were performed prior to the present enthusiasm for surgical intervention. The patients in these studies may differ from those selected for vein bypass surgery, but these differences are not readily apparent. Most patients in the natural history series were relatively young and presented with symptoms suggestive of angina pectoris; many of them would now be considered candidates for bypass surgery in the same institutions. Data from series reporting natural history of angiographically documented disease are summarized in Table 2 and depicted graphically in Figure 3. In all instances at least 50 percent obstruction was required to declare a vessel significantly diseased. Remarkable consistencies are noted. Patients with single-vessel coronary disease are at lowest risk with yearly mortality rates of 2 to 5 percent. Isolated left anterior descending disease is associated with subsequent mortality approximately twice that of isolated right coronary artery disease (Sheldon et al, 1973; Bruschke et al, 1973; Moberg et al, 1972; Lichtlen and Mocetti, 1972; Mocetti and Lichtlen, 1973) with single vessel circumflex lesions falling somewhere between the two. Two- and three-vessel disease are associated with a yearly mortality of 6 to 13 percent and 8 to 18 percent, respectively. Left main lesions carry the most ominous prognosis with 8 to 30 percent yearly mortality, many of these deaths occurring within a few weeks of the angiographic study. Mild (30 to 50 percent occlusive) disease in a second vessel associated with single vessel 50 percent or greater obstruction sig-

TABLE 1. Late Mortality Following Bypass Graft Surgery[a]

	NO. PTS.	LATE MORTALITY[b] PER YEAR (%)	PERIOD OF FOLLOW-UP
Hall et al (1974)	1,329	2.6	9–46 mos
Reul et al (1972a)	1,158	1.9	mean 16 mos
Sheldon et al (1972, 1974)	960	2.3 (1st yr) 1.4 (2nd yr) 0.7 (3rd yr)	22–60 mos
Cannom et al (1973, 1974) Alderman et al (1973)	400	4.8	mean 9.9 mos
Clark et al (1974)	340	1.4	1 yr
Adam et al (1972b)	316	2.7	mean 15.7 mos
Sewell (1974)	154	2.6	1 yr
Green (1972)	136	1.4	mean 13.4 mos
Seaquist et al (1972)	133	2.3	1 yr
Mittler et al (1974)	130	4.0	1 yr
Kennedy, personal communication	122	0.6	mean 14 mos
Collins et al (1973)	105	4.3	mean 8.9 mos
Hammond et al (1973a)	91	3.3	1 yr
Zeft et al (1972)	51[c]	4.0[c]	13–27 mos

[a] Adapted from Wilson: Heart and Lung 3:431, 1974.
[b] Excludes 30-day operative mortality.
[c] All patients with greater than 75 percent obstruction of the left main coronary artery.

TABLE 2. Mortality with Medical Management of Angiographically Documented Coronary Artery Disease[a]

	NO. PTS.	PERIOD OF FOLLOW-UP	YEARLY MORTALITY (%)[b]				
			1 Vessel	2 Vessel	3 Vessel	Left Main	Total[c]
Bruschke et al (1973)[d]	590	5–9 yrs	2.9	7.6	10.8	11.4	6.9
Moberg et al (1972),[d] Sheldon et al (1973)	476	6+ yrs	3.5	7.8	12.7		9.3
Lichtlen and Mocetti (1972, 1973)	231	mean 32.5 mos	3.7	6.7	12.6		7.8
Oberman et al (1972)	148	mean 20.3 mos	2.7	13.7	18.1		11.8
Lim et al (1972)[d]	119	5 yrs	2.3	5.8	8.9		5.7
Friesinger et al (1970, 1973)	103	mean 79 mos	1.5		7.4		4.6
Slagle et al (1972)	94	mean 15 mos	5.0	19.0	25.0		19.1
Amsterdam et al (1970b)	66	mean 26 mos	6.6	12.5	13.5		10.9
Pichard et al (1973)[d]	48	mean 72 mos				8.0	
Kaltenbach et al (1973)	34	mean 17 mos					14.0
Sehapayak et al (1972)	33	mean 28 mos					10.4
Kisslo et al (1973)	32	1 yr				25.0	
Blumchen et al (1973)	27	mean 37 mos	0.0		12.9		6.1
Basta et al (1971)	21	mean 33 mos			12.0		5.2
DeMots et al (1974)	16	18 mos				33.0	
Cohen et al (1972)	10	mean 25 mos				20.8	
Lavine et al (1972)	9	1 mo				33.3	

[a] *Adapted from Wilson: Heart and Lung 3:431, 1974.*
[b] *Death from proven or probable cardiac cause only when specified.*
[c] *Average yearly mortality (%) for all patients and entire period of observation.*
[d] *These series all reported from Cleveland Clinic. Some patients may be included in more than one series.*

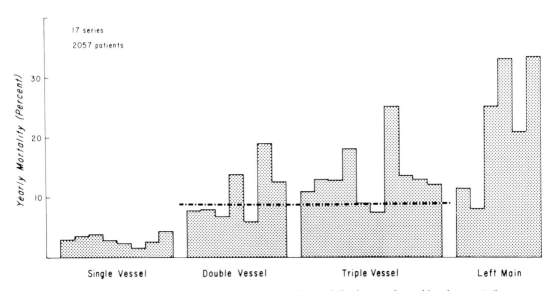

FIG. 3. The natural history of coronary artery disease following angiographic documentation. Values are based on 17 series (2,057 patients) listed in Table 2. Each level represents a mortality figure from a separate series. Larger series are positioned toward the left in each category. At least 50 percent obstruction was present in one, two, or all three major coronary arteries or in the left main coronary artery. The dashed horizontal line indicates a 9 percent yearly mortality figure thought representative of the data noted for two- and three-vessel disease (see text for details).

nificantly increases the mortality risk (Bruschke et al, 1973). Patients under age 40 reported by Lim et al (1972) are at slightly less risk than somewhat older patients reported by others from the experience of the same institution (Bruschke et al, 1973, Moberg et al, 1972). Natural history mortality also was relatively low among the young group of patients (mean age 41.4 years) reported by Friesinger et al (1970, 1973). The majority of patients in these series enjoyed well-preserved left ventricular function at the time of study and in some series (Moberg et al, 1972; Friesinger et al, 1973) left ventricular dysfunction was systematically excluded. In series where data with respect to left ventricular function were included, dysfunction was associated with significantly increased mortality risk (Bruschke et al, 1973; Lichtlen and Mocetti, 1972; Oberman et al, 1972; Amsterdam et al, 1970b; Slagle et al, 1972; Mocetti and Lichtlen, 1973; Murray et al, 1974). Series in which data were available on patients specifically noted to have normal left ventricular function (Bruschke et al, 1973; Moberg et al, 1972; Oberman et al, 1972; Friesinger et al, 1973; Murray et al, 1974) report total yearly mortality rates of 5.0 percent, 5.5 percent, 4.8 percent, 4.6 percent, and 2.7 percent in these patients. Data with respect to the presence of collaterals are inconclusive (Moberg et al, 1972; Lichtlen and Mocetti, 1972; Slagle et al, 1972; Mocetti and Lichtlen, 1973).

Survival statistics from patients followed conservatively after angiography (Table 2) and those treated by vein bypass (Table 1) may be compared (Fig. 4). The majority of patients undergoing surgery have had two- and three-vessel disease. Yearly mortality rates of 6 to 18 percent would be anticipated in similar patients treated medically (Table 2, Fig. 3). A figure of 9 percent has arbitrarily been chosen. Thirty-day surgical mortality in appropriately selected patients is 5 percent or less in most series, and this figure has been chosen. A figure of 3 percent per year late postoperative mortality has been selected as representative of the data in Table 1. The data from these series thus suggest (Fig. 4) that survival from one year onward in appropriate patients is favorably influenced by vein bypass surgery. Large-scale control studies are needed to confirm this tentative conclusion. Surgery directed toward improved survival in the carefully selected asymptomatic or mildly symptomatic patient emerges as a reasonable alternative where an established team with survival statistics equal to, or better than, those noted above is available. *The conclusion is inescapable that surgery, properly performed in the appropriately selected angina patient for the purpose of improving the quality of life, does not shorten life.* It should be noted that the statistics on which these conclusions are based, while largely representing experience in academic centers, do not solely reflect experience from one

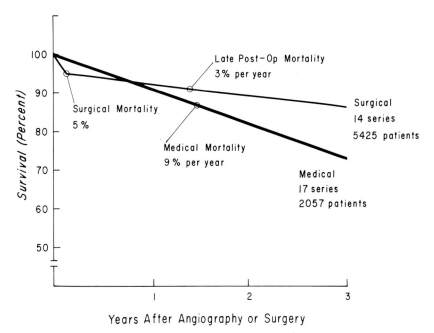

FIG. 4. Comparison of survival with medical and surgical management following angiographic definition. Data are from uncontrolled series containing similar patients (see Tables 1, and 2, Figure 3, and text for details). Adapted from Wilson: Heart and Lung 3:431, 1974.

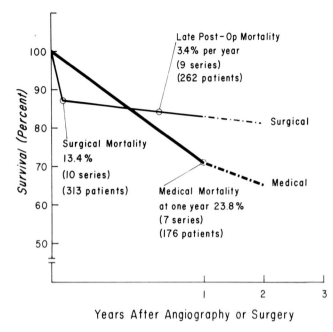

FIG. 5. Comparison of survival with medical and surgical management of patients with greater than 50 percent obstruction of the left main coronary artery. Data are from uncontrolled series containing similar patients (see Table 2 and text for details). Adapted from Wilson: Heart and Lung 3:431, 1974.

TABLE 3. Medically Treated Preinfarction Angina[a]

	NO. PTS.	HOSPITAL DEATHS (%)[b]	TOTAL DEATHS (%)	TOTAL NONFATAL MI (%)	PERIOD OF FOLLOW-UP
Vakil (1964)	190		10	27	3 mos
Gazes et al (1972, 1973)	140		18	12	1 yr
Krauss et al (1972)	100	1	26	8	mean 20 mos
See et al (1972)[c]	90	8	12	10	1 yr
Mulcahy et al (1970)	52		12	21	mean 4 yrs
Theroux and Campeau (1972)	44	3	3	19	1 mo
Scanlon et al (1973, 1974)[c]	40	25	25		? wks
Robinson et al (1972)[c]	38		18	32	mean 6 mos
Slagle et al (1972)[c]	34		29		mean 15 mos
Matloff et al (1974)	27	41	41		2 wks
Fischl et al (1973)[c]	23	0	33		mean 32 mos
Conti et al (1973)[c]	15	7	13	7	mean 10 mos
Favaloro (1973)	15	40	40		1 mo
Berk et al (1974)	14	22	22	42	1 mo
Ernst et al (1973)[c]	12		17	58	few mos

[a] *Adapted from Wilson: Heart and Lung 3:431, 1974.*
[b] *While hospitalized or within one month of diagnosis.*
[c] *Angiographic documentation.*

or two large referrral institutions and represent reasonable goals for competent teams anywhere. Increasing knowledge of factors related to operative mortality, graft closure, and induced changes in recipient coronary arteries may allow improved future patient selection and consequent improved late survival.

Figure 5 compares available data with respect to medical and surgical follow-up in patients with significant lesions of the left main coronary artery. The medical survival is based on seven series (Lavine et al, 1972; Cohen et al, 1972; Bruschke et al, 1973; Pichard et al, 1973; Kisslo et al, 1973; Scanlon et al, 1974a, DeMots et al, 1974) where conservative therapy followed angiographic documentation in a total of 176 patients. Mean mortality in the first year following angiography was 23.8 percent. High mortality in the weeks immediately following angiography is apparent in those series in which mortality at one month is specifically reported (Lavine et al, 1972; Bruschke et al, 1973). In series in which follow-up beyond the first year after angiography was specifically reported (Bruschke et al, 1973; Pichard et al, 1973; DeMots et al, 1974), attrition rates in the second and subsequent years are somewhat less than that during the first year. Deaths related to angiography are excluded from the medical series. The surgical data are based on reports of a total of 42 operative (30-day) deaths among 313 patients undergoing saphenous vein bypass surgery in ten series (Oldham et al, 1972; Lavine et al, 1972; Cohen et al, 1972; Pichard et al, 1973; Sharma et al, 1973; Kisslo et al, 1973; Scanlon et al, 1974a; Cohn and Collins, 1974; DeMots et al, 1974; Zeft et al, 1974). Patients with inadequate revascularization (only a single graft) in one series (Oldham et al, 1972) have been excluded. Follow-up to approximately one year was available in 262 surgical survivors with late deaths occurring in nine patients (Zeft et al, 1972; Lavine et al, 1972; Cohen et al, 1972; Pichard et al, 1973; Sharma et al, 1973; Scanlon et al, 1974a; Cohn and Collins, 1974; DeMots et al, 1974). It should be noted that coronary angiography alone in the presence of disease of the left main coronary artery is associated with significant mortality (15 deaths in 587 patients in 10 series) (Lavine et al, 1972; Cohen et al, 1972; Pichard et al, 1973; Sharma et al, 1973; Kisslo et al, 1973; Wolfson et al, 1973; Rosch et al, 1973; Scanlon et al, 1974a; DeMots et al, 1974; Battock et al, 1974; Zeft et al, 1974), and this 2.7 percent added risk must be considered in the

assessment of the surgical results. Figure 5 then represents a prediction of medical and surgical survival in a patient in whom coronary angiography has already been successfully performed and for whom a course of medical or surgical management must be selected. The surgical mortality is relatively high, nearly three times that for two- or three-vessel disease depicted in Figure 4. Late mortality after surgery is strikingly low, however, and not significantly greater than that noted in Table 1 and Figure 4. Mortality at one year with medical management is nearly three times the average figure for two- and three-vessel disease (Table 2, Fig. 3 and 4). Data are insufficient to make a definitive representation after the first year. No attempt has been made to depict the apparent increased risk during the few weeks following angiography. Despite the relatively high surgical mortality, the incidence of death in the medical series rapidly exceeds that in patients managed surgically and the evidence suggests that the survival curves will continue to diverge. In short, survival would appear to be significantly improved by vein bypass surgery in patients known to have significant disease of the left main coronary artery.

IMPACT OF BYPASS SURGERY ON SURVIVAL IN CRESCENDO ANGINA

Vein bypass has been used with increasing frequency in the treatment of the syndrome variously called crescendo, accelerated, unstable, or preinfarction angina. Reports from a large number of series document a surgical mortality of 7 to 8 percent among patients operated upon in the setting of increasingly frequent and more easily provoked anginal pain, often occurring at rest, but unassociated with evidence of demonstrable infarction (Wilson, 1974). Postoperative follow-up of at least 6 to 12 months is available in several series (Sustaita et al, 1973; Miller et al, 1973; Conti et al, 1973a; Conti et al, 1973b; Motlagh et al, 1972; Robinson et al, 1972; Wisoff et al, 1973; Bolooki et al, 1973a; Rahimtoola et al, 1973; Schroeder et al, 1973; Hammond and Poirier, 1974; Collins et al, 1974; Suzuki and Hardy, 1974; Bonchek et al, 1974) and suggests the yearly mortality rate following surgery for unstable angina is similar to the 2 to 4 percent figure noted for stable angina. Even severe left ventricular dysfunction in the setting of crescendo angina is not necessarily a contraindication, and normal function has been noted postoperatively in occasional patients in cardiogenic shock (without infarction) preoperatively (Sustaita et al, 1972). Most patients undergoing operation for preinfarction return to active asymptomatic life.

Widely varying results of conservative therapy in this syndrome make it difficult to assess the effect of surgery on survival. Medical series reported between 1964 and 1974 are listed in Table 3. One recent study (Fulton et al, 1972) was excluded because it consisted largely of patients not meeting criteria generally used in the medical and surgical series cited. When available, the mortality within one month of diagnosis or during hospitalization has been included. Several of the recent series include angiographic documentation of coronary artery anatomy. It is of interest that 19 percent of patients meeting clinical criteria for preinfarction angina in one recent series (Scanlon et al, 1973) had normal coronary arteriograms. The nonangiographic series undoubtedly contain significant numbers of such patients with consequent dilution of cardiac sequellae. All series in which follow-up was extended to several months or more after diagnosis document subsequent mortality in excess of 10 percent (Table 3). There is an equal additional incidence of nonfatal myocardial infarction. Increased mortality has been noted in patients with two- or three-vessel disease

(Robinson et al, 1972; See et al, 1972; Scanlon et al, 1974a; 1974b) or in those in whom angina continues to recur despite intensive therapy (Gazes et al, 1972; 1973). The prior presence of stable angina and the association of ECG changes with the accelerated anginal attacks appear also to correlate with even higher risk of subsequent infarction and death (Gazes et al, 1973). The degree to which observed mortality concentrated within the first month after diagnosis was highly variable.

Figure 6 attempts to compare the survival statistics from the unmatched medical (Table 3) and surgical series. A surgical mortality of 8 percent and late mortality following surgery of 3 percent per year has been used. A figure of 15 percent has been selected as a conservative representation of the mortality with medical therapy within one year of diagnosis (Table 3). One-third of this mortality (5 percent) arbitrarily has been assigned to the first month after diagnosis. On the basis of these preliminary and admittedly uncontrolled data, survival several months after the diagnosis of preinfarction or accelerated angina appears to be improved by surgical intervention. Prospective randomized studies are needed, particularly to define subset characteristics associated with greatest risk. The question of optimal timing of the bypass procedure requires further study (Theroux and Campeau, 1972; Theroux and Campeau, 1973; Fischl et al, 1973). The data

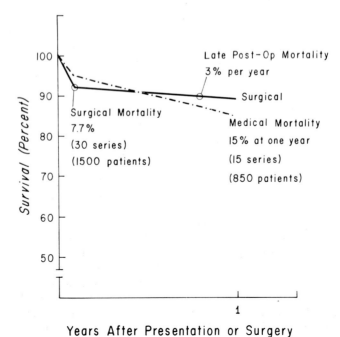

FIG. 6. Comparison of survival with medical and surgical management after presentation with accelerated angina. Data are from uncontrolled series (see Table 3 and text for details). Adapted from Wilson: Heart and Lung 3:431, 1974.

cited suggest that the risk of interim death by infarction exceeds the relatively small added risk of immediate surgery.

WHEN ANGIOGRAPHY?
WHEN SURGERY?
THE BASIS OF THE DECISION
TO INTERVENE

Limitation by symptoms and expectation of survival must be considered in the decision of whether, and when, to suggest surgery for a given patient. Relief of angina pectoris can be anticipated in a patient with "favorable" anatomy. The operation makes good sense physiologically and would appear to provide the increased myocardial oxygen delivery intended. For the active individual severely limited and made terribly unhappy by refractory angina pectoris, the decision to intervene surgically usually is an easy one. For many patients, however, the predicted impact of the surgery on survival assumes an important, if not central, role in the decision-making process. Survival alone, independent of symptomatic considerations, may be an indication for surgery in some individuals. Clinical, anatomic, and physiologic factors must all be considered in the prediction of surgical impact on survival (Table 4).

When should angiography be performed in the patient with known or suspected coronary artery disease? Information with respect to coronary anatomy and left ventricular function, obtained only by catheterization, is essential to the predicted impact of surgery on survival. In that this prediction may greatly influence the timing of surgical intervention, it would seem reasonable to obtain this information early, *as soon as the diagnosis is made,* in a patient who is in other respects a potential surgical candidate. The finding of a combination of factors suggesting a high likelihood of improved survival with surgery (that is, a young, otherwise healthy individual with three-vessel proximal disease, large distal vessels and runoff beds, and normal left ventricular function) argues for early surgical intervention, irrespective of symptomatic status or potential symptomatic response to medical management. Similar findings combined with a clinical presentation of accelerated or crescendo angina makes the argument for undelayed surgery more compelling. On the other hand, the finding of a combination of factors suggesting an equivocal or unpredictable impact of surgery on survival shifts the basis for management decisions to the patient's symptomatology: how limited he is; how unhappy he is with his limitations; and how well he responds to vigorous medical management. The decision for surgery may be postponed and periodically reconsidered. The definition of a combination of

TABLE 4. Will Surgery Enhance Survival?

	LESS LIKELY		MOST LIKELY
Clinical:	Pain-free	Stable angina	Accelerated or unstable angina
	Negative exercise testing		Marked ischemic ECG changes with low levels of exercise or with spontaneous pain episodes
	Recent MI		No preceding MI
	Over 65, additional pulmonary or systemic disease		Under 60–65, health otherwise excellent
Anatomic:	Isolated lesion of RCA	Isolated LAD lesion	Lesion L Main, 2- or 3-vessel disease
	Diffuse distal disease, small runoff bed, small distal diameter vessel		Greater than 70 percent proximal lesion with large distal vessels and runoff beds
Physiologic:	Severe LV dysfunction		Normal LV function
	Area distal to obstructive lesion is akinetic; there is ECG evidence of infarction in corresponding area		Normal wall motion or mild hypokinesia distal to obstructive lesion
	Other evidence to suggest scar, not ischemic dysfunction (see text)		Other evidence to suggest dysfunction is ischemic, not scar (see text)

After Wilson (1973).

factors for which surgery is unlikely to improve or likely to shorten survival, finally, allows the early commitment of both clinician and patient to vigorous medical management of his disease.

QUESTIONS MOST URGENTLY NEEDING ANSWERS

It is apparent that information gaps exist in our present state of knowledge in several critical areas. Investigative efforts directed at these unanswered questions should allow further refinement in patient selection and additional improvement in clinical results.

Undoubtedly, the most important information anticipated to appear in the near future are the results of *prospective randomized studies of medical and surgical management.* Preliminary reports of one study already have appeared (Mathur and Guinn, 1973), establishing the feasibility of such studies; several others are under way. The critical importance of these studies lies in the improved definition they will provide with respect to which sort of patient is likely to benefit most from surgery, particularly in terms of his prospects for survival. The relative weight of factors outlined in Table 4 remains incompletely defined in the absence of such studies. This additional information may allow the future recommendation of surgery in increasing numbers of patients on the basis of survival alone. Similarly, it may allow more vigorous pursuit of medical management in others, with the increased confidence that such management offers no less and perhaps greater chance for survival.

A major uncertainty in preoperative assessment lies in our *inability to distinguish between ischemia and scar* as a cause for segmental or diffuse abnormalities of left ventricular function. Scar is unimproved by revascularization and substantially increases operative risk. Functional improvement in viable ischemic muscle, on the other hand, is often dramatic, and risk may be increased when surgery is delayed. A reliable means of making this distinction preoperatively would enhance our ability to select patients most likely to benefit from the procedure. Promising possibilities mentioned above will need to be pursued and others explored.

What are the technical factors related to late graft occlusion and are they avoidable? More observations are needed relating late occlusion rates to vein graft size and methods employed in harvesting, preparing, and inserting the vein. *Is late vein occlusion a phenomenon largely limited to the initial 12 months after surgery and not a threat to long-term surviving grafts?* This observation is of extraordinary importance and requires further confirmation by other groups and after longer periods of graft function.

Further observations with respect to changes in recipient coronary arteries are pertinent. *How benign is proximal arterial obstruction in the presence of a functioning graft? How commonly does distal arterial occlusion accompany vein graft occlusion? What is the effect of the graft on the subsequent progression of distal disease in the recipient vessel?*

Further experience with the internal mammary artery direct anastomosis to the anterior descending of small diameter or runoff bed size may make operative intervention a viable alternative for some patients now inoperable. It remains to be seen whether transposed internal mammary grafts are deserving of widespread application.

The question of when to intervene surgically in the patient with accelerated or crescendo angina requires further study. The value of a period of stabilization utilizing Beta-blockade with or without heparin prior to surgery remains to be established. Should surgery be offered to the high-risk patient with continuing or recurrent pain following documented infarction? *Means of earlier definition of the infarction patient destined for progression to cardiogenic shock* may allow improved survival in such patients treated earlier with balloon assist and vein bypass surgery.

SUMMARY

Concepts with regard to aortocoronary bypass surgery are evolving rapidly. Near normal coronary flow is achieved in distal coronary beds where flow and pressure were severely compromised before surgery. Substantial flow persists a year or more following surgery and responds in a normal manner to increased myocardial oxygen need. The operation is highly successful in the relief of angina pectoris. Oxygen delivery is enhanced. Left ventricular function in some instances may be improved. This is particularly apparent when significant left ventricular dysfunction accompanies rest pain.

Surgical mortality has declined steadily, reflecting in part more complete knowledge of factors allowing better patient selection and increased recognition of the need for more complete revascularization when surgery is elected. Intraoperative myocardial infarction occurs in 5 to 20 percent. Relief of anginal pain is anticipated in survivors and only occasionally is due to infarction.

Postoperative patency rates are good and early occlusion by thrombus largely predictable from preoperative angiographic data. Late occlusion from subintimal hyperplasia occurs in perhaps 15 percent of grafts. It is rare after 12 to 18 months of patency. Increasing knowledge of factors related to early and late occlusion should lead to improved patient selection and operative technique with improved patency and function. Patients with nonvisualized or small distal arteries and limited runoff beds should be treated medically irrespective of their clinical presentation. Careful attention should be paid to the handling of the vein, and a vessel approximating the artery in size should be selected. Graft flow should be measured at surgery for its prognostic value and as a guide to further reoperation should late graft occlusion occur.

Progression of proximal narrowing to proximal occlusion in recipient coronary arteries is consistently observed in a substantial percentage of bypassed vessels. Consequences of this event are real, particularly when occlusion of the graft also occurs. Progression to occlusion distal to the point of bypass insertion has been less thoroughly documented and deserves intensive evaluation. Observed changes in recipient arteries disallow the concept that a bypass, ie a prophylactic one, "can do no harm."

Conclusions as to the impact of the surgical procedure on long-term survival in patients with stable angina are tentative and await the results of large-scale randomized prospective studies. Increasing information from unmatched but apparently similar natural history series with angiographic documentation (Table 2) and postoperative series reporting long-term follow-up (Table 1) strongly suggests that survival after one to two years is enhanced by surgery, at least in those patients with multivessel or left main proximal disease (Fig. 4 and 5). Certainly surgery does not statistically shorten life in the appropriately selected patient. Similar statements can be made with respect to the medical and surgical therapy of preinfarction angina (Fig. 6). These conclusions are based on nationwide experience and are not limited to two or three large referral centers.

The decision for, and timing of, surgery in patients with coronary artery disease must be based on considerations of both symptomatology and survival. Because the precise definition of coronary anatomy and left ventricular function is essential

to prediction of surgical impact on survival, coronary and left ventricular angiography should be performed early in the management of those patients who are in other ways potential surgical candidates.

Future investigative efforts should be directed toward several critical voids in our present knowledge. Controlled comparisons of substantial numbers of patients managed medically and surgically will allow better definition of patients most likely to be helped with surgery, particularly in terms of survival. Methods must be defined to distinguish left ventricular dysfunction due to scar from that resulting from ischemia. Further delineation of avoidable factors related to late occlusive changes in vein grafts may allow improved long-term patency. Additional long-term follow-up observations are needed to confirm initial conclusions that graft occlusion and coronary disease death are uncommon after the first anniversary of surgery. Further experience with direct anastomosis of the internal mammary to the small and questionably adequate anterior descending system may make operation feasible in patients now thought inoperable. The appropriate timing of surgery to achieve maximum survival in the patient with crescendo angina requires further study.

References

Adam M, Geisler GF, Lambert CJ, et al: Re-operation following clinical failure of aorta-to-coronary artery bypass vein grafts. Ann Thorac Surg 14:272, 1972

Al-Bassam MS, Hall RJ, Garcia E, et al: Survival of patients on various anti-thrombotic regimens following aortocoronary bypass surgery. Coronary Artery Medicine and Surgery Conference: Abstracts. Texas Heart Institute, Houston, Texas, February 21–23, 1974, p 68

Alderman EL, Matloff HJ, Wesler L, et al: Results of direct coronary artery surgery for the treatment of angina pectoris. N Eng J Med 288:535, 1973

Aldridge HE and Trimble AS: Progression of proximal coronary artery lesions to total occlusion after aortocoronary saphenous vein bypass grafting. J Thorac Cardiovasc Surg 62:7, 1971

Amsterdam EA, Iben A, Hurley EJ, et al: Saphenous vein bypass graft for refractory angina pectoris: Physiologic evidence for enhanced blood flow to the ischemic myocardium. Am J Cardiol 26:623, 1970a

Amsterdam EA, Most AS, Wolfson S, et al: Relation of degree of angiographically documented coronary artery disease to mortality. Ann Intern Med 72:780, 1970b

Anderson RP: Effects of coronary bypass graft occlusion on left ventricular performance. Circulation 46:507, 1972

Apstein CS, Kline SA, Leven DC, et al: Left ventricular function and graft patency following coronary artery-saphenous vein bypass surgery: Implications for surgical indications. Coronary Artery Medicine and Surgery Conference: Abstracts. Texas Heart

Institute, Houston, Texas, February 21–23, 1974, p 115

Arbogast R, Solignac A, Bourassa MG: Influence of aortocoronary saphenous vein bypass surgery on left ventricular volumes and ejection fraction. Am J Med 54:290, 1973

Banka VS, Bodenheimer H, Helfant RH: Value of coronary collaterals, pathologic Q waves and segmental location as determinants of reversibility of asynergy. Am J Cardiol 33:105, 1974

Barner HB, Kaiser GC, Codd JE, et al: Influence of diabetes on coronary graft flow. Circulation 46 (Suppl II):128, 1972

Bartel AG, Behar VS, Peter RH: Effects of aortocoronary bypass surgery on treadmill exercise. Circulation 46 (Suppl II):24, 1973a

Bartel AG, Behar VS, Peter RH, et al: Exercise stress testing in evaluation of aortocoronary bypass surgery—report on 123 patients. Circulation 48:141, 1973b

Bartley TD, Bigelow JC, Page VS: Aortocoronary bypass grafting with multiple sequential anastomoses to a single vein. Arch Surg 105:915, 1972

Battock DJ, Steele PP, Davis H: Left main coronary artery disease—is surgery always indicated? Am J Cardiol 33:125, 1974

Bemis CE, Gorlin R, Kemp HG, et al: Progression of coronary artery disease. Circulation 47:455, 1973

Benchimol A, Desser KB: Measurement of phasic aortocoronary bypass graft blood flow velocity in conscious man. Am J Cardiol 32:895, 1973

Bennett KR, Smith RO, Suzuki A, et al: The use of the potassium-45 myocardial scan in evaluating myocardial revascularization. Am J Cardiol 31:120, 1973

Bolooki H, Ghahramani A, Mallon S, et al: Long-term follow-up of patients with impending and early myocardial infarction treated by emergency myocardial revascularization. Circulation 48 (Suppl IV):147, 1973a

Bolooki H, Hallon S, Ghahramani A, Sommer L, et al: Objective assessment of the effects of aorto-coronary bypass operation on cardiac function. J Thorac Cardiovasc Surg 66:916, 1973b

Bolooki H, Robinson RM, Michie DD, et al: Assessment of myocardial contractility after coronary bypass grafts. J Thorac Cardiovasc Surg 62:543, 1971

Bonchek LI, Anderson RP, Rahimtoola SH, Bristow JD, Starr A: Unstable angina: Extended follow-up (1–4 years) after urgent bypass operation. Coronary Artery Medicine and Surgery Conference: Abstracts. Texas Heart Institute, Houston, Texas, February 21–23, 1974, p 117

Bourassa MG, Goulet C, Lesperance J: Progression of coronary arterial disease after aortocoronary bypass grafts. Circulation 48 (Suppl III): 127, 1973a

Bourassa MG, Lesperance J, Campeau L, et al: The nonprogressive nature of change in aortocoronary vein grafts. Am J Cardiol 31:122, 1973b

Bousvaros C, Chaudhry MA, Piracha AR: Progression of proximal coronary arterial lesions to total occlusions after vein graft surgery and its effects. Am J Cardiol 29:255, 1972a

Bousvaros C, Pirache AR, Chaudhry MA, et al: Increase in severity of proximal coronary disease after successful distal aortocoronary grafts. Circulation 46:870, 1972b

Bowyer AF: Myocardial revascularization surgery evaluated by multivariate analysis of exercise stress test data. Circulation 48 (Suppl IV):148, 1973

Brody WR, Angell WW, Kosek JC: Histologic fate of the venous coronary artery bypass in dogs. Am J Path 66:111, 1972a

Brody WR, Kosek JC, Angell WW: Changes in vein grafts following aortocoronary bypass induced by

pressure ischemia. J Thorac Cardiovasc Surg 64:847, 1972b

Brody WR, Rossiter SJ, Kosek JC, Lipton M, Angell WW: Atheroma production in autogenous venous aorto-coronary bypass grafts. Coronary Artery Medicine and Surgery Conference: Abstracts. Texas Heart Institute, Houston, Texas, February 21–23, 1974, p 8

Bruschke AVG, Proudfit WL, Sones FM: Progressive study of 590 consecutive nonsurgical cases of coronary disease followed 5–9 years. I. Arteriographic correlations. Circulation 47:1147, 1973

Buis B, Endlich B, Arntzenius AC: A technique to measure the diameter of coronary arteries and venous bypass grafts from 70 mm spot-films. Circulation 48 (Suppl IV):88, 1973

Campeau L, Elias G, Esplugas E, Lesperance J, Bourassa M: Left ventricular performance during exercise before and one year after saphenous vein graft surgery for angina pectoris. Circulation 48 (Suppl IV):53, 1973

Cannom DS, Miller C, Fogarty TJ, et al: Long-term follow-up of patients undergoing saphenous vein bypass surgery. Am J Cardiol 31:125, 1973

Cannon PJ, Dell RB, Dwyer EM: Regional myocardial perfusion rates in patients with coronary artery disease. J Clin Invest 51:978, 1972

Carlson RG, Kline S, Apstein C, et al: Lactate metabolism after aortocoronary vein bypass grafts. Ann Surg 176:680, 1972

Carlson RG, Lillehei CW: Reversal of abnormal myocardial metabolism (lactates) after coronary artery bypass grafts. Coronary Artery Medicine and Surgery Conference: Abstracts. Texas Heart Institute, Houston, Texas, February 21–23, 1974, p 3

Chatterjee K, Parmley WW, Sustaita H, et al: Influence of aortocoronary artery bypass on left ventricular asynergy. Am J Cardiol 29:256, 1972a

Chatterjee K, Parmley WW, Swan HJC, Sustaita H, Matloff J: Improved left ventricular asynergy and pump function after successful and uncomplicated direct myocardial revascularization. Coronary Artery Medicine and Surgery Conference: Abstracts. Texas Heart Institute, Houston, Texas, February 21–23, 1974, p 155

Chatterjee K, Swan HJC, Parmley WW, et al: Depression of left ventricular function due to acute myocardial ischemia and its reversal after aortocoronary saphenous vein bypass. N Engl J Med 286:1117, 1972b

Chatterjee K, Swan HJC, Parmley WW, et al: Influence of direct myocardial revascularization on left ventricular asynergy and function in patients with coronary heart disease. Circulation 47:276, 1973

Cheanvechai C, Effler DB, Loop FD et al: Emergency myocardial revascularization. Am J Cardiol 32:907, 1973

Christie LG, Achuff SC, Griffith LSC: Occlusive changes in coronary arteries after implant or vein bypass surgery. Circulation 48 (Suppl IV):52, 1973

Chychrota NN, Gau GT, Pluth JR, et al: Myocardial revascularization—comparison of operability and surgical results in diabetic and nondiabetic patients. J Thorac Cardiovasc Surg 65:856, 1973

Cline RE, Merrill AJ, Thomas CN, Armstrong RH, Stanford W: Symptomatic results of aortocoronary bypass compared with postoperative exercise performance. Coronary Artery Medicine and Surgery Conference: Abstracts. Texas Heart Institute, Houston, Texas, February 21–23, 1974, p 107

Cohen MV, Cohn PF, Herman MV, et al: Diagnosis and prognosis of main left coronary artery obstruction. Circulation 45 (Suppl I):57, 1972

Cohn LH, Collins JJ: Reduced mortality following revascularization surgery for left main coronary artery stenosis. Coronary Artery Medicine and Surgery Conference: Abstracts. Texas Heart Institute, Houston, Texas, February 21–23, 1974, p 39

Collins JJ, Laks H, Cohn LH: Prognosis after surgery for preinfarction angina. Coronary Artery Medicine and Surgery Conference: Abstracts. Texas Heart Institute, Houston, Texas, February 21–23, 1974, p 25

Conti CR, Brawley RK, Griffith LAC, Pitt B, et al: Unstable angina pectoris: Morbidity and mortality in 57 consecutive patients evaluated angiographically. Am J Cardiol 32:745, 1973a

Conti R, Brawley R, Pitt B, et al: Unstable angina: Morbidity and mortality in 57 consecutive patients evaluated angiographically. Am J Cardiol 31:127, 1973b

Conti CR, Pitt B, Gundel WD, et al: Myocardial blood flow in pacing-induced angina. Circulation 42:815, 1970

Darling RC, Linton RR, Razzuk MA: Saphenous vein bypass grafts for femoropopliteal occlusive disease: A reappraisal. Surgery 61:31, 1967

Dart GH, Scott S, Fish R, et al: Direct blood flow studies of clinical internal thoracic (mammary) arterial implants. Circulation 42 (Suppl II):64, 1970

Davidson GK, Gau GT, Davis GD: Early results of vein bypass grafts for coronary artery disease. Mayo Clin Proc 48:487, 1973

DeMots H, Rosch J, Bonchek LI, Anderson RP, Starr A, et al: Survival in left main coronary disease: The role of coronary angiography, coexisting coronary artery disease, and revascularization. Coronary Artery Medicine and Surgery Conference: Abstracts. Texas Heart Institute, Houston, Texas, February 21–23, 1974, p 48

Diethrich FB: Discussion of Grondin CM et al (Ann Thorac Surg 14:223, 1972)

Diethrich FB, Friedewald VE, Goldfarb D, et al: Intraoperative stress testing: An immediate physiologic assessment of myocardial revascularization. Chest 64:392, 1973

Dodek A, Kassebaum DG, Griswold HE: Stress electrocardiography in the evaluation of aortocoronary bypass surgery. Am Heart J 86:292, 1973

Dwyer EM, Dell RS, Cannom PJ: Regional myocardial blood flow in patients with residual anterior and inferior transmural infarction. Circulation 48:924, 1973

Effler DB, Favaloro RG, Groves LK, et al: The simple approach to direct coronary artery surgery—Cleveland Clinic experience. J Thorac Cardiovasc Surg 62:503, 1971

Emight LP, Marion AM, Daily PO, et al: Human coronary artery bypass grafts and left ventricular function. Surg 72:404, 1972

Favaloro RG: Clinical application of direct myocardial revascularization by saphenous vein graft technique. Heart & Lung 2:45, 1973

Favaloro RG: Discussion of Johnson WD et al (J Thorac Cardiovasc Surg 64:523, 1972)

Fischl SJ, Herman MV, Gorlin R: The intermediate coronary syndrome—clinical, angiographic, and therapeutic aspects. N Engl J Med 288:1193, 1973

Flemma RJ, Johnson WD, Lepley D, et al: Late results of saphenous vein bypass grafting for myocardial revascularization. Ann Thorac Surg 14:232, 1972

Friesinger GC, Humphries JD, Ross RS: Prognostic significance of coronary arteriography. In Kaltenbach M, Lichtlen P, Friesinger GC (eds): Coronary Heart Disease. Stuttgart, Georg Thieme, 1973, p 132

Friesinger GC, Page EE, Ross RS: Prognostic significance of coronary arteriography. Trans Assoc Am Phys 83:78, 1970

Fulton M, Duncan B, Lutz W, et al: Natural history of unstable angina. Lancet 1:860, 1972

Furuse A, Klopp EH, Brawley RK, Gott VL: Hemodynamics of aorta-to-coronary artery bypass. Ann Thorac Surg 14:282, 1972

Gander MP, Jansen C, Warehaus E, Huse W, Judkins MP: Internal mammary to anterior descending coronary anastomosis, evaluated postoperatively with high resolution arteriography and myocardial perfusion scanning. Circulation 48 (Suppl IV):90, 1973

Garcia E, Treistman B, El-Said G, et al: Treadmill evaluation of coronary artery bypass surgery. Circulation 46 (Suppl II):154, 1972

Gardner TJ, Brantigan JW, Perna AM, et al: Intramyocardial gas tensions in the human heart during coronary artery-saphenous vein bypass. J Thorac Cardiovasc Surg 62:844, 1971

Garrett HE, Dennis EW, DeBakey ME: Aortocoronary bypass with saphenous vein graft—seven year follow-up. JAMA 223:792, 1973

Gazes PC, Mobley EM, Faris HM, et al: Preinfarction angina—prospective study 10 year follow-up. Circulation 46 (Suppl II):23, 1972

Gazes PC, Mobley EM, Faris HM, et al: Preinfarction (unstable) angina—a progressive study 10 year follow-up. Circulation 48:331, 1973

Girodin CM, Lepage G, Gastonguay YR, et al: Aortocoronary bypass graft—initial blood flow through the graft and early postoperative patency. Circulation 44:815, 1971

Glassman E, Krauss KR, Weisinger B, Spencer FC: The effect of bypass grafting on the coronary circulation. Circulation 48 (Suppl IV):53, 1973

Gould R, Hamilton G, Lipscomb K, Kennedy W: Hemodynamics of coronary stenosis. Part II: Assessment of coronary flow reserve by dual isotope myocardial imaging in animals and man. Coronary Artery Medicine and Surgery Conference: Abstracts. Texas Heart Institute, Houston, Texas, February 21–23, 1974, p 58

Green GE: Internal mammary artery-to-coronary artery anastomosis: Three year experience with 165 patients. Ann Thorac Surg 14:260, 1972

Greene DG, Klocke FJ, Schimert GL, Bunnall IL, et al: Evaluation of venous bypass grafts from aorta to coronary artery by inert gas desaturation and direct flowmaker techniques. J Clin Invest 51:191, 1972

Griffith LSC, Achuff SC, Conti CR, et al: Changes in intrinsic coronary circulation and segmental ventricular motion after saphenous vein bypass graft surgery. N Engl J Med 288:589, 1973

Griffith LSC, Brawley RK, Hutchins GM: Morphology of the coronary artery bypass graft anastomosis. Am J Cardio 33:141, 1974

Grondin CM, Gastonguay YR, Lesperance J, et al: Attrition rate of aorta-to-coronary artery saphenous vein grafts after one year. Ann Thorac Surg 14:223, 1972

Grondin CM, Lesperance J, Bourassa MG, Pasternac A, et al: Serial angiographic evaluation in 60 consecutive patients with aorto-coronary artery vein grafts 2 weeks, 1 year, and 3 years after operation. J Thorac Cardiovasc Surg 67:1, 1974

Grondin CM, Meere C, Gastonguay Y, et al: Progressive and late obstruction of an aortocoronary venous bypass graft. Circulation 43:698, 1971

Groves LK, Loop FK, Silver GM: Endarterectomy as a supplement to coronary artery-saphenous vein bypass surgery. J Thorac Cardiovasc Surg 64:514, 1972

Guiney TE, Rubenstein JJ, Sanders CA, et al: Functional evaluation of coronary bypass surgery by exercise testing and oxygen consumption. Circulation 48 (Suppl III):141, 1973

Hairston P, Newman WH, Daniell HB: Myocardial contractile force as influenced by direct coronary surgery. Ann Thorac Surg 15:364, 1973

Hamaker WR, Doyle WF, O'Connell TJ, Gomez AC: Subintimal obliterative proliferation in saphenous vein grafts. Ann Thorac Surg 13:488, 1972

Hamby RI, Aintablian A, Tabrah F, Hartstein ML, Wisoff G: Determinants of reversibility of left ventricular function after aortocoronary bypass surgery. Am J Cardiol 33:142, 1974

Hamby RI, Wisoff BG, Kilker P, et al: Intractable angina pectoris in the 65 to 79 age group: A surgical approach. Chest 64:46, 1973

Hamilton GW, Lapin ES, Murray JA, Allen D: Evaluation of coronary artery surgery by 99Tc MMA myocardial perfusing imaging. Circulation 48 (Suppl IV):118, 1973

Hammermeister KE, Kennedy JW: The failure of successful saphenous vein bypass grafting to improve resting left ventricular performance in patients with chronic angina pectoris. Coronary Artery Medicine and Surgery Conference: Abstracts. Texas Heart Institute, Houston, Texas, February 21–23, 1974, p 63

Hammermeister KE, Kennedy JW, Hamilton GW, Stewart DK, et al: Aortocoronary saphenous vein bypass. Failure of successful grafting to improve resting left ventricular function in chronic angina. N Engl J Med 290:186, 1974

Hammond GL: Metabolic response of the myocardium to aortocoronary artery vein grafting. Circulation 42 (Suppl III):163, 1970

Hammond GL, Poirier RA: Early and late results of direct coronary reconstructive surgery for angina. J Thorac Cardiovasc Surg 65:127, 1973a

Hammond GL, Poirier RA: Graft patency and changes in coronary lesions and left ventricular function following saphenous vein grafting. Circulation 48 (Suppl IV):173, 1973b

Hammond GL, Poirier R: Acute surgical management and two year follow-up of 45 patients with preinfarction angina. Coronary Artery Medicine and Surgery Conference: Abstracts. Texas Heart Institute, Houston, Texas, February 21–23, 1974, p 24

Helton WC, Johnson FW, Hurnung J, Pyle RB, Amplatz K, et al: Treadmill exercise tests following coronary artery surgery. Coronary Artery Medicine and Surgery Conference: Abstracts. Texas Heart Institute, Houston, Texas, February 21–23, 1974, p 108

Itscoitz SB, Redwood DR, Graver LE, Reis RL, et al: Long-term durability of patent saphenous vein aortocoronary bypass grafts. Am J Cardiol 33:146, 1974

Jacob K, Chabot M, Saltiel J, Campeau L: Improvement of left ventricular asynergy following aortocoronary bypass surgery related to preoperative electrocardiogram and vectorcardiogram. Am Heart J 86:438, 1973

Jansen C, Judkins MP, Grames GM, Gander M, Adams R: Myocardial perfusion color scintigraphy with MAA. Radiology 109:369–380, 1973

Johnson WD: Surgical techniques of myocardial revascularization: an overview. Bull NY Acad Med 48:1146, 1972a

Johnson WD: The surgery everyone's talking about: Whom it's for and why. Medcom Learning Systems (Warner-Chilcott Labs):99, 1972b

Johnson WD, Auer JE, Tector AJ: Late changes in coronary vein grafts. Am J Cardiol 26:640, 1970a

Johnson WD, Flemma RJ, Manley JC, et al: The physiologic parameters of ventricular function as affected by direct coronary surgery. J Thorac Cardiovasc Surg 60:483, 1970b

Johnson WD, Hoffman JF, Flemma RJ, et al: Secondary surgical procedure for myocardial revascularization. J Thorac Cardiovasc Surg 64:523, 1972

Jones M, Conkle DM, Ferrons VJ, Roberts WC, Levine FH, et al: Lesions observed in arterial autogenous vein grafts. Circulation 48 (Suppl III):198, 1973

Kaiser GC: Discussion of Bittar N et al (J Thorac Cardiovasc Surg 64:855, 1972)

Kaiser GC, Barner HB, Willman VL, et al: Aortocoronary bypass grafting. Arch Surg 105:319, 1972

Kakos GS, Oldham HN, Dixon SH, et al: Coronary artery hemodynamics after aorta-to-coronary artery vein bypass. J Thorac Cardiovasc Surg 63:849, 1972

Kaplitt MJ, Frantz SR, Gandhi RK, Gross S, Beil AR: Use of methylprednisolone in improving long-term patency of vein grafts. Coronary Artery Medicine and Surgery Conference: Abstracts. Texas Heart Institute, Houston, Texas, February 21–23, 1974, p 69

Kay EB, Naraghipour H, Beg RA, DeManey M, et al: Limitation of coronary angiography as a criteria to bypass surgery. Am J Cardiol 33:147, 1974

Kern WH, Dermer GB, Lindesmith GG: The intimal proliferation in aortic-coronary saphenous vein grafts. Am Heart J 84:771, 1972

Kimbiris D, Lavine P, van den Broek H, et al: The evolution of coronary arterial pathology in patients with angina pectoris as determined by the coronary arteriogram. Am J Cardiol 29:273, 1972

Kirk ES, Lambretti JJ, Cohn LH, Collins JJ, Gorlin R: Low saphenous vein graft blood flow and absence of reactive hyperemia in non-occlusive coronary artery disease. Circulation 48 (Suppl IV):59, 1973

Kisslo J, Peter R, Behar V, Bartel A, Kong Yihong: Left main coronary artery stenosis. Circulation 48 (Suppl IV):57, 1973

Klima T, Milam JD: Pathology of aortocoronary artery autogenous saphenous vein grafts. Coronary Artery Medicine and Surgery Conference: Abstracts. Texas Heart Institute, Houston, Texas, February 21–23, 1974, p 37

Knobel SB, McHenry PL, Phillips JF, et al: Objective assessment of saphenous vein bypass grafts. Circulation 44 (Suppl II):187, 1971

Kremkau EL, Kloster FE, Neill WA: Influence of aortocoronary bypass on myocardial hypoxia. Circulation 44 (Suppl II):103, 1971

Langston M, Selzer A, Cohn K: Enhanced rate of progression of coronary disease due to aortocoronary bypass. Circulation 48 (Suppl IV):58, 1973

Lapin ES, Murray JA, Bruce RA: A new hypothesis to improve selection of patients for saphenous vein graft surgery. Am J Cardiol 31:144, 1972

Lavine P, Kimbiris D, Segal BL, et al: Left main coronary artery disease. Am J Cardiol 30:791, 1972

Leatherman LL, Rochelle DG, Dawson JT, et al: Coronary arteriography after coronary artery bypass surgery. Circulation 46 (Suppl II):181, 1972

Lesperance J, Bourassa MG, Biron P, et al: Aorta to coronary artery saphenous vein grafts—Preoperative angiographic criteria for successful surgery. Am J Cardiol 30:459, 1972a

Lesperance J, Bourassa MG, Saltiel J, et al: Late changes in aortocoronary vein grafts: Angiographic features. Am J Roentgen and Radiotherapy 116:74, 1972b

Lesperance J, Bourassa MG, Saltiel J, Campeau L, Grondin CM: Angiographic changes in aortocoronary vein grafts: Lack of progression beyond the first year. Circulation 48:633, 1973

Levin DC, Carlson RG, Baltaxe HA: Angiographic determination of operability in candidates for aortocoronary bypass. Am J Roentgen and Radiotherapy 116:66, 1972

Lichtlen P, Mocetti T: Prognostic aspects of coronary angiography. Circulation 46 (Suppl II):7, 1972

Lichtlen P, Mocetti T, Halter J, et al: Postoperative evaluation of myocardial blood flow in aorta-to-coronary artery vein bypass grafts using Xenon-residue detection techniques. Circulation 46:445, 1972

Lichtlen P, Mocetti T, Halter J, Gattiker K: Postoperative

evaluation of myocardial blood flow in aorta-to-coronary artery vein bypass grafts using the Xenon-residue detection technique. In Kaltenbach M, Lichtlen P, Friesinger GC (eds): Coronary Heart Disease. Stuttgart, Georg Thieme, 1973, p 286

Lim J, Proudfit WL, Sones FM: Prognosis of young men with coronary disease. Circulation 46 (Suppl II):60, 1972

McDonough JR, Danielson RA, Foster RK: Maximal cardiac output before and after coronary artery surgery in patients with angina. Am J Cardiol 33:154, 1974

McGowan RL, Martin ND, Zaret BL, Wall HP, Flamm MD: Rubidium-81 a new agent for myocardial perfusion scans at rest and exercise, and comparison with potassium-45. Am J Cardiol 33:154, 1974

Mahdi SA, Hall RJ, Garcia E, et al: Evaluation of the effects of antithrombotic therapy on survival following aortocoronary bypass surgery. Am J Cardiol 33:122, 1974

Malinow MR, Kremkau EL, Kloster FE: Occlusion of coronary arteries after vein bypass. Circulation 46 (Suppl II):23, 1972

Malinow MR, Kremkau EL, Kloster FE, et al: Occlusion of coronary arteries after vein bypass. Circulation 47:1211, 1973

Manley JC, Johnson WD: Effects of surgery on angina (pre- and post-infarction) and myocardial function (failure). Circulation 46:1208, 1972

Mathur VS, Guinn GA: Prospective randomized study of coronary bypass surgery: Preliminary report. Circulation 48 (Suppl IV):58, 1973

Matloff HJ, Alderman EL, Wexler L, et al: What is the relationship between the response of angina to coronary surgery and anatomical success? Circulation 48 (Suppl III):168, 1973

Maurer BJ, Oberman A, Jones WB, Kouchoukos NT, Reeves TJ: Clinical and angiographic follow-up of patients with saphenous vein bypass grafts. Circulation 48 (Suppl IV):196, 1973

Miller DC, Cannom DS, Fogarty TJ, et al: Saphenous vein coronary artery bypass in patients with "pre-infarction angina." Circulation 47:234, 1973

Miller SEP, Johnson WD, Tector AJ, et al: The effect of myocardial revascularization on anginal symptoms, ventricular function and exercise performance. Circulation 46 (Suppl II):24, 1972

Mitchel BJ, Adam M, Lambert CJ, et al: Ascending aorta-to-coronary artery saphenous vein bypass grafts. J Thorac Cardiovasc Surg 60:457, 1970

Moberg CH, Webster JS, Sones FM: Natural history of severe proximal coronary disease as defined by cineangiography (200 patients, 7 year follow-up). Am J Cardiol 29:282, 1972

Mocetti T, Lichtlen P: Prognostic aspects of coronary angiography based on a one to six year control. In Kaltenbach M, Lichtlen P, Friesinger GC (eds): Coronary Heart Disease. Stuttgart, Georg Thieme, 1973, p 142

Moran JM, Chen PY, Rheinlander HF: Coronary hemodynamics following aortocoronary bypass graft. Arch Surg 103:539, 1971

Moran SV, Tarazi RC, Urzua JU, et al: Effects of aortocoronary bypass on myocardial contractility. J Thorac Cardiovasc Surg 65:335, 1973

Motlagh FA, Pansegrau DG, Wilson HE: Direct myocardial revascularization for preinfarction syndrome. Circulation 46 (Suppl II):195, 1972

Murray JA, Chinn N, Peterson DR: Influence of left ventricular function on early prognosis in atherosclerotic heart disease. Am J Cardiol 33:159, 1974

Najmi M, Ushigama K, Blanco G, Adam T, Segal BL: Results of aortocoronary artery saphenous vein bypass surgery for ischemic heart disease. Am J Cardiol 33:42, 1974

Nener TPE, Ellis FH, Kirk ES: Intraoperative delineation

of ischemic and scarred myocardium by localized detection of ^{42}Potassium in dogs. Circulation 48 (Suppl IV):91, 1973

Oberman A, Jones WB, Riley CP, et al: Natural history of coronary artery disease. Bull NY Acad Med 48:1109, 1972

Oldham HN, Kong Y, Bartel AG, et al: Risk factors in coronary artery bypass surgery. Arch Surg 105:918, 1972

Parker FB, Neville JF, Hanson EL, Webb WR: Collateral pressures and flow in the preinfarction syndrome. Circulation 48 (Suppl IV):92, 1973

Parsonnet V, Gilbert L, Gielchinsky I: A prospective study of the causes for and prevention of aorto coronary bypass graft closure. Coronary Artery Medicine and Surgery: Abstracts. Texas Heart Institute, Houston, Texas, February 21–23, 1974, p 66

Piccone V, Sawyer P, LeVeen H, et al: The mechanism of anginal relief following direct cardiac revascularization. Chest 64:405, 1973

Pichard AD, Sheldon WC, Kasumitsu S, Effler DB, Sones FVH: Severe arteriosclerotic obstruction of the left main coronary artery: Follow-up results in 176 patients. Circulation 48 (Suppl IV):53, 1973

Pine R, Meister SG, Banka VS, et al: Detection of reversible ventricular contraction abnormalities with nitroglycerin: Correlation with post coronary bypass ventriculography. Circulation 48 (Suppl IV):104, 1973

Rahimtoola SH, Bonchek LI, Starr A, Anderson RP, Bristow JD: Late results after emergency aortocoronary bypass surgery for unstable angina. Circulation 48 (Suppl IV):205, 1973

Reddy PS, Mathews RH, O'Toole JD, Salerni R, Shaver JA: Reversibility of left ventricular asynergy assessed by post nitroglycerin left ventriculography. Coronary Artery Medicine and Surgery: Abstracts. Texas Heart Institute, Houston, Texas, February 21–23, 1974, p 56

Reul GJ, Morris GC, Howell JF, et al: Current concepts in coronary artery surgery. Ann Thorac Surg 14:243, 1972

Rickards A, Wright J, Balcon R: Observations on the effect of occlusion, nitroglycerin, and papaverine on coronary artery bypass grafts. Am J Cardiol 33:164, 1974

Ritchie J, Hamilton G, Murray J, Lapin E: Myocardial imaging with ^{99}Tc macro-aggregates: Clinical, hemodynamic, ECG, surgical, and autopsy correlations. Am J Cardiol 33:165, 1974

Robinson WA, Smith RF, Stevens TW, et al: Preinfarction syndromes: Evaluation and treatment. Circulation 46 (Suppl II):212, 1972

Rosch J, Bonchek L, Antonovic R, et al: Angiographic appraisal of vessel suitability for aortocoronary venous bypass graft surgery. Circulation 46 (Suppl II):213, 1972

Rosch J, DeMots H, Antonovic R, Rahimtoola SH, Judkins MP: Coronary arteriography in left main coronary artery disease. Circulation 48 (Suppl IV):209, 1973

Ross D, Sutton R, Dow J, et al: Venous graft surgery in treatment of coronary heart disease. Brit Med J 2:644, 1972

Rowe GE, Thompson JH, Stenlund RR, et al: A study of hemodynamic and coronary blood flow in man with coronary artery disease. Circulation 39:139, 1969

Saltiel J, Lesperance J, Bourassa MG, et al: Reversibility of left ventricular dysfunction following aortocoronary bypass grafts. Am J Roentgenol Radium Ther Nucl Med 110:739, 1970

Scanlon PJ, Nemickas R, Moran JF, et al: Accelerated angina pectoris—clinical, hemodynamic, arteriographic and therapeutic experience in 85 patients. Circulation 47:19, 1973

Scanlon PJ, Talano JV, Moran JF, Gunnar RM, Pifarre R: Main left coronary artery disease. Coronary Artery Medicine and Surgery Conference: Abstracts. Texas Heart Institute, Houston, Texas, February 21–23, 1974a, p 38

Scanlon PJ, Talano JV, Moran JF, et al: Preinfarction angina: Experience with 162 consecutive patients. Coronary Artery Medicine and Surgery Conference: Abstracts. Texas Heart Institute, Houston, Texas, February 21–23, 1974b, p 22

Scherer JL, Goldstein RE, Stinson RP, et al: Correlation of angiographic and physiologic assessment of coronary collaterals in patients receiving bypass grafts. Circulation 48 (Suppl IV):88, 1973

Schroeder JS, Berndt TB, Cannom DS, et al: Long-term results of surgery for unstable angina pectoris. Circulation 48 (Suppl IV):216, 1973

Schwartz L, Froggatt G, Couvey HD, Taylor K, Morch JE: Measurement of left anterior descending coronary arterial blood flow. Am J Cardiol 32:679, 1973

See JR, Cosby RS, Giddings JA, Mayo M: Medical management of acute coronary crises. Circulation 46 (Suppl II):318, 1972

Segal BL, Likoff W, van den Broek H, et al: Saphenous vein bypass surgery for impending myocardial infarction. JAMA 223:767, 1973

Sewell WH: Discussion of Flemma RJ et al (Ann Thorac Surg 14:232, 1972)

Sharma S, Khaja F, Henle R, Goldstein S, Easley R: Left main coronary artery lesions: Risk of catheterization, exercise test and surgery. Circulation 49 (Suppl IV):53, 1973

Sheldon WC, Rincon G, Effler DB: Vein graft surgery for coronary artery disease: Survival and angiographic results among the first one thousand patients. Circulation 46 (Suppl II):110, 1972

Sheldon WC, Rincon G, Effler DB, et al: Vein graft surgery for coronary artery disease—Survival and angiographic results in 1,000 patients. Circulation 48 (Suppl III):184, 1973

Siderys H, Pittman JN, Herod G: Coronary artery surgery in patients with impaired left ventricular function. Chest 61:482, 1972

Slagle RC, Bartel AG, Behar VS, et al: Natural history of angiographically documented coronary artery disease. Circulation 46 (Suppl II):60, 1972

Smith HC, Frye RL, Wood EH, et al: Sequential measurement of saphenous vein graft flows and dimensions. Circulation 46 (Suppl II):68, 1972a

Smith SC, Gorlin R, Herman MV, et al: Myocardial blood flow in man: Effects of coronary collateral circulation and coronary artery bypass surgery. J Clin Invest 51:2556, 1972b

Smullens SN, Wiener L, Kasparian H, et al: Evaluation and surgical management of acute evolving myocardial infarction. J Thorac Cardiovasc Surg 64:495, 1972

Solignac A, Campeau L, Bourassa MG: Regression and appearance of coronary collaterals in humans during life. Circulation 48 (Suppl IV):92, 1973

Staiman RI, Hammond GL: Histopathologic changes occurring in aortic coronary artery saphenous vein grafts. Coronary Artery Medicine and Surgery Conference: Abstracts. Texas Heart Institute, Houston, Texas, February 21–23, 1974, p 7

Sustaita H, Chatterjee K, Matloff JM, et al: Emergency bypass surgery in impending and complicated acute myocardial infarction. Arch Surg 105:30, 1972

Sustaita H, Chatterjee K, Matloff JM, Swan HJC: The rationale for surgery in preinfarction angina. Am J Cardiol 31:160, 1973

Suzuki A, Hardy JD: Surgery for impending myocardial infarction. Coronary Artery Medicine and Surgery Conference: Abstracts. Texas Heart Institute, Houston, Texas, February 21–23, 1974, p 47

Theroux P, Campeau L: Aorto-coronary vein graft surgery for unstable angina. Circulation 46 (Suppl II):229, 1972

Theroux P, Campeau L: The influence of timing of surgery on mortality and incidence of myocardial infarction following aortocoronary vein graft surgery in crescendo angina. Am J Cardiol 31:162, 1973

Trimble AS, Goldman BS, Morch JE, et al: Late hemodynamic evaluation of patients with aortocoronary bypass grafts. Coronary Artery Medicine and Surgery Conference: Abstracts. Texas Heart Institute, Houston, Texas, February 21–23, 1974, p 110

Tristani FE, Virinderjit SB, Maleki M: Angiographic evidence of competitive flow following aorta-coronary bypass surgery. Chest 64:409, 1973

Urschel HC, Razzuk MA, Wood RE, et al: Factors influencing patency of aorto-coronary artery saphenous vein grafts. Surgery 72:1048, 1972

Urschel HC, Razzuk MA, Wood RE: Factors influencing patency of aorto-coronary artery saphenous vein grafts. Coronary Artery Medicine and Surgery Conference: Abstracts. Texas Heart Institute, Houston, Texas, February 21–23, 1974, p 67

Van der Mark F, Frank HLL, Buis B, et al: Significance of blood flow measurements in implanted aorta-coronary bypass grafts. Circulation 46 (Suppl II):232, 1972

Verska JJ, Gosney WG, Walker WJ: Aortocoronary bypass in the diabetic patient. Am J Cardiol 33:174, 1974

Vladover Z, Edwards JE: Pathological changes in aortic-coronary arterial saphenous vein grafts. Circulation 44:710, 1971

Walker JA, Friedberg IID, Flemma RJ, et al: Determinants of angiographic patency of aortocoronary vein bypass grafts. Circulation 45 (Suppl I):86, 1972

Webb WR, Neville JF, Parker FB, Hanson EL: Collateral blood flows and pressures in coronary artery disease. Coronary Artery Medicine and Surgery Conference: Abstracts. Texas Heart Institute, Houston, Texas, February 21–23, 1974, p 161

Webb WR, Parker FB, Neville JF: Retrograde pressures and flows in coronary arterial disease. Ann Thorac Surg 15:256, 1973

Wechsler AS, Gill C, Rosenfeldt F, et al: Augmentation of myocardial contractility by aortocoronary bypass grafts in patients and experimental animals. J Thorac Cardiovasc Surg 64:861, 1972

Wilson WS: Aortocoronary saphenous vein bypass: A review of the literature. Heart and Lung 2:90, 1973

Wilson WS: Aortocoronary bypass II—An updated review. Heart and Lung 3:431, 1974

Wisoff BG, Kilker P, Harstein ML, et al: Surgical approach to impending myocardial infarction. J Thorac Cardiovasc Surg 65:523, 1973

Wolfson S, Grant D, Ross AM, Cohen LS: Risk of death related to coronary arteriography: Role of left coronary lesions. Circulation 48 (Suppl IV):88, 1973

Zeft HJ, Manley JC, Huston JH, et al: Direct coronary surgery in patients with left main coronary artery stenosis. Circulation 46 (Suppl II):50, 1972.

Zeft HJ, Manley JC, Huston JH, Tector AJ, et al: Left main coronary artery stenosis. Results of coronary bypass surgery. Circulation 49:68, 1974

2

"NATURAL" HISTORY OF SEVERE ANGINA PECTORIS WITH INTENSIVE MEDICAL THERAPY ALONE
When Should Surgery Be Considered?

Henry I. Russek

At the present time, there is no reliable index of prognosis applicable to patients with angina pectoris receiving optimal medical care. Proponents of bypass surgery frequently seek support of their views by citing ill-defined, inapplicable, or antiquated statistics in evidence of the allegedly poor response attending medical management. Often such data have been derived from nonrandom samples of patients, treated "casually" or inadequately by current standards, and weighted in the direction of clinical profiles at serious risk. Although a number of authors have reported on mortality rates in large groups of patients followed for one, two, or more decades (Table 1), the advent of modern drugs and new perspectives in management must raise serious doubt as to the relevance of such data to patient populations under treatment at the present time.

With no specific regimen of therapy, Zukel et al,[19] for example, reported the annual mortality rate in a large series of patients with angina pectoris to be only about 3 percent while Kannel and Freinleib[5] found the yearly attrition rate in

their patients at Framingham to be approximately 4 percent. Today, with modern therapeutic approaches consisting of dietary management, weight reduction, hypocholesterolemic drugs, control of hypertension and diabetes, curtailment of stress and tobacco, exercise training, and the use of such agents as propranolol and isosorbide dinitrate, it does not seem unreasonable to expect that the outlook has become more favorable. At the present time, however, we cannot be certain of the extent to which this may have occurred. The availability of comprehensive measures, even of established value, affords no assurance that the available therapeutics will be applied on a wide scale and in an effectual manner. The status of treatment for arterial hypertension in this country, for example, provides adequate insight into the wide gulf that may exist between the actual results of *casual* management and those potentially attainable under *optimal* therapy. A similar disparity may exist with respect to the management of angina pectoris. This is suggested by the fact that a large segment of the patients now being referred for bypass surgery have had medical care no better, and often worse, than that which prevailed 100 years ago. In a recent survey[17] of 200 patients admitted to hospital for surgical revascularization allegedly for intractable angina, 46 percent were found to have been treated with no other antianginal agent but nitroglycerin and even this drug had been frequently employed only to abort an attack rather than to prevent it. In many instances, ineffectual antianginal preparations had been prescribed or potent agents administered indiscriminately or improperly. Frequently, little effort had been expended by patient or physician to eliminate either precipitating factors for angina

TABLE 1. Mortality in Angina Pectoris

AUTHORS	ANNUAL MORTALITY (%)
Zukel and coworkers[19]	3
Kannel and associates[5]	4
Parker et al[10]	6
Block and coworkers[1]	6
Moberg et al[8]	6.4
	3.3 (1 vessel)
	6.7 (2 vessels)
	10.5 (3 vessels)
Sheldon and Associates[18]	8.8

pectoris or risk factors for atherosclerosis. In no single instance was the patient returned to the referring physician with a recommendation for more intensive medical management or was surgery deferred on this account. This narrow approach has not only contributed appreciably to the incidence of "refractory" patients but has also led to premature or needless referral for surgical revascularization. From such practices, neither the attending physician nor the cardiovascular surgeon can stand on firm ground in attempting to evaluate the indications or results of operative intervention.

It should be evident that even if accurate statistics were now available to indicate the average annual mortality rate in anginal patients receiving optimal medical care, the physician would gain little help in assessing prognosis for the individual case and in rendering a decision with regard to surgery. Just as average mortality rates for acute myocardial infarction tell little about the actual risk with a mild first attack or with a massive recurrent episode associated with cardiogenic shock, average annual attrition rates for patients with angina pectoris as a group must similarly mask the mortality risk prevalent in various clinical subsets of this syndrome. At the present time, therefore, there is urgent need not only to seek out clinical profiles that may identify anginal patients at varied risk but also to record the natural hazards in these categories under the best available medical care.

Since there are a variety of factors that are known to influence the prognosis in angina pectoris, the classification, intensive treatment, and follow-up of patients in relatively high and low risk categories could provide useful data for weighing the hazards of surgery against the natural consequences of the disease. Insight gained from long clinical experience has shown that among the major factors contributing to risk in this disorder are cardiac enlargement, congestive heart failure, multiple myocardial infarctions, hypertension, atrial fibrillation, valvular heart disease, and diabetes mellitus. Since patients suffering from severe angina pectoris frequently possess none of these poor prognostic signs, it seemed that it might be possible to identify "good-risk" subjects who, despite severe initial symptoms, could have excellent prospects under appropriate medical therapy for both dramatic clinical improvement and relatively long survival. It is of interest that similar classifications have proved useful in selecting patients for anticoagulant therapy in acute myocardial infarction.[11] Thus, we have reported that

the low morbidity and mortality in patients initially classified as "good risk" on the basis of clinical prognostic signs did not justify even the small hazard attending the use of anticoagulant drugs during the acute phase of myocardial infarction. In contrast, the reverse was found to be true for "poor-risk" patients. The question we sought to answer with respect to severe angina pectoris, therefore, was whether or not similar classification and follow-up could prove helpful in establishing criteria for or against surgical intervention. From the prospective study that was begun in November 1966 and has continued to the present time, useful data appear to be emerging.[12-16]

MATERIAL

In all, a total of 133 patients presenting with severe forms of angina pectoris, unresponsive to conventional treatment, have been followed under a well-defined and intensive therapeutic program. Their ages ranged from 29 to 80 years. Of the total, 102 patients were men and 31 were women. In each instance slight to moderate physical or emotional stress regularly evoked classic episodes of angina pectoris, which, until the time of study, could not be adequately controlled or prevented despite the customary use of nitroglycerin, long-acting nitrates, sedatives, and other measures. As a consequence, in many patients the activities of daily living, occupational performance, and even sleep were frequently disturbed. Alterations in life style also had had limited influence on disability in these patients. Among the measures tried were reduction in the speed of walking; reserving more time for dressing in the morning; a change in the manner of transportation; avoidance of overeating and of walking after meals or in cold weather; and the elimination of emotional outbursts, prolonged conversation, straining at stool, or watching competitive sports. The average number of nitroglycerin tablets used per day varied from 5 to 50 in these patients. None in the series had been treated with beta blocking agents prior to this study. The diagnosis was confirmed in each patient by an unequivocal history of the classic symptoms present for one year or more, typical ischemic electrocardiographic (ECG) patterns after exercise, previous episodes of myocardial infarction, or cinecoronary angiographic evidence of advanced disease. Within the three-month period preceding this study, 32 patients in the series had been studied by angiography and 26 of this number were found to have severe triple coronary artery disease. A history of one or more myocardial infarctions requiring hospitalization was elicited in 55 of the 133 patients and confirmed by electrocardiography. Seventeen in the series were on digitalis therapy prescribed for previous congestive heart failure. Eight suffered from other complications such as cerebrovascular insufficiency, previous stroke, or severe and uncontrolled diabetes. Twelve patients were over the age of 70 years.

CLASSIFICATION OF PATIENTS

Although all patients suffered from severe and refractory forms of angina pectoris, they were classified as "good risk" or "poor risk" at the time of their initial examinations on the basis of certain clinically recognized poor prognostic signs. Such classification was maintained unaltered throughout the period of study irrespective of events occurring during the course of follow-up. Thus a patient was considered to be a poor risk for relatively long survival if he presented any one of the following unfavorable criteria:

1. Congestive heart failure, past or present. This important prognostic sign was elicited by means of careful history to determine the occurrence of effort dyspnea, paroxysmal nocturnal dyspnea and edema, and by physical examination and roentgenography.
2. Significant enlargement of the heart. Clinical evidence of cardiac enlargement was presumed to be present when the maximal apical impulse was accentuated or diffuse and situated lateral to the midclavicular line and when the area of cardiac dullness on percussion extended well beyond 10 cm to the left of the midsternal line in the fifth interspace. In all instances confirmation was required by fluoroscopic and roentgenologic examination prior to final classification. From fluoroscopic study important information was also obtained concerning left ventricular function and asynergy.
3. Multiple myocardial infarctions. In all instances documentation of such events was obtained by careful history, reference to records of previous hospitalizations, and detailed electrocardiographic study. ,
4. Gallop rhythm. Each patient was auscultated sitting, supine, and after mild exercise in the left lateral position.

The presence of a protodiastolic (third) heart sound at the apex on auscultation was recorded as a sign of serious ventricular impairment.

5. Refractory hypertension. Levels of blood pressure persisting above 170 mm, systolic, and 100 mm, diastolic, despite adequate and vigorous therapy were considered to exert an adverse influence on prognosis.
6. Atrial fibrillation. In the presence of severe angina pectoris this arrhythmia with its impairment of stroke volume and potential for complications was deemed to be an unfavorable prognostic criterion.
7. Severe and uncontrolled diabetes. Patients refractory to vigorous therapy or uncooperative in its administration and showing persistent glycosuria and hyperglycemia were assumed to have a guarded prognosis.
8. Previous "stroke" or cerebrovascular insufficiency. This complication in the presence of severe angina pectoris was accepted as evidence of diffuse atheromatosis with poor outlook for survival.
9. Advanced age. Considering the limitations of the normal life span this was arbitrarily chosen as "over the age of 70."

Of the 133 patients in the series, 102 qualified as "good risk" by manifesting none of the predesignated unfavorable indices, while 31 were identified as "poor risk" on the basis of these criteria (Table 2). Fifteen of 26 patients with severe triple coronary artery disease on angiography were classified in the good-risk group because of the presence of good left ventricular function and no adverse clinical signs. All 11 with angiographic evidence of significant left ventricular asynergy also would have been classified as "poor risk" from the clinical criteria alone.

When judged by functional status (New York Heart Association Classification), 87 of the

TABLE 2. Classification and Characteristics of 133 Patients with Severe Angina Pectoris

	"GOOD RISK"	"POOR RISK"
Number	102	31
Average age	58.8	65.2
Over 70 years old	0	12
Congestive heart failure	0	17
Previous myocardial infarction	28	27
Other complications	0	8

patients were found to be in Class III and 46 were in Class IV.

Therapeutic Management

All patients were placed on a regimen designed to achieve or maintain optimum weight. Serum lipid abnormalities were treated by means of diet and often by hypocholesterolemic agents. Hypertension and diabetes were managed with appropriate drugs with the aim of careful control. Tobacco and stimulants were proscribed. Alterations in life style to minimize stress were adopted where feasible. When left ventricular function was not impaired, graduated exercise on a daily basis, always preceded by prophylactic medication, was encouraged.

Medicinal treatment in all cases consisted of the combined administration of propranolol and isosorbide dinitrate (ISDN). The dosage of propranolol was determined in each patient by careful titration to discover the amount needed to reduce resting heart rate to a frequency of 55 to 60 beats per minute. The daily dosage of propranolol varied from as little as 10 mg twice daily to 160 mg four times daily. Sixty-two percent of the patients required 40 mg, twenty percent 60 to 80 mg, ten percent 100 to 160 mg, and eight percent 20 mg or less, as a single dose three or four times daily. Isosorbide dinitrate was administered *sublingually* in a dosage varying between 2.5 and 10 mg, according to individual tolerance and response. Seventy-four percent of the patients took 5 mg of ISDN, six percent 2.5 mg, and twenty percent 10 mg as their usual sublingual dose. The dose of propranolol was taken orally *before* each meal and that of ISDN sublingually *after* each meal in order to obtain the longest possible period of synergistic activity during expected times of physical stress.[12-15] When congestive heart failure was detected or even suspected, digitalis and an oral diuretic were prescribed prior to the use (or continuation) of propranolol.

RESULTS

Clinical Manifestations

The striking clinical response to propranolol and isosorbide dinitrate observed among subjects in this series has been previously reported.[12-15]

In 90.2 percent of the 133 patients, marked amelioration of angina pectoris associated with significant increments in exercise tolerance have been documented by controlled observations. In these patients, there has been not only a reduction of 50 percent or more in the frequency of anginal episodes and in nitroglycerin requirements but also a striking increase in the ability to exercise without pain ($p < 0.01$). The favorable clinical responses correlate closely with improvement in ischemic ECG patterns evoked by standard exercise. In 50 percent of 62 patients so tested, there has been complete reversal of exercise ECG abnormalities when evaluations were performed during periods of combined pharmacologic activity of these agents (Fig. 1). It is of interest that no tendency has been observed toward an attenuation of effect with the passage of time.

Improvement in functional class following the administration of propranolol-isosorbide dinitrate therapy has been most significant (Table 3). Twenty of the 87 patients originally in Class III showed sufficient improvement to be grouped in Class I, while 63 shifted to Class II. Of the 46 patients in Class IV at commencement of this study, 18 were judged to be in Class II and 19 were in Class III after the institution of therapy.

Myocardial Infarction

Over the six-year period, 25 of the 102 "good-risk" patients suffered attacks of acute myocardial infarction, and of these, 19 recovered and 6 died. In the "poor-risk" group, myocardial infarction occurred in 24 patients and accounted for death in 17 of the 31 patients during the same period.

Mortality Rate

A total of 6 "good-risk" patients, followed from three to six years, have died. None of the 102 patients, followed for two years, died during the first year; two died the second year. One of the 100 surviving patients died during the third year. Two of the 94 patients, followed for four years, died; one of the 85 patients, followed for five years, died. A small number have been followed through the sixth year, during which there were no deaths. From the mortality rate experience in this study, the probability of death in "good-risk" and "poor-

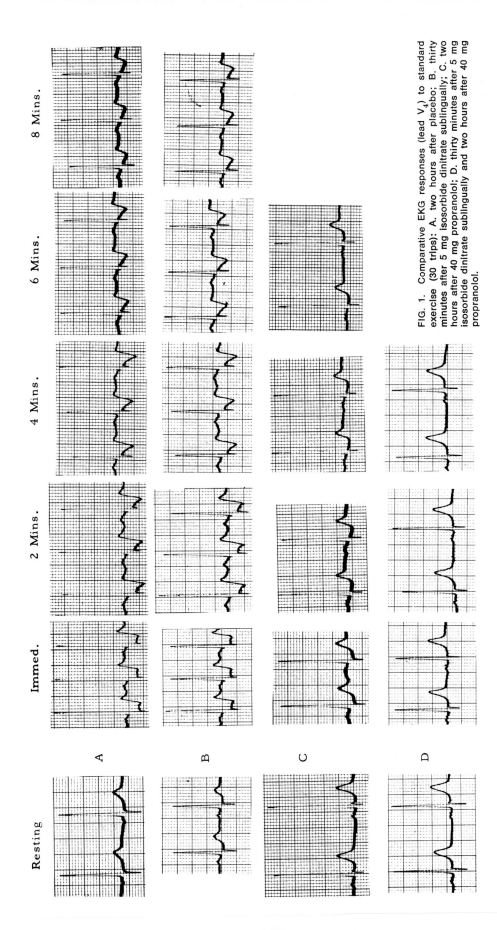

FIG. 1. Comparative EKG responses (lead V_4) to standard exercise (30 trips): A. two hours after placebo; B. thirty minutes after 5 mg isosorbide dinitrate sublingually; C. two hours after 40 mg propranolol; D. thirty minutes after 5 mg isosorbide dinitrate sublingually and two hours after 40 mg propranolol.

27

TABLE 3. Comparison of New York Heart Association Functional Class before and after Propranolol-ISDN Therapy

FUNCTIONAL CLASS	NO. PTS.	
	Pre Treatment	Post Treatment
I	–	20
II	–	81
III	87	23
IV	46	9

risk" patients has been plotted in Figure 2. It can be seen that 6 percent of "good-risk" patients may be expected to die by the end of fifth year of follow-up, indicating an average annual mortality rate of 1.2 percent for this group. In sharp contrast, in "poor-risk" patients it may be anticipated to approximate 25 percent. These differences are highly significant statistically $(p < .001)$. Although only one-third of our "poor-risk" patients survived to the end of the fourth year, it is of interest that none in this group died during the fifth year of observation. Since all of the survivors in the "poor risk" group were patients over the age of 70 with good left ventricular function and no adverse clinical signs, it seems apparent that old age *per se* should not have been used as one

of the indices for an unfavorable five-year prognosis. These data make it clear that overall mortality rates in any reported series will depend on the composition of the sample with respect to the numbers of "good-risk" and "poor-risk" patients.

DISCUSSION

The indications for surgical revascularization cannot be fully established until the fate of the patient with angina pectoris under optimal medical care has been clearly defined. Currently, two divergent views are readily found in the literature: (1) that angina pectoris is a highly lethal disease, and (2) that it is a benign disorder compatible with long survival in the majority of cases. In consonance with these respective philosophies, one finds bypass grafting endorsed as the therapeutic procedure of choice [4] or condemned as a needless, dangerous, and costly intervention.[2, 16]

Up to the present time there have been no available data to define the prognosis among anginal patients with varying clinical profiles under optimal medical therapy. The present study has shown that in carefully selected "good-risk" patients managed under a modern comprehensive

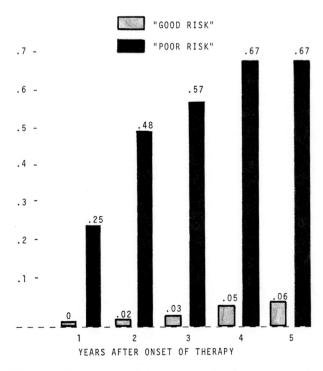

FIG. 2. Probability of death of patients under propranolol–isosorbide dinitrate therapy, according to clinical status. Gray bars represent "good risk" and black, "poor risk" patients.

medical regimen, the probability of death over a period of five years was only 6 percent, or approximately 1.2 percent a year. This rate of mortality is only slightly above that found in the general population in the same age groups. The significance of this observation is perhaps more meaningful when it is realized that it has been made in patients who, at the time of entry into this study, mere suffering from serious and refractory forms of angina pectoris often associated with severe two or three vessel disease but with relatively *normal* left ventricular function. Inasmuch as coronary bypass surgery in similar patients is associated with an immediate operative mortality rate ranging from 2.5 to 10 percent, as well as with a formidable incidence of nonfatal complications and graft failure, early and late,[3,7,9] these data make it difficult to justify surgical intervention unless disabling symptoms persist despite optimal medical care. The justification for any procedure in clinical medicine must be based on a clear demonstration of its capacity to improve the natural course of the disease for which it is employed whether through the alleviation of symptoms or the prolongation of life or both. But proof of such benefit is not enough unless it can also be shown that the overall improvement clearly outweighs the risks.

The relatively favorable outlook for "good-risk" patients in this study despite presenting symptoms of severe angina pectoris is undoubtedly related to comparatively normal left ventricular function in all cases. Although angiography was obtained in only 20 percent of these patients, careful clinical assessment in conjunction with fluoroscopic and roentgenographic study did disclose normal heart size and function in all subjects. In this regard, the use of other noninvasive measures may prove valuable to identify or confirm those believed to be at minimal risk. In any case, in the event that some "poor-risk" patients were inadvertently included in the "good-risk" group, the conclusions to be drawn from this study would assume even greater validity. While careful selection was undoubtedly a crucial factor, the total medical regimen directed at the removal of coronary risk factors and the utilization of propranolol in combination with isosorbide dinitrate to prevent recurrent bouts of coronary insufficiency may have played an important, although presently undefined, role in determining the excellent prognosis in these patients.

These findings should not be construed to mean that coronary artery pathology demonstable by coronary angiography has no prognostic importance. There is no conflict with the finding that morbidity and mortality is greater in patients with triple coronary artery disease than in those with single- or double-vessel involvement (Table 1).[8] It must be borne in mind, however, that triple coronary artery disease is also associated with a significantly higher incidence of congestive heart failure, cardiac enlargement, multiple infarctions, and asynergy. Consequently, since the major determinant of survival is the status of left ventricular function, the probability of death when such function is relatively normal may not be appreciably increased even in the presence of triple vessel disease (over a five-year period of intensive medical therapy).

When refractory angina pectoris is associated with impairment of left ventricular performance as observed in "poor-risk" patients of this series, the prognosis appears grave whether medical or surgical therapy is adopted. In spite of excellent symptomatic response to medical treatment in most cases, 25 percent of these "poor-risk" subjects died within the first year and 67 percent failed to survive to the end of the fourth year. Equally dismal, however, are the results of surgical therapy in which the immediate mortality rate has been reported to be as high as 40 percent or more with the chances of salvage relatively poor. In this category, too, therefore, operative intervention should be considered only after the most careful clinical assessment.

The overall mortality rate for the 133 patients in this series was approximately 4 percent per year, which is strikingly similar to that reported by Kannel and Freinleib[5] in the Framingham study. When it is realized, however, that all of the patients in the present investigation suffered from severe symptoms often associated with one or more previous myocardial infarctions, whereas those in the Framingham study were selected anginal subjects without prior infarction, significant benefit from intensive medical therapy is suggested. In this regard, careful attention to risk factors and the administration of propranolol and sublingual isosorbide dinitrate to prevent pain and ischemic changes could prove to be of paramount importance.

A review of the current literature indicates that operative mortality from bypass surgery throughout this country varies from as little as 0.8 percent[4] to as much as 20 percent.[6] The incidence of myocardial infarction and nonfatal major complications as the result of bypass procedures also seems to show considerable variability but is undoubtedly of appreciable significance in all series.

Obviously, the experience of the surgical team, the pre- and postoperative care, the manner of selection of patients, and the choice of operative procedure, are important determinants of the outcome. By analogy, it should not seem unreasonable to expect that under a wholly medical regimen, the prognosis in angina pectoris may also vary with the quality of care and the skill, patience, and fortitude of the attending physician.

The dramatic relief obtained in some patients from disabling angina pectoris following bypass surgery should not blind the practicing physician to the high price in morbidity and mortality that may be exacted by this intervention. In one large community hospital,[6] it was found that the patient submitted to bypass surgery had about two chances out of three of either dying, having no patent graft, or having a life-threatening postoperative complication. Even in the foremost surgical centers of this country where the operative mortality may be well under 5 percent, postoperative complications such as myocardial infarction, graft closure, pulmonary embolism, brain damage, hemorrhage, renal failure, serum hepatitis, and other nonfatal major disorders are not uncommon. Certainly these cases cannot be considered to have been aided by bypass surgery. Moreover, when a formidable risk is posed by an anatomical lesion in the coronary circulation, should surgery be considered the only recourse if the operative procedure itself is associated with an equal or greater immediate threat to life?

From these considerations, it is clearly evident that the consequences of today's optimal medical therapy must be compared with those from a cross-section of the various institutions now performing coronary bypass surgery. The risks of the procedure in its various settings could then be better gauged, the clinician would gain a more factual overview of the operation, and a more valid judgment could be reached in selecting the treatment of choice for the various clinical subsets of the disease.

SUMMARY AND CONCLUSIONS

A prospective study in 133 patients with severe angina pectoris has shown that the prospects for five-year survival are excellent in patients with good left ventricular function and no adverse clinical signs. The annual mortality rate in a group of 102 "good-risk" patients selected in this manner was actually only 1.2 percent. In sharp contrast the yearly attrition rate in subjects with poor left ventricular function and/or other adverse signs ("poor-risk" patients) approximated 25 percent. Marked amelioration of pain, increase in exercise tolerance, and improvement of ischemic exercise-electrocardiographic patterns were observed in 90.2 percent of the 133 patients in response to dosages of propranolol and sublingual isosorbide dinitrate, respectively, titrated for the individual patient.

It is concluded that:

1. Severe angina pectoris that is refractory to *casual* methods of management frequently responds to an intensive program of *optimal* medical care.
2. The favorable outlook in "good-risk" patients responding to modern medical therapy does not appear to indicate the need or justify the risk of surgical revascularization. Consideration for surgery seems waranted in this group primarily to improve the quality of life in the relatively small number of patients whose symptoms cannot be controlled by a comprehensive medical regimen.
3. The high mortality rate in "poor-risk" patients whether treated medically or surgically requires careful clinical assessment and meticulous selection of patients if lives are to be salvaged by surgical intervention.
4. The synergistic action of propranolol and sublingual isosorbide dinitrate when properly employed in the treatment of severe angina pectoris generally affords excellent control in cases previously refractory to traditional management.
5. It is only when medical therapy has been pursued with a high degree of enthusiasm and intensity of purpose that the attending physician can gain insight into the true indications for surgical intervention.

References

1. Block WJ, Crumpacker EL, Dry TJ, Gage RP: Prognosis in angina pectoris: Observations in 6,682 cases. JAMA 150:259, 1952
2. Burch GE: Coronary artery surgery—saphenous vein bypass (Editorial). Am Heart J 82:137, 1971
3. Corday E: Myocardial revascularization: Need for hard facts. JAMA 219:507, 1972
4. Hutchison JE, Green GE, Mekhjian HA, et al: Coronary bypass grafting in 476 patients consecutively operated on. Chest 64:706, 1973
5. Kannel WB, Feinleib M: Natural history of angina pectoris in the Framingham study. Am J Cardiol 29:154, 1972

6. Karnegas JN: Experience with the coronary artery bypass graft in a community hospital. Am Heart J 86:51, 1973

7. Lesperance J, Bourassa MG, Biron P, Campeau L, Saltiel J: Aorta to coronary artery saphenous vein grafts: Preoperative angiographic criteria for successful surgery. Am J Cardiol 30:459, 1972

8. Moberg CH, Webster JS, Sones FM: Natural history of severe proximal coronary disease as defined by cineangiography (200 patients, seven year follow-up). Am J Cardiol 29:282, 1972

9. Morris GC, Reul GJ, Howell JF, et al: Follow-up results of distal coronary artery bypass for ischemic heart disease. Am J Cardiol 29:180, 1972

10. Parker RL, Dry TJ, Willius FA, Gage RP: Life expectancy in angina pectoris. JAMA 131:95, 1946

11. Russek HI, Zohman BL: Limited use of anticoagulants in acute myocardial infarction. JAMA 162:922, 1957

12. Russek HI: Propranolol and isosorbide dinitrate synergism in angina pectoris. Am J Med Sci 254:406, 1967

13. Russek HI: Propranolol and isosorbide dinitrate synergism in angina pectoris. Am J Cardiol 21:44, 1968

14. Russek HI: New dimension in angina pectoris therapy. Geriatrics 24:81, 1969

15. Russek HI: Intractable angina pectoris. Med Clin North Am 54:333, 1970

16. Russek HI: Prognosis in severe angina pectoris: Medical versus surgical therapy. Am Heart J 83:762–768, 1972

17. Russek HI: Unpublished data, 1974

18. Sheldon WC, Rincon G, Effler DB, et al: Vein graft surgery for coronary artery disease—survival and angiographic results in 1,000 patients. Circulation 48 (Supp III): 184, 1973

19. Zukel WJ, Cohen BM, Mattingly TW, et al: Survival following first diagnosis of coronary heart disease. Am Heart J 78:159, 1969

3

ISCHEMIC CORONARY ARTERY DISEASE
DURING INFANCY AND CHILDHOOD

John A. Ogden and H. C. Stansel, Jr.

INTRODUCTION

Ischemic coronary arterial disease encountered during infancy, childhood, or adolescence is usually related to a congenital (or, rarely, acquired) structural abnormality of the coronary vasculature. The two most frequent congenital variations are anomalous origin of the left coronary artery from the pulmonary artery and coronary artery/cardiac chamber fistula. The clinical presentations vary considerably and are highly contingent upon the degree of physiologic aberration introduced by the anatomical variation. Additionally, there are less frequent congenital variations that may cause ischemic disease, either primarily or secondarily, such as hypoplasia of a major coronary arterial system (primary), or abnormal origin of the anterior descending artery from the right coronary artery in tetralogy of Fallot (secondary transection during ventriculotomy). There are many congenital variations of the coronary circulation that have no significant effect upon myocardial physiology during growth. Exemplary are separate origin of the circumflex and anterior descending arteries from the left aortic sinus (Fig. 1) or a single coronary artery.[1,2] However, such asymptomatic congenital variations may be significant later in the diagnosis and treatment of adult coronary arterial disease.[3]

Other forms of coronary circulatory compromise leading to ischemic change during infancy or childhood are rare. Occlusion of the proximal coronary artery may be caused by arterial wall changes in supravalvular aortic stenosis,[4,5] although the seven cases in our series all demonstrated marked coronary arterial dilatation (ectasia) and no symptoms or electrocardiographic changes indicative of ischemia.[6,7] Isolated cases of ischemia

or death have been attributed to calcification of the arterial wall,[8,9] periarteritis nodosa,[10] coronary artery endothelial fibroelastosis,[11] embolus,[6,12] syphilitic arteritis,[13] and atheroma formation.[14] One case of fibrous occlusion of the left coronary ostium causing symptoms of ischemia in a 14-year-old boy was corrected by a saphenous vein graft.[15]

EMBRYOLOGY

Implicit to an understanding of the pathophysiology of the various congenital variations of the coronary arteries is an appreciation of their development. During the sixth to seventh week of gestation, prior to the division of the truncus arteriosus into aorta and pulmonary artery, two endothelial communications ("buds," "outgrowths") develop between the lumen of the truncus and a primitive angioblastic epicardial network present in the atrioventricular, interatrial, and interventricular grooves, as well as circumferentially around the developing great vessels as a peritruncal ring (Fig. 2). Through a combination of genetic and physiologic control, certain regions of this angioblastic plexus evolve into dominant arteries, similar to the development of the blood supply to other organs or extremities, wherein multiple small-vessel systems, through growth and coalescence, become a characteristic adult pattern.[6,16] These developing epicardial vessels communicate with a developing myocardial vascular network that is partially derived from the primitive intertrabecular spaces. This myocardial network, in turn, communicates with the cardiac chambers through arteriosinusoidal and arterioluminal vessels and thebesian veins.

Variations in the coronary vasculature may arise through several mechanisms. Failure of the truncus arteriosus to be partitioned properly could cause the left coronary artery, or less frequently

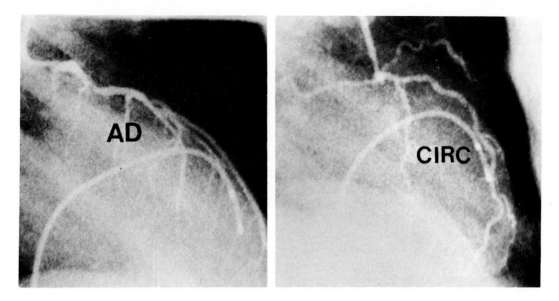

FIG. 1. Cine study showing separate origin of the left anterior descending (left panel) and circumflex (right panel) arteries from the left aortic sinus.

the right or both coronary arteries, to originate from the pulmonary artery, rather than the aorta. Failure of the normal arteriosinusoidal or arterioluminal vessels to decrease to capillary size would allow formation of a coronary artery–cardiac chamber fistula. Once intraluminal and intracardiac pressure changes occur following closure of the ductus arteriosus, significant shunts (left to right) may develop in both the aforementioned abnormalities. Failure of an aortic coronary "bud" to join the preexistent angioblastic plexus could allow formation of a single coronary artery. Failure of peripheral portions of the angioblastic epicardial network to evolve could cause hypoplasia or ab-

FIG. 2. Schematization of embryologic theory of coronary artery origin presented in detail in reference 6. A. A vascular network forms in the sites of the coronary arterial system, with a significant peritruncal anastomosis around the truncus. B. As the truncus divides into aorta and pulmonary artery, communications develop between the aorta and this vascular network (ie the coronary "buds"). C and D. Various portions of the vascular network coalesce to form the characteristic arteries, while other sections of the network regress (eg the primitive vessels over the right ventricular outflow tract).

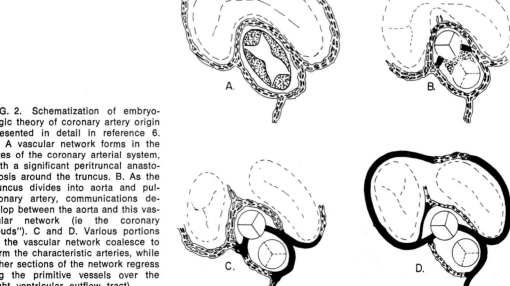

sence of specific branches. The timing of such "failures" would be a major factor in the degree of collateral formation.

ANOMALOUS ORIGIN OF THE LEFT CORONARY ARTERY FROM THE PULMONARY ARTERY

Anomalous origin of the left coronary artery from the pulmonary artery is the most common, as well as one of the most serious, of congenital coronary anomalies. Symptoms of myocardial ischemia may appear as early as two to three weeks of age, and there is an extremely high mortality rate during infancy. Wesselhoeft [17] recently reviewed the medical and pathophysiologic aspects of the lesion, but despite the increasing number of cases being described, some controversy still exists as to what type of surgical correction should be attempted, and at what age.[18-27] Perry [22] stated there were no long-term studies available to assess the morbidity and mortality of surgery, especially during infancy.

CASE MATERIAL

Forty-one patients were available for review, with all phases of the clinical syndrome represented. All were less than 10 years of age at symptom onset. There were 25 girls and 16 boys. Sixteen patients underwent surgery and are summarized in Table 1.

Ten patients had ligation of the left coronary artery at the origin from the pulmonary artery. Seven are doing well, but three continue to have angina with marked exertion, and two have stress electrocardiographic changes. Three patients, each less than one year of age, died following ligation. In four cases the preoperative diagnosis was mitral disease, and surgery was directed only at the mitral valve. All four died, with autopsy revealing the anomalous left coronary artery in each case. One patient had pericardial poudrage and showed no evidence of pericardial constriction two years later. Several cases warrant further description.

CASE 4:   *This black female, currently 25 years old, first had cardiac symptoms at four months of age. She was intermittently treated for congestive heart failure. Electrocardiography revealed left ventricular hypertrophy and strain patterns but never any acute ST or T changes. Cardiac catheterization at six years failed to produce a specific*

diagnosis. At eight years she began experiencing exertional chest pain. The electrocardiogram now showed ischemic changes. Catheterization was repeated at 16 years, revealing an anomalous left coronary artery. She underwent ligation. There was a significant improvement in her symptoms, but the electrocardiographic changes remained. Stress testing 18 months after surgery showed ST depression (2 mm) and T wave inversion. Nine years after ligation she was thoroughly reevaluated. She had chest pain only with significant exertion. The electrocardiogram showed T wave inversion in I, AVL, V1-V6, being similar to her previous tracings. Stress test showed a 2 mm ST depression (rate 175). Cardiac catheterization showed adequate left ventricular contraction (calculated ejection fraction—56 percent) and no mitral regurgitation (although there was prolapse of the posterior mitral leaflet). Selective right coronary arteriography showed a dilated, dominant right coronary artery with collateral filling of narrow left anterior descending and collateral branches. The left circumflex branch was poorly visualized (Fig. 3). This study is the longest postligation follow-up available to date and shows that adequate function may be obtained, although the circumflex artery showed severe regressive change.

CASE 7:   *At 16 years of age this girl had an attempted ligation of the left coronary artery. However, temporary occlusion resulted in severe ischemic changes and the procedure was discontinued. Because of continued exertional angina, a second thoracotomy was done (at age 20). Adhesions precluded external ligation, so she was placed on cardiopulmonary bypass and the ostium of the anomalous left coronary artery was oversewn without consequence. She is asymptomatic three years later, but electrocardiographic changes remain.*

CASE 14:   *This four-year-old girl experienced congestive failure from age two months and underwent prosthetic replacement of a severely stenotic mitral valve. She did well for a year but then developed signs of recurrent mitral stenosis. At surgery the prosthetic valve had been partially occluded by extension of the fibroelastotic process in the left ventricle. A second valve was inserted. She died two days later. Autopsy revealed the anomalous left coronary artery (Fig. 4).*

CASE 16:   *This 14-year-old girl had intermittent chest pain from six years of age. At 13 years she had an end-to-end saphenous vein graft from the aorta to the bifurcation of the left coronary artery. One year later she was asymptomatic, although electrocardiographic evidence of ischemia persisted. Arteriography showed mild right coronary dilatation. The saphenous vein graft was patent, but there was a constriction at the anastomosis, with post-stenotic dilatation of the*

TABLE 1. Summary of 16 Operated Cases

CASE	SEX	SYMPTOM ONSET	OPERATION		RESULTS
			Age	Procedure	
1	F	4 mos	6 mos	Ligation	Postoperative angina, death (1 mo)
2	F	4 mos	4 mos	Ligation	Angina for 2 mos; asymptomatic for 7 1/2 yrs
3	F	7 mos	22 mos	Plication of mitral valve	Postoperative death (1 day)
4	F	7 mos	16 yrs	Ligation	Continued exertional angina, ECG changes for 9 yrs
5	M	4 mos	9 yrs	Ligation	Residual mitral insufficiency 6 yrs later, asymptomatic
6	F	3 mos	5 yrs	Poudrage	Good 2 yrs later; lost to follow-up
7	F	5 mos	a) 16 yrs	Unsuccessful ligation	Continuing exertional angina
			b) 20 yrs	Ligation[b]	Asymtomatic 3 yrs later (ECG changes remain)
8	M	7 yrs[a]	8 yrs	Mitral prosthesis	Postoperative death (1 day)
9	M	3 mos	3 mos	Ligation	Postoperative death (1 day)
10	F	1 mo	16 mos	Ligation	Postoperative death (8 days)
11	M	3 mos	8 yrs	Mitral prosthesis	Postoperative death (5 days)
12	F	7 yrs	8 yrs	Ligation	Asymptomatic 9 yrs later
13	M	4 mos	a) 6 mos	Exploratory thoracotomy	Exertional angina
			b) 6 yrs	Ligation	Asymptomatic 6 yrs later
14	F	3 mos	a) 2 yrs	Mitral prosthesis	Recurrence of "mitral stenosis"
			b) 4 yrs	Mitral prosthesis	Postoperative death (2 days)
15	F	6 yrs	6 yrs	Ligation	Asymptomatic 8 yrs later
16	F	6 yrs	13 yrs	Saphenous graft	Stenosis/dilatation of graft 1 yr later, but asymptomatic

[a] Probable ischemic attacks during feeding as infant (less than 1 year), but no medical treatment (ie digitalis, diuretics) required.
[b] Ligation through pulmonary arteriotomy.

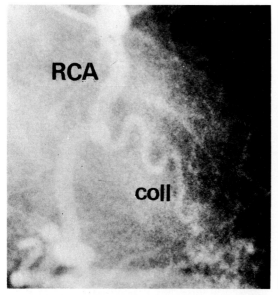
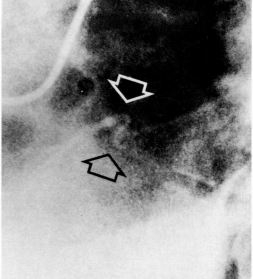

FIG. 3. Catheterization study nine years after ligation of the left coronary artery at the pulmonary artery. There is significant enlargement of the right coronary artery, with multiple collaterals to the small anterior descending artery. The circumflex artery visualized poorly (right frame).

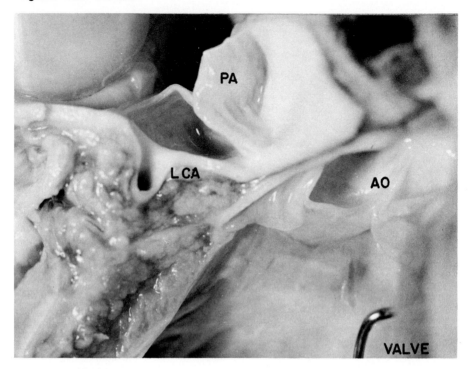

FIG. 4. Autopsy specimen showing prosthetic mitral valve and origin of the left coronary artery from the pulmonary artery.

proximal circumflex and anterior descending branches (Fig. 5).

DISCUSSION

Utilizing a comprehensive review [6] plus subsequently reported cases,[17-27] 294 cases were available for review. Of these, 176 (60 percent) died within the first year of life, while 106 underwent various surgical procedures.

Anomalous origin of the left coronary artery from the pulmonary artery has multiple clinical presentations, from anginal symptoms (ie feeding difficulty) during infancy, mitral insufficiency, sudden death, or an asymptomatic murmur. Initial reports led to the terms "infantile" and "adult" to describe the seemingly disparate groups. Later, the terms "transition phase" and "coronary steal phase" were added. However, this coronary anomaly should be conceived of as a dynamic lesion, and not a series of static phases. Most patients died within the first year of life (approximately 60 percent mortality), and those patients surviving beyond the first 6 to 12 months have all the features attributed to the "adult" phase, except chronological age. Therefore, the terms "infantile" and "adult" must be considered inapposite. It is suggested that they be replaced by the terms "im-

mature" and "mature" (Fig. 6). The concept of the "transition phase" should be retained, as this describes the critical period of collateralization between the right and left coronary systems. This phase appears to correlate with the closure of the ductus arteriosus and the decreasing fetal hemoglobin concentration (Fig. 7). The combination of decreased oxygen saturation and perfusion pressure in the left coronary system must stimulate collateral formation with the right coronary system. This is probably also an extremely time-dependent phase. If the rate of collateral formation cannot keep pace with increasing metabolic/circulatory demands, death undoubtedly results. The degree of right coronary predominance must also affect the dependence on collateralization. The separate phase of "coronary steal" should be deleted, since this is an integral portion of the mature phase and probably also exists to a lesser degree in the transition phase once the pressure in the pulmonary artery drops. The size of the shunt ("steal") is variable, just as the size of the left-to-right shunt varies in patients with coronary artery–cardiac chamber fistulas.

Electrocardiography showed anterolateral myocardial infarction in approximately 80 percent of the patients, no matter what the age or stage of disease.[6,17] There was considerable individual variation, which would be expected in view of the

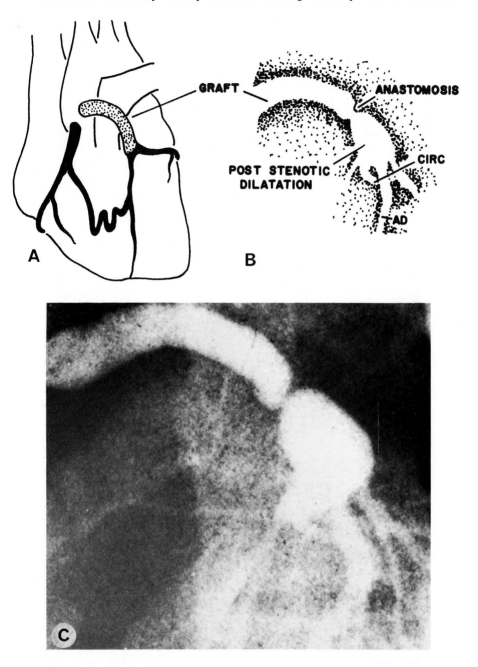

FIG. 5. Schematization (top) and cine study (bottom) of saphenous vein graft to anomalous left coronary artery. The vein graft had dilated; the anastomosis was constricted, and there was post-stenotic diltation.

variability of symptom severity. Most of the cases undergoing surgery showed very little change in the electrocardiographic patterns postoperatively, despite significant symptomatic improvement. This might be expected, since the infarcted ventricular wall is not resected. However, many have shown a significant improvement in the stress electrocardiogram.

Several methods were attempted to improve the anomalous circulation: aortopulmonary anastomosis, supravalvular pulmonary banding, pericardial poudrage, chemical deepicardialization, and cardiopneumopexy. None were particularly successful. Once the concept was well established that flow was from the right coronary artery to the left coronary artery and finally into the pulmonary

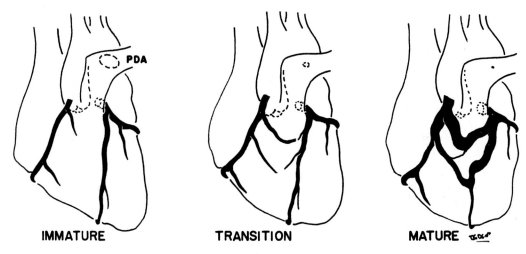

FIG. 6. Three phases of anomalous origin of the left coronary artery from the pulmonary artery (see text for details).

artery, ligation of the left coronary artery at the pulmonary arterial origin became the treatment of choice.

The results of ligation are summarized in Table 2. Sixteen of 30 infants less than 18 months of age at time of surgery survived (53 percent). In view of an overall morbidity of 60 percent (176 of 294 cases), this does not represent a significant improvement. However, 33 of 34 patients over 18 months survived surgery (97 percent), representing a significant improvement. Therefore, the operative success in ligation is contingent upon the degree of development of collateral circulation. If the communications are sparse, as in the

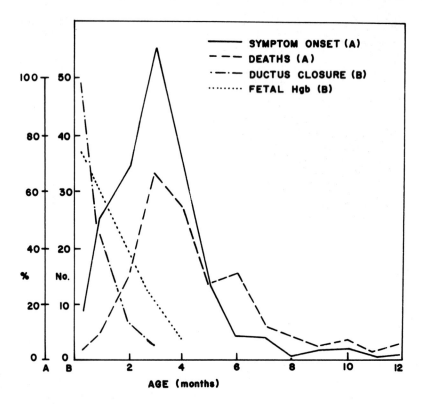

FIG. 7. Graphic analysis of onset of symptoms relative to normal sequence of ductus arteriosus closure, fetal hemoglobin decrease, and death rate during the first year of life in children with anomalous origin of the left coronary artery from the pulmonary artery.

TABLE 2. Operative Results

	CASES	SURVIVORS	
Operations	106	73	(69%)
Less than 18 months[a]			
All procedures	51	27	(53%)
Ligation only	30	16	(53%)
More than 18 months[a]			
All procedures	55	46	(84%)
Ligation only	34	33	(97%)
Anastomosis	10	10	(100%)

[a]*Age at time of surgery.*

immature and early transition phases, ligation may not prevent continued ischemia and death. In contrast, the improved collateralization of the late transition and mature phases enhances success significantly.

However, ligation has a significant disadvantage—the production of a single coronary circulation. Early attempts to create a two-vessel system by anastomosis of the left carotid, left subclavian, or aorta to the left coronary artery were unsuccessful. However, several recent reports indicate the insertion of a saphenous vein graft from the aorta to the left coronary artery may be beneficial.[20,21,23-27] The 10 reported cases have all survived. The most complete follow-up study, however, indicates the grafts may not remain patent, or may constrict at the anastomosis.[21] El-Said, et al,[21] recommended an end-to-side, rather than end-to-end, anastomosis to lessen the chance of anastomotic constriction.

Case 4 in the current series demonstrated marked regression of the size of the circumflex, and, less so, the anterior descending branches, a fact that might indicate technical difficulty if vascular anastomosis were considered in any of the postligation patients. Since virtually all the patients undergoing ligation after 18 months of age appear to have done as well as those undergoing saphenous graft, we could not currently recommend further surgery to create a two-vessel system in any of these patients, unless there is a significant worsening of symptoms.

With the exception of a successful subclavian–left coronary artery anastomosis under one year,[28,41] saphenous vein grafts have not been attempted in children under three to four years old. In view of the minimal improvement in mortality following ligation of the left coronary artery in this age group, we would concur with the recommendation that medical treatment be attempted until the patient is old enough to do a satisfactory anastomosis. If medical treatment does not tempo-

rize the situation, surgery should be done, with the aim being to anastomose, if feasible, and ligate, if anastomosis is not technically feasible.

CORONARY ARTERY/CARDIAC CHAMBER FISTULA

Well over 200 cases of communications between a coronary artery and a cardiac chamber have been described.[6,29-34] These abnormalities may cause myocardial ischemia and congestive heart failure because of decreased myocardial perfusion by the fistulous artery. Congestive failure appears to manifest primarily in young children (less than 4 years) and older adults with the lesion.[6,29,31,34]

CASE MATERIAL

Thirty-eight cases of coronary artery/cardiac chamber fistulas were reviewed. Eighteen of these occurred in children, and are summarized in Table 3. The sites of termination were the coronary sinus (2 cases), right atrium (3 cases), right ventricle (9 cases), pulmonary artery (3 cases), and left atrium (1 case). Eight patients had congestive failure (CHF) at some point in their clinical course. Ten patients had abnormal electrocardiograms, with all showing evidence of left or biventricular hypertrophy, and three showing evidence of myocardial ischemia.

Three patients with associated intracardiac abnormalities (pulmonary stenosis, atresia) died within the first year of life.

Surgery has been done in 13 patients and is planned in two others. Eleven patients had the involved artery (or arteries) ligated at the site of the fistula. One patient died postoperatively, during a sickle cell crisis. The other two operated patients had the artery ligated both at the site of fistula as well as at the aortic origin of the artery. In both cases there was massive dilatation of the involved right coronary artery, with epicardial collateral flow from the left anterior descending artery. Neither patient has had any difficulty postoperatively.

Two cases with ischemic complications will be discussed further:

CASE 2: *This female, now six years old, was first noted to have a murmur at five months. It was holosystolic over the precordium and had a diastolic component between the scapulae. An electrocardiogram showed right ventricular hypertrophy.*

TABLE 3. Coronary Artery–Cardiac Chamber Fistulas during Childhood

CASE	AGE[a]	SEX	ARTERY	TERMINATION	SBE	CHF	ECG[b]	SURGERY[c]	FOLLOW-UP/ COMMENTS
1	14	F	RCA (SNA)	CS	–	+	+	Ligation	Asymptomatic 8 yrs later
2	3	F	LCIR, LADCA	CS	–	–	+	Ligation	Asymptomatic 3 yrs later
3	7	M	LCA (SNA)	RA, type 2	–	–	–	Ligation	Asymptomatic 5 yrs later
4	7	F	RCA (SNA)	RA, type 2	–	–	–	Ligation	Asymptomatic 3 yrs later
5	10	F	RCA	RA, type 1	–	–	+	Ligation	Asymptomatic 2 yrs later
6	3	M	RCA (Post Desc)	RV-P, type 2	–	–	–	Ligation	Asymptomatic 4 yrs later
7	4	M	RCA	RV-P, type 1	–	+	+	Ligation[d]	Asymptomatic 3 yrs later
8	13	M	RCA	RV-P, type 1	–	–	–	Ligation[d]	Asymptomatic 5 yrs later
9	18 mos	F	LADCA	RV-P, type 3	–	–	–	Ligation	Death 8 mos later/sickle cell crisis
10	8	M	RCA/LCA	RV-P, type 1	–	–	–	Ligation	Asymptomatic 1 yr later
11	11	M	RCA	RV-P, type 1	–	+	+	Planned	Also has VSD
12	10 mos	F	LADCA	RV-S, type 3	–	+	+	–	Died after intracardiac surgery
13	3 mos	F	RCA/LADCA	RV-S, type 2	–	+	+	–	Found at autopsy
14	15	M	RCA	RV-I, type 3	–	+	+	Ligation	Fistula developed after ventriculotomy
15	7	F	LADCA	PA-P, type 1	–	–	–	Ligation	Asymptomatic 2 yrs later
16	8	M	RCA/LADCA	PA-P, type 3	–	+	+	Ligation	Asymptomatic 6 mos later/ECG normal
17	3	F	RCA	PA-S, type 1	–	+	+	–	Found at autopsy
18	7	F	LCIR	LA	–	–	–	Planned	–

[a] *Age in years, except as indicated in months, at time of initial evaluation.*
[b] *ECG findings primarily left ventricular hypertrophy.*
[c] *Ligation of artery at site of fistula, except those indicated by* [d].
[d] *Aortic origin.*
  RCA: right coronary artery; LCA: left coronary artery; LADCA: left anterior descending coronary artery; RA: right atrium; RV-P: right ventricle, no other cardiac defects; RV-S: right ventricle, associated cardiac defects; RV-I: right ventricle iatrogenic fistula (following ventriculotomy); PA-S: pulmonary artery, associated cardiac defects; SBE: subacute bacterial endocarditis; CHF: congestive heart failure.

Two months later, a definite continuous murmur was heard over the entire precordium. At 14 months cardiac catheterization showed a left-to-right shunt at the right atrial level. A pulmonary angiocardiogram (levophase) showed a dilated left circumflex artery entering the coronary sinus (Fig. 8.A). Electrocardiography showed biventricular hypertrophy. Two years later, prior to surgery, she was again catheterized. The left anterior descending artery was also communicating with the coronary sinus, along with the fistula from the left circumflex artery (Fig. 8.B). Selective catheterization of the uninvolved right coronary artery resulted in immediate cardiac arrest, implying inadequate myocardial perfusion from either left branch. Following recovery from resuscitation, she underwent ligation of each of the three fistulae into the coronary sinus. One year after ligation she was asymptomatic, but the electrocardiogram showed incomplete right bundle block, right ventricular hypertrophy, and mild ST depression. Eighteen months after surgery the electrocardiogram became normal.

CASE 16: At eight years this boy was noted to have a continuous murmur. This had never been described on previous examinations. His electro-cardiogram was normal. Six months later he began experiencing mild exertional dyspnea and an electrocardiogram showed nonspecific ST-T changes. Following arteriography and catheterization that showed a fistula into the pulmonary artery (Fig. 9), he underwent ligation of the fistula. The major arterial involvement was from the left anterior descending artery, although there was a smaller branch from the right coronary artery. Five months after surgery the stress electrocardiogram had returned to normal.

DISCUSSION

While most reports stress surgical closure of a coronary arterial fistula because of the possibilities of subacute bacterial endocarditis or congestive heart failure, these complications are described as relatively infrequent. Daniel [29] cited an incidence of congestive failure of 14 percent in 150 patients. However, the current study had 8 of 18 (45 percent) manifesting congestive failure, and recent reports summarizing fistula termination in either the coronary venous system [31] or the atria (right and left) [33] showed incidences of congestive fail-

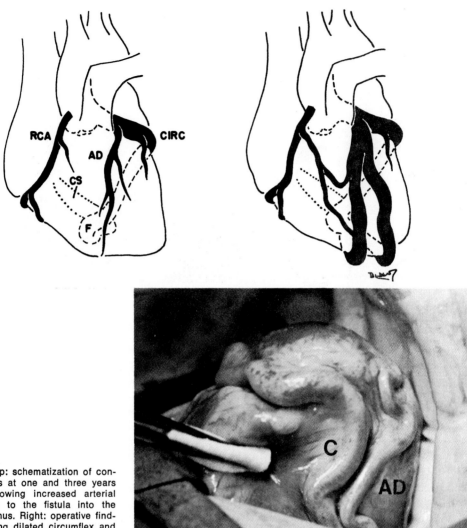

FIG. 8. Top: schematization of contrast studies at one and three years of age, showing increased arterial contribution to the fistula into the coronary sinus. Right: operative findings, showing dilated circumflex and anterior descending arteries.

ure, respectively, of 53 percent and 44 percent. There was significantly less failure in cases terminating in the right ventricle or pulmonary artery.[6] Thus, congestive failure should not be considered an uncommon complication of these fistulas.

Electrocardiographic changes are usually nonspecific and generally show only ventricular hypertrophy. Less frequently, ischemic changes may be found. Arrhythmias have been reported in several older patients. One patient in the current study had a cardiac arrest when the uninvolved right coronary artery was selectively catheterized. This complication undoubtedly occurred because the right coronary artery was perfusing the myocardium, while all the blood in the left coronary system went directly through the fistula. Flow studies in one case showed proximal coronary flow of 785 ml/min and shunt flow of 735 ml/min, leaving an effective myocardial flow of 50 ml/min.[33] It is interesting that cases with ischemia usually had major involvement through the left anterior descending artery.

The anatomy of these coronary arterial fistulas is extremely variable and is given in detail in several other communications.[6,31,33,34] It is imperative that the circulatory pattern be delineated prior to surgery. This allows for better specificity of approach.

Most fistulas have been ligated only at the site of the communication. When doing this, it is important that the area be temporarily clamped and the electrocardiogram monitored. There are several examples where this resulted in acute ischemic changes. Further dissection usually revealed a small arterial branch between the clamp and the fistula. Leaving such a small branch would allow the fistula to remain open and gradually enlarge. Several cases have been ligated concom-

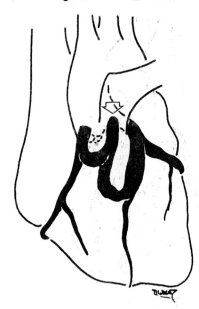
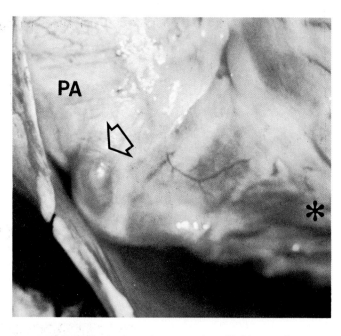

FIG. 9. Left: schematization of coronary arterial fistula to the pulmonary artery. Right: operative findings, showing coronary artery entering the pulmonary artery, with tortuous branch from the anterior descending artery (*).

itantly at the aorta. This may be necessary in massively dilated vessels. We have had one case of a death five years after distal ligation of a right coronary artery/coronary sinus fistula, with both old and fresh thrombosis of a still dilated right coronary artery.[31] Apparently closure of the fistula had removed the stimulus to collateral development from the left artery and perhaps even caused a regression of the collaterals that had developed. The dilated right artery never diminished in size and was prone to stagnation of flow. The several cases ligated at the aorta have not experienced any complications, undoubtedly because of good collateral flow. However, such double ligation does leave the patient with a single coronary system.

The morbidity and mortality of coronary arterial fistulas is thus significantly less than anomalous origin of the left coronary artery from the pulmonary artery. However, significant shunts may result in myocardial ischemia and congestive failure very easily, as blood flow is diverted from the smaller branches through the main branches into the fistula.

HYPOPLASIA OF THE CORONARY ARTERY

Hypoplasia of a proximal coronary artery may be associated with a single coronary artery. However, the single artery is usually completely dominant, covering all regions normally supplied by both right and left arterial systems, and the hypoplasia involves only a small segment of the proximal "absent" artery.[2] Three cases have been studied in which there was major arterial hypoplasia that was not associated with this characteristic "overgrowth" of the other artery usually seen in cases of single coronary artery.

CASE 1: *This two-day-old male died suddenly while feeding. There had been no prior indication of cardiac or respiratory distress. Autopsy revealed that the entire left coronary system was hypoplastic (Fig. 10.A). The left ventricle was also hypoplastic. The right coronary artery was normal sized. No significant anastomoses were noted.*

CASE 2: *This one-year-old male presented with symptoms compatible with a diagnosis of anomalous origin of the left coronary artery from the pulmonary artery. However, coronary arteriography revealed that the left coronary artery arose normally from the aorta. The circumflex branch visualized well, but the anterior descending branch had only a narrow stream of contrast material (Fig. 10.B). Three years later he had shown symptomatic improvement, although exertional angina still occurred. The electrocardiogram continued to show evidence of left ventricular ischemia. It is anticipated that he will require myocardial revascularization in the future.*

CASE 3: *This 14-year-old male had intermittent chest pain associated with physical exertion over the previous six months. Physical examination was*

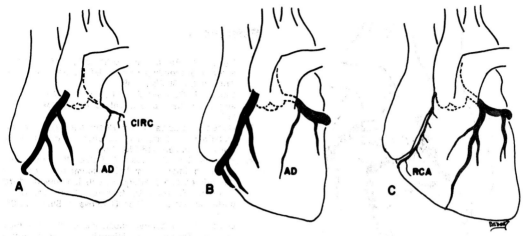

FIG. 10. Three cases of minor vessel hypoplasia. A. Entire left coronary artery. B. Only anterior descending branch. C. Right coronary artery. See text for details.

unremarkable. Electrocardiogram showed ST segment and T wave changes compatible with anterior myocardial ischemia. Aortic root injection showed a mildly dilated, dominant left coronary artery with a hypoplastic right coronary artery (Fig. 10.C). Two years later his symptoms still recur but have not significantly changed in severity. He may require a revascularization procedure in the future.

DISCUSSION

Hypoplasia of a major artery or branch may be a dominant factor in coronary disease affecting the child or young adult. Unfortunately, significant symptoms may not be present, and the child may die suddenly during increased physical exertion. McClellan and Jokl[35] reported several cases of hypoplasia of various coronary arteries in a series of sudden deaths in young athletes. Whiting[36] and Wainwright[37] each reported sudden death in adolescence associated with hypoplasia of the right coronary artery. Grossman and Burko[38] described an 18-year-old boy with chest pain attributed to hypoplasia of the right coronary artery. He finally underwent epicardial abrasion in an attempt to revascularize the myocardium over the right ventricular outflow tract. The result was satisfactory for two months, but symptoms and electrocardiographic changes recurred.

As more of these cases become available for long-term study, a better evaluation of the potential for surgical revascularization can be undertaken. Presently, only the severely symptomatic patient should be considered for these procedures. Allen et al[42] bypassed a proximal left coronary artery stenosis with a saphenous graft. Six months

later the patient had good filling of the anterior descending artery. One year later he was still asymptomatic.

CORONARY VASCULARITY IN TETRALOGY OF FALLOT

Tetralogy of Fallot, and less commonly ventricular septal defect, may be associated with abnormalities of the coronary circulation. The most common variation is increased vascularity over the right ventricular outflow tract, although less frequently a major artery supplying the left ventricle may arise from the right coronary artery (Fig. 11). This hypervascularity complicates ventriculotomy and may contribute significantly to postoperative ischemia, as illustrated by the following case:

This 14-year-old girl, who 10 years previously had undergone a left Blalock-Taussig shunt, underwent a complete repair of tetralogy of Fallot. During ventriculotomy several large epicardial vessels were avoided, but an aberrant artery within the right ventricular myocardium was inadvertently transected. After surgery she developed chest pain and electrocardiography showed an anterolateral myocardial infarction. A year later, after several episodes of congestive heart failure, she underwent resection of a left ventricular aneurysm, but died three days later.

Transection of a vessel crossing the right ventricular outflow tract may not necessarily be fatal. Most studies have shown that, while the area is hypervascular, the anterior descending branch or even the entire left coronary system infrequently arises from the right coronary ar-

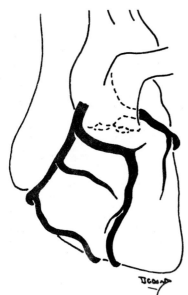

FIG. 11. Frequent pattern of vessel abnormality in tetralogy of Fallot, showing anterior descending artery originating from the right coronary artery.

tery.[6,39,40] Unfortunately, the few cases in which this branch has arisen from the right coronary system, and has been transected during surgery, have had a fatal outcome, usually preceded by evidence of massive left ventricular ischemia.

Adequate arteriographic evaluation of the coronary arteries as an integral part of the catheterization evaluation of tetralogy patients may help to delineate the types of circulatory abnormality and allow the surgeon more effectively to plan his ventriculotomy.

SUMMARY

Decreased perfusion of the myocardium in infancy and childhood is usually related to congenital abnormality of the coronary vasculature, with the three most common causes being (1) anomalous origin of the left coronary artery from the pulmonary artery, (2) coronary arteriovenous fistula, and (3) hypoplasia of a coronary artery or major branch (eg anterior descending).

ACKNOWLEDGMENTS

We would like to express our sincere gratitude to the many physicians whose case contributions made this study feasible.

References

1. Ogden J: Anomalous aortic origin: Circumflex, anterior descending or main left coronary arteries. Arch Pathol 88:323, 1969
2. Ogden J, Goodyer A: Patterns of distribution of single coronary artery. Yale J Biol & Med 43:11, 1970
3. Ogden J, Stansel H Jr: Roentgenographic manifestations of congenital coronary artery disease. Am J Roentgen 113:538, 1971
4. Price A, Lee D, Kagan K, Baker W: Aortic dysplasia in infancy simulating anomalous origin of the left coronary artery. Circulation 48:434, 1973
5. Peterson T, Todd D, Edwards J: Supravalvular aortic stenosis. J Thor Cardiovasc Surg 50:734, 1965
6. Ogden J: Congenital anomalies of the coronary arteries. Thesis, Yale University School of Medicine, 1968
7. Ogden J: Congenital variations of the coronary arteries. Am J Cardiol 25:474, 1970
8. Brown C, Richter I: Medial coronary sclerosis in infancy. Arch Pathol 31:449, 1941
9. Holm V: Arteriopathia calcificans infantum. Acta Paediatr Scand 56:537, 1967
10. Becker H, Kellerer K: Koronarerkrankungen im Sauglings—und Kleinkindesalter. Helv Paediatr Acta 24:474, 1969
11. MacMahon H, Dickinson P: Occlusive fibroelastosis of coronary arteries in newborn. Circulation 35:3, 1967
12. Arthur A, Cottom M, Evans R, Spencer H: Myocardial infarction in a newborn infant. J Pediatr 73:110, 1968
13. Goormaghtigh N, DeVos L, Blancquaert A: Ostial stenosis of coronary arteries in nine-year-old girl. Arch Int Med 95:341, 1955
14. Rigdon R, Willeford G: Sudden death during childhood with atheroma tubersum. JAMA 142:1268, 1950
15. Mullen C, El-Said G, McNamara D, Cooley D, Triestman B, Garcia E: Atresia of the left coronary ostium, repair by saphenous vein graft. Circulation 46:989, 1972
16. Ogden J: Origin of the coronary arteries. Circulation 38 (suppl. VI) 150, 1968
17. Wesselhoeft H, Fawcett J, Johnson A: Anomalous origin of the left coronary artery from the pulmonary trunk. Circulation 38:403, 1968
18. Ogden J: Surgical correction of congenital coronary defects. I. Anomalous origin of the left coronary artery from the pulmonary artery. Conn Med 34:626, 1970
19. Wright N, Baue A, Baum S, Blakemore W, Zinsser H: Coronary artery steal due to an anomalous left coronary artery originating from the pulmonary artery. J Thor Cardiovasc Surg 59:461, 1970
20. Cooley D, Hallman G, Bloodwell R: Definitive surgical treatment of anomalous origin of left coronary artery from pulmonary artery: Indications and results. J Thor Cardiovasc Surg 52:798, 1966
21. El-Said G, Ruzyllo W, Williams R, Mullins C, Hallman G, Cooley D, McNamara D: Early and late results of saphenous vein graft for anomalous origin of left coronary artery from pulmonary artery. Circulation 48:suppl 3:2, 1973
22. Perry L, Scott L: Anomalous left coronary artery from pulmonary artery. Circulation 41:1043, 1970
23. Gaisor R, Winters W, Glick H, Sandiford F, Chapman D, Morris G: Anomalous origin of left coro-

nary artery from pulmonary artery. Am J Cardiol 27:215, 1971

24. Reis R, Cohen L, Mason D: Direct measurement of instantaneous coronary blood flow after total correction of anomalous left coronary artery. Circulation 39:suppl 229:34, 1969

25. Summer G, Hendrix G: Surgical ligation of an anomalous left coronary artery arising from the pulmonary artery. Am Heart J 76:812, 1968

26. Dalton M, Arrington J, King S: Surgical treatment of adult-type anomalous origin of the left coronary artery from the pulmonary artery. Ann Thor Surg 7:333, 1969

27. Somerville J, Ross D: Left coronary artery from the pulmonary artery. Physiological considerations of surgical correction. Thorax 25:207, 1970

28. Meyer B, Stefanik G, Stiles Q, Lindesmith G, Jones J: A method of definitive surgical treatment of anomalous origin of left coronary artery. J Thor Cardiovasc Surg 56:104, 1968

29. Daniel T, Graham T, Sabiston D Jr: Coronary artery-right ventricular fistula with congestive heart failure: Surgical correction in the neonatal period. Surgery 67:985, 1970

30. Ogden J: Surgical correction of congenital coronary defects. II. Coronary artery: Cardiac chamber fistulas. Conn Med 35:168, 1971

31. Ogden J and Stansel H: Coronary arterial fistulas terminating in the coronary venous system. J Thor Cardiovasc Surg 63:172, 1972

32. Sabbagh A, Shocket L, Griffin T, Anderson R, Goldberg S, Fritz J, O'Hare J: Congenital coronary artery fistula. J Thor Cardiovasc Surg 66:794, 1973

33. Ogden J, Stansel H: The anatomic variability of coronary arterial fistulae termination in the right and left atria. Chest 65:76, 1974

34. Ogden J: Secondary coronary arterial fistulas. J Pediatrics 78:78, 1971

35. McClellan J, Jokl E: Congenital anomalies of coronary arteries as cause of sudden death associated with physical exertion. Am J Clin Path 50:229, 1968

36. Whiting W: Angina pectoris at age fourteen associated with rudimentary right coronary artery and rudimentary posterior cusp of mitral valve. Am Heart J 14:104, 1937

37. Wainright C: Sudden death asociated with hypoplasia of the right coronary artery. Cited in Grossman

38. Grossman L, Burko H: Diminutive coronary arteries and congenital coronary anomalies. J Tenn Med Assoc 61:687, 1968

39. Meng C, Eckner F, Lev M: Coronary artery distribution in tetralogy of Fallot. Arch Surg 90:363, 1965

40. Senning A: Surgical treatment of right ventricular outflow tract stenosis combined with ventricular septal defect and right-left shunt ("Fallot's Tetralogy"). Acta Chir Scandinav 117:73, 1969

41. Pinsky W, Fagan L, Kraeger R, Midd J, William V: Anomalous Left Coronary Artery. J Thorac Cardiovasc Surg 65:810, 1973

42. Allen H, Moller J, Formanek A, Nicoloff D: Atresia of the proximal left coronary artery associated with supravalvular aortic stenosis. J Thorac Cardiovasc Surg 67:266, 1974

4

SCANNING ELECTRON MICROSCOPY OF NORMAL AND ATHEROSCLEROTIC HUMAN CORONARY ARTERIES

ROBERT H. LISS and JOHN C. NORMAN

INTRODUCTION

The complex pathophysiologic factors that initiate coronary atherosclerosis are largely obscure and still discussed primarily in descriptive terms. It is clear, however, that the pathogenesis of the disease is centered in the tunica intima and is expressed most importantly at the blood-intimal interface. This chapter seeks to correlate historic pathologic data on the disease with scanning electron microscopic (SEM) observations of human coronary artery intimal surfaces. SEM provides a unique tool for the study and reconstruction of the sequence of surface changes in intimal topography during the atherosclerotic process.

Coronary atherosclerosis is a specific instance of the generalized disease that affects the intima and media of the coronary arteries and similarly, the aorta and the larger distributing arteries of man. Atherosclerosis is characterized by deposition of abundant lipid, protein, and calcium debris in the intima and media. These depositions take the form of focal thickenings or plaques of fibrins and fatty material.[7] Atherosclerotic changes may promote thrombosis and total occlusion of blood flow within a narrowed coronary artery with a resultant ischemia to the cardiac tissue supplied. Widespread, severe, often fatal complications frequently result from the advanced atherosclerotic lesions, but the severity of clinical findings do not always parallel the pathologic changes because of the focal nature of the disease and the irregularity with which complications develop.

An important difference between arteriosclerosis and atherosclerosis is made. According to French,[8] chronic arterial changes that occur in the smaller arteries in hypertension (diffuse hyperplastic sclerosis) or in the media of certain muscular arteries (medial or Mönckeberg's sclerosis) are characterized as arteriosclerosis; this term should not be used synonymously with atherosclerosis. In arteriosclerosis, the arterioles of many organs become thickened by hyaline protein substance, collagen, and increased numbers of myointimal and medial cells; in medial artery sclerosis (Mönckeberg) the media of major arteries become calcified and rigid with relatively little compromise of the diameter of the lumen. Atherosclerosis, on the other hand, is characterized by the fibrinous, fatty intimal plaques, which lead to a reduction in the diameter of the coronary artery lumen.[2]

The earliest lesions of coronary atherosclerosis begin in most individuals after the cessation of skeletal growth while clinical signs of the disease may not be manifest until later in life when occlusion or narrowing of the arteries is evident. The evolution of atherosclerosis involves a number of pathologic processes. Evidence for the initiation of the molecular events and the etiologic factors that culminate in the atherosclerotic process must be sought by study of nutritional, physiologic, environmental, and genetic factors. Clearly, no unified hypothesis on the genesis of atherosclerosis in man yet explains the complex interactions of the many factors involved in the initiation and promotion of the disease. It is clear, however, that the disease process centers in the intima and the expression of pathologic correlates of atherosclerosis is related to events at the blood-endothelial interface. The excellent review of French [8] on atherosclerosis, and his especial attention to the relation of the structure and function of the arterial intima and endothelium to the genesis of the disease, is perhaps the definitive summary of the way in which the tunica intima is modified and progresses through the successive pathologic changes of atherosclerosis.

The purpose of this chapter is not to discuss material on the genesis of coronary atherosclerosis that has been reviewed elsewhere,[15,17,19] rather, emphasis will be placed on correlating summary histopathologic observations of other investigators with scanning electron microscopic observations made on human coronary arteries. Since the pathology of atherosclerosis already has been characterized by light microscopy and transmission electron microscopy, this report will seek to relate these observations to representative scanning electron micrographs of progressive atherosclerotic changes at the intimal-blood interface in human coronary arteries.

HYPOTHESES FOR THE GENERATION OF ATHEROSCLEROSIS

Four principal hypotheses on the development of atherosclerotic plaques that relate to the scanning electron microscopic observations on topographic changes in coronary atherosclerosis have been summarized. They are (1) the alteration of the properties of the matrix, fibers, and cells of the coronary artery wall,[22] (2) filtration of plasma components from the lumen through the intima and media,[20] (3) formation of thrombi on the intimal surface of plaques and within plaques, from platelets and plasma proteins,[3,4] and (4) the implication of homocysteine derivatives in the initiation of hyperplasia of arterial cells.[12-14] These theories of atherosclerosis are relevant to intimal surface changes because irrespective of the etiologic factors, which are important in the genesis of the disease, they are all ultimately expressed as alterations in vessel wall properties, altered filtration of plasma constituents, and formation of thrombi. Yet, the factors that initiate the processes involved in atherosclerosis in man and in experimental models[10,11] are largely obscure at the molecular level.

Altered Matrix of Coronary Artery Wall

Virchow[22] was the first to recognize that deposition of mucoid substances within intima was among the first changes in the early atherosclerotic plaque. Later, others confirmed this temporal relationship, that alterations in the artery wall matrix precede lipid deposition, fibrosis, and calcification in the development of atherosclerotic plaques. This alteration in ground substance is generally considered to be of nutritional or metabolic origin. Whatever its cause, variations in the extent of matrix deposition would be expected to vary with location and structure of the artery wall—ie, ostia of branches and areas of high angulation. Furthermore, changes in amount and properties of intimal and medial matrix proteoglycans would be expected to alter the permeability and capacity for filtration of plasma components through the artery wall.

Filtration of Plasma Through Coronary Artery Wall

The relatively large amounts of cholesterol in advanced atherosclerotic plaques are believed to result from deposition of plasma lipids within the base of the lesion.[20,22] The protein component of plasma low density lipoprotein (LDL) can be demonstrated within developing plaques, and proteoglycan fractions extracted from aortic wall form relatively insoluble complexes with serum LDL fractions *in vitro*. Phospholipids are the most prominent lipid fraction deposited in early lesions, but cholesterol and esters accumulate in older lesions. The rate of filtration of plasma through intima is dependent on blood pressure, alterations in artery wall matrix, injury to endothelium, and other factors. This filtration process raises the possibility that plasma factors may be responsible for the alterations in arterial wall matrix and cellular hyperplasia prominent in early developing plaques.[1,9,21]

Thrombogenic Origin of Plaques

Deposits of fibrin and platelet-associated protein have been demonstrated within developing plaques by immunofluorescent methods.[23] Hemorrhages and thrombi, both recent and organized, are prominent processes occurring in well-developed plaques. Platelets, which are very rich in phospholipids and sulfated proteoglycans, have increased adhesiveness and susceptibility to aggregation in some patients with atherosclerosis. In areas of endothelial damage, large numbers of platelets adhere to the site of injury, eg, as produced by mechanical trauma, and lead to adherent thrombi at the site of injury. The effect of platelet constituents on endothelium and intima may lead to alteration of the matrix, cellular hyperplasia and changes in plasma filtration at the site of platelet adherence. Substances released from platelets during aggregation probably affect arterial wall matrix and cells adjacent to the site of endothelial injury.[6,18]

Homocysteine Theory of Atherosclerosis

The finding that accelerated arteriosclerosis occurs in two different but closely related inherited enzymatic disorders resulting in homocystinuria implicates homocysteine derivatives in the initiation of arteriosclerosis.[12-14] In cystathionine synthetase deficiency, plasma methionine and homocysteine are increased, but cystathionine is reduced in concentration. In methyl folate homocysteine transferase deficiency, plasma methionine is reduced, and both homocystine and cystathionine concentrations are increased. The association between homocystinemia and arteriosclerosis in these disorders suggests that some homocysteine derivative initiates arteriosclerotic plaques. Fibrous arteriosclerotic plaques can be produced in rabbits injected with methionine or homocysteine. Addition of these compounds to diet, however, only inhibits growth and feeding unless pyrodoxine is also given. Rabbits given homocysteine injections and fed cholesterol develop prominent deposition of lipid in fibrolipid plaques. Larger doses of injected methionine or homocysteine result in venous thrombosis and pulmonary embolism.

Methionine sulfur is converted to sulfate ester by enzymatic pathway, methianine $\rightarrow$ homocysteine $\rightarrow\rightarrow$ homomcysteic acid $\rightarrow\rightarrow$ PAPS $\rightarrow\rightarrow$ sulfate ester. The pathway requires ascorbic acid and is crucial to the synthesis of sulfated proteoglycan matrix of cartilage, artery wall, and other connective tissues. Present indications are that an oxidized form of homocysteic acid is the sulfate precursor that mediates the action of growth hormone by initiation of cell division and synthesis of matrix proteoglycans.

Initiation and evolution of arteriosclerotic plaques can be interpreted as an increased effect of oxidized homocysteine derivatives on the myointimal cells of arteries. The somatotrophic activity of these compounds is believed to initiate hyperplasia of arterial cells, as increased amounts are filtered through the arterial wall. Increased amounts of sulfated proteoglycans are synthesized and deposited by arterial cells because of conversion of fibrillar to a granular, highly sulfated matrix, and, as the lesion progresses, relatively insoluble cholesterol and cholesterol esters are deposited in the lesion as phospholipids and triglycerides are partially metabolized. Alterations at the intimal-blood interface, reflected by increased platelet adhesiveness in atherosclerosis and homocystinuria, may be related to deposition of the fibrin, initiation of thrombosis, and local growth stimulation in areas of endothelial injury, turbulence, or angulation of the artery wall.

SCANNING ELECTRON MICROSCOPIC OBSERVATIONS AND THE PATHOLOGY AND EVOLUTION OF CORONARY ATHEROSCLEROTIC LESIONS

French [5-7] has noted that atherosclerosis is not yet adequately understood in terms other than morphologic. Lesions in human coronary arteries, he reports, exhibit a wide morphologic diversity, ranging from such minimal intimal lesions as fatty streaks to overt fibrous plaques and advanced, occlusive lesions with thrombosis, intimal hemorrhage, or calcification.

In our studies, the minimal lesions observed in human coronary arteries consisted of focal thickenings of the intima scattered over the intimal surface of the artery. In Figure 1, a scanning electron photomicrograph of a focal intimal thickening, or fatty streak, is seen. The lesion consists of raised, parallel, regularly oriented surface elevations. The highly oriented lesions seem to predominate at the bifurcation points or orifices of branches of the coronary arteries. The specific, ordered orientation of the lesions at these points may be related to origins of high flow turbulence, high pressure, or marked angulation of the flow of blood through the coronary arteries. Fibrin and fibrin thrombi were not seen associated with these early lesions. The question is moot whether such intimal thickening or hyperplasia should be considered as an integral part of the atherosclerotic process, should be accepted as normal, or be viewed as precedent to the development of additional intimal lesions (ie, atherosclerosis).[8] Scanning electron microscopy of such minimal lesions demonstrates the focal distribution of lipid streaks adjacent to essential normal tunica intima; however, the appearance of these early lesions in the straight segments of the coronary arteries differs from those at bifurcations. Figure 2 is a scanning electron photomicrograph of a lipid streak whose gross appearance as a linear sudanophilic deposit is seen with SEM to be composed of more randomly, less organized substructure than the lesion

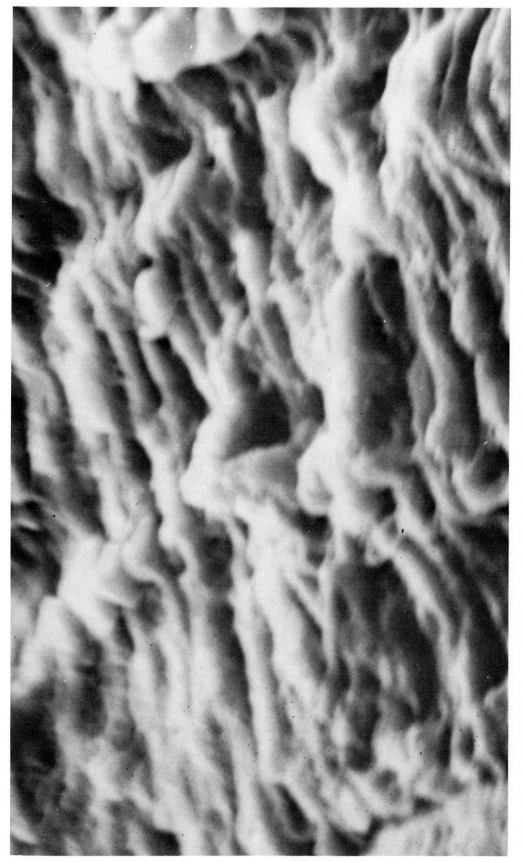

FIG. 1. The focal intimal thickening, or fatty streak, consists of raised, parallel, regularly oriented surface elevations at bifurcation points of the coronary artery. ×3300

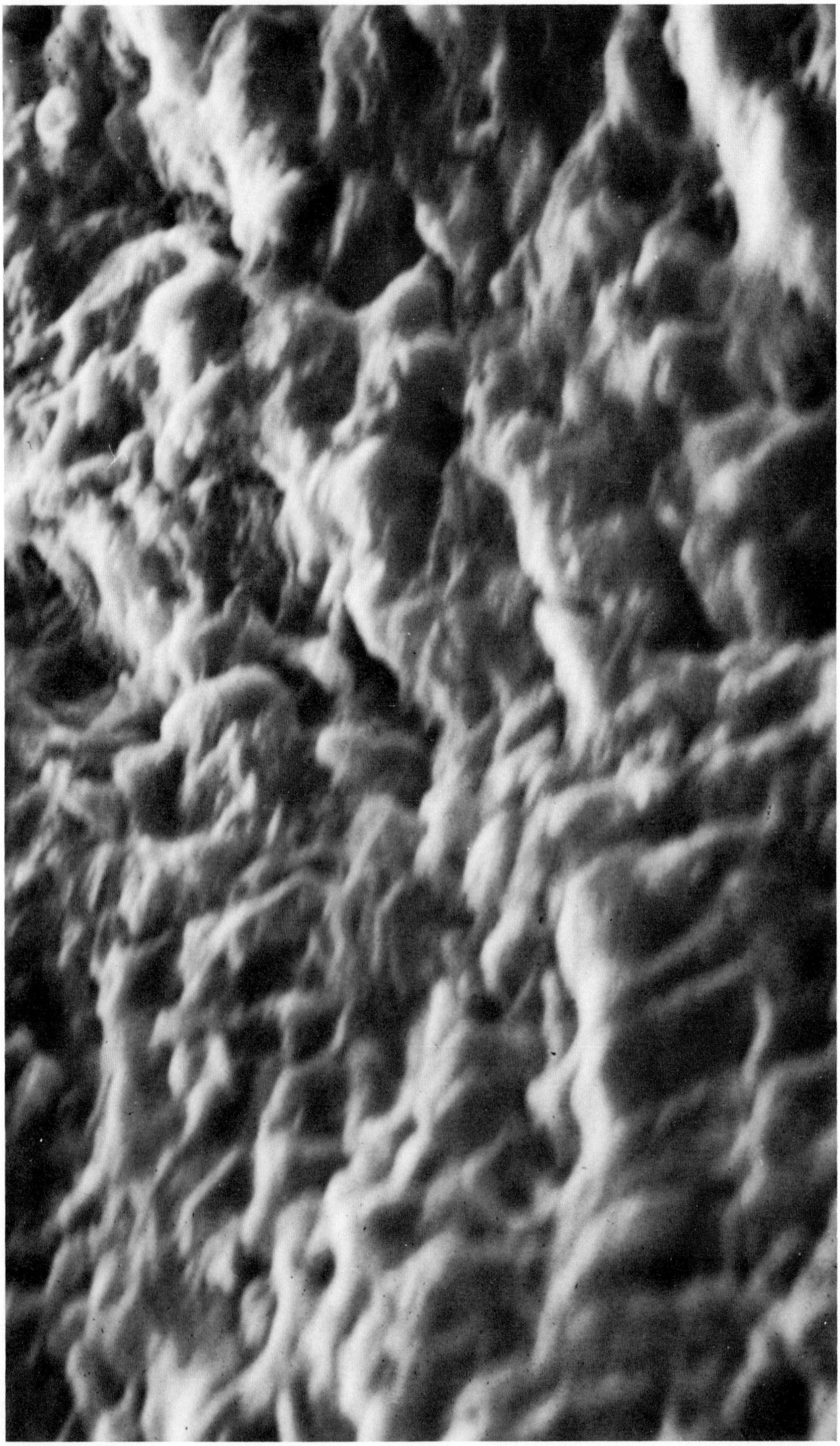

FIG. 2. Lipid streaks in straight segments of coronary arteries are less oriented than more linear arrays of this lesion near coronary artery branches. ×3300

in Figure 1. The general impression obtained in this study is that lipid streaks in straight segments of coronary arteries are less oriented than the more linear arrangements of this early lesion seen at or near coronary artery bifurcations.

The earliest definitive lesion of the intima seen in these studies is the fibrous or fibrolipid plaque. Histologically, fibrous plaques consist of (1) increased numbers of smooth muscle cells of intima and superficial layers of media, (2) degeneration, splitting, and fragmentation of internal elastic membrane, and (3) deposition of metachromatic matrix, increased numbers of collagen fibrils, lipid droplets, calcium salts, and fibrin. The lipid droplets may be free and extracellular, lying along elastic fibers, or located within foam cells or within smooth muscle cells. These early plaques are focal and scattered but are more frequently at vessel ostia. The gross appearance of an early plaque is slightly elevated grey or grey-tan well-circumscribed thickened area of intima. Such areas are seen in Figure 3. A number of red blood cells are seen lying on the intimal surface of this opened human coronary artery. Prominent projection along the surface correspond to the areas of plaque previously described. In Figure 4, a relatively normal appearing, plaque-free area of coronary artery intimal surface is seen. The apparent splitting of the intimal surface is a preparation artifact; noteworthy is the relatively smooth appearance of this lesion-free surface.

More advanced lesions observed in this study of human coronary arteries were the large swollen atheromas. Histologically, they consist of a thick fibrous cap containing dense collagen and hyperplastic smooth muscle cells. In these advanced atherosclerotic lesions, fatty elements predominate, and in the coronary arteries, fibrous tissue and calcification are prominent. Figure 5 shows a portion of an advanced atherosclerotic lesion, an atheroma, adjacent and continuous with a hyperplastic intimal layer. The topography of the fibrous, linearly oriented atheroma and the dense areas of extracted lipid are continuous with the coronary artery wall.

Progressive, degenerative changes may follow rupture of the atheroma and successive layers of mural thrombi may form, leading to fibrin deposition, organization, and further fibrosis. The plaque may become vascularized during organization, and the high pressure transmitted to these small vessels frequently leads to hemorrhage within the plaques. Thrombosis and infarction may develop because of sudden formation of a thrombus and total occlusion of blood flow within a narrowed coronary artery. Figure 6 shows a coronary artery totally occluded by thrombus. Recanalization of the thrombus is evident. However, as is seen at higher magnification in Figures 7 and 8, recanalization often results in incomplete channels; in serial scanning electron photomicrographs of occlusive thrombi, the incomplete nature of the canals in the thrombus mass can be established. Such gradual obliteration of coronary artery lumens by fibrocalcific sclerosis leads to increasing impairment of arterial circulation, ischemia in the heart tissues supplied, and loss of cardiac muscle function.

SUMMARY AND CONCLUSIONS

Etiologic factors important in coronary atherosclerosis are expressed as alterations in endothelial, intimal, and vessel wall properties. The complex pathophysiological factors responsible for the genesis of atherosclerosis are largely obscure and are discussed generally in morphologic terms. An exception is the homocysteine theory of arteriosclerosis,[12-14] which seeks to interpret the initiation and evolution of arteriosclerotic plaques as an increased effect of oxidized homocysteine derivatives on the myointimal cells of arteries.

While the molecular events that promote coronary atherosclerosis are obscure, as a pathologic process the disease involves the intima and intimal-blood interface of these arteries. The features of the tunica intima, the forces that affect the tissue and both the mechanical and chemical factors that influence the integrity of human coronary arteries with age have been reviewed.[8]

Recent interest in the correlation of historic data on coronary artery pathology with scanning electron microscopic observations provides new perspectives on the nature and development of the disease in man. Reconstruction of the sequence of surface alterations in progressive coronary atherosclerosis is possible through scanning electron microscopic characterization of intimal topography; moreover, the lesions can be staged by companion histopathologic methods. Such information makes possible subsequent *in situ* studies of the chemical composition of developing atherosclerotic lesions by energy dispensive analysis of x-rays (EDAX) techniques. This methodology can provide analytical information on the atomic composition of the same topographic lesion viewed with the scanning electron microscope and allows for a correlation between the qualitative observations of developing coronary atherosclerosis and quantitative assessment of associated chemical changes in the intimal surface. Such studies are

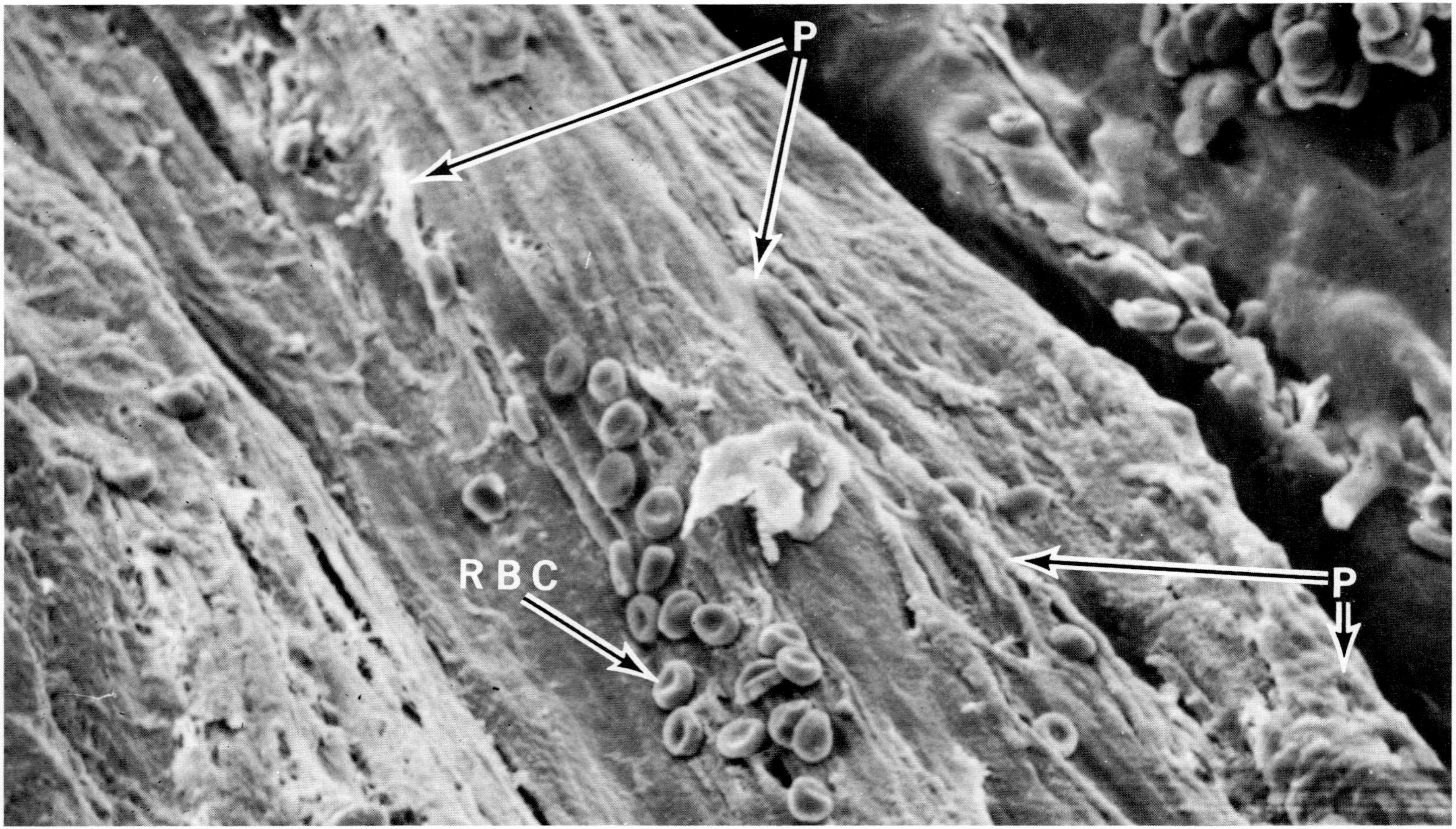

FIG. 3. The irregular appearance of the plaque (P) and red blood cells (RBC) on the intimal surface of this opened coronary artery are characteristic of early plaque lesions in human coronary arteries. ×500

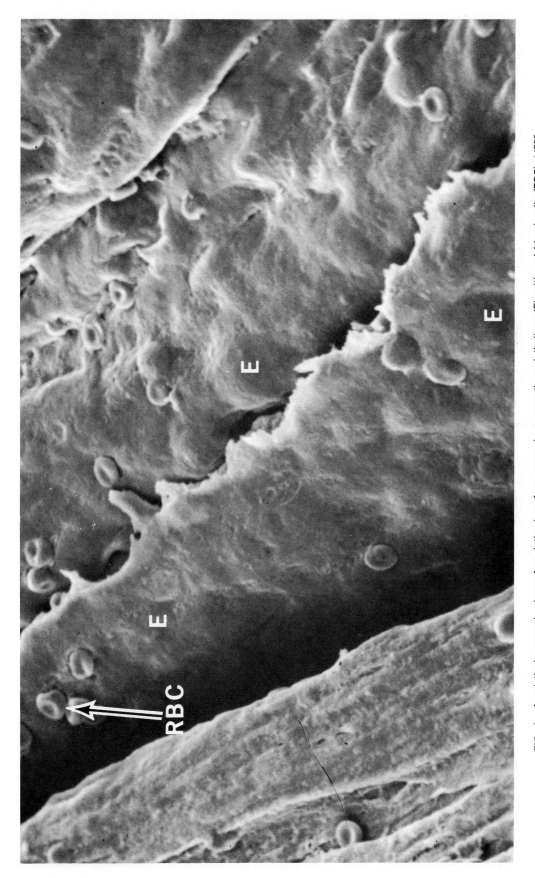

FIG. 4. A relatively normal, plaque-free intimal surface presents a smooth endothelium (E) with red blood cells (RBC). ×500

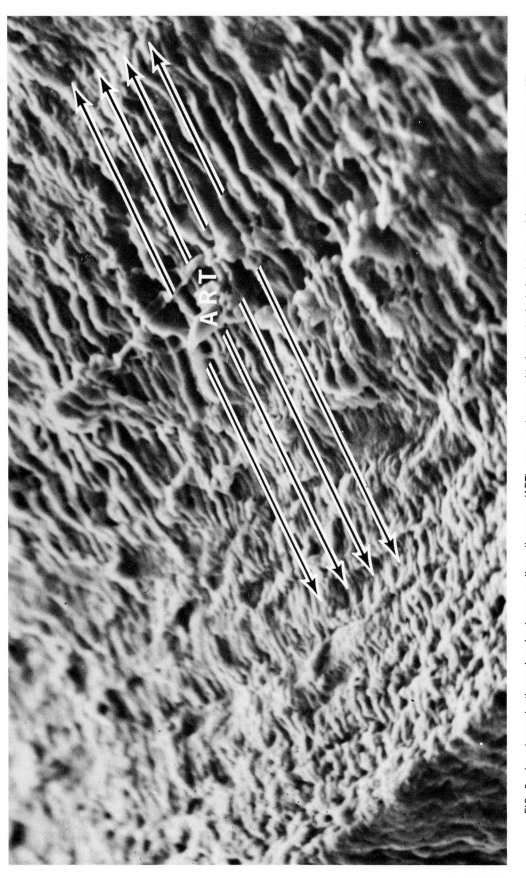

FIG. 5. In advanced atherosclerosis, large swollen atheromas (ART) are continuous with hyperplastic intimal layers of human coronary ateries. ×670

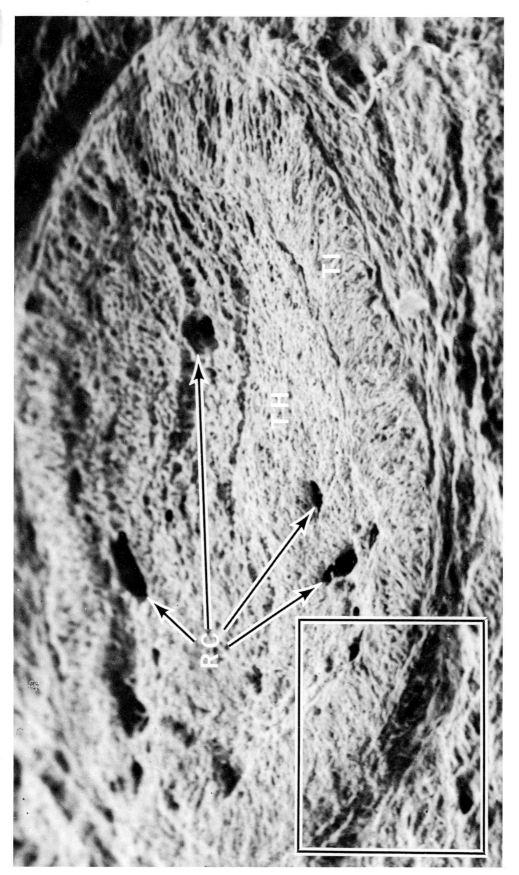

FIG. 6. A human coronary artery, totally occluded by thrombus (TH), is seen with evidence of recanalization (RC). Note the thickened tunica intima (TI). The area in the rectangle appears at higher magnification in Figure 7. ×150

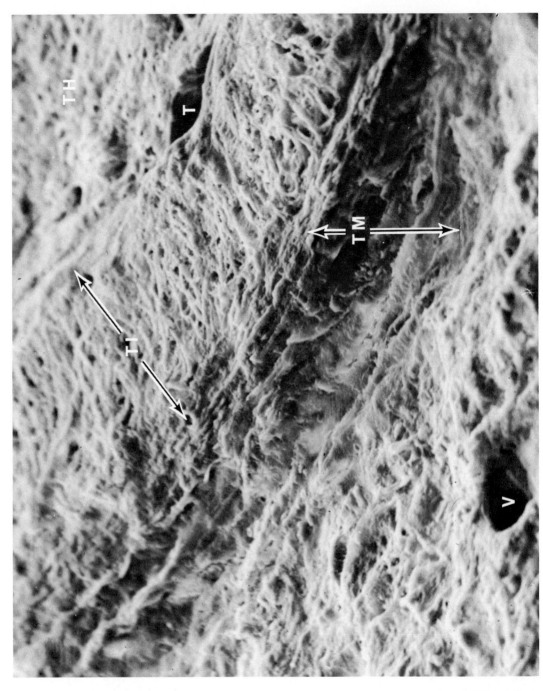

FIG. 7. The thickened tunica intima (TI), tunica media (TM), and a vessel in the adventitia (V) are seen. Thrombus (TH) fills the arterial lumen and recanalization at the thrombus-intimal junction (T) is seen. ×420

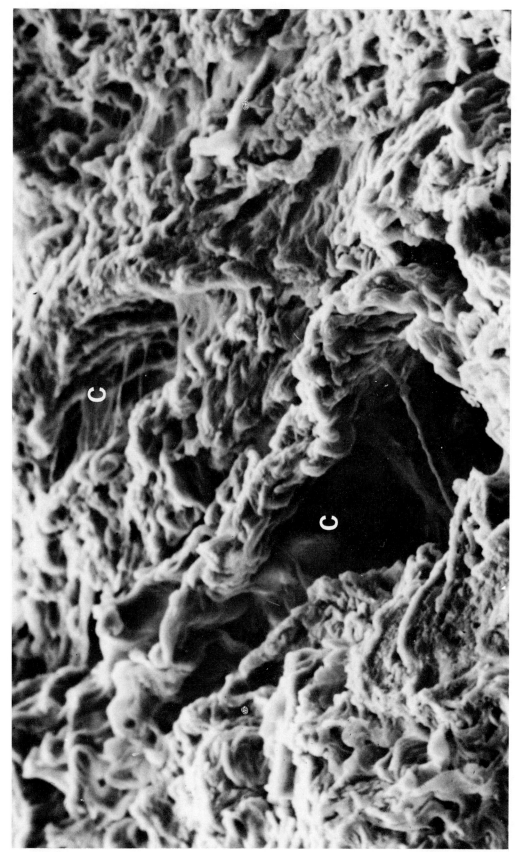

FIG. 8. The incomplete nature of most recanalizations (C) of thrombus can be established by serial scanning electron microscopic observations. ×670

in progress in our laboratory, and this approach to the problem of coronary atherosclerosis may provide an understanding of the pathology of coronary atherosclerosis beyond the current descriptive, morphologic terms.

ACKNOWLEDGMENTS

We are indebted to Dr. Kilmer S. McCully (Departments of Pathology, Massachusetts General Hospital and Harvard Medical School) for the benefit of his research expertise in atherosclerosis and his generous permission to quote from his lecture materials.

The authors are especially grateful to Mr. Raymond M. Cornish, Arthur D. Little, Inc., for his collaboration in the preparation of the scanning electron photomicrographs.

References

1. Abdulla YH, Adam CWM, and Morgan RS: Connective-tissue reactions to implantation of purified sterol, sterol esters, phosphoglycerides, glycerides and free fatty acids. J Pathol Bact 94:63, 1967
2. Crawford T: Morphological aspects in the pathogenesis of atherosclerosis. J Atheroscler Res 1:3, 1961
3. Duguid JB: Thrombosis as a factor in the pathogenesis of coronary atherosclerosis. J Pathol Bact 58:207, 1946
4. Duguid JB: Thrombosis as a factor in the pathogenesis of aortic atherosclerosis. J Pathol Bact 60:57, 1948
5. French JE: Atherosclerosis. In Jones, RJ (ed): Evolution of the Atherosclerotic Plaque. Chicago, University of Chicago Press, 1963, pp 15–28
6. French, JE: Atherosclerosis. In Chalmers DJ, Gresham GE (eds): Biological Aspects of Occlusive Arterial Disease. London, Cambridge Univ Press, 1964, pp 24–30
7. French JE, Jennings MA, and Florey HW: Morphological studies on atherosclerosis in swine. Ann NY Acad Sci 127:780, 1965
8. French JE: Atherosclerosis and the arterial Intlma. In Richter, GW and Epstein, MA (eds): Int Rev Exp Pathol NY, Academic Press, 1966, p 253
9. Hollander W: Recent advances in experimental and molecular pathology: Influx, synthesis, and transport of arterial lipoproteins in atherosclerosis. Exp Mol Pathol 7:248, 1967
10. Liss RH, Burg AW, et al: Ultrastructure and chemistry of bovine pseudoendothelia from implantable pumps. J Cell Biol 47:124, 1970
11. Liss RH, Huffman FN, Warren S, Norman JC: Electron microscopy and thermal analysis of neointima heated and irradiated *in vivo* for two years. Ann Thorac Surg 12:251, 1971
12. McCully KS: Homocysteine metabolism in scurvy, growth and atherosclerosis. Nature 231:391, 1971
13. McCully KS: Homocysteinemia and arteriosclerosis. Am Heart J 83:571, 1972a
14. McCully KS: Molecular basis for homocysteine-induced changes in proteoglycan structure In growth and arteriosclerosis. Am J Pathol 66:83, 1972b
15. Minkowski WL: The coronary arteries of infants. J Med Sci 214:623, 1947
16. Mitchell JRA and Schwartz CJ: Arterial Disease. Oxford, Blackwell, 1965
17. Moon HD: Coronary arteries In fetuses, infants, and juveniles. Circulation 16:263 1957
18. Morgan, AD: The Pathogenesis of Coronary Occlusion. Oxford, Blackwell, 1965
19. Neufeld HN, Wagenvoort CA, and Edwards JE: Coronary arteries in fetuses, infants, juveniles, and young adults. Lab Invest 11:837, 1962
20. Page IH: The Lewis A. Conner Memorial Lecture: Atherosclerosis: An Introduction. Circulation 10:1, 1954
21. Parker F: An electron microscopic study of experimental atherosclerosis. Am J Pathol 36:19, 1960
22. Virchow R: Gesammelte Abhandlungen zur Wissenschaftlichen Medicin. Meidinger Sohn, Frankfurt, 1856, pp 458–636
23. Walton KW and Williamson N: Histological and immunofluorescent studies on the evolution of the human atheromatous plaque. J Atheroscler Res 8:599, 1968

5

THE LONG-TERM FATE OF INTERNAL MAMMARY IMPLANTS AND BIOCHEMICAL OBSERVATIONS ON INDUCED ATHEROSCLEROSIS

Robert J. Gardner, William B. Cline,
Milton R. Hales, and Herbert E. Warden

INTRODUCTION

Although only occasionally used at present, indirect myocardial revascularization has the potential advantage of increasing coronary flow with the passage of time.

Late closure of aortocoronary bypass grafts usually is precipitated by decreased runoff due to a progression of atherosclerosis in the distal coronary arteries. In contrast, numerous implant-coronary anastomoses can develop with implant maturation, make the implant less dependent on one coronary artery or segment for distal flow, and thereby decrease late failure rates. In addition, many experimental and clinical studies have noted that the internal mammary artery is not a common site of atherosclerosis. This experimental study is primarily concerned with evaluation of the fate of internal mammary artery implants in the face of continued atherosclerosis. Secondarily, the serum lipid and arterial anatomic changes associated with induced atherosclerosis in the dog are documented.

METHODS

Ten unselected adult mongrel dogs weighing between 17.4 kg and 25 kg were anesthetized

Funded through a grant from the American Heart Association West Virginia Affiliate.

with intravenous sodium pentobarbital. An endotracheal tube was inserted and ventilation maintained with a positive pressure respirator. A left fifth interspace incision was made and the left internal mammary artery mobilized from its origin at the subclavian to the superficial epigastric junction. At this level the vessel was ligated, divided, and implanted in the anterolateral myocardium under the left anterior descending coronary artery. The myocardial tunnel was made approximately 3 centimeters long so that at least three freely bleeding intercostals were buried. A stainless steel jacketed ameroid constrictor was applied to the left anterior descending coronary artery about two centimeters from its origin. The right internal mammary artery was left undisturbed in its bed so that if physical or local factors were significant in atherogenesis, each animal would act as its own control.

Steiner and Kendall [12,13] were the first investigators to produce experimental atherosclerosis in the mongrel dog by thyroid suppression and a high cholesterol diet. Since then many modifications have duplicated this experimental preparation reliably and in a shorter time, usually by increasing the dietary cholesterol. We elected to utilize a method first developed by Page and Brown.[6] Essentially it consisted of a medical thyroidectomy and the administration of a high fat diet containing 20 percent cholesterol. During a pilot study two animals died prematurely of massive fatty infiltration of the liver, so choline was empirically added to the dietary regime and appeared to resolve the problem. Therefore, two weeks following the revascularization operation, thyroid function was ablated by intravenous I_{131}, 0.5 millicuries per kilogram of body weight. The animals were then fed a diet consisting of cholesterol, 20 gm; cooking oil,* 73 gm; cholic acid, 5 gm; thiouracil, 2 gm; and choline, 15 mg added to each one pound of canned dog food † daily. During a six-to-nine-month observation period the following determinations were made monthly: serum cholesterol,‡ serum triglycerides,§ serum total lipids, ‖ lipoprotein cellulose acetate electrophoresis,# hemoglobin, and fasting blood sugar.

In addition each animal underwent a four-hour glucose tolerance test during the fourth or fifth month on the diet. Three dogs were observed for six months, two for seven months, two for eight months, and the remaining three were followed for nine months before reoperation.

At the conclusion of the observation period the animals were reanesthetized and a median sternotomy was performed. Flow rates were determined in the internal mammary artery with an electromagnetic flow probe placed around the vessel near its entrance into the myocardial tunnel. In a similar fashion flow rates were measured in the left anterior descending coronary artery, the circumflex coronary artery, and the right coronary artery, in that order. If cardiac arrest occurred, resuscitative measures were instituted and appropriate medication was used as required to maintain the vital signs as near normal as possible.

After each flow study was completed the animal was sacrificed and an autopsy was done. The left internal mammary implant, the right internal mammary artery, and the coronary and systemic arteries were examined grossly and microscopically with H & E and Sudan stains. Elastic and connective tissue stains were done on selected sections. Sections of the internal mammary implant were taken midway between its origin and entrance into the myocardium and in its intramyocardial tunnel. Implant, right internal mammary, and coronary artery lesions were graded on a scale of 0 to 4+ based on the decrease in lumen size seen microscopically.

* Hydrogenated vegetable oil
† Rival Dog Food
‡ Huang method (SMA 12/60), 1961
§ Method of Royer and Ko, 1969
‖ Method of Zollner and Kirsch, 1961–1963
Method of Fletcher and Styliou, 1970

0   no atheromata
1+   minimal microscopic changes (no decrease in lumen size)
2+   moderate (lumen decreased up to 25 percent)
3+   moderately severe (lumen decreased from 25 to 50 percent)
4+   severe (lumen decreased more than 50 percent)

Abdominal aortic atheromata were grossly graded without staining based on the extent of intimal involvement.

0   no lesions
1+   minimal (5 to 10 percent)
2+   moderate (10 to 25 percent)
3+   moderately severe (25 to 75 percent)
4+   severe (75 to 100 percent)

RESULTS

The animals showed striking individual variations in responses to the atherogenic regimen in clinical appearance, blood chemistries, and the severity of the atherosclerotic lesions (Table 1). The serum cholesterol, triglycerides, and total lipids promptly began to rise within one month after the start of the special diet. Cholesterol levels reached a plateau after three months and total lipid values at about six months (Fig. 1). Serum cholesterol values ranged from 393 to 2,850 mg % and total lipids from 1,011 to 6,060 mg % in the 10 animals. Triglycerides varied from 24 to 402 mg % as the mean value slowly increased. Six animals developed an anemia of less than 75 percent of the preoperative hemoglobin value. The hypothyroidism and diet were poorly tolerated by five animals who became lethargic and lost more than 25 percent of their body weight. The anemia, weight loss, and lethargy were more prevalent in dogs developing very high cholesterol and total lipid values. Individual resistance to atherosclerosis was well shown by dog #2058 whose average cholesterol and total lipids were 1,238 and 3,115 mg % respectively. An example of extreme susceptibility to induced atherosclerosis is #2141 where individual cholesterol and total lipid values of 2,550 and 6,060 mg % were recorded.

Lipoprotein electrophoretic patterns are shown graphically in Figure 2. In general, beta lipoproteins rose steadily, chylomicra appeared at

TABLE 1. Average Serum Lipid Concentrations

VESSEL	CHOLESTEROL	TRIGLYCERIDES	TOTAL LIPIDS	ANEMIA	WT. LOSS	NO. MOS. ON DIET
1983	2303 ± 143^a	289 ± 28^a	4131 ± 445^a	yes	yes	8
1982	1997 ± 154^a	244 ± 25^a	2883 ± 202^a	no	no	6
1985	1590 ± 145^a	261 ± 32^a	3851 ± 387^a	no	no	9
1981	1672 ± 114^a	239 ± 15^a	3048 ± 168^a	no	yes	9
2058	1238 ± 141^a	137 ± 20^a	3115 ± 495^a	no	no	9
2174	1669 ± 178^a	188 ± 35^a	4073 ± 720^a	yes	no	7
2139	2096 ± 229^a	285 ± 46^a	4565 ± 561^a	yes	yes	7
2155	1390 ± 126^a	345 ± 31^a	2730 ± 284^a	yes	no	6
2105	1685 ± 134^a	170 ± 71^a	3089 ± 201^a	yes	yes	6
2141	2100 ± 144^a	309 ± 25^a	4493 ± 519^a	yes	yes	8
Cont.	167 ± 10^a	49 ± 5^a	556 ± 29^a	—	—	0

^{a}Standard error of the mean.

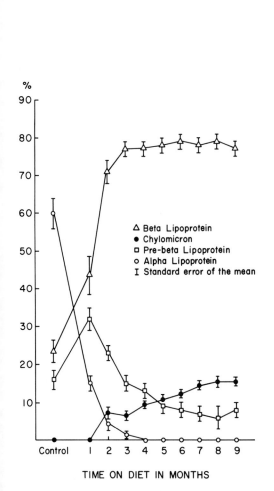

FIG. 1. Graph of lipid values.

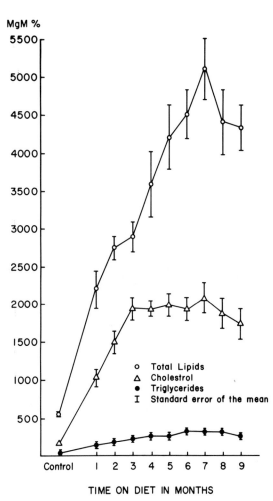

FIG. 2. Graph of lipoproteins.

TABLE 2. Flow Rates in cc/min

VESSEL	IMPLANT	LAD	CIRC	RCA	CARDIAC ARREST	NO. MOS. ON DIET
1983	2	10	52	84	no	8
1982	0	05	60	86?	yes	6
1985	0	00	65	80	no	9
1981	0	10	50	30?	yes	9
2058	2	30	50	60	no	9
2174	0	12	45	90	no	7
2139	0	18	40	75?	yes	7
2155	1	55	56	80	no	6
2105	0	00	48	60?	yes	6
2141	0	00	75?	45?	yes	8

two to three months, pre-beta particles progressively declined, and alpha lipoproteins rapidly disappeared from the serum. No animal developed overt diabetes mellitus, and the glucose tolerance test was normal in every instance. It was observed that fasting plasma when left to stand overnight in the refrigerator at 4 C formed a dense white band at the top of the tube consistent with the presence of chylomicrons. The remainder of the plasma was densely opalescent.

At reoperation, pronounced cardiac irritability was noted especially upon placement of the flow probe on the coronary arteries. Flow rates in the implant were negligible or zero. One animal

(2141) arrested as the probe was placed on the circumflex coronary artery; it was resuscitated but arrested again as the flow in the right coronary artery was being measured. Four more animals (1982, 1981, 2139, and 2105) developed ventricular fibrillation while the probe was on the right coronary artery. Although the animals were resuscitated long enough to complete the flow studies, the pulse rate and blood pressure were not stable and that cast considerable doubt on the significance of those measurements. Flow rates are summarized in Table 2. With these reservations in mind, it still was our impression that total coronary flow was reduced in all animals and that

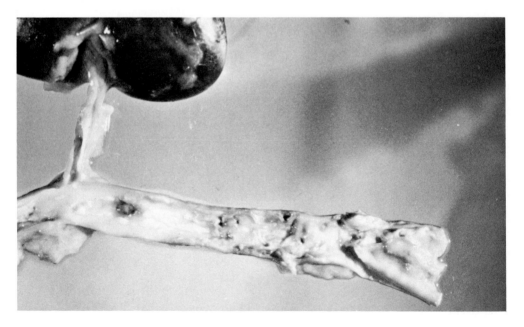

FIG. 3. This specimen illustrates that the distal abdominal aorta, iliacs, and femoral arteries are areas of predilection in canine atherosclerosis.

the cardiac irritability was a manifestation of severe ischemic heart disease.

Gross inspection of the heart invariably revealed a moderate to severe diffuse coronary atherosclerosis. Small vessels on the pericardial surface commonly were found to be severely diseased. The internal mammary implant was either occluded or presented a pinpoint lumen (Fig. 3). Of the systemic arteries, atherosclerotic changes were most frequent and severe in the terminal aorta, iliacs, and femoral arteries (Fig. 4). Small areas of the disease were commonly seen surrounding each orifice of the vessels originating from the thoracic and abdominal aorta. Scattered plaques were found in the subclavian, carotid, renal, and pulmonary arteries, on the aortic valvular cusps and the sinuses of Valsalva. There was minimal evidence of atherosclerotic change in the right internal mammary artery usually confined to a plaque at its origin. The severity of the anatomic changes is tabulated in Table 3.

Microscopic findings confirmed the impressions gained by gross inspection. A diffuse coronary atherosclerosis that was graded from moderate to severe and showed all stages of the disease was seen (Fig. 5–7). Lesions were seen in major coronary trunks, epicardial branches, and small vessels throughout the heart. The changes varied from infiltration with foam cells, large cholesterol clefts, fibrosis, severe intimal thickening, destruction of the internal elastic membrane and of the media, intramural hemorrhage, and in some cases complete occlusion of the vessel. The right internal mammary artery was either free of disease or had minimal involvement (Fig. 8, 9). The implants, both extra and intramyocardially, were severely affected or occluded and uniformly showed the most severe atherosclerosis of any of the vessels

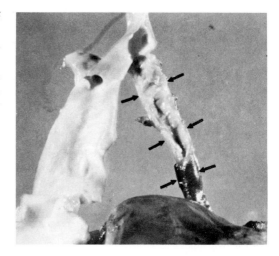

FIG. 4. The internal mammary implant is outlined by arrows. Note the severe atherosclerotic changes in the extramyocardial portion of the implant and the sparing of the thoracic aorta and subclavian artery.

examined (Fig. 10–12). Microscopic examination of the large vessels, including the aorta, did not reveal the extensive atherosclerotic abnormalities seen in the coronary arteries or the internal mammary implant.

COMMENT

Experimentally, Creech and Jordan et al[1] were the first to focus attention on the direct relationship between dietary and serum cholesterol concentrations and the severity and rapidity of the atherogenesis. Although Suzuki and Kim[14] have shown it is possible to produce atheromatous lesions in dogs without adding cholesterol to the

TABLE 3. Degrees of Atherosclerosis

VESSEL	ABDOM. AORTA	CORON.	RT. INTER. MAMM.	EXTRAMYOCARD. IMPLANT	INTRAMYOCARD. IMPLANT	NO. MOS. ON DIET
1983	++	+++	+	occl.	occl.	8
1982	++	+++	0	+++	++++	6
1985	+++	+++	+	+++	++++	9
1981	++++	+++	+	++++	occl.	9
2058	++	+++	0	+++	++++	9
2174	++	++++	+	++++	occl.	7
2139	++++	++++	+	++++	occl.	7
2155	++	++	+	++++	++++	6
2105	++++	+++	0	+++	++++	6
2141	++++	++++	+	occl.	occl.	8

diet, hypothyroidism was induced and a high fat diet was utilized in their study. The resulting atherosclerosis required 36 months to develop and was only mild to moderate in severity. As demonstrated in this study and the reports of others, thyroid suppression combined with a high-fat, high-cholesterol diet rapidly results in the development of atherosclerosis in the major arteries including the coronaries. The hyperlipoproteinemia produced by this method involves an elevation of the beta lipoproteins, which carry mainly cholesterol, and of the chylomicra, which are composed almost entirely of triglycerides. Since evaluation was performed by electrophoresis, it is possible that the pre-beta band is increased, as a lipoprotein is known that migrates on electrophoresis like a beta lipoprotein but floats in the ultracentrifuge like a pre-beta lipoprotein. The intensely cloudy serum is consistent with markedly elevated serum triglycerides carried by pre-beta or beta lipoproteins or by the chylomicron fraction. Assessment of the net and combined effects of lipids on atherogenesis is a complicated matter. Clinical studies suggest that each lipid component makes an independent con-

tribution to atherosclerosis and the severity rises in proportion to the number of lipid abnormalities present. The profound abnormalities required experimentally to produce serum lipid changes make clinical and experimental comparison impossible.

The experiments of Kelly, Taylor, and Haas [5] were among the first to point out the importance of physical and local factors in atherosclerosis. Sabiston and Smith et al [8] have shown that hypertension accelerates the atherosclerotic process. Sako,[9] Friedman,[3] and Scott and Mogan et al [10] have shown that autogenous vein grafts placed in the arterial system are very susceptible to atherosclerosis. Stevenson and Mann et al [11] have observed increased segmental deposition of atheromata by reversing abdominal aortic segments. In all of the above studies, hypercholesterolemia was essential for accelerated atherogenesis. In summary, most authors agree that atherosclerosis is the result of systemic metabolic changes and local factors such as operative trauma, turbulence, fixation of arteries by branching, and disturbance of laminar flow. Our observations of severe atherosclerosis in an internal mammary implant and minimal dis-

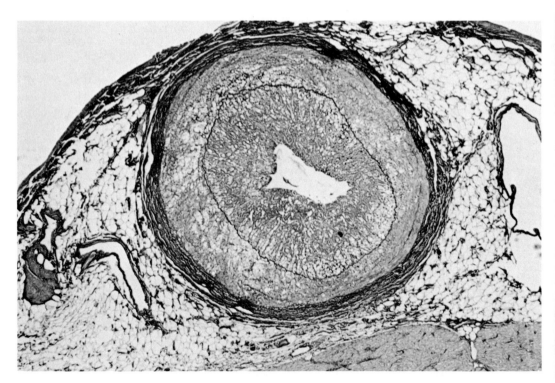

FIG. 5. Right coronary artery with severe atheromatous degeneration. Foam cell infiltration is evident in the intima and media. The internal elastic membrane is intact. Note the small vessel to the left almost occluded by atheroma. Elastic stain ×25

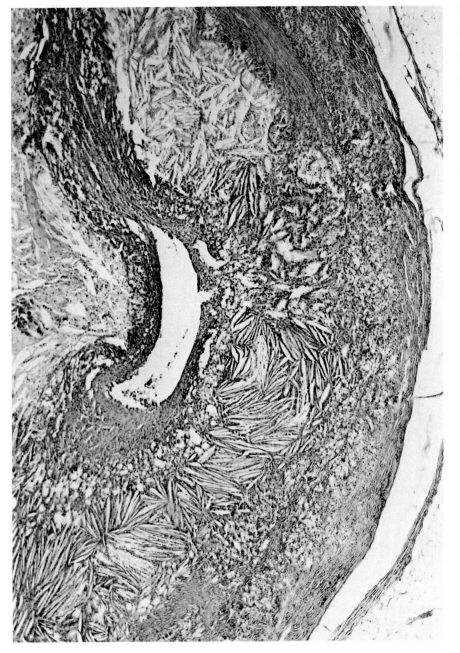

FIG. 6. Photomicrograph of the left anterior descending coronary artery demonstrating massive cholesterol clefts. H & E ×87

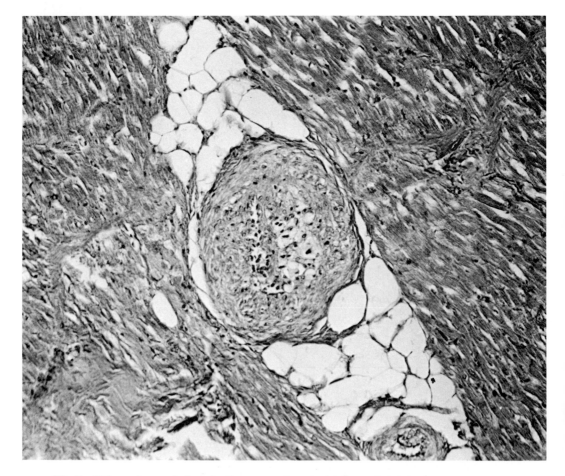

FIG. 7. This small vessel deep in the myocardium is totally occluded by the atherosclerotic process. The vessel measures 250 microns. Small-vessel disease is typical of coronary artery disease in the dog and does not resemble the ordinary clinical coronary atherosclerosis. H & E ×100

ease in an undisturbed internal mammary artery in the presence of hyperlipidemia strongly supports the concept that local factors are important in atherogenesis.

It should be emphasized that it is not possible to conclude that results of this study can be transposed to humans because of the highly artificial experimental circumstances. The results do emphasize the metabolic and mechanical components involved in the atherosclerotic process in both animals and man.

We have concluded that in the dog the internal mammary artery when implanted in the myocardium will not withstand the stress of induced atherogenesis. The hyperlipidemia and the local vascular alterations that result from moving the artery to a new location combine to predis-

pose the vessel to extensive atherosclerotic lesions. Whether the local factors responsible are simple mechanical trauma to the arterial wall, turbulence, or the inevitable decrease in flow associated with implanting a systemic artery into the myocardium, or a combination of these factors, is unknown at this time.

SUMMARY

An experimental study designed to assess the long-term fate of internal mammary artery implants in dogs on a standard atherogenic regimen has been performed. Alterations resulting from the regimen consisted of a marked elevation of serum cholesterol, triglycerides, and total lipids.

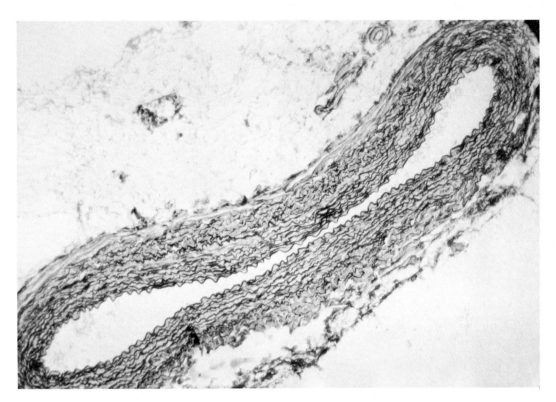

FIG. 8. Photomicrograph of the right internal mammary artery. No atherosclerotic changes are seen. Elastic stain ×21

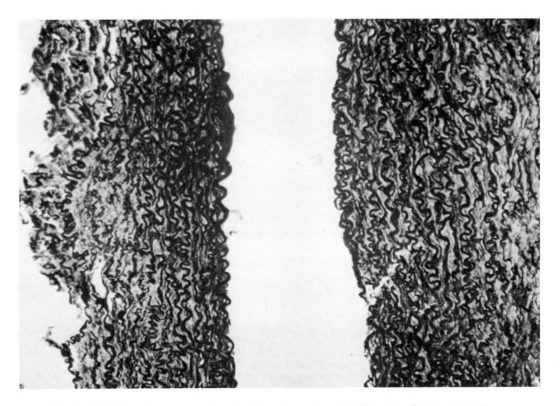

FIG. 9. Right internal mammary artery showing a trace of medial thickening. Elastic stain ×50.

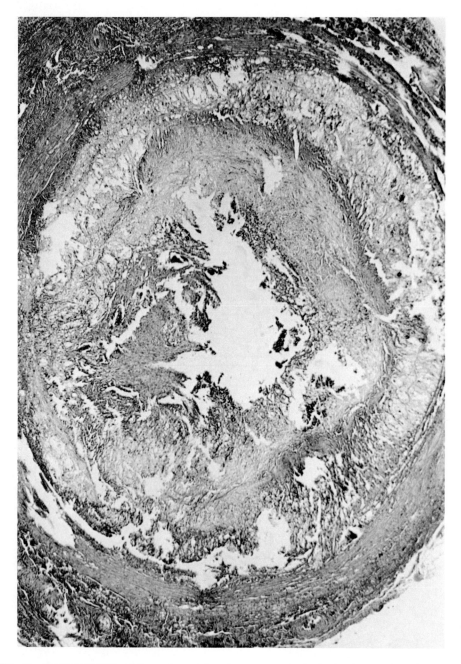

FIG. 10. Extramyocardial portion of an internal mammary implant showing moderately severe atherosclerosis. H & E ×25

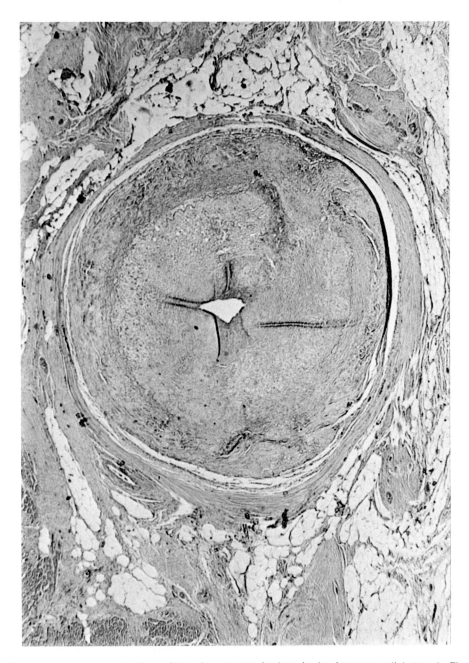

FIG. 11. Photomicrograph of an internal mammary implant in its intramyocardial tunnel. The vessel although severely diseased still is patent and has the largest lumen of all the implants in this study. H & E ×25

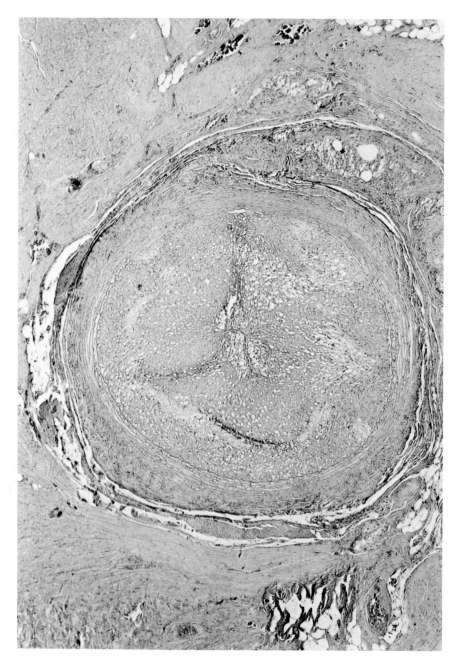

FIG. 12. Internal mammary implant that is completely closed by atherosclerosis. There was no evidence of hemosiderin or thrombus in any of the occluded implants. H & E ×25

The hyperlipoproteinemia represented essentially an increase in the beta lipoproteins and chylomicrons. Pre-beta and alpha lipoproteins decreased or disappeared from the serum of these animals.

A severe atherosclerosis was produced in the internal mammary implants and the coronary arteries. The right internal mammary artery, which was not involved in operative dissection, had only minimal or no atherosclerotic changes.

References

1. Creech OJ, Jordan GL, DeBakey ME, Overton RA, Halpert B: The effect of chronic hypercholesterolemia on canine aortic transplants. Surg Gynecol Obstet 101:607, 1955
2. Fletcher MJ, Styliou MH: A simple method for separating serum lipoproteins by electrophoresis on cellulose acetate. Clin Chem 16:362, 1970
3. Friedman M: Spontaneous atherosclerosis and experimental thromboatherosclerosis. Arch Pathol 76:115, 1963
4. Huang TC, Chen CP, Wetler V, Raftery A: A stable reagent for the Libermann-Burchard reaction: Application to rapid serum cholesterol determination. Anal Chem 33:1405, 1961
5. Kelly FB Jr, Taylor CB, Hass GM: Experimental atherosclerosis: Localization of lipids in experimental lesions of rabbits with hypercholesteremia. Arch Pathol 53:419, 1952
6. Page IH, Brown HB: Induced hypercholesterolemia and atherogenesis. Circulation 6:691, 1952
7. Royer ME, Ko H: A simplified semiautomated assay for plasma triglycerides. Anal Biochem 29:405, 1969
8. Sabiston DA, Smith GW, Talbert JL, Gutelius J, Vasko JA: Experimental production of canine coronary atherosclerosis. Ann Surg 153:12, 1961
9. Sako Y: Susceptibility of autologous vein grafts to atheromatous degeneration. Surg Forum 247, 1961
10. Scott HW, Morgan CV, Bolasay BL, et al: Experimental atherosclerosis in autogenous venous grafts. Arch Surg 101:677, 1970
11. Stevenson SE, Mann GV, Younger R, Scott HW Jr: Factors influencing the segmental deposition of atheromatous material. Arch Surg 84:49, 1961
12. Steiner A, Kendall FE: Atherosclerosis and arteriosclerosis in dogs following ingestion of cholesterol and thiouracil. Arch Pathol 42:433, 1946
13. Steiner A. Kendall FE: Production of arteriosclerosis in dogs by cholesterol and thiouracil feeding. Am Heart J 28:34, 1949
14. Suzuki M, Kim H: Induction of atherosclerosis in dogs without added cholesterol in the diet. Abstract 335, FASEB, Atlantic City, NJ, April 1972
15. Zollner N, Kirsch K: Uber die quantitative bestimmung von lipoiden (mikromethode) mittels der vielen naturlichen lipoiden (allen bekannten plasmalipoiden) gemeinsamen sulfphosphavanillin-reaktion. Zeitschrift fur die Gesamte Experimentelle Medizin 135–136:545, 1961–63

6

ATHEROMA PRODUCTION IN AUTOGENOUS VENOUS AORTOCORONARY BYPASS GRAFTS

WILLIAM R. BRODY, STEPHEN J. ROSSITER, JON C. KOSEK, MARTIN LIPTON, and WILLIAM W. ANGELL

The widespread application of autogenous saphenous vein segments for bypass of atherosclerotic coronary artery disease has stimulated research efforts to determine the long-term histologic fate of such grafts. Because of the low mortality and the apparent success of these grafts clinically, there have been few opportunities to examine postoperatively many human specimens to assess the long-term structural alterations.

Several reports of canine coronary bypass with autogenous vein grafts in normolipidemic dogs have documented arteriosclerotic changes. An important question remains concerning what happens to these grafts in the hyperlipidemic host: Can atherosclerotic changes be induced, and, if so, is the vein graft more or less susceptible to the development of atherosclerotic lesions than the host arterial circulation?

This chapter describes experimental coronary artery bypass performed in dogs with both normal and markedly elevated serum lipid levels, and compares the histologic changes in the venous bypass grafts between the two groups.

EXPERIMENTAL METHODS

Twenty-eight mongrel dogs were placed into two dietary groups (Table 1) as described below. All animals in both groups underwent coronary artery bypass and were sacrificed from 1 to 24 months postoperatively. At the time of sacrifice or death, specimens of the vein graft, aorta, and

coronary arteries of the animal were examined by light microscopy. Sudan stains were employed to confirm the presence or absence of lipid deposits in the grafts. Angiography and electron microscopy of the vein grafts were performed in selected animals.

Operative Procedure

Animals were anesthetized with intravenous pentobarbital, paralyzed with succinylcholine after intubation, and placed on a positive pressure ventilator. A three-inch segment of cephalic vein of the foreleg was dissected free, care being taken to avoid traumatizing the vessel wall, and side branches were ligated with #4–0 silk ligatures. After removal, the vein was temporarily stored in a solution of heparinized saline.

A left lateral thoracotomy was performed through the fourth intercostal space, and routine cardiopulmonary bypass was employed with a bubble oxygenator. The heart was fibrillated with cold saline instilled in the pericardial well, and after the left anterior descending (LAD) coronary artery in its middle third was isolated, a longitudinal arteriotomy was created and the aorta cross-clamped. The vein graft was then anastomosed end-to-side to the LAD with a running suture of #6–0 silk. Next, the aortic cross-clamp was removed, and the remaining end of the vein segment was anastomosed end-to-side to the ascending aorta with #5–0 silk. The LAD was then ligated proximal to the takeoff of the first septal perforating branch, the heart defibrillated, and cardiopulmonary bypass stopped. Heparinization was reversed with protamine sulfate.

Dr. Brody was supported by a fellowship from the Bay Area Heart Research Committee.

TABLE 1. Experimental Groups

GROUP	NO. PATENT/ TOTAL NO.	DURATION (mos)	DEGREE OF FIBROSIS (medial and intimal)	ATHERO-SCLEROSIS (incidence)	SERUM CHOLESTEROL (average, mg%)
I	13/16	1–24	1+ to 4+	0	171
IIA	3/5	2–3	1+ to 2+	0	346
IIB	5/5	3	1+ to 2+	60%	600
IIC	2/2	21	3+ to 4+	100%	–

Diet

All Group I animals received the standard laboratory kennel diet. Group II dogs received the standard kennel diet, except for a three- to four-month period, when they were placed on an atherogenic diet. This diet [20] consisted of a two-pound portion of canned dog food (Kal-Kan registered trademark) to which had been added a 100 gram mixture containing 20 gms of cholesterol, 73 gms of cooking oil (cottonseed oil), 5 gms of cholic acid, and 2 gms of thiouracil. Serum cholesterol levels in Group II were measured biweekly. Contrary to most other atherogenic regimens, thyroid ablation, either surgically or with I^{131}, was *not* employed.

As shown in Table 1, Group IIA animals were started on the atherogenic diet for one month preoperatively and were maintained on this diet for three months postoperatively. Group IIB animals were started on the diet on the second postoperative day, and maintained for three months. Group IIC animals were begun on the atherogenic regimen 18 months postoperatively and continued for three months.

RESULTS

A summary of the results is shown in Table 2. The average fasting lipid levels for the normal diet animals (Group I) were

Cholesterol   171 ± 40 mg% (mean ± s.d.)
Triglycerides 94 ± 64 mg%

The corresponding values for the atherogenic diet animals (Group II) were

Cholesterol   397 ± 222 mg%
Triglycerides 160 ± 91 mg%

These differences between Groups I and II are statistically significant (p < 0.005).

Within Group II there were marked differences between groups. The cholesterol levels ranged from 201 to 2,144 mg percent, with mean values of 346 mg percent for Group IIA and 600 mg percent for Group IIB. While fasting levels were not available for Group IIC, random samples in this latter group ranged between 300 and 2000 mg percent. Individual animals varied markedly in their susceptibility to develop hyperlipidemia while on the diet, and differences between Groups IIA and IIB may be explained at least partly on this basis. In addition, all Group II animals showed highest lipid levels between the first and second months on the diet, with a gradual decline in subsequent months. Because Group IIA animals were started one month preoperatively on the diet, their lipid levels during the entire postoperative period were lower than the Group IIB animals, which were started immediately postoperatively.

Eighty-one percent of the Group I grafts were patent at the time of sacrifice, compared with 83 percent for Group II. Both occlusions in the atherogenic animals were in Group IIA.

Histologic Alterations

The detailed structural alterations in the Group I grafts have been described in considerable detail elsewhere [3] and will be summarized briefly.

TABLE 2. Summary of Results

EXPERI-MENTAL GROUP	NO. ANIMALS	DIET	
		Preoperative	Postoperative
I	16	regular	regular
IIA	5	atherogenic for 1 mo	atherogenic for 3 mos
IIB	5	regular	atherogenic for 3 mos
IIC	2	regular	regular for 18 mos then atherogenic for 3 mos

The long-term changes in the Group I vein grafts consist of medial fibrosis and intimal fibrosis. Medial fibrosis results from the metaplasia of smooth muscle cells to fibrocytes with subsequent collagen deposition. Intimal fibrosis, also called intimal fibrous proliferation, is a collagenous thickening of the intimal layer in association with cushions of proliferating cells (the myointimal cells). While medial fibrosis appears within the first few weeks after surgery, intimal fibrosis occurs usually after the first month and appears to be progressive.

All animals in both Group I and Group II showed at least some degree of intimal thickening by myointimal cells and fibrous tissue, roughly proportional in degree and extent to the postoperative duration. In no case was the intimal fibrosis severe enough to cause appreciable stenosis.

Medial fibrosis was also evident in all grafts. Its degree was variable and was independent of the postoperative duration. Though not consistently present, there was an inverse correlation between the degree of medial fibrosis and intimal fibrosis. Figure 1 demonstrates these medial and intimal changes in a vein graft from a Group I animal.

In the hyperlipidemic group, intimal fibrous thickening was greatly increased over Group I grafts of similar duration. In contrast, the degree of medial fibrosis was not appreciably different between groups.

In addition to the fibrotic changes, 50 percent of the patent Group II grafts showed marked atherosclerotic changes. Of the involved grafts, none was in Group IIA, while three out of five Group IIB grafts and both of Group IIC grafts showed marked atheromatous degeneration. None of the hyperlipidemic animals showed any evidence of atherosclerosis in either the aorta or coronary arteries.

Lipid was not present in any Group I grafts but was present to some degree in all of the Group II grafts. The degree of lipid deposition did not clearly correlate with postoperative duration, degree of hyperlipidemia, or time of induction of the hyperlipidemia. With fat stains, fine droplets of lipid were present in both myocytes of the media and myointimal cells of the thickened intima, and larger deposits and foam cells were found chiefly within the intima. In five Group II grafts, the lipid deposits constituted well-developed atheromata, with grossly evident yellow plaques, and histologic demonstration of degenerating fat-laden cells, phagocytic ingestion of lipid, and abscess-like extracellular deposits of lipid and cellular debris (Fig. 2–4).

The extent of lipid deposition was usually, though not invariably, proportional to the degree of intimal thickening, and the sites with greatest intimal thickening contained the most lipid.

DISCUSSION

The results of this experiment can be stated succinctly:

1. Autogenous vein grafts used for coronary artery bypass appear to be susceptible to the development of atherosclerotic lesions;
2. In all cases, the degree of atherosclerotic involvement of the vein grafts was significantly greater than that of the host's arterial circulation;
3. These grafts were susceptible to accelerated atheroma formation even if the hyperlipidemic state was not induced until 18 months postoperatively.

The most striking finding of these experiments is that severe atherosclerotic lesions were induced within three months, with the host arterial circulation remaining essentially uninvolved.

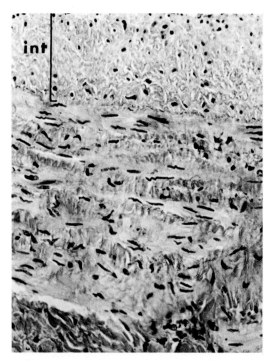

FIG. 1. Group I vein graft demonstrating intimal thickening with fibrosis and myointimal cell proliferation without evidence of lipid deposition. H. & E ×200

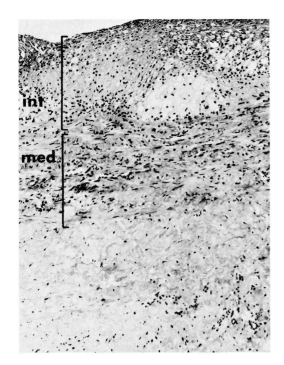

FIG. 2. Group II vein graft demonstrating atherosclerotic changes. Note marked intimal thickening and presence of foam cells. H & E ×100

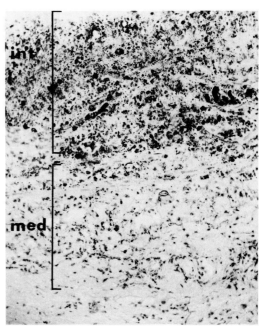

FIG. 3. Group II vein graft, documenting lipid deposition in media and intima with Sudan stain. H & E ×100

The behavior of vein grafts in hyperlipidemic animals has been reported by several investigators for carotid, aortic, and femoral arterial bypass. Sako[19] used vena caval grafts in the abdominal aorta and showed that, while these grafts did develop atheromata, they were no more susceptible than the host arterial circulation. Penn, Schenk, et al,[17] using external jugular or femoral veins for carotid or femoral arterial bypass, reported that such grafts were resistant to atherosclerotic change. By contrast, most other investigators found increased susceptibility of venous grafts to atheroma formation. Rivkin, Friedman, et al[18] induced atheromata at sites of thrombus formation in external jugular vein grafts to the abdominal aorta, showing that the vein grafts took up four times as much cholesterol in the plaques than did a corresponding site on the host aorta. Wyatt and Gonzales[23] and Scott, Morgan, et al[20] reported increased atheroma formation in vein grafts used for carotid, aortic, or femoral artery bypass. Scott's data support the concept that the degree of atherosclerotic involvement is proportional to the degree of hypercholesterolemia.

The data in this experiment support the thesis that vein grafts undergo atherosclerotic changes at an accelerated rate over the host arterial circulation. The fact that Group IIA grafts

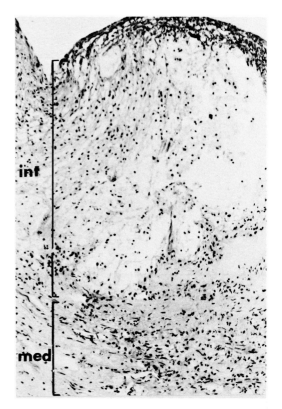

FIG. 4. Group II vein graft with atheromatous abscess. There is marked intimal thickening with abscess-like deposition of extracellular lipid and cellular debris. H & E ×100

did not show frank atherosclerosis appears to be related to the lower cholesterol and triglyceride levels in this group as compared with Group IIB. Further data are needed, therefore, to make any comparative statements regarding atherogenic susceptability between Groups IIA, IIB, and IIC.

Histologically, the atherosclerotic lesions in the vein grafts resemble those seen in "spontaneous" arterial atherosclerosis.[11] The typical lesions develop in the vein when it is subjected to arterial pressure. In a series of experiments, Friedman [11] interchanged aorta and vena cava in hyperlipidemic animals; the result was atherosclerotic change in the vena caval graft but no atherosclerosis in the aortic graft placed in the venous circulation. Interruption of the vasa vasorum, which occurs whenever the vein is removed from its connective tissue bed for use as a free graft, does not appear to influence the development of atherosclerosis. Wyatt and Gonzales [23] used *in situ* external jugular vein grafts (intact vasa vasorum) for carotid artery bypass and found that these grafts developed atherosclerosis to a degree similar to the free venous grafts.

The behavior of vein grafts for coronary artery bypass under normal serum lipid conditions has been well documented experimentally.[5,2,15,13] The pathologic alterations include changes in the media and the intima. The changes are summarized by the terms *medial fibrosis* and *intimal fibrous proliferation*. Experimental data [2] support the concept that the medial fibrosis arises from vein ischemia, resulting from interruption of the vasa vasorum, while the fibrous intimal proliferation occurs whenever the vein graft is subjected to arterial pressure (Fig. 5).

Sites of foam cell accumulation appear to be localized in those segments of the vein graft associated with intimal fibrous proliferation. In experiments on the arterial circulation, Flaherty, Ferrans, et al [9] showed that when the arteries are

exposed to increased shear stress (created by increasing the velocity of blood flow through the vessel), both lipid deposition and intimal proliferation occurred. In the vein graft, it is probably the elevated tensile stress (wall tension) rather than shear stress that appears to induce these same lesions, although tensile stress and shear stress have not been independently controlled in reported experiments. The fact that the hyperlipidemic animals showed more marked intimal fibrous thickening than the normal lipid group indicates that the lipid contributes to this lesion in addition to the elevated wall tension.

Clinical experience with saphenous vein grafts for peripheral arterial bypass has produced collaborative evidence of atherosclerotic graft degeneration. While it was initially thought that such grafts were resistant to atherosclerotic changes,[6] recent evidence points toward the contrary. Szilagyi, Elliot, et al [21] reported pathologic follow-up on several hundred saphenous vein grafts for femoral-popliteal bypass and found that 80 percent of grafts in place for more than two years showed evidence of atherosclerosis.

While several reports have documented severe intimal fibrosis in human vein grafts for coronary bypass,[12,14,16,22] only one case of atherosclerosis has been reported.[4] The latter case showed foam cells and lipid deposits in the intima of a thrombosed vein graft. By extrapolating the experimental results and Szilagyi's findings, however, it seems quite likely that atherosclerotic degeneration will be noted in long term coronary bypass vein grafts.

The implications of graft atherosclerosis, however, are not clear. Whether such changes will be progressive and whether they represent a more serious threat to graft patency than intimal fibrosis alone needs to be investigated. Control of serum lipids in post-bypass patients would seem prudent. The efficacy of other measures (eg, anti-platelet aggregation agents) to modify the response of the vein graft to elevated wall tension remains to be demonstrated.

References

1. Beebe HG, Clark WF, DeWeese JA: Atherosclerotic change occurring in an autogenous venous arterial graft. Arch Surg 101:85, 1970
2. Brody WR, Kosek JC, Angell WW: Changes in vein grafts following aortocoronary bypass induced by pressure and ischemia. J Thor Cardiovasc Surg 64:487, 1972
3. Brody WR, Angell WW, Kosek JC: Histologic fate of the venous coronary artery bypass in dogs. Am J Pathol 66:111, 1972
4. Brynjolfsson G: Pathologic changes in venous coronary bypass. Lab Invest 26:472, 1972

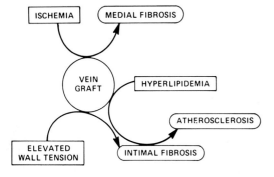

FIG. 5.   Pictorial representation of vein graft changes.

5. Dedomenico M, Sameh AA, Berger K, Wood SJ, Sauvage LR: Experimental coronary artery surgery. J Thor Cardiovasc Surg 56:617, 1968

6. DeWeese JA: Discussion of paper by Scott HW, Morgan CV, et al. Arch Surg 101:682, 1970

7. DeWeese JA, Robb CG: Autogenous venous bypass grafts five years later. Ann Surg 174:346, 1971

8. Ejrup B, Hiertonn T, Moverg A: Atheromatous changes in autogenous venous grafts: Functional and anatomical aspects. Case report. Acta Chir Scand 121:211, 1961

9. Flaherty JT, Ferrans VJ, Pierce JE, Carew TE, Fry DL: Localizing factors in experimental atherosclerosis. In Likoff W, Segal BL, Insull W, Moyer JH (eds): Atherosclerosis and Coronary Heart Disease. NY, Grune and Stratton, 1972, p 40

10. Flemma RJ, Johnson WD, Lepley D, et al: Late results of saphenous vein bypass grafting for myocardial revascularization. Ann Thorac Surg 14:232, 1972

11. Friedman M: Spontaneous atherosclerosis and experimental thromboatherosclerosis. Effect of arterial and venous environments. Arch Path 76:571, 1963

12. Grondin CM, Meere C, Castonguay Y, Lepage G, Grondin P: Progressive and late obstruction of an aorto-coronary venous bypass graft. Circulation XLIII:698, 1971

13. Hirose T, Marshall D: A comparative study of the direct internal mammary-to-coronary artery anastomosis and the aortocoronary vein bypass graft. Ann Thorac Surg 16:471, 1973

14. Johnson WD, Auer JE, Tector AJ: Late changes in coronary vein grafts. Am J Cardiology 26:640, 1970

15. Jones M, Conkle DM, Ferrans VJ, et al: Lesions observed in arterial autogenous vein grafts. Light and electron microscopic evaluation. Circulation, Supplement III to Vols XLVII and XLVIII, p III-198, 1973

16. Lesperance J, Bourassa MG, Saltiel J, Campeau L, Grondin CM: Angiographic changes in aortocoronary vein grafts: Lack of progression beyond the first year. Circulation XLVIII:633, 1973

17. Penn I, Schenk E, Robb C, DeWeese J, Schwartz S: Evaluation of the development of athero-arteriosclerosis in autogenous venous grafts inserted into the peripheral arterial system. Circulation, Supplement I to vols 31 and 32, p I-192, 1965

18. Rivkin LM, Friedman M, Byers SO: Thromboatherosclerosis in aortic venous autografts: A comparative study. Br J Exp Pathol 44:16, 1963

19. Sako Y: Susceptibility of autologous vein grafts to atheromatous degeneration. Surg Forum 12:247, 1961

20. Scott HW, Morgan CV, Bolasny et al: Experimental atherosclerosis in autogenous venous grafts. Arch Surg 101:677, 1970

21. Szilagyi DZ, Elliot JP, Hageman JH, Smith RF, Dall'olmo CA: Biologic fate of autogenous vein implants as arterial substitutes: Clinical, angiographic, and histopathologic observations in femoral-popliteal operations for atherosclerosis. Ann Surg 178:232, 1973

22. Vlodaver Z, Edwards JE: Pathologic changes in aortic-coronary arterial saphenous vein grafts. Circulation XLIV:719, 1971

23. Wyatt AP, Gonzales IE: Atheromatous lesions in arterialized vein grafts: An experimental study. Br J Surg 56:193, 1969

7

LIPID AND CONNECTIVE TISSUE METABOLISM IN HYPERTENSIVE BLOOD VESSELS

Irving M. Madoff, Dieter M. Kramsch, Marilyn A. Colombo,
Margaret F. DiModica, and William Hollander

INTRODUCTION

There is substantial evidence in man and experimental animals that a sustained elevation of arterial blood pressure, regardless of its cause, aggravates and accelerates atherosclerosis.[6,20,22,28] A number of investigators have studied coronary atherosclerosis in autopsy material from normotensive and hypertensive man and have concluded that coronary atherosclerosis is more severe in hypertensive than in normotensive man. The actual mechanism by which hypertension aggravates atherosclerosis has not been established. However, available evidence appears to indicate that the changes in connective tissue metabolism and endothelial permeability associated with atherosclerosis are augmented by hypertension.[11] Although hypertension can aggravate atherosclerosis, it is not clear that hypertension *per se*, in the absence of other atherogenic factors, can cause atherosclerosis.

Previous studies by our laboratory in experimental hypertension of coarctation of the aorta [11,13,14] gave rise to the concept that many of the changes in the structure and metabolism of the arterial wall associated with hypertension are largely due to the physical stress placed on the arterial wall by a high level of arterial pressure. In these short-term studies it was found that the salt, water, and acid mucopolysaccharide content of the hypertensive portion of the coarcted aorta was significantly increased as compared to the findings in control animals, while the content of these constituents in the relatively normotensive aortic segment below the coarctation was normal or reduced.

Supported in part by USPHS Grant HL 13262.

Although the biochemical changes in the aorta were striking, they were not accompanied by morphological changes of atherosclerosis. In the present study, the experimentally induced hypertension was studied for a longer period of time to determine whether prolonged hypertension might induce further metabolic changes in the arterial wall and lead to complicating atherosclerosis.

METHODS

Procedure

Coarctation of the thoracic aorta was produced in adult mongrel dogs. The dogs were anesthetized with sodium pentobarbital, and pulmonary ventilation was maintained with an intratracheal tube and a mechanical insufflator. An incision was made anteriorly and laterally along the fifth left intercostal space. The thoracic aorta was exposed and completely occluded by a Derra clamp at its mid-portion for 15 minutes. During this time the walls of the occluded aorta were stenosed by sutures for a distance of about 2.5 cm. A supporting band of nylon was drawn around the coarcted portion and sutured without further constriction of the vessel. The stenosis caused approximately a 75–90 percent decrease in the cross-sectional area of the aorta. After completion of the operation, a thrill was palpable in the thoracic aorta distal to the coarctation. The plasma renin activity was determined, as described previously,[14,30] by the rat bioassay method. The coarcted dogs and the 15 matched control dogs were maintained on a standard diet of Purina Dog Chow with daily supplements of ground beef. The dogs were sacrificed with intravenous pentobarbital from one to two years after the surgical coarctation. A complete autopsy was done. The thoracic aorta was dissected and removed immediately after sacrifice. Segments of the descending thoracic aorta proximal to the coarctation and distal to the coarctation were excised and analyzed separately. The same thoracic aortic segments were analyzed in the matched control dogs. The adventitia was stripped from the arterial segments to be analyzed. The fresh specimens were blotted of adhering blood, weighed, and then frozen.

Biochemical Analyses

The arterial tissue was minced and extracted into chloroform methanol, 2:1 (v/v) according to the method of Folch et al.[7] Aliquots of the extract were used to determine cholesterol, triglycerides, and phospholipids as described previously.[13] The delipidated aortic tissue was extracted with 0.1 N NaOH for 50 minutes at 95 C according to the method of Lansing and coauthors.[16] After cooling, the solution was neutralized with equal volumes of 0.1 N HCl and was maintained at 4 C for a minimum duration of 4 hours. The samples were centrifuged at 3,000 rpm for 20 minutes in order to separate the sedimented elastin fraction from the supernatant. The supernatant, which contained alkali hydrolysates or aortic collagen, was further hydrolyzed in sealed ampoules with 6 N HCl at 106 C for 24 hours. The hydroxyproline content of the acid hydrolysates was determined by the method of Bergman and Loxley.[1] A factor of 7.46 was used to convert the hydroxyproline values to collagen. This factor is based on an average hydroxyproline content of 13.5 percent in mammalian collagen.

The elastin fraction was desiccated, and the dry weight was determined. The protein content of the fraction was measured from a small portion by the Kjeldahl method.

The acid mucopolysaccharides in the arterial wall were determined by a slight modification of the method of Sirek et al.[24]

RESULTS

Arterial Blood Pressure

Immediately after the surgical narrowing of the thoracic aorta, the thoracic aortic blood pressure proximal to the coarctation rose on the average of 34/15 mmHg above control values. In the thoracic aorta distal to the coarctation, the blood pressure fell on the average of 20/5 mmHg and resulted in a marked reduction of the pulse pressure below the coarcted site. After the coarctation, the cuff systolic blood pressure in the forelimbs progressively rose and reached a definite hypertensive level in one week after the operation. At this time the cuff systolic blood pressure was 212 ± 9 SE as compared to the preoperative value of 149 ± 5 SE.

The intra-arterial pressures simultaneously measured in the carotid and femoral arteries of the control and coarcted dogs at the time of sacrifice are shown in Table 1.

In comparison with the arterial pressures of the control dogs, the coarcted dogs developed a significant elevation of blood pressure in the carotid artery and presumably in the thoracic aorta proximal to the coarctation. The rises in carotid, systolic diastolic, and mean blood pressures averaged 40, 37, and 38 mmHg above control levels, respectively. In the femoral artery, and presumably in the thoracic aorta distal to the coarctation, the systolic blood pressure fell significantly. The decrease in femoral systolic blood pressure averaged 31 mmHg below control values, while the diastolic blood pressure showed a slight and insignificant rise. As a result of these changes, there was a striking decrease of 39 mmHg in the femoral arterial pulse pressure (Fig. 1) without a significant change in the mean femoral arterial pressure. Similar decreases in systolic and pulse

TABLE 1. Comparison of Carotid and Femoral Arterial Pressure in Control and Coarcted Dogs at Time of Sacrifice

	BODY WEIGHT (kg)	CAROTID ARTERIAL PRESSURE		FEMORAL ARTERIAL PRESSURE	
		Systolic (mmHg)	Diastolic (mmHg)	Systolic (mmHg)	Diastolic (mmHg)
Control dogs	26.5 ± 5.3	158 ± 16	102 ± 12	160 ± 19	100 ± 11
Coarcted dogs	27.2 ± 5.8	$198^a \pm 22$	$139^a \pm 15$	$129^a \pm 12$	108 ± 15

Values represent the mean and standard deviation.
[a]*Significantly different from control values (P < 0.01).*

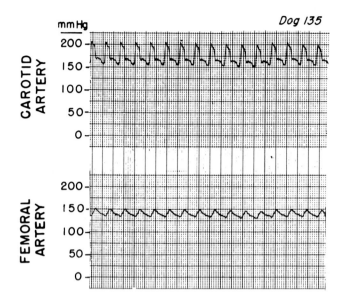

FIG. 1. Carotid and femoral arterial pressures simultaneously measured in a dog with coarctation of the aorta.

pressures were assumed to occur in the thoracic aorta distal to the coarcted site. The body weights of the control and coarcted dogs were comparable (Table 1).

Plasma Renin Activity

The typical changes in peripheral plasma renin activity following surgical coarctation are shown in Figure 2. Immediately following the surgical narrowing of the thoracic aorta an increase in renin activity was detected in the plasma of the peripheral and renal veins. Thereafter, plasma renin activity increased steadily and reached a maximal level in 24 to 48 hours after the coarctation. These changes in renin activity were associated with a marked fall in the mean blood pressure

distal to the coarctation. In one to two weeks after surgery, the plasma renin activity had returned to control levels even though the blood pressure proximal to the coarctation had risen to hypertensive levels. Plasma renin continued to be normal up to the time of sacrifice.

Cardiovascular Complications of Aortic Coarctation

Most of the coarcted dogs developed transient ischemic paralysis of the hind legs, which disappeared in 1 to 2 days after the coarctation operation. A number of dogs developed additional complications and were excluded from the study. These complications were associated with severe hypertension and included acute pulmonary

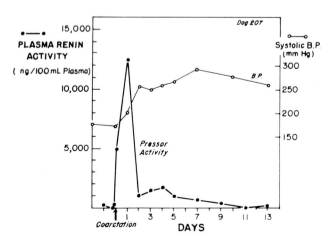

FIG. 2. Changes in plasma renin activity following surgically induced coarctation of the thoracic aorta.

TABLE 2. Composition of Aorta in Normal and Coarcted Dogs

	UPPER THORACIC AORTA		LOWER THORACIC AORTA	
	Normal Dog	Coarcted Dog	Normal Dog	Coarcted Dog
Cholesterol (mg/g dry wt.)	5.8 ± 1.2	5.6 ± 1.4	4.6 ± 0.7	4.4 ± 0.5
MPS[a] (mg/g dry wt.)	7.2 ± 0.4	$9.5^b \pm 0.5$	6.1 ± 0.4	$4.7^b \pm 0.3$
Collagen (mg/100 mg dry wt.)	13.9 ± 1.0	$17.5^b \pm 1.2$	14.8 ± 1.3	15.2 ± 1.4
Elastin (mg/100 mg dry wt.)	42.2 ± 2.5	$55.7^b \pm 2.3$	40.4 ± 1.8	42.4 ± 2.0

Values represent the mean and standard deviation.
[a]*MPS: Acid mucopolysaccharides.*
[b]*Significantly different from normal control values (P < 0.01).*

edema, congestive heart failure, dissecting aneurysm, aortic rupture, and thrombosis of the coarcted site. All the coarcted dogs, including those selected for study, were autopsied and found to have anatomical evidence of enlargement of the left ventricle. The arteries above the coarctation were thickened while the wall thickness of the arteries below the coarctation appeared normal. None of the dogs were found to have macroscopic or microscopic evidence of atherosclerosis above or below the coarctation.

Lipid Content of Aorta

The lipid content of the normal and coarcted aorta are compared in Table 2. The total MPS content of the aorta was calculated as the sum of its major constituents; hexuronic acid, hexosamine, and sulfate in milligram per gram of dried defatted tissue. As compared with the control values, the contents of MPS in the hypertensive segment of the coarcted aorta was significantly increased by about 32 percent. This increase of MPS appeared to be due to an increase in the sulfated MPS. The MPS in the normotensive aortic segment of the coarcted dogs also changed significantly but in an opposite direction. The MPS content in this portion of the aorta showed decreases of about 23 percent below control values, which appeared to be due to a decrease in the sulfated MPS.

Fibrous Protein Content of the Aorta

The collagen and elastin content of the aorta of coarcted dogs and of the corresponding aortic segments of control dogs are compared in Table 2. The hypertensive portion of the coarcted aorta contained significantly more fibrous proteins than did the control aorta. The increase in the collagen and elastin content averaged 26 percent and 32 percent above control values, respectively. In contrast to these findings, the content of collagen and elastin in the relatively normotensive segment of the coarcted aorta was not significantly different from that of the normal aorta.

DISCUSSION

The overall evidence indicates that the hypertension of coarctation of the aorta is primarily a Goldblatt type of hypertension. The observations that support the renal origin of the hypertension include the following: (1) constriction of the aorta above (but not below) the renal arteries is followed by a gradual rise of the blood pressure to hypertensive levels; (2) the transplantation of the kidneys to the neck is followed by a return of the blood pressure to normotensive levels[23] and the changes in plasma renin following the surgical coarctation are similar to those reported following experimental renal (Goldblatt) hypertension.[3]

The present findings, in support of previous studies,[11-14] provide strong evidence for a direct mechanical effect of a high level of blood pressure on the structure and function of the arterial wall. As compared to the corresponding aortic segment of normal dog, the hypertensive segment of the aorta *above* the coarctation contained significantly increased amounts of acid mucopolysaccharides, collagen, and elastin. The relatively normotensive segments below the coarctation contained normal amounts of collagen and elastin, and significantly reduced amounts of acid mucopolysaccharides. In contrast to these findings, the cholesterol content of the aorta above and below the coarcted site showed no significant changes, suggesting that hypertension may have a direct effect on the connective tissue metabolism of the arteries without necessarily altering the metabolism of lipids in these vessels.[11]

It is not clear from the present studies that hypertension *per se,* in the absence of other atherogenic factors, can cause atherosclerosis since the vascular changes produced by the experimental hypertension did not result in the development of atherosclerosis. The arterial changes characteristic of hypertension involve primarily the media and include (1) increased thickness and rigidity of the arteries, (2) hyperplasia and hypertrophy of arterial smooth muscle cells, (3) increased deposition of acid mucopolysaccharides, collagen and elastin in the arteries, and (4) increase in the arterial content of sodium, chloride, potassium, calcium, and water.[5,11,13,14,26,29] Proliferation of smooth muscle cells and connective tissue also occurs in atherosclerosis, but these changes are focal, mainly involve the intima, and are accompanied by deposition of lipid, chiefly free, and ester cholesterol.

In addition to mechanical factors, there is a growing interest in the role of vasoactive agents and chemical mediators of injury or inflammation in accelerating atherosclerosis and hypertensive vascular disease. Certain of these agents also have been implicated in the pathogenesis of hypertension and include catecholamines, renin, and prostaglandins. A number of experimental studies indicate that high plasma levels of catecholamines, renin, and angiotensin can alter the metabolism of the arterial wall and produce vascular damage that may be potentiated by mineralocorticoids and diets high in sodium content.[8-10,19] In rabbits intravenous infusions of norepinephrine have been reported to produce atherosclerosis.[17] Constantinides and Robinson as well as Robertson and Khairallah [4,21] have shown that angiotensin may increase the permeability of the arterial intima by causing contraction of the endothelial cells and opening of the interendothelial junctions. Similar effects of serotonin, histamine, and bradykinin on small vessels have been described.[18] Prostaglandins also have been reported to play a role in vascular permeability and inflammation.[15,27] However, there is conflicting evidence about the precise nature of their involvement. In the present study there was no evidence that the renin-angiotensin system played a role in the observed aortic changes since these changes were limited mainly to the hypertensive segment of the coarcted aorta. Furthermore, the plasma renin levels returned to normal during the chronic phase of the hypertension.

CONCLUSION

There is both clinical and experimental evidence that the injury of blood vessels by hypertension is due in part to the direct mechanical effects of a high level of arterial pressure on the arterial wall. The present studies were undertaken to study the mechanical effects of hypertension on the structure and metabolism of the arterial wall in dogs with hypertension of coarctation of aorta. The dogs were sacrificed at one and two years after surgical production of coarctation of the midthoracic aorta. Following surgery, the blood pressure proximal to the coarctation became markedly elevated (198/139) while the mean blood pressure distal to the coarctation remained at about normotensive levels (129/108). These changes in blood pressure were associated with initial increases in plasma renin activity. As compared to the corresponding aortic segment of normal dog, the hypertensive segment of the aorta above the coarctation contained significantly increased amounts of collagen and elastin and significantly reduced amounts of acid mucopolysaccharides. In contrast to these findings, the cholesterol, triglyceride, and phospholipid content of the aorta above and below the coarcted site showed no significant changes. None of the coarcted animals showed atherosclerotic changes in the blood vessels.

The findings indicate that a high level of arterial pressure has a direct mechanical effect on the connective tissue metabolism of the arteries without necessarily altering the metabolism of lipids in these vessels or causing atherosclerosis.

References

1. Bergman I, Loxley R: Lung tissue hydrolysates: Studies of the optimum conditions for the spectrophotometric determination of hydroxyproline. Analyst 94:575, 1969
2. Boucher R, Veyrat R, De Champlain J, Genest J: New procedures for measurement of human plasma angiotensin and renin activity levels. Can Med Assoc J 90:194, 1964
3. Brown TC, Davis JO, Olichney MJ, Johnston CI: Relation of plasma renin to sodium balance and arterial pressure in experimental renal hypertension. Circ Res 18:475, 1966
4. Constantinides P, Robinson M: Ultrastructural injury of arterial endothelium. II. Effects of vasoactive amines. Arch Pathol 38:106, 1972
5. Crane WAJ, Dutta LP: The utilization of tritiated thymidine for deoxyribonucleic acid synthesis by the lesions of experimental hypertension in rats. J Pathol Bacteriol 86:83, 1963

6. Deming QB, Mosbach EH, Bevans M, Daly MM, et al: Blood pressure, cholesterol content of serum and tissue and atherogenesis in the rat. J Exp Med 107:581, 1958

7. Folch J, Lees M, Stanley GHS: A simple method for the isolation and purification of total lipids from animal tissues. J Biol Chem 226:497, 1957

8. Giese J: Acute hypertensive vascular disease: I. Relation between blood pressure changes and vascular lesions in different forms of acute hypertension. Acta Pathol Microbiol Scand 62:481, 1964

9. Hollander W, Yagi S, Kramsch DM: In vitro effects of vasopressor agents on the metabolism of the vascular wall. Circulation 30 (Suppl II): II-1, 1964

10. Hollander W, Kramsch DM, Yagi S: The metabolism of norepinephrine in arteries. Trans Assoc Am Physicians 77:210, 1964

11. Hollander W, Madoff IM, Kramsch DM, Yagi S: Arterial wall metabolism in experimental hypertension of coarctation of the aorta. Hypertension 13:191, 1965

12. Hollander W, Kramsch DM, Yagi S, Madoff IM: Metabolic and hemodynamic factors in the increased salt and water content of hypertensive arteries. International Club on Arterial Hypertension. Expansion Scientifique Française, Paris 1: 305, 1966

13. Hollander W, Kramsch DM, Farmelant M, Madoff IM: Arterial wall metabolism in experimental hypertension of coarctation of the aorta of short duration. J Clin Invest 47:1221, 1968

14. Hollander W: Hypertension, antihypertensive drugs and atherosclerosis. Circulation 48:1112, 1973

15. Kaley G, Weiner R: Prostaglandin E_1: A potential mediator of the inflammatory response. In Ramwell P, Shaw JE (eds): Prostaglandins. Ann NY Acad Sci 180:338, 1971

16. Lansing AI, Rosenthal TB, Alex M, Dempsey EW: The structure and chemical characterization of elastic fibers as revealed by elastase and by electron microscopy. Anat Rec 114:555, 1952

17. Lorenzen PH, Garbarsch C, Mathiessen ME: Ar-

teriosclerosis in rabbit aorta induced by noradrenaline. Atherosclerosis 12:125, 1970

18. Majino G, Gilmore V, Leventhal M: On the mechanisms of vascular leakage caused by histamine-type mediators. Circ Res 21:833, 1967

19. Masson GMC, Mikasa A, Yasuda H: Experimental vascular disease elicited by aldosterone and renin. Endocrinology 71:505, 1962

20. McGill HC Jr: The geographic pathology of atherosclerosis. Lab Invest 18:463, 1968

21. Robertson AL, Khairallah PA: Effects of angiotensin II and some analogues on vascular permeability in the rabbit. Circ Res 31:923, 1972

22. Robertson WB, Strong JP: Atherosclerosis in persons with hypertension and diabetes mellitus. Lab Invest 18:538, 1968

23. Scott W Jr, Collins HA, Langa AM, Olsen NS: Additional observations concerning the physiology of the hypertension associated with experimental coarctation of the aorta. Surgery 3:445, 1954

24. Sirek OV, Schiller S, Doriman A: Acid mucopolysaccharides in aortic tissue of the dog. Biochem Biophys Acta 83:148, 1964

25. Skinner SL, McCubbin JW, Page IH: Control of renin secretion. Circ Res 15:64, 1964

26. Tobian L, Binion J: Artery wall electrolytes in renal and DCA hypertension. J Clin Invest 13: 1407, 1954

27. Vane JR: Inhibition of prostaglandin synthesis as a mechanism of action for aspirin-like drugs. Nature (New Biol) 231:232, 1971

28. Wakerlin GE, Moss WG, Kiely MS: Effect of experimental and renal hypertension on experimental thiouracil-cholesterol atherosclerosis in dogs. Circ Res 5:426, 1957

29. Wolinsky H: Response of the rat aorta media to hypertension. Circ Res 26:507, 1970

30. Yagi S, Kramsch DM, Madoff IM, Hollander W: Plasma renin activity in hypertension associated with coarctation of the aorta. Am J Physiol 215: 605, 1968

8

CONSEQUENCES OF REPERFUSION FOLLOWING ACUTE CORONARY OCCLUSION

Samuel Meerbaum, Tzu-Wang Lang, Costantino Costantini,
Jules Osher, Herbert Gold,
John Friedman, and Eliot Corday

One of the recommended interventions aimed at saving the jeopardized myocardium after coronary occlusions is to provide reperfusion of the affected distal zone by saphenous vein coronary bypass. Current controversy centers on the advisability of and criteria for coronary revascularization in acutely evolving myocardial infarction.[28] The success of such an intervention is critically related to an understanding of the physiological mechanisms that influence myocardial viability both during periods of ischemia and subsequent restoration of perfusion. In order to provide data on the progressive hemodynamic, metabolic, and morphologic derangements following coronary occlusions, and also to assess the effectiveness of reperfusion, improved experimental models and sophisticated measurements are required.

In spite of extensive investigations, some of which are reviewed in this paper, much debate persists with regard to the limits of myocardial viability following complete coronary occlusions. Reperfusion following experimental acute occlusion of coronary arteries was most often studied by using some form of acute or chronic open-chest procedure. The anterior descending (LAD) or circumflex (LCF) branches of the left coronary artery were ligated for periods from several minutes to six hours, following which reperfusion was instituted and continued for hours, days, or weeks.

The results were generally analyzed through histopathologic and histochemical analysis of ischemic tissue samples taken from the excised hearts. Using differing species and divergent preparations and methodologies, investigators reported that acute occlusions lasting 45 minutes or less seldom led to extensive myocardial necrosis. While longer temporary occlusions result in regional infarction, there is little unanimity as to the location, types, and extent of tissue damage, or its implication in terms of left ventricular contractility, myocardial metabolism, and hemodynamics. This is not surprising when one considers the multiplicity of factors that might alter myocardial function and viability, including the prevailing coronary collateral circulation. Recently, several investigators reported significant benefits of reperfusion after three to five hours of acute occlusion of a major coronary artery.[11,12] However, evidence has also been presented that reperfusion may cause development of a characteristic hemorrhagic infarction.[6] Reperfusion tends to cause persistent arrhythmias, which frequently lead to ventricular fibrillation.[1]

Although it is clearly important to determine whether reperfusion is beneficial or harmful when applied at specific levels of cardiac function, very limited data are available on its effects on cardiac metabolic and contractile function. Correlation of simultaneously measured regional and global cardiac function should help elucidate the relationship of functional alterations to morphologic changes. A recent study of reperfusion after three hours of LAD occlusion in open-chest dogs [20] employed correlations of epicardial ST segment mapping and tissue CPK determinations with histologic findings, along with observations of regional wall motions.

Supported in part by Grant HL 15834–01 and under the Myocardial Infarction Research Program from the National Heart and Lung Institute of the National Institutes of Health. Further support is acknowledged from Mr. Berle Adams, the Abe and Muriel Lipsey Charitable Foundation, and Mr. Norman Levin.

In the present study, we used a closed-chest model, which features intracoronary balloon occlusion of coronary arteries and permits simultaneous determination of myocardial metabolism in the ischemic and nonischemic regions, in addition to other measurements of global left ventricular function.[8] This model is being applied in studies of the progressive alterations following differing periods of coronary occlusion and reperfusion.[23] The current study reports on the consequences of a three-hour acute occlusion of the proximal left anterior descending coronary artery and subsequent reperfusion over a five-hour period.[19]

INTRACORONARY BALLOON OCCLUSION: REPERFUSION MODEL

We have developed a closed-chest model with reversible intracoronary occlusion for study of the consequences of acute coronary occlusion and reperfusion.[8] The model has now been applied in approximately 200 dogs and is suitable for anesthetized and conscious preparations. Figure 1 illustrates schematically the methodology employed during a closed-chest study of left anterior descending (LAD) coronary artery occlusion.

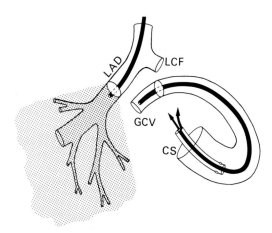

FIG. 1. Schematic representation of the model of coronary artery occlusion and reperfusion in the closed-chest preparation. Intracoronary occlusion of the proximal LAD, and brief temporary obstruction of the GCV, is by means of double lumen balloon catheters. Reperfusion is achieved by deflation of the LAD balloon catheters. Blood is simultaneously sampled from the CS, which drains the nonoccluded zone perfused by the LCF, and from the GCV draining the occluded zone through the center lumen of the catheter distal to the GCV balloon. Measurements can also be performed through the center lumen of the LAD balloon catheter distal to the coronary occlusion. From Am J Cardiol 33:51, 1974

Coronary artery or branch occlusion is performed with a double lumen intracoronary balloon catheter. This catheter is maneuvered under fluoroscopic control until the desired occlusion site is reached, eg, within the proximal LAD. The balloon is filled with 50 percent (weight/volume) Hypaque® (Winthrop Laboratories) to aid in its visualization and is inflated to achieve occlusion of the coronary artery. Coronary angiography and measurement of pressure distal to the occlusion serve as a check on the completeness and permanence of the occlusion. Reperfusion at a preselected time is performed simply by deflating the intracoronary balloon.

To assess the regional metabolic function of coronary occluded and nonoccluded segments of the left ventricle, a second double lumen balloon catheter is passed through or alongside a coronary sinus (CS) catheter until it is deep within the great cardiac vein (GCV) and its balloon is in the proximity of the LAD occlusion. Temporary obstruction of the GCV separates the venous compartments serving the LAD and LCF perfused zones of the left ventricle. Simultaneous blood sampling from the GCV through the center lumen of the balloon catheter and from the CS (through a separate catheter) permits determination of regional myocardial metabolism. When coronary sinus thermodilution flow measurements are performed without and then with similar brief separation of the venous compartments, data on mixed coronary sinus and regional venous drainage permit assessment of coronary flow from the occluded and nonoccluded regions.

The center lumen of the intracoronary balloon catheter provides direct communication with the region distal to the coronary occlusion. This facilitates blood sampling and pressure or flow measurements from this zone. In addition, a platinum wire passed through the center lumen of the catheters allows measurement of an intracoronary quasiepicardial ECG in the ischemic as well as in the noninvolved myocardium. The double lumen balloon catheters are now being used by us in studies of selective infusions of pharmacologic agents directly into the ischemic zone.

METHODS AND PROCEDURES

The reperfusion study was carried out in seven anesthetized closed-chest mongrel dogs weighing 30–35 kg. Anesthesia was with morphine (2 mg/kg intramuscularly) followed 30 minutes later by pentobarbital (15 mg/kg intravenously), with supplemental doses as required to maintain a continuous state of light anesthesia. A Harvard respirator provided artificial respiration through a cuffed endotrachial tube. An initial dose of heparin (5 mg/kg) was followed by hourly supplementation at 2 mg/kg. Blood volume depleted by blood sampling and fluid losses was replenished by infusion of physiological saline at a rate of 75–100 cc/hour. Instrumentation and balloon catheter placement were accomplished in the closed chest. Hemodynamic and regional metabolic measurements were carried out in sham dogs and following acute proximal LAD occlusion and reperfusion.

Heart rate and cardiac rhythm were determined from a precordial electrocardiogram (V-4). A tip transducer (Bio-Tech Instruments, Pasadena, California) was introduced into the left ventricle for measurement of left ventricular pressure and left ventricular end-diastolic pressure. The maximal rate of left ventricular pressure rise was obtained by electrical differentiation. Aortic root pressure and pressure distal to the point of coronary occlusion were measured by means of Statham P23Db transducers. Cardiac output was determined with a Swan-Ganz thermodilution catheter. Coronary sinus flow was measured by the Ganz thermodilution technique.

Blood gases (pO_2, pCO_2) and pH were monitored throughout the experiment. Simultaneous aortic and regional venous blood samples were obtained from the CS and GCV in the presence of temporary short GCV balloon occlusion. Hemoglobin and oxygen saturation were measured to provide data for computation of regional oxygen extraction in the coronary occluded and nonoccluded regions, as well as global left ventricular oxygen consumption. Blood lactates were determined by the Hans-Jurgens-Hohorst technique. Blood potassium was measured by flame photometry.

After periods of LAD occlusion and reperfusion, gross and microscopic examinations were made of the excised hearts to assess myocardial damage. The area of gross infarction was delineated and tissue sections from the occluded and nonoccluded zones were prepared for light microscopy, using standard and specialized stains.

Electrocardiograms and hemodynamic data were recorded on an eight-channel Electronics for Medicine unit at paper speeds of 50 and 100 mm/sec. Statistical results of measurements were expressed as mean ± standard error of the mean. Significance was established by means of Student t-tests.

Following control measurements, acute occlusion of the proximal LAD was performed

through inflation of the intracoronary balloon at the tip of a 4F double lumen catheter (Edwards Laboratories, Santa Ana, California). Deflation of this balloon and retraction of the intracoronary catheter into the aorta provided total reperfusion of the coronary artery. At regular intervals throughout three hours of LAD occlusion and five hours of reperfusion, measurements were carried out of regional myocardial metabolism and coronary flow, as well as of global left ventricular contractile function and hemodynamics.

RESULTS

Figure 2 presents a statistical summary of hemodynamic and regional metabolic data in seven closed-chest dogs during a preocclusion control period, three hours of proximal LAD occlusion, and five hours of reperfusion. Hemodynamics are shown as percent changes from preocclusion control. The accompanying legend indicates the control levels as follows: heart rate (HR) in beats/min; peak systolic aortic pressure (SP) in mm Hg; left ventricular end-diastolic pressure (EDP) in mm Hg; left ventricular end-diastolic pressure (EDP) in mm Hg; maximal isovolumetric rate of rise in left ventricular pressure (dP/dt) in mm Hg/sec; cardiac output (CO) in liters/minute; systemic vascular resistance (SVR) in dynes sec cm^{-5}; cardiac stroke work (SW) in g·m/beat; and total coronary sinus flow (CSF) in ml/min.

Regional metabolic data during control, coronary artery occlusion, and subsequent reperfusion are reported for the myocardial segments perfused by the LAD and LCF coronary arteries respectively. These are based on simultaneous regional blood sampling from the GCV and CS respectively, during brief occlusion of the great cardiac vein (GCV) balloon. Arteriovenous lactate balance is given as $(A/V)/A \times 100$ in percent, potassium balance (A-V) in mEq/L, and percent oxygen extraction as A-V oxygen percent saturation. Coronary sinus flow measurements and left ventricular myocardial oxygen consumption determinations were performed in five of the seven dogs,

The asterisk (*) indicates significance ($p < 0.05$) relative to preocclusion control. The dot (·) represents significance of reperfusion measurements as compared with values at the end of three hours of LAD occlusion. Trends and data of four individual experiments are presented in Figures 3–6. Results of histopathologic study of tissue samples from the reperfused region will be briefly reviewed.

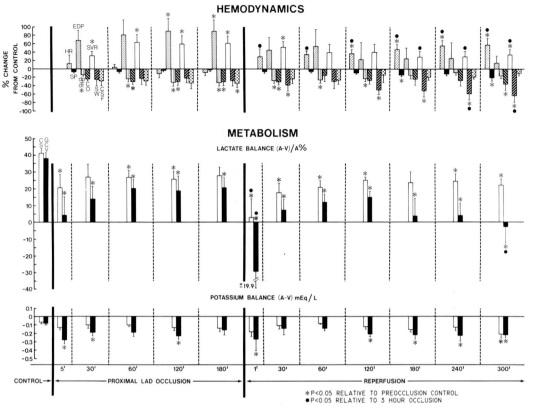

FIG. 2. Composite statistical summary (seven dogs) of hemodynamic and metabolic measurements (lactate and potassium balances) during a control period, three hours of occlusion, and five hours of reperfusion. The top bar graph indicates percent changes from preocclusion control. Control measurements were HR, 109 beats/min; SP, 136 mm Hg; EDP, 6 mm Hg; dP/dt 2740 mm Hg/sec; CO, 3.3 L/min; SVR, 2720 dynes sec cm^{-5}; SW, 47 g•m m/beat; CSF, 179 ml/min. Significant alterations during the occlusion period were a rise in EDP and SVR, while CO, dP/dt, SW, and CSF decreased. Reperfusion resulted in a further significant decrease of SW and increased heart rate. SP, CO, SVR, and EDP diminished while dP/dt improved. Five minutes after coronary occlusion there is a change from normal to significantly deranged lactate extraction in both the occluded and nonoccluded segment. Early reperfusion exhibits a major lactate washout from both segments. Five hours of reperfusion results in further metabolic deterioration as evidenced by lactic acid production in the occluded zone, although the coronary flow has returned toward normal. Potassium balance exhibits a large potassium loss from the occluded area and a smaller loss from the non-occluded zone almost immediately after occlusion. Significant potassium loss continued after reperfusion. From Am J Cardiol 33:71, 1974

Hemodynamics

Heart rate rose 13 percent above control at 30 minutes after LAD occlusion but at the end of three hours declined to 8 percent below pre-occlusion control. A significant rise in heart rate occurred following reperfusion, reaching 57 percent above control at five hours of reperfusion. Reperfusion caused arrhythmias in six dogs, consisting principally of sinus tachycardia, multifocal premature systoles, slow ventricular rhythm, intermittent and sustained ventricular tachyarrhythmias (Fig. 3).

Peak systolic pressure dropped 6 percent below control within five minutes of LAD occlusion, following which it remained stable throughout the three-hour occlusion period. Reperfusion caused a gradual decrease in this pressure, until it was 21 percent below preocclusion control. In five of the seven dogs, five hours of reperfusion resulted in a substantial reduction in peak systolic pressure, with two reaching shock levels (ie both systolic pressure and cardiac output more than 30 percent below control). Figure 4 illustrates such an individual experiment.

Left ventricular end-diastolic pressure was 6 mm Hg in control and rose 89 percent over three hours of LAD occlusion. Reperfusion resulted in a general decrease in LVEDP to near control levels.

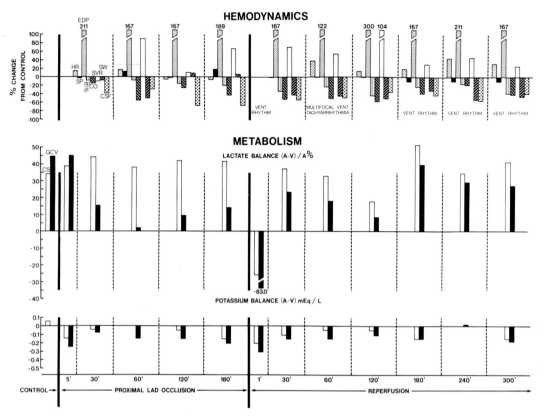

FIG. 3. Hemodynamics and regional metabolism were measured during control, over three hours of proximal LAD occlusion and five hours of reperfusion. Occlusion exhibits significant depression of the cardiac output and coronary sinus flow, while LVEDP and systemic vascular resistance are significantly increased. Reperfusion is characterized by persistent arrhythmias and further derangement in cardiac function. The coronary occluded zone shows a deranged lactate metabolism and potassium loss during the occlusion period, a major washout immediately following reperfusion, and fluctuating metabolism during the reperfusion period.

Maximal LV dP/dt dropped over three hours of LAD occlusion to 33 percent below control. Immediately following balloon deflation there was a slight improvement, but after five hours of reperfusion max LV dP/dt was still 17 percent below control.

Cardiac output was reduced 30 percent after 3 hours of occlusion. Immediately after reperfusion, cardiac output rose to 11 percent below control but subsequently dropped further during five hours of reperfusion to 36 percent below control. Following reperfusion, two animals sustained a 55–65 percent drop in cardiac output (Fig. 4) and developed shock. Two other dogs that did not develop hypotension had a drop in CO of 41 and 51 percent respectively (Fig. 5).

Systemic vascular resistance rose 16 percent immediately after occlusion and increased further to 63 percent above control after three hours of occlusion. During five hours of reperfusion, resistance fluctuated downwards to 33 percent above control.

Cardiac stroke work was reduced after three hours of LAD occlusion and decreased further to 64 percent below control at the end of the five-hour reperfusion period. This was usually associated with a rise in heart rate. The two animals that developed a shock state sustained a marked decrease in SW to 84 percent and 88 percent below control.

Coronary sinus flow was measured in five dogs. It dropped to 21 percent below control early in the LAD occlusion period. At the end of three hours, it was reduced to 36 percent below control. After 30 minutes of reperfusion, coronary sinus flow was 24 percent below control, and five hours after reperfusion, it was still 11 percent below preocclusion control.

Metabolism

LACTATE BALANCE (A-V)A × 100 (PERCENT). Preocclusion lactate extraction levels were 39 and 41 percent, respectively in

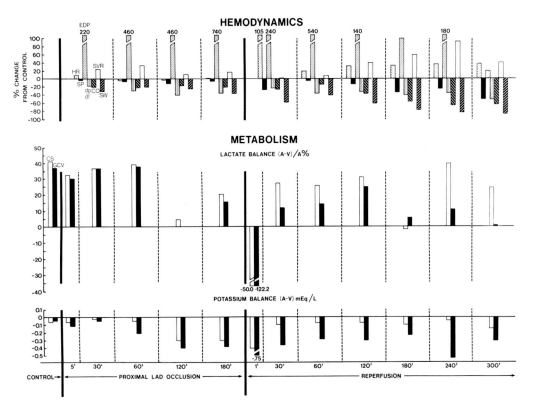

FIG. 4. Measurement of hemodynamics, lactate and potassium balances in an individual dog during control, following three hours of LAD occlusion and five hours of reperfusion. In the late occlusive period there is a large potassium loss from both occluded and nonoccluded zones. With reperfusion, a large lactate and potassium washout occurred. The potassium loss from the occluded segment continued over five hours of reperfusion. Shock supervened three hours after onset of reperfusion, as exhibited by a decrease of 40 percent in SP and 50 percent in CO. From Am J Cardiol 33:75, 1974

the occluded and nonoccluded segments. Five minutes after LAD occlusion there was a significant decrease in the occluded region lactate balance to 4 percent, ie to near-production levels. The nonoccluded artery segment also exhibited a significant early decrease in lactate extraction to 21 percent. Three hours after occlusion, lactate balance in the occluded zone rose to 21 percent and in the nonoccluded to 28 percent. Immediately upon reperfusion, there was a marked drop in lactate balance to −30 percent in the occluded zone and to +3 percent in the nonoccluded region. These sudden changes are thought to represent washout of accumulated metabolites. After five hours of reperfusion, the previously occluded zone exhibited a −3 percent lactate production, while the nonoccluded zone showed a 22 percent lactate extraction.

Three dogs revealed substantial reduction of lactate balance in the nonoccluded zone during the three-hour LAD occlusion period (Fig. 6). During the same period, all seven dogs demonstrated severe derangement of lactate metabolism

in the occluded zone, with three exhibiting lactate production (Fig. 6). Following five hours of reperfusion, six out of the seven dogs had substantial lactate production in the previously occluded area, and all seven indicated reduction of lactate extraction in the nonoccluded region (Fig. 6).

POTASSIUM BALANCE (A-V) (mEq/L). Five minutes of LAD occlusion resulted in a significant potassium loss from the occluded zone (− 0.28 mEq/L) (Fig. 3, 5). The change in the nonoccluded myocardium was nonsignificant. During the remaining occlusion period, a lesser rate of potassium loss occurred in the occluded zone (ranging from − 0.16 to − 0.23 mEq/L). Immediately after reperfusion there was a significant loss of potassium from both zones, probably indicating a washout phenomenon. Thereafter, the previously occluded area continued to lose potassium.

REGIONAL OXYGEN PERCENT EXTRACTION (A-V). During the three-hour LAD occlusion there was evidence of a slight (5 percent) increase in oxygen extraction in both

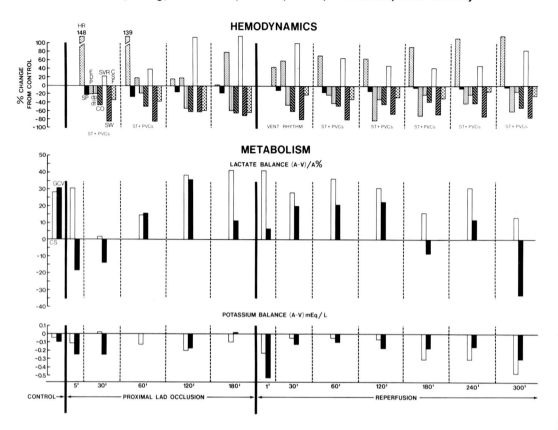

FIG. 5. Measurements of hemodynamics, lactate and potassium balances in a dog during control, three hours of LAD occlusion, and five hours of reperfusion. HR increased shortly after occlusion, while systemic pressure, CO, CSF, and SW diminished. At the same time lactate production and potassium loss occurred in the occluded area, with deranged lactate extraction in the nonoccluded zone. The metabolic derangements improved temporarily during the subsequent occlusion period. At the end of three hours the SVR increased, while dP/dt, CO, SW, and CSF were further reduced. Following reperfusion there was a washout of potassium, particularly from the occluded zone. Ventricular rhythm, sinus tachycardia with frequent PVCs supervened throughout the perfusion period. During the last three hours there was further deterioration in hemodynamic parameters, with increased HR and SVR. At five hours of reperfusion, major lactic acid production supervened in the occluded segment and metabolic derangements were noted in both zones.

the occluded and nonoccluded regions of the left ventricle. Except for a decreased extraction seen immediately upon reperfusion, the slightly increased extraction in both zones was maintained throughout the five-hour period of reperfusion.

TOTAL MYOCARDIAL OXYGEN CONSUMPTION. Total myocardial oxygen consumption dropped progressively over the three-hour period of occlusion, from a mean control value of 10.1 to 6.7 ml/min/100 gm. During reperfusion, total oxygen consumption gradually increased to 9.8 ml/min/100 gm.

Histopathology

Six of seven animals exhibited infarction in the anterior left ventricular wall and the anterior apex. In the two that developed hypotension, infarcts were also seen in the posterior left ventricle. Cellular necrosis and fragmentation of myofibrils was most pronounced in the shock dogs. Intramyocardial vascular congestion (hyperemia), microthrombi and hemorrhages accompanied the infarctions.

SURVEY OF STUDIES OF TEMPORARY OCCLUSION AND REPERFUSION

It is interesting to review the past efforts to define myocardial viability following temporary coronary occlusion. The earliest studies led to a widely accepted critical period of 20 minutes for ischemic tissue viability in the absence of significant collateral blood supply. Subsequently, it ap-

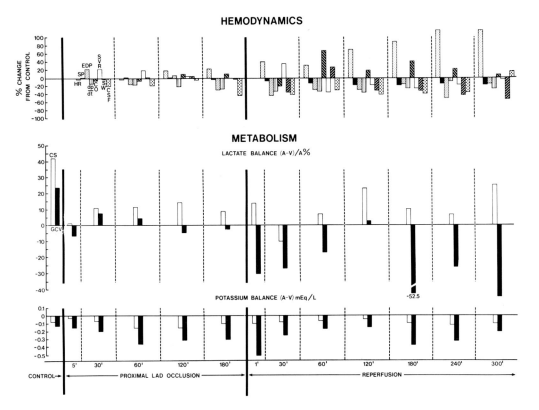

FIG. 6. Hemodynamic and regional metabolic measurements in control, during three hours of occlusion and five hours of reperfusion. LAD occlusion resulted in significant metabolic derangements in both occluded and nonoccluded zones, with major potassium loss and lactate production in the occluded region. Reperfusion exhibited early washout of lactic acid and potassium, and subsequent substantial deterioration of the lactate balance in the occluded segment and persisting derangement in the nonoccluded zone. From Am J Cardiol 33:74, 1974

peared that acute occlusion of major coronary arteries might generally cause infarction after 45 minutes and could be tolerated for three to four hours, with substantial return of myocardial function and reversal of myocardial injury following short or longer periods of reperfusion. These experimental studies used differing preparations, modes of occlusion, and means of analysis, and the investigators' interpretations and conclusions varied accordingly.

Blumgart, Gilligan, et al [4] performed open-chest dog studies of temporary occlusion of the LAD and LCF coronary arteries in order to establish the duration of localized ischemia necessary to produce irreversible damage of myocardial infarction. The primary tool was electrocardiographic analysis, but chemical changes in the myocardium and pathologic manifestations were also examined. In surviving animals, a 5- to 20-minute acute occlusion showed no gross evidence of myocardial infarction, although there were electrocardiographic changes typical of myocardial ischemia. Reestablishment of flow frequently led to ven-

tricular fibrillation. Reperfusion following occlusions lasting 25 to 45 minutes presented gross evidence of some infarction, borne out by subsequent microscopic examination. The irreversible damage due to 45 minutes' occlusion was found to be as extensive as that noted with an occlusion lasting several weeks.

Jennings, Somers, et al [14] presented interesting data on myocardial necrosis following temporary occlusion in a large number of open chest dogs. The circumflex coronary artery was occluded about 1.5 cm from the origin of the left coronary artey. ECG alterations were followed over periods of occlusion lasting from 0 to 60 minutes, followed by measurements during early reperfusion, and, again, after one to eight days. The excised hearts were examined for gross signs of necrosis, and thin sections of the middle of the posterior papillary muscle were subjected to metabolic and electron-microscopic studies. Arrhythmias and ventricular fibrillation were minimized by slowing the reperfusion and more gradual reoxygenation. Little if any necrosis was found in the myocardium up to 20 minutes of occlusion. Some necrosis was noted in all dogs with occlusions lasting between 20 to 60 minutes, and with 60 minutes of occlusion the myocardial damage was about the same as with permanent occlusion.

Fischer and Edwards[10] added more data on myocardial necrosis in open-chest dogs after occluding and reperfusing the proximal LAD. The period of observation following acute coronary occlusion ranged from 20 minutes to six hours. Reperfusion lasted from three to seven days before sacrificing the dogs for gross and microscopic examinations. All dogs that experienced occlusions for periods greater than 45 minutes exhibited the same type of infarction and pathological response as those that had permanent occlusions.

Bolooki, Rooks, et al[5] reported on ventricular function during temporary (10 to 60 minutes) and permanent acute occlusions of the proximal LAD. Functional data were also obtained one hour after reperfusion. The surviving dogs had their chests closed and were sacrificed seven days later for microscopic study. Forty minutes of ischemia produced histologic changes of myocardial infarction comparable to those of permanent occlusion of the coronary artery. Marked depression of the left ventricular function ensued whenever the ischemic event lasted more than 15 minutes. One-hour reperfusion did not correct left ventricular dysfunction after occlusion periods of more than 15 to 20 minutes, although myocardial damage was somewhat delayed.

Torok, Toth, et al[30] acutely occluded the LAD just distal to the septal branch and studied the effects of restoration of circulation following temporary occlusions of one, two, three, or four hours in open-chest dogs. In the animals that survived, the chest was closed and progressive reperfusion changes in ECG and aortic pressure were observed over a period of days. Persistent arrhythmias and frequent VF were encountered following reperfusion. After several minutes of reperfusion, the affected region exhibited subepicardial hemorrhages, and after four hours of occlusion and subsequent reperfusion, the entire LV wall was infiltrated with extravasated blood. All the hearts showed signs of infarction, but the one-hour occlusion infarction was patchy and alternated with intact myocardium. After one to two hours of coronary ligation, ischemic myocardial changes were equivalent to those caused by permanent occlusions and could not be reversed by reperfusion. On the other hand, mortality in the reperfused dogs was 10 to 30 percent in contrast with 60 to 70 percent for permanent occlusion. This latter improvement was attributed to reper-

fusion washing out dangerous myocardial metabolite accumulations. The implication was that even though reperfusion may not reduce the ischemic zone damage, it could be important in salvaging the remaining threatened myocardium.

O'Brien, Carroll, et al[24] occluded the proximal LAD for either one or two hours, with reperfusion measurements extending over two hours. Rb86 uptake and histochemical analysis of ischemic and nonischemic myocardial samples were employed to delineate perfusion and oxidative activity. It appeared that one-hour occlusion and two hours' reperfusion provided definite reversibility of metabolic injury, and longer reperfusion after two hours of occlusion was thought to reverse the injury. In an appended discussion, Jatene described experimental infarcts in dogs and pointed to the scar of infarction remaining with 30 days' reperfusion after a three-hour occlusion. Reperfusion was held responsible for a transformation from a normal anemic to a hemorrhagic type of infarct.

Bloor and White[3] studied, in conscious dogs, early reperfusion alterations in the reactive hyperemia and coronary blood flow response to nitroglycerin. LCF coronary occlusions lasted 2 to 72 hours and reperfusion extended up to four days. With occlusions up to two hours, early reperfusion exhibited little deviation from control, but with a six-hour occlusion the hyperemia and nitroglycerin response of early reperfusion were significantly reduced. These early reperfusion responses were absent with occlusions lasting more than 24 hours. However, a one-day reperfusion period caused a partial return of the response, and two to five days of reperfusion brought about a full return to control, indicating that these particular effects of reperfusion were only temporary.

McNamara[22] investigated the myocardial viability in open-chest monkeys after temporary acute LAD occlusions lasting one to five hours. Cineventriculography, surface pH, epicardial ECG mapping, and postmortem histology were used to assess viability. With three hours' LAD ligation, 70 percent of the animals showed functional improvement and/or reduction or infarct within the first hour of reperfusion. Forty-five percent of the monkeys with four-hour ligations showed similar benefits after one-hour reperfusion. Histologic evidence of infarction was present in all these cases, but the infarct size was significantly smaller when compared with permanently ligated animals. No early reperfusion improvements were, however, evident after five-hour ligations. The conclusion was that with up to four-hour ligations there exists large potentially salvageable peripheral zone of ischemic nonfunctional myocardium that is significantly benefited by reperfusion.

Ballo and Snow [2] carried out electronmicroscopic ultrastructural studies on myocardial biopsies to determine the effects of a 24-hour reperfusion following acute coronary occlusions in dogs. After a 120 minutes of ischemia, the zone from which biopsies were taken was noncontractile and exhibited epicardial ECG injury potentials. Ultrastructural evidence of myocardial derangements included disruption of mitochondrial matrix and sarcoplasmic reticulum, loss of glycogen and disorganization of myofibrillar structure. After 24 hours of reperfusion, tissue samples from this zone indicated substantial repair of these ultrastructural changes. There were no thrombi and little evidence of vascular alterations except for endothelial edema.

Krug et al [16,17,18] described, in a series of papers, experiments on cats in which the proximal LAD coronary artery was occluded for periods up to 180 minutes with subsequent reperfusion extending up to six hours. Permanent occlusion was also studied (10 days). Acridine orange labeling and green dye techniques were used to delineate the ischemic regions of the myocardium and study their perfusability. Hydrogen ion concentration, enzyme histochemistry, and histology were studied to assess recognizable changes in the myocardial tissue. Blood CPK and SGOT were examined.

Typical transmural infarcts were seen with permanent occlusion. Temporary occlusions of 45 to 120 minutes exhibited increasingly larger areas of ischemic derangement, particularly in the subendocardial layer, but these shrank considerably in the first hour of reperfusion. Histologic examination on the tenth day indicated patchy necrosis with 60 minute occlusion. With 90–120 minute occlusion, portions of the ischemic zone could not be adequately reperfused and morphologic study indicated irreversible myocardial damage in this zone. Three hours of occlusion followed by reperfusion generally resulted in transmural infarction, which was as extensive as that in the permanent occlusion. Relieving the work of the heart by a heart-lung machine during reperfusion did not change these results. The major conclusion was that irreversible myocardial damage begins to occur after 75 to 90 minutes of LAD occlusion and that blood flow disturbances during the early reperfusion period may play a significant role in the development of necrosis.

Maroko, Ginks, et al [20] described the effects of a 24-hour reperfusion on local myocardial function and the extent of myocardial necrosis following three hours of proximal LAD occlusion in open-chest dogs. Over the three-hour occlusion period, epicardial ST segment elevations were monitored. The chest was then closed and reopened 24 hours after the occlusion for CPK determinations and histologic study of transmural specimens from the occluded and nonoccluded region, in which epicardial electrocardiograms had been previously recorded. Based on correlation of ST segment, CPK and histology, reperfusion after the three-hour occlusion showed much reduced incident of abnormal histology (43 percent versus 97 percent for permanent occlusion). One hour of reperfusion was shown to reverse the paradoxical movement of the left ventricle wall.

Ginks, Sybers, et al [11] extended the above investigation in dogs to one week of reperfusion following a three-hour proximal LAD coronary artery occlusion. Epicardial ECG segment elevations and enzymatic and histologic assessment of myocardial damage after one week were employed for analysis. Sixty-four percent of the acutely injured zone was infarcted in permanent occlusion control dogs, whereas only 10 percent of the injured zone was infarcted in the seven-day reperfusion animals. In contrast with permanent occlusion, animals subjected to seven days of reperfusion after three hours of occlusion exhibited little CPK depletion or evidence of myocardial cell necrosis.

Symes, Arnold, et al [29] investigated in cats the effects of early revascularization following acute myocardial infarction secondary to proximal LAD occlusions lasting 30 minutes, two hours, and four hours. Hemodynamic parameters such as LVEDP and maximal LV dP/dt were observed. Coronary occlusions resulted in immediate significant cardiac dysfunction, which then persisted throughout the period of ischemia. With occlusions lasting two hours, measurements at 30 minutes' reperfusion showed no improvement, but a return to control was noted after six weeks. Four-hour occlusion failed to respond to reperfusion in terms of hemodynamics. While reperfusion following 30 minutes' occlusion showed no evidence of myocardial damage, four-hour temporary occlusion as well as permanent occlusion exhibited fibrous scar tissue in the affected zone. Chronic inflammation and disruption of myocardial fibrils were noted. Lesser effects occurred with a two-hour occlusion. Reperfusion arrhythmias were attributed to washout of intracellular constituents or to increased levels of catecholamines or free fatty acids.

Puri [25] studied coronary reperfusion by measuring regional contractility with strain-gauge-tipped probes and tissue adenosine triphosphate and creatine phosphate content by regional tissue biopsy analysis. Reperfusion after up to 45 minutes of LAD occlusion resulted in prompt return of contractility and 95 percent to 100 percent of ATP and CP. After occlusions lasting one, two, or three hours, contractility returned only after two weeks of reperfusion, during which period ATP recovery was 91 percent, 81 percent, and 73 percent, respectively, while CP values were 95 percent, 90 percent, and 85 percent. It thus appeared that extended reperfusion periods were required, but that major recovery of myocardial energetics could be achieved even after a three-hour LAD occlusion.

Several studies reported the incidence of ventricular fibrillation following reperfusion. Thus, Sewell, Koth, et al [27] described temporary LAD occlusions in open-chest dogs lasting up to 40 minutes and reported that six of 31 animals developed ventricular fibrillation within 20 seconds of reperfusion. He stated that no fatalities occurred in 11 dogs in which the release of the ligature was intermittent. Arnulf and Martin [1] indicated that sudden resumption of circulation in coronary vessels after occlusion may cause ventricular fibrillation. They ascribed this tendency to rapid changes in metabolic unbalance, particularly of potassium and lactic acid.

A series of further papers on reperfusion following coronary occlusion were presented during the 23d Scientific Session of the American College of Cardiology.[13,15,21,31] The general conclusions are in accord with the above studies. At the same meeting, discussion of clinical revascularization in acute infarction indicated concern that hemorrhagic infarction may ensue during reperfusion instituted within several hours of the acute event. Contrasting instances of favorable results achieved with surgery in acute infarction might be associated with benefits derived through cardiopulmonary bypass assist employed during the revascularization procedure.

Interpretation of Reperfusion Data

In the prior studies, temporary coronary occlusion or reperfusion were performed in the open chest, even though extended duration reperfusion and permanent occlusion entailed subsequent closing of the chest and continued observation for days or weeks before the animals were sacrificed. Generally, conclusions were based on histologic and histochemical assessment, with more recent correlative studies of epicardial ECG

ST segments and tissue CPK measurements. Very limited data are available on the hemodynamic alterations of reperfusion. There is no literature on the progressive alterations of regional and global myocardial metabolism. No studies exist on the functional effects of reperfusion following intracoronary occlusions in the closed chest.

The problem of assessing the critical time factor in myocardial viability was recognized by most of the investigators, as was the significance of such data to surgical revascularization during an acute infarction. An apparent discrepancy exists, however, in conclusions relative to the magnitude of this critical viability period. Some studies indicate that as little as 45 minutes of acute proximal LAD occlusion in dogs results in irreversible myocardial damage, which is as extensive as that experienced after permanent occlusion. Other investigations, in contrast, report that the dysfunction and myocardial injury of similarly instituted temporary occlusions in dogs lasting two or three hours can be substantially reduced by short or long periods of reperfusion. Additional studies in monkeys indicate an even longer period of myocardial viability. Many investigators noted that reperfusion frequently leads to serious arrhythmias and a higher incidence of ventricular fibrillation. Persisting arrhythmias might cause functional derangements, which could severely compromise the myocardium during reperfusion. There is also growing evidence that acute reperfusion after periods of coronary occlusion can lead to hemorrhagic myocardial damage. The above quantitative discrepancies of reperfusion results may be due to one or more of several factors such as (1) differences and variability in anatomy of coronary vessels and intercoronary collaterals, (2) effects of open- versus closed-chest preparations, including different heart rates, anesthesia, heparinization, and so on, (3) specific modes and sites of coronary occlusions, (4) incidence and treatment or nontreatment of postreperfusion arrhythmias, (5) size of the ischemic zone and derangements encountered in the nonoccluded region, and (6) type of measurements and analytical techniques used in arriving at conclusions.

Our data were obtained in a novel closed-chest preparation that is believed to provide physiologically valid and comprehensive functional data. The results define the progressive alteration in hemodynamics and regional metabolism during three hours of intracoronary balloon occlusion of the proximal LAD five hours of reperfusion. The primary conclusions that we can draw from our data are these: (1) after a three-hour acute proximal LAD occlusion, hemodynamics and metabolic function were significantly depressed in both the coronary occluded and nonoccluded regions; (2) subsequent five hours of reperfusion failed to improve cardiac function and led to further derangements in both hemodynamics and regional metabolism; (3) two out of seven dogs developed shock; (4) six out of seven dogs exhibited reperfusion arrhythmias of varying severity; and (5) histologic studies of reperfused regions of the myocardium showed evidence of hemorrhagic damage.

More extended reperfusion periods, and reperfusion after shorter occlusions, are currently being studied. We believe that a three-hour acute occlusion of the proximal LAD in dogs is associated with ischemic damage, ultrastructural alterations, metabolite accumulations, and functional derangements in both the coronary occluded and nonoccluded regions. These derangements may sensitized the myocardium so that a sudden reperfusion, with its accompanying hyperemia, metabolite washout, and ventricular arrhythmias, may lead to further deterioration in function as well as development or extension of hemorrhagic infarction. If the reperfused ischemic zone was extensive, and the nonoccluded region undergoes significant functional derangements as well, vicious cycles may set in leading to the development of cardiogenic shock. Hence, we would conclude that, to be effective, reperfusion following an acute occlusion in the dog should commence early, eg, two hours after occlusion. Alternately, a more gradual and longer reperfusion, or reperfusion supplemented with appropriate pharmacological or circulatory assist support, might provide extension of the critical time of myocardial viability and thus improve the effectiveness of revascularization in acute infarction.

Several authors, including Cohn et al, Scanlon et al, and Favaloro et al,[7,9,26] have reported on clinical revascularization 3 to 12 hours following acute infarctions. At this time, there appears to be no generalized criterion that could precisely establish how long an ischemic myocardium can be preserved for surgical intervention. It is reasonable to expect a dependence on such factors as the initial general physiological condition of the patient, the state of his coronary vasculature including its collaterals, the extent of ischemia resulting from imbalance between myocardial energy demands and supply through occluded or restricted coronary vessels, myocardial alterations that have already taken place, the duration of the ischemic or infarction event, and the method as well as effectiveness of restoration of coronary

blood flow. Nonetheless, it is interesting to note that the bulk of the animal experimentation, involving several species, tends to support the concept that acute total occlusion of a major coronary artery lasting from two to six hours are very likely to lead to myocardial damage, which may not be reversed by reperfusion. More research and development is required to provide a mode of reperfusion (eg gradual or with pharmacological or mechanical assist) that could avoid the observed rapid metabolite washout, prevent the severe and often lethal arrhythmias, minimize the hemorrhagic damage to the previously occluded region, and counteract the metabolic derangements in this as well as in the nonoccluded segment of the heart. It is believed that the acutely infarcting myocardium requires the indicated earliest revascularization because there is not enough time for the development of normal compensatory mechanisms, such as coronary collateralization and ventricular hypertrophy. To avoid major extension of the infarct and to escape the vicious cycles of cardiogenic shock, revascularization in acute infarction should be applied within hours (perhaps less than three hours) of the event, and when diagnostic evidence indicates a substantial proportion of salvageable though injured myocardium.

References

1. Arnulf G, Martin CL: Fibrillation ventriculaire au cours du rétablissement circulatoire dans les artères coronaires. Arch Mal Coeur 66:869, 1973
2. Ballo JM, Snow JA: The effects of reestablishment of effective coronary perfusion on acutely ischemic myocardium in dogs. Lab Invest 26:470, 1972
3. Bloor CM, White FC: Coronary artery reperfusion: Early effects on coronary hemodynamics. Am J Cardiol 31:121, 1973
4. Blumgart HL, Gilligan DR, Schlesinger MJ: Experimental studies on the effect of temporary occlusion of coronary arteries. II. The production of myocardial infarction. Am Heart J 22:374, 1941
5. Bolooki H, Rooks JJ, Viera CE, et al: Comparison of the effect of temporary or permanent myocardial ischemia on cardiac function and pathology. J Thorac Cardiovasc Surg 56:590, 1968
6. Breshnahan GF, Shell WF, Ross J Jr: Deleterious effects of reperfusion in evolving myocardial infarction. Circulation 45-46:II-13, 1972
7. Cohn LH, Gorlin R, Collins JJ: Aorto-coronary bypass for acute myocardial infarction. Paper presented to Am Assoc for Thor Surg, Los Angeles, 1972
8. Corday E, Lang TW, Meerbaum S, et al: A closed chest intracoronary occlusion model for the study of regional cardiac function. Am J Cardiol 33:49, 1974
9. Favaloro RG, Effler DB, Cheanvechai C, et al: Acute coronary insufficiency (impending myocardial infarction) and myocardial infarction. Surgical treatment by saphenous vein graft technique. Am J Cardiol 28:598, 1971
10. Fisher SM, Edwards WS: Tissue necrosis after temporary artery occlusion. Am Surg 29:617, 1963

11. Ginks WR, Sybers HD, Maroko PR, et al: Coronary artery reperfusion. II. Reduction of myocardial infarct size at one week after the coronary occlusion. J Clin Invest 51:2717, 1972
12. Hamer J: Discussion to Brachfeld N: Maintenance of cell viability. Circulation 39–40:IV-216, 1969
13. Jarmakani JM, Cox JL, Graham TC, Hackel DB: Coronary hemodynamics and myocardial perfusion after reestablishing coronary flow in experimental myocardial infarction. Am J Cardiol 33:146, 1974
14. Jennings RB, Sommers HM, Smyth GA, et al: Myocardial necrosis induced by temporary occlusion of a coronary artery in the dog. Arch Pathol 70:82, 1959
15. Kane J, Murphy M, Bissett J, Doherty J, Straub K: Does restoration of blood flow preserve acutely ischemic myocardium? Am J Cardiol 33:146, 1974
16. Krug A: The extent of ischemic damage in the myocardium of the cat after permanent and temporary coronary occlusion. J Thorac Cardiovasc Surg 60:242, 1970
17. Krug A: Myokardennekrosen nach Permanentem oder Temporarein Koronararterienverschluss mit und ohne Herzentlastung durch Extrakorporale Zirkulation. Arch Kreislaufforschung 67:326, 1972
18. Krug A, de Rochemont WM, Korb G: Blood supply of the myocardium after temporary coronary occlusion. Circ Res 19:57, 1966
19. Lang TW, Corday E, Gold H, et al: Consequences of reperfusion following coronary occlusion: Effects on hemodynamic and regional myocardial metabolic function. Am J Cardiol 33:69, 1974
20. Maroko PR, Libby P, Ginks WR, et al: Coronary artery reperfusion. I. Early effects on local myocardial function and the extent of myocardial necrosis. J Clin Invest 51:2710, 1972
21. Mathur VS, Guinn GA: Early revascularization in acute infarction, help or hazard: A randomized study. Am J Cardiol 33:156, 1974
22. McNamara JJ, Soeter JR, Suehiro GT, Morgan AL: Myocardial viability after transient ischemia. Am J Cardiol 31:146, 1973
23. Meerbaum S, Lang TW, Corday E, et al: Progressive alterations of cardiac hemodynamic and regional metabolic function following acute coronary occlusion. Am J Cardiol 33:60, 1974
24. O'Brien CM, Carroll M, O'Rourke PT, et al: The reversibility of acute ischemic injury to the myocardium by restoration of coronary flow. J Thorac Cardiovasc Surg 64:840, 1972
25. Puri PS: Coronary reperfusion: Correlation between recovery of contractility and high energy phosphates. Physiologist 16:426, 1973
26. Scanlon PJ, Nemickas R, Tobin JR, et al: Myocardial revascularization during acute phase of myocardial infarction. JAMA 218:207, 1971
27. Sewell WH, Koth DR, Higgins CE: Ventricular fibrillation in dogs after sudden return of flow to the coronary artery. Surgery 38:1050, 1955
28. Swan HJC, Chatterjee K, Corday E, et al: Myocardial revascularization for acute and chronic coronary heart disease. Ann Intern Med 79:751, 1973
29. Symes JF, Arnold IMF, Blurdell PE: Early revascularization of the acute myocardial infarction: The critical time factor. Can J Surg 16:275, 1973
30. Torok B, Toth I, Temes G, et al: Mortality after restoration of circulation following temporary coronary ligation. Acta Chirurgica Academia scientiarum Hungaricae 12:57, 1971
31. Verrier R, Corbalan R, Bown B: Analysis of vulnerability changes during acute coronary occlusion and release. Am J Cardiol 33:174, 1974

9

RESTORATION OF BLOOD FLOW AND PRESERVATION OF ACUTELY ISCHEMIC MYOCARDIUM: A CONTINUING CONTROVERSY

James Kane, Marvin Murphy, Joe Bissett, James Doherty, and Karl Straub

INTRODUCTION

Although now practiced across the country as treatment for chronic incapacitating angina, the coronary bypass operation and its role in the relief of acute ischemia—ie, impending or acute myocardial infarction—is controversial. Most of the controversy centers on whether or not blood flow restored to an area of acutely ischemic myocardium will result in a return of function. Previous studies [19] have shown that a coronary artery may be ligated for up to three hours without causing necrosis. There are recent indications, however, that reperfusion alters the metabolism of ischemic myocardium and may even hasten necrosis.[4,14] Clearly, the optimal time for reperfusion of acutely ischemic myocardium and its effect on cardiac metabolism are not yet well established.

Most previous experimental studies have been done on dogs. Because of the well-documented differences in canine and human circulation,[8] it is questionable whether or not these results are readily applicable to myocardial infarction in man. The pig, however, has a major coronary distribution, a collateral circulation, and a blood supply to the conduction system that is virtually identical to that of man.[12,18] Because of these anatomic similarities between the hearts of pigs and men, we have chosen the pig as our experimental model.

In cardiac muscle the mitochondria, which make up at least 20 percent by dry weight of the cell,[16] consume oxygen for the production of ATP through oxidative phosphorylation. ATP is then used by the myocardium as its energy source for contraction and other cellular functions.[6] Previous studies [1] have suggested that mitochondria are very susceptible to hypoxia. Thus, mitochondrial failure may be the mechanism by which irreversible changes take place in ischemic myocardium.[11]

The purpose of this study was to examine the effects of ischemia and reperfusion on mitochondrial function and to determine how long the myocardium can be ischemic before reversal by reperfusion is no longer possible. In addition, regional blood flow was estimated by distribution of a radioactive isotope (^{3}H digoxin) and a vital dye (alphazurine 2G).

METHODS

Thirty mature farm pigs of both sexes, weighing from 70 to 120 pounds, were fasted for 18 hours and then anesthetized with 6 percent phenobarbital intravenously. A tracheostomy was performed, and respirations maintained with a Harvard pump using room air supplemented with 100 percent O_2 to maintain the arterial PaO_2 over 100. A midline sternal splitting thoracotomy was performed, and the heart was suspended in a pericardial cradle thus exposing the anterior surface of the heart and the distribution of the left anterior descending coronary artery. Central aortic pressure was monitored using a polyethylene catheter from the femoral artery. Left ventricular pressure was monitored by a pigtail catheter positioned retrograde across the aortic valve from the carotid artery. These pressures, with lead II of the electrocardiogram, were displayed and recorded on an Electronics for Medicine DR8 recorder.

The anterior descending coronary artery was dissected free from the epicardium and myocardium at its midportion after the first or second diagonal branch. Predictably, occlusion of the left anterior descending coronary artery at this point resulted in a septal, apical, and left ventricular free wall infarction area of ischemia estimated to involve 25 to 30 percent of the left ventricular mass. The artery was occluded with a nontraumatic rubber ligature that could easily be released without apparent residual damage to the vessel. Complete occlusion in each case was evident by the appearance of a nonpulsatile, nondistended artery distal to the occlusion, nondistended veins draining the ischemic area, and by the cyanosis and bulging of the ischemic segment that occurred within seconds of ligation. The coronary vein was preserved and not ligated.

Ventricular arrhythmia secondary to coronary occlusion was treated with lidocaine or DC countershock using an American Optical defibrillator set at 30 to 50 watt seconds. Although no attempt was made to heparinize the animals, 1,000 to 2,000 units of heparin was placed in each liter of flush solution for the arterial lines.

The coronary artery was occluded in each animal for intervals that varied from 15 minutes to 180 minutes. At the end of each occlusion period, the ligature was released, and the ischemic tissue reperfused for two hours. Four animals had a 180-minute occlusion without reperfusion.

Within 10 minutes of release of the ligature, 0.5 to 1.0 mg of ^{3}H digoxin was injected intravenously to serve as a blood flow marker and perhaps, as a measure of cell viability in the area of ischemia.[2,9] Serial blood samples were obtained at intervals of 5, 10, 15, 30, 60, 90, and 120 minutes to establish serum turnover curves of tritiated digoxin.

At the end of each two-hour reperfusion, 2.5 to 5.0 cc of 10 percent alphazurine 2G blue dye was injected intravenously in order to identify areas of the myocardium that were not perfused. This dye stained perfused tissue a vivid blue and was not taken up by ischemic tissue.

Immediately after injection of the dye, the heart was removed from the chest and taken to the cold room, where samples were excised from the normal and reperfused areas of the left ventricle using the surface anatomy and dye staining as guidelines.

The tissue samples were minced and homogenized by methods similar to those previously outlined.[23] Briefly, mitochondria were separated

and suspended in a medium containing 0.25 molar sucrose, 0.001 molar neutralized EDTA, 0.01 molar tris buffer at pH 7.4, 7.5 millimolar potassium phosphate at pH 7.4, and 0.01 molar substrate in a final volume of 3 ml. The two substrates used were neutral sodium salts of glutamic acid (0.01 molar) or of pyruvic acid (0.01 molar) plus L malic acid (0.005 molar). The latter combination was referred to as malate. Oxidative phosphorylation studies were done in duplicate by the polarographic method[5] and were completed within 80 to 90 minutes of sacrifice of the animals. Twenty micromole increments of ADP were added to each reaction mixture to give a rapid burst of state-3 respiration. In each experiment, mitochrondria from the normal areas of the left ventricle were tested simultaneously with mitochondria from the reperfused area. Indices obtained were as follows:

1. Mitochrondrial oxygen consumption in microatoms of oxygen consumed per milligram of mitochondrial protein per minute during state-3 respiration; this is a measure of electron transport capability.[22]

2. ADP:O ratio, the ratio of micromoles of ADP phosphorylated to atoms of oxygen consumed; this is a measure of the efficiency of ATP production.[15]

3. The respiratory control ratio (RCR) or the ratio of oxygen consumed in the presence of ADP to oxygen consumed after complete phosphorylation of the ADP; this is a measure of tightness of coupling of phosphorylation to respiration.[15]

Mitochondrial protein was determined by a standard method,[17] with attempts made to achieve 2 mg/ml of mitochondrial protein. ADP assays were determined spectrophotometrically.[3] Tissue and serum ^{3}H digoxin levels were measured as previously described.[20]

RESULTS

Within seconds following coronary occlusion, myocardium supplied by the left anterior vessel ceased contracting, became cyanotic, and bulged. This persisted throughout the occlusion. Arterial blood pressure, heart rate, and left ventricular end-diastolic pressure were not significantly different from control values in most of the animals.

Following release of the ligature and reper-

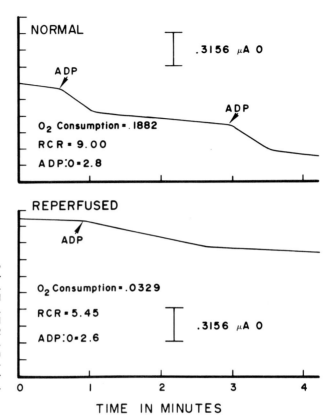

FIG. 1. Mitochondrial O_2 consumption, using glutamate, after 60 minutes of coronary occlusion and two hours of reperfusion. Mitochondrial O_2 consumption from normal left ventricle is shown in the upper panel. Addition of 20 micromoles of ADP induced a rapid burst of state-3 respiration (0.1882 μA O/mg mitochondrial protein per minute). Twenty μmoles of ADP induced a much slower rate of O_2 consumption in mitochondria from reperfused left ventricle (lower panel), 0.0329 μA O/mg mitochondrial pattern per minute.

fusion, the distal left anterior descending coronary artery became distended, and the epicardium lost its cyanosis within 30 seconds to one minute of release. The reperfused epicardium became hyperemic when compared to normal areas of the left ventricle. Bulging of the involved segment also diminished within 30 seconds to one minute. The muscle, however, became akinetic and firm rather than regaining contractile function. Reperfusion for two hours did little to change the akinesis or firmness.

Following removal of the heart, the reperfused area could be recognized by its firm texture as opposed to the soft and pliable normal myocardium, or the myocardium from hearts with 180-minute occlusions and no reperfusion, which also remained soft and pliable.

Figure 1 shows the effect of 60 minutes of coronary occlusion and two hours of reperfusion on mitochondrial oxygen consumption by mitochondria from normal and reperfused myocardium. Addition of 20 micromoles of ADP induced a rapid burst of state-3 respiration in normal mitochondria with an oxygen consumption of 0.1882 microatoms of oxygen per milligram of mitochondrial protein per minute. In the reperfused mitochondria, addition of the same amount of ADP

resulted in a much lower rate of oxygen consumption, or 0.0329 microatoms of oxygen per milligram of mitochondrial protein per minute. In this animal, the respiratory control ratio was decreased, but the ADP:O ratio was essentially the same. The effect of different occlusion times on mitochondrial oxygen consumption by mitochondria from normal and reperfused areas of the left ventricle using glutamate substrate is shown in Figure 2. After only 15 to 30 minutes of occlusion time, there was a slight decrease in oxygen consumption in the reperfused mitochondria ($P < 0.05$).[*] By 60 minutes, the difference was highly significant ($P < 0.001$). Further impairment was evident with longer occlusion times. As shown in Figure 3, malate substrate gave similar results. Figure 4 shows the results of different times of occlusion on the respiratory control ratio again using glutamate substrate. Although there was little difference after a 15-to-30-minute occlusion, occlusion times longer than 60 minutes resulted in a significant decrease in the respiratory control ratio ($P < 0.001$). ADP:O ratios, a measure of efficiency of ATP production, were not sig-

* Student's t test

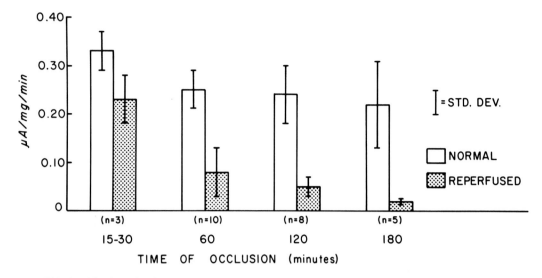

FIG. 2. Mitochondrial O$_2$ consumption, using glutamate substrate during state-3 respiration in 26 animals. Mitochondria from normal areas of the left ventricle (clear bars) are compared with mitochondria from reperfused areas (dotted bars). Occlusion time was 15 minutes to 180 minutes. All animals had a 120-minute reperfusion.

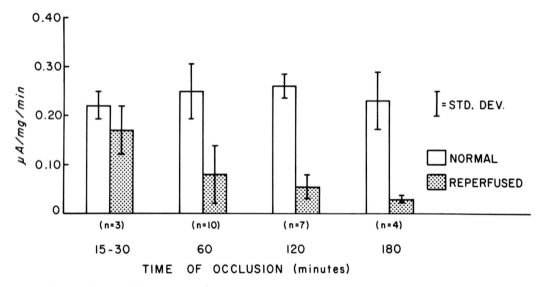

FIG. 3. Mitochondrial O$_2$ consumption using malate substrate during state-3 respiration in 25 animals. Mitochondria from normal areas of the left ventricle (clear bars) are compared with mitochondria from reperfused areas (dotted bars). Occlusion time was 15 minutes to 180 minutes. All animals had a 120-minute reperfusion.

nificantly different* even with occlusions of up to three hours (Fig. 5). The decreased rate of oxygen consumption in the presence of ADP with normal ADP:O ratios suggests that there is inhibition of oxidative phosphorylation or a block in electron flow rather than uncoupling of oxi-

dative phosphorylation. That reperfusion itself may have contributed to this inhibition of oxidative phosphorylation is shown in Figure 6. Oxygen consumption of mitochondria from normal and reperfused tissue is compared with mitochondria from animals that had the same length of occlusion (180 minutes) but did not have the two-hour reperfusion period. Note that with either glutamate or malate substrate, mitochondrial function

* One-way analysis of variance

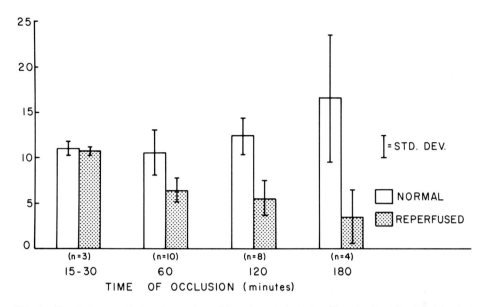

FIG. 4. Respiratory control ratios using glutamate substrate in 25 animals. Mitochondria from normal areas of the left ventricle (clear bars) are compared with mitochondria from reperfused areas (dotted bars). Occlusion time was 15 minutes to 180 minutes. All animals had a 120-minute reperfusion.

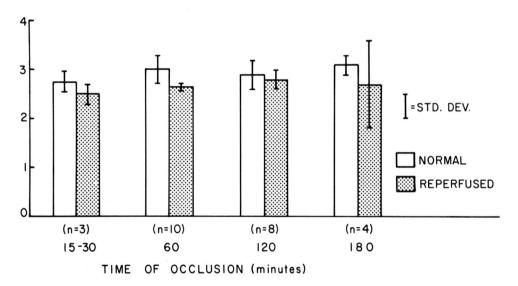

FIG. 5. ADP:0 ratios using glutamate substrate in 25 animals. Mitochondria from normal areas of the left ventricle (clear bars) are compared with mitochondria from reperfused areas (dotted bars). Occlusion time was 15 minutes to 180 minutes. All animals had a 120-minute reperfusion.

was worse in the reperfused tissue ($P < 0.005$). This suggests that after a three-hour coronary occlusion, further damage took place during reperfusion.

After reperfusion there was also an altered distribution of ^3H digoxin as shown in Figure 7. Although there was little difference in the 15-to-30-minute group, following 60 minutes or more of coronary occlusion there was a highly signifi-

cant decrease in tritiated digoxin concentration in the reperfused tissue ($P < 0.001$).

DISCUSSION

These results demonstrate a severe metabolic derangement in myocardium that has been made ischemic for more than 60 minutes and then

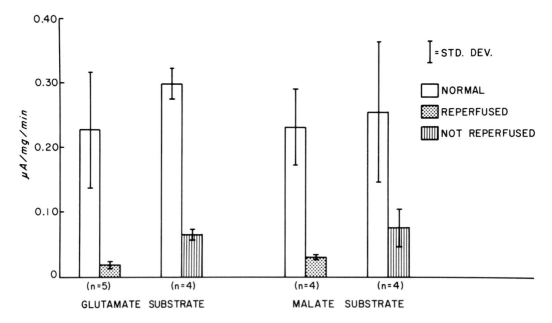

FIG. 6. O_2 consumption during state-3 respiration of mitochondria from normal areas of the left ventricle (clear bars) and mitochondria from left ventricle, which had a 180-minute occlusion and 120 minutes of reperfusion (dotted bars), are compared to mitochondria from animals that had 180 minutes of occlusion, but no reperfusion (striped bars) using glutamate and malate substrates.

reperfused for two hours. There was marked functional impairment of mitochondria isolated from the reperfused area as compared to mitochondria from a normal left ventricle. Occlusion times greater than 60 minutes appear to result in irreversible changes. The near normal ADP:O ratios with a decreased oxygen consumption suggest that oxidative phosphorylation was inhibited

rather than uncoupled or that there was a block in electron transport.

Our results agree with those reported by other investigators. Ekholm et al [7] reperfused dog hearts after 10 and 20 minutes of ischemia and found little change in mitochondrial ultrastructure or function. Krug,[13] using cats in reperfusion experiments, found that there were ischemic

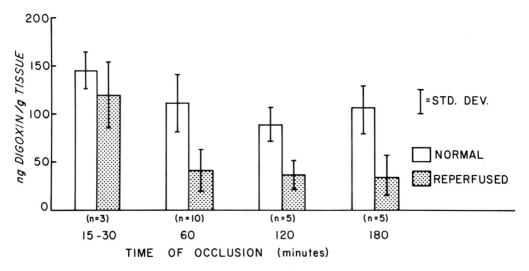

FIG. 7. ^3H digoxin concentration (ng digoxin/g wet tissue) in normal (clear bars) and reperfused (dotted bars) myocardium is compared in 23 animals, which had 15 minutes to 180 minutes of coronary occlusion and 120 minutes of reperfusion.

areas in the inner layers of the heart that could not be reperfused after coronary ligations of 30 to 45 minutes. He suggested that damage occurred after release of the ligature and that there were secondary disturbances in blood flow during the reperfusion period. Copeland et al [6] showed that there was morphologic change in dog heart mitochondria after 45 minutes of anoxia and that this morphologic change was not reversed by up to seven hours of reperfusion. Anoxic periods less than 45 minutes, followed by reperfusion, resulted in some improvement. They suggested that mitochondria were very sensitive to anoxia and that irreversible myocardial cell damage to anoxia was secondary to mitochondrial failure. Jennings et al [10] likewise noted ultrastructural change and marked functional abnormalities in mitochondria from ischemic dog papillary muscle after a 60-minute coronary occlusion. The morphologic change included mitochondrial swelling, disruption of cristae, loss of matrical density, accumulation of granules, and increased fragility of the mitochondria. These damaged mitochondria were unable to carry out oxidative phosphorylation even after addition of various co-factors. They concluded that after 60 minutes of ischemia the mitochondria were damaged irreversibly. These experiments did not involve a reperfusion period. Lang and Corday [14] have reported profound changes in hemodynamics, metabolic function, and morphologic structure in dog hearts after three hours of coronary occlusion followed by five hours of reperfusion. They concluded that reperfusion may not reverse hemodynamic and metabolic disorders induced by three hours of occlusion and that reperfusion may even have a detrimental effect, accelerating necrosis and the deterioration of function. Bresnahan et al,[4] using serial serum CPK measurements, likewise found that reperfusion for 24 hours after a five-hour coronary occlusion in dogs caused extension of the infarction in many of the animals. Reperfusion was associated with gross myocardial hemorrhages especially in the center of the ischemic area. They concluded that reperfusion of an evolving myocardial infarction may sometimes be deleterious.

In our study, impairment of mitochondrial oxygen consumption correlated with the gross functional appearance of the involved myocardium as well as the altered distribution of ^{3}H digoxin, and the poor uptake of alphazurine 2G dye. The failure of reperfused tissue to accumulate ^{3}H digoxin and the vital dye may simply indicate a failure to restore blood flow to the area, or it may be a further reflection of cellular damage. Other investigators have also reported a marked

alteration of ^{3}H digoxin by infarcted and ischemic left ventricles.[2] They have suggested that ^{3}H digoxin is a marker of regional blood flow. Similar patterns of distribution have been shown with radioactive microspheres injected into the circulation.[2] Parker et al [21] have also demonstrated that there is actually an increase in resistance to blood flow during reperfusion indicative of further pathological changes with restoration of blood flow. Although our study did not attempt to measure ^{3}H digoxin in the concentration in the inner and outer layers of the left ventricular wall, it was evident from staining by the alphazurine dye that there was a marked defect in regional blood supply to the middle layers. The epicardium and endocardium generally stained evenly after reperfusion. These findings indicate a disturbance in circulation, especially to the innermost layers of the left ventricular wall, which persists and may even progress after reperfusion.

In summary, this study shows that an acute coronary occlusion of 60 minutes results in damaged mitochondria which were not improved by two hours of reperfusion. Reperfusion after 180 minutes of occlusion may hasten or accelerate myocardial necrosis as evidenced by mitochondrial function, which was worse in reperfused tissue than in tissue not reperfused. There was also a marked alteration in the distribution of ^{3}H digoxin and alphazurine 2G dye following reperfusion, which indicates disturbances in regional circulation to the reperfused area.

References

1. Aschenbrenner R, Zak A, Cutilletta AF, Rabinowitz M: Degradation of mitochondrial components in rat cardiac muscle. Am J Physiol 221:1418, 1971
2. Beller GA, Smith TW, Wood WB: Altered distribution of tritiated digoxin in infarcted canine left ventricle. Circulation 46:572, 1972
3. Bergmeyer HU: Methods of enzymatic analysis. New York and London, Academic Press, 1965, pp 573–77
4. Bresnahan GF, Roberts R, Shell WE, Ross J Jr, Sobel BE: Deleterious effects due to hemorrhage after myocardial reperfusion. Am J Cardiol 33:82, 1974
5. Chance B, Williams GR: Respiratory enzymes in oxidative phosphorylation. J Biol Chem 217:383, 1955
6. Copeland J, Kosek JC, Hurley EJ: Early functional and ultrastructural recovery of canine cadaver hearts. Circulation (II) 37:188, 1968
7. Ekholm R, Kerstell J, Olsson R, Rudenstam CM, Svanborg A: Morphologic and biochemical studies of dog heart mitochondria after short periods of ischemia. Am J Cardiol 22:312, 1968
8. Hood WB: Salvage of myocardium in acute ischemia. Circulation 43:11, 1971
9. Hopkins BE, Taylor RR: Digoxin distribution in the dog's left ventricle in the presence of coronary

artery ligation. J Molecular and Cellular Cardiol 5:197, 1973

10. Jennings RB, Herdson PB, Sommers HM: Structural and functional abnormalities in mitochondria isolated from ischemic dog myocardium. Lab Invest 20:548, 1969

11. Jennings RB, Kaltenbach JP, Sommers HM: Mitochondrial metabolism in ischemic injury. Arch Path 84:15, 1967

12. Kong Y, Chen JT, Zeft HJ, Whalen RE, McIntosh HD: Natural history of experimental coronary occlusion in pigs: A serial cine angiographic study. Am Heart J 77:45, 1969

13. Krug A: The extent of ischemic damage in the myocardium of the cat after permanent and temporary coronary occlusion. Am J Cardiol 33:69, 1974

14. Lang TW, Corday E, Gold H, et al: Consequences of reperfusion after coronary occlusion. Effects on hemodynamic and regional myocardial metabolic function. Am J Cardiol 33:69, 1974

15. Lindenmayer GE, Sordahl LA, Harigaya S, et al: Some biochemical studies on subcellular systems isolated from fresh recipient human cardiac tissue obtained during transplantation. Am J Cardiol 27:277, 1971

16. Lindenmayer GE, Sordahl LA, Schwartz A: Reevaluation of oxidative phosphorylation in cardiac mitochondria from normal animals and animals in heart failure. Circ Res 23:439, 1968

17. Lowry OH, Rosenbrough NJ, Farr AL, Randall RJ: Protein measurement with the folin phenol reagent. J Biol Chem 193:265, 1951

18. Lumb G, Singletary HP: Blood supply to the atrioventricular node and bundle of His: A comparative study in pig, dog, and man. Am J Path 41:65, 1962

19. Maroko PR, Libby P, Ginks WR, et al: Early effects on local myocardial function and the extent of myocardial necrosis. J Clin Invest 51:2710, 1972

20. Murphy ML, Doherty JE: Comparison of heart size and serum concentration as determinants of digoxin tissue concentration in the normal and hypertrophied rabbit heart. Am J Cardiol 31:47, 1973

21. Parker PE, Downey HR, Bashour FA: Coronary hemodynamics in reperfused myocardium. Clin Res 21:815, 1973

22. Schwartz A, Wood JM, Allen JC, et al: Biochemical and morphologic correlates of cardiac ischemia. Am J Cardiol 32:46, 1973

23. Sobel BE, Jequier E, Sjoerdsma A, Lovenberg W: Effects of catecholamines and adrenergic blocking agents on oxidative phosphorylation in rat heart mitochondria. Circ Res 19:1050, 1966

10

THE EFFECTS OF REPERFUSION ON MYOCARDIAL VIABILITY

Harold Haston, Gregory T. Smith, Samuel M. Sims,
John R. Soeter, and J. Judson McNamara

INTRODUCTION

Therapeutic modalities utilized in the management of patients with evidence of acute myocardial ischemia place emphasis on limitation of infarct size after coronary occlusion.[12] Development of cardiogenic shock and refractory ventricular tachyarrhythmias are related to increasing infarct size.[16,17] Salvage of ischemic myocardium improves both the immediate prognosis of the patient and adds to future cardiac reserve. Following coronary occlusion, myocardial viability in the resulting ischemic area is most dependent upon oxygen available and oxygen requirement of that area.[12] Myocardial reperfusion directly increases oxygen supply and has been shown effective in decreasing infarct size.[7] Recent clinical reports of myocardial revascularization in patients with acute ischemic injury indicate a significant improvement in survival if surgical intervention is initiated early;[16,17] however, criteria for selection of patients and the appropriate timing for revascularization have not been well-defined. The purpose of this study was to examine in primates the effects of coronary reperfusion on myocardial viability after varying periods of ischemia.

METHODS

Studies were carried out in 31 primates (*macaca cynamolugus*) weighing 3–7 kg and anesthetized with phencyclidine hydrochloride (0.8–1.0 mgm/kg). Respiration was controlled with a volume respirator (Harvard Apparatus Co., Millis, Mass.) and anesthesia was maintained with sodium thiopental. A left anterolateral thoracotomy was performed and the heart was suspended in a pericardial cradle. A snare was placed around the left anterior descending coronary artery just distal to the main diagonal branch. A catheter with an I.D. of 3.25 mm was placed in the left ventricle by direct puncture of the apex and attached to a Statham pressure transducer (Model P23AA) to monitor left ventricular pressure. Femoral pressure and limb lead EKG were also recorded. Epicardial EKG's were taken with a unipolar electrode fashioned from stainless steel wire at 10 predetermined anatomically reproducible points on the anterior surface of the left ventricle. All variables were recorded on a Gould Brush Mark 260 recorder system with ECG coupler (Model 11430101, Gould, Inc., Cleveland, Ohio). Intraventricular pressure was attached to a differentiating circuit and both intraventricular pressure and the first derivative, dP/dt, were displayed on a Tektronix Model 564 storage oscilloscope and recorded at 100 mm/sec.

The animals were divided into five ligation groups according to duration of coronary occlusion that was maintained for one hour, two hours, four hours, six hours, or permanently with six animals in each group. In one control animal, the snare was not tightened during the experiment. Epicardial ECG's were taken before occlusion, 10 minutes, and hourly following occlusion until ligature release. Further recordings were made 20 minutes, one hour, and two hours post reperfusion. ST segment elevation (ST ↑), R + S wave amplitude (RS), and Q wave amplitude were measured for mapping points greater than 2 mV ST elevation over baseline preligation values. Each parameter was summated (ΣST ↑, ΣRS, ΣQ) over the mapping points. These summations reflected evolving injury to the myocardium during periods of occlusion and reperfusion.

Myocardial contractility was measured by determination of contractile element velocity (Vce) as described by Mason from simultaneously displayed LVP and dP/dt curves on the oscilloscope. The formula

$$Vce = \frac{dP/dt}{KP}$$

was used for calculation where P = developed isometric ventricular pressure and the series elastic constant $(K) = 32$ muscle length.[25] Curves were taken of two beats per time period and averaged. Paired points on both LVP and dP/dt curves were taken at two msec intervals during the period of isovolumic contraction for calculation of Vce. Computer analysis of Vce and isovolumic pressure curves was used for linear extrapolation of max-Vce at zero load (Vmax.) Peak dP/dt, peak Vce, and Vmax were determined prior to coronary occlusion, 10 minutes post occlusion, and hourly until ligature release. Following reperfusion, measurements were made at 20 minutes, one hour, and two hours.

Animals were maintained seven days, whereupon each parameter was again measured in a similar fashion. The heart was then excised and placed in 10 percent formalin. Ten transverse sections of equal thickness were made along the long axis of the left ventricle. Two slides were made of each section and stained with hematoxylin-eosin and Gomoritrichrome. Previous reports have described the morphological changes of myocardial ischemia and necrosis.[10] Histological findings in this study agree with Cox's description of an area of patchy necrosis surrounding a central necrotic infarct.[5] Planimetry of each section was carried out to determine the area of central infarct (A_I), area of patchy necrosis (A_P), and area of total left ventricle (A_V). Summating A_V for all 10 sections (ΣA_V) provided an expression of total left ventricular myocardial volume. Similarly, the total volumes of A_P and A_I were estimated by summating corresponding values of each in all ten sections $(\Sigma A_P$ and $\Sigma A_I)$. Percentage of infarcted ventricle is expressed by the ratio $\Sigma A_I / \Sigma A_V$. The ratio of patchy necrosis to infarction was reflected by $\Sigma A_P / \Sigma A_I$ and total injury to the left ventricle by $(\Sigma A_I + \Sigma A_P)/\Sigma A_V$.

RESULTS

Following coronary occlusion an area of cyanosis appeared immediately on the anterior surface of the left ventricle and demonstrated marked paradoxical motion during systole. The cyanotic area was found to correspond to the area of acute ischemia as mapped by epicardial ECG changes. Previous studies in the dog report similar findings.[13]

ST segment elevation changes were summated $(\Sigma ST \uparrow)$ over the 10 epicardial recording points and are shown in Figure 1. After coronary occlusion, $\Sigma ST \uparrow$ increased rapidly, reaching maximal elevation at one hour. Following this peak value, $\Sigma ST \uparrow$ declined gradually during the period of occlusion. Comparison of the decline in $\Sigma ST \uparrow$ ($\Sigma ST \uparrow$ decline) between ligation groups is plotted in Figure 2 as a percentage of max $\Sigma ST \uparrow$ expressed as 100 percent. The $\Sigma ST \uparrow$ decline was proportional to duration of occlusion; however, the rate of voltage loss decreased with increasing duration of occlusion. Reperfusion significantly alters the time course of $\Sigma ST \uparrow$ decline, producing a rapid return of $\Sigma ST \uparrow$ to preligation values.

Changes in epicardial R+S wave amplitude (ΣRS) are shown in Figure 3. Loss of EMF is demonstrated in Figure 4 as a percentage of preligation ΣRS amplitude expressed as 100 percent in all groups. The decrease ΣRS is proportional to increasing duration of occlusion, though the rate of voltage loss decreases with increasing periods of ischemia. Reperfusion resulted in very little restoration of ΣRS amplitude; however, it seemed to prevent further decline in ΣRS in all groups except those reperfused after six hours of ischemia. Mean values and standard error data for each group are presented in Table 1.

The ΣQ wave depth taken from epicardial recording points increased in all groups except one-hour ligations. No significant difference was noted between the ligation groups.

Quantification of actual infarct size by histological examination and expressed as a percent of the left ventricle is shown in Figure 5. Infarct size increased significantly from the one-hour ligation group 12.8 ± 3.9 percent $(\overline{X} \pm SEM)$ to 24.3 ± 2.5 percent in the four-hour group $(p < .05)$ and 30.6 ± 2.5 percent in the six-hour group $(p < .01)$. A significant increase was also noted from the two-hour group 15.2 ± 2.9 percent to the four-hour group $(p < .05)$ and to the six-hour group $(p < .01)$. Figure 6 shows a rapid decrease in the ratio of patchy necrosis (ΣA_P) to central infarct (ΣA_I) with increasing periods of ischemia up to six hours. The chronic ligation group had a wide range in variability resulting in a lower mean value than the six-hour ligation group. Total injury of the left ventricle

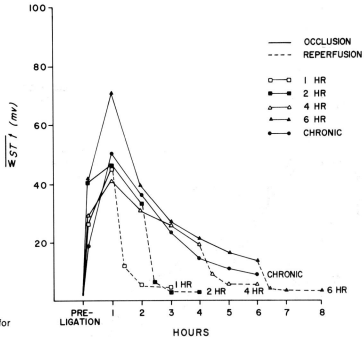

FIG. 1. Observed mean $\Sigma ST \uparrow$ for each ligation group.

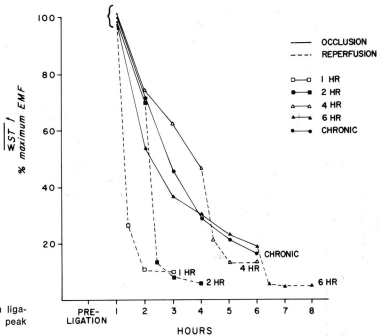

FIG. 2. Mean $\Sigma ST \uparrow$ for each ligation group as a percent of peak elevation.

$(\Sigma A_I + \Sigma A_P)/\Sigma A_V$ expressed as a percentage in Figure 7 demonstrates increasing histologic damage with longer periods of ischemia. The six hour group (36.5 ± 3.0 percent) was significantly higher than reperfusion after one hour = $22.4 \pm$ 5.2 percent ($p < .01$), and four hours = 27.4 ± 2.5 percent ($p < .05$).

Myocardial contractility was evaluated by calculation of Vmax from curves of Vce and isovolumic pressure for each animal at the specified

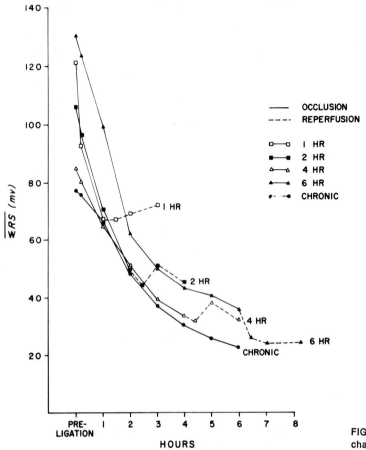

FIG. 3. Observed   mean ΣRS changes for each ligation group.

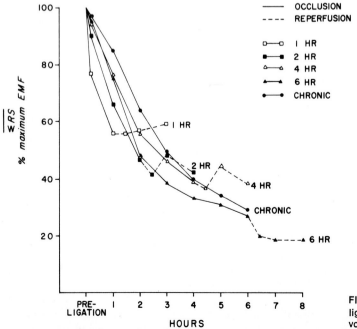

FIG. 4. Mean ΣRS changes for each ligation group as a percent of peak voltage (preligation).

TABLE 1. Mean Values and Standard Error Data

LIGATION GROUP	N	PRE-LIGATION	POSTOCCLUSION 10 min	1 hr	2 hr	3 hr	4 hr	5 hr	6 hr	POSTREPERFUSION 20 min	1 hr	2 hr
ΣRS												
1 hr occl.	6	121.0 ± 21.5	92.4 ± 13.3	67.0 ± 6.7						67.6 ± 9.0	68.9 ± 9.5	71.5 ± 8.4
2 hr occl.	6	105.6 ± 16.9	95.6 ± 12.8	70.1 ± 7.3	49.8 ± 6.2					43.6 ± 7.8	51.0 ± 9.2	45.0 ± 8.4
4 hr occl.	6	84.9 ± 10.2	80.0 ± 15.9	64.7 ± 13.8	50.7 ± 15.2	39.2 ± 13.7	33.17 ± 11.10			31.4 ± 11.0	37.9 ± 4.9	32.3 ± 5.5
6 hr occl.	6	130.5 ± 15.4	123.9 ± 15.9	99.1 ± 16.5	61.7 ± 10.9	50.1 ± 8.3	43.1 ± 6.1	40.7 ± 7.48	35.5 ± 4.29	25.8 ± 4.6	23.9 ± 5.3	24.6 ± 4.9
Chronic	6	77.3 ± 11.2	75.2 ± 7.7	65.5 ± 7.2	49.7 ± 6.5	37.3 ± 5.7	30.1 ± 3.8	25.9 ± 3.4	22.6 ± 3.5			
ΣST↑												
1 hr occl.	6	3.3 ± 1.6	26.8 ± 7.1	45.4 ± 5.7						12.0 ± 5.3	5.1 ± 1.9	4.5 ± 1.4
2 hr occl.	6	1.3 ± 1.2	40.2 ± 9.8	46.8 ± 8.3	32.8 ± 7.0					6.0 ± 3.8	3.8 ± 2.3	3.0 ± 1.8
4 hr occl.	6	4.0 ± 1.3	29.4 ± 5.9	41.6 ± 7.9	31.1 ± 9.4	26.0 ± 7.2	19.6 ± 4.03			9.0 ± 2.9	5.4 ± 2.6	5.5 ± 2.5
6 hr occl.	6	4.9 ± 1.0	41.7 ± 10.9	71.9 ± 11.9	39.2 ± 6.3	26.5 ± 2.7	22.0 ± 3.9	16.7 ± 1.6	13.9 ± 2.3	4.1 ± .9	3.6 ± .9	3.7 ± .9
Chronic	6	2.0 ± 1.0	19.3 ± 3.7	50.6 ± 9.4	36.6 ± 6.4	23.1 ± 3.9	14.8 ± 3.3	11.0 ± 2.2	8.8 ± 1.8			

Mean ± SEM (mv) for grouped data used in constructed Figures 1.A and 2.A. N equals the number of animals in each ligation group.

TABLE 2. Group Data for Max Vce and Vmax

LIGATION GROUP	PRE-LIGATION	POSTOCCLUSION 10 min	1 hr	2 hr	3 hr	4 hr	5 hr	6 hr	POSTREPERFUSION 20 min	1 hr	2 hr	7 day
Vmax												
1 hr occl.	2.21 ± 0.07	2.13 ± 0.21	2.28 ± 0.10						—	2.33 ± 0.09	2.53 ± 0.09	2.34 ± 0.19
2 hr occl.	2.64 ± 0.21	2.41 ± 0.17	2.28 ± 0.12	2.47 ± 0.14					2.47 ± 0.21	2.50 ± 0.20	2.68 ± 0.20	2.44 ± 0.15
4 hr occl.	2.65 ± 0.08	2.13 ± 0.17	2.32 ± 0.11	2.56 ± 0.02	—	2.43 ± 0.21			2.20 ± 0.03	2.17 ± 0.20	2.35 ± 0.13	2.54 ± 0.47
6 hr occl.	2.24 ± 0.09	1.96 ± 0.29	2.16 ± 0.04	2.27 ± 0.03	2.39 ± 0.05	2.23 ± 0.02	2.36 ± 0.08	2.39 ± 0.06	2.26 ± 0.13	2.46 ± 0.07	2.31 ± 0.09	2.30 ± 0.17
Chronic	2.55 ± 0.14	2.47 ± 0.17	2.47 ± 0.10	2.39 ± 0.09	2.37 ± 0.11	2.16 ± 0.11	2.44 ± 0.31	2.41 ± 0.10				2.19 ± 0.08
MAX Vce												
1 hr occl.	1.83 ± 0.08	1.62 ± 0.21	1.82 ± 0.12						—	1.98 ± 0.11	2.11 ± 0.11	1.52 ± 0.14
2 hr occl.	2.82 ± 0.53	2.29 ± 0.32	1.96 ± 0.16	2.36 ± 0.41					2.39 ± 0.39	2.29 ± 0.23	1.99 ± 0.21	1.99 ± 0.17
4 hr occl.	2.74 ± 0.39	1.86 ± 0.12	2.11 ± 0.07	2.50 ± 0.16	—	2.23 ± 0.25			2.02 ± 0.12	2.10 ± 0.39	2.15 ± 0.27	2.13 ± 0.63
6 hr occl.	1.98 ± 0.24	1.54 ± 0.22	1.74 ± 0.03	1.94 ± 0.03	1.97 ± 0.08	1.87 ± 0.03	2.00 ± 0.05	2.03 ± 0.07	1.78 ± 0.03	2.07 ± 0.11	1.96 ± 0.08	1.99 ± 0.51
Chronic	2.18 ± 0.06	1.95 ± 0.14	2.09 ± 0.17	2.05 ± 0.05	2.11 ± 0.14	1.92 ± 0.14	2.01 ± 0.19	2.07 ± 0.16				1.75 ± 0.10

Mean ± SEM (ML/sec).

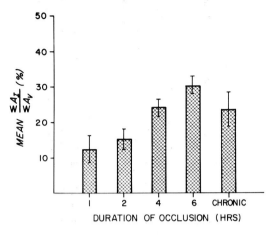

FIG. 5.   Central infarct size as a percent of left ventricle for each ligation group. Mean ± SEM.

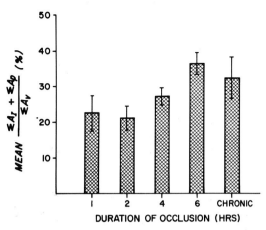

FIG. 7.   Total injury (patchy necrosis + central infarct) as a percent of left ventricle. Mean ± SEM.

times. Group data for maxVce and Vmax are given in Table 2. Figures 8 and 9 represent the maxVce and Vmax for each group and time period, respectively. Following coronary occlusion, an initial drop is seen in all groups followed by prompt recovery of both maxVce and Vmax. Reperfusion had no significant effect on Vmax in any ligation group. Determination of both maxVce and Vmax taken seven days later were unchanged over preligation values.

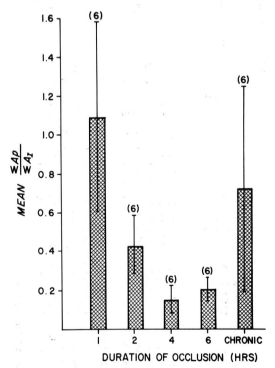

FIG. 6.   Ratio of patchy necrosis to central infarct size for each ligation group. Mean ± SEM.

DISCUSSION

Following acute coronary occlusion, the myocardium supplied by that vessel becomes ischemic and cell death begins within 20 minutes if perfusion is not restored.[10] The severity of ischemia, however, is not uniform within this area. Various histologic patterns of ischemia and necrosis can be demonstrated as a function of time and coronary artery distribution.[5] Characteristically, an area of central severe ischemia progresses to infarction if occlusion is maintained longer than 60 minutes. A peripheral zone of less severe ischemia exists that is composed of potentially viable myocardium.[5] Continued lack of coronary perfusion to an area results in progression of the central necrotic zone at the expense of the marginally ischemic myocardium.[16,17] Salvage of this marginal ischemic zone could result in significant reduction of total infarct size. The survival of these ischemic cells depends upon a critical balance between myocardial oxygen supply and demand.[12] Increased myocardial oxygen consumption results in increased ischemic injury, as seen after administration of iso-proteronol, digitalis, glucagon, bretylium, and with tachycardia. Conversely, decreasing myocardial oxygen consumption results in decreased ischemic injury.[13] Myocardial reperfusion results in reduction of ischemic injury;[7] however, the exact time course of its effect has not been established.

Previous reports have utilized epicardial ECG mapping to characterize the extent of ischemic injury.[11] This has the distinct advantage of eliminating some animal variability because of

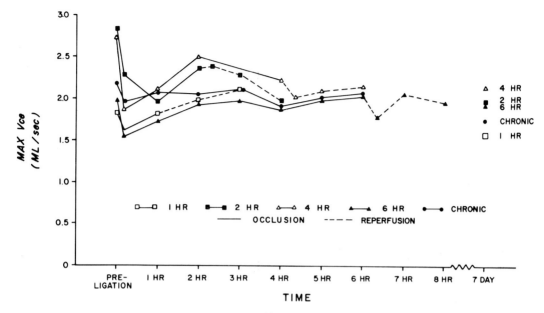

FIG. 8. Time course of changes in maximum contractile element velocity (Vce). Points represent mean values for each ligation group.

variations in coronary artery distribution. Myocardial CPK depletion,[13] serum CPK isoenzyme elevation,[22] myocardial lactate extraction,[21] and reactive coronary bed hyperemia[2] have also been used in estimation of ischemic myocardial injury. Reperfusion after three hours of ischemia has been shown to decrease the area of injury.[7] Bloor, White[2] and Bresnahan[3] found increased CPK levels if reperfusion was carried out after five hours of ischemia, suggesting a deleterious effect of late reperfusion. The purpose of this study was to elucidate further the effect reperfusion had on ischemic myocardium.

EFFECTS OF REPERFUSION ON EPICARDIAL ECG CHANGES

Rapid increase in the $\Sigma ST \uparrow$ following coronary occlusion (Fig. 1) in all ligation groups is representative of an increasing area of ischemia. Myocardial necrosis within this area progresses with increasing duration of ischemia and is reflected electrophysiologically in the $\Sigma ST \uparrow$ decline (Fig. 4). Reperfusion at any point in the time course of ischemic injury reverses these parameters returning $\Sigma ST \uparrow$ to baseline levels rapidly and preventing further EMF loss (ΣRS decline). This data correlates well with previous studies of $\Sigma ST \uparrow$ changes[13] and EMF loss[6] as a function of ischemic time. Clinical reports have shown similar results though the time course is altered in that $\Sigma ST \uparrow$ decline is more gradual.[18]

EFFECTS OF REPERFUSION ON INFARCT SIZE

Histological assessment of infarct size ($\Sigma A_I / \Sigma A_V$) in this study is represented in Figure 5, which demonstrates increasing necrosis with increasing periods of ischemia. A significant difference has been shown between early and late reperfusion of ischemic myocardium. Increasing infarct size as a result of reperfusion is based on the theory that hemorrhage into the ischemic area further reduces the oxygen supply to the edematous marginally viable cells of the peripheral zone of ischemia. The cells in this "twilight zone" might otherwise remain viable receiving blood supply through collateral vessels.[12] Evidence presented in this study substantiates this theory as shown by increased areas of injury ($\Sigma A_I + \Sigma A_P$)/ΣA_V in the four- and six-hour ligation groups (Fig. 7) compared to the one- and two-hour groups. Progression of necrosis in the area of ischemia expands with time at the expense of the peripheral zone of ischemia. Areas of patchy necrosis decrease relative to the expanding central infarct ($\Sigma A_P / \Sigma A_I$).

Data presented here indicate that early reperfusion produces smaller infarcts and smaller areas of total injury than permanently ligated animals. However, variability in coronary artery distribution makes it difficult in small sample size groups to assess statistical significance between these groups. Variable coronary patterns will pro-

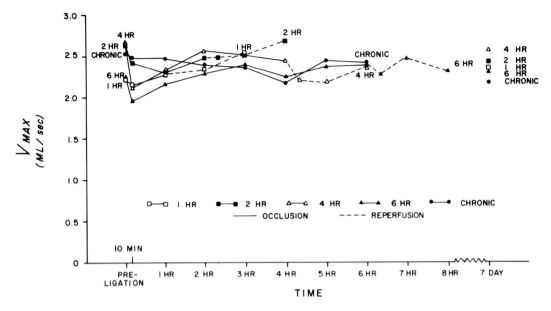

FIG. 9.   Time course of changes in maximum velocity of contraction extrapolated to zero load (Vmax). Points represent mean values for each ligation group.

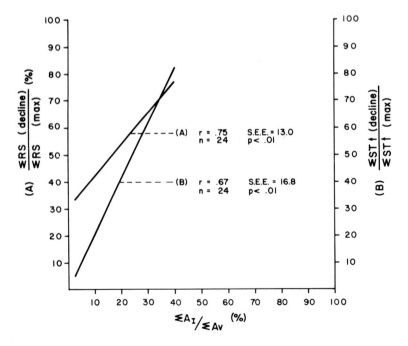

FIG. 10.   Regression lines comparing electrocardiographic indices of the progression of infarction to the observed histologic infarct size. r: correlaton coefficient; S.E.E.: standard error of estimate; n: number of animals.

duce different areas of ischemia dependent upon the collateral blood supply. Ideally, comparison of the infarct size to the total ischemic area would eliminate some of the animal variability; however, accurate determination of the size of ischemic area by epicardial ECG mapping was not possible because of significant but variable infarction of the intraventricular septum.

CORRELATION OF ECG CHANGES WITH INFARCT SIZE

In an effort to examine the influence of variable coronary artery distribution among animals on the observed histological changes, the indices $\Sigma ST\uparrow$ decline/$\Sigma ST\uparrow$ max and ΣRS decline/ΣRS max were determined just prior to ligature release for each animal. Each voltage determination ($\Sigma ST\uparrow$ decline, $\Sigma ST\uparrow$ max, ΣRS decline, ΣRS max) is dependent on the size of the ischemic area, whereas the indices are not. Thus, these indices would be expected to correlate with the area of infarction relative to the area of ischemia. This minimizes variations from animal to animal, due to variations in coronary artery distribution, which result from expressing infarct size as a percent of total left ventricle. The good correlation of these indices and actual observed infarct size (Fig. 10) indicates that variability in infarct size from animal to animal due to variations in coronary distribution is nearly eliminated by expressing infarct size as a percent of the total ischemia area.

EFFECTS OF REPERFUSION ON MYOCARDIAL CONTRACTILITY

Measurement of myocardial contractility can be made that is independent of load, thereby assessing the effects of acute ischemia on myocardial muscle function as opposed to myocardial pumping efficiency.[20] Determination of maximum velocity of contraction (maxVce) and extrapolation to zero load (Vmax) for each animal demonstrated a significant decrease in both parameters immediately following coronary occlusion, ($p < .05$ n = 22) from preligation to one hour postocclusion. This was followed by a rapid return to preligation values, as shown in Figure 9. Reperfusion had no effect on either Vmax or maxVce. Similar findings were noted in dogs where coronary reperfusion

one hour after occlusion resulted in further decrease in ventricular function.[1] One explanation of these findings is that there is a compensatory increase in contractility in the noninfarcted myocardium.[9] If the area of acute ischemia is small relative to the ventricle, then no significant change would be expected in the contractile state (Vmax). Myocardial contractility has been found to be a good index of ventricular function in patient studies[8] and can be used as a sensitive means of comparing ventricular function between patients.[14] Clinical reports of myocardial revascularization in patients with acute ischemia demonstrated marked improvement in Vmax following surgery.[4] Comparison of changes in myocardial contractility following acute coronary occlusion in the experimental animal with a normal heart and significant myocardial reserve cannot be made with changes in contractility in man where generalized coronary artery disease may have critically reduced myocardial reserve, thus limiting any ability to a compensatory increase in contractility in non-infarcted myocardium.

SUMMARY

The effects of reperfusion following acute coronary occlusion on myocardial viability have been studied in 31 primates with variable periods of myocardial ischemia. The time course of epicardial ST segment elevation, decrease of EMF (R+S wave amplitude), and the progression of infarction within the area of ischemia have been demonstrated. Reperfusion up to four hours following coronary occlusion resulted in smaller infarcts compared to permanently ligated animals and to those animals reperfused after six hours. Although an initial decrease was noted in myocardial contractility following coronary occlusion, no significant change was produced by reperfusion.

Recent clinical reports of early myocardial revascularization in patients with acute ischemia or infarction have shown a significant increase in the survival rate in a high risk group of patients.[4,16,17,19,21,23] In view of a slower rate of decline of $\Sigma ST\uparrow$ in man,[18] conceivably infarction within the area of ischemia may progress at a slower rate than that demonstrated in experimental animals. This represents good evidence that early reperfusion does alter the size of the ischemic area and limits the size of infarction in man.

References

1. Banka VS, Chadda KD, Meister SG, Helfant RH: Limitations of myocardial revascularization in restoration of regional contraction abnormalities produced by coronary occlusion. Am J Cardiol 31:118, 1973 (abstract)
2. Bloor CM, White FC: Coronary artery perfusion: Early effects on coronary hemodynamics. Am J Cardiol 31:121, 1973 (abstract)
3. Bresnahan GF, Shell WE, Ross John Jr, Roberts R, Sobel BE: Deleterious effects of reperfusion in evolving myocardial infarction. Circulation 45: 13 (Supplement II), 1972 (abstract)
4. Chatterjee K, Swan HJC, Parmley WW, et al: Depression of left ventricular function due to acute myocardial ischemia and its reversal after aortocoronary saphenous-vein bypass. N Engl J Med 286:1117, 1972
5. Cox JL, McLaughlin VW, Flowers NC, Horan LG: The ischemic zone surrounding acute myocardial infarction: Its morphology as detected by dehydrogenase staining. Am Heart J 76:650, 1968
6. Cox JL, Daniel TM, Boineau JP: The electrophysiologic time-course of acute myocardial ischemia and the effects of early coronary artery reperfusion. Circulation 48:971, 1973
7. Ginks WR, Sybers HD, Maroko PR, et al: Coronary artery reperfusion: II. Reduction of myocardial infarct size at 1 week after the coronary occlusion. J Clin Invest 51:2717, 1972
8. Hermann HJ, Singh R, Dammann JF: Evaluation of myocardial contractility in man. Am Heart J 77:755, 1969
9. Hood WB: Experimental myocardial infarction. III. Recovery of left ventricular function in the healing phase: Contribution of increased fiber shortening in noninfarcted myocardium. Am Heart J 79:531, 1970
10. Jennings RB: Early phase of myocardial ischemic injury and infarction. Am J Cardiol 24:753, 1969
11. Maroko PR, Libby P, Ginks WR, et al: Coronary artery reperfusion I. Early effects on local myocardial function and the extent of myocardial necrosis. J Clin Invest 51:2710, 1972
12. Maroko PR, Braunwald E: Modification of myocardial infarction size after coronary occlusion. Ann Intern Med 79:720, 1973
13. Maroko PR, Kjekshus JK, Sobel BE, et al: Factors influencing infarct size following experimental coronary artery occlusions. Circulation 43:67, 1971
14. Mason DT, Spann JF, Zelis R: Quantification of the contractile state of the intact human heart. Am J Cardiol 26:248, 1970
15. Mirsky I, Pasternac A, Ellison RC: General Index for the assessment of cardiac function. Am J Cardiol 30:483, 1972
16. Mundth ED, Buckley MJ, Leinbach RC, et al: Surgical intervention for the complications of acute myocardial ischemia. Ann Surg 178:379, 1973
17. Mundth ED, Buckley MJ, Leinbach RC, et al: Myocardial revascularization for the treatment of cardiogenic shock complicating acute myocardial infarction. Surgery 70:78, 1971
18. Reid PR, Taylor DR, Kelly DT, et al: Myocardial infarct extension detailed by precordial ST segment mapping. N Engl J Med 290:123, 1974
19. Scanlon PJ, Nemickas R, Tobin JR, et al: Myocardial revascularization during acute phase of myocardial infarction. JAMA 218:207, 1971
20. Siegel JH, Sonnenblick EH: Isometric-time tension relationship as an index of myocardial contractility. Circulation Res 12:597, 1963
21. Smullens SN, Wiener L, Kasparian H, et al: Evaluation and surgical management of acute evolving myocardial infarction. J Thorac Cardiovasc Surg 64:495, 1972
22. Sobel BE, Bresnahan GF, Shell WE, Yoder RD: Estimation of infarct size in man and its relation to prognosis. Circulation 46:640, 1972
23. Sustaita H, Chatterjee K, Matloff JM, et al: Emergency bypass surgery in impending and complicated acute myocardial infarction. Arch Surg 105: 30, 1972
24. Wolk MJ, Keefe JF, Bing OHL, Finkelstein LJ, Levine HJ: Estimation of Vmax in auxotonic systoles from the rate of relative increase of isovolumic pressure: (dP/dt)kP. J Clin Invest 50: 1276, 1971
25. Yeatman LA, Parmley WW, Sonnenblick EH: Effects of temperature on series elasticity and contractile element motion in heart muscle. Am J Physiol 217:1030, 1969

II

EARLY AND LATE MYOCARDIAL RESPONSES TO REVERSIBLE ANOXIA

Frank B. Cerra, Thomas Z. Lajos,
Mario Montes, and John H. Siegel

INTRODUCTION

With the continued application of coronary artery bypass surgery and cardiac assist devices to the clinical conditions of preinfarction angina and acute myocardial infarction, it becomes of paramount importance to define quantitatively the time sequence of ischemic injury and the point of reversibility; and to correlate the structural changes with the observed functional observations during this time-sequence.[7,12,13] Many experimental approaches have been attempted, ranging from coronary artery ligation to the injection of plastic microspheres. These preparations, however, (1) do not allow precise control of collateral flow, (2) do not consistently produce localized transmural changes, (3) do not utilize an anatomically defined segment of myocardium for study, (4) do not separate the local from the systemic effects of myocardial injury, and (5) are not generally available for use as chronic models in studying reversibly applied ischemia.[4,8,12,14,16]

To circumvent these experimental limitations, a new *in vivo* isolated myocardial-pedicle preparation was developed in dogs that enables the quantitative assessment of reversibly applied myocardial insults in acute and chronic preparations.[6] Using this preparation, varying lengths of anoxia were applied to the defined, vascularly isolated, anatomic segments, each anoxic period being immediately followed by revascularization. By using

appropriate monitors, the structural and functional responses of the myocardium were correlated, in the absence of systemic effects, both acutely and four weeks after the anoxic episode.

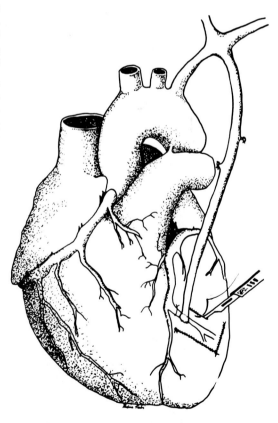

FIG. 1. Internal mammary artery anastomosis to second diagonal branch of left anterior descending coronary artery. The pedicle construction is in progress. Reprinted through courtesy of Annals of Thoracic Surgery.

Supported by United Health Fund Grant CL-BGH-72 and by Grant HL-15676 from the National Heart and Lung Institute.

PREPARATION AND DEVELOPMENT OF THE METHODOLOGY

Vascularized Pedicles

In 13 dogs, anesthesia was induced with pentobarbitol and, after intubation, positive pressure ventilation was maintained with 98 percent oxygen and 2 percent carbon dioxide. A left thoracotomy was performed, and the left mammary artery was dissected to its origin, and its branches were ligated. After fashioning a pericardial basket, the second diagonal branch of the left anterior descending coronary artery was isolated at its take-off. Care was taken to preserve the two veins adjacent to the diagonal, as they and the Thebesian veins were the only venous drainage for the pedicle to be constructed. The mammary artery was then anastomosed in an end-to-side fashion to the second diagonal using an interrupted technique with 7–0 suture. The second diagonal was ligated proximal to the anastomosis, while that distally served as the sole arterial inflow for a transmural myocardial pedicle formed by a simultaneous incision and suture technique (Fig. 1). After stay sutures were placed at corners outlining a rectangular portion of myocardium around the second diagonal, a transmural incision was made with a hook knife. The incision was then extended to each stay suture, except in the area of anastomosis and was immediately followed

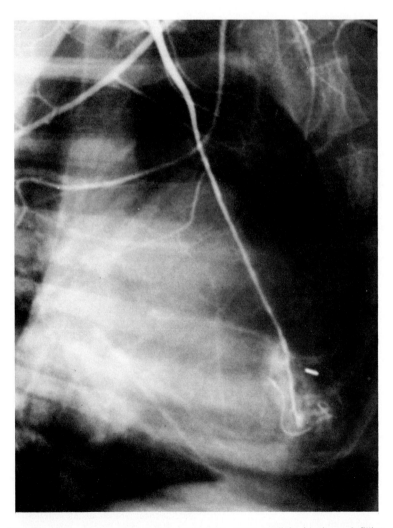

FIG. 2. Cineangiogram frame demonstrating mammary artery, pedicle blush, and filling of great cardiac vein and coronary sinus. No contrast is present in peripedicle myocardium. A wire suture partially outlines the surface of the pedicle. Reprinted through courtesy of Annals of Thoracic Surgery.

by a continuous running suture. The procedure was performed on a beating heart, without cardiopulmonary bypass.

The pedicles measured 2.5 to 4.5 cm on a side and comprised 10–15 percent of the left ventricle by weight. There was no evidence of hypokinesis, akinesis, or dyskinesis. Limb and right atrial EKG's were identical to control tracings. Mammary artery flow after pedicle formation measured 10–15 ml/min. When Walton-Brodie strain gage arches were sutured to a pedicle and reference area and the pedicle was then constructed, there was no significant change after stabilization in either the strain gage response or the development of left ventricular pressure as monitored through an apical cannula.

The chest was closed in a routine manner;

a chest tube was left in place for several hours. There were no postoperative fluid or exercise restrictions. The structural and functional integrity of the preparations was evaluated three to six weeks.

Four dogs underwent selective cineangiography. When contrast material was injected into the left mammary artery, a pedicle blush appeared and was immediately followed by filling of the great cardiac vein at the pedicle level. No contrast material appeared in the peripedicle myocardium (Fig. 2). Selective left coronary artery injection demonstrated good filling of the anterior descending and circumflex branches, with no contrast material appearing in the pedicle.

Surgery was repeated in all 13 dogs. The mammary artery was patent in all, with a flow of

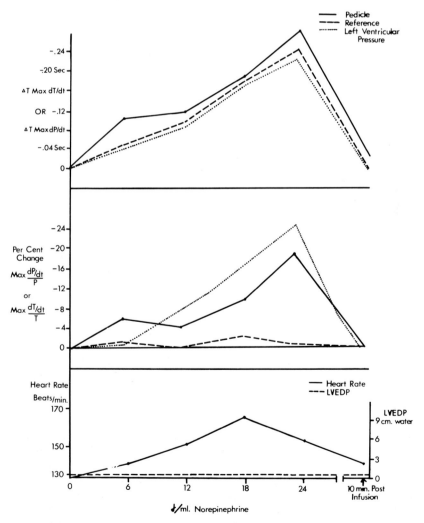

FIG. 3. Simultaneous strain gage responses following norepinephrine infusion. A decrease in Δt max dP/dt or dT/dt, or an increase in percent change in max dP/dt or dT/dt reflects an increase in myocardial contractility. Reprinted through courtesy of Annals of Thoracic Surgery.

10–15 ml/min. In six dogs, Walton-Brodie strain gage arches were sutured to a pedicle and a reference area, and a 3 cm metal cannula was inserted through the apical dimple into the left ventricular cavity for monitoring the development of cavitary pressure. Simultaneous recordings were taken, using either right atrial or Lead II EKG as a timing reference. In three dogs, norepinephrine infusion-response curves were plotted, using infusion concentrations of 0 to 30 r/min. The pedicle and reference myocardium responded concurrently, with return to control parameters within 10 minutes after cessation of the infusion. Enddiastolic pressure remained normal (Fig. 3).

In one dog, a bolus of norepinephrine (40 r) was released in the right atrium and simultaneous recordings taken. The reference gage responded first, followed 1.05 seconds later by the pedicle gage, both contributing to the development of left ventricular pressure (Fig. 4).

A hydrogen infusion wash-out curve was performed and revealed a nutrient flow of 60 ml/100 Gm tissue, a value within normal range for this study.[5]

Multiple tissue sections were taken from pedicle, peripedicle, and reference areas in six dogs and submitted for light and electronmicroscopic analysis. Hematoxylin and eosin and Masson Trichrome staining demonstrated a 1 to 3 mm scar encompassing the pedicle with no abnormal fibrous tissue within the pedicle or the peripedicle myocardium. Electronmicrograph sections were indistinguishable from control specimens (Fig. 5).

Devascularized Pedicles

In 10 dogs, totally devascularized pedicles were created by using the simultaneous incision and suture technique to encompass an area of myocardium. No vascular anastomosis was performed. Selective left ventriculograms 6 and 12 months later demonstrated dyskinesis in the devascularized area. On serial sectioning of these grossly scarred areas, dense fibrous tissue was found with a thin layer of surviving myocardium subendocardially and subepicardially.

A new canine preparation for quantitatively investigating the myocardial response to reversible ischemia, both acutely and chronically, was thus devised. It has the advantages of (1) not altering overall ventricular function; (2) allowing the study of a precisely defined segment of myocardium; (3) separating local from systemic effects of myocardial dysfunction; (4) making chronic

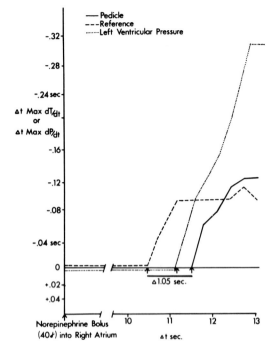

FIG. 4. Norepinephrine bolus released into the right atrium resulted in differential strain gage responses, the reference responding first followed 1.05 seconds later by the pedicle. Reprinted through courtesy of Annals of Thoracic Surgery.

preparations readily available; and (5) controlling the influence of collateral circulation.

THE INITIAL RESPONSE TO ACUTE ANOXIA

Eighteen additional canine preparations were divided into three groups of six dogs each. Group I received 15 minutes of pedicle anoxia (mammary artery occlusion) followed by 30 minutes of revascularization. Group II received 30 minutes with 30 minutes of revascularization; and Group III had 60 minutes of pedicle anoxia and 60 minutes of revascularization. Walton-Brodie strain gage arches were sutured to the pedicle and a reference area of myocardium near the marginal branch of the circumflex coronary artery. A stiff metal cannula was inserted through the apical dimple to monitor the development of left ventricular cavitary pressure. Additional cannulas were placed for monitoring central venous pressure, aortic root pressure and the right atrial electrocardiogram. During each anoxic and revascularization period, EKG, strain gage responses, cardio-

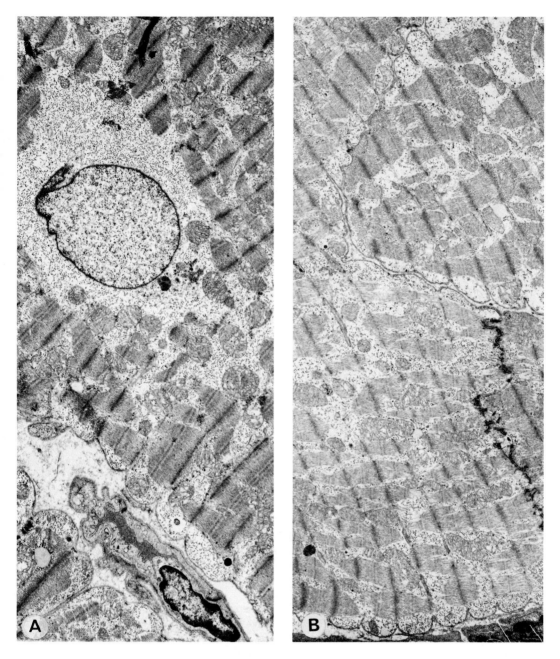

FIG. 5. Electronmicrographs from control (A) and from a pedicle six weeks after formation (B). Gluteraldehyde-osmium fixation with epon imbedding. ×6300

green dye curves, and arteriovenous oxygen saturation differences ($A\text{-}VO_2$) were monitored.[9,10] Biopsies for electronmicroscopy (EM) were taken from pedicle and reference areas before and during anoxia, and following revascularization.

Within 90 seconds of the onset of anoxia, all pedicles became cyanotic and dyskinetic; pedicle strain gage response (Δt to Max dT/dt)[11] markedly decreased while the reference gage (Δt to Max dT/dt)[11] remained at, or nearly at, control levels. Cardiac output, left ventricular pressure development (Δt to Max dP/dt),[11] dynamic cardiac mixing time (tm, reflecting overall myocardial contractility),[9] dynamic dispersive time (td, reflecting pulmonary mean transit time),[9] and $A\text{-}VO_2$ changed little during anoxia or during revascularization. With revascularization, mammary artery flow demonstrated a hyperemic phase of 18-24 ml/min and then stabilized at 6–10 ml/min within 10–15 minutes after initiation of revascularization.

Group I: Fifteen Minutes Reversible Anoxia (Acute Changes)

Pedicle function and color returned within three minutes of revascularization. Pedicle strain gage function had returned to control level by 30 minutes of revascularization (Fig. 6).

The electron micrographs during anoxia revealed generalized glycogen depletion and mitochondrial swelling, as well as some intercellular edema. After revascularization, all changes returned to control levels (Fig. 5), with no evidence of perivascular hemorrhage (Fig. 7.A and B).

Group II: Thirty Minutes Reversible Anoxia (Acute Changes)

The pedicle response to anoxia was the same as Group I. After revascularization, however, there was gross return of color, but incomplete return of function. The pedicle contractility gradually improved, so that at the end of 30 minutes of revascularization it was at −60 percent of control level (Fig. 8). There was little change in C.O., tm, td, or $A\text{-}VO_2$.

The biopsies during anoxia revealed generalized severe glycogen depletion, intercellular edema, and mitochondrial swelling. In addition, there were *focal* areas of mitochondrial degeneration; of myofibril fragmentation, and disappearance; and of minimal ectasia of the T-tubular

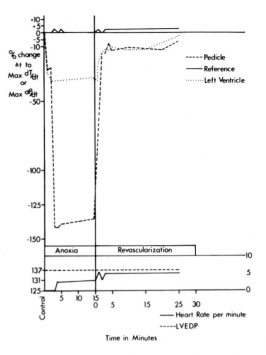

FIG. 6. Contractility response in percent change in Δt to max dT/dt or dP/dt during 15 minutes of anoxia and 30 minutes of revascularization. The pedicle rapidly returns to control level. Reprinted through courtesy of Journal of Surgical Research.

and endoplasmic reticular systems. After revascularization, glycogen returned and mitochondrial swelling disappeared. The other morphologic changes persisted, including some intercellular edema. No vascular alterations were noted (Fig. 9.A and B).

Group III: Sixty Minutes Reversible Anoxia (Acute Changes)

The pedicle remained cyanotic and dyskinetic throughout the sixty-minute revascularization period. There was little return of pedicle contractility, it remaining at about −150 percent of control. C.O., tm, td, and $A\text{-}VO_2$ changed insignificantly from control (Fig. 10).

EM's after anoxia revealed *generalized* glycogen depletion and mitochondrial degeneration. There were large areas of myofibril fraying, fragmentation, and disappearance, together with moderate to marked ecstasia of the T-tubular and endoplasmic reticular systems. Revascularization produced some decrease in mitochondrial swelling, but with otherwise persistent changes. No vascular abnormalities were demonstrable (Fig. 11.A and B).

In the absence of the effects of systemic hypotension and collateral circulation, the response of an anatomically defined area of myocardium to acute, reversible, anoxic insults was precisely investigated. The earliest detectable ultramicroscopic changes were those of generalized severe glycogen depletion, mitochondrial swelling, and interstitial edema. These were completely reversible after 15 minutes of anoxia, and to a large extent following 30 minutes of normothermic anoxia. With 30 minutes of anoxia, however, there were focal areas of irreversible myofibril and mitochondrial damage. Sixty minutes of anoxia produced severe generalized damage to all structures except the sarcolemma and blood vessels.

The glycogen stores and mitochondria seem to be the most sensitive to acute, reversible anoxia, while the sarcolemma and blood vessels seem to be most resistant. This pattern of injury is somewhat different than that observed using other preparations. With coronary artery ligation techniques, the earliest changes detected were those of mild glycogen depletion, and some interstitial edema and myofibril band changes after 15 to 20 minutes of occlusion. With longer periods of arterial ligation, progressively more muscle became involved with differing degrees of mitochondrial, myofibril, and tubular degeneration, there being considerable variability with respect to the location and extent of the injury produced.[1,10,12,13]

Myocardial contractility returns to control

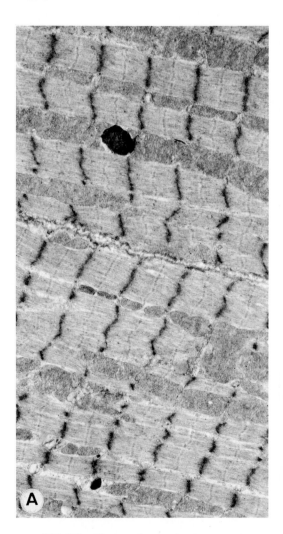 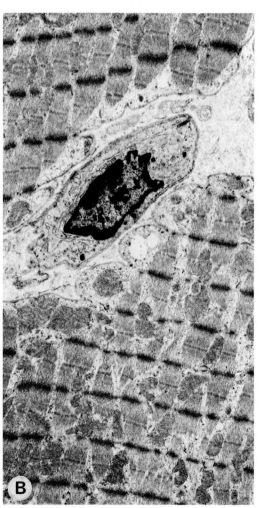

FIG. 7.A. Electronmicrograph after 15 minutes of pedicle anoxia, demonstrating generalized glycogen depletion and mitochondrial swelling and some intercellular edema. ×6300, gluteraldehyde-osmium fixation, epon imbedding. B. Electronmicrograph after 15 minutes of pedicle anoxia and 30 minutes of revascularization. All changes have returned to control (Fig. 5.A) ×6300, gluteraldehyde-osmium fixation, epon imbedding. Reprinted through courtesy of Journal of Surgical Research.

levels after 15 minutes of pedicle anoxia, while there is little recovery after 60 minutes. Thirty minutes produces a partial persistent loss of the contractile function. It is of note that in all cases there was no evidence of hemorrhage or hemorrhagic infarction following revascularization. This finding, as well as the contractile response, correlates well with the observed ultrastructural aberrations. Other investigations have reported return of contractile function four hours after coronary artery ligation. The influence of collateral flow in healthy animal hearts, however, was an influential and uncontrolled variable.[14,15]

THE CHRONIC RESPONSE TO ACUTE ANOXIA

Twelve additional animals with myocardial-pedicle preparations were divided into three groups of four dogs each. Group 1 received 15 minutes of pedicle anoxia; Group II 30 minutes; and Group III 60 minutes. In each case, following the anoxic period, the pedicle was immediately revascularized, the chest closed, and the dog allowed to recover. Four weeks postoperatively, each was reoperated upon. Mammary artery flow was determined and gross observations recorded. The strain gages and monitoring devices were applied as previously described. Biopsies were taken from the pedicle and a reference area for electron microscopy. After baseline recordings, norepinephrine infusion-response curves were performed, using concentrations of 6 to 24 r per minute. At each steady state, C.O., tm, td, ejection time, A-VO$_2$, and total peripheral resistance were determined. Transmural biopsies through the pedicle and peripedicle muscle tissue were then taken for serial sectioning and special staining for fibrous tissue. During the reoperation, a balanced electrolyte solution was infused at a constant rate of 3 ml/min.

In all preparations, the mammary artery was patent. Left ventricular end-diastolic pressure was within normal limits, as was the C.O., cardiac index, tm, td, and the A-VO$_2$. During the norepinephrine infusion, the indices also remained within normal range, although the C.O. and total peripheral resistance generally increased and the tm and td generally decreased.

Group I: Fifteen Minutes of Pedicle Anoxia (Late Response)

On gross inspection, there was no hypokinesis, akinesis, or dyskinesis. Patency of all mam-

mary arteries was observed. During norepinephrine infusion, the pedicle contractility responded as well as the refence myocardium and the development of left ventricular pressure. Following norepinephrine, there was a moderate depression of all contractility parameters (Fig. 12).

Light microscopic analysis demonstrated the pedicle to be encompassed by scar tissue. The pedicle and peripedicle tissue was normal in morphology. Lie and Masson staining failed to reveal any evidence of abnormal fibrosis (Fig. 13). Electronmicrographs were unchanged from control (Fig. 14).

Group II: Thirty Minutes of Pedicle Anoxia (Late Response)

There was no gross evidence of kinetic abnormality. All mammary arteries were patent. The pedicle responded to the same magnitude as the reference myocardium and left ventricular pressure during the norepinephrine infusion. There was, again, a moderate depression of contractility parameters after the cessation of the drug infusion (Fig. 15).

These pedicles were also surrounded by a zone of scar tissue in the incision and suture line. The peripedicle tissue had normal light and elec-

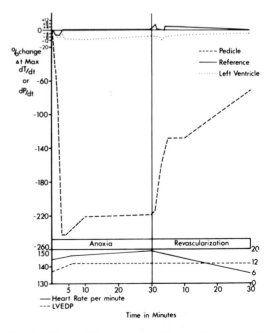

FIG. 8. Contractility response following 30 minutes of anoxia and 30 minutes of revascularization. The pedicle contractility gradually returned to within −60 percent of control level. Reprinted through courtesy of Journal of Surgical Research.

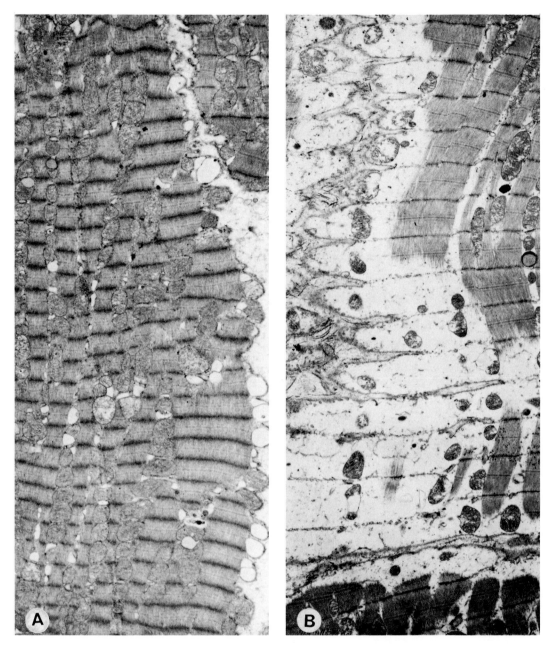

FIG. 9.A. Electromicrograph following 30 minutes of anoxia. Generalized glycogen depletion and the focal degenerative changes are noted. Gluteraldehyde-osmium fixation, epon imbedding, ×6300. B. Electronmicrograph following 30 minutes of anoxia and 30 minutes of revascularization, demonstrating the persistence of the focal mitochondrial, myofibril, and tubular degenerative changes. Gluteraldehyde-osmium fixation, epon imbedding, ×6300. Reprinted through the courtesy of Journal of Surgical Research.

tronmicroscopy. The myocardial pedicle itself had several areas of focal scarring within the surrounding normal muscle tissue. These areas were estimated to comprise 10 to 15 percent of the total pedicle volume. In the perimetry of these areas of fibrous tissue, some capillary proliferation was noted. Masson and Lie stains confirmed these

findings, with occasional positivity of the Lie and staining of the fibrous foci by Masson (Fig. 16).

Electronmicrographs demonstrated focal collagen replacement, corresponding to the focal fibrosis on light microscopy. In sections where muscle tissue was present, the myofibril ultrastructure was generally well preserved. Some areas at

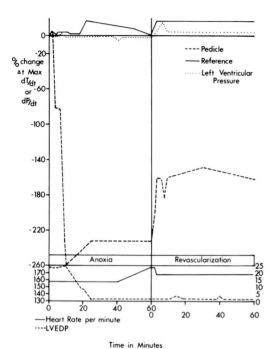

FIG. 10. Contractility response after 60 minutes of
pedicle anoxia and 60 minutes of revascularization.
There was little return of pedicle function. Reprinted
through the courtesy of the Journal of Surgical Research.

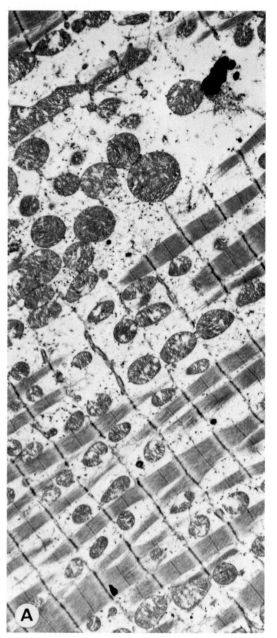

FIG. 11.A. Electronmicrograph after 60 minutes of pedicle anoxia demonstrating severe generalized degenerative changes. Gluteraldhyde-osmium fixation; epon imbedding, ×6300

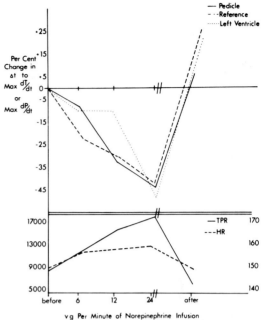

FIG. 12. Contractility response to norepinephrine infusion four weeks after 15 minutes of pedicle anoxia. The pedicle responds as well as the reference gauge and left ventricular pressure development.

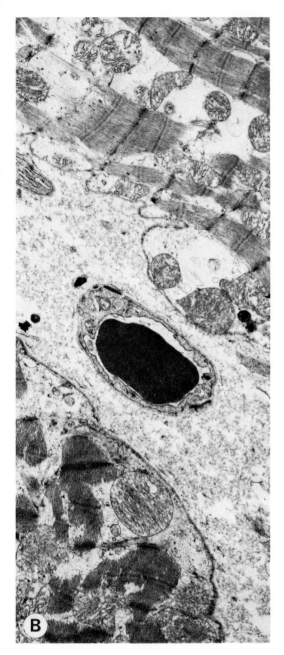

FIG. 11.B. Electronmicrograph after 60 minutes of pedicle anoxia and 60 minutes of revascularization illustrating persistence of the ultrastructural aberrations. Gluteraldehyde-osmium fixation, epon imbedding, ×6300. Reprinted through courtesy of Journal of Surgical Research.

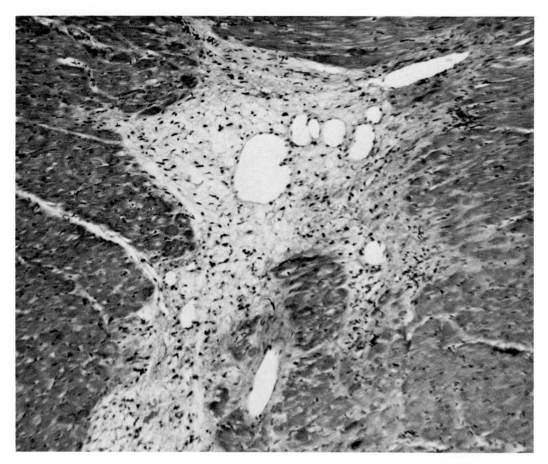

FIG. 13. Light microscopy demonstrating normal morphology of pedicle (L) and peripedicle tissue (R). Aside from the incision and suture scar, no abnormal fibrosis was observed. Masson stain, ×10

the periphery showed vacuolization and the formation of myelin bodies. There was cristae degeneration in some mitochondria; occasional fragmentation of the intercalated discs, and some mild ectasia of the T-tubular and endoplasmic reticular systems. The vascular structures were unremarkable (Fig. 17).

Group III: Sixty Minutes of Pedicle Anoxia (Late Response)

The pedicles were grossly akinetic or dyskinetic. Flow was present in all mammary arteries. During the norepinephrine infusion-response curves, there was little to no response from the pedicle. However, the reference myocardium and left ventricular pressure development demonstrated a good response. Postnorepinephrine depression of contractile parameters was also observed (Fig. 18). In addition, the EKG demonstrated a left bundle branch block pattern during the infusion, but with return to normal conduction with the cessation of infusion.

Light microscopy demonstrated that the pedicles were outlined by a zone of scar tissue. The peripedicle muscle was normal. Within the pedicle, however, there were many large, sometimes confluent, areas of scar extending from the epicardium to the endocardium. Inflammatory infiltration was present, with macrophages, 3+, lymphocytes, 1+, and rare plasma cells. It was estimated that 80 to 85 percent of the pedicle volume was replaced by fibrous tissue. Adjacent to these areas was proliferating young connective tissue with capillaries (4+). In between these large areas of necrosis were small islands of normal muscle. In other areas, however, myocytolysis and hypertrophied muscle tissue were observed. Lie stain was negative for reaction (Fig. 19).

Electronmicrographs confirmed the light microscopy and revealed large areas of complete organelle replacement by collagen matrix. There were occasional myofibrils and mitochondria of relatively normal morphology, but most demonstrated severe degenerative changes, as did the T-tubular and endo-plasmic reticular systems. Glycogen was absent. Sarcolemmal and vascular struc-

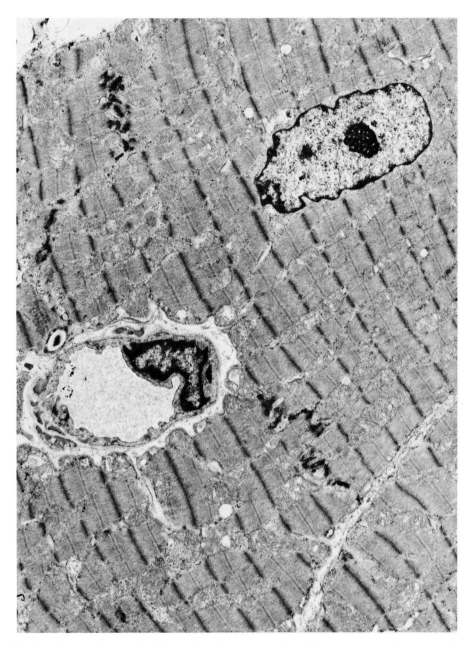

FIG. 14. Electronmicrograph of the pedicle four weeks after 15 minutes of anoxia was applied. The ultrastructure is unchanged from control (Fig. 5A and B). Gluteraldehyde-osmium fixation, epon imbedding, ×6300

tures were intact. Intercalated discs were fragmented (Fig. 20).

SUMMARY AND DISCUSSION

Four weeks after 15 minutes of reversible anoxia was applied to the isolated myocardial pedicle, normal function, morphology, and ultrastruc-

ture were present. After 30 minutes, the functional characteristics were unaltered from control myocardium. There was, however, morphologic and ultrastructural evidence of significant damage, mainly limited to focal areas of myofibrils, mitochondria, and tubular systems. With 60 minutes of anoxia, there is little or no function demonstrable four weeks later. This finding correlates well with the light and electronmicrographic find-

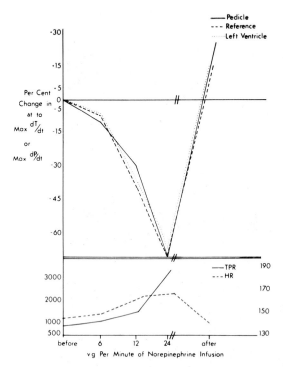

FIG. 15. Contractility response to norepinephrine four weeks after 30 minutes of pedicle anoxia. There is little difference in the pedicle, reference, and left ventricular pressure responses.

FIG. 16. Light micrograph of the pedicle myocardium demonstrating focal scarring within surrounding normal myocardium. Hematoxylin-eosin staining, ×10

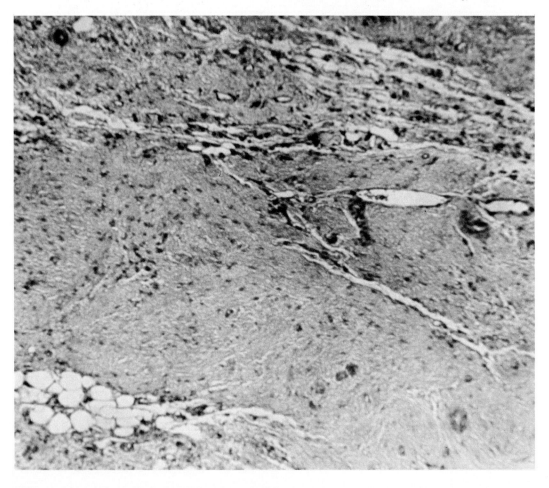

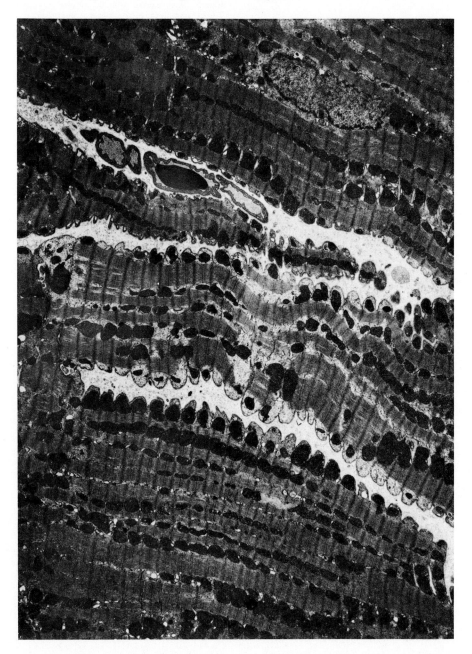

FIG. 17. Electonmicrograph of the pedicle four weeks after 30 minutes of reversible anoxia. The ultrastructure is generally well preserved, with a few focal areas of fibrosis, tubular ectasia, and cystic mitochondrial degeneration. Gluteraldehyde-osmium fixation, epon imbedding, ×6000

ings of large, sometimes confluent, areas of transmural replacement of muscle tissue by scar tissue. Blood vessel systems, however, remain intact.

The morphologic findings were somewhat similar in trend to those reported by some authors [2,3,4,14] using reversible occlusion of a coronary artery and examination of the posterior papillary muscle one to seven days after the occlu-

sion episode. Up to 15 to 20 minutes of occlusion produced little or no irreversible injury. With longer periods of occlusion, progressively more necrosis occurred, eg, with 60 minutes of occlusion, up to 85 percent of the papillary muscle had changes present. It is interesting to note, however, that in the longer follow-up preparations, the percent involvement decreased from 85 to 60 percent

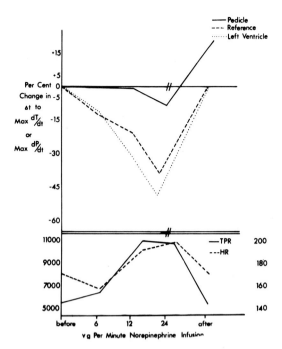

FIG. 18. Contractile response during norepinephrine infusion four weeks after 60 minutes of pedicle anoxia. There was little or no pedicle response.

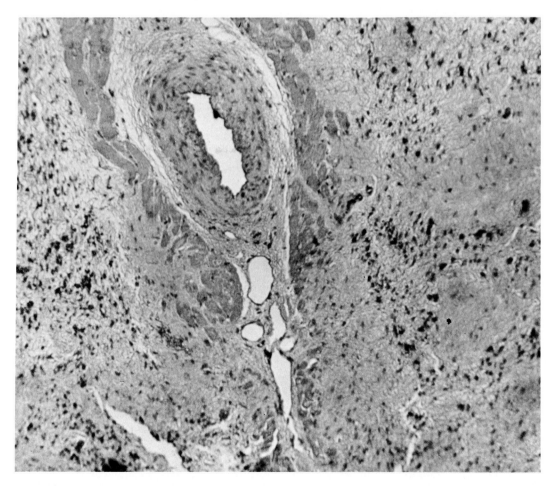

FIG. 19. Light micrograph four weeks after 60 minutes of pedicle anoxia demonstrating the large areas of dense scarring within the pedicle. Some normal muscle was also observed between the large areas of scarring. Hematoxylin-eosin staining, ×10

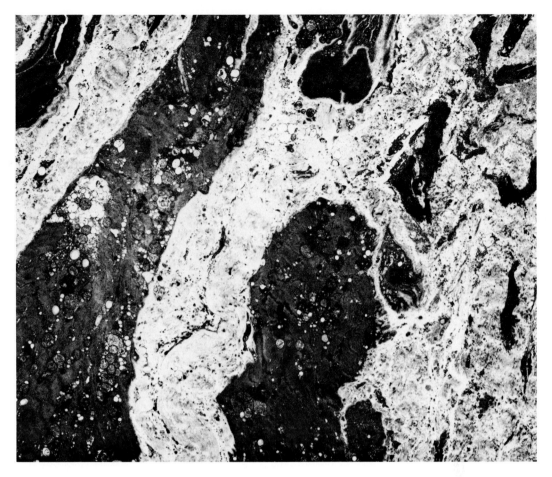

FIG. 20. Electronmicrograph from the pedicle four weeks after 60 minutes of pedicle anoxia. There is nearly complete organelle replacement by collagen and macrophages. Gluteraldehyde-osmium fixation, epon imbedding, ×6000

after 60 minutes of occlusion. This presumably reflects the influence of collateral flow in healthy canine myocardium, whose influence is unchecked in their particular preparation.[1,4] In contrast, with 60 minutes of reversible anoxia in the absence of collateral flow using the myocardial-pedicle preparation, complete transmural fibrosis is present in all preparations by four weeks after anoxic insult. After 30 minutes of oxygen deprivation, function returns to normal, but focal areas of fibrosis ensue.

The functional result also differed quite markedly from that in the coronary artery ligation preparation. In the ligation model, contractility returned to control level after up to two hours of reversible coronary artery occlusion.[14] This discrepancy probably reflects the influence of unimpaired collateral flow in a normal heart as well as the absence of a defined, anatomic, transmural, myocardial segment for both control and experimental manipulation.

In summary, a new preparation was utilized to quantitate the myocardial, functional, and ultrastructural response to reversibly applied anoxic insults. This preparation utilized an anatomically defined transmural, myocardial segment whose arterial blood supply is isolated from the rest of the coronary circulation. The local effects of myocardial anoxia can be investigated in the absence of the systemic effects; preparations are readily available for chronic study.

When 15 minutes of reversible anoxia are applied to the segment, functional and ultrastructural alterations occur that are completely reversed by 30 minutes of revascularization and remain reversed after four weeks of follow-up. After 30 minutes of anoxia, initially there is partial return of function and persistent ultrastructural changes. Four weeks after the insult, function has returned to control level, but focal areas of infarction persist with fibrous tissue replacement. Sixty minutes of acute anoxia produced permanent loss of function in the pedicle segment. This correlated well with the morphologic and ultrastructural findings of large areas of transmural fibrosis with little intervening normal muscle.

The organelle most sensitive to oxygen deprivation appears to be the mitochondria. The T-tubular and endoplasmic reticular systems and some myofibrils seem to be next; while the sarcolemma, intercalated discs, and blood vasculature appear to be the most resistant.

The development of this myocardial preparation provides a tool for evaluating the potential protective effects of various pharmacologic and mechanical measures on ischemic myocardium.

References

1. Cerra FB, Lajos TZ, Montes M, Siegel JH: Structural-functional correlates of reversible myocardial anoxia. J Surg Res, vol. 16, 1974
2. Farrens VJ, Roberts WC: Myocardial ultrastructure in acute and chronic hypoxia. Cardiology 56:144–60, 1971
3. Jennings RB, Baum JH, Herdson PB: Fine structural changes in myocardial ischemic injury. Arch Path 79:135–43, 1965
4. Jennings R, Sommers H, Smyth G, Flach H, Linn H: Myocardial necrosis induced by temporary occlusion of the coronary artery in the dog. Arch Path 70:84, 1960
5. Klocke FJ, Rosing DR, Pittman DE: Inert gas measurement of coronary blood flow. Am J Cardiol 23:548, 1968
6. Lajos TZ, Cerra FB, Montes M, Siegel, JH: A chronic experimental model for reversible myocardial anoxia. Ann Thoracic Surg 17:20–35, 1974
7. Mundth ED, Buckley MJ, Austen G: Myocardial revascularization during postinfarction shock. Hospital Practice pp. 113–23, Jan 1973
8. O'Beid A, Smulyan H, Gilbert R, Eich R: Regional metabolic changes in the myocardium following coronary artery ligation in the dog. Am Heart J 83:189, 1972
9. Siegel JH, Farrell E, Goldywyn RM, Friedman HP: The surgical implications of physiologic patterns in myocardial infarction shock. Surgery 72:121–41, 1972
10. Siegel JH, Farrell E, Lewin IL: Quantifying the need for cardiac support in human shock by a functional model of cardiopulmonary vascular dynamics with special reference to myocardial infarction. J Surg Res 13:166, Oct 1972
11. Siegel JH, Sonnenblick EH, Judge RD, Wilson WS: The quantification of myocardial contractility in dog and man. Cardiology 45:189–220, 1964
12. Skinner DB, Davis WG, Camp TF: Left circumflex coronary artery division in dogs given supportive treatment. Ann Thor Surg 7:243, 1969
13. Sustaita H, Chatterjee K, Matloff JM, et al: Emergency bypass surgery in impending and acute myocardial infarction. Arch Surg 105:30, 1972
14. Symes JF, Arnold MF, Blundell PE: Early revascularization of the acute myocardial infarction: The critical time factor. Can J Surg 16:275–83, July 1973
15. Tomada H, Parmley WW, Fujimura S, Matloff J: Effects of ischemia and reoxygenation on regional myocardial performance in the dog. Am J Physiol 221:1718–21, Dec 1971
16. Weber KT, Malinin TI, Dennison BH, et al: Experimental myocardial ischemia and infarction. Am J Cardiol 29:793, 1972

12

THE ROLE OF HYPEROSMOLAL MANNITOL IN THE TREATMENT OF MYOCARDIAL ANOXIA

James Christodoulou, Charles Smithen, Robert Erlandson, Thomas Killip, and Norman Brachfeld

INTRODUCTION

During prolonged oxygen deprivation, cell-swelling induced by electrolyte and water shifts is further aggravated by intracellular accumulation of osmotically active particles contributed by tissue metabolites and ultimately by autolytic breakdown of protein.[10] The physiological significance of such changes may be expressed with particular detrimental effects in the myocardium. Myocardial cellular swelling may dilute intracellular contents and lead to palpable firmness of the ventricular wall. Reduction in ventricular compliance caused by high membrane tensions can seriously impair hemodynamic performance.

Recent studies by Willerson et al[14] demonstrated a beneficial action of elevated osmolality in protecting ischemic myocardium against the potential deleterious effects of increased cell volume. Its mechanism of action, however, is not completely understood. These studies were designed to evaluate the effects of an obligatory extracellular hyperosmolal agent (mannitol) during anoxia under the controlled conditions provided by the isolated perfused isovolumic nonrecirculating Langendorff rat heart preparation. Hemodynamic, metabolic, and ultrastructural studies were performed to explore its mechanism of action and form the subject of this report.

MATERIALS AND METHODS

Seventy-nine isolated rat hearts were perfused utilizing a modified Langendorff apparatus.

Supported by U.S.P.H.S. Contract PH 43–67–1439.

Male Sherman rats weighing 250 to 290 gm were used and allowed to feed ad lib on Wayne Lab chow. Rats were killed by axial fracture, and the heart was rapidly removed and immediately placed in chilled saline. Contractions ceased within five seconds and the heart was then mounted on an aortic cannula.

Experimental Design

The effects of hyperosmolal mannitol were compared to buffered perfusion during three sequential periods: (1) 15 minutes of paced aerobic perfusion (control), (2) 15 minutes of unpaced anoxic perfusion (anoxia), (3) 15 minutes of paced aerobic perfusion (recovery). At the termination of each period, left ventricular hemodynamics were measured and samples of perfusate were taken across the coronary vascular bed for total lactate and glucose determinations using an automated assay technique. A second series of hearts were studied after being compressed by a Wollenberger clamp and assayed for tissue levels of glycogen and high-energy phosphates using standard laboratory methods.

To determine the effect of hyperosmolality when introduced after anoxia had been established, an additional group of seven hearts were perfused with isosmolal buffer during the control and anoxic periods and with the hyperosmolal solution during the recovery phase.

A third series of 16 hearts were similarly perfused, and after each study period, samples were taken for ultrastructural studies. For electron microscopic examination, the cardiac apex was excised while still beating and immediately immersed in buffered 2 percent acrolein and 5 percent glutaraldehyde for 1.5 hours and postfixed in buffered osmium tetroxide.[11] After dehydration, specimens were embedded in Maraglas-D.E.R. 732 epoxy resin.[3] Thin sections were stained by uranyl acetate and examined in a Siemens Elmiskop 101 electron microscope; thick (1μ) sections for light microscopic examination were stained with toluidine blue.

Rat Heart Apparatus

The apparatus used was a modification of the orthodox rat heart perfusion apparatus (Fig. 1). A tandem system was used to permit rapid exchange of perfusate varied as to osmolality and pO_2. Perfusate was pumped from a substrate reservoir to a bubbling reservoir for appropriate gas exchange. The bubbling reservoir was set to deliver at a fixed perfusion pressure of 75 mm Hg. Perfusate reached the heart by retrograde flow through a temperature control coil. All glass-

ware was jacketed, and buffer solutions were maintained at 37 C.

A modification of the method of Kadas and Opie[7] was used to assess ventricular function. Left ventricular pressure was obtained after left atrial appendectomy and insertion of a small latex balloon catheter. The balloon was inflated (diastolic pressure–atmosphere pressure) and ventricular pressure and dP/dt were recorded on a Sanborn Model 8800 multichannel system using a Statham P23D transducer. A stab wound in the wall of the left ventricle prevented accumulation of thebesian drainage. Heart rate was maintained constant at 300 beats/minute during aerobic perfusion by external bipolar ventricular pacing. Coronary sinus flow was monitored directly by collection of fluid draining from the right heart. Arterial samples were drawn from the aortic cannula.

PERFUSATES. The control perfusate consisted of modified Krebs-Ringer-bicarbonate

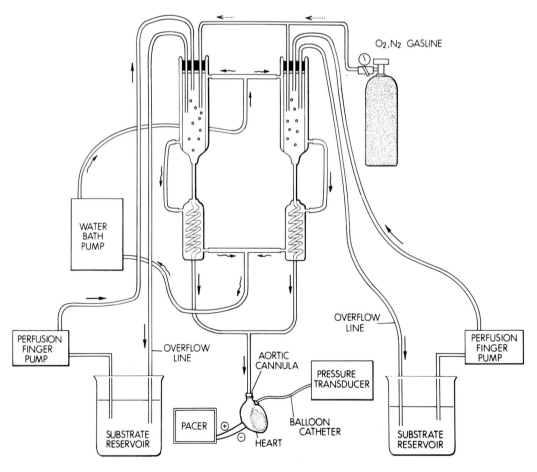

FIG. 1. Modified Langendorff rat heart perfusion apparatus. A retrograde, nonrecirculating, externally paced tandem system is diagramed allowing for isovolumic ventricular contraction by inflation of a latex balloon catheter.

(KRB) buffer containing 5 mM glucose, 0.1 mM Na lactate, and 25 milliunits of glucagon-free insulin/ml solution (osmolality = 290 mOsm). The experimental perfusate differed by the addition of 13 gm mannitol/liter perfusate (osmolality = 350 mOsm).

During aerobic studies perfusate pO_2 was maintained at 550 ± 10 mm Hg by gassing with 95 percent O_2 −5 percent CO_2. For anoxic studies, solutions were bubbled with 95 percent N_2 −5 percent CO_2 yielding a fluid pO_2 of 50 mm Hg with the pH maintained at 7.4.

STATISTICAL ANALYSIS. Group means are presented with the standard error of the mean as the index of dispersion. Statistical analysis was performed using Student's t-test for independent and paired observations.

RESULTS

Hemodynamics

During control aerobic perfusion, hyperosmolality did not significantly affect left ventricular systolic peak pressure. Active contraction ceased soon after onset of anoxia, and pressures could not be recorded. Although during the recovery period neither series of hearts reached preanoxic performance levels, those perfused with mannitol showed significant improvement over those perfused with KRB alone. Isosmolal perfusate pressures reached 68 percent of aerobic controls (127 ± 5 mm Hg → 86 ± 6 mm Hg), whereas hyperosmolal perfusate pressures were 77 percent of control (132 ± 5 mm Hg → 102 ± 7 mm Hg, $p < 0.01$) (Fig. 2).

Enhanced performance was more evident when the first derivative of the ventricular pressure curve was analyzed (Fig. 3). With KRB, mean recovery values of dP/dt were only 50 percent of control (3513 ± 328 mm Hg/sec → 1758 ± 172 mm Hg/sec) whereas hyperosmolal perfusion increased dP/dt to 79 percent of control aerobic perfusion (3817 ± 2.5 mm Hg/sec → 2998 ± 234 mm Hg/sec, $p < 0.01$).

Improved recovery was also demonstrable when hyperosmolality was induced at the termination of the anoxic period. Under these circumstances of recovery, peak systolic pressure was 86 percent (141 ± 6 mm Hg → 121 ± 4 mm Hg, $p < 0.01$) and left ventricular dP/dt 81 percent (4165 ± 402 mm Hg/sec → 3360 ± 311 mm Hg/ sec, $p < 0.01$) of aerobic controls.

Coronary flow during aerobic perfusion with isosmolal buffer was 11.9 ± 0.7 ml/min, rose markedly at the onset of anoxia to 19.2 ± 2.4 ml/min, and then fell to 8.4 ± 0.9 ml/min with cessation of contractile activity at the end of the anoxic period. During recovery, flow rate decreased to 7.12 ml/min, which did not differ significantly from aerobic control when total flow was corrected for heart work. The presence of mannitol did not significantly affect these flow rates.

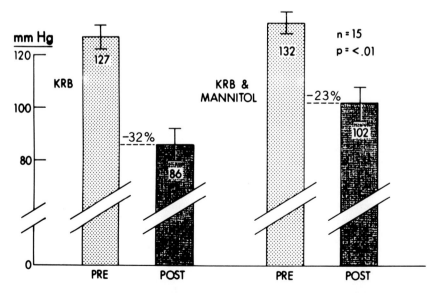

FIG. 2. Effect of mannitol on left ventricular systolic peak pressure. A significant difference in systolic pressure is noted with mannitol when the aerobic period ("pre": prior to anoxia) is compared with the recovery period ("post": after anoxia).

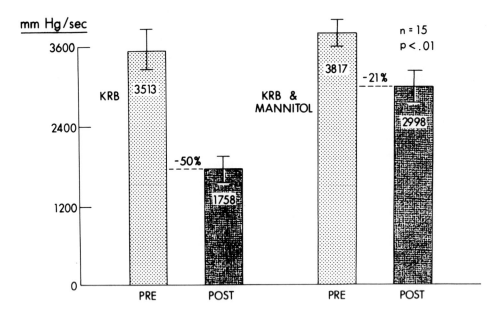

FIG. 3. Effect of mannitol on left ventricular maximum dP/dt. Maintenance of ventricular function during reoxygenated recovery is noted with mannitol.

Carbohydrate Metabolism

Mean lactate production during aerobic isosmolal perfusion with KRB alone was 0.57 ± 0.16 m moles/min. Production increased to 3.05 ± 0.53 m moles/min during anoxic perfusion with a switch to an aerobic metabolism and returned to approach control during the reoxygenated recovery period (0.78 ± 0.13 m moles/min) (Fig. 4). The use of the hyperosmolal perfusate did not alter lactate metabolism at any phase of the study. Production was 0.81 ± 0.12 m moles/min in period (I), 3.04 ± 0.26 m moles/min in period (II) and 1.07 m moles/min in period (III) (p = NS).

Glucose consumption did not differ significantly at either level of osmolality. With isosmolal buffer, consumption was 61 ± 13 m moles/min during control aerobic perfusion and remained at 61 ± 17 m moles/min despite total cessation of contractile activity during anoxia. With aerobic recovery, consumption fell to 36 ± 20 m moles/min. During hyperosmolal perfusion, glucose consumption was 59 ± 11 m moles/min in period (I) 54 ± 13 m moles/min in period (II) and 40 ± 10 m moles in period (III) (P = NS).

Tissue glycogen concentration was 103 ± 11 μ moles/g dry wt. during aerobic perfusion with isosmolal buffer. During anoxic perfusion it fell to 41 ± 5 μ moles/gdw and remained close to this level during aerobic recovery (43 ± 4 μ moles/gdw) (Fig. 5). Hyperosmolality per se did not affect glycogen concentration. It was 93 ± 10 μ moles/g dry wt. during period (I), 37 ± 1 μ moles/gdw during period (II), and 47.7 ± μ moles during period (III) (p = NS).

Tissue High-Energy Phosphate

Hyperosmolality did little to alter the depletion of myocardial high-energy phosphate during anoxia nor its repletion during reoxygenated recovery. Creatine phosphate (CP) levels of 28.1 ± 1.4 μ moles/gdw during isosmolal aerobic perfusion fell to negligible levels (0.3 ± 0.1 μ moles/gdw) during anoxia and rose to 20.6 ± 3.0 μ moles/gdw. CP concentrations obtained with hyperosmolal buffer were (I) 29.4 ± 6.5, (II) 0.2 ± 0.05, and (III) 24.6 ± 3.0 μ moles/gdw (P = NS) (Fig. 6). Tissue ATP concentrations showed a qualitatively similar change. With isosmolal buffer, ATP levels were (I) 20.1 ± 1.3, (II) 10.1 ± 1.1, (III) 8.47 ± 1.2 μ moles/g dry wt. Hyperosmolal perfusion did not significantly improve this balance nor did it significantly alter ADP or AMP concentrations (Fig 7.)

Myocardial Tissue Water Content

The presence of hyperosmolal mannitol significantly affected total tissue water content during all three phases of perfusion (Fig. 8). Tissue wet/dry weight ratio with isosmolal perfusion

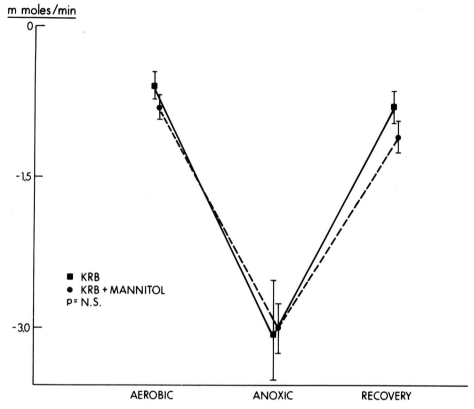

FIG. 4. Comparison of total lactate production during the three perfusion periods. No significant differences are noted with mannitol perfusion.

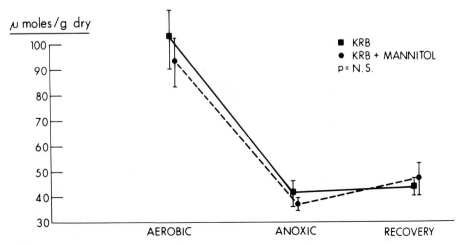

FIG. 5. Comparison of tissue glycogen levels with and without mannitol present. No significant difference between the two perfusates are observed during the three periods of study.

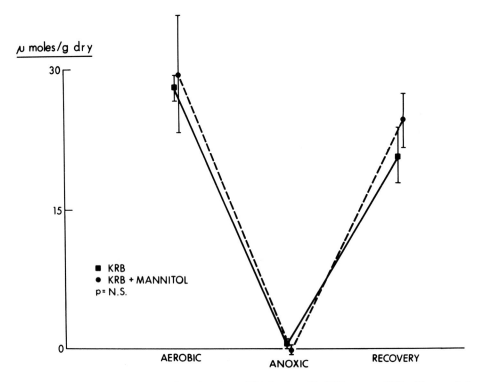

FIG. 6. Comparison of tissue creatine phosphate (CP) levels with KRB versus KRB with mannitol. Total depletion of CP is seen in both groups during anoxia and a similar degree of high-energy phosphate repletion is noted during recovery.

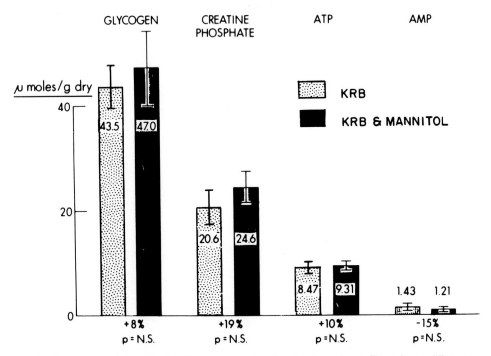

FIG. 7. A summary of tissue metabolic studies during the recovery phase. There is no difference in glycogen, creatine phosphate, ATP, AMP with or without mannitol.

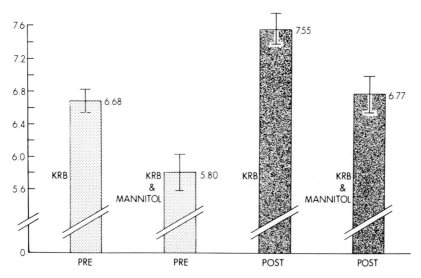

FIG. 8. Effect of mannitol on myocardial water content as judged by wet weight/dry weight ratios. Mannitol totally prevented the increase in wet weight/dry weight ratio seen in its absence during anoxic perfusion. Note also the decrease in the ratio when mannitol is present during the aerobic period.

during period (I) was 6.68 ± 0.41, rose to 7.48 ± 0.56 (p < 0.01) during anoxia and remained elevated throughout the recovery period (7.55 ± 0.17). Hyperosmolal perfusion reduced the ratio during aerobic perfusion (5.80 ± 0.26). Myocardial water content during anoxic perfusion was significantly less than that with isosmolal buffer and remained fixed during recovery (6.77 ± 0.19, p < 0.01). A similar change toward control levels was also noted when mannitol was added only during the recovery period.

Electron Microscopic Studies

The submicroscopic appearance of rat myocardium after aerobic perfusion was unremarkable in both the KRB- and mannitol-treated groups and revealed only scattered degenerative foci (Fig. 9 and 10). After anoxic perfusion with KRB, severe ultrastructural changes were noted (Fig. 11). Marked mitochondrial edema, vacuolization, disruption of cristae, and extraction of the matrix to an electron-lucent configuration were observed. Myofibrillar swelling, focal myolysis, fusion, and contraction were also evident. Varying degrees of subsarcolemmal edema, junctional disruption of the intercalated disc, and focal endothelial cell changes were also observed with only minimal improvement noted following reoxygenated perfusion (Fig. 12).

The presence of hyperosmolal mannitol during anoxia significantly reduced the severity of the aforementioned mitochondrial and myofibrillar al-

terations (Fig. 13), and ultrastructure often appeared to be indistinguishable from normal controls in sections taken during the recovery period (Fig. 14).

DISCUSSION

The importance of intracellular volume regulation has been emphasized by Leaf,[9] and the physiologic significance of cell swelling has recently been reviewed.[10] His postulation that intracellular edema may play a critical role during acute oxygen deprivation and that prevention of cellular swelling might have a beneficial effect on organ function is provocative and has stimulated much current interest.

In both brain and kidney, infusion of hyperosmolal solutions has been shown to improve function following an ischemic insult.[1,5] The demonstration by Willerson et al[14] of reversal of depressed ventricular function in the postcoronary ligated dog heart extended these observations to the myocardium and suggested a new therapeutic modality for the treatment of acute myocardial infarction. Improved ventricular performance was associated with a reduction in the area of ischemic injury as detected by epicardial ST segment maps and by an increase in both total and collateral coronary blood flow. It was suggested the induced obligatory extracellular hyperosmolality improved regional perfusion by a reduction of endothelial cell swelling and an increase in patency of ar-

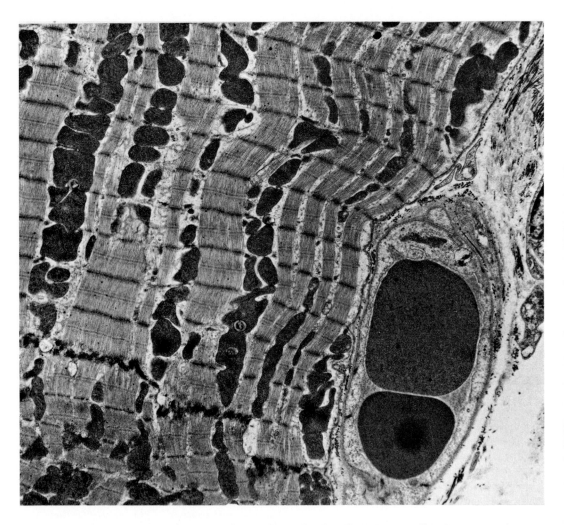

FIG. 9. Normal rat heart fixed immediately after extirpation. Normal myocardial ultrastructure is observed. Myofibrils and mitochondria are in register and the intercalated disc is well defined. ×7400

terioles and capillaries or by a direct reduction in coronary arteriolar resistance. Other studies by Caulfield et al[2] have demonstrated marked mitochondrial swelling and distortion of cristae following acute hypoxia in mammalian papillary muscle. These ultrastructural changes were prevented by increasing the ambient osmolality, and it was postulated that improved myocardial function during hypoxia resulted from enhanced oxidative phosphorylation and energy production by the maintenance of mitochondrial conformation.

Our results are in agreement with those of Willerson et al[14] and demonstrate improved recovery of hemodynamic function following anoxia in the isolated perfused rat heart when perfusate osmolality was raised by 60 milliosmoles either before or after an anoxic insult. We were, however, unable to demonstrate any differential increase in

total coronary flow during hyperosmolal perfusion at either high or low pO_2.

These findings may be explained by the use of different animal models and experimental design. In the absence of formed blood elements, capillary entrapment was, of course, not possible. Furthermore, a reversal of capillary and arteriolar endothelial cell-swelling sufficient to improve flow might well have been masked by the gross nature of the coronary flow measurement utilized or by the marked arteriolar vasodilatation induced by acute anoxia. Silicone rubber injection studies of the microcirculation (not illustrated) also failed to demonstrate any difference in vessel caliber during hyperosmolal perfusion.

If enhanced regional perfusion or an improvement in oxidative phosphorylation due to maintenance of mitochrondial structure did ac-

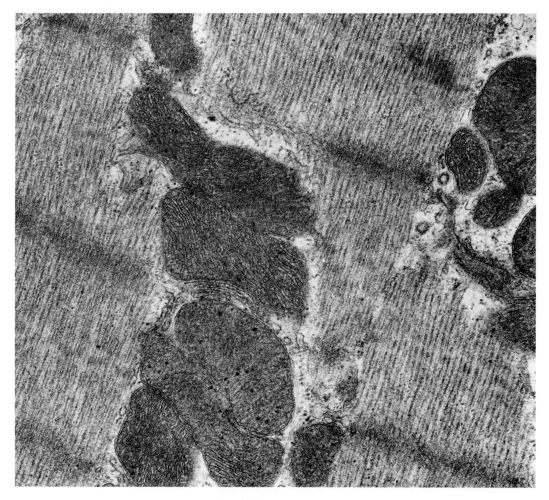

FIG. 10.   Isolated rat heart control aerobically perfused with mannitol. Note the dense pleomorphic mitochondria with rows of closely packed cristae. ×36000

count for the effects of hyperosmolal mannitol, the severe effects of anoxia on carbohydrate metabolism and high-energy phosphate production should have been partially prevented. In fact, there was no significant biochemical improvement noted with mannitol during anoxia after recovery. ATP and CP stores remained depleted and glucose and glycogen utilization depressed. Thus, the improvement in hemodynamic performance induced by hyperosmolality did not appear to be related to a similar improvement in myocardial energetics.

It was of note that mannitol appeared to be protective against severe ultrastructural damage even in myocardial samples taken immediately after anoxia despite the almost total depletion of tissue ATP and glycogen stores noted in both KRB and mannitol-treated groups. Thus, significant dissociation between preservation of mitochondrial

and myofibrillar structure and their functional capability was present in this model, as emphasized in a recent review by Ferrans and Roberts.[4] These findings are in contrast to those of other investigators utilizing isolated subcellular systems where maintenance of mitochondrial form was generally associated with preservation of organelle function.[6,12]

Koch-Weser[8] has suggested that the inotropic effect of hyperosmolality was related to loss of fiber water with a relative increase in intracellular Ca^{++} concentration in those areas of the muscle fiber in which Ca^{++} plays an essential role in excitation-contraction coupling. This passive increase in Ca^{++} concentration might be particularly important during oxygen deprivation where intracellular calcium is markedly diluted and the normal contractile response to this ion, already bur-

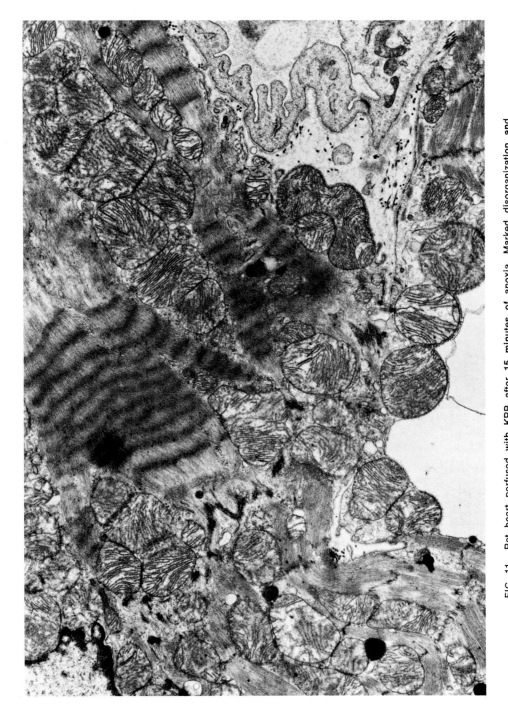

FIG. 11. Rat heart perfused with KRB after 15 minutes of anoxia. Marked disorganization and edema of cellular constituents is observed. Mitochondrial swelling, disruption of cristae, and extraction of matrix is seen. Myofibrillar fusion, contraction bands, and dense bodies are seen in the sarcoplasm. ×11600

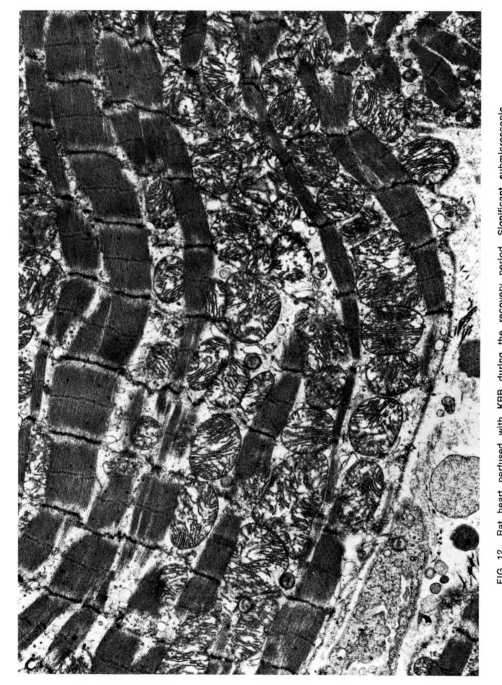

FIG. 12. Rat heart perfused with KRB during the recovery period. Significant submicroscopic alterations persist despite reoxygenation. Swelling of mitochondria and the subsarcolemma, fraying of myofilaments and focal endothelial cell changes are still evident. ×12000

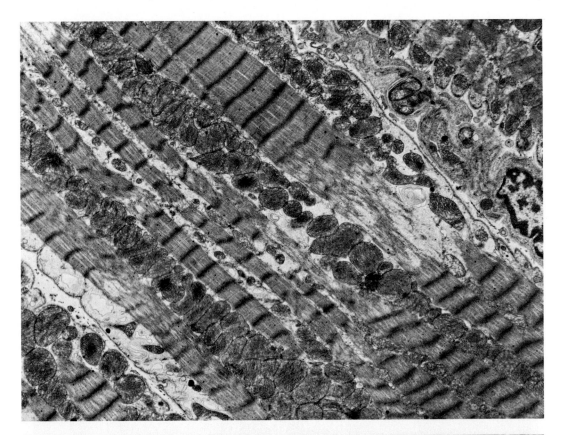

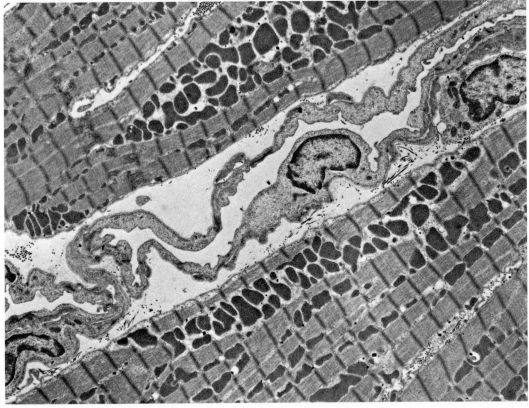

FIG. 13. Top left: Rat heart treated with mannitol after 15 minutes of anoxia. A substantial reversal of the previously described mitochondrial and myofibrillar alterations is seen, although foci of severe subcellular change are also present. ×6500

FIG. 14. Bottom left: Rat heart perfused with mannitol during reoxygenated recovery following acute anoxia. A striking improvement in submicroscopic conformation is noted appearing almost identical to control hearts. ×6000

dened by competition with hydrogen ion for contractile binding sites, is lessened. This hypothesis is supported by Willerson's studies [14] of the inotropic effect of hyperosmolality in isolated cat papillary muscles during increasing Ca^{++} concentrations. Prior elevation of Ca^{++} above a critical level abolished the inotropic action.

A direct osmotic effect on myocardial tissue water content appears to be a primary factor in the mechanism of action of hyperosmolal mannitol. There was a positive correlation between reduction in wet/dry weight ratio and enhanced mechanical performance during the improved recovery of period II when mannitol was present and osmolality raised. This effect may reflect an improvement in compliance due to a reduction in tissue water content, a more favorable intracellular milieu due to stabilization of subcellular membranes and/or a passive increase in Ca^{++} concentration as cell volume is reduced.

It was of interest that despite a significant reduction in myocardial water content during the aerobic control period, no improvement in ventricular function resulted. This suggests that there is an optimal myocardial cell volume at which maximum function is obtained; further reduction in cell size will not induce additional improvement. At the critical volume, crowding of cell constituents may occur and friction between parallel sliding contractile elements may result.

Thus, these findings would support the thesis that mannitol protects myocardium deprived of oxygen resulting in maintenance of structural integrity and improvement of hemodynamic performance. Further investigation of the mode of action of hyperosmolal agents in improving left ventricular function following anoxia or ischemia is required. The clinical applicability of an agent that acutely increases serum osmolality and expands extracellular fluid volume during or following an episode of myocardial ischemia remains to be determined.

References

1. Ames A, Wright RL, Kowada M, Thurston JM, Majno G: Cerebral ischemia: the no-reflow phenomenon. Am J Pathol 52:437, 1968
2. Caulfield JB, Willerson JT, Weisfeldt ML, Powell WL: Effect of mannitol on mitochondrial morphology in hypoxic myocardium. In Dhalla NS (ed): Myocardial Metabolism, Vol 3. Baltimore, University Park Press, 1974, p 753
3. Erlandson RA: A new Maraglas, DER 732, embedment for electron microscopy. J Cell Biol 22:704, 1964
4. Ferrans VJ, Roberts WC: Myocardial ultrastructure in acute and chronic hypoxia. Cardiol 56: 144, 1971/72
5. Flores J, DiBona D, Beck C, Leaf A: The role of cell swelling in ischemic renal damage and the protective effect of hypertonic solute. J Clin Invest 51:118, 1972
6. Hackenbrock CR: Chemical and physical fixation of isolated mitochondria in low energy and high energy states. Proc Natl Acad Sci 61:598, 1968
7. Kadas T, Opie LH: Isolated perfused rat heart adapted for simultaneous measurement of left ventricular contraction, electrocardiogram and metabolism of 14C-labelled substrates. J Physiol (Lond) 167:6, 1963
8. Koch-Weser J: Influence of osmolality on contractility of mammalian myocardium. Am J Physiol 204:957, 1963
9. Leaf A: Regulation of intracellular fluid volume and disease. Am J Med 49:291, 1970
10. Leaf A: Cell swelling—a factor in ischemic tissue injury. Circulation 48:455, 1973
11. Sandborn E, Koen PJ, McNabb JD, Moore G: Cytoplasmic microtubules in mammalian cells. J Ultrastruct Res 11:123, 1964
12. Weinbach EC, Garbus J, Sheffield HG: Morphology of mitochondria in the coupled, uncoupled and recoupled states. Exp Cell Res 46:129, 1967
13. Willerson JT, Crie JS, Adcock RC, Templeton GH, Wildenthal K: The influence of calcium on the inotropic effect on cardiac muscle of hyperosmolar agents. (Abstract) Clin Res 21:460, 1973
14. Willerson JT, Powell WJ, Guiney TE, Stark JJ, Sanders CA, Leaf A: Improvement in myocardial function and coronary blood flow in ischemic myocardium after mannitol. J Clin Invest 51:2989, 1972

13

SHIFTS IN MYOCARDIAL LDH ISOZYME PATTERNS DURING CHRONIC CARDIAC ISCHEMIA IN MAN

Graeme L. Hammond, Joseph Lewis,
Bernardo Nadal-Ginard, and Clement L. Markert

Cardiac muscle, which contains a highly developed mitochondrial apparatus for aerobic metabolism, poorly tolerates acute periods of hypoxia or anoxia. Under normal conditions, breakdown of substrate in the Krebs Cycle produces hydrogen ions that are delivered to the cytochrome system with the generation of ATP, CO_2, and H_2O and the subsequent release of energy (Fig. 1).

During periods of acute anoxia, or when energy demands exceed oxygen supply, the heart, like other muscle tissue, is able to rely on the anaerobic breakdown of glucose as a source of energy.[1] During anaerobic glycolysis, the conversion of glyceraldehyde-3-phosphate to 1-3-diphosphoglycerate requires the removal of hydrogen ions from glyceraldehyde-3-phosphate. These hydrogen ions are attached to coenzyme nicotinamide adenine dinucleotide (NAD) and so converts oxidized NAD to reduced $NADH_2$.

However, in order for glycolysis to proceed in the absence of oxygen, $NADH_2$ must itself be oxidized so that a fresh supply of NAD is again free to accept hydrogen ions from glyceraldehyde-3-phosphate. This occurs at the last step of the glycolytic pathway, ie, the conversion of pyruvate to lactate. This reaction, which is mediated by LDH, causes the hydrogen ions on $NADH_2$ to be delivered to pyruvic acid with the formation of lactic acid and oxidized NAD (Fig 2). The purpose of lactic acid, therefore, is to provide a temporary reservoir for the storage of hydrogen ions until oxygen again becomes available. Because of the adverse effect on rhythm and contractility, however, the accumulation of lactic acid in cardiac muscle has much more serious consequences than its accumulation in skeletal muscle. The enzyme responsible for the conversion of pyruvic acid to lactic acid, and its possible role in chronic cardiac ischemia, is the subject of this chapter.

Lactate dehydrogenase is distributed in virtually all vertebrate cells in five isozymic forms. The physiochemical analysis of LDH shows that it is a tetramer composed of four equal sized subunits. These tetramers can be dissociated into the A + B (or M + H) polypeptides. Combinations of these two monomeric subunits into the tetramers generates the standard LDH pattern of isozymes:[2]

LDH-1	LDH-2	LDH-3	LDH-4	LDH-5
A_0B_4	A_1B_3	A_2B_2	A_3B_1	A_4B_0

Tissues relying primarily on aerobic metabolism, such as the heart, have a preponderance of LDH-1 or B subunits, whereas cells that have a great capacity for anaerobic metabolism, such as skeletal muscle, have predominantly LDH-5 or A subunits (Fig 3). Since the relative amounts of these isozymes are a function of the relative rates of synthesis and degradation, it is conceivable that changes in the cellular environment such as protracted tissue ischemia, could induce shifts in the relative concentrations of these isozymes in order to favor anaerobic metabolism.

METHOD

Ten patients undergoing aortocoronary artery saphenous vein bypass grafts had small muscle specimens which were excluded by the left ventricular drain stitch examined. Care was taken to avoid inclusion of scar tissue in the sample. To serve as controls, left ventricular myocardial specimens were also obtained at post-mortem

Supported by a grant from the Fanny E. Ripple Foundation and the National Science Foundation.

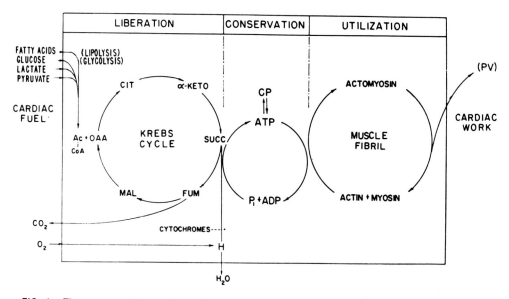

FIG. 1. The energy pathway of aerobic metabolism. From Olson and Piatnek: Conservation of energy in cardiac muscle. Ann NY Acad Sci 72:466, 1959.

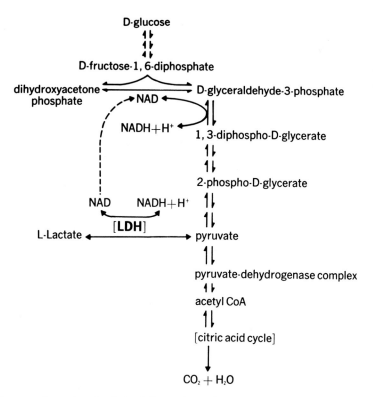

FIG. 2. Energy pathway for glycolysis. Scheme shows the points where NAD is reduced to $NADH_2$ and where $NADH_2$ is oxidized to form NAD and lactic acid. The latter step is mediated by LDH.

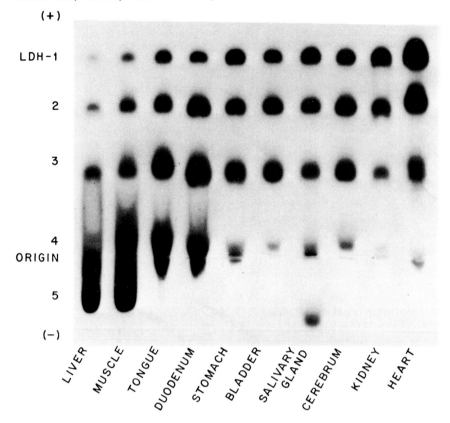

FIG. 3. Zymogram showing LDH profile of various organs. Those with a well-developed oxidative energy delivery system having more LDH-1 while those with a less well-developed oxidative system having more LDH-5.

examination from 10 previously healthy trauma victims. The age distribution was 16 to 38 years (mean 28 years), and no evidence of cardiac injury was apparent at autopsy. The specimens were homogenized in phosphate buffer, and the soluble proteins were separated by centrifugation. The supernatant, containing LDH, was electrophoresed on a cellulose acetate membrane, and the five isozymes were identified by a tetrazolium staining procedure.[3] Quantitative measurements of each isozyme were then made by spectrophotometric scanning of the stained isozymes and the proportion of A and B subunits calculated.

RESULTS

The percentages of each subunit, A or B, for the control and experimental groups, are presented in Table 1. The mean percentage of A monomers in the total LDH sample for control hearts was 12.9 percent (sd 3.1) while the percentage for ischemic hearts was 17.0 percent (sd 4.7) with a p value of 0.04. This represented a

TABLE 1. The Percentage of A and B Subunits of LDH in Control and Ischemic Hearts

SUBJECT	CONTROL GROUP		ISCHEMIC GROUP	
	A Units	B Units	A Units	B Units
1	12.0	88.0	17.2	82.8
2	10.0	90.0	18.5	81.5
3	12.2	87.8	17.4	82.6
4	10.0	90.0	12.8	87.2
5	15.4	84.6	21.0	79.0
6	12.5	87.5	10.0	90.0
7	15.0	85.0	15.3	84.7
8	10.0	89.2	18.0	82.0
9	11.4	88.6	13.4	86.6
10	20.0	80.0	27.0	73.0

mean increase of 33.6 percent in A subunits in ischemic hearts when compared to controls (Fig. 4).

DISCUSSION

While the synthesis of LDH subunits is under genetic control and seems fixed once ma-

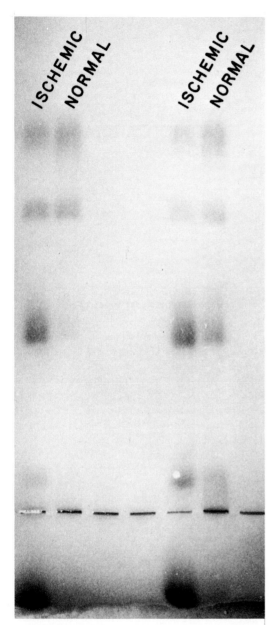

example, it is recognized that the isozymic distribution of mammalian heart LDH in the relatively hypoxic conditions of fetal life lies predominantly in the A band (LDH-5) or that which functions best in the presence of large amounts of lactate.[4] At birth, however, when an adequate oxygen supply becomes readily available, the distribution of isozymes shifts toward the LDH-1 form, or that characteristic of the aerobic pattern.

The LDH-1 form, found in tissues operating primarily by aerobic metabolism, is readily inhibited by accumulations of lactic acid and thus converts little pyruvate to lactate. In the heart, this is of crucial importance and, in fact, helps insure the survival of the species.

The question is whether, under the powerful stress of severe, chronic ischemia, the fully developed adult heart can revert to a system of glucose metabolism that will favor lactic acid production. This question is far too complex to be answered by this experiment. However, since energy produced by the Krebs Cycle is restricted in hypoxia and, since glycolysis cannot proceed without some method of hydrogen ion disposal, it follows that the heart, in order to maintain viability for itself and its parent organism, would need to adapt.

The data derived from this experiment lends support to the theory that, under the influence of prolonged stimuli, gene function in cardiac muscle can be reprogramed in such a way that continued muscle function is made possible. Interestingly, the observed shifts in LDH isozyme composition show only a partial shift toward that of greater lactic acid production. The contracting cells of the ischemic heart apparently attempt to achieve a balance between enough energy production for survival but not so much that survival is jeopardized by lactic acid accumulation.

References

FIG. 4. Photograph of a cellulose acetate membrane with typical zymogram showing control heart on the right and ischemic heart on the left.

turity of the cell is achieved, it is possible that cellular environment might induce changes in gene activity to produce shifts in isozyme patterns to facilitate a more efficient use of substrate. For

1. Cornblith M, Randle PJ, Parmeggiani A, and Morgan ME: Regulation of glycogenolysis in muscle. J Biol Chem 238:1592–97, 1963
2. Markert CL, Whitt GS: Molecular varieties of isozymes. Experientia 24:977, 1968
3. Markert CL, Moller F: Multiple forms of enzymes: tissue ontogenetic and species specific patterns. Proc Nat Acad Sci 45:753, 1959
4. Zinkham WH, Blanco A, Kupchyk L: Isozymes: biological and clinical significance. Pediatrics 37: 120–31, 1966

14

METABOLIC INFLUENCES UPON HYPOXIC CARDIAC FUNCTION: EFFECT OF GLUCOSE AND GLYCOLYSIS ON CONTRACTILITY

CARL S. APSTEIN

INTRODUCTION

Hypoxia is the heart's "energy crisis." The myocardium responds to the oxygen shortage by increasing the rate of glycolysis with an increased utilization of glucose and glycogen, and production of lactic acid. The effect of the accelerated glycolytic rate is to increase the rate of adenosine triphosphate (ATP) synthesis by this anaerobic pathway; thus more ATP can be synthesized without increasing oxygen consumption. However, in order to generate this additional ATP, the myocardial cell may pay the price of intracellular acidosis due to the increased formation of lactate.

Nevertheless, despite the presence of ischemia, glycolysis does not approach its theoretical maximum in the myocardial cell (Opie, 1970). This limitation on the glycolytic rate may be a protective mechanism that prevents an excess of intracellular acidosis from occurring, or it may be a consequence of a feedback regulation that is beneficial under physiologic, well-oxygenated conditions but is actually self-defeating when the heart becomes hypoxic, a "turning-off" of glycolysis at a time when the heart needs it the most in order to generate ATP.

The evidence to date suggests that with myocardial hypoxia the benefit of an increased ATP synthesis, with an acceleration of glycolysis, outweighs the deleterious effects of acidosis, and the net result is one of increased contractility. However, if tissue lactic acidosis becomes too severe, the net effect may be a loss of contractility. The purpose of this chapter is to review some studies relating to this question.

EFFECT OF INCREASED MYOCARDIAL GLYCOGEN

An increase in substrate for the glycolytic pathway is generally associated with better hypoxic cardiac performance. The presence of large amounts of myocardial glycogen, which is an endogenous substrate for glycolysis, is associated with increased tolerance to hypoxia. Turtle hearts, which have considerably more glycogen than mammalian hearts, are particularly resistant to hypoxic deterioration (Bing et al, 1972). When rat hearts were treated with reserpine to increase their glycogen content, they tolerated hypoxia better than controls (Scheuer and Stezoski, 1970). Secondly, when iodoacetate, which blocks glycolysis, is added to turtle ventricular muscle strips or rat papillary muscle, the tolerance to hypoxia is markedly diminished (Bing et al, 1972).

The effect of hypoxia on turtle and rat heart isolated muscle in the presence and absence of glucose and iodoacetate is shown in Figure 1. The panel on the left shows that when turtle heart ventricular strips were made hypoxic, developed tension fell to about 50 percent of the prehypoxic control value after 60 minutes (Bing et al, 1972). The addition of glucose did not affect the performance of the turtle heart muscle. However, blocking glycolysis with iodoacetate resulted in a rapid fall in developed tension. The panel on the right shows the effect of hypoxia on rat papillary muscle. The rat papillary did not perform as well as the turtle heart muscle even when 100 mg percent glucose was added. In the absence of glucose, the rat heart muscle functioned more poorly, and

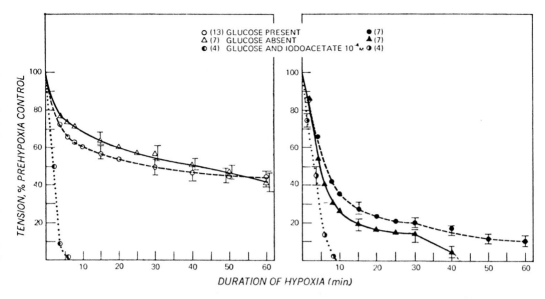

FIG. 1. Effect of Hypoxia on Tension Development in Isolated Turtle Ventricular Strips (left panel) and Rat Papillary Muscle (right panel). At time = 0 the muscle bath was switched from 95 percent O_2 — 5 percent CO_2 to 95 percent N_2 — 5 percent CO_2 (from **Bing** et al, 1972).

when iodoacetic acid was added, there was a rapid fall in tension, as in the turtle heart.

Thus, this study showed that both the turtle and rat heart are dependent upon glycolysis with hypoxia since blocking glycolysis with iodoacetate led to rapid deterioration in both species. The greater glycogen content of the turtle heart appeared to give it the ability to tolerate hypoxia better than the rat heart, which had less endogenous glycolytic substrate.

EFFECT OF INCREASED EXOGENOUS GLUCOSE CONCENTRATION

Further elucidation of the effect of glycolytic substrate on hypoxic cardiac muscle comes from papillary muscle studies where the exogenous glucose concentration was increased (Apstein and Levine, 1972). The experimental question was whether a high exogenous glycolytic substrate (glucose) in the rat papillary muscle preparation could substitute for the high endogenous glycolytic substrate (glycogen), which is native to the turtle.

The results of this study are summarized in Figure 2. Rat papillary muscles were incubated in either 100 (□) or 400 mg percent (O) glucose, or 100 mg percent glucose plus 300 mg percent

mannitol (Δ); in this last group equiosmolar mannitol was substituted for the additional glucose in order to separate any osmotic effect of the additional glucose from a metabolic one.

After a control period, the muscles were made severely hypoxic by gassing the muscle baths with 95 percent N_2 —5 percent CO_2, so that the bath pO_2 was less than 5 mm Hg. The muscles were kept hypoxic for two hours and then reoxygenated.

The higher glucose level (400 mg percent) allowed for significantly better tension development during hypoxia and with reoxygenation. Substitution of equiosmolar mannitol for the additional glucose did not increase contractility. Thus with 400 mg percent glucose, the papillary muscles maintained 24 percent of tension development after two hours of severe hypoxia, and recovered to 75 percent of control levels with reoxygenation. The most striking effect of the higher glucose concentration was to preserve the functional integrity of the papillary muscle during the two hours of hypoxia. Thus recovery with reoxygenation was more dramatic compared to controls, than maintenance of developed tension during hypoxia.

Isolated rat papillary muscles characteristically develop contracture or rigor with severe hypoxia. Figure 3 shows the effect of glucose concentration and mannitol on contracture tension,

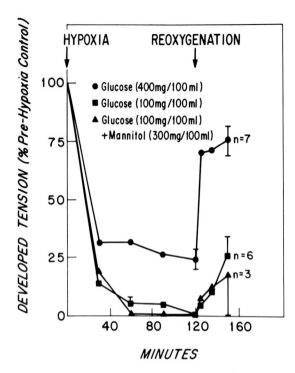

FIG. 2. Effect of Glucose and Mannitol on Developed Tension in Isolated Hypoxic Rat Papillary
Muscles (after Apstein and Levine, 1972). Rat papillary muscles were incubated in 400 mg percent glucose (O), 100 mg percent glucose ($\square$), or 100 mg
percent glucose and 300 mg percent mannitol ($\triangle$).
At time = 0 the bath gassing mixture was switched
from 95 percent O_2 — 5 percent CO_2 to 95 percent
N_2 — CO_2 to induce severe hypoxia ($pO_2 < 5$). After
two hours the bath was reoxygenated. The higher
glucose concentration resulted in greater tension
development during hypoxia and after reoxygenation.
Substitution of equiosmolar mannitol for the additional glucose had no significant effect.

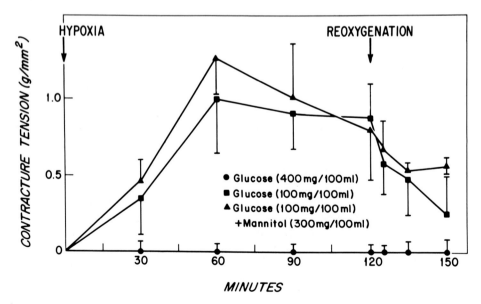

FIG. 3. Effect of Glucose and Mannitol on Contracture Tension (after Apstein and Levine, 1972).
Symbols and protocol are those of Figure 2. The 400 mg percent glucose concentration completely
prevented the development of contracture; substitution of equiosmolar mannitol for the additional
glucose did not provide any protection against contracture.

which is the increase in resting tension that occurs during the hypoxic period. Hypoxia was associated with significant development of contracture with 100 mg percent glucose (□), but with 400 mg percent glucose as substrate (O) no contracture occurred. Substitution of mannitol for the additional glucose (Δ) did not provide any protection against the development of contracture.

Reoxygenation resulted in partial reversal of contracture. The rate of decline of contracture tension with reoxygenation was not affected by mannitol. Comparison with Figure 1 shows that contracture development is associated with poor recovery following reoxygenation. The muscles in 100 mg percent glucose, with or without mannitol, all developed severe contracture and had poor recovery with reoxygenation; in contrast, muscles in 400 mg percent glucose did not develop contracture and had good recovery with reoxygenation.

Thus the effect of increasing the exogenous glucose concentration from 100 mg percent to 400 mg percent, an increase that could be tolerated clinically, was to sustain partial tension development during two hours of severe hypoxia, to protect the heart from contracture during hypoxia, and to increase markedly the recovery of tension development with reoxygenation. Despite the added glucose, however, developed tension of the rat papillary muscle with hypoxia was only half as great as with the hypoxic turtle heart muscle strip.

Thus, these studies on the rat papillary muscle provide evidence that increasing the glycolytic substrate increases the tolerance of cardiac muscle to hypoxia. The fact that equiosmolar mannitol did not provide any benefit to the papillary muscles suggests that the benefit of the added glucose was due to a metabolic rather than osmotic mechanism. However, we could not prove this hypothesis since the minute size of these papillary muscles precluded metabolic measurements of their glycolytic rate.

However, anaerobic glycolysis has been correlated with hypoxic ventricular performance (Weissler et al, 1973). These workers studied rat hearts that were perfused with glucose concentrations from 50 to 500 mg percent with and without insulin. Figure 4 shows the effect of adding insulin (100mH/ml) to a substrate of 200 mg percent glucose under anaerobic conditions. The rate of glycolysis increased, as manifested by the increased rate of lactate production. Hemodynamic measurements made simultaneously with this metabolic intervention showed that the increased lactate production was associated with a higher level of left ventricular systolic pressure and left ventricular dP/dt. Thus, in these experiments, the increase in glycolysis caused by insulin resulted in improved hemodynamic performance under anaerobic conditions, suggesting that the increased glycolytic synthesis of ATP had a beneficial effect that outweighed any increased acidosis associated with the increase in lactate production.

The effect of increasing the perfusate glucose concentration, in the presence of insulin, on the anaerobic rate of glycolysis (as manifested by the rate of lactate production) and on simultaneous anaerobic left ventricular pressure development is shown in Figure 5 (after Weissler et al, 1973).

Maximum left ventricular performance is achieved at an exogenous glucose level of 100 mg percent. However, lactate production continues to rise at higher glucose concentrations, suggesting that above a certain level of glycolysis the additional increase in glycolytic ATP may be balanced by the deleterious effect of the acidosis associated with the increase in lactate production. An alternative explanation would be that the additional ATP generated is used for processes other than contractility, such as for fatty acid synthesis.

Hence, the evidence thus far would indicate that increasing anaerobic glycolysis is beneficial to myocardial performance, with the qualification that above a certain level, an increased glycolytic rate does not progressively increase contractility.

EFFECT OF ISCHEMIA VS. HYPOXIA

Further evidence that too much glycolysis is not good for the oxygen-deprived heart comes from studies in the isolated rat heart that was made ischemic by decreasing the coronary flow (Rovetto et al, 1973) in contrast to the previous work cited (Weissler et al, 1973), where coronary flow had been maintained, and coronary perfusate pO_2 was reduced (hypoxia).

A major consequence of the ischemic mechanism was to decrease the wash-out of tissue lactate, with intracellular lactate levels increasing markedly during the ischemic period. After eight minutes of ischemia, tissue lactate had increased sixfold and left ventricular performance had markedly diminished. Adding insulin and high glucose levels increased glycolysis and increased tissue lactate concentrations but did not affect ventricular performance (Rovetto et al, 1973).

In summary, the studies reviewed demonstrate that increasing glycolytic metabolic support

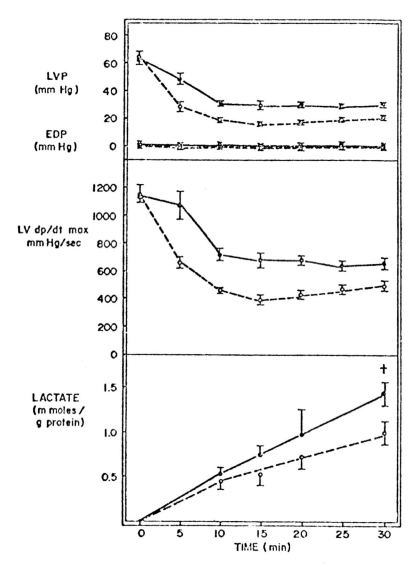

FIG. 4. Effect of Insulin on Glycolysis and Contractility in the Isolated Perfused Rat Heart (from Weissler et al, 1973). At time = 0 the rat heart is switched from an oxygenated perfusate to an anaerobic one. Glucose (200 mg percent) is present as substrate with insulin (100 mU/ml, solid line) or no insulin (dashed line). The presence of insulin increased the glycolytic rate, as manifested by the increase in lactate production; the increased glycolysis was associated with better ventricular pressure development and dP/dt.

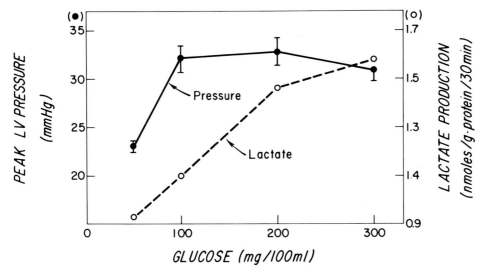

FIG. 5. Effect of Glucose Concentration on Anaerobic Glycolysis and Contractility (after Weissler et al, 1973). Isolated rat hearts were made anaerobic as in Figure 4. Glucose was provided, at the concentrations shown, in the presence of insulin (100 mU/ml). Maximum left ventricular pressure development occurs at a glucose concentration of 100 mg percent. Further increases in the level of provided glucose increase the rate of lactate production but do not significantly affect hemodynamic performance.

increases contractility in the oxygen-deprived myocardium. However, above a certain rate of glycolysis, no further increase in contractility occurs. The failure of contractility to parallel glycolytic rate at higher glycolytic fluxes may be due to accumulation of tissue lactate and acidosis. The net effect of glycolysis on the oxygen-deprived myocardium may depend on the extent of coronary flow that removes the glycolytic end-product, lactic acid.

References

Apstein CS, Levine HJ: Protective effect of moderate hyperglycemia in myocardial hypoxia. Circulation (Suppl II to V, 45 and 46): II-125, 1972

Bing OHL, Brooks WW, Inamdar AN, and Messer JV: Tolerance of isolated heart muscle to hypoxia: turtle vs. rat. Am J Physiol 223:1481, 1972

Opie LH: The glucose hypothesis: relation to acute myocardial ischemia. J Mol Cell Cardiol 1:107, 1970

Rovetto MJ, Whitmer JT, and Neely JR: Comparison of the effects of anoxia and whole heart ischemia on carbohydrate utilization in isolated working rat hearts. Circ Res 32:699, 1973

Scheuer J, Stezoski SW: Protective role of increased myocardial glycogen stores in cardiac anoxia in the rat. Circ Res 27:835, 1970

Weissler AM, Altschuld RA, Gibb LE, Pollack ME, and Kruger FA: Effect of insulin on the performance and metabolism of the anoxic isolated perfused rat heart. Circ Res 32:108, 1973

15

REVERSAL OF ABNORMAL MYOCARDIAL METABOLISM (LACTATES) AFTER CORONARY ARTERY BYPASS GRAFTS

Robert G. Carlson, Nadya Keller,
and C. Walton Lillehei

INTRODUCTION

Successful coronary artery bypass grafts were demonstrated by electromagnetic flow meter studies (Fig. 1) and by postoperative angiography (Fig. 2). Initial graft patency was 92 percent at two weeks, and 90 percent of these patent grafts remained patent at one year (Carlson, Baltaxe, et al, 1971).

There has been some doubt as to the significance of blood flow and angiographic studies. Myocardial lactate metabolism has been considered an objective parameter for determining successful revascularization of the myocardial cells. In this study arterial and coronary sinus lactate levels were measured at rest and during electrical pacing of the right atrium. Successful patent coronary artery bypass grafts were associated with more "normal" postoperative lactate levels compared with "abnormal" levels during preoperative stress testing. Occlusion of a graft was associated with lactate levels failing to return toward normal.

METHOD

Patients with coronary artery disease and normal controls were subjected to cardiac stress by means of right ventricular or right atrial pacing. They were selected by clinical history, electrocardiogram (ECG), and angiographic evidence of coronary artery disease and myocardial ischemia. Patients with atypical signs and symptoms in whom the ECG at rest and after ergometric stress testing had been proved equivocal were also included.

TIMING OF STUDIES

Patients were sedated mildly on the evening prior to study and one hour before catheterization. Sodium citrate solution (0.5 percent) in isotonic saline by slow catheter drip was the sole anticoagulant used. Routine right and left heart catheterizations were performed. The catheters were placed in the midportion of the coronary sinus, the left ventricle, the right atrium, and the aorta in order to permit sampling and pacing, along with pressure and flow recording, during the study. Aortic pressure and ECG were monitored throughout the study (Fig. 3). Arterial and coronary sinus samples were drawn at rest for determination of glucose and lactate controls. Pacing was begun after 35 minutes of steady state performance and was raised to the original threshold, or to 2 to 2.5 times the resting ischemic state. Sampling was repeated at 3, 6, 9, and 15 minutes of pacing. Cardiac output and ventricular pressures were determined intermittently during the increased rate. Lactate determinations were performed by the Auto Analyser method of Apstein, Puchner, et al (1970). The determination of lactate is based on its enzymatic conversion to pyruvate in the presence of nicotinamide adenine dinuclueotide (NAD+), diphospho-pyridine nucleotide (DPN+), and lactic dehydrogenase (LDH). The fluorescence of the NADH (DPNH) produced by this reaction is measured

FIG. 2 Facing page: Angiogram 2 weeks post-operative shows quadruple coronary artery bypass with 2 veins (one side-to-side LAD and end-to-side circumflex lateral marginal, and the other side-to-side right and end-to-side posterior marginal).

FIG. 1. Electromagnetic blood flows recorded at coronary artery bypass graft operation. The median blood flow was 65 ml per graft. The distal runoff appears to determine the amount of blood flow. Larger flows were noted in coronary arteries supplying larger areas of myocardium and when the least amount of myocardial scarring was present. The blood flow was similar with vein grafts, direct internal mammary artery anastomoses, or when 1 vein was anastomosed to 2 coronary arteries (end-to-side and side-to-side). Maximum mammary artery flow was 120 ml/minute whereas maximum vein graft flow was 250 ml/minute.

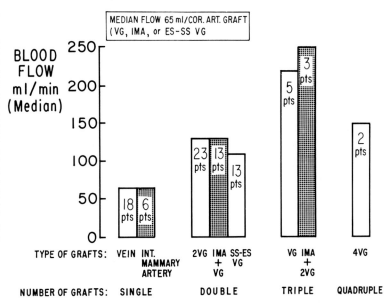

MEDIAN FLOW 65 ml/COR. ART. GRAFT
(VG, IMA, or ES-SS VG

BLOOD FLOW ml/min (Median)

TYPE OF GRAFTS: VEIN | INT. MAMMARY ARTERY | 2VG | IMA + VG | SS-ES VG | VG IMA + 2VG | 4VG

NUMBER OF GRAFTS: SINGLE | DOUBLE | TRIPLE | QUADRUPLE

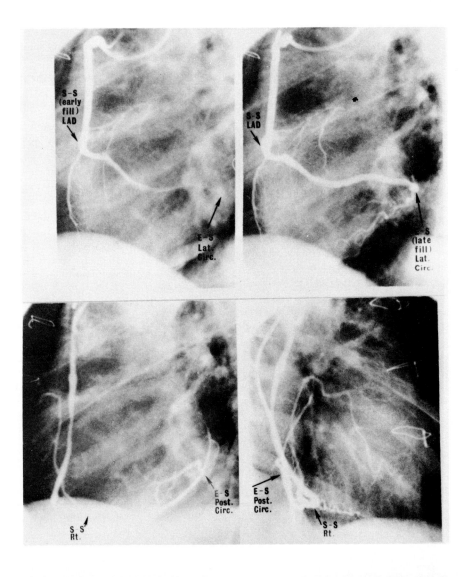

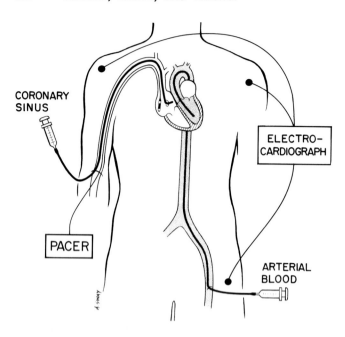

FIG. 3. Model for lactate measurements during rest and ventricular work produced by right atrial electrical pacing. Left ventricular and coronary sinus catheters are placed for aspirating blood samples. Ischemic changes are recorded on the electrocardiogram. From Carlson et al (1972).

after excitation of the molecule by a 355 mμ light source. Immediate initial deproteinization of the aspirated blood sample is imperative. This is accomplished by mixing equal amounts of sample solution with 0.6 N perchloric acid (PCA). The denaturized sample then can be refrigerated and stored until processed in the Auto Analyzer. The coefficient of variation of duplicate plasma determinations is less than 2 percent. A sample of only 0.03 ml is required if the specimen has been previously deproteinized with 0.6 N PCA. Glucose determinations were made also.

In electrocardiographic studies the amount of ST depression was measured as an index of myocardial ischemia.

The patients were restudied at 48 hours, two weeks, and three or six months postoperatively. The 48-hour postoperative study was performed using a temporary epicardial wire, a transatrial coronary sinus catheter and a radial artery cannula (Gianelli, Conklin, et al, 1968). The disposable Landé-Edwards membrane oxygenator provided effective, safe, total cardiopulmonary support during the revascularization operations (Carlson, Landé, et al, 1973).

PATIENT SELECTION

Control Subjects

Two patients with normal coronary arteriograms had normal lactates at rest and after pacing.

Preoperative Coronary Artery Disease

There were 11 patients who had a mean age of 50 years. All but one were males. In six, metabolic lipid disorders could be demonstrated. In only one was the ECG within normal limits. Eight demonstrated changes that were diagnostic of previous myocardial infarction or of myocardial ischemia. Five presented with a clinical history of myocardial infarction. In three, voltage changes of left ventricular hypertrophy were noted. All patients showed moderately severe degenerative changes in the coronary cineangiogram (over 75 percent stenosis).

Postoperative Coronary Artery Bypass Vein Grafts

The postoperative group was composed of six patients with studies prior to and following bypass surgery. Preoperative electrocardiographic abnormalities of the ischemic type were present in all six; three of these showed a previous myocardial infarction and one, a positive ergometric stress test. In two patients, the ECG was within normal limits. Angiography revealed significant multivessel disease in all. The ventriculogram was normal in half of this group. Multiple vein grafts were placed in all patients. Postoperative angiography demonstrated that the grafts remained patent in all but two patients. One had an occluded graft to a large left anterior descending coronary artery but a patent small right coronary artery graft. The other had a reverse situation—the patent graft supplied a large LAD and the occluded graft a small right coronary artery distribution.

RESULTS

Preoperatively, the heart rate was increased by pacing 2 to 2.5 times the resting rate, or else to the onset of angina. Hemodynamic studies of cardiac index and "effort" index increased with pacing in almost all patients indicating increased cardiac external work and increased oxygen demand as previously reported (Beer, Keller, et al, 1972). Pacing caused an immediate significant increase in lactate production, which was related to the severity of the coronary artery disease as evaluated clinically (symptoms, electrocardiograms, coronary arteriograms, and hemodynamic or symptomatic response to pacing).

Under resting-fast conditions the aortocoronary sinus levels (A-CS) indicated normal lactate extraction in all but one of 13 patients and were comparable to normal controls. With the onset of pacing, mean A-CS levels indicated lactate production in eight of eleven (73 percent) of the patients with angiographic evidence of coronary artery disease. In both normals (100 percent), and in 3 of 11 (27 percent) patients with angiographic evidence of coronary artery disease, the lactates continued to be extracted normally (Fig. 4). Such changes in extraction-production due to the progressive increase in CS lactate concentrations after onset of pacing exceeded controls by 95 percent within 10 minutes (p < 0.01).

Postoperative studies were completed on five patients after angiographic and clinically successful aortocoronary artery bypasses with reversed saphenous vein grafts. Each patient had two vein grafts, anastomosed between the ascending aorta and the left anterior descending coronary artery, and the right coronary artery. The first patient, in whom lactates were tested 48 hours postoperatively, had an occluded vein graft to a small but dominant right coronary artery when selective angiograms were performed two weeks postoperatively. The other nine vein grafts were patent at angiography performed two weeks to two months postoperatively. Each patient with patent grafts had clinical relief of angina. The patient with one occluded and one significant patent graft had decreased, but definitely persistent, angina.

Electrocardiographic onset of ST depression

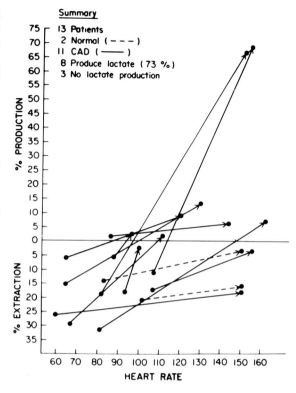

FIG. 4. Lactate metabolism before operation. During ventricular pacing note the ischemic lactate production in 8 to 11 (73 percent) patients with coronary artery disease. Note normal lactate extraction during pacing in the two normal patients and in 3 to 11 (27 percent) patients with significant coronary artery disease confirmed by angiography. From Carlson et al (1972).

correlated fairly well with the onset of angina during preoperative pacing. Postoperatively, the absence of angina during pacing correlated well with the absence of ST depression and the absence of lactate production.

CASE REPORTS

Example: Return of ST Depression and Lactate Production to Normal

CASE 1: *P. McD., a 61-year-old man with angina and prior myocardial infarction, received a double-vein bypass graft. Preoperatively the arterial coronary sinus lactate difference indicated 41 percent extraction at rest and 8 percent production during electrical pacing to a rate of 150. Two weeks postoperatively the lactates showed normal extraction of 47 percent during pacing at a heart rate of 150. Ischemic ST changes present preoperatively were absent postoperatively.*

Example: Correlation of Lactate Improvement with One Occluded and One Patent Vein Graft

CASE 2:   F.D., *a 48-year-old man with angina and two prior myocardial infarctions, had 6 percent lactate extraction at rest and 4 percent production during pacing before operation. Two days after double-vein bypass operation, 8 percent of the lactate was extracted both at rest and during pacing. Two weeks postoperatively, selective angiography indicated a patent vein graft to the large left anterior descending coronary artery but an occluded vein graft to the small but dominant right coronary artery.*

Example: Angiographic and Metabolic Improvement

CASE 3:   H.G., *a 61-year-old male, had a four-year history of shortness of breath on exertion. Five years prior to admission, he was hospitalized for 43 days for a well-documented myocardial infarction. Progressive shortness of breath now occurred with minimal exertion and was associated with severe episodes of anginal pain. Six months earlier he was hospitalized for severe chest pain. The SGOT enzyme elevation confirmed clinical evi-*

dence of a second myocardial infarction. Five to six daily episodes of progressive angina persisted until his present hospital admission. Physical examination was normal. The serum cholesterol level was elevated to 287 mg/100 ml and triglycerides to 178 mg/100 ml. The electrocardiogram suggested a healed posterior myocardial infarction. Right and left heart catheterization was performed preoperatively. Pacing to a rate of 150/minute resulted in anginal pain, a rise in left ventricular end-diastolic pressure, ST segment depression in the lateral precordial leads and arterial-coronary sinus lactate production. Coronary angiography demonstrated double vessel stenosis. The patient underwent double aortocoronary bypass with reversed saphenous vein autografts. His postoperative course was uneventful. Two weeks later, pacing at 150/minute resulted in no angina and no ST segment depression. The patient could walk a mile and climb a flight of stairs without symptoms during the following year. Vein graft angiograms two weeks and six months postoperatively were normal.

CASES 4 and 5:   *Two other patients, J.S., 47 years old, and C.R., 54 years old, had similar histories of angina and prior myocardial infarctions; they were treated by successful double aortocoronary artery bypasses with vein grafts. Their lactate studies are outlined with the other examples (Fig. 5).*

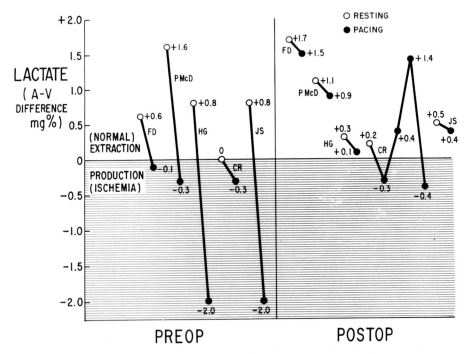

FIG. 5.   Individual preoperative and postoperative artery coronary sinus lactate differences in 5 patients during rest (control) and right ventricular pacing (ischemic stress). Note preoperative pacing produces ischemic lactate levels, whereas postoperatve levels show normal extraction except in part of one study (C.R.) From Carlson et al (1972)

The average values of these five pre- and postoperative lactate studies are diagramed (Fig. 6). Note the production of lactate in all five patients during preoperative pacing. Postoperative pacing resulted in continued normal lactate extraction in four patients. The fifth patient, C.R., had both lactate extraction and production at various times during postoperative pacing.

Example: Correlation of Angiograms and Metabolism. (Occluded Graft Associated with Angina and Failure of Lactate "Improvement")

CASE STUDY: *A 46-year-old male, had progressive angina following a questionable myocardial infarction 1.5 years prior to admission for coronary artery bypass graft. Resting electrocardiogram was normal. Selective coronary arteriogram indicated an occluded right coronary artery with good retrograde filling of the distal right. The anterior descending coronary was occluded prior to the first septal branch. The distal LAD filled retrograde from the circumflex artery. The latter vessel was jeopardized by severe stenosis of the proximal large lateral marginal artery, and mild stenosis of the proximal circumflex artery. The ventriculogram showed normal contractility. The left ventricular end-diastolic pressure was normal (11 mm Hg).*

On November 6, 1970, two vein grafts were anastomosed to the LAD and the right coronary. Postoperative angiography indicated a patent vein graft to the LAD but an occluded vein graft to
the right coronary artery. The circumflex artery was not bypassed. (During the past three years, we would have performed a triple graft).

Lactate studies were performed preoperatively, three days postoperatively, and six months postoperatively (Fig. 7). Failure of "improvement" of lactate production during pacing was recorded postoperatively. Persistent angina, ST elevations with exercise to a heart rate of 125, and lactate production were similar before and six months after bypass operation. We interpret these results to indicate that inadequate (occluded grafts) or incomplete surgery (omitting circumflex graft) was the cause of postoperative ischemia.

DISCUSSION

Theory: Lactate Metabolism

The primary metabolic disturbance in myocardial anoxia or ischemia is related to an inadequate supply of oxygen to convert substrates into carbon dioxide and water and a shift to an anaerobic metabolism, with the end product being lactic acid. The heart normally extracts 20 to 40 percent of the lactic acid in the arterial blood converting it into CO_2 and water, but during anoxia this pathway is no longer available and lactic acid is produced by the heart either from endogenous glycogen or from glucose (Case, Nasser, et al, 1969). Production of lactic acid by the anoxic or ischemic heart has been shown in man during angina (Krasnow and Gorlin, 1963). Effective myocardial revascularization would be expected to reverse this anaerobic metabolism.

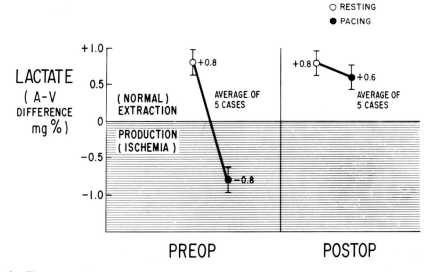

FIG. 6. The average lactate study in 5 patients demonstrated ischemic production of lactate during preoperative pacing but normal lactate extraction during postoperative pacing. From Carlson et al (1972).

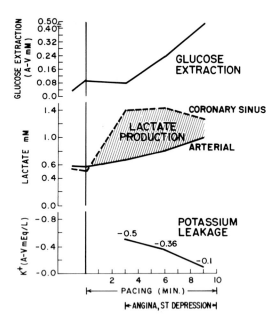

FIG. 7. The failure of lactate improvement toward normal aerobic metabolism was associated with an occluded coronary artery bypass graft.

Opie et al (1971) discussed the value of measuring lactates in the evaluation of coronary artery ischemia. Forrester, Gorlin, and associates demonstrated that heart rate increased by electrical pacing has minimal effects upon other hemodynamic indices and arterial substrate concentrations, thus providing a considerable advantage over exercise and isoproterenol as a relatively uncomplicated form of myocardial stress (Forrester, Helfant, et al, 1971).

Revascularization procedures are aimed at restoring flow to ischemic tissue; they clearly have nothing to offer a zone of necrotic tissue in the infarction. The potential contribution of the surgical treatment of coronary insufficiency, therefore, should be evaluated most properly in functional terms. Coronary cineangiography offers an invaluable tool for visualizing the vascular changes that are causal to this degenerative process. It also permits the surgeon to determine the patency of the bypass, but it cannot provide an answer to the critical question of whether there has been an improvement in the adequacy of myocardial oxygenation. When considered in these terms, it is evident that correction of a hemodynamic abnormality is not synonymous with improvement in nutritional vascular supply to ischemic tissue. Electrocardiographic stress testing and functional parameters calculated from data obtained at car-

diac catheterization come closer to the mark but remain several stages removed and are reflections of what is occurring at the cellular level.

We are primarily concerned with restriction of coronary vascular reserve: Studies performed during a loading stress permit us to make some quantitative estimation of this reserve, regardless of the method utilized. *Surprisingly little information can be obtained from studies performed at rest. Atrial pacing has proven particularly valuable in studies of myocardial metabolism.* Electrically stimulated increases in heart rate represent a significant myocardial stress but have minimal effects on hormonal and neural factors and on arterial substrate concentration (Forrester, Helfant, et al, 1971). When pacing exhausts coronary reserve, and neither coronary flow nor oxygen extraction can be increased to meet the demands of the stress, an ischemic state is established. Normal metabolic pathways for energy production no longer prove adequate and the cell must switch metabolic gears. An enhancement of anaerobic glycolysis, of glycogenolysis, and of changes in fatty acid metabolism occurs and is reflected in the blood perfusing the ischemic tissue. Maximal anaerobic metabolism may make a significant contribution to the maintenance of viability of the borderline ischemic cell although it cannot maintain the adenosine triphosphate requirement of the normally working heart (Most, Gorlin, et al, 1972). Direct surgical revascularization of the ischemic myocardium is clearly an attractive approach to a difficult problem facing the physician today.

SUMMARY

Techniques for the objective evaluation of the degree of myocardial ischemia are discussed in relation to the applicability of the saphenous vein aortocoronary bypass procedure for myocardial revascularization. These methods apply equally as diagnostic means of establishing the existence of myocardial ischemia in patients who demonstrate equivocal signs, symptoms, electrocardiographic, or angiographic findings. The importance of stress loading to determine reduction in coronary vascular reserve is emphasized. Metabolic studies permitted us to define those patients with angina pectoris who have signs of significant myocardial ischemia (Brachfield, Apstein, et al, 1973).

Left ventricular coronary sinus lactic acid levels were measured during a resting (control) and an electrically paced (ischemic stress) state to angina or to a heart rate of 2 to 2.5 times normal. Preoperatively, lactates in 13 patients averaged 0 to 8 mg/100 ml extraction at rest and 0.8 mg/100 ml production during pacing. Double aortocoronary artery bypass with vein grafts were performed for symptoms of angina or prior myocardial infarction. Two days to two months postoperatively, five patients averaged 0.8 mg/100 ml lactate extraction at rest and 0.6 mg/100 ml extraction during pacing. Postoperative relief of angina and improvement in ST depression correlated well with angiographic evidence of vein graft patency and aerobic lactate extraction. Severe ischemic changes noted in one postoperative patient were associated with an occluded vein graft.

The studies have provided a framework for the objective evaluation of patients considered for remedial surgery.

References

Apstein CC, Puchner E, and Brachfeld N: Improved automatic lactate determination. Anal Biochem 38: 20, 1970

Beer N, Keller N, Kline S, Tarjan E, Carlson RG, and Brachfeld N: The cardiac hemodynamic and metabolic responses to coronary arterio-venous bypass surgery. Am J Cardiol 29:252, 1972

Brachfeld N, Apstein CW, Beer N, Keller N, Carlson RG, and Kline S: Myocardial metabolic response to revascularization. In Corday E and Swan HJC (eds): Myocardial Infarction—New Perspectives in Diagnosis and Management. Baltimore, William and Wilkins Co, 1973, pp 344–56

Carlson RG, Baltaxe H, Levin D, Apstein C, Brachfeld N, Killip T, and Lillehei CW: Surgical treatment of coronary artery insufficiency. NY State Med 71:14, 1721–26, 1971

Carlson RG, Lande AJ, Landis B, Rogoz B, Baxter J, Patterson RH Jr, Stenzel K, and Lillehei CW: The Landé-Edwards membrane oxygenator during heart surgery. J Thorac Cardiovasc Surg 66:6, 894–905, 1973

Carlson RG, Kline S, Apstein C, Scheidt S, Brachfeld N, Killip T III, and Lillehei CW: Lactate metabolism after aorto-coronary arteryvein bypass grafts. Ann Surg 176:680–85, 1972

Case RG, Nasser MH, and Crampton RS: Biochem aspects of early myocardial ischemia. Am J Cardiol 24:766, 1969

Forrester JS, Helfant RH, Pasternac A, Amsterdam EA, Most AS, Kemp HG, and Gorlin R: Atrial pacing In coronary artery disease. Am J Cardiol 27:237, 1971

Gianelli S, Jr, Conklin EF, Ayres SM, Mueller H, and Gregory J: Coronary sinus cannulation at surgery for postoperative myocardial metabolic studies. Ann Thorac Surg 5:371, 1968

Krasnow N, and Gorlin R: Myocardial lactate metabolism in coronary insufficiency. Ann Intern Med 59:781, 1963

Most AS, Gorlin R, Soeldner JS: Glucose extraction by the human myocardium during pacing stress. Circulation 45:92, 1972

Opie LH et al: Value of lactates. Europ J Clin Invest 1:295, 1971

16

CLINICAL INTRAOPERATIVE CORONARY ARTERY SAPHENOUS VEIN BYPASS PRESSURE-FLOW RELATIONSHIPS

Keith Reemtsma, Eduardo N. Parodi, David Bregman,
Richard N. Edie, Frederick O. Bowman, Jr.,
and James R. Malm

The advent of myocardial revascularization surgery [6,7,8,14] has created the need for an increased understanding of alterations in coronary artery pressure-flow patterns. The present study was designed to investigate three areas of clinical intraoperative coronary artery hemodynamics:

1. The flow capacity of the coronary arterial system distal to a saphenous bypass graft. This is a function of perfusion pressure and arterial resistance. The estimate of flow at varying coronary perfusion pressures permits an estimate of the capacity of the coronary vascular bed at physiologic levels.
2. The determination of the relation between right and left saphenous vein graft peak flows and the aortic pulse trace. This would establish whether the saphenous vein graft has modified the normal phasic coronary flow pattern.
3. The effects of unidirectional dual-chambered intraaortic balloon pumping on intraoperative coronary graft flows. The flows were evaluated before and during assisted circulation.

METHODS AND MATERIALS

Sixty-two vein grafts in 38 patients were studied at the Columbia-Presbyterian Medical Center between November 1971 and March 1973. The saphenous veins were obtained from the distal lower extremity. Cardiopulmonary bypass was established using a nonhemic prime and a Temptrol bubble oxygenator.* The distal end-to-side saphenous vein coronary artery anastomosis was performed under hypothermic anoxic arrest or induced ventricular fibrillation using a continuous suture technique.[5] A coronary artery perfusion cannula was then inserted in the proximal end of the saphenous vein graft (Fig. 1). Oxygenated blood from the heart-lung machine was perfused through the graft using a calibrated occlusive roller pump. The graft flow was increased in increments of 20 ml/minute until the mean pressure in the perfusion line reached 90 to 100 mm Hg. Electromagnetic flow probes † were placed around the vein grafts, and flows were measured simultaneously by both the roller pump and the flow probe. The increments in flow were correlated with the observed pressure changes within the system. A pressure-flow curve was constructed.[15] A representative pressure-flow curve is illustrated in Figure 2. The proximal aortic-saphenous vein anastomosis was then completed and cardiopulmonary bypass was discontinued. Electromagnetic flow probe measurements were then repeated with the functioning bypass graft, and simultaneous mean pressure was recorded. Similar pressure-flow studies were performed before and after the use of Papaverine in nine of these patients. Papaverine (10 mg) was injected directly into the vein graft during a continuous recording period.

Supported in part by National Institutes of Health Research Grant #HL 12738

* Bentley Laboratories, Inc., Santa Ana, Calif.
† Carolina Medical Electronics, Winston-Salem, N.C.

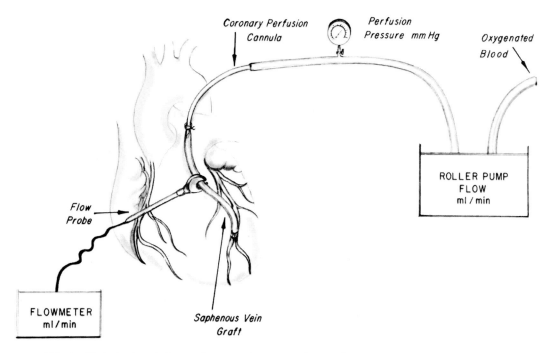

FIG. 1. Method of perfusing saphenous vein graft during cardiopulmonary bypass. The perfusion cannula is inserted in the proximal end of the saphenous vein graft. An electromagnetic flow probe was placed around the vein graft and flow was measured simultaneously by both the probe and the roller pump. These measurements were then correlated with pressure changes within the system.

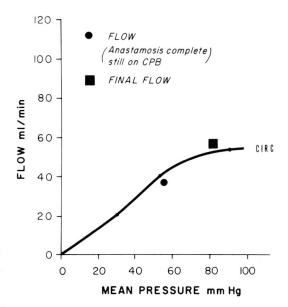

FIG. 2. An example of a pressure-flow curve for the circumflex coronary artery graft. The curve was constructed by increasing perfusion pressure in 30 mm Hg increments. The heavy black dot represents the final mean graft flow after the completion of the proximal anastomosis while the patient is still on cardiopulmonary bypass. The black square denotes the observed mean graft flow off bypass when the patient was hemodynamically stable. Note that when both of these flows are plotted on the pressure-flow curves they correlate nearly 100 percent.

In a separate study, after the termination of cardiopulmonary bypass, phasic flow patterns were observed in 12 additional patients (20 grafts) by means of an electromagnetic flow probe. Right and left graft flow tracings were recorded simultaneously with the aortic pulse pressure curve. The timing of the peak graft flow was related to the phase of the cardiac cycle.[9]

Similar flow measurements in coronary grafts were recorded in five patients[4] during intraoperative unidirectional dual-chambered balloon pumping.*[1,2,3] The balloon was inserted through a 10-mm Dacron side arm graft through the common femoral artery and was positioned in the aorta just distal to the left subclavian artery. Left radial pulse was monitored continuously, and right and left coronary flows were measured with and without intraaortic balloon pumping.

RESULTS

The correlation of the predicted mean saphenous vein bypass graft flow from the pressure-flow curve constructed by this method with the observed saphenous vein flow at the completion of

* Datascope System 80, Datascope Corp., Paramus, N.J.

cardiopulmonary bypass can be seen in Figure 3. All of the 62 graft flows measured cluster around the 100 percent correlation line, with a correlation coefficient of 0.931. This observation demonstrates the accuracy with which one can predict the final saphenous vein graft flow, before the proximal coronary anastomosis is completed. The average mean graft flow in this group of patients, after the termination of cardiopulmonary bypass, was 70ml/minute for the right coronary artery (range: 15 to 200 ml/minute); in the left anterior descending coronary artery it averaged 66ml/min (range 15 to 120 ml/minute); and in the left circumflex coronary artery the average was 58ml/min (range: 20 to 200 ml/minute) (Fig. 4). The administration of Papaverine into the saphenous vein graft resulted in an increase in coronary graft flow of 0 to 35 ml/minute, which was confirmed by both calibrated roller pump and electromagnetic flow probe recordings.

Two clinical examples, which illustrate the usefulness of intraoperative pressure-flow determinations, are presented. Figure 5 illustrates the pressure-flow curve constructed in a 63-year-old man whose angiocardiogram revealed two 70 per-

cent and 80 percent stenoses of his dominant right coronary artery with a good distal right coronary vessel. In addition, he had 60 percent stenosis between the second and third diagonal branches of his left anterior descending coronary artery. The final saphenous vein coronary graft flow, prior to the closure of his chest, fell exactly on the constructed pressure-flow curve. Evaluation of the patient's preoperative angiocardiogram, in conjunction with the intraoperative pressure-flow curve constructed, indicated that the patient had an excellent distal coronary artery bed and that his revascularization would be successful. This indication was borne out by the patient's benign postoperative course.

Figure 6 illustrates the pressure-flow curve constructed in a 42-year-old hypertensive male with severe diffuse triple vessel coronary artery disease and a left ventricular aneurysm. His preoperative clinical course was complicated by recurrent bouts of angina pectoris, a myocardial infarction, and severe congestive heart failure. The cardiac catheterization data revealed marked dilatation of the left ventricle associated with a massive apical aneurysm. In addition, there was

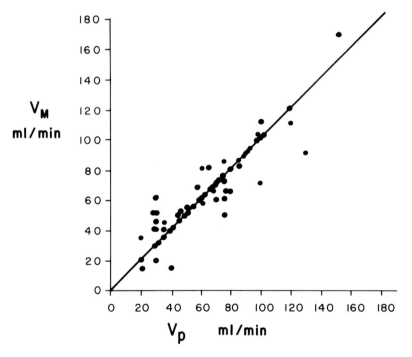

FIG. 3. The predicted mean saphenous vein bypass graft flow is plotted against the observed saphenous vein graft flow at the completion of cardiopulmonary bypass. The black line represents 100 percent correlation between the measured flow and the predicted flow (correlation coefficient: 0.931). The black dots to the right of the 100 percent correlation line denote final flows that were smaller than predicted flows, while those to the left indicate flow at the completion of cardiopulmonary bypass greater than predicted. Vp: predicted flow (mean coronary graft flow with the roller pump, while on cardiopulmonary bypass); Vm: measured flow (mean coronary graft flow measured by electromagnetic flow probe, at the termination of cardiopulmonary bypass).

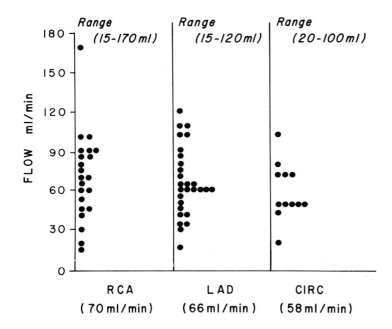

FIG. 4. Mean graft flows in the 38 patients (62 grafts), at the termination of cardiopulmonary bypass. RCA: right coronary artery; LAD: left anterior descending coronary artery; CIRC: circumflex coronary artery.

severe diffuse triple vessel coronary artery disease with poor distal runoff. Urgent surgery was performed, and, after resection of the ventricular aneuysm, saphenous vein grafts were anastomosed to both the left circumflex and right coronary arteries. The low graft flows measured following cardiopulmonary bypass could be predicted on the basis of his constructed pressure-flow curves. Technical limitations to graft flow were therefore ruled out, and low flow in this patient was related to poor runoff with a low-capacity coronary bed. The patient was felt to have a poor prognosis, which was confirmed by a complicated postoperative course associated with intractable ventricular tachyarrhythmias and death.

Phasic flow recordings were made at the termination of cardiopulmonary bypass, when the patient was hemodynamically stable, in 12 additional patients (20 grafts) underdoing aortocoronary saphenous vein bypass grafting (Fig. 7).

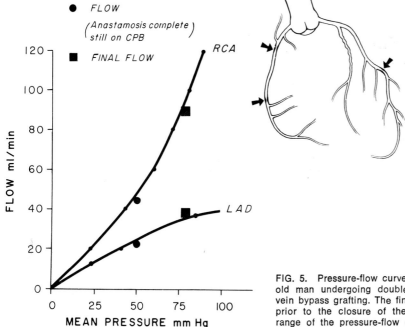

FIG. 5. Pressure-flow curves constructed in a 63-year-old man undergoing double aortocoronary saphenous vein bypass grafting. The final graft flow in both grafts, prior to the closure of the chest, falls in the upper range of the pressure-flow curve.

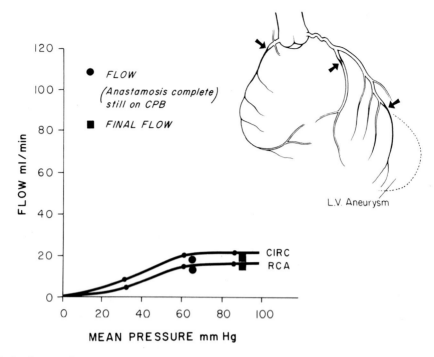

FIG. 6.   Pressure-flow curves constructed in a 42-year-old man with severe diffuse triple coronary artery disease, complicated by a ventricular aneurysm. The flattened contour of these curves correlates significantly with the poor runoff seen angiographically.

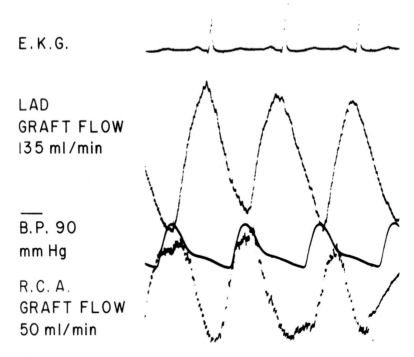

FIG. 7.   Phasic flow patterns in left anterior descending coronary artery (LAD) and right coronary artery (RCA) grafts in a patient undergoing aortocoronary saphenous vein bypass revascularization. Mean blood pressure was measured at the aortic root. The peak phasic flow in the LAD occurs in diastole, but in the RCA the peak flow occurs during systole.

Saphenous vein graft phasic flow patterns consistently showed that peak flow in the left coronary graft occurred during diastole, while peak flow in the right coronary graft occurred primarily during systole.

Coronary graft flow was recorded with and without the effects of counterpulsation with a unidirectional dual-chambered intraaortic balloon pump in five patients. Flows were measured in the patient's vein grafts at the completion of cardiopulmonary bypass (Fig. 8 and 9). There was a 117 percent increase in mean coronary graft flow during intraaortic balloon pumping. The peak increase in coronary graft flow occurred coincident with the diastolic augmentation phase of intraaortic balloon pumping. This diastolic augmentation of flow was seen in both the right and left graft flow tracings.

DISCUSSION

Saphenous vein graft flow is usually measured by an electromagnetic flow probe, at the termination of cardiopulmonary bypass, when the patient is hemodynamically stable.[12,13,16] This technique, though valuable, may leave the surgeon in the undesirable position of reexploring the anastomoses as a consequence of low flow within the graft.[16]

By our previously described method of constructing a pressure-flow curve[15] and correlating direct pressure-flow measurements through the proximal saphenous vein graft with subsequent electromagnetic flow probe confirmation at the termination of cardiopulmonary bypass, the surgeon can determine if the final low graft flow is due to a technical problem or if it is related to poor runoff. This method can therefore be used to aid the surgeon during the operative procedure.

The management of recurrent angina in conjunction with demonstrated graft occlusion[17,18] is influenced by knowledge of the pressure-flow curve. If a patient with a pressure-flow curve demonstrating the existence of a large distal coronary vascular bed has graft occlusion, reoperation is indicated. By the same criteria, reoperation is contraindicated in the presence of a curve indicating a poor coronary vascular bed capacity.

The difference in the phasic flow patterns between the right and left coronary artery grafts was consistent with previously described flow patterns.[9,10,11] This indicates that these phasic flow patterns are not altered either by coronary artery disease or by bypass grafting. In accordance with these findings, the proximal anastomosis of the right coronary artery graft should be constructed to promote systolic flow and hopefully also to reduce both the turbulence at the anastomosis and the possibility of late graft closure. In a

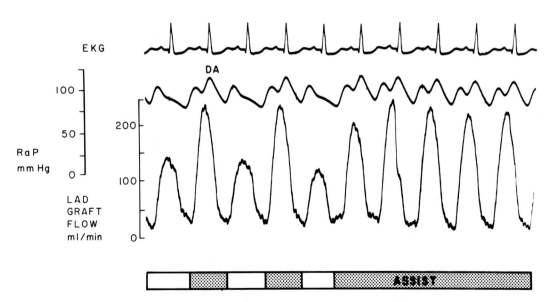

FIG. 8. Unidirectional dual-chambered intraaortic balloon pumping in a patient assisted after aortocoronary bypass graft surgery. With every other beat assisted, there is doubling of the Left Anterior Descending Coronary Artery graft flow. Tracing speed 25 mm/second. EKG: electrocardiogram; RaP: radial artery pressure; LAD: left anterior descending coronary artery; DA: diastolic augmentation.

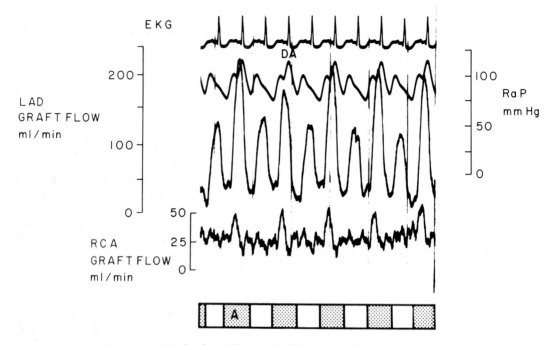

FIG. 9. Unidirectional dual-chambered intraaortic balloon pumping in a patient assisted after aortocoronary bypass surgery. There is a 100 percent increase in both coronary artery vein graft flows during intraaortic balloon pumping. The patient is assisted on every other beat. Tracing speed 10 mm/second. EKG: electrocardiogram; RaP: radial artery pressure; LAD: left anterior descending coronary artery; RCA: right coronary artery; A: assisted period; DA: diastolic augmentation.

similar fashion, the proximal anastomosis of the left coronary graft should be constructed to promote diastolic flow.

Finally, in relation to the use of unidirectional dual-chambered intraaortic balloon pumping, the data clearly indicate that coronary graft flow increases an average of 117 percent after the termination of cardiopulmonary bypass during balloon pumping.[4] It is interesting to observe that the peak flow in both the right and left coronary artery grafts occurs during diastole, which is in contrast to the phasic flow pattern described above for the right coronary artery.

SUMMARY

1. A simple and accurate intraoperative method for saphenous vein coronary artery pressure-flow measurements is described. The pressure-flow curve constructed by this method gives us an early estimate of the patency of the distal anastomosis and resistance in the coronary bed. The predicted flow from this curve correlates well with the graft flow at the termination of the surgical procedure. These flow curves are good indices of the potential flow capacity of the distal coronary bed.

2. The peak right coronary artery graft flow occurs mainly during systole and the flow in the left coronary artery graft peaks in diastole. These flows are physiologically normal in relation to the cardiac cycle.

3. During intraoperative unidirectional dual-chambered intraaortic balloon pumping, phasic graft flows are modified with the peak flow in both right and left coronary artery grafts occurring during diastole. An increase in coronary graft flow during unidirectional intraaortic balloon pumping of 117 percent was recorded.

References

1. Bregman D, Goetz RH: A failsafe cardiac assist system for intra-aortic balloon pumping. Trans Am Soc Artif Intern Organs 18:505, 1972
2. Bregman D, Goetz RH: Clinical experience with a new cardiac assist device—the dual-chambered intra-aortic balloon assist. J Thorac Cardiovasc Surg 62:577, 1971
3. Bregman D, Kripke DC, Goetz RH: The effect of synchronous unidirectional intra-aortic balloon pumping on hemodynamics and coronary blood

flow in cardiogenic shock. Trans Am Soc Artif Intern Organs 16:439, 1970

4. Bregman D, Parodi EN, Reemtsma K, and Malm JR: Abstracts: Coronary Artery Medicine and Surgery Conf., Houston, Tex, Feb 21–23, 1974

5. Cooley DA, Dawson JT, Hallman GL, Sandiford FM, Wukasch DC, Garcia E, Hall RJ: Aortocoronary saphenous vein bypass. Results in 1,492 patients, with particular reference to patients with complicating features. Ann Thorac Surg 16: 380, 1973

6. Cooley DA, Hallman GL, Wukasch DC: Myocardial revascularization using combined endarterectomy and vein bypass autograft: technique and results. Int Surg 56:373, 1971

7. Favaloro RG, Effler DB, Groves LK, Sheldon WC, Sones Jr FM: Direct myocardial revascularization by saphenous vein graft. Ann Thorac Surg 10:97, 1970

8. Favaloro RG, Effler DB, Groves LK, Sheldon WC, Shirey EK, and Sones Jr FM: Severe segmental obstruction of the left main coronary artery and its divisions: surgical treatment by the saphenous vein graft technique. J Thorac Cardiovasc Surg 60:469, 1970

9. Gregg DE: Phasic blood flow and its determinants in the right coronary artery. Am J Physiol 119:580, 1937

10. Gregg DE: Phasic changes in flow through different coronary branches. In Moulton FR (ed): Blood, Heart and Circulation. Washington, D.C.,

American Association for the Advancement of Science, publication 13, 1940, pp 81-93

11. Gregg DE: The Coronary Circulation in Health and Disease. Philadelphia: Lea & Febiger, 1950

12. Grondin CM, Castonguay YR, Lespérance J, Bourassa MG, Campeau L, Grondin P: Attrition rate of aorta-to-coronary artery saphenous vein grafts after one year. Ann Thorac Surg 14:223, 1972

13. Grondin CM, Lesperance J, Bourassa MG, Pasternac A, Campeau L, Grondin P: Serial angiographic evaluation in 60 consecutive patients with aorto-coronary vein grafts 2 weeks, 1 year, and 3 years after operation. J Thorac Cardiovasc Surg 67:1, 1974

14. Johnson WD, Flemma RJ, Lepley DJ: Determinants of blood flow in aortic-coronary saphenous vein bypass grafts. Arch Surg 101:806, 1970

15. Merker C, Parodi EN, Bowman FO Jr, Malm JR, Reemtsma K: Saphenous vein coronary artery pressure flow measurement. Simple operating room method. NY State J of Med, March 1, 1973

16. Urschel HC, Razzuk MA, Wood RE, Paulson DL: Factor influencing patency of aortocoronary artery saphenous vein grafts. Surgery 72:1048, 1972

17. Vlodaver Z, Edwards JE: Pathologic analysis in fatal cases following saphenous vein coronary arterial bypass. Chest, 64:555, 1973

18. Walter JA, Friedberg HD, Flemma RJ, Johnson WD: Determinants of angiographic patency of aorto-coronary vein bypass grafts. Circulation 45, 46:86, 1972

17

THE FUNCTIONAL STATE OF THE CORONARY VASCULAR SYSTEM AFTER AORTA-TO-CORONARY BYPASS SURGERY

Robert S. Reneman and Merrill P. Spencer

INTRODUCTION

The beneficial effect of aorta-to-coronary bypass grafts has been demonstrated in several studies. Patent grafts can improve left ventricular function (Manley et al, 1970; Rees et al, 1971; Rutherford et al, 1972), enhance blood flow to the ischemic myocardium (Amsterdam et al, 1970), and enhance aerobic metabolism (Beer et al, 1972). On the other hand increase in severity of proximal coronary artery disease, even to total occlusion (Aldridge and Trimble, 1971; Bousvaros et al, 1972), and regression of intercoronary collateral vessels (Cibulski et al, 1973) have been reported after successful grafts. These observations might explain the finding of Rees and coworkers (1971) that left ventricular function can deteriorate, as compared to preoperative function, when the graft becomes occluded. These findings indicate that, beside their obvious beneficial effects, bypass grafts can create unfavorable situations that are difficult to predict. Therefore, more information is required about the functional state of the coronary vasculature after aorta-to-coronary bypass surgery.

Changes in diastolic reactive hyperemia (DRH) and the instantaneous flow tracing have been proposed as a method to evaluate the coronary vascular system (Reneman and Spencer, 1972). In the present study mean (MBF) and instantaneous (IBF) blood flow through aorta-to-

Supported by the Institute of Environmental Medicine and Physiology, Seattle, Washington, and Netherlands Organization for the Advancement of Pure Research (ZWO).

coronary bypass grafts were measured and the amount of DRH was determined at the completion of the surgical procedure. Special attention was paid to the systolic component of graft flow since animal experiments have shown that the amount of systolic blood flow in the left coronary artery is mainly determined by the inotropic state of the left ventricle (v d Meer and Reneman, 1973). We also investigated whether or not there was a correlation between MBF and, respectively, mean arterial pressure (MAP) and heart rate (HR), both of which are known to be important determinants of coronary blood flow.

METHODS

In 160 patients MBF and IBF through 264 aorta-to-coronary bypass grafts were measured and the DRH-response to a 10-second occlusion was determined. In 258 cases the stenosis was bypassed by a saphenous vein graft and in 6 cases by an internal mammary artery. Patients with single and multiple grafts were included in this study. In case of multiple saphenous vein bypasses, aorta-to-coronary anastomoses were made either by Y-grafts or grafts with separate orifices in the aorta. When Y-grafts were used, the flow to separate arteries was determined by measuring on one leg of the graft. In six cases one leg of the graft was anastomosed to two coronary arteries. Total cardiopulmonary bypass was employed during the period of graft anastomosis. In most cases ventricular fibrillation and mild hypothermia (26–30 C) were induced during the bypass procedure.

The EKG was derived from limb leads. HR was determined from the R-R intervals of the EKG. Arterial blood pressure was measured in millimeters of mercury through a polyethylene catheter in the radial or brachial artery connected to a Statham * pressure transducer (P23 Db or P 23 AA). The blood flow through the grafts was measured with an electromagnetic flow probe (Carolina Medical Electronics †) that was connected to a 240 Hz square-wave or a 500 Hz pulsed-field electromagnetic flowmeter (Carolina Medical Electronics). Zero flow was determined by occlusion of the graft distal to the probe. Mean flow was obtained by RC-damping. The flow probes were calibrated either on bypass grafts after the anastomosis with the aorta or on excised venous segments. In the latter case the veins were perfused with blood and surrounded by air to simulate the circumstances of measuring on implanted grafts. The amount of DRH was calculated from the increase in peak diastolic flow over the initial value following release of the 10-second occlusion and was expressed in percentage of the initial value (percent DRH). The EKG and the analogue pressure and flow signals were recorded on a multichannel recorder (Offner Type R ‡).

The initial measurements were performed under stable hemodynamic conditions 14–30 minutes after cardiopulmonary bypass had been discontinued. In 41 patients the measurements were repeated on 51 grafts 20–164 minutes later, just before closing the thorax. Seven patients had a re-thoracotomy 17 hours to 13 days after the first operation because of complications not related to the graft implantation. In these patients the measurements were repeated on 12 grafts during the reoperation.

Student's t-test was used for the evaluation of statistical significances between the values obtained during the first and second measurements and between the values obtained during the first and second surgical procedure. The correlation coefficients of MBF versus MAP and HR were calculated and the significance of the correlation determined.

RESULTS

Flow measurements were made on grafts to the anterior descending branch (n = 106), the circumflex branch (n = 16), and the marginal branch (n = 5) of the left coronary artery (LAD,

* Statham Instruments, Inc., Los Angeles, Calif.
† Carolina Medical Electronics, Inc., Winston-Salem, N.C.
‡ Beckman Instruments, Inc., Offner Division, Schiller Park, Ill.

LC, and LMg, respectively) as well as on grafts to the main stem (n = 56), and the posterior descending branch (n = 23) of the right coronary artery (RM and RPD, respectively). The remaining measurements (n = 58) were performed on grafts supplying more than one coronary artery. The average values and standard deviations of MAP, HR, MBF, and the amount of DRH in 160 patients are presented in Table 1. When more than one series of measurements was made intraoperatively in one patient, only the last measurements were included in the table. The average MBF through grafts supplying more than one coronary artery was lower than the total average MBF to these arteries, when each artery was perfused by a separate graft.

The amount of systolic flow was usually high in grafts to the right coronary artery (Fig. 1, first row) and low in grafts to the left coronary artery (Fig. 1, third row) but in several cases a low systolic flow component was seen in grafts to the RPD (Fig. 1, second row) and a high systolic flow component in grafts to the left coronary artery (Fig. 1, fourth row).

DRH was present in approximately 80 percent of the measurements. The amount of DRH varied considerably and was 20 percent or less in 40 of the 264 determinations. A marked reactive hyperemia response is shown in Figure 2. During reactive hyperemia, the increase in diastolic flow was usually more pronounced than the increase in inflow at the end of isovolumic contraction, enlarging the peak-to-peak amplitude of the instantaneous flow tracing. The increase in systolic flow shifted the tracing from the base line. In the following, we will refer to these kinds of instantaneous flow curves as dilated instantaneous tracings since they represent a dilated coronary vascular bed.

DRH was absent or inconsiderable in combination with normal (Fig. 3), dilated (Fig. 4), and damped (Fig. 5) instantaneous flow tracings. To our standards damped instantaneous tracings are characterized by a low peak-to-peak amplitude, a shift of the tracing from the base line, and a slow flow increase in early diastole. When the instantaneous tracing appeared damped and no DRH was present, the MBF through the graft could be within normal range (Fig. 5, top half). In the patient shown in this figure, the anastomosis of the graft with the ascending aorta was found to be too narrow. Repair of the anastomosis resulted in improved flow with a dilated but acceptable instantaneous tracing, an increase in MBF and appearance of DRH (Fig. 5, bottom half).

TABLE 1. Average Values and Standard Deviations of Mean Arterial Pressure,
Heart Rate, Mean Flow through Graft, and Amount of Diastolic Reactive Hyperemia
in 160 Patients with Aorta-to-Coronary Bypass Grafts, and Percentage of Measurements
in Which DRH Was Present

RECIPIENT ARTERY	N	MAP (mmHg)		HR (BEATS/MIN)		MBF (ML/MIN)		DRH (%)[a]		DRH (% present)
		$\overline{x}$	s	$\overline{x}$	s	$\overline{x}$	s	$\overline{x}$	s	
LAD	106	96.6	16.4	93.5	18.6	81.3	51.0	38.7	31.2	85
LC	16	95.0	15.1	100.9	21.0	68.1	31.4	41.3	28.6	81
LMg	5	89.4	6.4	92.2	16.7	33.4	24.9	14.6	23.9	40
RM	56	98.1	17.9	92.1	18.7	82.8	59.6	67.7	63.4	88
RPD	23	96.3	14.0	88.5	21.2	69.2	48.0	68.9	68.1	83
Combinations										
LAD + Dg	23	96.0	11.2	103.1	20.4	121.2	54.5	36.1	37.2	83
LAD + LC	5	91.0	12.7	121.2	12.4	98.9	53.2	33.8	26.4	80
RM + LC	17	90.8	15.4	117.1	17.0	132.3	38.1	28.5	17.2	82
RM + LVE + LC	6	99.0	27.3	116.7	20.5	156.8	46.0	12.7	15.3	67
RPD + LC	7	103.0	19.8	93.5	15.9	114.3	33.1	41.3	29.2	86

[a]*Percentage increase in peak diastolic flow over the initial value.*

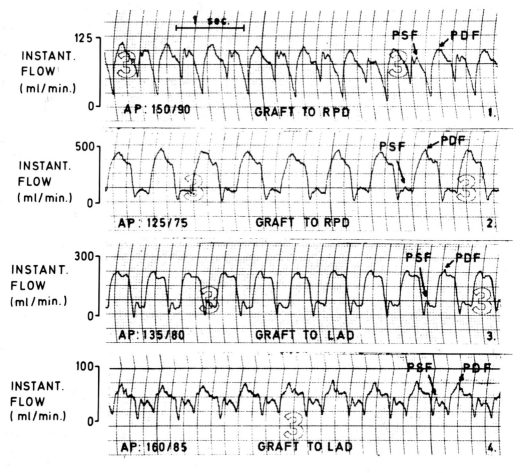

FIG. 1. Instantaneous flow tracings of saphenous vein bypass grafts to the RPD and LAD with high and low systolic flow components. PSF: peak systolic flow; PDF: peak diastolic flow; AP: arterial blood pressure.

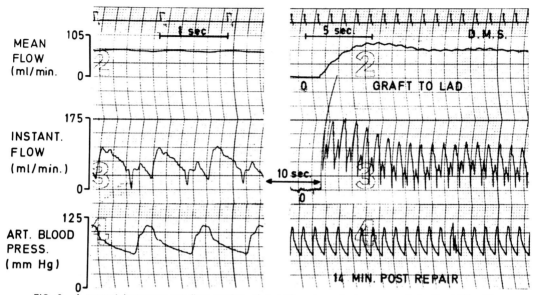

FIG. 2. A normal instantaneous flow tracing of a saphenous vein bypass graft to the LAD with marked diastolic reactive hyperemia (DRH).

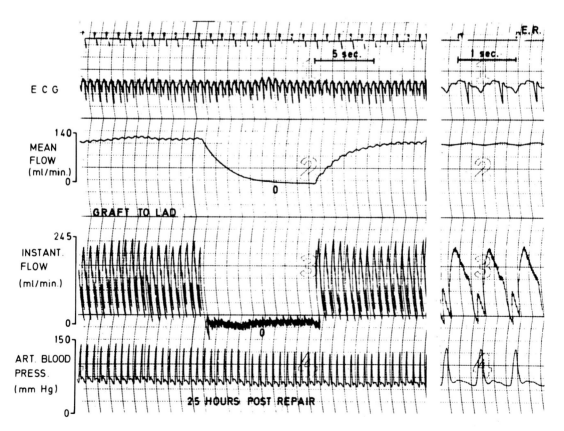

FIG. 3. A normal instantaneous flow tracing of a saphenous vein bypass graft to the LAD without DRH.

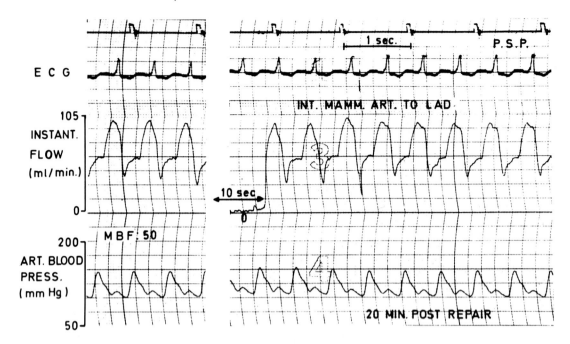

FIG. 4. A dilated instantaneous flow tracing of an internal mammary artery graft to the LAD without DRH.

Occlusion of the coronary artery, proximal to the anastomosis with the bypass graft, often increased the amount of graft DRH or elicited a DRH response in the graft that was not present before the anastomosed artery was occluded (Fig. 6). The latter phenomenon especially occurred when the instantaneous flow tracing looked normal or showed evidence of backflow in systole, which disappeared when the flow in the proximal artery was interrupted. MBF through the bypass graft usually increased after occlusion of the proximal artery (Fig. 6).

In patients with two bypasses, the blood flow through one graft often increased when the other one was occluded (Fig. 7).

In 41 patients the measurements were repeated intraoperatively on 28 grafts to the LAD, 16 grafts to the RM, and 7 grafts to the RPD. No signficant changes could be detected between the first and second MAP determinations. HR was significantly (P < 0.005) lower in the second series of measurements only when the LAD was the recipient artery. In all three groups MBF was lower and the amount of DRH higher in the second series of measurements than in the first one. The decrease in MBF was significant (P < 0.05) in two groups, and the increase in DRH was significant (P < 0.005) in one group. Repetition of the measurements usually showed that the dilated instantaneous flow tracings became normal or looked less dilated than during

the first recording. In several patients, however, dilated tracings were still present just before closing the chest. In the seven patients who had a re-thoracotomy, no significant differences could be detected between the data obtained from the measurements during the reoperation and the data obtained from the last measurements during the first surgical procedure. In one patient the instantaneous tracing was still dilated 22 hours after implantation of the graft.

The correlation coefficients of MBF versus MAP and HR are shown in Table 2. The correlation coefficients were low (r maximally 0.37 and 0.46) in spite of some significant correlations (P < 0.05). No better correlation coefficients could be obtained when only the data from the last measurements during the first surgical procedure were evaluated.

TABLE 2. Correlation Coefficients of MBF versus MAP and HR

RECIPIENT ARTERY	N	MAP–MBF	HR–MBF
		r	r
LAD	106	0.16	0.41[a]
LC	16	0.37	0.12
RM	56	0.27[a]	0.32[a]
RPD	23	0.01	0.46[a]

[a]P < 0.05

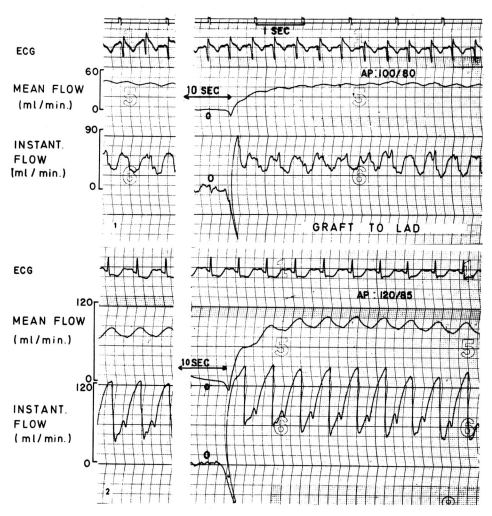

FIG. 5. Top: ECG and a damped instantaneous flow tracing of a saphenous vein bypass graft to the LAD without DRH. Bottom: Same graft after repair of the anastomosis with the ascending aorta: a dilated, but acceptable instantaneous tracing with DRH (adapted from Reneman and Spencer: Ann Thorac Surg 13:477–87, 1972).

DISCUSSION

In the present study the diastolic part of the reactive hyperemia is used to evaluate the coronary vascular system since this part is due to vasodilatation alone, while the systolic part results not only from vasodilatation, but also from a local decrease in intramyocardial pressure (v d Meer et al, 1970; v d Meer and Reneman, 1973). Therefore, DRH is a better estimate of the coronary flow reserve than is systolic reactive hyperemia. An occlusion of 10 seconds was used, since occlusions of this duration were found to be sufficient to elicit a maximal DRH response (Olsson and Gregg, 1965; v d Meer, 1972). The presence of DRH means that the coronary system can meet circumstances that are associated with an increase in oxygen demand. Although DRH was present in approximately 80 percent of the determinations, one must realize that the amount of DRH could be small: 20 percent or less in 40 of the 264 measurements. The actual flow reserve, however, will probably be higher than the amount of DRH suggests since some of the hyperemia responses were determined during vasodilatation, while collateral circulation and flow through the proximal artery will mask a maximal DRH response.

Marked DRH suggests that the graft provides the main blood supply. A normal instantaneous flow tracing without DRH or with an inconsiderable amount of DRH, on the other hand, indicates that there is circulation through paths other than the graft—for example, through

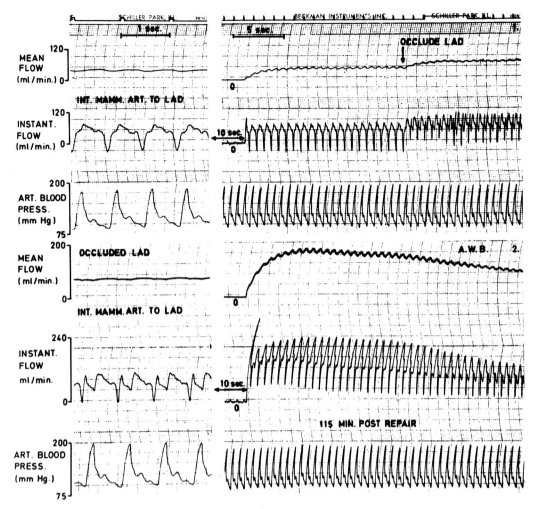

FIG. 6. Flow tracings of an internal mammary artery graft to the LAD with evidence of back-flow in systole without DRH (top). After occlusion of the LAD, proximal to the anastomosis with the graft, MBF increases and the backflow in systole disappears (top). When the LAD is occluded, a DRH response can be elicited in the graft (bottom).

well-developed collaterals or through the anasto-mosed coronary artery or both. Evidence of func-tional flow through the anastomosed coronary artery is given by the fact that occlusion of the artery proximal to the anastomosis often increased the amount of graft DRH or elicited a DRH re-sponse in the graft that was not present before the artery was occluded. Moreover, the MBF through the graft usually increased after inter-ruption of the flow in the proximal artery. John-son et al (1970b) showed that functional col-lateral circulation can be present between the perfusion areas of various grafts. Further evidence for functional anastomoses between the grafts is given by the fact that the blood flow through one graft can increase when another one is occluded.

Implantation of a bypass graft in an area with well-developed collateral circulation and/or

functional flow through the anastomosed coronary artery does not benefit the patient since the im-provement in myocardial blood flow is minimal under these circumstances (Smith et al, 1972). The presence of back flow, which disappeared after occlusion of the proximal artery, indicates that part of the blood in the grafts is flowing to and fro when there is a functional flow through the proximal artery. The partition of flow between the proximal artery and the graft depends, under these circumstances, on the graft-to-artery diameter ratio (Overton et al, 1973) and the degree of stenosis present in the proximal artery (Furuse et al, 1972). Therefore, the net forward flow through these grafts can decrease the amount of flow through the proximal artery, increasing the severity of proximal coronary disease (Aldridge and Trimble, 1971; Bousvaros et al, 1972).

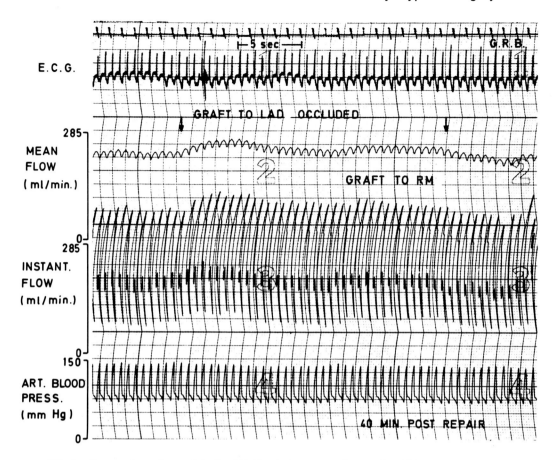

FIG. 7. Flow tracings of a graft to the RM. The instantaneous flow tracing looks dilated. Occlusion of the graft to the LAD results in an increase in blood flow in the graft to the RM.

DRH can also be diminished or absent as a result of a critical stenosis proximal or distal to the site of measurement. In this situation the MBF through the graft is usually in the normal range, but the instantaneous tracing appears damped (Reneman and Spencer, 1972; this study). This is in agreement with previous animal experiments in which reactive hyperemia (Elliot et al, 1968, and Khouri et al, 1968), and especially DRH (v d Meer and Reneman, 1972), was found to be more sensitive to constriction of a coronary artery than mean coronary blood flow. Therefore, a critical coronary artery stenosis can be overlooked by recording MBF alone and can lead to the erroneous conclusion that an adequate coronary repair has been accomplished.

HR and MAP are known to be important determinants of coronary blood flow. The low correlation coefficients of MBF versus HR and MAP, therefore, suggest that in patients with coronary artery disease the maximum coronary blood flow is mainly determined by the distal runoff.

The wide range of MBF values, which has

also been described by other investigators (Johnson et al, 1970a), can be explained by various degrees of vasodilatation and/or local variations in intramyocardial "pressure." Diminished dilatation of the coronary vasculature can probably be held responsible for the decrease in MBF and the increase in the amount of DRH in the period between the first and second measurements since the dilitated instantaneous tracings became normal during this period or appeared less dilated during the second recording. The fact that in several patients the instantaneous tracing was still dilated and DRH was absent or significantly diminished several hours after implantation of the graft, even after 22 hours, demonstrates that restoration of the normal rest tone of the coronary vascular bed can be slow. It would be interesting to know whether in these patients a normal rest tone, and therefore a normal autoregulation, can be obtained after the blood flow has been compromised for several years.

The amount of systolic coronary blood flow is mainly determined by the size of the area in the myocardium in which during systole the "pressure" is lower than the pressure in the ascending aorta, and by the magnitude of the systolic pressure difference between the ascending aorta and this myocardial area. Therefore, normally, the systolic flow component in grafts supplying the right ventricle is large and that in grafts supplying the left ventricle is small. A low systolic flow rate in grafts to the right coronary artery indicates that this artery mainly supplies the left ventricle. Recent animal experiments have shown that the area in the myocardium of the left ventricle, in which the pressure is lower during systole than the pressure in the ascending aorta, increases when negative inotropic changes are induced and decreases when the inotrophy is influenced positively (v d Meer and Reneman, 1973). Consequently the systolic flow component in grafts to the left coronary artery will be low when the left ventricle contracts vigorously and high when the left ventricle contracts weakly. That elongation of the graft (Greenfield et al, 1972) can be considered as an important cause of the transient flow increase during systole is not very likely because there is no reason for grafts to the right coronary artery to elongate more than grafts to the left coronary artery.

The present study shows that following the implantation of the bypass graft, valuable information can be obtained about the functional result of the surgical procedure and the functional state of the coronary vasculature by measuring heart rate, mean arterial pressure, and mean and instantaneous blood flow though the graft and by determining the diastolic creative hyperemia response to a 10-second occlusion of the graft. However, follow-up studies are necessary to determine the true significance of the observed findings at their true value.

SUMMARY

Mean (MBF) and instantaneous blood flow through 264 bypass grafts were measured electromagnetically, and the diastolic reactive hyperemia response to a 10-second occlusion was determined in 160 patients. Heart rate and mean arterial pressure were also assessed. The first measurements were made 14 to 30 minutes after discontinuation of the cardiopulmonary bypass. In 41 patients the measurements were repeated intraoperatively after 20 to 164 minutes. In seven patients who had a re-thoracotomy, the measurements were repeated from 17 hours to 13 days later. There was a wide range in MBF values,

which can be explained by various degrees of vasodilatation and/or local variations in intramyocardial pressure. In spite of some significant correlations, the correlation coefficients of MBF versus MAP and HR were low, indicating that MBF is mainly determined by the distal runoff. The amount of systolic blood flow can indicate whether or not a graft to the right coronary artery supplies mainly the right or mainly the left ventricle or whether a graft to the left coronary artery supplies weakly or vigorously contracting muscle.

Although DRH was present in approximately 80 percent of the measurements, the amount of DRH could be small: 20 percent or less in 40 of the 264 measurements. The presence of DRH indicates that grafts can participate in increased myocardial oxygen supply. DRH was inconsiderable or absent in combination with normal, dilated, or damped instantaneous tracings. A normal instantaneous tracing without DRH suggests well-developed collateral circulation and/or functional flow through the proximal coronary artery, while marked DRH indicates that the graft is the main supply. In several patients, vasodilatation was still present during the last measurements, even 22 hours after implantation of the graft. A damped instantaneous tracing without DRH suggests a critical stenosis, which can be overlooked by recording MBF alone.

ACKNOWLEDGMENTS

We are indebted to the cardiovascular surgical teams of Drs. Sauvage, Mansfield, Wood, and Share and Drs. Thomas, Jones, Edmark, Starney, and Carson of the Providence Hospital in Seattle for their assistance in obtaining the data, and to Mr. Dony for the statistical evaluation of our results. Special appreciation is given to Risa Lavizzo and Richard Turner for technical assistance.

References

1. Aldridge HE and Trimble AS: Progression of proximal coronary artery lesions to total occlusion after aorta-coronary saphenous vein bypass grafting. J Thorac Cardiovasc Surg 62:7–11, 1971
2. Amsterdam EC, Iben A, Hurley EJ, et al: Saphenous vein bypass graft for refractory angina pectoris: physiologic evidence for enhanced blood flow to the ischemic myocardium. Am J Cardiol (abstract) 26:623, 1970
3. Beer N, Keller N, Apstein C, et al: The cardiac hemodynamic and metabolic responses to coronary arterio-venous bypass surgery. Am J Cardiol (abstract) 29:252, 1972
4. Bousvaros G, Piracha AR, Chaudhry MA, et al:

Increase in severity of proximal coronary disease after successful distal aortocoronary grafts: Its nature and effects. Circulation 46:870–79, 1972

5. Cibulski AA, Lehan PH, Timmis HH, and Hellems HK: Regression of intercoronary collateral vessels in mongrel dogs after coronary bypass grafting. Am J Cardiol 31:480–83, 1973.

6. Elliott EC, Jones EL, Bloor CM, Leon AS, and Gregg DE: Day-to-day changes in coronary hemodynamics secondary to constriction of circumflex branch of left coronary artery in conscious dogs. Circ Res 22:237–50, 1968

7. Furuse A, Klopp EH, Brawley RK, and Gott VL: Hemodynamics of aorta-to-coronary artery bypass. Ann Thorac Surg 14:282–92, 1972

8. Greenfield JC, Rembert JC, Young WG, et al: Studies of blood flow in aorta-to-coronary venous bypass grafts in man. J Clin Invest 51:2724–35, 1972

9. Johnson WD, Flemma RJ, and Lepley D: Determinants of blood flow in aortic-coronary saphenous vein bypass grafts. Arch Surg 101:806–10, 1970a

10. Johnson WD, Flemma RJ, Manley JC, and Lepley D: The physiologic parameters of ventricular function as affected by direct coronary surgery. J Thorac Cardiovasc Surg 60:483–89, 1970b

11. Khouri EM, Gregg DE, and Lowensohn HS: Flow in the major branches of the left coronary artery during experimental coronary insufficiency in the unanesthetized dog. Circ Res 23:99–109, 1968

12. Manley JC, Johnson WD, Flemma RJ, and Lepley D: Direct myocardial revascularization: postoperative assessment of ventricular function at rest and during ergometer exercise. Circulation, Suppl III, 41 & 42:181, 1970

13. Meer v d JJ: Myocardial ischemia and epicardiectomy. An experimental study. Thesis, University of Groningen, The Netherlands.

14. Meer v d JJ, and Reneman RS: An improved technique to induce a standardized functional stenosis of a coronary artery. Eur Surg Res 4:407–18, 1972

15. Meer v d JJ, and Reneman RS: The relation of intramyocardial pressure (IMP) to coronary blood flow (CBF), 7th Eur Conf Microcirculation, Aberdeen 1972, Part I. Bibl anat 11:151–57, Basel, Karger, 1973

16. Meer v d JJ, Reneman RS, Schneider H, and Wieberdink J: A technique for estimation of intramyocardial pressure in acute and chronic experiments. Cardiovasc Res 4: 132–40, 1970

17. Olsson RA and Gregg DE: Myocardial reactive hyperemia in the unanesthetized dog. Am J Physiol 208:224–30, 1965

18. Overton JB, Smith JC, Robel SB, et al: Origin of downstream flow in non-obstructed coronary arteries. Arch Surg 107:764–70, 1973

19. Rees G, Bristow JD, Kremkau EL, et al: Influence of aortocoronary bypass surgery on left ventricular performance. N Engl J Med 284:1116–20, 1971

20. Reneman RS and Spencer MP: The use of diastolic reactive hyperemia to evaluate the coronary vascular system. Ann Thorac Surg 13:477–87, 1972

21. Rutherford BD, Gau GT, Danielson GK, et al: Left ventricular haemodynamics before and soon after saphenous vein bypass graft operation for angina pectoris. Br Heart J 34:1156–62, 1972

22. Smith SC, Gorlin R, Herman MV, Taylor WJ, and Collins JJ: Myocardial blood flow in man: effects of coronary collateral circulation and coronary artery bypass surgery. J Clin Invest 51:2556–65, 1972

18

COLLATERAL BLOOD FLOWS AND PRESSURES IN CORONARY ARTERY DISEASE

Watts R. Webb, E. Lawrence Hanson,
Frederick B. Parker, Jr., and John F. Neville, Jr.

Operative studies have been performed to evaluate antegrade and retrograde flows and pressures in the coronary arteries distal to obstructive lesions. Theoretical considerations and hemodynamic studies have demonstrated that an artery must be narrowed at least 50 percent before a change occurs in the distal pressure or flow, and often this does not become significant until the obstruction is 75 percent or more. Our previous observations indicated that collateral to a coronary artery is not demonstrable by coronary arteriography until there is at least a 90 percent proximal occlusion.[10] Studies made at the time of arteriotomy for grafting can evaluate the volume of collateral flow for alleviating angina or preventing infarction.

METHODS

Antegrade and retrograde pressures and flows were obtained from 197 vessels in 96 patients during operations for coronary artery revascularization. This included 80 antegrade measurements and 117 retrograde measurements. While both studies could usually be obtained in the proximal right coronary artery and left anterior descending artery, vessels on the posterior aspect of the heart often could be cannulated in only one direction.

The coronary artery was cannulated in both antegrade and retrograde directions with a no. 16 gauge plastic catheter through the arteriotomy, which was to be used for the graft anastomosis (Fig. 1). Free flow from the catheter was collected for 15 seconds with the end of the catheter held at the same level as the coronary artery. Pressures were obtained by attaching the catheter to a pressure transducer. The coronary artery diameter was determined by passing calibrated probes in both directions.

After the bypass graft had been completed, an electromagnetic flow meter probe was used to measure blood flow through the graft with and without occlusion of the recipient vessel proximal to the anastomosis (Fig. 2). This allowed evaluation of the flow passing both antegrade and retrograde into the grafted coronary artery since much flow often passed into branches of the coronary artery distal to the obstruction but proximal to the site of anastomosis.

Pressures could again be obtained postoperatively by inserting a 25-gauge needle into the completed vein graft, (1) with the graft open to be certain that graft pressure was the same as aortic pressure; (2) with the proximal graft occluded to measure pressure in the recipient coronary artery distal to the obstruction, which, in general, should correlate with the antegrade pressure; and (3) with both the proximal graft and the proximal recipient vessel completely occluded, which should correlate with the retrograde pressure.

Pressures and flows were recorded during cardiopulmonary bypass when the mean aortic pressure was maintained at 65 to 70 mm Hg. Postoperative measurements were made only after the aortic systolic pressure had reached at least 110 mm Hg.

OBSERVATIONS

Antegrade flow and pressure measurements are summarized in Table 1 and retrograde measurements in Table 2. Antegrade pressures and

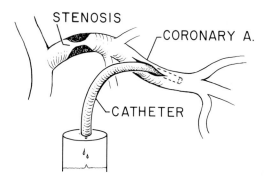

FIG. 1. Cannulation of coronary artery through arteriotomy for recording retrograde flow or for measuring pressure by connecting to a pressure transducer.

TABLE 1. Antegrade Measurements

PERCENT STENOSIS	NUMBER STUDIES	PRESSURE		FLOW	
		Range	Mean	Range	Mean
95+	23	30–100	54	0.0–28	10
85–95	34	30–100	69	0.0–40	15
70–85	20	20–100	83	3.0–66	33
50–70	3	73–100	91	4.5–30	22

TABLE 2. Retrograde Measurements

PERCENT STENOSIS	NUMBER STUDIES	PRESSURE		FLOW	
		Range	Mean	Range	Mean
95+	34	25–80	45	0–27	7.0
85–95	47	15–75	34	0–16	3.2
70–85	33	10–55	30	0–8	1.7
50–70	3	25–40	34	0–5	2.0

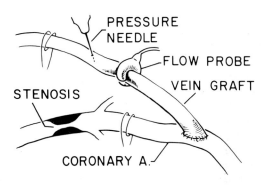

FIG. 2. Flow probe around the graft measures flow with all vessels open or, if proximal coronary artery snare is occluded, flow into distal bed with proximal contribution excluded. Initially pressure is recorded with all vessels open. If the proximal graft is occluded, the pressure is that in the coronary artery distal to the stenosis (antegrade pressure). Occlusion of both graft and proximal coronary artery yields retrograde pressure in the coronary artery to confirm pregrafting records obtained as shown in Figure 1.

flows through an obstructive segment of the artery were roughly inversely proportional to the degree of occlusion. The arterial graft obstructions were classified into categories of 95 percent or greater, 85 to 95 percent, 75 to 85 percent, and less than 70 percent. With obstructions greater than 95 percent, the mean antegrade pressure through the obstruction averaged 54 percent of the aortic pressure and in only one instance was greater than 60 percent of the aortic pressure. This was in a lesion thought to be an eccentric plaque where the estimation of arteriographic narrowing is difficult. In lesions of less magnitude, there was a similar inverse relationship between the degree of stenosis and the mean pressure correlation with aortic pressure.

Flow in an antegrade fashion was severely compromised in vessels with 95 percent stenosis and similarly low at the 85 percent stenosis range. In only three instances was grafting performed on a vessel with less than 70 percent obstruction. The antegrade flow was less than 30 cc in each one of these and since flow in these patients after grafting ranged from 90 to 120 cc per minute, it is probable that these stenoses were underestimated from the angiocardiogram. Similarly, in all patients, subsequent flow through the graft was much higher than the antegrade flow measured at the initial arteriotomy, suggesting that the stenosis had been producing significant reduction of the potential flow to the distal coronary artery.

Retrograde pressure showed much more variability, but in this larger series of patients, in contradistinction to our earlier study,[10] there was a reasonable correlation of retrograde pressure with the degree of proximal stenosis. Thus, patients with a 95 percent stenotic lesion had a mean retrograde pressure of 45 percent of the aortic pressure, though below this level of stenosis the mean pressure in all patients was roughly one-third that of the aortic pressure.

Similarly, the highest retrograde flows were in those patients with greater than 95 percent stenosis, with a range of 0 to 27 ml per minute and a mean of 7 ml per minute. If those patients with the preinfarction syndrome are excluded, the mean flow would be 12 ml per minute, since the preinfarction group—even though having from 90 to 99 percent stenosis—had a retrograde flow less than 2.5 ml per minute.

An interesting subgroup in the study is comprised of those 18 patients with preinfarction syndrome.[5] None of these had less than 90 percent stenosis and the mean antegrade pressure was 52 percent, essentially the same as the total group. Antegrade flow was likewise comparable. Retrograde pressure averaged only 32 percent of aortic pressure compared to 45 percent in the main group and retrograde flow only 2.5 ml per minute with eleven of these patients having no demonstrable retrograde flow.

Collaterals were not evident by coronary arteriography in any patient of this entire series who was judged to have less than 90 percent stenosis of the parent vessel. Virtually all patients with 95 percent stenosis had collaterals except in the group with the preinfarction syndrome. Of these 18 patients—all having at least 90 percent stenosis—only four had any collaterals. We feel that this reflects the rather sudden progressive occlusion in the preinfarction syndrome, which in large measure accounts for the sudden increased symptomatology since there is little or no protection with collateral retrograde flow.

DISCUSSION

This method of measurement of pressures and flows in the coronary artery distal to a point of obstruction affords basic data hitherto unavailable in patients with coronary stenosis. There are some limitations in measuring flows and pressures in this fashion since side branches are open that may either dissipate the pressure or, by collateral flow, enhance the pressure. In some patients, for example, where there was total proximal stenosis, the distal antegrade pressure might be higher than the retrograde pressure. In these vessels, there were usually prominent intersegmental collaterals from the proximal vessel to the poststenotic segment. This, among other things, suggests that collateral flow from the proximal artery via intersegmental collaterals around an obstructive lesion, may be more effective than retrograde collateral flow to a distal portion of the artery. It was of interest that this phenomenon was seen only in the left anterior descending coronary artery, which ordinarily has many more sources of collateral flow than the right or left circumflex coronary artery.

On some occasions, pressure distal to a high-grade obstruction was identical to that of the aortic pressure. If the vessel distal to an obstruction has no side branches for runoff for flow coming through the obstruction, the measurement becomes the equivalent of a wedge pressure and, therefore, measured aortic pressure. Undoubtedly, when the distal vessel is not obstructed by the measuring catheter, pressure is much lower.

The above method of measuring flow also has the inherent error of measuring antegrade or retrograde flow higher than exists in the normal state since the resistance of the distal arterial bed has been removed. The 16-gauge catheter itself probably does not offer a restricting influence, since flow at usual arterial pressures can be as high as 400 ml per minute through this size of catheter. It would seem, in fact, that this resistance is less than that of the distal arterial bed and thus flows may be regarded as maximal rather than minimal.

The accuracy, however, of the flows as measured by the catheter method is demonstrated by several cases in which retrograde flow was collected from the vein graft after it had been anastomosed to the coronary artery. In this situation, the distal arterial bed offers "normal" resistance, while, of course, the vein graft offers very minimal resistance. In these cases, flow through the vein graft, which primarily represents antegrade flow through the partially obstructed vessel, very closely approximated the antegrade flow obtained by the catheter technique. Differences seen have been compatible with the differences in aortic pressure at the particular time of measurement.

These measurements of pressures and flows distal to obstructing lesions confirm previous concepts that these are rarely altered if the arterial obstruction is less than 75 percent. It is important to note that even though pressures may be normal, flows nonetheless may be reduced. This occurs because autoregulation of the distal arterial bed can maintain a relatively normal pressure if the flow is not too greatly reduced, just as systemic blood pressure can be maintained at relatively normal levels in spite of a severely reduced cardiac output.

The very limited volume of retrograde flow, which in none of the vessels we have studied ever exceeded 27 ml per minute, has been somewhat surprising. In addition, this represents retrograde flow when the antegrade pressure has been removed and may be higher than occurs in normal circumstances. There have been no other direct measurements to our knowledge, but our results correlate fairly well with those of Yokoyama and Sakakibara,[11] who found that retrograde flow through patent internal mammary artery implants with collateral flow varied from 0.3 to 5 ml per minute. In these implants, the retrograde pressure, which averaged about 80 mm Hg, was much higher than we found in the distal coronary artery. Similarly, Sabiston, Fauteux, and Blalock[6] found retrograde flow through patent internal mammary artery implants to have a maximum of 5.5 ml per minute with a retrograde pressure varying from 80 to 100 mm Hg. None of these results support the conclusion of Sewell that coronary collaterals rated as 4+ angiographically will carry as much blood as a normal unoccluded coronary artery.[7] His conclusions, however, were not based on direct flow measurements but only on angiograms and corrosion casts.

In none of these patients was collateral circulation demonstrated by arteriography when the obstruction was less than 90 percent, and usually only minimal collateral was evident if the obstruction was less than 95 percent. Also, in those patients with no collateral blood, retrograde flow averaged less than 3 ml per minute. In this regard, retrograde blood-flow measurements correlated well with the angiographic interpretations. Similarly, in an analysis of 100 arteriograms, Gensini and DaCosta[3] were not able to demonstrate collaterals to those coronary arteries having an obstruction of less than 90 percent. It is also of great interest that they found that in 37 patients with severe obstructive coronary arterial disease but with well-developed collateral circulation, only five had EKG changes. On the other hand, 10 patients with severe obstruction and no noted collaterals all showed EKG changes suggestive of myocardial ischemia. This correlates with our studies of patients with preinfarction syndrome who all had very high grade stenosis (greater than 90 percent) but only four of the 18 had any evidential collaterals. These observations suggest that minimal retrograde flow is adequate to maintain the viability of tissue or even to prevent angina though it may not be adequate for the functional needs of stressed myocardium.

Blumgart, Zoll, et al[1] over 30 years ago stressed the existence and pathologic significance of collateral anastomoses within the coronary circulation. These potential communications are probably congenitally determined,[4] and do not become demonstrable or functional except on the demand of a severe perfusion gradient.[9] Our observations and those of Gensini and DaCosta indicate that a truly significant perfusion gradient does not develop until the degree of stenosis exceeds 90 percent and probably requires 95 percent obstruction for maximal development of collaterals. Sewell's observations based on 372 patient years of followup on 104 patients with mammary artery implants further suggest the importance of developing collaterals.[8] In these patients, there was an inverse correlation between the extent of collateral circulation that developed between the internal mammary pedicles and the degree of obstruction of the coronary arterial system. Also, long-term survival was directly proportional to the number of functioning implants *with collaterals* in each patient.

The excellent experiments of Furuse, Klopp, et al,[2] demonstrated that when a graft is anastomosed to a normal coronary artery, the distribution of flow between the graft and the coronary artery will be proportionate to their respective diameters (which largely determines resistance). The total flow through the distal arterial bed will remain the same whether through the coronary artery, through the graft, or through both. This is true because autoregulation of the distal arterioles determines the magnitude of total flow. In all our patients, after 30 seconds of occlusion of the graft post-bypass, there was a sharp transient rise in flow reflecting the autoregulation of the distal coronary artery bed and pinpointing the site of control as being here. Since all patients had significant stenosis of the proximal grafted coronary artery the measured graft flow represents the major portion of the flow. Also, almost invariably there was demonstrable flow from the graft into that segment of the coronary artery proximal to the anastomosis and distal to the stenosis. This was true even in those instances when the antegrade pressure in the coronary artery was systemic. Even in those stenotic arteries in which antegrade pressure as measured above was not reduced, the antegrade flow appeared to be limited because flow through the graft was always much greater than flow preoperatively through the partially obstructed artery. This likewise emphasizes the importance of the autoregulation of the distal arterial bed.

Comparison of the elective group of patients with the preinfarction syndrome group was very revealing. Although antegrade pressure, antegrade flow, and retrograde pressure correlated quite well between the two groups, retrograde flow showed a significant difference, which depended on the presence or absence of coronary collaterals. Even though the degree of high-grade proximal obstruction may be the same, there was much less blood available to the distal arterial bed in the preinfarction group. This suggests a more dangerous situation in the preinfarction patients, who presumably have rapid progression of the proximal obstruction and thus have not had time to develop the protection of collateral vessels found in the elective group. This lack of developed collaterals in the preinfarction must limit the oxygen available and undoubtedly places the viability of the myocardium in greater jeopardy.

References

1. Blumgart HL, Zoll PM, Freedberg AS, Gilligan DR: Experimental production of inter-coronary arterial

anastomoses and their functional significance. Circulation 1:10, 1941

2. Furuse A, Klopp EH, Brawley RK, Gott VL: Hemodynamics of aorta-to-coronary artery bypass. Ann Thorac Surg 14:282, 1972

3. Gensini GG, DaCosta BCB: The coronary collateral circulation in living man. Am J Cardiol 24:393, 1969

4. James TN: Anatomy of the coronary arteries and veins. In JW Hurst and RB Log (eds): The Heart. NY, Blakiston Div, McGraw-Hill, 1966, p 635

5. Parker FB Jr, Neville JF Jr, Hanson EL, Webb WR: Retrograde and antegrade pressures and flows in pre-infarction syndrome. Circulation (Suppl I) 49: 122–26, 1974

6. Sabiston DC, Fauteux JP, Blalock A: An experimental study of the fate of arterial implants in the left ventricular myocardium. Ann Surg 145:927, 1957

7. Sewell WH: Basic factors relating to the experimental production of collateral channels to the coronary arteries. Surg Forum 12:223, 1961

8. Sewell WH: Relationships between coronary deaths and collateral from mammary artery pedicles. Ann Thorac Surg 9:301, 1970

9. Sheldon WC: On the significance of coronary collaterals. Am J Cardiol 24:303, 1969

10. Webb WR, Parker FB Jr, Neville JF Jr: Retrograde pressures and flows in coronary arterial disease. Ann Thorac Surg 15:3, March 1973

11. Yokoyama M, Sakakibara S: Blood flow measurements in internal mammary artery implanted into the myocardium. Ann Thorac Surg 13:155, 1972

19

REACTIVE HYPEREMIC TESTING IN SURGICAL MANAGEMENT OF CORONARY ARTERY DISEASE

David B. Skinner, W. E. Elzinga,
and Hugoe R. Mathews

Surgical treatment for acute myocardial ischemia or infarction is now a reality. The decision remains difficult as to whether a bypass graft or an infarctectomy may be the better procedure (Cohn, Gorlin, et al, 1972; Mundth, Buckley, et al, 1973). Follow-up coronary cinearteriograms demonstrate a substantial rate of bypass graft occlusions (Bourassa, Lesperance, et al, 1972). Factors such as anastomotic narrowing, distal coronary artery occlusions, and inappropriate selection of site for the coronary anastomosis are implicated as contributing to early and late graft occlusions. Results of surgery from acute myocardial infarction might be improved if a method were available in the operating room to guide the surgeon in the choice of bypass graft versus infarctectomy, to predict the likelihood of long-term patency of bypass grafts, and to detect and correct factors that might contribute to graft occlusions. Studies of coronary artery peak reactive hyperemic response in 118 canine experiments suggest that this test may be valuable for these purposes.

PEAK REACTIVE HYPEREMIC RESPONSE

Immediately after release of a brief coronary artery occlusion, a temporary increase in flow normally occurs, representing dilatation of the vascular bed in response to transient ischemia (Olsson and Gregg, 1965). In the myocardium,

this hyperemic response following a 10-second test occlusion is reproducible in a given vessel under constant conditions and is easily measured in the operating room or laboratory (Matthews, Skinner, et al, 1971). The coronary artery to be studied is dissected sufficiently to place an electromagnetic flow probe of appropriate size around the vessel. A snare is passed around the vessel several millimeters distally. Zero flow is recorded by distal vessel occlusion. After a steady-state baseline flow is recorded, the snare is applied to occlude the vessel for exactly 10 seconds. After releasing the snare, the greatest increase in flow rate above baseline flow is calculated as the peak reactive hyperemic response (PRHR) (Fig. 1), by calculating the area under the flow curve recording until baseline flow is again reached. The total increase in volume of flow may also be measured. In the normal canine heart, a 10-second occlusion of either the left anterior descending (LAD) or left circumflex coronary artery (LCCA) causes a more than twofold increase in coronary flow, which gradually falls to baseline levels during the ensuing minute.

MODEL FOR ISCHEMIA AND INFARCTION

The effects on myocardial histology of temporary occlusions of the LAD from 15 minutes to six hours duration were studied in 16 dogs. In an additional 11 dogs, the effects on myocardial histology of one-hour temporary occlusion of the LCCA were investigated. A snare occluded the selected coronary artery for a measured time and was released to reestablish coronary blood flow.

This research was supported in part by Grants #HL-11831 and #HL-15717, from the National Institutes of Health, Department of Health, Education and Welfare.

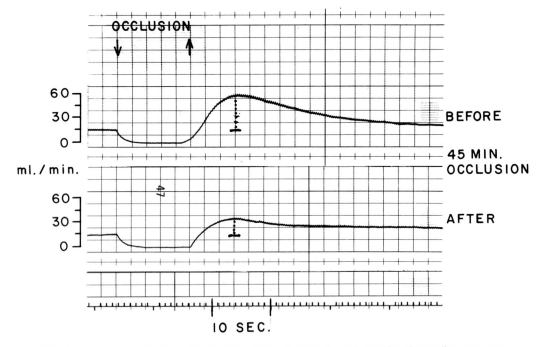

FIG. 1. Electromagnetic flowmeter tracings obtained from the left anterior descending coronary artery before and after 45 minutes of ligation. To the left of each tracing, the level of stable baseline mean coronary flow is shown to be comparable at both times. Following a 10-second occlusion during which zero flow is recorded, release of the ligature results in flow increased above baseline levels (reactive hyperemia). The largest increase in flow after release of the occlusion compared to baseline flow determines the value of the peak hyperemic response (PRHR). From Matthews, Skinner, et al, 1971.

Animals were supported as needed during the immediate recovery period. Hearts were defibrillated when necessary. The dogs were sacrificed after one to two weeks, and the hearts were studied for the degree of infarction. In four animals with LAD occlusions of 15 minutes or less, the myocardium appeared normal microscopically. In four animals with occlusions of 30 and 45 minutes, patchy myocardial necrosis to subendocardial infarction was noted. In eight animals in which the LAD was occluded for one hour or more, extensive infarction was observed in each (Matthews, Skinner, et al, 1971). Ten of 11 of the dogs in which the LCCA had been occluded showed myocardial infarction at autopsy even though satisfactory flow had been reestablished immediately after the 60 minutes' occlusion.

In 12 dogs, both coronary arteries were temporarily occluded by snares at their origins from the aorta, and the systemic circulation of the animals was supported by mechanical ventricular assistance (Skinner, 1971). In two dogs having bilateral coronary occlusion for 15 minutes, normal myocardial function resumed after release of the snares and the animals survived.

When sacrificed a week later, the myocardium was normal histologically. In four dogs with double coronary occlusions for 30 minutes, heart function resumed in each, but none survived more than six hours after intensive postoperative support was discontinued. In four dogs with 45 minutes of double coronary occlusion, none survived longer than three hours after restoration of the circulation, and the heart of one animal did not function at all. After 60 minutes of coronary occlusion, both dogs had no myocardial function (Matthews, Skinner, et al, 1971).

These experiments demonstrated that myocardium deprived of its blood flow for less than 30 minutes recovered completely after revascularization, whereas canine myocardium deprived of blood flow for 60 minutes progressed to irreversible infarction in spite of revascularization. Intermediate degrees of damage were observed in animals with occlusions for 30 and 45 minutes. In subsequent experiments, the effects on coronary artery flow and PRHR of ischemia from 15 or 20 minutes of temporary occlusion and infarction caused by one hour or more of coronary occlusion were studied.

EFFECTS OF ISCHEMIA AND INFARCTION ON CORONARY ARTERY FLOW AND PRHR

In 61 mongrel dogs of both sexes, the effects of temporary occlusion of the LAD or LCCA ranging from five minutes to six hours were studied (Matthews, Skinner, et al, 1971; Elzinga, Skinner, et al, 1974). Employing pentobarbital anesthesia and endotracheal mechanical ventilation with room air, a left thoracotomy was performed. The selected coronary artery was dissected at its origin and a Biotronex electromagnetic flow probe was applied. A snare was placed distally for vessel occlusion. Another Biotronex electromagnetic flow probe was placed on the pulmonary artery to measure cardiac output using the end diastolic flow plateau as the zero flow level. Polyethylene catheters were inserted into the aorta and vena cava to monitor pressures. Flow and pressure signals were recorded on a direct writing recorder. Electrocardiogram was monitored. In addition to mean and pulsatile coronary artery flow, PRHR was measured several times during the control period. Hematocrit, arterial blood gases, pH, and body temperature were measured at intervals during experiments. After baseline levels had been stable for at least 30 minutes, the coronary artery was occluded by the snare for the desired period of time. After release of the occlusion, pressure and flow measurements were made frequently for up to four hours.

After release of the snare, coronary flow was promptly reestablished and increased markedly above baseline levels in all animals. By one hour after release of the occlusion, coronary flow in both the LAD and LCCA returned to baseline levels in all animals with either an ischemic or infarction injury.

In 39 dogs studied following LCCA occlusions of 20, 60, or 120 minutes, flow measurements were continued for four hours after release of the occlusion (Elzinga, Skinner, et al, 1974). At one hour, the flow in all three groups was equal to baseline flow. In five dogs following 20 minutes of LCCA occlusion, flow remained at the baseline level throughout the four hours' observation period. However in the animals with 60- or 120-minute occlusions, flow fell after one hour. In the second, third, and fourth hours, coronary artery flow to the revascularized area was significantly less than baseline flow and less than

flow observed the same times following a 20-minute occlusion. Four hours after LCCA reopening, mean flow for animals with 60- or 120-minute occlusions averaged only 55 percent of control levels, and in several dogs LCCA flow following revascularization was near zero. In 80 percent of the dogs, the normal pulsatile flow pattern had changed to a nonpulsatile pattern by the fourth hour after revascularization. Flow during cardiac diastole was markedly reduced. Among these dogs with acute myocardial infarction, the mean arterial pressure dropped approximately 20 mm Hg from the baseline level four hours after revascularization.

These experiments demonstrated that coronary artery flow was elevated immediately after revascularization of either an ischemic or infarcted area, and normal levels of coronary flow could be observed as long as one hour after revascularization regardless of the eventual fate of the myocardium. With more prolonged observation, a significant difference in flow was observed between animals with an occlusion causing only ischemia, and animals with an occlusion sufficient to cause infarction in spite of the successful revascularization. Early measurements of coronary artery flow within one hour after revascularization were of no value in predicting success for the restoration of myocardial viability.

In contrast, the PRHR test readily differentiated within the first hour after revascularization those animals in which an infarction would occur from those in which the ischemia was reversible. In animals with one hour or more vessel occlusion, the PRHR was markedly reduced or absent in the early minutes after restoration of blood flow. One hour after opening the vessel, the PRHR was reduced an average of 64 percent from the baseline PRHR. This was true in animals with either LAD or LCCA occlusion. On the other hand the PRHR following a 15-minute occlusion of the LAD was reduced only 13 percent from control levels one hour after revascularization. Following 20 minutes of LCCA occlusion, the PRHR was reduced only 20 percent from preocclusion levels when studied one hour after vessel reopening (Table 1).

In terms of flow the peak coronary artery flow following a 10-second test occlusion always increased at least 50 percent above baseline coronary flow in animals destined to have a full recovery of the myocardium. In hearts destined to progress to infarction in spite of revascularization, the peak increase in hyperemic flow during the first hour after revascularization was less than 30

TABLE 1. PRHR Versus Occlusion Time in Dogs

OCCLUSION (min)	NO. DOGS	PERCENT REDUCTION IN PRHR	HISTOLOGY
1–15	4 (LAD)	13	normal
20	7 (LCCA)	20	normal
30	2 (LAD)	39	patchy necrosis
45	2 (LAD)	58	subendocardial necrosis
60–120	38 (LCCA)	64	extensive infarction
60–360	8 (LAD)	63	extensive infarction

percent above the baseline level of coronary flow just prior to the 10-second vessel occlusion (Table 2). This simple test of observing the level of increase after a 10-second test occlusion accurately differentiated between myocardium that could recover and myocardium that would progress to infarction in spite of revascularization.

EFFECTS OF CRITICAL STENOSIS ON CORONARY ARTERY FLOW AND PRHR

In addition to the severity of myocardial ischemia or fibrosis, other factors such as severe narrowing of a distal coronary artery or a narrow anastomosis between a bypass graft and coronary artery might affect the PRHR. To evaluate this, PRHR, LCCA flow, and aortic blood pressure were measured at varying degrees of LCCA stenosis in 18 mongrel dogs (Elzinga and Skinner, 1974). Electromagnetic flow probes were placed around the LCCA at its origin and around the pulmonary artery, and zero flow was determined. A specially designed coronary constricting device was loosely positioned around the LCCA distal

to the flow probe and snare. Baseline levels of LCCA flow, PRHR, cardiac output, electrocardiogram, and aortic blood pressure were recorded. The screw in the coronary constrictor device was turned at intervals to cause a gradual occlusion of the LCCA. Measurements were repeated after each step of the vessel occlusion. At the point at which the coronary artery diameter had been reduced by an average of 74 percent, and the area had been reduced by an average of 93 percent as determined by later x-ray studies, critical stenosis was achieved. At this point, further reduction in diameter caused a marked drop in coronary flow. At critical stenosis, mean LCCA flow was reduced from baseline levels of 42 cc per minute to 34 cc per minute. A change in the pattern of pulsatile coronary artery flow was observed in each dog at the point of critical stenosis. Average diastolic flow decreased significantly from 81 to 52 cc per minute and a significant increase occurred in systolic flow from 24 to 38 cc per minute. At critical stenosis, the PRHR was nearly abolished, 94 to 99 percent reduced compared to control PRHR levels. The reduction in PRHR proceeded linearly during vessel constriction. At critical stenosis, no significant changes were seen in mean aortic blood pressure or cardiac output. Isoelectric T-waves in Lead II of the ECG were noted in each dog at the point of critical stenosis.

These studies demonstrate that coronary flow is maintained near baseline levels by peripheral vascular regulation in spite of vessel narrowings up to 75 percent in diameter. The level of resting coronary artery flow is not a good guide to the patency of anastomosis or the adequacy of the distal run-off beyond a bypass graft. The PRHR test, by acutely reducing the resistance in the distal myocardial vascular bed, provides a measure of maximum flow rate through a coronary vessel or bypass graft and thus is highly sensitive to vessel narrowing. The PRHR test provides a better guide to patency of anastomoses and run-off than does simple measurement of coronary artery flow.

TABLE 2. PRHR as Percent Coronary Flow

	LCCA OCCLUSIONS		
	20 Min	60 Min	120 Min
Baseline	210	172	220
1 hr	201	100[a]	129[a]
2 hrs	179	74[a]	108[a]
3 hrs	180	72[a]	102[a]
4 hrs	179	62[a]	99[a]

[a]*p < .001 compared to baseline and p < .05 or less compared to 20-minute value at same time.*

CONCLUSIONS

The PRHR test provides a measure of the maximum volume of coronary artery flow that can be perfused into the myocardium. Two factors control this. The distal myocardial vascular bed must be able to dilate in response to transient ischemia. Inability to dilate as in the case of myocardial infarction results in reduced PRHR. Secondly, the diameter of the distal coronary vessel or anastomosis between a bypass graft and coronary artery must be of sufficient size to permit a doubling of resting coronary flow in response to lowered peripheral resistance. The PRHR test when applied in the operating room during revascularization of acutely ischemic myocardium provides useful information of several types. A low PRHR response to a 10-second test occlusion suggests that (1) the myocardium being revascularized is already infarcted and will not benefit from the procedure, or (2) that collateral circulation to the distal myocardial bed is sufficient to prevent an ischemic response to the 10-second test occlusion, or (3) that fibrosis in the distal myocardial bed is so extensive that the myocardium cannot respond to the ischemic challenge, or (4) that the anastomosis between the bypass graft and coronary artery is flow-limiting, or (5) that the distal coronary artery bed contains points of narrowing that prevent maximal coronary flow. Any of these factors should cause concern and suggest that the operation will fail to improve myocardial function. For this reason a coronary arteriogram should be obtained on the operating table to assess technical factors that might be improved in the bypass graft, or to determine whether a more distal anastomosis might bypass a critical stenosis in the peripheral coronary artery. If the problem appears to be in the myocardial vascular bed rather than in the vessels, consideration should be given to an infarctectomy if the patient's infarction appears to be life-threatening.

References

Bourassa MG, Lesperance J, Campeau L, Simard P: Factors influencing patency of aortocoronary vein grafts. Circulation 155:I-79, 1972

Cohn LH, Gorlin R, Herman MV, Collins JJ: Aortocoronary bypass for acute coronary occlusion. J Thorac Cardiovasc Surg 64:503, 1972

Elzinga WE, Skinner DB, Dutka M, Gott VL: Coronary blood flow and myocardial reactive hyperemia in the ischemic dog heart (submitted for publication)

Elzinga WE, Skinner DB: Hemodynamic characteristics of critical stenosis in canine coronary arteries (submitted for publication)

Matthews HR, Skinner DB, Pitt B: Reactive hyperemia following coronary occlusion as a measurement of myocardial viability. Current Topics in Surgical Research vol 3:39, 1971

Mundth ED, Buckley MJ, DeSanctis RW, Daggett WM, Austen WG: Surgical treatment of ventricular irritability. J Thorac Cardiovasc Surg 66:943, 1973

Olsson RA, Gregg DE: Myocardial reactive hyperemia in the unanesthetized dog. Am J Physiol 208:224, 1965

Skinner DB: Experimental and clinical evaluations of mechanical ventricular assistance. Am J Cardiol 27:146, 1971

20

HEMODYNAMICS OF CORONARY STENOSES AND THEIR CLINICAL EVALUATION

Lance Gould, Kirk Lipscomb,
and Glen Hamilton

INTRODUCTION

Angina pectoris and myocardial infarction usually indicate severe anatomic stenosis of one or more coronary arteries. Traditionally, the symptoms of coronary disease are thought to result from reduced blood flow relative to myocardial metabolic requirements, a consequence of intraluminal narrowing that is visualized by coronary arteriography. However, measurements of coronary blood flow in man by indicator techniques are normal in the presence of advanced coronary disease, even during exercise.[1,2] In experimental preparations resting coronary flow remains normal even with severe stenosis.[3,4,5,6] Thus, despite the traditional view, measurements of coronary blood flow have provided few diagnostic or quantitative insights into the hemodynamics of coronary lesions.

This chapter explains the reasons for these apparent discrepancies. It describes the hemodynamic consequences of coronary constrictions on resting and maximal coronary flow, on pressure gradients across stenosis at rest and under "stress" conditions, on stenosis resistance, on distal coronary pressure, and on regional myocardial perfusion. The effects of multiple lesions in series on flow, resistance, and distal coronary pressure are also presented. In addition, the data demonstrate the physiologic basis and clinical application of a new approach for quantifying the hemodynamic consequences of coronary narrowing. The approach utilizes the concept of coronary flow reserve. It provides a quantitative assessment, independent of arteriographic interpretation, of the hemodynamic effects of coronary stenoses before they become severe enough to reduce resting coronary flow or cause myocardial infarction.

METHODS

Animal studies: Black Labrador or German Shepherd dogs were anesthetized with sodium pentobarbital and morphine sulfate. Respiration was maintained with a Harvard ventilatory pump through a cuffed endotracheal tube and blood gases kept normal by volume adjustment or supplemental oxygen. Through a left thoracotomy the proximal 2.0 cm of the left circumflex and/or anterior descending coronary arteries were dissected clean. Appropriately sized, perivascular, electromagnetic flow transducers (Zepeda) were implanted on the circumflex and anterior descending arteries. A snare occluder attached to a machinist's micrometer was placed distal to each flow transducer. Each snare could be tightened by small precise amounts according to the 0.01 mm micrometer scale. A small Teflon catheter (Bardic 1968-7) was inserted into the coronary artery lumen distal to the constrictor in order to record circumflex pressure. In some dogs a second coronary constrictor and catheter were implanted more distal in the same artery in order to study the effects of two stenoses in series. Catheters were placed in the left atrium for injection of macroaggregated albumin and into the aorta for the measurement of pressure. A preformed Cordis coronary catheter with added side holes and shaped for dogs, or a standard Sones coronary catheter, was inserted through the left carotid. Neither the coronary catheters nor flow transducers interfered with resting or maximal coronary flow.[6]

All measurements were recorded on an Electronics for Medicine DR-12 recorder at paper speeds of 10 to 25 mm per second. Aortic and coronary pressures were measured with either a Statham P-23Db or a Bio-Tec BT-70 pressure transducer. Coronary flows were measured with a Zepeda, dual channel, square wave, electromagnetic flowmeter operating at 450 and 600 Hz.

Experimental procedure was as follows: Dogs were heparinized. Occlusive zero baseline for the electromagnetic flowmeter was established. Under fluoroscopy the tip of the coronary catheter was positioned at the orifice of the main left coronary artery so that the circumflex and anterior descending branches could be equally filled with contrast media. As demonstrated previously,[5] intra-coronary sodium and meglumine diatrizoate (Hypaque-M, 75 percent) causes maximal, transient, coronary hyperemia of three to seven times resting basal flow, a response equivalent to the hyperemia following 10 seconds of complete occlusion. Because of these effects, contrast media were utilized as a convenient means of repetitively stimulating maximal flow. A fixed dose of contrast (4 to 5 cc) was injected sufficient for fluoroscopic opacification of both coronary branches comparable to that seen in clinical coronary arteriography, and the resulting hyperemic flow was measured in both coronary branches. One or both of the constrictors were then tightened in 10 to 30 sequential steps and the hyperemic response to contrast was measured at each step. Percent diameter stenosis was calculated for each step by the following equation:

$$\text{percent stenosis} = 100 \left(\frac{\text{micrometer reading at no lesion-reading at each step}}{\text{total micrometer excursion}} \right)$$

The maximal flow response following contrast, or coronary flow reserve, was measured for the circumflex and anterior descending arteries in the presence of various combinations of stenoses. The absolute and relative distribution of flow to the left anterior descending and circumflex arteries were also determined by flowmeter for comparison to corresponding measurements by myocardial imaging.

With various degrees and combinations of stenoses on one or both arteries, regional distribution was determined by injection of tagged macroaggregated albumin in the following fashion: [99m]Technetium or [131]Iodine macroaggregated albumin (MAA) was injected into the left atrial catheter during the hyperemia following contrast. After completing an experiment, the animal was sacrificed and its heart was removed. The left ventricle was dissected free and opened by cutting

from base to apex along the anterior descending artery. The resulting specimen was placed flat with the endocardial surface down and imaging performed with a Nuclear Chicago Gamma Camera using a pinhole collimator. From 50,000 to 100,000 count scintiphotos were obtained of both ^{99m}Tc MAA and ^{131}I MAA using a pulse-height analyzer with a 20 percent window. Myocardium supplied by the circumflex was in the center of the specimen surrounded by myocardium supplied by the anterior descending (photo in Fig. 13, below). Heart imaging was done on postmortem specimens of dogs in order to measure regional flow distribution as accurately as possible without the compromising problems of counting geometry in the intact animal. Small region-of-interest windows of equal size were then placed over contiguous areas of ventricular myocardium supplied by the left anterior descending (LAD) or circumflex (CIRC) coronary arteries. Counts from each region-of-interest were collected for two minutes and relative flow expressed as percent of total ventricular counts. [99m]Tc counts were corrected for ^{131}I cross talk by counting a ^{131}I standard of the same geometric shape as the left ventricular sample. Data were analyzed by a PDP-8 computer. Correlation curves and equations were obtained by least squares fitting to a power series or exponential equation.

Human studies: Patients were studied during routine diagnostic coronary arteriography by the Judkins technique. After systemic heparinization and completion of diagnostic left coronary arteriography, the catheter was flushed with saline to remove contrast and coronary flow was allowed to stabilize for two minutes. In the basal state, 0.5 to 1.5 mCi of [113m]Indium MAA (30,000 particles, 20 to 40 microns diameter) was injected into the left coronary. Five cc of Hypaque-M, 75 percent was then injected and six seconds later 1.5 mCi of ^{99m}Tc MAA was injected. Images of ^{99m}Tc and [131]In were obtained with a gamma camera using a medium-energy collimator in anterior, posterior, lateral, left and right anterior oblique, and left posterior oblique views. Images were analyzed visually from scintiphotographs and also stored on magnetic tape for subsequent data processing.

RESULTS AND DISCUSSION

Coronary Flow Reserve

In the resting basal state, the variability of distal coronary vascular bed resistance is sufficient to prevent experimental analysis of pressure-flow relationships across stenoses of the proximal or major coronary arteries. With maximal coronary bed vasodilatation, however, pressure-flow relationships across proximal stenoses and across the distal coronary vascular bed may be separately analyzed. In our animal studies, transient maximal vasodilatation was produced while measuring coronary flow, aortic pressure, and coronary pressure distal to a variable constrictor. Intracoronary injection of Hypaque-M, 75 percent in dogs in doses adequate for coronary cine angiography caused a transient 3 to 5 fold (4.1 ± 1.0) increase in coronary flow which peaked at 6 seconds and slowly returned to normal over three minutes.[5] The magnitude of this response was equal to that following a 10 second coronary occlusion, considered to be a maximal stimulus for hyperemia.[7] Because of this effect, Hypaque was utilized as a convenient means of repetitively producing coronary vasodila-

tation and maximal coronary flow. Injection of Hypaque thus served as a "stress" equivalent for studying coronary pressure-flow-resistance characteristics because it increased flow to as great or greater an extent than found during extreme exercise.[8,9]

Figure 1 shows an example of the effects of Hypaque on flow in a normal coronary artery and in the same artery with an 82 percent diameter narrowing. The stenosis did not reduce resting flow but did impair the flow increase that normally occurs with vasodilatory stimulus, such as exercise or, in this case, intracoronary injection of Hypaque. The extent to which coronary flow increases over basal flow rates is a direct measure of coronary flow reserve. Stenosis places an upper limit on this increase. For example, in Figure 1 in the upper panel, flow increased approximately four times over basal flow rates and coronary flow reserve was therefore four. In the lower panel

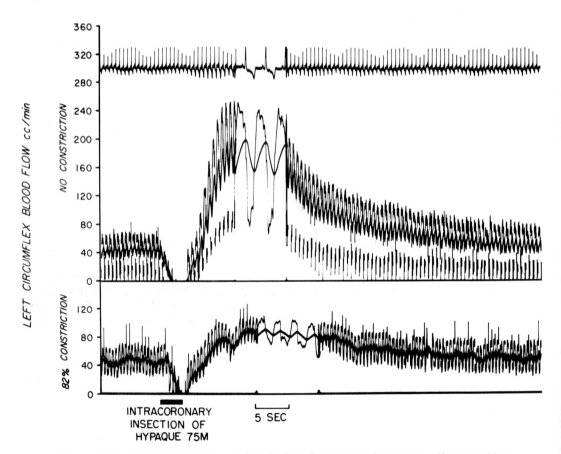

FIG. 1. The hyperemic flow response of the left circumflex following intracoronary Hypaque with no constriction (upper tracing) and with an 82 percent diameter narrowing of the circumflex coronary artery (lower tracing). The constriction reduces phasic variation but does not reduce mean resting flow. Maximal flow is greatly reduced, however. Heavy lines indicate mean flow. The paper speed is 5 mm/second and 25 mm/second. Hypaque 75M refers to Hypaque-M, 75 percent, Winthrop Laboratories brand of sodium and meglumine diatrizoate (from Ref. 5).

the increase in flow (or hyperemic response) was only 1.5 times baseline, indicating a corresponding reduction in coronary flow reserve.

Conditions that increase basal coronary flow also impair coronary flow reserve by reducing the potential flow increase available to meet additional myocardial oxygen demands.[5,10] For example, hypertrophy, anoxia, increased after-load and heart rate, anemia, volume overload, and thyrotoxicosis increase basal coronary flow. As a consequence, coronary flow reserve is "used" up, leaving little potential increase in the face of new metabolic demands by the myocardium. Coronary flow reserve is particularly impaired with the combination of stenosis, which reduces the upper flow limit, and one of these conditions, which increases the basal flow.

Figure 2 shows the effect in one dog of progressive coronary stenosis on resting coronary flow and on the maximum flow or hyperemic response following Hypaque (coronary flow reserve). Flows are expressed as ratios to baseline control coronary flow so that results from multiple experiments may be statistically compared. Resting flow was not affected until an 85 percent diameter narrowing, whereas maximum flow and coronary flow re-

serve were affected by a 45 percent constriction. Coronary flow reserve disappeared at 93 percent stenosis, a point at which resting flow began to fall. Figure 3 shows a composite of 12 experiments presented in the same format. It demonstrates that resting flow remained normal but coronary flow reserve was progressively impaired with stenoses above 45 percent diameter narrowing.

The importance of assessing coronary flow reserve is further illustrated by Figures 4 to 10. The data indicate that the impairment of coronary flow reserve correlates closely and quantitatively with the pressure-flow-resistance characteristics of coronary stenoses. In these figures, coronary flow reserve or the hyperemic response is again expressed as a ratio to control resting flow. Figure 4 shows the correlation between coronary flow reserve (hyperemic response) and resting mean pressure gradient across coronary constrictions. The dotted line indicates the relationship for a single stenosis. The solid line indicates the relationship to total pressure gradient across two stenoses in series. Figure 5 relates coronary flow reserve (hyperemic response) to distal coronary pressure beyond single and double stenoses in series. The correlations are good regardless of the

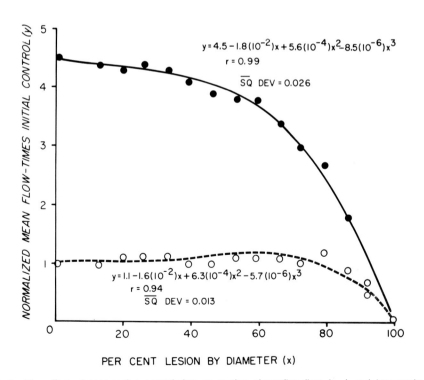

$$y = 4.5 - 1.8(10^{-2})x + 5.6(10^{-4})x^2 - 8.5(10^{-6})x^3$$
$$r = 0.99$$
$$\overline{SQ}\ DEV = 0.026$$

$$y = 1.1 - 1.6(10^{-2})x + 6.3(10^{-4})x^2 - 5.7(10^{-6})x^3$$
$$r = 0.94$$
$$\overline{SQ}\ DEV = 0.013$$

PER CENT LESION BY DIAMETER (x)

FIG. 2. The effect of progressive constriction on resting circumflex flow (- - -) and hyperemic response (——) to intracoronary Hypaque (coronary flow reserve) in a single experiment. Percent diameter narrowing is on the horizontal axis. Mean resting and hyperemic flows are expressed as ratios to control baseline flow (from Ref. 6).

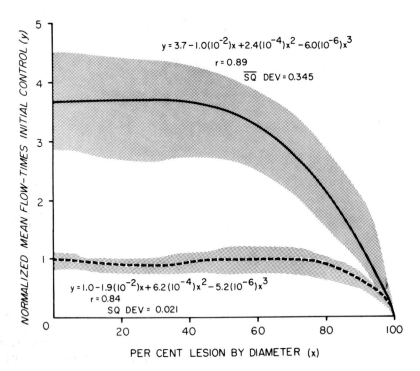

FIG. 3. The relationship of percent diameter circumflex constriction to resting mean flow (- - -) and hyperemic response (——) following Hypaque (coronary flow reserve) in 12 consecutive dogs. Flows are expressed as ratios to control resting mean values at the beginning of each experiment. The shaded area indicates the limits of the relationships plotted for individual dogs. r: correlation coefficient; SQ DEV: mean square of deviations (from Ref. 5).

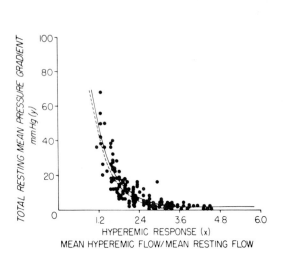

FIG. 4. Relationship of resting pressure gradient to coronary flow reserve (hyperemic mean flow after contrast/resting mean flow before contrast). The solid line and data points are for total pressure gradient across two stenoses in series. The dashed line is for the pressure gradient across a single stenosis shown for comparison (from Ref. 6).

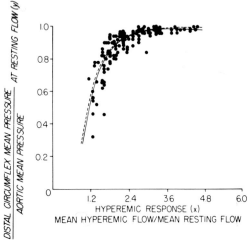

FIG. 5. Relationship of distal circumflex pressure at resting conditions to coronary flow reserve (hyperemic mean flow after contrast/resting mean flow before contrast). Distal circumflex pressure is expressed as a ratio of circumflex pressure/aortic pressure. The solid line and data points are for circumflex pressure distal to two stenoses in series. The dashed line is for circumflex pressure distal to a single stenosis shown for comparison (from Ref. 6).

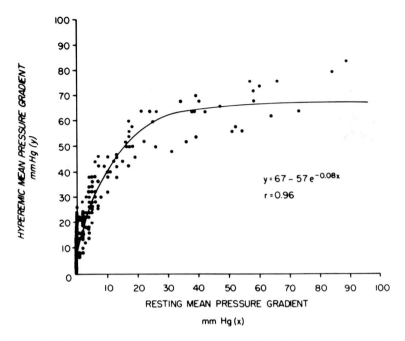

FIG. 6. Relationship between pressure gradient across a stenosis at resting conditions and the gradient at maximal flows that occur during hyperemia or heavy exercise.

number of stenoses because coronary flow reserve depends on the total or combined pressure-flow effects of lesions rather than the specific pathologic anatomy. As demonstrated by these figures, the relationships held true regardless of the geometric

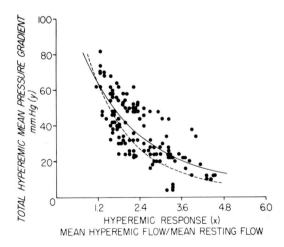

FIG. 7. Relationship of maximal pressure gradient at maximal hyperemia to coronary flow reserve (hyperemic mean flow after contrast/resting mean flow before contrast). The solid line and data points are for total pressure gradient across two stenoses in series during hyperemia. The dashed line is for pressure gradient across a single stenosis shown for comparison (from Ref. 6).

dimensions, anatomy, or number of lesions in an artery.

A pressure gradient present across a constriction at resting conditions increases under stress conditions when flow rises. This point is illustrated by Figure 6, which shows the relationship of the resting pressure gradient to that measured at maximal flow during hyperemia. Because of this fact, the relationship between coronary flow reserve and the greatest pressure gradient across a stenosis at maximal flows was also investigated. The results are shown in Figure 7. There is a good correlation between coronary flow reserve (hyperemic response) and the maximal gradient developed across single or double stenoses in series.

The clinical implications of this observation are illustrated in Figure 8, showing the relationship between coronary flow reserve (hyperemic response) and distal circumflex pressure during peak hyperemia when distal pressure dropped to much lower values than at resting flows. These curves in comparison to Figure 5 show that for any given reduction in coronary flow reserve, the distal coronary pressure was much lower during hyperemic flow than at resting flow. The solid line, indicating double stenoses in series, is similar to that for a single stenosis. Thus, if coronary vasodilatation develops during exercise in the presence of a stenosis that restricts coronary

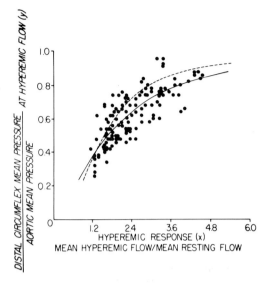

FIG. 8. Relationship of distal circumflex pressure at maximal flow to coronary flow reserve (hyperemic mean flow after contrast/resting mean flow before contrast). The solid line and data points are for circumflex pressure distal to two stenoses in series. The dashed line is for circumflex pressure distal to a single stenosis shown for comparison (from Ref. 6).

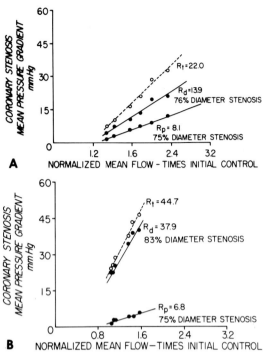

FIG. 9.A. Representative regression lines relating normalized mean circumflex flow to stenosis gradient across a proximal (R_p) and distal (R_d) stenosis separately and to total gradient across both stenoses together (R_t). The slope of each regression line is resistance. Numerical values of proximal stenosis resistance (R_p), distal stenosis resistance (R_d), and total resistance of both together (R_t) are shown. Total resistance calculated separately from total pressure gradient-flow relationships always equals the sum of the resistances for each individual stenosis (from Ref. 6). B. Same relationships described in A. However, the distal stenosis is more severe than in A. Total resistance is still equal to the sum of each individual resistance in series (from Ref. 6).

inflow, coronary perfusion pressure falls dramatically.

Coronary Stenosis Resistance

Since the pressure gradient across a constriction depended on the flow through it, a single parameter characterizing all pressure-flow effects was required for systematic comparisons or analysis of different coronary lesions. Coronary stenosis resistance is a calculated variable which fulfilled this criterion, as demonstrated in Figures 9.A and 9.B. These figures show regression lines correlating pressure and flow for each of two stenoses in series; the slope of the regression line is defined as resistance. It is indicated by R_p (proximal stenosis resistance) and R_d (distal stenosis resistance) for two constrictions in series. The total resistance across both stenoses (R_t) was calculated separately from the relationship between normalized flow and total pressure gradient. It is equal to the sum of the resistances calculated independently for each of the stenoses in series. Figure 9.B illustrates the same pressure-flow relationships and resistances with a more severe distal constriction. The slope of the regression line characterizing this more severe distal stenosis is much steeper than before, indicating a greater gradient for a given flow. Again, total resistance calculated separately across both stenoses is equal to the sum of resistances calculated separately for each stenosis. We analyzed 125 pairs of stenoses in series in this manner. In every instance total resistance determined independently from total gradient-flow relationships equaled the sum of the two individual resistances calculated separately.

The close relationship between coronary flow reserve (hyperemic response) and coronary stenosis resistance is shown in Figure 10. As resistance increased, coronary flow reserve (hyperemic response) diminished. The solid line, indicating the relationship for double stenoses in series, is only slightly different from that for a single constriction. The minor differences are a reflection of the shape or sharpness of the "break point" at hyperemic responses of about 2.4 rather than any basic differences in the relationships.

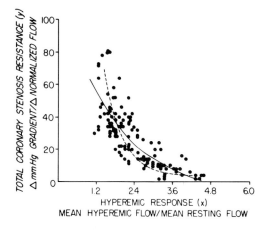

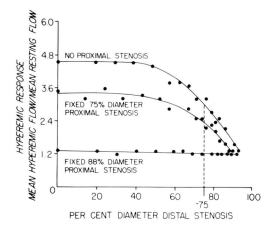

FIG. 10. Relationship of total coronary stenoses resistance to coronary flow reserve (hyperemic mean flow after contrast/resting mean flow before contrast). The solid line and data points are for total resistance across two stenoses in series. The dashed line is for resistance of a single stenosis shown for comparison (from Ref. 6).

FIG. 11. Relationship of hyperemic responses (coronary flow reserve) to progressive circumflex stenosis with no proximal stenosis, with a fixed 75 percent diameter proximal stenosis, and with a fixed 88 percent diameter proximal stenosis in one dog. The upper curve is typical for progressive single stenosis as shown in Figure 2. The middle curve shows that an additional fixed, 75 percent diameter proximal stenosis reduces all hyperemic responses. The lower curve shows this relationship with a fixed 88 percent diameter proximal stenosis, which is severe enough to prevent significant flow increases over baseline in response to contrast (from Ref. 6).

Multiple Stenoses in Series

It is a common clinical maxim that coronary hemodynamics are determined by the most severe lesion in a coronary artery. The data presented indicate that this concept is imprecise. Pressure gradients and resistances of stenoses in series are clearly additive. The effects of stenoses in series on flow are more complex. In some circumstances this maxim may be appropriate. For example, an 80 percent diameter stenosis did not reduce resting coronary flow in our studies; if in series with a 95 percent stenosis, which did affect resting flow, the more severe lesion determined entirely the effects on resting flow. Similarly, a 30 percent diameter stenosis did not reduce coronary flow reserve; if in series with a 60 percent diameter stenosis, which did reduce coronary flow reserve, the more severe lesion also determined entirely the effects on hyperemic flow. However, if both lesions were separately severe enough to reduce flow, their effects in series were cumulative and the most severe lesion did not determine all the effects on flow. For example, in Figure 11 the coronary flow reserve (hyperemic response) associated with two 75 percent diameter stenoses in series was more impaired than with one stenosis alone. Although not shown, two 95 percent stenoses in series reduced resting flow more than one alone. Thus, the maxim that the most severe lesion determines the hemodynamic effects of stenoses is accurate only under restricted circumstances related to severity of lesions and extent to which flow is elevated over basal resting levels.

In our studies the calculated resistance of an anatomically fixed proximal stenosis was observed to decrease slightly as the distal constrictor was tightened and as distal resistance increased markedly. An example of this observation is illustrated in Figure 12, showing resistances of each of two stenoses in series; the proximal constriction was anatomically fixed at 75 percent narrowing while the distal constriction was progressively increased from zero. As the resistance of the distal constriction increased from less than one up to 42, the resistance of the fixed proximal stenosis decreased from approximately 10 to 5. This decrease to 50 percent of the initial resistance was a relatively small change compared to the greater than 4000 percent increase in distal resistance but was consistently found. On the average, the resistance of the anatomically fixed proximal stenosis decreased to 60 percent of its initial value as the distal stenosis increased by an average of 3400 percent. The explanation for this observation is difficult to prove but turbulence occurring downstream from a stenosis diminishes or disappears if a more severe, distal constriction is added.[11] Elimination of downstream turbulence and the kinetic energy loss associated with it theoretically reduced the energy loss, and therefore pressure

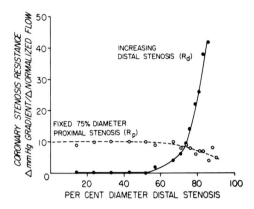

FIG. 12. Relationship of the coronary stenosis resistance of a fixed 75 percent diameter proximal stenosis to that of a progressive distal stenosis in series. As distal constriction increases, distal stenosis resistance (R_d) rises. However, the resistance of the anatomically fixed 75 percent proximal stenosis (R_p) decreases slightly in comparison to the large increase in distal resistance, probably because the distal stenosis eliminates proximal turbulence (from Ref. 6).

loss, across the proximal stenosis. This decreased pressure gradient for any given flow was reflected as a slightly decreased resistance even though the proximal stenosis was anatomically fixed.

Regional Myocardial Perfusion

Regional coronary perfusion in the resting state remains normal despite relatively severe coronary stenosis.[5] An example of myocardial flow distribution of a dog's left coronary artery in the presence of an 80 percent circumflex stenosis is shown in Figure 13. At rest (prior to hyperemia), regional perfusion was uniform despite an 80 percent circumflex constriction as shown by the upper left panel. During hyperemia induced by Hypaque, there was a marked increase in perfusion of myocardium supplied by the normal left anterior descending (LAD) artery. However, myocardium within the circumflex distribution failed to demonstrate comparable hyperemia due to the constriction. Thus, flow distribution with an 80 percent stenosis was normal at rest but showed marked abnormalities during hyperemia because of a limited coronary flow reserve of the circumflex artery. The myocardial image was quantitatively analyzed from a number of small, equal-sized region-of-interest areas distributed over myocardium supplied by anterior descending and circumflex arteries. The location and size of the areas of interest for this example are demonstrated in

the drawing of Figure 13. The number of counts recorded from each small area of myocardium was divided by the total number of counts from the entire left ventricle and represents the percent of total left ventricular flow for the various areas of the myocardium at rest and during hyperemia. The open squares of the graph are a quantitative display of the visual image showing normal regional perfusion at rest despite severe circumflex narrowing. Following a vasodilatory stimulus, as shown by the solid squares, the percent flow increased markedly to areas in the LAD distribution but changed little in the circumflex distribution. It was this relative or maldistribution of flow during hyperemia that caused an abnormal image under hyperemic "stress."

The visual and quantitative differences illustrated in Figure 13 were also expressed as the ratio of counts over myocardium supplied by the anterior descending (LAD counts) to counts over the myocardium supplied by the circumflex (CIRC counts) before and after hyperemic stimulus. These ratios were averaged for all experiments and the results are shown in Figure 14. The mean data in Figure 14 were obtained with a mean left circumflex constriction of 85 percent diameter narrowing. At resting flow, before Hypaque, the maximal ratio of peak LAD counts/mean CIRC counts was 1.0 ± 0.2, indicating uniform flow distribution. However, after Hypaque this ratio increased to 2.3 ± 0.5 ($p < 0.001$), indicating markedly abnormal flow distribution. In extensive animal testing, regional malperfusion during hyperemia as quantified by myocardial imaging was very accurate quantitatively when compared to simultaneous measurements by electromagnetic flowmeter.

Clinical Application

The application of these principles to the evaluation of patients at present utilizes the gamma camera to image myocardial regional perfusion in the resting and hyperemic states. As detailed in methods, patients were studied by left intracoronary injection of [113m]Indium macroaggregated albumin in the resting state and ^{99m}Tc macroaggregated albumin during the hyperemia that follows intracoronary injection of Hypaque-M, 75 percent. After completion of coronary arteriography, myocardial images were obtained in multiple views at the two different energy levels appropriate for [113m]In and [99m]Tc. Scintiphotographs of

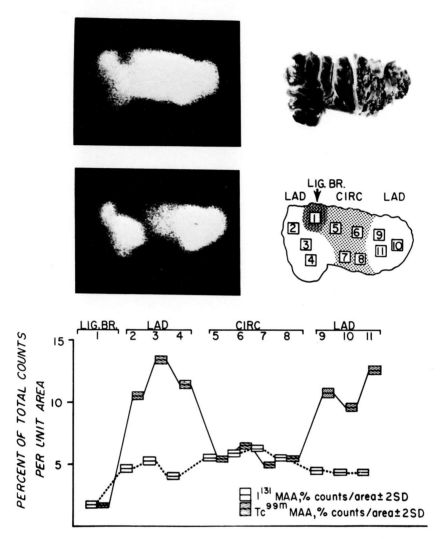

FIG. 13. Left ventricular regional flow distribution in a dog at rest and during hyperemia in the presence of 80 percent circumflex constriction. The dissected, opened left ventricle was positioned endocardium down for postmortem myocardial imaging as pictured on the upper right. The circumflex distribution is in the center of the specimen surrounded by myocardium supplied by the anterior descending. The ^{131}I image on the upper left shows normal resting regional perfusion despite 80 percent circumflex constriction. During the hyperemia induced by intracoronary Hypaque, a [99mTc] image on the lower left shows abnormal regional perfusion due to a normal hyperemic response in the anterior descending but lack of response in the constricted circumflex. The location of small, equal-sized, region-of-interest areas are indicated by the drawing on the lower right corresponding to the photographed specimen above. Counts for each region-of-interest area, expressed as percentage of total ventricular counts (percent of total ventricular flow), are plotted on the vertical axis of the graph with its corresponding location on the ventricle indicated by number on the horizontal axis. The graph is a quantitative, rather than visual, demonstration of regional coronary flow distribution. Lig. Br. refers to a very small coronary branch ligated during transducer implantation (from Ref. 5).

BEFORE CONTRAST   AFTER CONTRAST

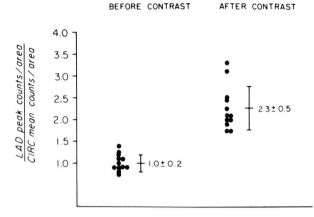

FIG. 14. Left ventricular regional flow distribution in 12 consecutive dogs before and after hyperemic stimulus in the presence of an average 85 percent circumflex constriction. On the vertical axis is shown the ratio of counts from myocardium supplied by the anterior descending (LAD counts) to counts from myocardium supplied by the constricted circumflex (CIRC counts). The ratios are significantly different with P < 0.001, demonstrating normal flow distribution at rest but markedly abnormal distribution during hyperemia (from Ref. 5).

myocardial images were visually interpreted and stored in digital form on magnetic tape for subsequent processing and reproduction, as for the examples presented subsequently. As shown in Figure 15, in the left posterior oblique view (LPO) the myocardial image of the left coronary distribution has a triangular shape. The top corner of the triangle corresponds to the origin of the coronary arteries; the left or anterior border of the image corresponds to the LAD distribution and the right or posterior border corresponds to the circumflex distribution; the inferior border corresponds to the posterior descending (PDA) distribution of the right coronary artery.

Figure 16 illustrates a clinical study on a patient in whom coronary arteriography demonstrated a 60 percent stenosis of the LAD and total occlusion of the right coronary, which filled retrograde from the LAD. In the LPO view, regional perfusion at rest was normal and uniform as shown in the left panel, indicating satisfactory flow to circumflex, LAD and right coronary distribution. However, during contrast-induced hyperemia, regional perfusion was markedly abnormal with a

relative cut in flow to areas supplied by the LAD (anterior or left border) and PDA (inferior). The circumflex region (posterior or right border) received most of the increase in coronary flow. Thus, the LAD stenosis had no hemodynamic significance in the resting state but under "stress" conditions at high flow rates caused significant regional malperfusion of a large segment of ventricular myocardium.

Figure 17 demonstrates the findings in a patient with a 50 percent stenosis of the mid-circumflex. In the LPO view, regional perfusion was normal at rest, as shown in the left panel. However, during the hyperemia induced by contrast media, regional perfusion became markedly abnormal with a relative cut in flow to the circumflex distribution (posterior or right border). As in the previous example, the circumflex lesion in this case had no hemodynamic consequences at

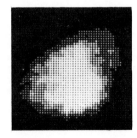
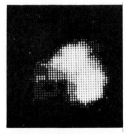

FIG. 16. Patient RAD. Coronary arteriography showed a 60 percent diameter stenosis of the anterior descending; the occluded right coronary filled from the LAD. A myocardial image in the LPO view using ^{113m}Indium MAA at rest showed normal regional distribution (left). A myocardial image by ^{99m}Tc MAA during the hyperemia following intracoronary contrast injection showed decreased perfusion to myocardium supplied by the anterior descending due to restricted coronary flow reserve of the LAD caused by the stenosis (right).

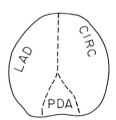
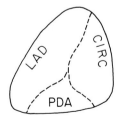

FIG. 15. Anatomy of myocardial regional perfusion as visualized by myocardial imaging in left anterior oblique view (left) and left posterior oblique view (right). LAD is left anterior descending; CIRC is left circumflex; PDA is the posterior descending branch of the right coronary artery.

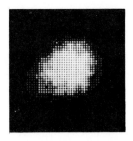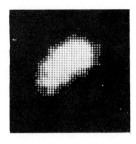

FIG. 17. Patient LEN. Coronary arteriography revealed a 50 percent diameter mid-circumflex stenosis. Regional flow distribution by ^{113m}Indium MAA was normal under resting conditions (left). Regional flow distribution by ^{99m}Tc MAA during hyperemia was decreased in the area distal to the mid-circumflex due to restriction on coronary flow reserve caused by the stenosis (right).

rest but caused gross malperfusion under "stress" conditions at elevated flow rates. There have been no ill effects arising from hyperemic perfusion studies.

Myocardial images of regional distribution during coronary hyperemia or at rest portray relative flow differences between various regions and do not show absolute changes in flow. For example, in animal experiments, if both the circumflex and anterior descending arteries were progressively constricted to the same degree, the hyperemic flow response became equally impaired in both and no regional maldistribution occurred despite an absolute decrease in the hyperemic responses of both vessels. Similarly in patients with balanced stenoses affecting LAD and circumflex flow equally, myocardial images may show uniform regional perfusion at rest and during hyperemia. Thus, while coronary arteriography indicates the anatomy of coronary stenoses, myocardial images of regional distribution at rest and during hyperemia indicate their hemodynamic significance.

Limitations of Indicator Dilution Techniques for Measuring Coronary Flow

All indicator dilution techniques require (1) delivery of an indicator, usually an inert gas, to the myocardium and (2) a record of the disappearance or clearance of the indicator from the myocardium over time. Coronary flow is calculated from the characteristics of the clearance curve utilizing equations whose validity assumes or requires (1) monoexponential disappearance rates, (2) constant mean flow during the period of clearance, and (3) flow-limited tissue exchange.

The many indicator techniques described differ only as to type of indicator, route of delivery, and means of recording the disappearance rate. All methods share the same basic assumptions and limitations to a greater or lesser extent. Routes of delivery include inhalation (N_2O, H_2), intravenous($Rb^{84}Cl$, $Rb^{86}Cl$, I^{131}-antipyrine), intraventricular (K^{85}), selective intracoronary (Xe^{133}, K^{85}, I^{125} antipyrine), intramyocardial (Xe^{133}, Na^{24}) injection or infusion. Recording methods include precardial counting, coronary sinus, and arterial blood sampling. Units of flow are usually expressed as cc/minute per 100 gm of myocardium. These units are not equivalent to measuring absolute coronary flow in cc/minute divided by an independently determined mass or volume of distribution for the indicator. The volume of distribution of the indicator is unknown and cannot be independently determined. Flow by clearance techniques is therefore not a measure of arterial flow comparable to "flow through a pipe" in cc/minute. Hypothetically for example, the coronary artery of a 100 gm heart having a clearance flow of 100 cc/minute/100 gm delivers an absolute flow of 100 cc/minute. By comparison the coronary artery of a 200-gm heart with the same flow per 100 gm delivers an absolute flow of 200 cc/minute. If the 200-gm heart were subjected to removal of half its mass, as by coronary occlusion with infarction, the flow to the remaining half would still be 100 cc/minute/100 gm, and therefore unchanged compared to the normal heart. However, the absolute flow in cc/minute would be reduced by half compared to the normal heart.

The limitations of clearance techniques for measuring coronary flow arise from the three assumptions necessary for calculating coronary flow from the disappearance curve. The most problematic of these assumptions is that the disappearance curve is monoexponential and results from homogeneous flow with identical rates of indicator delivery and clearance throughout the myocardium. Myocardial perfusion in coronary disease is now known to be heterogeneous with diseased areas of the myocardium having different clearance curves than normal or less diseased areas. Poorly perfused areas of myocardium demonstrate prolonged clearance of low concentrations of indicator. Consequently, standard recording periods using standard techniques, which do not sensitively detect small concentrations of indicator, fail to account for the low flow to diseased areas of myocardium. Flow measurements are therefore strongly biased by areas of normal or high flow and values are erroneously high. This error is particularly exaggerated at high flow rates (exercise, hyperemia) where normal perfusion increases much more than in diseased areas of myocardium.

Several excellent reports [12-15] demonstrate that standard techniques of indicator delivery and sampling introduce errors of over 50 percent in calculated resting coronary flow in the presence of heterogeneous flow. These errors are greatest with delivery of indicator over standard short periods of time (or by bolus injection), with standard short sampling times (3 to 10 minutes) and with standard analytical techniques or precordial counting which are insensitive to prolonged washout of low concentrations of indicator from slowly perfused regions. The errors are least with prolonged delivery and sampling times (three hours) and with very sensitive analytical techniques such as gas chromatography. However, with prolonged delivery and sampling times, coronary flow is more likely spontaneously to vary and introduce errors by violating the second assumption of constant flow.

These limitations are illustrated by an extensive literature. For example, coronary flows by nitrous oxide desaturation with units of cc/minute/100 gm myocardium are within normal limits in severe aortic valve disease,[16] severe coronary artery disease,[17] hypertension and congestive failure.[18] Normal or insignificantly reduced values are also found in coronary artery disease by techniques using Xenon[133,19-21] Krypton[85,22] Rubidium[86] chloride,[23] and Rubidium[84] chloride,[24,25] although data on the latter are not consistent.[26] In contrast to their inaccuracy in coronary disease, these methods do detect changes from normal in diseases with altered metabolic demands or oxygen transport such as thyrotoxicosis[27] and severe anemia.[28]

The Rubidium[84] chloride method expresses flow in units of cc/minute per whole heart. However, Rubidium uptake and clearance are not linearly related to absolute flow and vary greatly depending on the adequacy of myocardial oxygenation, absolute flow rates, coronary transit time, and effects of sympathetic amines[25,26,29-31] with errors up to 50 percent compared to an independent standard, such as a rotameter.[30] As a result, the term coronary "nutrient" flow has been applied to the results obtained by this method.[25,26,32] However, it does not correspond to absolute coronary artery flow in cc/minute. The method utilizing T-1824 bound to albumin and tritiated water is a method for measuring absolute left coronary artery flow.[33] However, it is applicable only to the left coronary artery, is invalid in the presence of heterogeneous flow or right to left collaterals, and requires a six-minute continuous infusion selectively into the left main coronary. Forty percent of studies were rejected due to technical difficulties.

It has been postulated that coronary flows in patients with coronary disease are within normal limits because they are measured at rest [21] rather than because of limitations in methodology. With exercise stress, coronary flow rates should theoretically be abnormal in coronary patients because of the limited capacity for increasing flow through stenotic coronary arteries. One study using Rubidium[84] chloride supports this hypothesis,[34] but five others found no difference in the coronary flow response of normal and coronary patients during exercise or pharmacologic stress by clearance methods of measuring flow.[2,22,35-38] Such discrepancies further emphasize the importance and limitations of methodology. It is therefore not surprising that the correlation between severity of coronary disease by arteriography correlates poorly with coronary flow measured by indicator dilution techniques.[38]

The problems indicated above have been avoided to some extent by using a multiple-crystal scintillation camera, which records disappearance curves over multiple areas of the myocardium, as opposed to single precordial counters used previously.[39] However, the sensitivity of this approach for identifying nonocclusive or subcritical lesions has not been demonstrated. Another approach that circumvents some of these difficulties employs myocardial imaging of ^{43}K at rest and during exercise.[40] The method is particularly appealing because it is noninvasive and may be performed on an outpatient basis. However, there are technical problems that also limit its applicability as currently described. ^{43}K is not readily available to most laboratories and the resolution of the myocardial images are presently inferior to those obtained by direct intracoronary injection of labeled macroaggregated albumin. Furthermore, in the presence of localized coronary disease-causing angina pectoris, the patient may not tolerate sufficient exercise (or pacing) to stress the surrounding areas of normal myocardium or increase flow in those areas comparable to that seen during pharmacologic hyperemia. For these reasons, myocardial imaging before and during hyperemia induced by intracoronary contrast media or comparable agents appears to be more sensitive and accurate than the ^{43}K technique. They are applicable, however, only during coronary arteriography.

SUMMARY

Resting coronary blood flow and regional perfusion are normal despite relatively severe coronary stenoses. Maximal coronary flow or coronary flow reserve is impaired by relatively mild stenoses before resting flow is affected. Assessment of coronary flow reserve and regional perfusion during maximal hyperemia provides a means of evaluating in patients the hemodynamic effects of coronary stenoses before they become severe enough to reduce resting flow or cause myocardial infarction.

References

1. Messer JV, Wagman RJ, Levine HJ, Neill WA, Krasnow N, Gorlin R: Patterns of human myocardial oxygen extraction during rest and exercise. J Clin Invest 41:725–42, 1962
2. Holmberg SW, Serzysko W, Varnauskas E: Coronary circulation during heavy exercise in control subjects and patients with coronary disease. Acta Med Scand 190:465–80, 1971
3. Eckstein RW: Effect of exercise and coronary artery narrowing on collateral circulation. Circ Res 5:230, 1957
4. Elliot EC, Jones EL, Bloor CM, Leon AS, Gregg DE: Day to day changes in coronary hemodynamics secondary to constriction of circumflex branch of left coronary artery in conscious dogs. Circ Res 22:237–50, 1968
5. Gould KL, Lipscomb K, Hamilton, GW: A physiologic basis for assessing critical coronary stenosis: instantaneous flow response and regional distribution during coronary hyperemia as measures of coronary flow reserve. Am J Cardiol 33:87–94, 1974
6. Gould KL, Lipscomb K: Effects of coronary stenoses on coronary flow reserve and resistance. Am J Cardiol (in press, 1974)
7. Olsson RA, Gregg DE: Myocardial reactive hyperemia in the unanesthetized dog. Am J Physiol 208:224–30, 1965
8. Khouri EM, Gregg DE, Rayford CR: Effect of exercise on cardiac output, left coronary flow and myocardial metabolism in the unanesthetized dog. Circ Res 17:427–37, 1965
9. Van Citters RL, Franklin DL: Cardiovascular performance of Alaska sled dogs during exercise. Circ Res 24:33–42, 1969
10. Marchetti GV, Noseda V, Visioli O: Myocardial blood flow in experimental cardiac hypertrophy in dogs. Cardiovasc Res 7:519–27, 1973
11. Robbins SL, Bentov I: The kinetics of viscous flow in a model vessel. Lab Invest 16:864–74, 1967
12. Klocke FJ, Koberstein RC, Pittman DE, Bunnell IL, Green DG, Rosing DR: Effects of heterogenous myocardial perfusion on coronary venous H_2 desaturation curves and calculations of coronary flow. J Clin Invest 47:2711–24, 1968
13. Klocke FJ, Rosing DR, Pittman DE: Inert gas measurement of coronary blood flow. Am J Cardiol 23:548–55, 1969
14. Klocke FJ and Wittenberg SM: Heterogeneity of coronary blood flow in human coronary artery disease and experimental myocardial infarction. Am J Cardiol 24:782–90, 1969
15. Sapirstein LA, Ogden E: Theoretic limitations of the nitrous oxide method for the determination of regional blood flow. Circ Res 4:245–49, 1956
16. Rowe GG, Afonso S, Lugo JE, Castillo CA, Boake WC, Crumpton CW: Coronary blood flow and myocardial oxidative metabolism at rest and during exercise in subjects with severe aortic valve disease. Circulation 32:251–57, 1965
17. Rowe GG, Thomsen JH, Stenlund RD, McKenna DH, Sialer S, Corliss RJ: A study of hemodynamics and coronary blood flow in man with coronary artery disease. Circulation 34:139–42, 1969
18. Bing RJ, Hammond MM, Handelsman JC, Powers SR, Spencer FC, Eckenhoff JE, Goodale WT, Hafkenschiel JH, Kety SS: The measurement of coronary blood flow, oxygen consumption, and efficiency of the left ventricle in man. Am Heart J 38:1–24, 1969
19. Ross RS, Veda K, Lichten PR, Rees JR: Measurement of myocardial blood flow in animals and man by selective injection of radioactive inert gas into the coronary arteries. Circ Res 15:28–41, 1964
20. Bernstein L, Friesinger GC, Lichtlen PR, Ross RS: The effect of nitroglycerin on the systemic and coronary circulation in man and dogs. Circulation 33:107–16, 1966
21. Homberg S, Paulin S, Prerousky I, Varnauskas E: Coronary blood flow in man and its relation to the coronary arteriogram. Am J Cardiol 19:486–91, 1967
22. Parker JO, West RO, DiGiorgi S: The effect of nitroglycerin on coronary blood flow and the hemodynamic response to exercise in coronary artery disease. Am J Cardiol 27:59–65, 1971
23. Donato L, Bartolomei G, Giordani R: Evaluation of myocardial blood perfusion in man with radioactive potassium or rubidium and precordial counting. Circulation 24:195–203, 1964
24. Cohen A, Gallagher JP, Luebs ED, Varga Z, Yamanaka J, Zaleski EJ, Blumchen G, Bing RJ: The quantitative determination of coronary flow with a position emitter (Rb84). Circulation 32:636–49, 1965
25. Cohen A, Zaleski EJ, Baleiron H, Stock TB, Chiba C, Bing RJ: Measurement of coronary blood flow using rubidium 84 and the coincidence counting method. Am J Cardiol 19:556–62, 1967
26. Cowan C, Duran P, Corsini G, Goldschlager N, Bing RJ: The effects of nitroglycerine on myocardial blood flow in man. Am J Cardiol 24:154–60, 1969
27. Rowe GG, Huston JH, Weinstein AB, Tuchman H, Brown JF, Crumpton CW: The hemodynamics of thyrotoxicosis in man with special reference to coronary blood flow and myocardial oxygen metabolism. J Clin Invest 35:272–76, 1956
28. Bhatia ML, Manchanda SC, Roy SB: Coronary hemodynamic studies in chronic severe anaemia. Br Heart J 31:365–74, 1969
29. Mack RE, Nolting DD, Hogancamp CE, Bing RJ: Myocardial extraction of Rb 86 in the rabbit. Am J Physiol 197:1175–77, 1959
30. Moir TW: Measurement of coronary blood flow in dogs with normal and abnormal myocardial oxygenation and function. Comparison of flow measured by a rotameter and by Rb 86 clearance. Circ Res 19:695–99, 1966
31. Conn HL: Use of external counting techniques in studies of the circulation. Circ Res 10:505–10, 1962
32. Tillich G, Mendona L, Bing R: Total and nutrient coronary flow. Supp I to Circ Res 38 and 39, I 148–53, 1971

33. Klassen GA, Agarwal JB, Tanser PH, Woodhouse SP, Marpole D: Blood flow and tissue space of the left coronary artery in man. Circ Res 27:185–95, 1970

34. Knoebel SB, Elliott WC, McHenry PL, Ross E: Myocardial blood flow in coronary artery disease. Correlation with severity of disease and treadmill exercise response. Am J Cardiol 27:51–58, 1971

35. Messer JV, Wagman RJ, Levine HJ, Neill WA, Krasnow N, Gorlin R: Patterns of human myocardial oxygen extraction during rest and exercise. J Clin Invest 41:725–42, 1962

36. Cohen LS, Elliott WC, Klein MD, Gorlin R: Coronary heart disease, clinical, cinearteriographic and metabolic correlations. Am J Cardiol 17:153–68, 1966

37. Sullivan JM, Gorlin R: Effects of epinephrine on the coronary circulation in human subjects with and without coronary artery disease. Circ Res 21:919–23, 1967

38. Schwartz L, Froggatt G, Covvey HD, Taylor K, Morch JE: Measurement of left anterior descending coronary arterial blood flow. Technique, methods of blood flow analysis and correlation with angiography. Am J Cardiol 32:679–85, 1973

39. Cannon PJ, Dell RB, Dwyer EM: Measurement of regional myocardial perfusion in man with ^{133}Xenon and a scintillation camera. J Clin Invest 51:964–77, 1972

40. Zaret BL, Strauss HW, Martin ND, Wells HP, Flamm MD: Noninvasive regional myocardial perfusion with radioactive potassium. N Engl J Med 288:809–12, 1973

21

RESPONSE OF THE SYSTOLIC TIME INTERVALS TO EXERCISE STRESS TESTING

Alan B. Miller and Robert C. Bahler

The prevalence of ischemic heart disease, including coronary atherosclerosis, has led to extensive investigations into the natural history, prognosis, and early diagnosis of this disorder. Data concerning the natural history of coronary artery disease indicate increasing mortality and morbidity based on the extent of coronary disease and the number of vessels involved. Consequently there has been more emphasis placed on methods that can accurately identify individuals with early or latent ischemic heart disease in an effort to alter the natural course through recent techniques of myocardial revascularization.

Indirect measures of cardiac function were introduced long before the advent of cardiac catheterization. It is interesting to note that in the present era of widespread availability of direct assessment of both hemodynamic parameters and the coronary circulation, there has been a flurry of activity in the area of indirect evaluation of cardiac function. Two such indirect methods are exercise testing and the external measurement of systolic time intervals.

Historically, the use of exercise as a diagnostic aid in ischemic heart disease began with Master over 40 years ago. Recent modifications have created almost a subspecialty within the field of cardiology (Blomqvist, 1971). The classic indication for stress testing is in the evaluation of individuals with atypical chest pain. Rhythmic exercise produces an increase in all parameters that determine myocardial oxygen consumption including heart rate (HR), contractility, and left ventricular wall tension. An exercise test can therefore provide a controlled stress on the cardiovascular system and the physiologic response can be observed. Various methods of stress testing are available today. The single load type is exemplified by the Master two-step. This method has been criti-

ficient workload for some subjects and exceeds the cized on the basis that it does not provide a sufficient cardiac reserve of others. Consequently, multistage tests were devised utilizing either the bicycle ergometer or the treadmill. These methods based on stepwise increments in workload, provide a means of increasing myocardial oxygen demand in a linear fashion. In this manner a quantitative estimate of physical work capacity can be obtained or a reduction in cardiac reserve can be detected.

The validity of the results utilizing graded exercise tests have been measured against direct studies of cardiac function obtained at cardiac catheterization and a positive correlation has been established (Roitman, Jones, et al, 1970). Recently however, investigators have critically evaluated the reliability of exercise testing in the evaluation of ischemic heart disease (Redwood and Epstein, 1972). They concluded that available exercise techniques are not adequate. That is, there are numerous subjects with documented ischemic heart disease but essentially negative stress tests as well as individuals with abnormalities on stress testing but normal cardiac catherizations.

It would seem logical that further evaluation of cardiac function in addition to the parameters monitored during stress testing (HR, blood pressure [BP], electrocardiographic [EKG] response) might enhance the diagnostic potential. The resting phases of systole have recently been measured in a quantitative fashion in various types of heart disease and were found to correspond well with the directly measured parameters (Weissler and Garrard, 1971; Martin, Shaver, et al, 1971). We have tried to correlate the results of a standard exercise protocol utilizing the bicycle ergometer with the response of the systolic time intervals (STI) to exercise in a consecutive group of subjects referred for exercise testing.

METHODS

Subjects were studied in the exercise physiology laboratory in the postabsorptive state. Informed consent was obtained prior to the stress test. A 12-lead resting EKG was obtained on each subject. Resting STIs were then obtained (Hewlett Packard Polybeam Recorder) by the simultaneous measurement of the EKG, phonocardiogram, and carotid artery pulse (Fig. 1). The EKG clearly delineated the onset of ventricular depolarization (initial septal forces). The microphone for the phonocardiogram was carefully placed to record the initial high-frequency components of the second heart sound (S2). The carotid pulse tracings in our laboratory were obtained through an air displacement system connected to a P-23-DB Statham transducer. The following phases of systole were determined: total electrical mechanical systole or QS2—measured from the onset of the QRS complex to the initial high frequency vibrations of S2; left ventricular ejection time or LVET—measured from the onset of the carotid pulse upstroke to the dicrotic notch; the preejection period or PEP—the difference between the QS2 and the LVET. A correction for heart rate was used to convert the measured interval to a corrected interval for QS2 (QS2c) and LVET (LVETc) (Weissler and Garrard, 1971). No correction was utilized for the preejection period (Whitsett and Naughton, 1971). The intervals were recorded at 200 mm/second with 40-msec time lines. Following the resting STIs, each subject pedaled an upright bicycle ergometer at increasing workloads with intermittent rest periods (three-minute exercise, two-minute rest). Target heart rates were 85 percent of the age-predicted maximum. During the test a CM-5 lead was continuously monitored and blood pressures were recorded with a standard sphygmomanometer at each work level. End points for terminating the test included attaining the target heart rate, severe fatigue, angina, ventricular arrhythmias, intraventricular, or atrioventricular conduction defects,

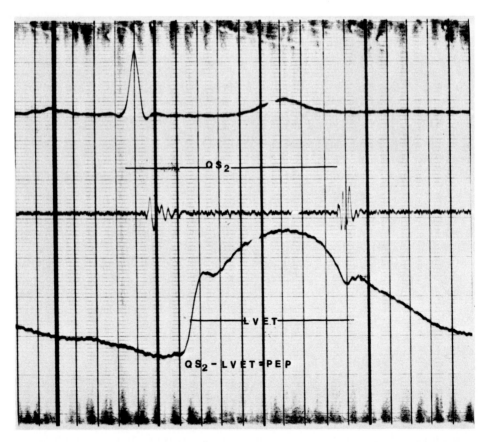

FIG. 1. Typical tracing of the phases of systole obtained in our laboratory. QS2 = total electrical mechanical systole; LVET = left ventricular ejection time; PEP = preejection period. Paper speed is 200 mm/second and intervals are measured to the nearest 2.5 msecs.

and the development of marked ST segment change. EKG and BP monitoring were continued for five minutes during recovery. Immediately upon termination of the test, repeat supine STIs were obtained. The postexercise recording could be accomplished within 30 seconds of peak exercise.

Criteria for an Abnormal Test

Electrocardiographic changes consisting of a downsloping or flattened ST segment depressed at least 1 mm and 0.08 seconds duration were interpreted as ischemic. If the ST segment was depressed 1 mm but was upward sloping, this was considered to be a form of "J"-point depression. The development of more than 10 premature ventricular contractions (PVCs) or coupled PVCs during exercise also indicated an abnormal test. The systolic blood pressure responses were recorded at each level of exercise and compared to a group of normal responders. Significant upward deviation from the normal slope, consistent with the development of an abnormal afterload also constituted an abnormal response to exercise (Miller and Naughton, 1973). Symptoms during the test of typical angina relieved by the cessation of exercise and without associated objective changes in the EKG or BP also connoted an abnormal response. An estimate of myocardial oxygen consumption (MVO2) at each workload level was derived from the formula: $2 \times Kp\text{-}m + 300/wt(kg) = MVO2$ in ml/kg/minute, where Kp-m is the workload in kilopound-meters. Physical work capacity was expressed in METs, where one MET is a metabolic equivalent consisting of a resting MVO2 of 3.5 ml/kg/minute (Miller and Naughton, 1973). Normal individuals should be able to increase their MVO2 to a level at least seven times the resting state (seven METs) in response to submaximal stress testing.

Abnormal Systolic Time Interval Response

As has been noted in previous investigations, the most consistent and reliable parameter that indicates an abnormal systolic time interval response to exercise is a prolongation of the LVETc postexercise (Whitsett and Naughton, 1971; Pouget, Harris, et al, 1971; Harris, Aytan, et al, 1973). We have utilized an increase of more than 5 msec in the postexercise LVETc to indicate an abnormal response.

Cardiac catheterization was performed on 22 of the study group. Left ventriculograms were

analyzed in the 30-degree right anterior oblique projection. Selective coronary arteriograms using the Sones technique, were obtained on 35-mm film with a Picker image intensifier and filming at 60 frames/second. Significant coronary obstruction was defined as 75 percent or greater narrowing in any major vessel.

RESULTS

The subjects were divided into groups based on both their exercise test results and systolic time interval responses (Fig. 2). Group I subjects had abnormal stress tests and abnormal STI responses; group II contained those with normal stress tests but abnormal STI responses; group III were those with normal STI and exercise responses. A subgroup comprised those subjects undergoing cardiac catheterization in group II.

Study Population

All of the study group, 28 men and 23 women, were referred to the Cleveland Metropolitan General Hospital exercise laboratory for evaluation of cardiac symptoms or physical work capacity. Group I was significantly older (mean 52.6 years) than the other groups (group II: mean 44.1 years; group III: 42.4 years) (p < 0.05) (Fig. 3.A). All groups were approximately equally divided regarding smoking habits and general level of physical activity. Three individuals were taking digitalis at the time of the study, which did not affect the stress test results. None of the subjects had been taking propranolol within 48 hours of the study.

Stress Test Results

Nineteen subjects fulfilled the criteria for an abnormal stress test (Table 1). Six (31.6 percent) underwent cardiac catheterization, and sig-

TABLE 1. Abnormal Exercise Responses

ABNORMALITY	NO. SUBJECTS	PERCENT
ST segment (1 mm; 0.08 secs)	9	47.3
Ventricular Arrythmias (More than 10 PVCs/min)	1	5.3
Angina	2	10.5
Abnormal Systolic BP Response	7	36.9
Total	19	

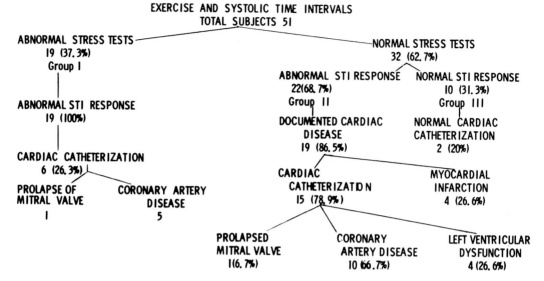

FIG. 2. Overall results of the study. Only two subjects in group III underwent cardiac catheterization and both were normal.

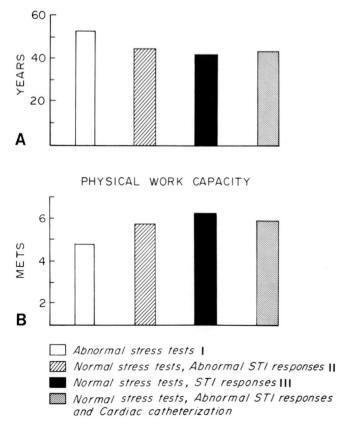

AGE OF SUBJECTS

PHYSICAL WORK CAPACITY

☐ *Abnormal stress tests* I

▨ *Normal stress tests, Abnormal STI responses* II

■ *Normal stress tests, STI responses* III

▤ *Normal stress tests, Abnormal STI responses and Cardiac catheterization*

FIG. 3.A. Age of the study population. Group I is significantly older (p < 0.05). In this and Figures 3.B, 4, 5, 7, and Table 1, a subdivision of group II, those individuals who underwent cardiac catheterization with normal exercise tests but abnormal systolic time Interval responses, is added for comparison. B. Physical work capacity. Group I has a lower physical work capacity compared to the other groups (mean METs).

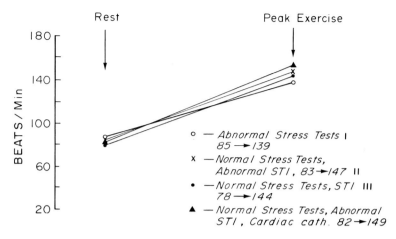

FIG. 4. Mean heart rate response. All the groups overlapped in both resting and peak heart rates.

nificant coronary artery disease was seen in five, and one had a prolapsing mitral valve.

HEART RATE RESPONSE. There is considerable overlap noted in the average resting heart rate in all of the groups, but the mean peak exercise heart rate was somewhat lower in the group with the abnormal stress tests (group I: 139 beats/minute; group II: 147 beats/minute; group III: 144 beats/minute) (n.s.) (Fig. 4).

BLOOD PRESSURE RESPONSE. Resting systolic BPs were slightly higher in group I (mean 131 mm Hg versus group II, 113 mm Hg and group III, 117 mm Hg) ($p < 0.05$) as was the mean systolic BP response (group I, 176 mm Hg; group II, 151 mm Hg; and group III, 153 mm Hg) ($p < 0.05$) (Fig. 5). Seven of the group I individuals developed a marked increase in sys-

tolic pressure during exercise when compared to a group of normals (Fig. 6). Diastolic blood pressures were not analyzed except to note that no subject had a resting diastolic blood pressure greater than 100 mm Hg. The mean postexercise change was not significant in any of the groups.

SYMPTOMS. Only two patients in group I developed angina without objective EKG changes.

PHYSICAL WORK CAPACITY. Physical work capacity was lower in group I (mean 4.8 METs; group II, 5.7 METs; group III, 6.2 METs) ($p < 0.05$) (Fig. 3.B).

ELECTROCARDIOGRAPHIC CHANGES. Ten subjects developed objective EKG changes at peak exercise, nine exhibited ST segment depression consistent with ischemia, and one developed

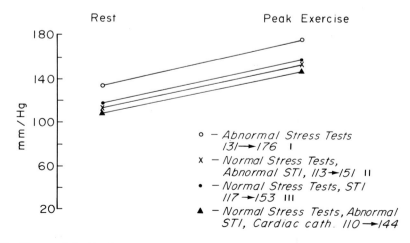

FIG. 5. Mean systolic blood pressure response. The higher systolic blood pressures as noted in group I may be due to the composition of that group.

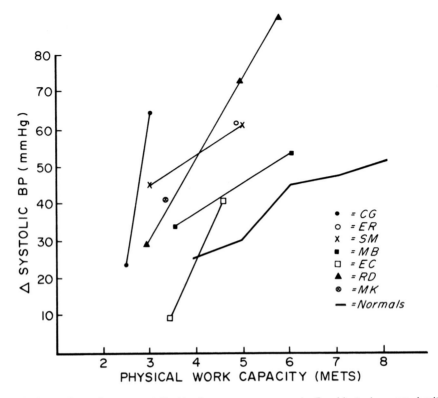

FIG. 6. Comparison of mean systolic blood pressure response in 7 subjects in group I with a group of normal individuals (normal curve from Miller, Naughton, et al). The change (Δ) in blood pressure at each work level is plotted against physical work capacity in METs. Some subjects only achieved one work level (eg, subject E.R.).

frequent PVCs. None of the subjects developed intraventricular or atrioventricular conduction disturbances.

Systolic Time Intervals (Figure 7)

LVETc. All of the 19 subjects with an abnormal stress test (group I) as well as 22 (68.7 percent) of those with normal tests demonstrated a prolongation of LVETc postexercise. This is in contrast to the shortening observed in each of the 10 other subjects with normal stress tests ($p <$ 0.005) (Table 2). Nineteen of the group II subjects (86.5 percent) had documented cardiac disease: 4 had myocardial infarctions, and 15 had abnormalities on cardiac catheterization (Table 3).

QS2c. Considerable overlap is noted between all groups in the resting and postexercise QS2c although the mean values of group III were greater when compared to the other groups ($p < 0.005$). However, a directional change on an individual basis was not noted.

PEP. There were no significant differences between the groups in the resting intervals or postexercise response.

ELECTROCARDIOGRAPHIC CORRELATIONS. Each subject with a definitely abnormal resting EKG—that is, previous myocardial infarction, intraventricular conduction delays, ST-T changes consistent with ischemia, or A-V conduction disturbances—had an abnormal systolic time interval response to exercise.

TABLE 2. **Mean Left Ventricular Ejection Time (msecs)**

	REST	POST EXERCISE	CHANGE
Abnormal stress tests: Group I (19 subjects)	390 ± 4.5	405 ± 4.1	+15 ± 2.5
Normal stress tests, abnormal STI response: Group II (22 subjects)	387 ± 4.0	407 ± 3.5	+21 ± 3.2
Normal stress test and STI response: Group III (10 subjects)	401 ± 6.4	386 ± 3.7	−14 ± 5.3

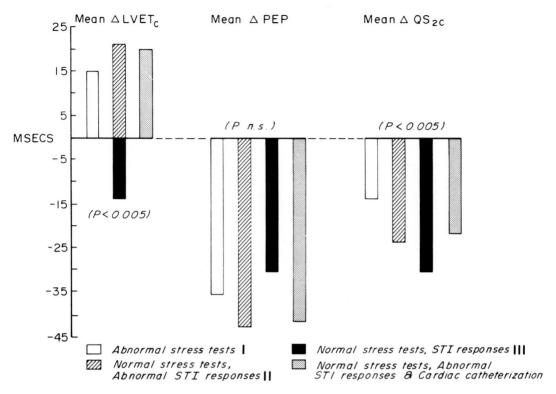

FIG. 7. Mean systolic time interval responses in all groups. A directional change is noted only in LVETc (Δ = post-exercise change).

Cardiac Catheterization (Table 3)

Twenty-three subjects underwent cardiac catheterization. Two individuals in group III had a normal study. All of the other subjects (6 or 26.3 percent from group I, 15 or 78.9 percent from group II) demonstrated either significant coronary artery disease or abnormal left ventricular function including two with prolapsing mitral valves.

DISCUSSION

Although an excellent correlation between an abnormal stress test and the response of the STI to exercise has been noted in this study, it is apparent that a significant number of subjects with cardiac disease have a normal response to submaximal graded exercise testing. The addition of the STI measurement to the basic exercise protocol has facilitated the identification of this group of individuals and provides the clue to the presence of latent ischemic heart disease.

The mechanisms of the STI changes noted postexercise have been previously described (Pouget, Harris, et al, 1971) and involve an understanding of the response of the normal heart to exercise. Rhythmic exercise causes catecholamine release, which through betaadrenergic receptors increases myocardial contractility. Also, the increase in venous return elicited by exercise may provide an increase in end diastolic myofiber length and increased contractility through the Starling mechanism. Consequently the rate of rise of the intraventricular pressure is more rapid and the time required for the left ventricular end diastolic pressure to rise to aortic diastolic levels prior to ejection is diminished. This is reflected in the short-

TABLE 3. Mean STI Response (± SEM),
Subjects with Normal Stress Tests,
Abnormal STI Response, and
Cardiac Catheterization (15)

	LVETc	PEP	QS2c
Rest	388 ± 3.2	118 ± 5.6	536 ± 6.4
Postexercise	408 ± 5.0	76 ± 5.3	527 ± 4.8
Change	+20 ± 5.0	−42 ± 3.7	−13 ± 4.0

ened PEP postexercise noted in all subjects. Some investigators have found that patients who develop angina during exercise testing demonstrated an even greater abbreviation of the preejection period compared to a group of normals. This has been attributed to an abnormal increase in left ventricular end diastolic pressure during exercise and an excess level of catecholamines (Pouget, Harris, et al, 1971).

The most consistent STI response noted in this study that clearly suggests abnormal cardiac function was the directional change of postexercise LVETc. The left ventricular ejection time is determined by several factors. It varies directly with stroke volume, cardiac output, venous return and afterload, and inversely with inotropic factors—that is, myocardial contractility. Rhythmic exercise causes an increase in all of these parameters, and as they have opposite effects on LVETc in the normal individual, since contractility is increased somewhat disproportionately, the left ventricular ejection time should shorten slightly after exercise. A marked prolongation in postexercise LVETc, however, is consistently noted in each of the subjects with abnormal stress tests, and in those with cardiac-catheterization-proven ischemic heart disease. This occurs because of two mechanisms. The first is related to an abnormal increase in afterload, which is frequently observed in patients with ischemic heart disease. Seven subjects in group I exhibited an inordinately elevated systolic blood pressure response to stress, and this probably contributed in part to the increase in postexercise LVETc. The most important factor, however, is left ventricular dysfunction, which exists as localized hypokinesis or asynergy, or frank dyskinesis in patients with obstructive coronary vascular disease, and as diffuse hypokinesis or abnormal left ventricular hemodynamics in patients with cardiomyopathy. With the abnormal contraction pattern, ejection time is prolonged. The stroke volume is maintained, but the inotropic response of the ischemic heart is not adequate and so LVETc lengthens in the face of an increased venous return.

Normally, QS2c should shorten postexercise as a reflection of increased contractility. As noted, the postexercise response in group III (normals) showed a significantly greater abbreviation of QS2c (mean values) although there was overlap noted individually. The failure of QS2c to shorten normally in response to exercise is a manifestation of the failure of LVETc to shorten. If the postexercise QS2c prolonged, this was invariably associated with concomitant lengthening of LVETc and left ventricular dysfunction.

It is important to realize that the postexercise STI response cannot distinguish between the various etiologies of ischemic heart disease. This term is used to encompass cardiac disease characterized by a disparity between myocardial oxygen supply and demand and excludes valvular and congenital abnormalities. Generally this definition pertains to coronary artery disease and myocardiopathies or disorders of left ventricular function without coronary atherosclerosis. The subjects with prolapsed mitral valve syndromes in this study are included in this category of left ventricular abnormalities, as has been recently suggested (Liedtke, Gault, et al, 1973).

Utilizing indirect assessment in the form of the postexercise STI response to gauge left ventricular function, one can study the effects of various pharmacological interventions on left ventricular performance. Investigators (Harris, Aytan, et al, 1973) have shown that nitrites can reverse left ventricular dysfunction in patients with exercise-induced angina pectoris. This is manifested by a "normalization" of the postexercise STI response or a shortening of LVETc, which had previously lengthened in response to exercise. This post-nitrite reversal of left ventricular dysfunction has also been demonstrated at cardiac catheterization as a reversal of asynergy noted on the left ventricular angiogram in patients with coronary artery disease (Mathews, Sudhaker, et al, 1974).

In conclusion, the combination of two methods of indirect assessment of cardiac function may provide a more accurate method of detecting patients with latent ischemic heart disease and should prove useful in the selection of asymptomatic individuals with EKG abnormalities, coronary risk factors, or atypical chest pain for coronary arteriography.

ACKNOWLEDGMENTS

The authors would like to express their appreciation to Miss Gladys Heckman, RN, Miss Hannah Januscovic, RN, and Mrs. Eileen Spak for technical assistance; the Medical Photography Department at Cleveland Metropolitan General Hospital and the Medical Communications Department at University Hospital of Jacksonville for assistance with charts and figures; and Mrs. DeAnne Miller for typing the manuscript.

References

Blomqvist CG: Use of exercise testing for diagnostic and functional evaluation of patients with arteriosclerotic heart disease. Circulation 44:1120–36, 1971

Harris WS, Aytan N, Pouget JM: Effects of nitroglycerin on responses of the systolic time intervals to exercise. Circulation 47:499–508, 1973

Liedtke AJ, Gault JH, Leaman DM, Blumenthal MS: Geometry of left ventricular contraction in the systolic click syndrome: characterization of a segmental myocardial abnormality. Circulation 47:27–35, 1973

Martin CE, Shaver JA, Thompson ME, Reddy PS, Leonard JJ: Direct correlation of external systolic time intervals with internal indices of left ventricular function in man. Circulation 44:419–31, 1971

Mathews RG, Sudhaker PR, O'Toole JD, et al: Reversibility of left ventricular asynergy assessed by post-nitroglycerin left ventriculography. Abst Am J Cardiol 33:156, 1974

Miller AB, Naughton J, Gorman P: Left axis deviation: diagnostic contribution of exercise stress testing. Chest 63:159–64, 1973

Pouget JM, Harris WS, Mayron BR, Naughton JP: Abnormal responses of the systolic time intervals to exercise in patients with angina pectoris. Circulation 43:289–98, 1971

Redwood DR, Epstein SE: Uses and limitations of stress testing in the evaluation of ischemic heart disease. Circulation 46:1146–54, 1972

Roitman D, Jones WB, Sheffield LT: Comparison of submaximal exercise ECG test with coronary cineangiogram. Ann Int Med 72:641–48, 1970

Weissler AM, Garrard CL: Systolic time intervals in cardiac disease. Mod Concepts Cardiovasc Dis 40:1–8, 1971

Whitsett TL, Naughton J: The effect of exercise on systolic time intervals in sedentary and active individuals and rehabilitated patients with heart disease. Am J Cardiol 27:352–58, 1971

22

THE TREADMILL EXERCISE TEST: DIAGNOSTIC
ACCURACY IN CORONARY ARTERY DISEASE

Efrain Garcia, Antoine Nasrallah,
Yousef Goussous, and Robert J. Hall

The treadmill exercise test (TET) is a non-invasive technique widely employed in the clinical diagnosis and evaluation of patients with coronary artery disease (CAD) and various syndromes of chest pain. Redwood and Epstein, 1972[7] have pointed out the limitations of the test in regard to detecting abnormalities in patients in whom advanced CAD is demonstrated angiographically. Controversy still exists [3-6] concerning the sensitivity and specificity of the test when the results of TET are correlated with angiographic findings by means of selective coronary cinearteriography. Utilizing the most commonly accepted criterion (1 mm ST segment depression) for positivity, investigators have reported the sensitivity of the test to range from 48 percent to 84 percent (true positive responses), while the specificity has ranged from 80 percent to 100 percent (true negative).[4-6,8]

METHODS

The results of the treadmill exercise test were correlated with angiographic findings in 392 patients who were referred to our institution for evaluation of chest pain. Only patients with normal resting ECG, nonspecific ST-T changes, or previous myocardial infarctions were included. Patients excluded were those in whom the resting ECG demonstrated left ventricular hypertrophy, conduction disorders such as complete left or right bundle-branch block, Wolff-Parkinson-White syndrome, or those currently receiving digitalis.

Of the total series, 191 patients demonstrated an abnormal ECG, with previous myocardial infarctions documented in 153 patients and nonspecific ST-T changes in 38. A multistage exercise protocol [1] was utilized and a modified 12-lead ECG was recorded before, during and for ten minutes after exercise.[1] Patients continued the exercise until they developed angina, severe exhaustion, significant arrhythmias or conduction disorders, characteristic ST changes, or if the heart rate reached at least 85 percent of the predicted maximum. A positive response was reflected by 1 mm of linear, or downsloping ST segment depression occurring after exercise. ST elevation after exercise was also considered an abnormal response when it occurred in the presence of a normal resting ECG.[3] Linear ST depression greater than 0.5 mm but less than 1.0 mm was interpreted as a borderline response.

Selective coronary arteriography was performed according to the Sones' technique,[9] and the severity of the coronary artery disease (CAD) was judged by the angiographic scoring methods of Friesinger and associates.[2]

RESULTS

Among the 392 patients, 68.1 percent (267/392) had significant CAD with a coronary artery score (CAS) greater than two. A positive response on the TET was recorded in 62.5 percent (167/267), a borderline response in 11.2 percent (30/267), and a negative result in 26.7 percent (70/267) (Fig. 1). The sensitivity of the test increased significantly with the severity of disease, since 84 percent (52/62) (Fig. 2) of patients with a CAS greater than 10 and 81.8 percent (18/22) of patients with main left coronary artery lesions had a positive TET (Fig. 3). Conversely, a negative result was frequent in patients with mild CAD in whom a negative TET was demonstrated in 52 percent (28/54) of those

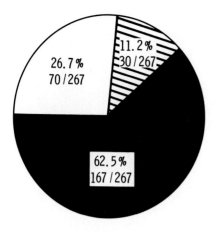

FIG. 1. Incidence of abnormal treadmill exercise test response in 267 patients with significant coronary artery disease (coronary artery score greater than 2); 62.5 percent of the patients had an abnormal response.

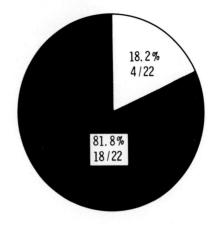

FIG. 3. Incidence of abnormal treadmill response in 22 patients with significant disease in the main left coronary artery.

with a CAS of less than five. Of patients with moderately severe disease—that is, a CAS of 6 to 10, only 59 percent (76/129) produced a positive TET response (Fig. 4).

ST segment elevation was rarely seen in patients with a normal resting ECG (less than 1 percent), while it was common (27.4 percent) in patients who had experienced a previous myocardial infarction (Fig. 5). Other investigators have reported a slightly higher incidence of ST elevation [3] following exercise, although in general it is recognized to be an infrequent occurrence. When present, ST elevation is almost always indicative of severe CAD. ST segment elevation on the ECG recorded after exercise in patients with previous myocardial infarctions and Q-wave de-

formity in the resting ECG are frequently associated with abnormalities of left ventricular wall motion such as akinesis or dyskinesis.

SPECIFICITY

Of 125 patients with a CAS of one or less (no significant CAD), 80.8 percent (101/125) demonstrated a negative TET, 12.8 percent (16/125) showed a borderline response, and only 6.4 percent (8/125) had a false-positive TET. If 1 mm of ST depression can be indicative of a positive response, 93.7 percent of the patients without CAD had a true negative response. (Fig. 6).

Of the eight patients with a false-positive result, 18.4 percent (7/38) had an abnormal resting ECG, while only 1.1 percent (1/88) had a normal resting ECG (Fig. 7). This finding is unfortunate since the test is *least specific* in patients with nonspecific abnormalities in the resting ECG and syndromes of atypical chest pain. False-positive results were not influenced by the incidence of male or female sex, which included 5.2 percent (3/57) women and 7.3 percent (5/68) men (Fig. 8).

SUMMARY

Our data show that the sensitivity of the multistage treadmill exercise test correlates well with the severity of CAD. A positive response was demonstrated by only 62.5 percent of all patients who had significant disease. The sensitivity of the test increased markedly with the severity of the disease, and a positive response was obtained in

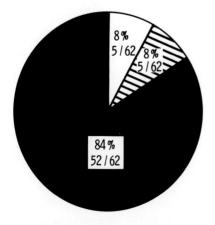

FIG. 2. Incidence of abnormal treadmill response in 62 patients with advanced coronary artery disease (coronary artery score greater than 10).

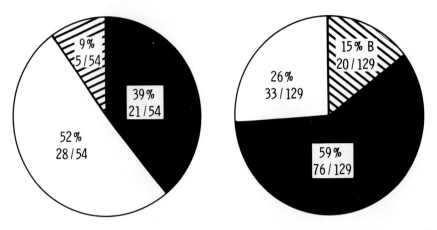

FIG. 4. Results of treadmill test in patients with a coronary artery score of 2–5 (left) and patients with a score of 6–10 (right).

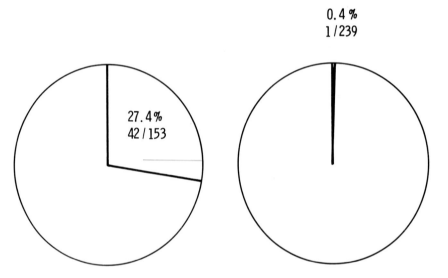

FIG. 5. Incidence of ST segment elevation in the treadmill exercise test; 27.4 percent of 153 patients with previous myocardial infarctions demonstrated ST elevation (left), while it occurred in less than 1 percent of 239 patients with a normal resting ECG (right).

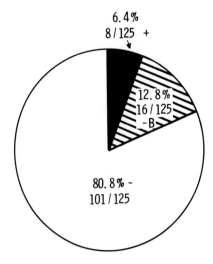

FIG. 6. Specificity of treadmill exercise test In 125 patients with no angiographic evidence of significant coronary artery disease.

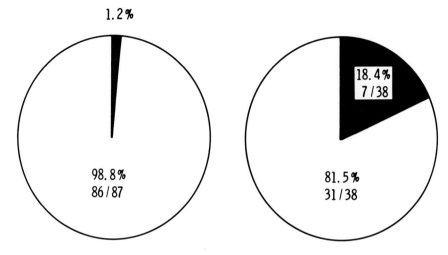

FIG. 7. Incidence of false-positive treadmill responses in patients with normal resting ECG (left) compared with those who had an abnormal resting ECG (right).

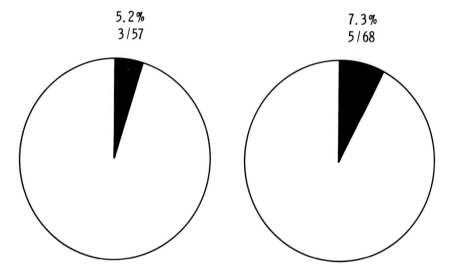

FIG. 8. Incidence of false-positive treadmill response in 57 men (left) and 68 women (right).

84 percent of the patients with severe obstructive disease as demonstrated by an angiographic CAS greater than 10 and 81.8 percent of patients with main left coronary artery lesions. The test was specific in 93.7 percent of all patients without CAD where a true negative result was obtained. A false-positive response was observed in 6.3 percent of all patients and was more common in those with an abnormal resting ECG (18.4 percent) and very rare in those with a normal resting ECG (1.1 percent).

A 1 mm linear, or downsloping ST segment depression is the most acceptable diagnostic criterion for abnormality of the treadmill exercise test in that the slight increase in sensitivity ob-

tained by a lesser degree of depression of the ST segment is outweighed by a loss of specificity.

References

1. Ellestad MH, Allen W, Wan MK, et al: Maximal treadmill stress testing for cardiovascular evaluation. Circulation 39:517, 1969
2. Friesinger GC, Page EE, Ross RS: Prognostic significance of coronary arteriography. Trans Assoc Am Physicians 83:78, 1970
3. Hegge F, Quna N, Burchell, H: The correlation of S-T segment elevations and axis shifts in graded treadmill exercise tests with coronary anteriographic findings (abstract). Circulation 29:269, 1972
4. Kassenbaum DG, Sutherland KI, Judkins MP: A

comparison of hypoxemia and exercise electrocardiography in coronary artery disease. Am Heart J 75:759, 1968

5. Martin CM, McConahay DR: Maximal treadmill exercise electrocardiography: Correlations with coronary arteriography and cardiac hemodynamics. Circulation 46:956, 1972

6. Mason RE, Likar E, Bienn RO et al: Multiple lead exercise electrocardiography. Experience in 107 normal subjects, and 67 patients with angina pectoris, and comparison with coronary cinearteriography in 84 patients. Circulation 36:517, 1967

7. Redwood D, Epstein S: Uses and limitations of stress testing in the evaluation of ischemic heart disease. Circulation 46:1115, 1972

8. Roitman D, Jones WB, Sheffield LT: Comparison of submaximal exercise ECG test with coronary cineangiocardiogram. Ann Intern Med 72:641, 1970

9. Sones FM Jr, Shirey ED: Cine coronary arteriography. Mod Concepts Cardiovasc Dis 31:735, 1962

23

ACCURACY OF DISCRIMINANT FUNCTION ANALYSIS IN PREDICTING CORONARY ARTERY DISEASE FROM PARAMETERS OF THE MULTISTAGE EXERCISE TEST

John F. Moran, Firouz Amirparviz, Patrick J. Scanlon, Rimgaudas Nemickas, James V. Talano, Rolf M. Gunnar, and John R. Tobin, Jr.

The multistage exercise test is a safe, noninvasive, and easily repeatable test of cardiac function that has achieved widespread acceptance (Detry, 1973; Adams, 1972; Blomqvist, 1971; Simonson, 1970; Goldbarg, 1970). Yet studies that have compared ischemic ST segment responses in exercise with cineangiographically demonstrated coronary artery disease have shown a great range of correlation between the two tests and, therefore, a great range in the diagnostic accuracy of exercise testing for ischemic heart disease (Redwood and Epstein, 1972). The degree of sensitivity (true positives) and specificity (true negatives) is related to the type and level of exercise as well as the ST segment criteria used to define an abnormal test (Bruce and Hornsten, 1969).

Angina pectoris is the result of an imbalance between myocardial oxygen supply and demand. If the diagnostic accuracy of the exercise test is dependent on the production of ischemia then it should be enhanced at higher cardiac workloads (Friesinger and Smith, 1972). In patients with coronary artery disease the heart rate and the heart-rate blood pressure product measured during exercise have been shown to vary directly with the magnitude of ST segment depression (Detry, Piette, Brasseur, 1970). Therefore, in addition to ST segment changes an analysis of these hemodynamic parameters during exercise may add to the diagnostic accuracy of the test.

Supported in part by USPHS HL05971-02.

The purpose of this study was to evaluate various types of ST segment changes in addition to 1-mm flat or downward-sloping ST segment depression, which would increase the diagnostic accuracy of the exercise electrocardiogram (Simonson, 1970). A discriminant function analysis was performed on the hemodynamic parameters to define those parameters, which were more important in accurately classifying patients as normal or abnormal by the exercise test. Coronary arteriography defined the normal and abnormal patients. A group of 186 consecutive patients who were referred for evaluation of angina-like chest pain and who underwent cardiac catheterization, coronary angiography, and stress exercise electrocardiograms form the study group.

METHODS

From May 1969 to December 1972, approximately 1,200 patients underwent cardiac catheterization and coronary angiography at Loyola University Medical Center. Of this group, 225 patients had a multistage exercise test by the method of Doan et al (1965) on a Quinton treadmill as part of their cardiovascular work-up. Thirty-nine patients in this group were eliminated because of valvular lesions, intraventricular conduction defects, atrial fibrillation, cardiomyopathy, and the use of digitalis. The remaining 186 patients formed the study group. There were 145 males and 41 females in the study group.

All patients were exercised in a fasting state after a resting 12-lead electrocardiogram was taken. The resting ECG was again recorded when the patient was standing for a baseline prior to exercise. A 45-second period of hyperventilation was performed and the standing baseline ECG repeated. The lead system used to record the ECG was the precordial electrocardiogram described by Abarquez et al (1960) with minor modifications. The minor modifications still allowed for an approximation of the orthogonal lead system. This ear-ensiform precordial lead system has been described as being very sensitive to ischemic ST segment depression (Blackburn, 1967).

Our modification placed the leads in the following positions—right arm at the base of the neck, left arm over the ensiform process, left leg at V_6, chest (V) at V_4, and the right leg at the V_4R position. Recordings of the ECG were made successively at the following lead selector switch positions: AVR (base of neck), AVL (ensiform), AVF (V_6), and V (V_4). One-minute recordings were made from the lead showing the largest R-wave, and all four leads were recorded at the end of each three-minute stage. Blood pressure was recorded by the cuff method every three minutes. All of the exercise ECGs were reviewed independently by two of the authors. Differences of opinion were decided by a third author (Blackburn et al, 1968). Interobserver variation was small (10 cases in the 186 were disputed). The exercise test was stopped for symptomatic reasons. Chest pain, especially if progressive, generalized fatigue, dyspnea, leg weakness, arrhythmias, inappropriate changes in blood pressure or heart rate, and light-headedness were all reasons for discontinuing the test. No patient was stopped in exercise because of ST segment depression. The ST-T-waves of the exercise ECG were classified as normal or abnormal according to one of the following six patterns.

1. 1.0 mm flat or downward-sloping ST segment depression persisting for 0.08 seconds.
2. 0.5 mm flat or downward-sloping ST segment depression persisting for 0.08 seconds;
3. upsloping ST segments that are still 1 mm or more below the baseline 0.08 seconds after the S-wave.
4. "U"-shaped ST segment depression where there is 1 mm or more ST depression 0.08 seconds after the S-wave.
5. J-junction depression more than 2 mm that is not a T-wave, and
6. isolated T-wave inversion.

All exercise ECG tests were first examined for the number one ST-T wave abnormality listed above, and these were separated from the whole group. The remaining exercise tests were then screened again for the ST-T-wave abnormalities listed above, numbers 2 through 6.

Coronary arteriography was performed on all 186 patients by the method of Sones. All of the cinearteriograms were considered adequate for interpretation. Significant coronary obstruction was defined as an area showing greater than 60 percent obstruction. The vessels included for study were the right coronary artery, the main left coronary artery, the left anterior descending artery and its diagonal branch, and the left circumflex artery and its obtuse marginal branch. A total of six vessels was evaluated. Normal patients as shown by coronary angiography numbered 99 and abnormals totaled 87 patients. These normal patients represented about half of all the normal patients studied in our laboratory during this period. Left ventricular angiography was performed in 160 patients in the 30 degree right anterior oblique position. A gross assessment of the left ventricular contractility was made in all of these patients.

The data were keypunched onto IBM cards. Means, standard deviations (SD), standard errors of the means (SEM), and the Student's t-test were carried out with standard programs on an IBM 1622 computer. Coronary arteriography was used to determine the normal and abnormal groups. Then standard programs on the IBM 1622 computer weighed the following parameters from the exercise ECG—age, sex, resting heart rate, resting systolic blood pressure, resting diastolic blood pressure, maximal heart rate in exercise, maximal systolic blood pressure, the maximal blood pressure-heart rate product, duration of exercise on the treadmill, and any ST segment change of the above. A discriminant function analysis was used to weigh all of these factors in an attempt to decide which parameters were more important in classifying an individual patient as normal or abnormal (Rao, 1952; Cornfield, 1964).

RESULTS

Figure 1 illustrates the types of ST segment changes that were evaluated. Table 1 is a summary of the results of patient classification by type of ST segment change. Seventy patients were classified as abnormal by the first criterion, ie 1.0 mm flat or downward-sloping ST segment depres-

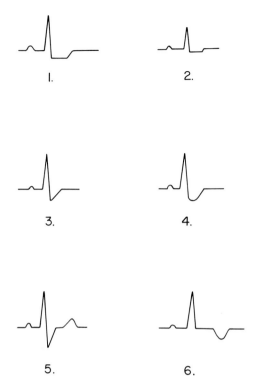

FIG. 1.   Types of ST Segment Changes Evaluated.

four actually had coronary artery disease (80 percent).

The means and standard error of the means of the ages and the hemodynamic parameters of the exercise electrocardiogram for the normal and abnormal groups by coronary arteriography are shown in Table 2. Of the 99 arteriographically normal patients, 64 were males, and 35 were females. Of the 87 arteriographically abnormal patients, 81 were male and six were female. As can be seen in Table 2 the means of age, resting heart rate, resting systolic and diastolic blood pressure, maximal heart rate in exercise, and the duration of exercise are all significantly different in the arteriographically normal and abnormal groups.

The 87 patients with abnormal coronary arteriograms can be classified according to the number of coronary vessels that were significantly obstructed. Twenty-three patients had single-vessel disease, while 14 had two vessels significantly obstructed. Fifty of the 87 patients had three or more coronary arteries with major obstructions. Forty-eight patients had collateral coronary circulation, and 47 showed left ventricular contraction abnormalities as judged qualitatively from the left ventricular cineangiogram. The vast majority of patients with collateral coronary circulation and left ventricular dysfunction by angio-

sion. Of these 70 patients, 52 actually had abnormal coronary arteriograms. The remaining 116 patients were then reexamined by the ST-T segment criteria listed as numbers 2 through 6. By these criteria an additional 36 patients were classified as abnormal, but only 14 actually had an abnormal coronary arteriogram (39 percent). The remaining 80 patients were then classified as normal while 59 patients actually had normal coronary angiograms.

The diagnostic accuracy of the ST-T wave criteria 2 through 6 varied from 11 percent to 80 percent. ST segments that were flat or downward sloping and 0.5 mm depressed were found in six patients but only two had coronary artery disease. Criterion number 3, of an upsloping ST segment that is still 1.0 mm depressed 0.08 seconds after the S-wave, was found in five patients but only two had disease of the coronary arteries. "U"-shaped ST segment depression of 1.0 mm for 0.08 seconds classified 11 patients as abnormal while five had coronary artery obstructions. Criterion number 5, J-junction depression of 2 mm or more was found in nine patients, but only one patient had disease of the coronary arteries. T-wave inversion in exercise was found in five patients and

TABLE 1.   Angiography Results Versus Patient Classification by Type of ST Segment Change

EXERCISE ECG	PATIENTS CLASSIFIED	CORONARY CINE ANGIOGRAPHY	
		Normal	Abnormal
1. 1 mm ST seg. depression, flat or down	70	18 (26%)	52 (74%)
Normal	80	59 (75%)	21 (25%)
2. 0.5 mm ST seg. depression, flat or down	6	4 (67%)	2 (33%)
3. 1.0 mm ST seg. depression, up-sloping	5	3 (60%)	2 (40%)
4. "U"-shaped ST seg. depression, ↓1.0 mm for 0.08 sec	11	6 (55%)	5 (45%)
5. J-junction depression > 2 mm	9	8 (89%)	1 (11%)
6. T-wave inversion	5	1 (20%)	4 (80%)
Total	186	99	87

TABLE 2. Angiography Results Versus Age and Exercise Testing Results

	CORONARY ANGIOGRAPHY		P
	Normal N = 99	Abnormal N = 87	
Age	47 ± 0.8 yrs	51 ± 0.9 yrs	< 0.001
Rest HR	84 ± 1.4 beats/min	78 ± 2 beats/min	< 0.02
Rest BP	125 ± 2 mmHg	131 ± 2	< 0.04
	84 ± 1	87 ± 1	< 0.05
Max HR	151 ± 2/min	138 ± 2/min	< 0.001
Max BP	163 ± 3 mmHg	169 ± 3	ns
	87 ± 1	91 ± 2	ns
BP X HR	24.5 ± 0.3 X 10^3	23.5 ± 0.3 X 10^3	ns
Duration of Exercise	6.8 ± 0.4 mins	4.9 ± 0.3 mins	< 0.001

gram had three or more coronary arteries significantly diseased.

Many of the parameters of the exercise electrocardiogram show a statistically significant difference when the coronary arteriographic normal and abnormal groups are compared (Table 2). Because of these significant differences, the hemodynamic parameters of resting heart rate, resting blood pressure, maximal heart rate and blood pressure in exercise, the maximal double product (maximal heart rate × maximal blood pressure), and the duration of exercise were added to age, sex, and any ST segment change. These were then submitted to a linear discriminant function analysis. The F coefficients for these 11 factors are shown in Table 3. By a process of systematic deletion, the analysis showed that sex, maximal heart rate in exercise, the double product, the duration of exercise, and ST segment changes were important in classifying patients as normal or abnormal by the exercise electrocardiogram.

Each of the 11 factors in Table 3 was next evaluated for each of the 186 patients in the study. The sum of these 11 factors as they were found in each of the patients generated a discriminant function for each individual patient. If the individual discriminant function was less than zero, it was

normal. If greater than zero, it was abnormal. These individual values are compared to coronary arteriographic findings in Table 4. The sensitivity (true positives) is 80.5 percent and the specificity (true negatives) is 76.8 percent. This means that the discriminant function classified 70 of 87 (80.5 percent) patients as abnormal while the criterion of 1.0 mm flat or downward-sloping ST segment classified 52 of 87 (60 percent) as abnormal. The discriminant function labeled 76 of 99 (76.8 percent) as normal, but the absence of 1.0 mm flat or downward-sloping ST segment depression labeled 81 of 99 patients (82 percent) as normal. The overall percentage of correctly classified patients by discriminant function analysis was 78.6 percent.

The discriminant function analysis appears to be helpful in classifying patients as normal or abnormal by exercise testing. The analysis suggests that the factors of sex, maximal heart rate in exercise, the double product, and the duration of exercise in addition to ST segment depression are the more important characteristics in the classification of patients. Therefore, an examination of these factors in the misclassified patients was done (Table 1).

Eighteen patients with normal coronary arteriograms developed 1.0 mm flat or downward sloping ST segment depression in exercise (false negatives). Twelve of these patients were female

TABLE 3. F Coefficients of 11 Factors

FACTOR	F COEFFICIENT
Age	5.09
Sex	46.46
Rest HR	0.18
Rest syst BP	2.00
Rest diast BP	3.52
Max HR	6.40
Max syst BP	1.21
Max diast BP	0.10
Double product (BP X HR)	3.82
Duration of exercise	8.36
ST segment changes	22.76

TABLE 4. Classification by Discriminant Function

ANGIOGRAPHIC DIAGNOSIS	NORMAL	ABNOR- MAL	% COR- RECTLY CLASSI- FIED
Normal (N = 99)	76	23	76.8
Abnormal (N = 17)	17	70	80.5
Total	93	93	78.5

and six were male. The average maximal heart rate was 154 beats/minute with a range of 125 to 177 beats/minute. The average double product was 25.9×10^3 and the duration of exercise was 5.4 minutes with a range of 1.8 to 8.2 minutes. These values can be compared with their respective values in the angiographically normal group in Table 2.

Twenty-one patients with coronary artery disease by cinearteriograms were classified as normal by their ST segment response on the exercise electrocardiogram (Table 1). Twenty of these 21 patients were male and one was female. The average maximal heart rate for this subgroup was 139 beats/minute with a range of 91 to 188 beats/minute. The average double product was 24.1×10^3 and the average duration of exercise was 6.1 minutes with a range of 1.4 to 10.6 minutes. The number of coronaries obstructed in this subgroup of 21 patients varied from one- to five-vessel disease. Eight of the 21 patients had single-vessel disease: four had right coronary artery obstructions, two had left circumflex artery disease, and two had left anterior descending artery narrowings. Three of these eight patients had collateral coronary circulation. The average maximal heart rate for this group of eight patients with single-vessel disease was 145 beats/minute. Four patients had two-vessel coronary disease, and nine patients had three or more coronary artery obstructions.

Thirty-six patients were classified as abnormal by the ST-T segment criteria listed as numbers 2 through 6 in Table 1. Twenty-two of these patients had normal coronary arteriograms (61 percent). The average maximal heart rate for these 22 patients was 156 beats/minute with a range of 120 to 177 beats/minute. The average double product was 25.8×10^3 and the average duration of exercise was 7.4 minutes, with a range of 1.8 to 15.2 minutes. These average values should be compared to the respective averages in the arteriographically normal group in Table 2. The average values for these arteriographically normal subgroups are close to the averages of the arteriographically normal group as a whole. This is especially true for maximal heart rate in exercise; however, there is a wide range of response in maximal heart rate as well as duration of exercise.

DISCUSSION

The use of the discriminant function analysis in this group of 186 patients improved overall diagnostic accuracy from 133 of 186 (71.5 percent), correctly classified by 1.0 mm flat or downward-sloping ST segment depression, to 146 of 186 (78.5 percent) correctly classified by discriminant function. Sensitivity (true positives) was increased from 52 of 87 abnormal patients (60 percent) to 70 of 87 abnormals (80.5 percent) comparing 1.0 mm flat or downward-sloping ST segment depression to the discriminant function analysis, respectively. Specificity (true negatives), however, was not much different by these two approaches: 81 of 99 normal patients (82 percent) by the absence of 1.0 mm flat ST segment depression and 76 of 99 normals (78.5 percent) by the discriminant function classified correctly.

The use of 1.0 mm flat or downward-sloping ST segment depression remained the best single criterion of an abnormal exercise electrocardiogram as noted previously (Simonson, 1970). Other types of ST-T-wave changes were not helpful because of the large number of false-positives found. Isolated T-wave inversion is uncommon in exercise but was quite accurate, predicting four of five patients as having coronary artery disease in our study. Although the number of patients is small, Smith (1969) had comparable results in 10 of 11 patients when he used the vectorcardiogram. However, Smith (1969) did not have coronary arteriograms in these patients. Since isolated T-wave inversion is as common as ischemic ST segment depression in resting electrocardiograms and is frequent in anoxemia tests, its general lack of predictive value in the exercise test may be in part due to the ECG display (Simonson, 1970). This needs more study.

The increase in diagnostic accuracy with the use of discriminant function analysis of all factors of the exercise test is in agreement with the relationship of maximal heart rate and double product to ST segment depression (Detry, 1970). However, the increase in overall diagnostic accuracy was small, only 7 percent improvement. Sex, maximal heart rate in exercise, double product, and duration of exercise were all helpful, but there was an area of overlap with the normal patients.

This can best be appreciated by an examination of the misclassified patients by ST segment depression. There were 18 false positive patients with an average maximal heart rate of 154 beats/minute and a range of 125 to 177 beats/minute. There were 21 false-negative patients with an average maximal heart rate of 139 beats/minute and a range of 91 to 188 beats/minute. The ranges for duration of exercise in the 18 false positive patients and 21 false negative patients were 1.8 to 8.2 minutes and 1.4 to 10.6 minutes, respectively. Although these differences were statistically significant, they can only be considered clues to classification of any individual patient from a clinical viewpoint because of the overlapping range of numbers. This range of values may also account for the relatively small (7 percent) increase in overall diagnostic accuracy by the discriminant function analysis.

The large number of females in the false positive group (12 of 18) is unexplained. These women probably represent examples of the syndrome of anginalike chest pain and normal coronary arteriograms (Waxler et al, 1971). These authors felt the syndrome had a benign prognosis in a series of 100 women followed up to 2.5 years.

The group of 21 false negative patients is also of great concern. Nine of these patients had severe three-vessel coronary disease but eight patients had single-vessel disease. Rothbaum et al (1974) have recently suggested that patients with extensive coronary artery disease may normalize their ST-T segments in exercise. However, a sample exercise electrocardiogram they presented showed an exercise heart rate of approximately 125 beats/minute. Three of our nine patients with three-vessel coronary disease developed maximal heart rates of 158, 167, and 188 beats/minute. Still the cancellation of ischemic ST segment vectors in exercise by ischemia in the ventricular wall opposite an old infarction is an important concept in explaining false negative patients.

The eight false negative patients with single-vessel disease are somewhat more difficult to understand. These patients as a subgroup exercised well, developing an average maximal heart rate of 145/minute, average duration of exercise of 6.8 minutes, and double product of 26.2×10^3. They were all males. The fact that six of the eight obstructed vessels were the right coronary artery (four) or left circumflex artery (two) may suggest our lead system isn't as sensitive as we thought for inferior or lateral wall ischemia (Blackburn, 1967). Only three of these eight patients had collateral coronary circulation, and two of these three had a left anterior descending artery lesion. In our study as well as others (Helfant et al, 1971), collateral coronary circulation is best related to severe coronary artery disease.

The correlation between the multistage exercise test and cinecoronary arteriograms is not perfect. But it is relatively good considering the two techniques are examining different facets of the problem of myocardial ischemia: The exercise test measures physiologic function and the coronary arteriogram delineates coronary artery anatomy. The use of discriminant function analysis in this group of 186 patients has led to a greater understanding of the diagnostic accuracy of the exercise test.

CONCLUSIONS

1. 1.0 mm flat or downward-sloping ST segment depression is probably the best single criterion for abnormal exercise ECG and coronary artery disease.
2. T-wave inversion needs more study.
3. Sex, maximal heart rate in exercise, double product, and duration of exercise are helpful, in addition to ST segment changes, as clinical clues to the classification of patients as normal or abnormal by the exercise test.
4. The prevalence of females in the false positive group is unexplained.
5. False negatives are mostly male patients.

ACKNOWLEDGMENT

The authors wish to acknowledge the statistical assistance of Mr. Jack M. Becktel of the Research Support Center, Veterans Administration Hospital, Hines, Illinois.

References

1. Abarquez RF, Freiman AH, Reichl F, Ladue JS: The precordial electrocardiogram during exercise. Circulation 22:1060, 1960
2. Adams CW (ed): Symposium on Exercise and the Heart. Am J Cardiol 30:713, 1972
3. Blackburn H, Blomqvist G, Freiman A, et al: The exercise electrocardiogram: differences in interpretation. Am J Cardiol 21:871, 1968
4. Blackburn H, Taylor HL, Okamoto N, et al. Standardization of the exercise electrocardiogram: a systematic comparison of chest lead configurations employed for monitoring during exercise. In Karvonen MJ and Barry AJ (eds): Physical Activity and the Heart. Springfield, Charles C. Thomas, 1967, p 101
5. Blomqvist CG: Use of exercise testing for diagnostic and functional evaluation of patients with arteriosclerotic heart disease. Circulation 44:1120, 1971
6. Bruce RA, Hornsten TR: Exercise stress testing in evaluation of patients with ischemic heart disease. Prog Cardiovasc Dis 11:371, 1969
7. Cornfield J: Discriminant functions. Proceedings of the 6th IBM Medical Symposium, Poughkeepsie, NY, 1964
8. Detry JMR: Exercise testing and training in coronary heart disease. Baltimore, Williams and Wilkins, 1973
9. Detry JMR, Piette F, Brasseur LA: Hemodynamic determinants of exercise ST segment depression in coronary patients. Circulation 42:593, 1970
10. Doan AE, Peterson DR, Blackburn JR, Bruce RA: Myocardial ischemia after maximal exercise in normal men: a method for detecting latent heart disease. Am Heart J 69:11, 1965

11. Friesinger GC, Smith RF: Correlation of electro-cardiographic studies with arteriographic findings with angina pectoris. Circulation 46:1173, 1972

12. Goldbarg AN, Moran JF, Resnekov L: Multistage electrocardiographic exercise tests: principles and clinical applications. Am J Cardiol 26:84, 1970

13. Helfant RH, Vokonas PS, Gorlin R: Functional importance of the human coronary collateral circulation. N Engl J Med 284:1277, 1971

14. Rao CR: Advanced Statistical Methods in Biometric Research. New York, John Wiley and Sons, 1952

15. Redwood DR, Epstein SE: Uses and limitations of stress testing in the evaluation of ischemic heart disease. Circulation 46:1115, 1972

16. Rothbaum DA, Noble RJ, McHenry PL, Anderson GJ: Normalization of the electrocardiogram during angina pectoris in patients with subendocardial infarction (abst). Am J Cardiol 33:167, 1974

17. Simonson E: Electrocardiographic stress tolerance tests. Prog Cardiovasc Dis 13:269, 1970

18. Smith RF: Quantitative exercise stress testing in the naval aviator population and in the projected Apollo spacecraft experiment MO-18. In Blackburn H (ed): Measurement in Exercise Electrocardiography. Springfield, Charles C. Thomas, 1969

19. Waxler EB, Kimbris D, Dreifus LS: The fate of women with normal coronary arteriograms and chest pain resembling angina pectoris. Am J Cardiol 28:25, 1971

24

AN ASSESSMENT OF RISKS AND CAUSES OF DEATH IN ASSOCIATION WITH CORONARY ARTERIOGRAPHY

Timothy Takaro, Herbert N. Hultgren, and Katherine M. Detre

This is a progress report of a continuing investigation into the causes of deaths occurring in association with coronary arteriography at a group of cooperating Veterans Administration Hospitals, with an assessment of the risks of this now common diagnostic procedure. The background of this study has been previously described.[45,46]

The clinical records, coronary arteriograms, catheterization data, and autopsy reports of eight additional deaths were reviewed, analyzed, and added to the earlier series. The incidence of this complication in the cooperating hospitals was reassessed, and the current literature on this subject reviewed.

RESULTS

During the five-year period from 1969 through 1973, 4,532 coronary arteriograms were reported on arteriography logs by participating hospitals. There were 56 deaths that occurred in association with the procedure (1.2 percent). All but four patients died within one week of the arteriogram, and 41 of the 56 patients died within 24 hours of the arteriogram.

In addition to the 56 cases reported on the arteriography logs, 18 cases from other hospitals not participating in the VA Cooperative Study were contributed for this analysis. Clinical characteristics and causes of death were analyzed for the total number of 74 cases. Autopsies were available in 62 of them.

CLINICAL CHARACTERISTICS

These were all male patients. The majority of them were between 40 and 60 years of age and were being considered for surgery in most instances (68 percent) because of angina pectoris. Uncertainty of diagnosis was the indication for arteriography in six cases; and postoperative studies were being conducted in eight. Other indications were congestive failure or cardiomegaly, and possible ventricular aneurysms in five. In another five cases the indication for arteriography was not discernible from the record.

A history of myocardial infarction was apparent in 48 patients (65 percent). There was electrocardiographic evidence of old infarcts, or of myocardial ischemia, as well as positive stress tests in 90 percent of the patients. Of the 49 patients in whom ventriculography had been performed, a significant abnormality in size, contractility, or ejection fraction was noted in 28 (57 percent). Evidence of significant coronary atherosclerosis by angiography or autopsy was noted in 72 of 74 patients (97 percent); and in 35 of the 52 patients (67 percent) in whom coronary arteriography had been completed, there was involvement of the three major vessels. Thus, significant coronary occlusive disease was the common denominator in almost every case.

CAUSES OF DEATH

The causes of death were acute coronary occlusion in 37/74 (50 percent); acute cardiac arrhythmia in 9/74 (12 percent); acute myocardial infarction without evidence of acute occlusion in eight; cerebral vascular accident in four; complications involving the femoral arterial cannulation site in four; and unidentified causes in 11 (Table 1). One patient died of septicemia four days after the procedure.

TABLE 1. Causes of Death

	NO. CASES	PERCENT
Acute coronary occlusion	37	50
Acute cardiac arrhythmia	9	12
Acute myocardial infarction	8	11
Cerebral vascular accident	4	5
Complications of femoral cannulation site	4	5
Septicemia	1	1
Unidentified cause	11	15
Total	74	

Acute coronary occlusion was identified either angiographically or anatomically, or by both means. Angiographic evidence of acute occlusion was accepted if complete occlusion of a vessel noted to be patent earlier in the same arteriographic procedure was demonstrated angiographically. Anatomic evidence was accepted if fresh thrombus was recognized at surgery, autopsy, or both.

Thirty of this group of 37 patients (81 percent) succumbed within six hours of arteriography—the rest survived up to nine days. In eight patients in this group, an acute myocardial infarction could also be identified at autopsy, mostly among patients who survived over 10 hours. In 15, a "catheter embolus" as previously described by Price et al, was recognized on histologic sections.[33]

Seven of eight patients in whom an acute myocardial infarction (without an acute occlusion) was identified lived for 12 hours or more (up to 13 days). In the remaining nine patients with a sudden acute cardiac episode, neither an acutely occluding lesion nor an acute myocardial infarction could be identified at autopsy. All of these patients died within 24 hours of arteriography. The cause of death was classified as "acute cardiac arrhythmia."

Four patients died of the consequences of a cerebrovascular accident that occurred during the procedure. These patients lived from two to nine days after angiography. Three of the four patients who died of complications of the femoral cannulation site succumbed from cardiac causes during or after corrective surgery on the femoral artery.

In 34 of the 37 patients who sustained an acute coronary occlusion at arteriography, the transfemoral technique had been used, and there had been at least one change of catheters, prior to the acute episode, with as many as three or more changes of catheter in many cases. In three instances, the fatal episode occurred after change of catheters, but before the injection of any contrast material; and in seven patients, only a small test injection in or near the left coronary orifice had been made. In over half the cases, concomitant or associated studies, such as combined right and left heart catheterizations, implant arteriography, cardiac output studies, or exercise testing with catheters in place, had delayed the selective coronary injections and prolonged the procedure. In some instances, an excessive number of injections had been made (23 in one case), and in many instances, episodes of hypotension prior to the fatal episode were observed. In nearly every instance (32/37) (85 percent), the left coronary artery was being catheterized at the time of the acute episode.

DISCUSSION

The incidence of fatal complications was so low in the early years of coronary arteriography, when the transbrachial technique was used almost exclusively, and even later when the transfemoral technique was introduced, that coronary arteriography quickly gained acceptance as a safe diagnostic procedure.[19,21,38,42,44] Beginning in 1971, however, there was reported an unmistakable increase in the incidence of fatal complications, which seemed to be related to increasing use of the transfemoral approach.[1,2,6,7,20,31,47]

This disparity between the fatality rates of the two techniques was noted by several authors[2,6,20,31,45] (Table 2) and is borne out by this study. The transfemoral method was easier to learn, since the familiar Seldinger technique was used—passing preformed catheters into the ascending aorta via the femoral arteries. This avoided a brachial arteriotomy, with its attendant complications, which can be substantial even in experienced hands.[5,25] Because coronary arteriography

TABLE 2. Coronary Arteriography: Influence of Technique on Mortality

	TRANS-BRACHIAL		TRANS-FEMORAL	
	No. Pts.	Inci-dence	No. Pts.	Inci-dence
Kaltenbach and Lichtlen (1971)	1,367	0.4	431	0.9
Chahine, Herman, Gorlin (1972)	413	0.0	478	2.0
Petch, Sutton, Jefferson (1973)	111	0.0	248	1.5
Adams, Fraser, Abrams (1973)	24,124	0.13	22,780	0.78
VA Coop Study (1973)	1,670	0.25	2,852	1.8

using this method seemed to be a simple extension of visceral arteriography by the transfemoral percutaneous technique, it quickly gained wide popularity.

In the ascending aorta, however, and with the use of multiple changes of catheters, the procedure proved to be more dangerous. A major reason for the danger seems to be due to the mechanism of sudden coronary (or cerebral) arterial occlusion caused by emboli originating from thrombotic material on guidewires or catheters. As will be seen, the guidewire is an essential element in this mechanism.

The deposition of a platelet-fibrin film on catheters and guidewire surfaces promptly after exposure to the blood stream has been well-recognized.[11,13,17,27,28] Not so well appreciated is the ease with which this film can be stripped off a wire by the closely fitting catheter tip, or removed from the outside surface of a catheter by the arterial wall at the puncture site, as the catheter is exchanged for another.[18,41] In the second instance, the guidewire remains in the artery during this exchange, acting as a nidus for the "withdrawal" clot to cling to; then it is not swept away as it would be if the wire were not left in place (Fig. 1). In these two ways, material adherent to the

guidewire may be transferred to the catheter tip, and, unless it fragments and is swept away downstream, it may be transported into the aortic arch and ascending aorta. Its presence is ordinarily undetectable by pressure tracings, and cannot be removed by repeated flushing, because the material adheres to the outside surface of the catheter. If any of this material breaks off in the aortic arch or the ascending aorta and embolizes to the brain, a cerebral vascular accident may be the result (Fig. 2). If the material is pulled off the catheter tip and swept into the coronary artery as the catheter tip nears a coronary orifice, where the direction of blood flow relative to the catheter tip is the reverse of that to which the catheter has been exposed on its journey through the aorta, a coronary embolus results.[3,8,12,32,33,34,39,45] This may trigger a serious arrhythmia or an acute myocardial infarction or both. In a heart with compromised circulation from disease the result can be fatal. The material is not often recognized at autopsy, probably because it fragments so easily, and may also be readily dislodged, either spontaneously, or by vigorous efforts at resuscitation. In those instances in which it has been recognized at surgery or at autopsy (Fig. 3), such emboli of presumably catheter or wire origin can be

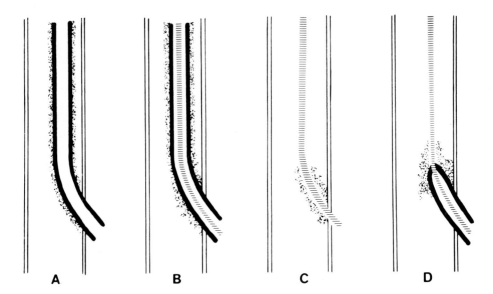

FIG. 1. Diagrammatic representation of one mechanism postulated for the formation and propagation of "catheter emboli." A. Catheter (heavy black lines) passing through wall of artery (fine double lines) and lying in arterial lumen. The intraarterial portion of the catheter is covered by a fine deposit of platelets, here exaggeratedly thick (stippled layer). B. A guidewire has been inserted into the lumen of the catheter, which is now being withdrawn from the artery. The layer of platelets is being wiped off the catheter by the arterial wall and is accumulating at the arterial puncture site. C. The thrombotic platelet material remains adherent to the puncture site and around the retained guidewire. D. This material is being wiped off the guidewire by the tip of the next catheter inserted into the artery. This material adheres now to the tip of this second catheter. Reproduced from Takaro, et al: Acute coronary occlusion following coronary arteriography: mechanisms and surgical relief. Surgery 72:1018, 1972, The C. V. Mosby Company.

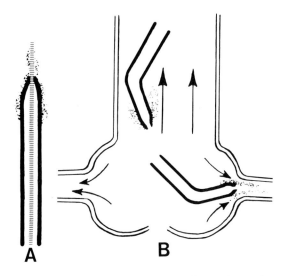

A   **B**

FIG. 2A. Diagrammatic representation of another mechanism for the formation and propagation of "catheter emboli." Thrombotic material deposited on an intraarterial guidewire (stippled) is shown being wiped off guidewire by the tip of an advancing catheter (heavy black lines). B. The catheter tip (upper black heavy lines) is now in the ascending aorta, with the adherent thrombotic material streaming in the direction of blood flow (vertical arrows). Embolization from this position can result in a cerebral vascular accident. In the lower right, the catheter tip is near a coronary arterial orifice. Blood flow (curved arrows) now causes thrombotic material to stream toward the coronary arteries and to cause coronary embolization, even without injection of contrast material. Reproduced from Takaro, et al: Acute coronary occlusion following coronary arteriography: mechanisms and surgical relief. Surgery 72:1018, 1972. The C.V. Mosby Company.

lism from catheters and guidewires. Since guidewires are not ordinarily used in the transbrachial technique, and with the absence of an indwelling guidewire, changes of catheter do not usually permit the accumulation of thrombotic material at the brachial arteriotomy site, coronary and cerebral embolism, and the resulting fatalities are much less common using the transbrachial approach.

The incidence of fatalities associated with coronary arteriography in our own study has decreased sharply in the past two years (Fig. 6). This decrease was accompanied not only by a rise in the total volume of coronary arteriograms reported but also by a relative increase in the number of arteriograms performed using the transbrachial technique. Whereas in the first three

identified as a mass of tightly packed coils or cords of aggregated platelets, with little fibrin and few red cells, occluding a coronary artery in which an atherosclerotic lesion, if any, is not the predominant feature (Fig. 4).[33] The material occasionally extends into a side branch. This characteristic histologic appearance and its extension into side branches helps to distinguish it from in situ thrombi seen in patients dying suddenly with coronary arterial occlusive disease.[35] Another distinguishing feature between patients dying with coronary embolism at coronary arteriography and those dying with acute myocardial infarction is the difference in survival time after the acute episode, as reported by Roberts and by Spain (Fig. 5).[35,36,43] The bulk of the sudden deaths associated with coronary arteriography occurred within six hours of the procedure, in contrast to the patients dying of their disease alone. This suggests a different pathogenesis for the "fresh thrombus" found in coronary arteries of patients following arteriography, and supports the concept of embo-

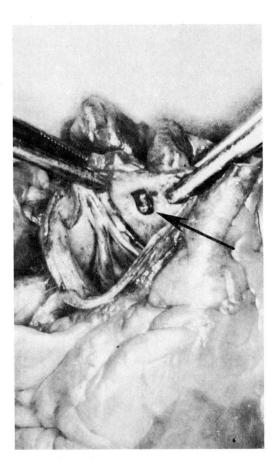

FIG. 3. Gross specimen of a "catheter embolus" (arrow) lodged in the left coronary arterial orifice of a patient who died within 15 minutes of the acute episode. This patient had had 2 changes of catheter, with the use of the transfemoral Seldinger technique, prior to the acute episode. Reproduced from Takaro, et al: Acute coronary occlusion following coronary arteriography: mechanisms and surgical relief. Surgery 72: 1018, 1972, The C.V. Mosby Company.

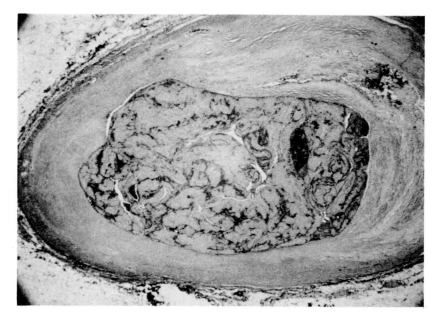

FIG. 4. Histologic section through a coronary embolus, in a patient who died in association with coronary arteriography, showing characteristic appearance of coiled masses of platelets, with few red cells and little fibrin, in an artery with little evidence of severe atherosclerosis. (Trichrome Stain, ×25). Reproduced from Takaro et al: Acute coronary occlusion following coronary arteriography: mechanisms and surgical relief. Surgery 72:1018, 1972. The C.V. Mosby Company.

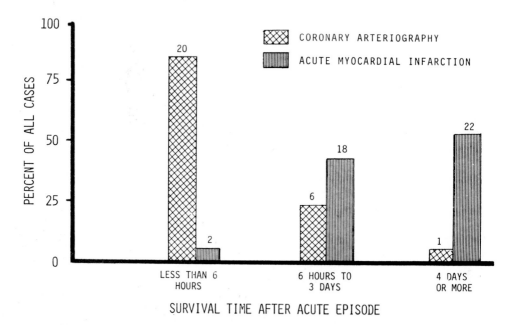

FIG. 5. Relative distribution of survival times after acute episode in all cases (27) in which "fresh thrombus" was reported at autopsy following coronary arteriography (this report) compared with 42 cases of coronary thrombosis found at autopsy following acute myocardial infarction (Roberts and Buja, 1972). Numbers over each column refer to numbers of patients in each group.

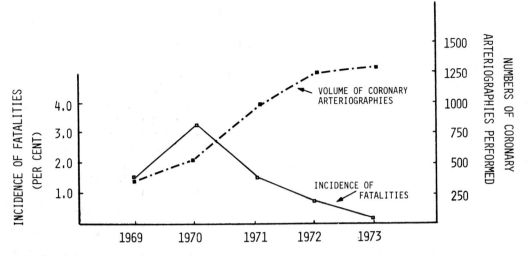

FIG. 6. Graph showing yearly collective coronary arteriographic volume and collective incidence of fatalities in association with coronary arteriography (up to two weeks) in cooperating hospitals. Declining incidence in the last two years was associated not only with increasing volume, but also with increasing use of the transbrachial technique, and of full heparinization with the transfemoral technique (see text).

years of the study period, more than twice as many transfemoral procedures were done as transbrachial, in the last two years, approximately equal numbers of both techniques were reported. In addition, in almost all hospitals continuing to use the transfemoral technique 5,000 to 10,000 units of heparin are now being administered at the beginning of the procedure.

The incidence of fatalities in association with the transbrachial method in this study was 0.25 percent (four deaths in approximately 1,670 procedures); whereas for the transfemoral it was 1.8 percent * (52 in approximately 2,852 procedures). In five hospitals performing 100 procedures or more per year, mortality ranged from 0 to 2.3 percent. In four others with only half of this volume, the mortality rate spanned exactly the same range: 0 to 2.3 percent. However, several other hospitals with the lowest reported volumes recorded the highest mortality rates. This supports the findings of Adams, Fraser, and Abrams that hospitals reporting low coronary arteriographic volumes reported the highest mortality rates.[2]

There is accumulating evidence suggesting that systemic heparinization may be useful in preventing thromboembolic complications. In this study, in no instance has a "catheter embolus" been identified in a fully heparinized patient.

Nelson et al[29] found that systemic heparinization (5,000 units injected into the abdominal aorta at the beginning of the procedure) resulted

in no thromboembolic complications in 76 cases, against six major thrombotic or embolic complications in 51 patients (11.8 percent) without the use of heparin. Reversal with protamine was advocated. We presented evidence to suggest that 5,000 units may not provide adequate protection,[46] and Nelson subsequently reported using 10,000 units with each procedure.[30] Wallace et al also reported that systemic heparinization significantly decreased the complications of angiography due to thrombosis.[48]

Luepker[24] in a randomized prospective controlled study involving 82 patients, found that systemic heparinization (100 units/Kg BW I-V immediately prior to femoral artery puncture) was associated with no loss of distal pulses, and minimal reduction in blood flow by impedance plethysmography, compared with loss of distal pulses in 10 percent (4/40) and measurably diminished blood flow 24 hours after catheterization in 7/40 nonheparinized patients. Protamine was used (0.5 mgm/K).

Walker et al[47] reported a series of 155 patients subjected to coronary arteriography, in whom heparin (3,000 to 7,000 units) was injected into the abdominal aorta as the catheter was introduced. There were two thromboembolic complications and one death; as compared with 135 patients in whom heparin was used only in the flush solution (2,500 u/liter) with 24 thromboembolic complications and five deaths (3.5 percent). Each group had one hemorrhagic complication and protamine was not used. Subsequently, all the participants in that study adopted the use

* p < 0.001

of heparin systematically. There were no further thromboembolic episodes.

Conceivably, use of heparin in dosages approximating 10,000 units might be hazardous when transseptal catheterization techniques are combined with coronary arteriography, because of the possibilities of puncture of the pericardial cavity, with subsequent bleeding and cardiac tamponade. The remote possibility of coronary arterial perforation by a catheter tip should also be mentioned but must occur extremely rarely.[26] Hemorrhage at the femoral puncture site is readily controlled by appropriately administered pressure and by careful observation, and it is readily managed if it does occur.

Other possible mechanisms that could cause deaths at coronary arteriography include acute aneurysm,[9] air embolism, and occlusion or mechanical obstruction of the coronary arteries by the catheter. Dislodgement of a mural thrombus and embolization to the coronary or cerebral circulation has also been suggested, but we have not been able to identify such a case.

We were able to uncover only three anatomically proven cases of coronary subintimal dissection at coronary arteriography or left heart catheterization.[22,42,45] Cases showing stasis or retention of contrast material during arteriography have been assumed by others (and also by us, initially) to represent subintimal dissection.[4,15] We have concluded on the basis of this study, however, that most such arteriographic appearances instead represent coronary arterial embolization from catheters and guidewires, with stasis of contrast material in the acutely occluded segment of vessel.

Air embolism has been observed occasionally at coronary arteriography but has not been shown to be responsible for fatality to our knowledge.

Temporary complete occlusion of an orifice end-on by the tip of the catheter ("wedging" of the catheter tip) can usually be recognized by damped pressures and can be quickly corrected by removing the catheter from the orifice. It easily results in a serious arrhythmia. Partial occlusion of a side-orifice, such as the circumflex, by a catheter inadvertently positioned subselectively in the left anterior descending artery, may also occur but is not as readily recognizable as "wedging." If coronary blood flow is already precarious because of severe atherosclerosis, the additional reduction of flow by a catheter either through "wedging" or obstructing a branch orifice, may result in a serious cardiac arrhythmia, or in further ischemic damage, and, occasionally, in death. The indirect form of mechanical obstruction to flow (occlusion of a side orifice) was recognized in one case and was

the only instance of a sudden death after coronary arteriography that occurred in a fully heparinized patient. On the other hand, "wedging" or the appearance of it, at some time during the procedure, was recognized in nearly one-third of the fatalities reported here.

All of the fatalities we collected could not be adequately explained, even after careful analysis. Since Petch and his colleagues did not observe fresh thrombus in any of their six fatal cases, they postulated a vasovagal mechanism with the transfemoral technique that apparently was not operative with the transbrachial technique.[31] We find it difficult to accept this hypothesis. Hildner points out the possibility of coincidental death of very sick patients from the natural course of the disease; therefore, the arteriographic procedure should not be made to bear the blame.[16] This must certainly be considered, and electrocardiography and enzyme studies prior to arteriography have been recommended to try to identify a "silent" myocardial infarction.

PREVENTION OF FATAL COMPLICATIONS

At least four factors can be recognized that seem to be related to the risk of coronary arteriography. The survey by Adams, Fraser, and Abrams brings some of these into sharp focus.[2] Recognition of these factors, which are interrelated, should result in diminished risk. Other published reports, as well as our more recent experience, support this view.[14,23,47] The factors are the extent of the patient's disease, the arteriographic technique used, the skill and experience of the angiographer, and the duration of the procedure.

The more precarious the patient's coronary circulation, the less tolerable will be the brief moments of diminished coronary blood flow caused by the catheter, the contrast material, or the episodes of hypotension that may occur from whatever cause. The worse the patient's left ventricular function, the greater the opportunity, presumably, for stagnation of blood flow (especially in the peripheral vessels) and for deposition of platelets and fibrin on catheters and wires.

The transbrachial technique is associated with a lower mortality rate in almost all comparative series (Table 2). "A catheter embolus" has not been recognized in any patient in whom this avenue was used. Fully heparinizing a patient, however, also reduces and apparently may eliminate this hazard of the transfemoral technique, since we have not observed this complication in a fully heparinized patient.

The skill and experience of the operator are obviously of great importance. With minimal trauma at the femoral arterial puncture site, less thrombotic material may be expected to accumulate. With a rapid procedure of short duration there is less time for the deposition of platelets on catheters and wires. Advancing a catheter over a guidewire when it is positioned in the ascending aorta or aortic arch should be avoided because of the special hazard of "catheter emboli" in these locations. With prompt recognition and correction of untoward events, such as "wedging" of the catheter, episodes of hypotension, chest pain, or electrocardiographic changes, more serious consequences can be avoided. Increased experience will lead to judicious early discontinuance of a procedure that is not going well.

Finally, the wisdom of prolonging the procedure by performing additional studies, some of them of undoubted physiologic value, is to be seriously questioned, especially in a laboratory that has an appreciable fatality rate. The possible value to the patient or to other patients, of obtaining data, must be weighed against the added risk to the individual patient of prolonging the procedure. An optimal risk-benefit ratio for each individual patient should be the constant aim of the angiographer.

TREATMENT

The surgical treatment of acute coronary occlusion occurring in association with coronary arteriography has been reported from a number of centers.[3,8,10,34,39] Combining reported instances from the literature with our own experience, emergency surgery was carried out in 36 cases. In 29, saphenous vein bypass grafts were done, with 10 survivors. Success seems to have been related to the presence or absence of cardiogenic shock and to the promptness with which surgical intervention was undertaken. In the remaining patients, cardiopulmonary bypass alone, or embolectomy alone, or valve replacement were done (with concomitant vein grafting in one instance). There were no survivors in this group. In a few patients, an acute myocardial infarction associated with an acute coronary occlusion sustained at coronary arteriography was treated conservatively, with survival. The difficulty of predicting which patients will do well without surgery under these circumstances is real. Clearly, prevention is much more effective than treatment.

SUMMARY AND CONCLUSIONS

In a cooperative study involving 18 hospitals, over a five-year period, the incidence of fatalities occurring in association with coronary arteriography was 1.2 percent. It was 1.8 percent in 2,852 procedures using the transfemoral technique and 0.25 percent in 1,670 procedures using the transbrachial approach. With the use of full heparinization by angiographers continuing to use the transfemoral technique, and increased use of the transbrachial technique, the overall incidence of fatalities has decreased to 0.4 percent for the past two years.

The deposition of platelets and fibrin upon catheter and guidewire surfaces and the subsequent transfer of this material to additional catheters used in the procedure with its consequent embolization to carotid and coronary vessels seems to have been responsible for the earlier, higher mortality. Effective anticoagulation has apparently had a significant influence on this mechanism, because it has not been identified as a cause of death since full heparinization has been used. Other factors affecting the risk of coronary arteriography are judged to be the extent of the patient's disease, the skill and experience of the operator, and the duration of the procedure. When all of these factors are optimal, the risk of the procedure is small but, in most centers, measurable. For these reasons, coronary arteriography should be undertaken only when indicated by the expectation that the findings may contribute significantly to the patient's management, and then only by carefully trained physicians.

ACKNOWLEDGMENTS

The active help and cooperation of present and former participants in the VA Cooperative Study of Surgery for Coronary Arterial Occlusive Disease and of cardiologists in other VA Hospitals, are gratefully acknowledged. They are *Ann Arbor*: Thomas A. Preston and Majid Mesgarzadeh; *Augusta*: Horace Killam; *Brooklyn*: Eugene Thompson; *Buffalo*: David C. Dean, Italo Besseghini, and Andrew A. Gage; *Cleveland*: Cathel Macleod and Berian Davies; *Dallas*: William Shapiro; *Hines*: William Meadows and Roque Pifarre; *Lexington*: Robert Class; *Little Rock*: Marvin Murphy; *Long Beach*: Nolan Resnick, Harold

March, John C. Kern, and Edward A. Stemmer; *Los Angeles*: Maylene Wong; *Madison*: James Thomsen; *Minneapolis*: Carl S. Alexander, James P. Lillehei, and Kyuhyun Wang; *New York*: Martin Dolgin; *Oteen*: Robert G. Fish, William Nelson, Norman Sollod, Stewart Scott, Charles Dart, Jr.; *Palo Alto*: James Pfeifer, William W. Angell, and Robert Wuerflein; *Salt Lake City*: Theofilos Tsagaris; *San Francisco*: Harold March, Richard Sanderson, and Albert D. Hall; *Seattle*: J. Ward Kennedy; *Washington*: Gerald I. Shugoll, Ross Fletcher, and Jerry A. Snow; *West Roxbury*: David Littman and Robert Morse.

We owe a special debt to Doctor H. Preston Price, chief, Laboratory Service, VA Hospital, Oteen, N.C., for reviewing all of the histologic sections made available to us for this study, and to the many pathologists in cooperating hospitals who generously submitted both autopsy protocols and histologic sections.

References

Abrams HL: Coronary arteriography: complications and indications. In Questions and Answers, JAMA 219: 917–18, 1972

Adams DF, Fraser DB, Abrams HL: Complications of coronary arteriography. Circulation 48:609–18, 1973

Berger RL, Wong J, Messer JV: Coronary embolectomy for acute coronary occlusion. Am J Surg 123:726–28, 1972

Braunwald, E: Deaths related to cardiac catheterization. Supplement III to Circulation, 37 and 38:III-23, May 1968

Campion BC, Frye RL, Pluth JR, Fairbairn JF, Davis GD: Arterial complications of retrograde brachial arterial catheterization. Mayo Clinic Proceedings 46:589–92, 1971

Chahine RA, Herman MV, Forlin R: Complications of coronary arteriography comparison of the brachial to the femoral approach (Abstract). Ann Intern Med 76:862, 1972

Cheng TO: Editorial: Fatal thromboembolism following selective coronary arteriography. Chest 62:1–2, 1972

Cohn LH, Gorlin R, Herman MV, Collins JJ: Aorto-coronary bypass for acute coronary occlusion. J Thorac and Cardiovasc Surg 64:503–9, 1972

Cooley DA, Wukasch DC, Hallman GL: Acute dissecting ascending aortic aneurysm resulting from coronary arteriography: successful surgical treatment. Chest 61:317–19, 1972

Danielson GK: Discussion of paper by Cohn, et al. J Thorac and Cardiovasc Surg 64:510, 1972

Formanek G, Frech RS, Amplatz K: Arterial thrombus formation during clinical percutaneous catheterization. Circulation 41:833–39, 1970

Giddings JA, See JR, Lewis RD, Cosby RS: Thromboembolism following coronary arteriography. Chest 61:235–39, 1972

Glancy JJ, Fishbone G, Heinz ER: Nonthrombogenic arterial catheters. Am J Roentgen 108:716, 1970

Green GS, McKinnon CM, Rosch J, Melvin P: Complications of selective percutaneous transfemoral coronary arteriography and their prevention. Circulation 45:552–57, 1972

Haas JM, Peterson CR, Jones RC: Subintimal dissection of the coronary arteries. Circulation 38:678–83, 1968

Hildner FJ, Javier RP, Ramaswamy K, Samet P: Pseudocomplications of cardiac catheterization. Chest 63: 15–17, 1973

Jacobsson B, Bergentz SE, Ljungqvist U: Platelet adhesion and thrombus formation on vascular catheters in dogs. Acta Radiol (Diagn) 8:221–27, 1969

Jacobsson B, Paulin S, Schlossman D: Thromboembolism of leg following percutaneous catheterization of femoral artery for angiography—symptoms and signs. Acta Radiol (Diagn) 8:97–108, 1969

Judkins MP: Percutaneous transfemoral selective coronary arteriography. Radiol Clin North Am 6: 467–92, 1968

Kaltenbach M, Lichtlen P: Coronary Heart Disease. Stuttgart, Germany, Georg Thieme Verlag, 1971, pp 19–29

Kasparian H, Lehman JS: Coronary arteriography in myocardial ischemia. Radiol Clin North Am 3:453, 1967

Kitamura K, Gobel FL, Wang Y: Dissection of the left coronary artery complicating retrograde left heart catheterization Chest 57:587, 1970

Lebowitz WB, Lucia W: Complications of selective percutaneous transfemoral coronary arteriography (Abstract). Circulation 48 (Suppl 4):90, 1973

Luepker RV, Bouchard RJ, Burns R, Warbasse JR: Systemic heparinization during percutaneous femoral artery catheterization (Abstract). Circulation 48 (Suppl 4):89, 1973

Machleder HI, Sweeney JP, Barker WF: Pulseless arm after brachial artery catheterization. Lancet 1:407–9, 1972

Morettin LB, Wallace JM: Uneventful perforation of a coronary artery during selective arteriography—a case report. Am J Roentgen 110:184–88, 1970

Nachnani GH, Lessin LS, Motomiya T, Jensen WN: Scanning electron microscopy of thrombogenesis on vascular catheter surfaces. N Engl J Med 286: 139–40, 1972

Nejad MS, Klaper MA, Steggerda FR, Gianturco C: Clotting on the outer surfaces of vascular catheters. Radiology 91:248–50, 1968

Nelson RM, Osborne AG: Systemic heparinization for percutaneous catheter arteriography. Circulation, Suppl II, 42 and 44 (Abstract):205, 1971

Nelson RM: Personal communication, 1972

Petch MC, Sutton R, Jefferson KE: Safety of coronary arteriography. Br Heart J 35:377–80, 1973

Pifarre R, Spinazzola A, Nemickas R, Scanlon PJ, Tobin JR: Emergency aortocoronary bypass for acute myocardial infarction. Arch Surg 103:525–28, 1971

Spain DM, Bradess VA: Sudden death from coronary heart disease. Chest 58:107–10, 1970

Takaro T, Dart CH Jr, Scott SM, Fish RG, Nelson WM: Coronary arteriography—indications, techniques, complications. Ann Thorac Surg 5:213–21, 1968

Takaro T, Pifarre R, Wuerflein RD, et al: Acute coronary occlusion following coronary arteriography: mechanisms and surgical relief. Surgery 72:1018–29, 1972

Takaro T, Hultgren HN, Littmann D, Wright EC: An analysis of deaths occurring in association with coronary arteriography. Am Heart J 86:587–97, 1973

Walker WJ, Mundal SL, Broderick HG, et al: Systemic heparinization for femoral percutaneous coronary arteriography. N Engl J of Med 288:826–28, 1973

Wallace S, Medellin H, de Jongh D, Gianturco C: Systemic heparinization for angiography. Am J Roentgen 116:204, 1972

25

REVIEW OF INTRAOPERATIVE CORONARY ANGIOGRAPHY IN AORTOCORONARY BYPASS SURGERY

Martin J. Kaplitt, Stephen L. Frantz, Anthony J. Tortolani, Frederic A. Newman, Harry L. Stein, and Stephen J. Gulotta

INTRODUCTION

The use of high-quality intraoperative cine-angiography for the evaluation of coronary bypass surgery was first described and reported by Diethrich et al in September 1972.[1,2,3] Since July 1972, we have utilized the same system for evaluating aortocoronary bypass grafts, and this report will review the technique, its application, and the results in the first 50 consecutive cases.

MATERIAL AND METHODS

With the development of a surgical anesthesia console, much of the equipment surrounding the operating table during open-heart surgery was consolidated and centralized in one area, facilitating the installation of a highly mobile, ceiling-mounted X-ray C-Arm (Fig. 1). This C-Arm could be rapidly positioned over the patient during open-heart surgery and fluoroscopy and 70-mm film could thus be easily and safely obtained. The technique employed in all cases was standard. The operative procedure was planned on the basis of anatomic findings seen on preoperative coronary angiography. The patient was placed on cardiopulmonary bypass, and either one or more coronary bypass grafts were performed, with or without endarterectomy. When the procedure was completed, the patient was taken off cardiopulmonary

Excerpts of this chapter reprinted from C.V. Supplement to Circulation, 1974, with permission from AHA.

bypass and his condition stabilized. At this time an 18-gauge catheter was inserted into the graft, either through a side branch or by direct puncture. Polyethylene tubing, with heparinized saline, was connected to a syringe of contrast media (Renografen 76) and 5 cc were injected under conditions of fluoroscopy. If no obvious technical errors (points of stenoses) were seen, a second injection was completed and 70-mm X-ray film was obtained. The film was developed within four minutes and brought into the operating room for more careful inspection. On two occasions ventricular fibrillation occurred during injection of contrast media, but the heart was easily defibrillated with one low-voltage shock. After review of the X-rays, the catheter was removed from the graft, protamine was given to neutralize heparin, and electromagnetic flowmeter (EMF) studies were conducted.

RESULTS

Fifty patients underwent aortocoronary bypass surgery, and either a single or double bypass procedure was performed. A total of 26 anterior descending grafts and 34 right coronary grafts were performed. Mean flows ranged from 15 cc per minute to 150 cc per minute in the right coronary grafts, and 26 cc per minute to 90 cc per minute in the anterior descending grafts (Table 1). Intraoperative coronary angiography performed on each graft was evaluated as an individual result. They were analyzed with regard to three critical factors: *size of recipient coronary artery, severity and distribution of disease,* and *distribution of flow* (Table 2). Technical errors with respect to the coronary anastomosis were de-

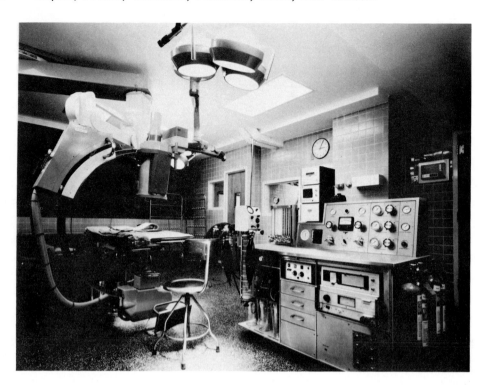

FIG. 1. Operating room designed for coronary artery surgery (see text). Reprinted from Cardio-vascular Surgery Supplement to Circulation, 1974, with permission from AHA.

tected during initial fluoroscopy or discovered on 70-mm X-rays, and corrections were made prior to the final angiogram. In two instances a technical error was noted. One error was seen on fluoroscopy and was found to represent a kink of the vein at the site of the anastomosis. This required repositioning of the vein graft but did not require resuturing of the anastomosis. In the second instance, a good result was assumed on fluoroscopy, but on review of the 70-mm angiograms, a filling defect was seen at the distal site of the coronary anastomosis. EMF studies demonstrated a flow of 50 cc/minute, but after an initial protamine dose, the graft thrombosed. This required resuturing of the anastomosis on cardiopulmonary bypass. Repeat angiography demonstrated correction of this technical error (Fig. 2).

On review of the individual angiograms, the three critical factors listed above were found to be of most significance in correlating each angiogram with the electromagnetic flow studies conducted at the time of surgery. In order to appreciate more clearly the significance of the intraoperative findings and to correlate these findings with the preoperative angiograms, a system of classification was developed based on the three critical factors. This system of classification subdivides the factors of size (S), location of disease (L), and distribution of flow (D) into a category into which each of the intraoperative angiograms could fall (Table 3). On review of the angiograms, it became quite evident that the variation in the quality of these intraoperative X-rays was most closely associated with the blood flow rates

TABLE 1. Review of 50 Consecutive Cases

	NO.	MEAN FLOWS	
		Mean	Range
Rt. bypass	24	73	15–150
LAD bypass	38	60	29–90

Reprinted from Cardiovascular Surgery Supplement to Circulation, 1974, with permission from AHA.

TABLE 2. Intraoperative Angiograms Classification (I–IV)

FACTORS DETERMINING CLASSIFICATION

1. Size of recipient coronary artery
2. Severity and distribution of disease
3. Distribution of flow

Reprinted from Cardiovascular Surgery Supplement to Circulation, 1974, with permission from AHA.

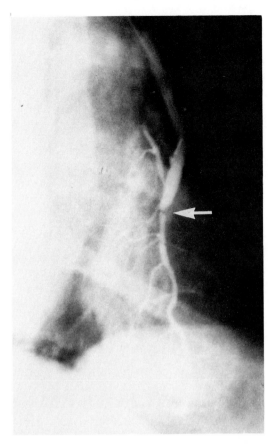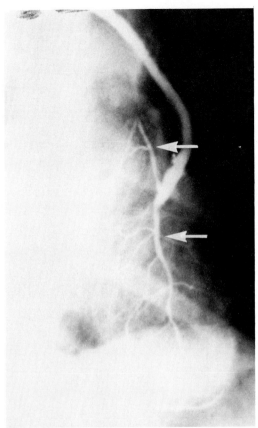

FIG. 2. Intraoperative angiogram demonstrating stenosis at distal suture line (left, arrow). Intra-
operative angiogram after correction (right) demonstrates enhanced disribution of flow (arrows).
Graft flow increased from 45 cc to 60 cc/minute (see text). Reprinted from Cardiovascular Surgery
Supplement to Circulation, 1974, with permission from AHA.

TABLE 3. Method of Classification

A. Size
    1. 2 mm or greater
    2. 1.5 mm or greater
    3. Less than 1.5 mm

B. Severity and Distribution of Disease
    1. No significant disease other than primary lesion
    2. Other disease present but not hemodynamically
        significant
    3. Diffuse disease

C. Distribution of Flow
    1. Fills entire vessel system
    2. Good distribution but less than entire system
    3. Limited distribution

Class I: all 1's
Class II: two 1's and one 2
Class III: two or more 2's
Class IV: one 3

*Reprinted from Cardiovascular Surgery Supplement to
Circulation, 1974, with permission from AHA.*

through the grafts, not with the radiologic technique. With this in mind, each of the angiograms
was grouped into either Class I, II, III, or IV.
Using this classification, any intraoperative angiogram could be subdivided according to an S, L, D
system (Fig. 3 and 4). After classifying all of
the angiograms, the intraoperative flow studies
were correlated with each graft according to classification, and the results were tabulated, as seen
in Table 4. It is apparent that flow rates coincide
closely with classification. The clinical results
(follow-up to one year) in most patients parallels
both the classification and flow rates. It is of interest that of 50 consecutive patients, 31 had
triple vessel involvement (RCA, LAD, and Circumflex) and 10 had main left coronary disease
(eight with triple vessel involvement). With respect to ventricular function, 30 had normal ventricular function, four showed mild impairment,
12 moderate impairment, and four severe impairment. There were no operative mortalities, and

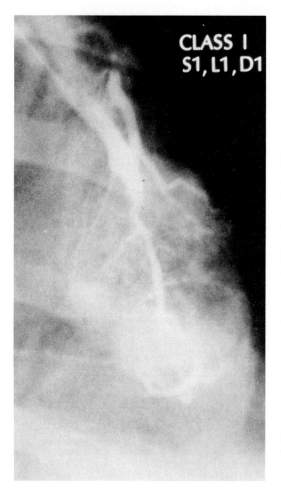

FIG. 3. Class I intraoperative angiogram according to S, L, D classification. Flow through this graft was 90 cc/minute (see text). Reprinted from Cardiovascular Surgery Supplement to Circulation, 1974, with permission from AHA.

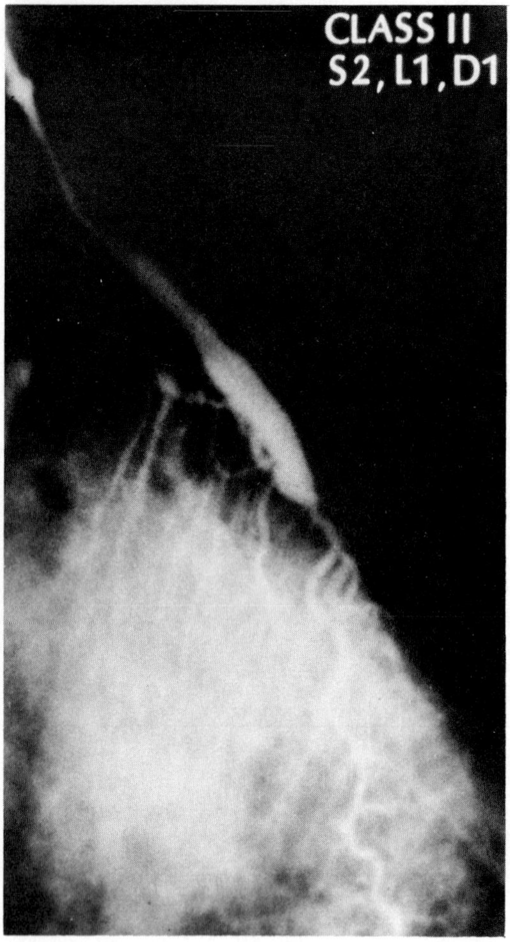

FIG. 4. Class II intraoperative angiogram according to S, L, D classification. Graft flow was 80 cc/ minute (see text). Reprinted form Cardiovascular Surgery Supplement to Circulation, 1974, with permission from AHA.

TABLE 4. Intraoperative Angiograms Classification (I–IV)

CORRELATION WITH GRAFT FLOWS		AVERAGE MEAN FLOW	
Class	No.	LAD	RT
I	18	88	100
II	25	61	66
III	13	46	50
IV	6	31	22

Reprinted from Cardiovascular Surgery Supplement to Circulation, 1974, with permission from AHA.

in follow-up to one year, there have been no mortalities. In none of these patients were more than two grafts performed. There were six patients who developed Q-wave infarctions on the electrocardiogram; however, all infarctions were in the distribution of a grafted vessel. In each case, the recipient artery was either a Class III or Class IV vessel. In those patients where only one bypass was performed and the intraoperative angiogram was judged to be a Class IV, return of preoperative symptoms was common. In contrast, however, those patients who demonstrated a Class I intraoperative angiogram, in either one or both grafts, did exceptionally well clinically with no return of symptoms and negative treadmill stress tests. In patients who have had more than one coronary artery bypass, the clinical result has followed the

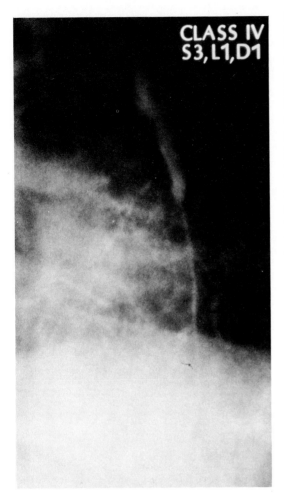

CLASS IV
S3, L1, D1

FIG. 5. Intraoperative angiogram of Class IV vessel. Flow through this graft was 40 cc/minute. Reprinted from Cardiovascular Surgery Supplement to Circulation, 1974, with permission from AHA.

the placement of the critical angle sutures. Additionally, flow rates have been taken in coronary bypass grafts, and flows of 40 cc per minute or more have been considered as generally representative of a good result.[4] These two techniques have been relied upon most often to insure the best technical result possible. It was surprising, therefore, to find that a patient could have a 50-cc-per-minute flow measured in the vein graft with patency of the graft as seen in Figure 2, but still have a filling defect that could cause ultimate thrombosis of the graft. The usual surgical techniques were performed on the particular patient seen in Figure 4, with successful passage of a small dilator, both antegrade and retrograde. This case demonstrated that even subtle errors can occur and escape notice. Note that on the repeat angiogram, the distribution of flow is significantly enhanced.

Our experience has further confirmed that bypass grafts that are flowing in the high range (approximately 60 cc per minute or more) are very likely to be successful both with respect to patency and clinical follow-up. Questionable clinical results and lower patency rates were seen in those cases where grafts demonstrated a flow of less than 60 cc's per minute. Intraoperative angiograms of these grafts fall into either a Class III or IV category, and a review of these angiograms clearly demonstrates why these poor results could have been anticipated (Fig. 5). Many of these grafts close either early in the postoperative period or within the first six months. Without intraoperative angiography closure of grafts with such flows would have been difficult to understand. More often than not, surgical techniques would have become suspect.

It was the intraoperative angiograms of the Class IV group that were most startling and clearly documented the fact that technical success with respect to the anastomosis was in no way indicative of a successful surgical procedure. Up to this time a flow of 40 cc per minute obtained at the time of surgery was presumed to indicate an acceptable result with the anticipation of benefit to the patient. On reviewing Class IV intraoperative angiograms, however, it became obvious that flows in the range of 30 to 40 cc per minute (assuming no technical error) represent a severely restricted runoff that precluded successful revascularization. It would certainly appear from these findings that if we hope to extend successful surgery to the Class IV category, our attention should not be directed to alternate surgical techniques that focus attention on the particular tube graft used for bypass, but rather on techniques to

expected course for the more favorable coronary artery. For example, when a patient had revascularization of a Class II anterior descending coronary artery and a Class IV right coronary artery, the expected clinical course followed the Class II vessel.

DISCUSSION

Technical errors in vascular surgery will result in failure of the surgery either immediately or early in the postoperative period. One of the standard techniques for avoiding technical problems related to anastomosis has been the use of small dilators passed through both the apex and base of an end-to-side anastomosis, subsequent to

expand the restricted runoff bed itself (counter-pulsation, vasodilators).

After a comparison of preoperative and intraoperative angiograms and correlation with flow rates, it became apparent that the preoperative films could be categorized and classified according to the same criteria as were used for the intraoperative studies. With few exceptions this classification can indicate those patients who are likely to have the best clinical results. One exception to this has been noted when a vessel is totally occluded and fills only from intercoronary collateral sources. Here an accurate assessment (of vessel diameter or potential distribution) cannot always be made from the preoperative film. It has become clear to us that a simple but meaningful "surgical" classification of coronary arteries, should be developed to enable a more critical evaluation of the usefulness of surgical intervention and as a basis for comparison from one patient to the next or from one center to another.

In view of experiences demonstrating adverse affects of vein grafting,[5] it is important to distinguish those arteries likely to be successfully bypassed from those likely to be unworthy of a bypass. It is, therefore, our impression that if we are to anticipate better mortality and morbidity following aortocoronary bypass surgery, we should look toward a more realistic preoperative assessment of the vessels to be bypassed rather than a "complete revascularization." In reviewing our series of patients, we have found that the mortality and morbidity on the one hand and benefits derived from surgery on the other, have not differed markedly from the best reported series despite the use of only one or two bypass grafts in cases of multiple vessel involvement and altered ventricular function. While multiple-vessel grafting may be indicated in those situations where all of the vessels to be bypassed are of good quality, in many other instances a method of classifying the vessels preoperatively would lead to a more physiologic revascularization.

SUMMARY

Fifty consecutive patients had intraoperative coronary angiography performed following aortocoronary bypass surgery. The intraoperative angiograms were correlated with graft flow studies, and a system of classification was developed. This system of classification was found to be applicable to the preoperative angiograms and provides a simple and realistic method of determining good candidates for bypass surgery.

References

1. Diethrich EB et al: Immediate assessment of coronary bypass grafts using operative arteriography—correlation with pressure gradients and flow studies. Chest 62:361, 1972
2. Diethrich EB, et al: Intraoperative coronary arteriography. Am J Surg 124:815, 1972
3. Diethrich EB: And the war goes on. Chest 68:83, 1973
4. Walker AJ, Friedberg DH, Flemma RJ, et al: Determinants of angiographic patency of aorto-coronary bypass grafts. Circulation (Supplement 1)45: 86, 1972
5. Vlodaver Z, Edwards JE: Pathologic analysis in fatal cases following saphenous vein coronary arterial bypass. Chest 64:555, 1973

26

MYOCARDIAL IMAGING WITH INTRACORONARY TECHNETIUM MAA: CLINICAL, HEMODYNAMIC, AND HISTOLOGIC CORRELATES
Potential Role in Revascularization Surgery

James L. Ritchie, Glen W. Hamilton, John A. Murray,
Eugene Lapin, and David Allen

INTRODUCTION

The expanding role of coronary revascularization procedures dictates increasing attention to optimal methods for identifying segments of myocardium that should be revascularized. Since the success of aortocoronary bypass grafting depends in large measure on the presence of an adequate distal capillary bed as shown by Johnson et al (1970), techniques providing direct information about this bed may be useful. Myocardial imaging with labeled microemboli allows assessment of the integrity of regional capillary perfusion as the particles lodge in a uniform manner related to arteriolar or precapillary blood flow (Schelbert et al, 1971). The technique is safe in humans (Endo et al, 1970; Schelbert et al, 1971) if strict attention to quality control in particle size and number of particles is observed. This review details our experience with this technique and compares the results of myocardial imaging with the hemodynamic, clinical, surgical, and autopsy findings.

METHODS

All patients with proven or suspected ischemic heart disease undergoing coronary arteriography were candidates for the study and none were excluded because of symptoms. The experimental nature of the study was fully explained to each patient, who signed a special consent form approved by the University of Washington Committee on Human Investigation.

Patients with associated valvular disease or cardiomyopathy were excluded from this analysis. All patients had a complete history and physical exam, ECG, and unless contraindicated, a maximal treadmill exercise test as described by Bruce (1971). Patients were additionally assigned a clinical index of probability of past infarction as follows: (1) None—no clinical or ECG evidence, (2) Possible—episodes of severe pain, no ECG changes, (3) Probable—clinical history of infarction, negative or equivocal ECG, and (4) Definite—clinical history plus ECG Q-waves. Coronary arteriography was performed by either the Sones or Judkins technique. Following arteriography, catheter position was ascertained and radiographic contrast medium flushed from the catheter. Following a two-minute delay (to minimize the effects of previous contrast material on coronary flow), 1–1.5 mCi of Technetium-99m labeled macroaggregated albumin (Tc MAA) was injected into one or both coronaries over 1 to 3 seconds and flushed in with 3 to 5 cc of saline. Subsequently, the remainder of the catheterization was completed including left ventricular biplane angiography utilizing 0.75 to 1 cc/kilo of Hypaque 75-M and large filming at 12 frames/second. Following catheterization, patients were taken to the Nuclear Medicine Laboratory where 100,000 count Polaroid scintiphotos of the myocardium were taken in the anterior, right and left anterior oblique, and left lateral and left posterior oblique views, using a low-energy, 1000-parallel-hole collimator. Imaging time was one to two minutes per view. Technetium MAA was prepared by the stannous chloride method as described by Allen et al (1973) such that 90 percent of particles were between 20 and 40 μ in diameter with none exceeding 100 μ. A total of 30,000 to 60,000 particles was injected per coronary artery. Twelve patients had injections of both coronary arteries, 33 had injections of the left coronary only, and six of the right coronary only.

Contraction plot abnormalities were assessed by the method of Hamilton et al (1972) as follows: I—normal, II—borderline abnormal, III—definite hypo- or akinesis, IV—dyskinesis, and V—generalized hypo- or akinesis. Ejection fractions were determined from volumes calculated by the area-length method (Dodge et al, 1960).

Images were interpreted in a subjective fashion by two independent observers without knowledge of arteriographic findings. Standards of normality were subsequently established from patients with normal arteriographic findings. Images were later reinterpreted; inter- and intraobserver concurrence was complete except in two cases that were assigned interpretations by consensus. Statis-

tical analyses were performed with the Student's t-test for unpaired data.

RESULTS

Fifty-one patients had myocardial images; 26 were normal and 25 were abnormal. There were no ECG changes, intracoronary pressure changes, or other identifiable adverse effects from the intracoronary injection of Tc MAA.

Myocardial Images

Figure 1 shows a normal left coronary image, a normal right coronary image, and a normal image when both coronaries are injected. The normal left coronary image is elliptical in the anterior and lateral views, and spherical in the left anterior oblique (LAO). The left ventricular cavity may be seen in the latter view as a central lucency. In patients with a dominant right coro-

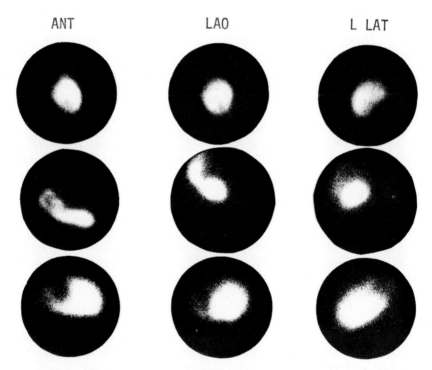

ANT   LAO   L LAT

FIG. 1. Normal myocardial images. Top: Normal image with left coronary artery injection only. Image is elliptical in the anterior and lateral views, spherical in the LAO. The central lucency is the left ventricular cavity; decreased activity is seen in the inferior diaphragmatic region corresponding to perfusion from the posterior descending coronary. Middle: Normal image with right coronary artery injection only. The appearance is that of a "ball and tail" configuration, the ball representing inferior diaphragmatic myocardium, the tail right ventricle. Bottom: Both right and left coronary arteries injected. The inferior myocardium is now perfused fully and the image is spherical in the LAO view, a rim of right ventricular activity is seen anteriorly in this view. ANT: anterior; L LAT: left lateral; LAO: left anterior oblique.

LAO   LAO   LAO

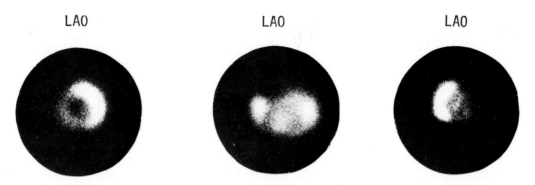

FIG. 2. Abnormal myocardial images: Perfusion defects are seen as regions of decreased or absent activity. Left: decreased activity in the septum secondary to anteroseptal infarction (left coronary injection; totally occluded LAD). Middle: decreased inferior activity secondary to diaphragmatic infarction (left and right coronary injection; totally occluded RCA). Right: decreased lateral activity secondary to posterolateral infarction (left coronary injection; totally occluded circumflex coronary artery). LAO: left anterior oblique.

nary system (all three patients in Figure 1), the left coronary image shows decreased activity in the inferior diaphragmatic region corresponding to perfusion from the posterior descending branch of the right coronary artery. This is usually best seen in the left anterior oblique view. The right coronary image shows a "ball and tail" distribution, the ball representing flow to the inferior diaphragmatic portion of the left ventricle and the tail to the right ventricular myocardium. When both arteries are injected, the image appears spherical in the LAO view as the inferior septum is perfused; a less dense rim of activity representing right ventricular myocardium is usually seen anteriorly on the LAO view.

Regional decreases in myocardial flow were seen as areas of diminished or absent activity. Figure 2 illustrates myocardial perfusion defects involving the anteroseptal, inferior diaphragmatic, and posterolateral portion of the left ventricle. These regions correspond to lesions of the left anterior descending, right, and circumflex coronary arteries respectively.

Correlation of Myocardial Images with Angina, Exercise Tolerance, and Exercise ST Depression

Forty-nine patients had anginal symptoms as a criterion for selection and thus there was no correlation between angina and the presence or absence of a scan abnormality. A positive ST segment response to exercise was defined as down-sloping or horizontal depression for at least 60 msec; positive and negative responses were evenly distributed between patients with and without scan abnormalities. Duration of performance on

the treadmill was significantly different in the two groups. Those with scan defects had a mean FAI * of 52 ± 18 percent ($p < 0.05$) (Fig. 3).

Correlation with History of Myocardial Infarction

All 19 patients clinically classified as definite or probable previous myocardial infarction (class 3 or 4) had an abnormal image when the area of infarction had been scanned (Fig. 4). Similarly, patients with normal scans had little or no evidence for past infarction (class 1 or 2). Considering only the presence or absence of a diagnostic ECG Q-wave, no patients with a normal scan had a Q-wave. Most patients (19/25) with scan defects had corresponding Q-waves. As shown in Figure 5, all patients with diagnostic Q-waves had abnormal myocardial images.

Correlation with Hemodynamic Data

The mean systolic ejection fraction was significantly lower in the group with scan defects (43 ± 14 percent versus 61 ± 10) percent than in those with normal images, $p < 0.001$ (Fig. 3). As a group, contraction plots were significantly more abnormal in those with abnormal images. Twenty of 21 patients with normal images had normal or borderline contraction plots (I or II) while 14 of

* FAI or functional aerobic impairment is an index of the percent difference from normal when compared to age, activity, and sex-matched controls of symptom-limited maximal oxygen consumption as described by Bruce (1971).

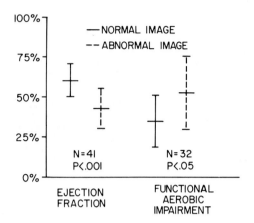

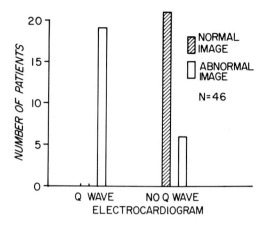

FIG. 3. Ejection fraction and functional aerobic impairment were both significantly reduced in the groups with scan defects (noted as the mean ± 1 standard deviation).

FIG. 5. The presence or absence of abnormal ECG Q-wave in patients with normal images and patients with image defects; an abnormal Q-wave was one of at least 0.04 seconds duration.

24 patients with abnormal images had clearly abnormal contraction plots (III, IV, or V).

Correlation with Coronary Arteriogram

The percent coronary stenosis of the arterial system scanned is compared to the presence or absence of a scan defect in Figure 6. All 19 patients with stenoses of 75 percent or less had normal images. Approximately equal numbers of patients with stenoses of 76 percent to 99 percent had normal and abnormal scans. Nineteen of 21 patients with complete occlusions had scan defects. Two patients with complete occlusion but no other ECG contractile plot or clinical evidence of infarction had normal images.

Correlation with Surgical and Histologic Data

Two patients expired within 60 days of myocardial imaging. Each had had ECG Q-wave, contractile plot and clinical evidence for infarction and each had scan defects in the area of expected infarction. At autopsy each had old infarctions; one an inferior transmural scar of 1.5 × 1.5 cm, the other a transmural apical scar of 1.5 × 1.5 cm with an associated 6 × 8 cm subendocardial septal scar (Fig. 7, top row). An additional patient had ECG, clinical, and contractile plot evidence for an anteroseptal infarction and underwent aneurysmectomy; he had an extensive anteroseptal scan defect with no detectable activity in this region of the scan (Fig. 7, bottom row)—histologic exam

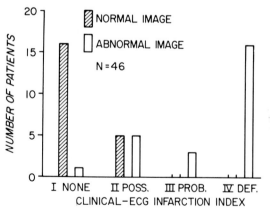

FIG. 4. Clinical—ECG Infarction Index is a clinical assessment of post myocardial infarction as follows: I: none, no clinical or ECG evidence; II: possible, episodes of severe pain, no ECG changes; III: probable, clinical history of infarction and negative or equivocal ECG, and IV: definite, clinical history plus ECG Q-waves.

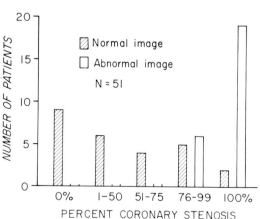

FIG. 6. The percent diameter stenosis of the most severely affected coronary artery that was imaged.

ANT   LAO   L LAT

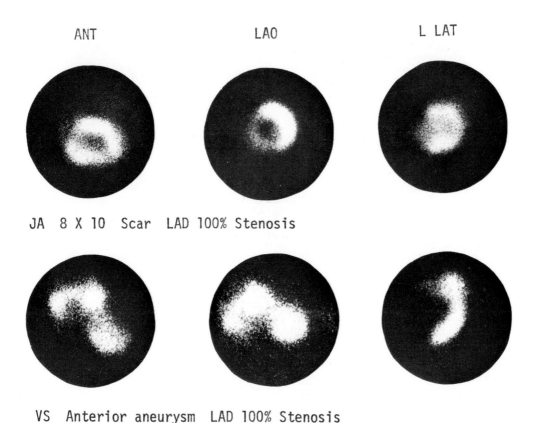

JA 8 X 10 Scar LAD 100% Stenosis

VS Anterior aneurysm LAD 100% Stenosis

FIG. 7. Patient JA: small apical transmural infarction and extensive subendocardial septal infarction at autopsy; image shows marked decrease in activity of apex and septum. Patient VS:
extensive anteroseptal transmural infarction documented at aneurysmectomy; image shows total
absence of activity in anteroseptal myocardium. ANT: anterior; LAO left anterior oblique; L LAT:
left lateral; LAD: left anterior descending.

of the resected tissue showed transmural scarring without associated viable muscle.

A comparison of scan findings and findings at surgical inspection was possible in 14 patients. All four patients with normal scans had normal ventricles at surgery. Eight patients had evidence of scarring at surgery and had corresponding myocardial image defects. One patient with a scan defect on left coronary injection had angiographic collateral to this region and a normal ventricle at surgery. One patient had scarring of the inferior myocardium related to right coronary occlusion; his left coronary scan had been normal.

DISCUSSION

Wagner et al (1969) and Tow et al (1966) have validated the principle of the microemboliza-tion technique and shown that particles of 10 to 60 μ diameter will lodge in the arterioles or capillaries of the vascular bed injected in a pattern proportionate to relative regional blood flow.

Fortuin et al (1971) extended these observations to the heart, utilizing left atrial injections in ex-perimental animals and showed that activity in 10 gram samples from the left ventricular free wall and septum were identical with only minor differences between the circumflex and left an-terior descending beds. Although incomplete mix-ing of particles is a potential problem with intra-coronary injection, Schelbert et al (1971) have shown uniform particle distribution by histologic exam following intracoronary injections in the dog. In this series, a single case was encountered in which the circumflex or left anterior descending coronary was selectively injected with MAA re-sulting in an apparent perfusion defect. Repeat catheterization and MAA injection of the alternate artery gave a normal composite image. This case was readily recognized by angiographic streaming of dye into one or the other artery; Jansen et al (1973) have also noted a small percentage of cases in which apparent image defects are created but recognized by selective streaming of angio-graphic dye.

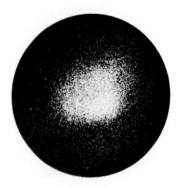 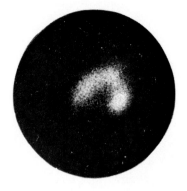

FIG. 8. Left: This patient has a normal resting left lateral image. Right: ten seconds following hyperemia and injection with a second isotope, there is a marked inferior defect. The patient had a complete right coronary occlusion with collateral perfusion from the left anterior descending coronary, which was 50 percent occluded.

An additional crucial technical factor is the timing of the MAA injection with respect to injection of radiographic contrast medium. Gould et al (1974) from this laboratory have shown in the experimental animal that intracoronary contrast media increases coronary flow an average of fourfold in the 6 to 10 seconds immediately following injection and that coronary flow remains elevated to a lesser degree for several minutes. If MAA injection is performed during this hyperemic flow period, marked changes in regional perfusion may occur (Fig. 8). Coronary flow returned to within 10 to 15 percent of baseline at the end of two minutes in that study and all MAA injections in this clinical study were made at least two minutes after the last intracoronary contrast injection.

The major conclusion of this study is that regional perfusion defects generally correlate with myocardial scarring secondary to infarction. This was most definitively established by histologic examination or direct visual inspection at surgery. The presence of ECG Q-waves, clinical history, contraction pattern abnormalities, reduced functional aerobic impairment, and lowered ejection fractions provided additional evidence. Only three patients had abnormal images without other evidence of infarction. In one only the left coronary artery was imaged and marked angiographic collateral from the right coronary to this region was present. A second patient had a scan defect associated with a distal circumflex occlusion and no other evidence of infarction or identifiable collateral to this area. This probably represented an infarction not detectable by other means; a large autopsy study by Horan et al (1971) has shown that infarctions in the posterobasal myocardium are commonly electrocardiographically silent. A final patient with a perfusion defect but without

other evidence of infarction had several 80 to 90 percent stenoses in the region of the scan defect, associated rest pain, and resting ST and T-wave changes by ECG. Presumably he had sufficient resting flow maldistribution that a defect was identifiable.

The finding that perfusion defects occurred primarily in patients with infarction agrees with findings obtained by Weller, et al (1972) in experimental animals. They showed that angiographically complete branch occlusions gave perfusion defects only when infarctions were produced. These results differ from those of Ashburn et al (1971) in which perfusion defects were identified in all cases with a greater than 75 percent coronary stenosis. This may in part be explained by their inclusion of more patients with severe resting flow abnormalities as in our single "preinfarctional" case. Alternatively, some of the defects in that series may have been induced by the temporal proximity of radiographic contrast medium to that of the radionuclide injection.

In this series the scanning technique was more sensitive than the ECG alone in predicting region of myocardial scar. Imaging was similar to contraction plot in the detection of regional abnormalities. Some contraction plot abnormalities may, however, be overlooked in single plane angiographic studies (Cohn et al, 1972); additionally, the type of reference system used in diagramming contraction plots may give disparate results. Chaitman et al (1973) have shown that one reference system detected wall motion abnormalities in 84 percent of patients with infarctions, a second method detected abnormalities in only 42 percent of this same group. These and related problems with available techniques suggest that imaging may provide more sensitive and more direct information about regional perfusion. One postoperative study by Gander et al (1973) has shown that regions of dysynergy were largely corrected by revascularization when the myocardial scan was normal; in those cases with scan defects in the region grafted, there was generally no improvement in myocardial contractility. Further studies of this nature to determine the efficacy of revascularization procedures appear warranted. At present, the long-term value of the myocardial imaging technique is uncertain, but promising.

References

Allen DR, Cheney FW, Nelp WB, Hartnett DE: Critical assessment of changes in the pulmonary circulation following injection of lung scanning agent (MAA). J Nuc Med 14:375, 1973

Ashburn WL, Braunwald E, Simon AL, Peterson KL, Gault SR: Myocardial perfusion imaging with radioactive-labelled particles injected directly into the coronary circulation of patients with coronary artery disease. Circulation 44:851, 1971

Bruce RA: Exercise testing of patients with coronary heart disease. Ann Clin Res 3:323, 1971

Chaitman BR, Bristow JD, Rahimtoola SH: Left ventricular wall motion assessed by using fixed external reference systems. Circulation 48:1043, 1973

Cohn PF, Gorlin R, Adams DF, et al: Biplane versus single plane left ventriculography in patients with coronary artery disease. Circulation 46 (Supplement IV):6, 1972 (abstract)

Dodge HT, Sandler H, Ballew DW, et al: The use of biplane angiocardiography for measurement of left ventricular volume in man. Am Heart J 60:762, 1960

Endo M, Yamazaki T, Kouno S, Hiratsuka H, et al: The direct diagnosis of human myocardial ischemia using 131I-MAA via the selective coronary catheter. Am Heart J 80:498, 1970

Fortuin NJ, Kaihara S, Becker LC, Pitt B: Regional myocardial blood flow in the dog studied with radioactive microspheres. Cardiovasc Res 5:331, 1971

Gander MP, Jansen C, Wareham E, Huse W, Judkins MP: Internal mammary to anterior descending coronary anastomosis—evaluated postoperatively with high resolution arteriography and myocardial perfusion scanning. Circulation 48 (Supplement IV):90, 1973 (abstract)

Gould KL, Lipscomb K, Hamilton GW: A physiologic basis for assessing critical coronary stenosis: instantaneous flow response and regional distribution during coronary hyperemia as measures of coronary flow reserve. Am J Cardiol 32:87, 1974

Hamliton GW, Murray JA, Kennedy JW: Quantitative angiocardiography in ischemic heart disease. Circulation 45:1065, 1972

Horan PLG, Flowers NC, Johnson JC: Significance of the diagnostic Q wave of myocardial infarction. Circulation 43:428, 1971

Jansen C, Judkins MP, Grames GM, Gander M, Adams R: Myocardial perfusion color scintigraphy with MAA. Radiology 109:369, 1973

Johnson WD, Flemma RJ, Lepley D: Determinants of blood flow in aortic-coronary saphenous vein bypass grafts. Arch Surg 101:806, 1970

Schelbert HR, Ashburn WL, Covell JW, et al: Feasibility and hazards of the intracoronary injection of radioactive serum albumin macroaggregates for external myocardial perfusion imaging. Invest Radiol 6:379, 1971

Tow D, Wagner HN, Lopez-Majans V, et al: Validity of measuring regional pulmonary arterial blood flow with macroaggregates of human serum albumin. Am J Roentgenol Radium Ther Nucl Med 96:664, 1966

Wagner HN, Rhodes BA, Sasaki Y, Ryan JP: Studies of the circulation with radioactive microspheres. Invest Radiol 4:374, 1969

Weller DA, Adolph RJ, Wellman HN, Carroll RG, Kim O: Myocardial perfusion scintigraphy after intracoronary injection of 99mTc-labelled human albumin microspheres. Circulation 46:963, 1972

27

RISK FACTORS IN PREMATURE CORONARY ARTERY DISEASE

Paul K. Hanashiro, Miguel E. Sanmarco, H. P. Chin, Ronald H. Selvester, and David H. Blankenhorn

The development of premature coronary artery disease involves a complex interplay of hereditary factors, metabolic alterations, and the individual's life-style. Although specific mechanisms have not been delineated, extensive prospective and retrospective studies have demonstrated that the incidence of coronary artery disease increases in the presence of conventional risk factors.[1-13] Moreover, combinations of risk factors further increase the risk of coronary artery disease.[14-16] The difference in incidence is most marked in the younger age groups.[4] This is probably because varying combinations of risk factors play a major role in accelerating the disease process. These risk factors are familial history of coronary artery disease, glucose intolerance, high serum cholesterol, high serum triglycerides, smoking, obesity, and hypertension.

The purpose of this report is to discuss the prevalence of these risk factors in a large number of patients who sustained a coronary event before the age of 50. Such profiling would serve to characterize the coronary-prone members of the population before manifestations of coronary artery disease occur.

METHODS

As part of a study of progression of atherosclerosis, 94 men with premature coronary artery disease were evaluated for seven coronary risk factors. These were as follows:

1. Smoking: 20 or more cigarettes per day
2. Family (any blood relative) history of coronary artery disease.
3. Abnormal intravenous glucose tolerance test (IVGTT): K_w = the rate constant of glucose disapparance in percent per minute; a value less than 0.91 was considered diabetic; a value of 0.91 to 1.1 was considered borderline; a value greater than 1.1 was considered normal.
4. High serum triglycerides: a value greater than 150 mg percent was considered abnormal.
5. High serum cholesterol: a value greater than 250 mg percent was considered abnormal.
6. Overweight: 15 percent greater than ideal weight (Metropolitan Life Insurance tables) was considered overweight.
7. Hypertension: a systolic blood pressure greater than 160 mm Hg and/or a diastolic blood pressure greater than 90 mm Hg recorded on two or more occasions was considered abnormal.

The criteria for the diagnosis of premature coronary artery disease were as follows:

1. Documented myocardial infarction by two of these three indicators in men under age 50:
   a. clinical history
   b. enzyme changes consistent with myocardial infarction
   c. electrocardiographic and/or vectorcardiographic evidence of myocardial infarction.
2. Sixty percent narrowing in one or more coronary arteries demonstrated by coronary arteriography.

The patients ranged from 33 to 52 years with a mean of 45.5. Eighty-nine percent were between 40 and 49 years of age. From the time of myocardial infarction to the time of evaluation, the range was two months to 17 years with a mean of three years. Eighty-five percent had one myocardial infarction and 15 percent had two myocardial infarctions prior to the time of evaluation. The IVGTT and lipid analyses were performed after an overnight fast of 12 to 16 hours. Twenty-five grams of glucose were injected and serial samples were drawn from another site for one hour. Cardiac catheterization and coronary arteriograms were performed for quantitation of coronary atherosclerosis and degree of left ventricular dysfunction.

RESULTS

The mean values for the group for individual risk factors are shown in Table 1. Only the values for smoking, IVGTT, and serum triglycerides were abnormal. However, a mean of 3.9 total risk factors was compiled for each person. The percentage of abnormality of the individual risk factors is indicated graphically in Figure 1 in decreasing order. Cigarette smoking was the highest, followed by family history of coronary artery disease, abnormal IVGTT, abnormal serum

TABLE 1. Values of the Mean, Standard Error of the Mean, and Range for Seven Risk Factors in 94 Patients with Premature Coronary Artery Disease

FACTOR	MEAN	SEM	RANGE
Cigarettes per day	28	2.05	0–80
FBS mg%	100	3.24	70–312
K_w	1.01	0.04	0.25–2.8
Cholesterol mg%	247	6.29	130–461
Triglycerides mg%	205	14.98	49–998
Percent Overweight	14	1.46	0–77
Systolic BP mmHg	130	2.10	90–225
Diastolic BP mmHg	87	1.41	50–140
Total Risk Factors per Patient	3.9	0.12	1–7

triglycerides, overweight, abnormal serum cholesterol, and hypertension. Although the prevalence of heavy smoking was highest, it was always observed in combination with other risk factors. This was also the case for the family history of coronary artery disease, hypertension, and overweight. Thus, no one factor was an overriding one, and most patients had multiple risk factors in varying combinations.

Table 2 shows the results of the IVGTT.

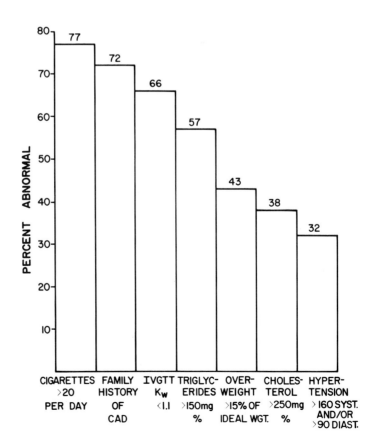

FIG. 1. Percent abnormal of individual risk factors in 94 patients with premature coronary artery disease.

TABLE 2. Results of the IVGTT in 94 Patients with Premature Coronary Artery Disease

FBS $<$ 110 mg%	86%
FBS $>$ 110 mg%	14%
K_W = $>$ 1.1	34%
K_W = 1.1–.91	19%
K_W = $<$ .91	47%
Abn K_W =	66%
Known Diabetics	8%

Only 14 percent had an abnormal fasting blood glucose prior to the test. However, 8 percent were known diabetics prior to the test, leaving only 6 percent of the total group with an abnormal fasting blood glucose that was previously undetected. Forty-seven percent of the patients had a diabetic response to the IVGTT. Nineteen percent had a borderline response. These observations indicated that the fasting blood glucose was not a reliable indicator for glucose intolerance. Table 3 shows the lipid analyses. Thirty-eight percent of the patients had serum cholesterol values greater than 250 mg percent. Fifty-seven percent had high serum triglycerides greater than 150 mg percent. Only 12 percent had high cholesterol as the only lipid abnormality, and 33 percent had high triglycerides as the only lipid abnormality. Twenty-six percent had both lipid abnormalities. Thus, there was a total of 71 percent of the patients with one or both lipid abnormalities. Phenotyping of the lipoprotein patterns by electrophoresis showed equal numbers of the Type II and Type IV hyperlipoproteinemias.

A combined analysis of the IVGTT and lipid abnormalities is shown in Table 4. Ninety-two percent of the patients had one or a combined metabolic abnormality, and only 8 percent had no carbohydrate or lipid abnormality. Scattered numbers of abnormal and normal lipid abnormalities were observed in patients with an abnormal IVGTT as well as in patients with a normal IVGTT. Twenty-one percent had an abnormal IVGTT alone, and 26 percent had a lipid abnormality alone. These data indicate an increased

TABLE 3. Results of Lipid Analyses in 94 Patients with Premature Coronary Artery Disease

I.	Cholesterol $>$ 250 mg%	38%
	Triglycerides $>$ 150 mg%	57%
II.	Cholesterol abnormality alone	12%
	Triglyceride abnormality alone	33%
	Mixed abnormalities	26%
III.	Total lipid abnormality	71%
IV.	Normal	29%

TABLE 4. Combined Analysis of IVGTT and Lipids in 94 Patients with Premature Coronary Artery Disease

(percent abnormal)

LIPID ANALYSIS	IVGTT K_W			
	Diabetic ($<$.91)	Borderline (.91–1.1)	Normal ($>$1.1)	Total
Cholesterol[a]	6	1	5	12
Triglycerides[b]	12	11	10	33
Mixed[a,b]	10	5	11	26
Normal lipids	19	2	8	29
Total	47	19	34	100

[a] $>$ 250mg%
[b] $>$ 150mg%

prevalence of abnormal metabolism of carbohydrate and lipids in premature coronary artery disease, which may be present singly or in combinations of abnormalities.

Figure 2 is a histogram of the total risk factors per person. The mean total was 3.9. There was no consistent pattern of risk factors noted. Another histogram is also displayed of comparable subjects. The men were between the ages of 44 and 49 with no evidence of coronary artery disease who had similar risk factors evaluated. The mean total risk factor in this group was 1.8. It is apparent that there is a qualitative risk factor difference between the two groups.

The majority of patients had two or more significant lesions in the coronary arteries: 59 percent having three vessels, and 21 percent having two vessels involved. Only 20 percent had one vessel involved. As shown in Figure 3, the degree and severity of coronary artery involvement was not correlated with the total risk factors or the kinds of risk factors. Severe three-vessel involvement was observed with one and two total risk factors. On the other hand, single-vessel involvement was also observed with five and six total risk factors.

DISCUSSION

The results of our study suggest that premature coronary artery disease in males is multifactorial, with most patients having multiple risk factors. Our observations are consistent with those of Hatch et al,[17] who reported that patients with premature coronary artery disease had higher total risk factors than their controls. Additionally, these investigators, as well as Walker and Gregoratos,[18]

FIG. 2. Histogram of total abnormal risk factors in 94 patients with premature coronary artery disease and 50 subjects without coronary artery disease.

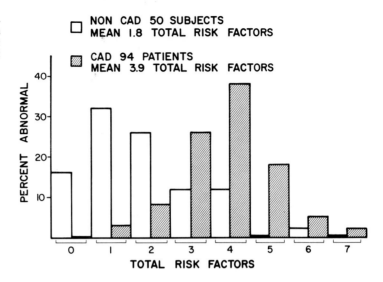

NON CAD 50 SUBJECTS
MEAN 1.8 TOTAL RISK FACTORS

CAD 94 PATIENTS
MEAN 3.9 TOTAL RISK FACTORS

and Gertler and White,[19] have shown the association of a positive family history of coronary artery disease, metabolic abnormalities, and the influence of the individual's "life-style," namely smoking, obesity, and hypertension as the major contributors to premature coronary artery disease.

The prevalence of metabolic alterations in our patients are consistent with reports of other investigators.[20-25] The important insight we have gleaned is that a single metabolic abnormality does not act as a major cause of premature coronary artery disease alone, but does so along with other risk factors including other metabolic alterations. The exceptions are diabetes and xanthomatous Type II hyperlipoproteinemia. There were only three patients in our study who were in these categories. One patient was a diabetic with two-vessel disease and two patients had xanthomatous Type

II hyperlipoproteinemia without other risk factors but with severe three-vessel disease.

An important observation that needs to be underscored is the increased alteration of glucose metabolism in patients with premature coronary artery disease. The fasting blood glucose of this study group was of little help in screening these abnormalities. Although the close association of diabetes or glucose intolerance with premature coronary artery disease had been reported,[23-25] many of the patients had no prior diagnostic work-up other than a fasting blood glucose after their myocardial infarctions. Thirty-nine percent of the patients had a past history of diabetes in the family.

The majority of the patients had severe coronary artery disease with 80 percent having multiple vessel involvement. The degree and severity

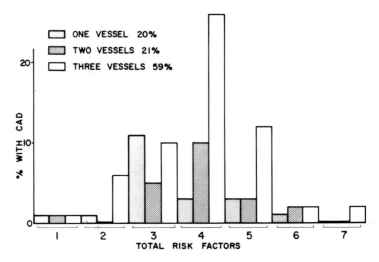

ONE VESSEL 20%
TWO VESSELS 21%
THREE VESSELS 59%

FIG. 3. Severity of coronary artery disease compared with total number of risk factors.

of the coronary artery disease with the total number of risk factors and/or type of risk factors were not clearly related in our study. The lack of correlation of risk factors with the severity of the coronary artery disease was also reported by Heinle et al [24] and Kimbiris, et al.[26]

From this study it seems germane to consider profiling each person with premature coronary artery disease for these risk factors and to "normalize" as many of these as possible with vigorous therapeutic interventions. Prophylactic screening of populations for the identification of high-risk individuals would also be a contribution in the reduction of premature coronary artery disease by the institution of early intervention trials for the high-risk individual.

SUMMARY

The results of our study suggest that premature coronary-artery disease in men is multifactorial, with most patients having multiple risk factors. Moreover, there seems to be a complex interplay of hereditary factors, metabolic alterations, and the individual's "life-style." No one factor seems to be an overriding one. These patients also tend to have severe coronary artery disease with multiple vessels involved by the time the clinical manifestations are first observed.

References

1. Keys A, Aravanis C, Blackburn H, et al: Probability of middle-aged men developing coronary heart disease in five years, Circulation, 45:815, 1972
2. Fowler NO: Clinical Diagnosis, Circulation, 46: 1079, 1972
3. Kannel WB, Gordon T, and Schwartz MJ: Systolic versus diastolic blood pressure and risk of coronary heart disease. The Framingham Study, Am J Cardiol, 27:335, 1971
4. Truett J, Coonfield J, and Kannel W: A multivariate analysis of risk of coronary heart disease in Framingham, J Chronic Dis, 20:511, 1967
5. Kannel WB, Castelli WP, Gordon T, et al: Serum cholesterol, lipoproteins, and the risk of coronary heart disease, The Framingham study, Ann Intern Med, 74:1, 1971
6. Hammond EC, Garfinkel L, and Seidman, H: Longevity of parents and grandparents in relation to coronary heart disease and associated variables. Circulation, 43:31, 1971
7. Ostrander D, Jr, Neff BJ, Block, WD, et al: Hyperglycemia and hypertriglyceridemia among persons with coronary heart disease, Ann Intern Med, 67: 34, 1967
8. Gertler MM, White PD, Cady LD, and Whiter HH: Coronary Heart Disease—A Prospective Study, Am J Med Sci, 35:377, Oct 1964
9. Kannel WB, Dawber TR, Kagan A, et al: Factors of risk in the development of coronary heart disease-six year follow-up experience. The Framingham Study, Ann Intern Med, 55:33, 1961
10. Mulcahy R, and Hickey N: Cigarette smoking habits of patients with coronary heart disease, Br Heart J, 28:404, 1966
11. Epstein FH: Hyperglycemia: A risk factor in coronary heart disease, Circulation, 36:609, 1967
12. Falsetti HL, Schnatz JD, Greene DG, & Bunnell IL: Serum lipids and glucose tolerance in angiographically proved coronary artery disease, Chest, 58:111, 1970
13. Chapman M, Coulson AH, Clark VA, & Borun ER: The differential effect of serum cholesterol, blood pressure and weight on the incidence of myocardial infarction and angina pectoris, J Chron Dis, 23:631, 1971
14. Stamler J: Acute myocardial infarction—progress in primary prevention, Br Heart J, 33 Supplement 145, 1971
15. Dick TBS and Stone MC: Prevalence of three cardinal risk factors in a random sample of men and in patients with ischaemic heart disease, Br Heart J, 35:381, 1973
16. Tibblin G: Risk factors in coronary heart disease. Advances in Cardiology, 4:123, 1969
17. Hatch FT et al: A study of coronary heart disease in young men. Characteristics and metabolic studies of the patients and comparison with age-matched healthy men. Circulation, 33:679, 1966
18. Walker W & Gregoratos G: Myocardial infarction in young men. Am J Cardiology, 19:339, 1967
19. Gertler MM & White PD: Coronary Heart Disease in Young Adults—Monograph. Cambridge, Mass., Harvard University Press, 1954
20. Carlson Lars A: Serum lipids in men with myocardial infarctions, Acta Med Scand, 167:399, 1960
21. Gertler MD et al: Ischemic heart disease. Insulin, carbohydrate, and lipid interrelationships. Circulation, 46:103, 1972
22. Tzagournis M, Seidensticker JF, Hamwi GJ: Serum insulin, carbohydrate, and lipid abnormalities in patients with premature coronary heart disease, Ann Intern Med, 67:42, 1967
23. Tzagournis M, Chiles R, Ryan JM, and Skillman TG: Interrelationships of hyperinsulinism and hypertriglyceridemia in young patients with coronary heart disease. Circulation, 38:1156, 1968
24. Heinle RA, Levy RI, Frederickson DS, and Gorlin R: Lipid and carbohydrate abnormalities in patients with angiographically documented coronary artery disease, Am J Cardiol, 24:178, 1969
25. Herman MV and Gorlin R: Premature coronary artery disease and the preclinical diabetic state, Editorial, Am J Med, 38:481, 1965
26. Kimbiris D, et al: Devolutionary pattern of coronary atherosclerosis in patients with angina pectoris. Coronary arteriographic studies, Am J Cardiol, 33:7–11 (Jan) 1974

28

CLINICAL ARTERIOGRAPHIC CORRELATIONS IN ASYMPTOMATIC MEN POST INFARCTION

Miguel E. Sanmarco, Paul K. Hanashiro,
Ronald H. Selvester, and David H. Blankenhorn

Selective coronary arteriography has provided a new perspective in the understanding of patients with ischemic heart disease. The incidence and severity of the coronary arterial lesions in symptomatic patients (angina, congestive failure, and so on) has been the subject of several reports.[9,15,16] There is little information available, however, concerning the arteriographic changes in young asymptomatic men or the possible value of the various risk factors in predicting the severity of the coronary artery lesions.

This report will discuss the results of arteriographic and ventricular function studies in 70 asymptomatic men with clinical and/or electrocardiographic evidence of myocardial infarction. This knowledge assumes vital importance in the understanding of the results of any proposed intervention to modify the course of the disease (diet, exercise, reduction of risk factors, surgery, and so on).

In January 1972 a prospective study of men with premature atherosclerosis (40 to 50 years of age) was instituted at the University of Southern California to ascertain the possible effects of vigorous exercise and weight reduction on the progression of the atheromatous lesion. Of the 94 patients studied since that time, 70 were totally asymptomatic and form the basis of this report.

CASE MATERIAL AND METHODS

All patients had a complete history and physical examination, routine laboratory studies, and chest roentgenograms.

Supported in part by USPHS Grant HL 14138.

Lipid determinations and intravenous glucose tolerance tests were performed in each patient after a 12-hour overnight fast.[2,10] The rate of glucose disappearance in percent per minute was calculated and a value of less than 0.91 was considered abnormal.

Electrocardiogram and Vectorcardiogram: Double-gain, double-speed electrocardiograms, and Cube and McFee VCGs were obtained on all patients. The infarction was located in one of 12 segments as previously described [19] and sized from 1 to 8 cm.

Treadmill Exercise Test: each patient underwent a treadmill exercise test, as described by Doan and coworkers [4] and modified by Sheffield and coworkers.[20] The test was terminated at 85 percent of the predicted maximum heart rate. Other reasons for terminating the test were (a) progressive angina (not present in any patient in this study); (b) severe shortness of breath; (c) rhythm disturbances, particularly coupled or multifocal premature ventricular contractions; (d) a conduction abnormality; and (e) lightheadedness or muscular exhaustion. Simple bipolar leads were positioned on the chest to approximate an orthogonal lead orientation. Electrocardiographic tracings were recorded at 50 mm per second chart speed to facilitate measurements. ST segment depression was considered abnormal if there was at least 0.1 mv J-point depression precipitated by exercise combined with a down-sloping or flat ST segment lasting for 0.08 seconds from the J-point. A test was considered indeterminate if a satisfactory level of tachycardia was not achieved or if there were other causes to invalidate the "abnormal" ECG response such as left ventricular hypertrophy, resting ST depression, bundle branch block, or digitalis effect.

Cardiac Catheterization and Angiography: Each patient underwent diagnostic right and left catheterization and biplane cine ventriculography. Left ventriculograms were calibrated with a grid system to calculate ventricular volumes. Selective coronary arteriography was performed using 35 mm cine at 60 frames per second. The cineangiograms were taken in multiple projections and in some instances following nitroglycerin.

For the purposes of this study, a vessel was considered involved when it had luminal narrowing of 60 percent or more of the linear dimension. An arteriographic score as suggested by Friesinger and associates [7] was calculated in each patient.

Left ventricular function was determined from the cine ventriculogram. The left ventricular end-diastolic and end-systolic volumes and ejection fraction were calculated by the area-length method of Dodge et al [5] modified for single plane calculations.[18] The extent of left ventricular dysfunction (hypokinesis or akinesis) was measured from the ventriculogram (using a digitizer-computer system) and expressed as a percent of the left ventricular surface area.

RESULTS

The distribution of coronary lesions appears in Table 1. Of the 70 patients, 39 had disease in all three vessels (56 percent). One- and two-vessel disease were found in 17 and 14 patients, respectively; the left anterior descending and right coronary artery were most commonly involved either alone or in combination. The left main was involved in three patients, all of whom had severe triple-vessel disease.

A pattern that has received little attention thus far is what we have termed "left main equivalent" disease. This is illustrated in Figure 1 and consists of significant narrowing in the left anterior descending and circumflex coronary artery, just at the bifurcation or before any significant branches. This combination was found in five patients in the present study. The arteriographic score for all the patients is shown in Figure 2.

Table 2 depicts the degree of coronary artery narrowing in each one of the major vessels. Of a total of 210 vessels, there were 80 complete occlusions (an incidence of 38 percent) and an additional 27 with greater than 80 percent narrowing (13 percent).

The incidence of complete occlusion of at least one vessel was very high in this study. Sixty-five patients had complete occlusion of at least one artery, 11 men had complete occlusion of two major arteries, and there were three patients in whom the three major arteries were totally occluded.

Metabolic Abnormalities: Figures 3 and 4 show the distribution of patients with single-, double-, or triple-vessel disease according to the lipid abnormality and glucose tolerance test. The high incidence of triple-vessel disease was the same in all groups, although it appears slightly higher in those with Type II or mixed hyperlipidemia. Table 3 illustrates the cholesterol levels and the incidence of one-, two-, and three-vessel disease. Serum cholesterol exceeded 250 mg percent in 25 patients and exceeded 300 mg percent in six patients, five of which had triple-vessel disease.

ECG-VCG Abnormalities: The ECG-VCG was abnormal in 68 of the 70 patients. Sixty-seven had evidence of an old myocardial infarction and one showed left ventricular hypertrophy. In two instances, the ECG-VCG was entirely within normal limits. Figure 5 illustrates the angiographic findings in relation to the ECG-VCG abnormalities. There were 23 patients with anterior myocardial infarctions, and in those the incidence of

TABLE 1. Distribution of Coronary Lesions

NO. VESSELS WITH 60% NARROWING	COMBINATION	NO. PTS.
One	LAD	9
	Cx	3
	RCA	5
Two	LAD and Cx	3
	LAD and RCA	10
	Cx and RCA	1
Three	LM, LAD, Cx, and RCA	3
	LAD, Cx, and RCA	36

LAD: left anterior descending; Cx: left circumflex artery or main marginal branch; RCA: right coronary artery; LM: left main coronary artery.

TABLE 2. Degree of Luminal Narrowing

	NORMAL OR <50%	60–75%	80–95%	100%
LM	67	3	0	0
LAD	10	24	9	27
Cx	25	16	10	19
RCA	15	13	8	34

LM: left main; LAD: left anterior descending; Cx: circumflex; RCA: right coronary artery.

JG 49 M

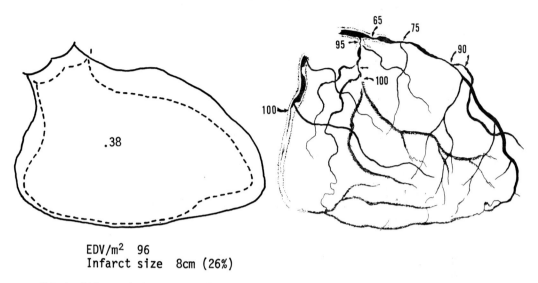

EDV/m² 96
Infarct size 8cm (26%)

FIG. 1. RAO ventriculogram and diagram of the coronary arteries in a patient with significant narrowing at the bifurcation of the left main coronary artery ("left main equivalent"). Severe disease is present in all vessels. A large inferior infarction is present with an ejection fraction of 0.38.

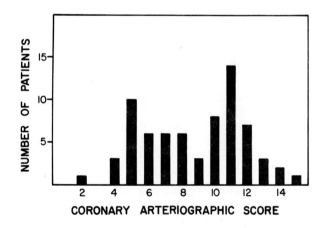

FIG. 2. Coronary arteriographic score for all patients (see text).

TABLE 3. Cholesterol Levels and Incidence of One-, Two-, and Three-Vessel Disease

CHOLESTEROL LEVELS (Mg%)	NO. PTS.	NO. VESSELS INVOLVED		
		One	Two	Three
150–99	17	7	3	7
200–49	28	6	6	16
250–99	19	4	4	11
300–49	2	0	1	1
350–99	1	0	0	1
>400	3	0	0	

TABLE 4. Vectorcardiographic Prediction of Coronary Lesion

VCG LOCATION	NO. PTS.	COMPLETE OCCLUSION OF APPROPRIATE ARTERY		
		LAD	CX	RCA
Anterior-superior	23	19 (82.6%)		
Posterior	10		10 (100%)	
Inferior				26 (90%)

LAD: left anterior descending; CX: circumflex; RCA: right coronary artery.

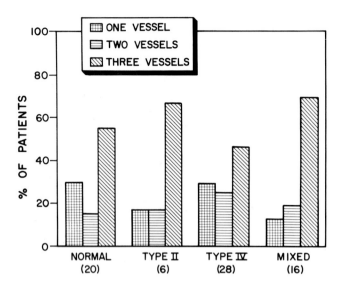

FIG. 3. Degree of coronary vessel involvement in relation to lipid abnormalities. The numbers in parenthesis indicate the number of patients in each group.

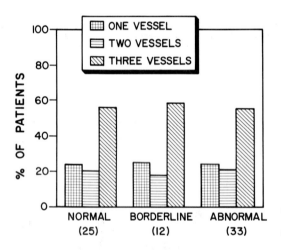

FIG. 4. Degree of coronary vessel involvement in relation to the rate of glucose disappearance (K). The numbers in parenthesis indicate the number of patients in each group. Normal K > 1.1; borderline 0.91 to 1.1; abnormal < 0.91.

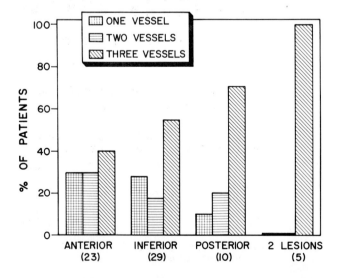

FIG. 5. Degree of coronary vessel involvement in relation to location of the myocardial infarction by ECG-VCG. The numbers in parenthesis indicate the number of patients in each group.

one-, two-, and three-vessel disease was approximately the same. Thirty-nine patients had either inferior or posterior MI, and of those almost two-thirds had triple-vessel disease. Of the five patients who had ECG evidence of two separate infarctions, all showed severe involvement of all three vessels. The vectorcardiogram predicted which vessel was occluded with approximately 90 percent accuracy (Table 4). Of the 23 patients with evidence of anterior MI, 19 had complete occlusion of the left anterior descending. Ten patients had evidence for posterior infarction on the vectorcardiogram, and all had complete occlusion of the circumflex or marginal branch. Of the 29 patients with inferior myocardial infarction, 26 had complete occlusion of the right coronary artery. As suspected from this high correlation, the vectorcardiogram predicted the location of the hypokinetic or akinetic segment with the same degree of accuracy.

ECG-VCG Sizing: In general, vector sizing by published criteria tended to overestimate small infarctions and underestimate large akinetic areas. A linear correlation between the electrocardiographic-vectorcardiographic sizing of infarction and the ventriculographic estimate yielded a correlation coefficient of 0.685 (p < 0.001).

Treadmill Exercise Test: Figure 6 demonstrates the angiographic findings in relation to the treadmill exercise test. The treadmill test was positive in 37 patients, indeterminate in 12, and negative in 21. Of the 21 patients with a negative exercise test, 10 (47 percent) had one-, five (23 percent) had two-, and six (30 percent) had three-vessel disease. Conversely, if the test was positive,

37 patients (73 percent) showed triple vessel disease.

The incidence of a negative test (false negative) for the total group was 30 percent. A negative test was present in 10 of the 17 patients with single-vessel, five of the 14 with two-vessel, and six of the 39 with three-vessel disease. The incidence of false negatives is therefore 59 percent, 35 percent, and 15 percent for one-, two-, and three-vessel disease, respectively.

A severe degree of ST depression (more than 0.3 m) was seen in 15 of the 37 patients who had a positive exercise test. Fourteen had triple coronary disease, and over 50 percent had either left main or "left main equivalent" disease. This is illustrated in Figure 7. All eight patients in this series with left main or "left main equivalent" had this highly positive exercise test.

Left Ventricular Function (Table 5): Thirty-six patients (51 percent) had infarctions that involved less than 10 percent of the left ventricular myocardium. A definite area of hypokinesis or small akinetic segment was seen on either the RAO or LAO ventriculogram in 26 of these, while in 10 patients, the ventriculogram was entirely normal. None of the hemodynamic measurements in this group of patients differs significantly from normal, although there is a tendency for a larger end-diastolic volume and end-diastolic pressure and a slightly reduced ejection fraction. In 18 patients (26 percent) the damage involved between 10 and 20 percent of the left ventricular surface area, and in all of these, there was definite akinesis. While the cardiac index and stroke index were also normal in this group,

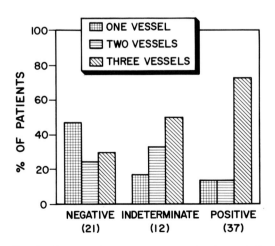

FIG. 6. Degree of coronary vessel involvement in relation to treadmill exercise test (see text). The numbers in parenthesis indicate the number of patients in each group.

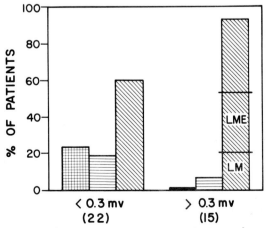

FIG. 7. Degree of coronary vessel involvement in relation to degree of ST depression on the treadmill exercise test (see text). The numbers in parenthesis indicate the number of patients in each group.

TABLE 5. Infarct Size Versus Left Ventricular Function

| | INFARCT SIZE (% SURFACE AREA) | | |
	Small (<10%)	Medium Size (10–20%)	Large (>20%)
Number of patients	36	18	16
CI (3.3 ± 0.6)	3.2 ± 0.7	3.0 ± 0.4	2.7 ± 0.4[b]
SI (42 ± 6)	42 ± 7	39 ± 4	36 ± 6[b]
LVEDP (7 ± 2)	9 ± 4[a]	13 ± 4[b]	17 ± 5[b]
SI/EDP (6 ± 1.6)	4.9 ± 1.4[a]	3.2 ± 1.4[b]	2.2 ± 0.5[b]
EDV/m² (71 ± 10)	80 ± 15[a]	95 ± 10[b]	116 ± 10[b]
EF (.69 ± 0.05)	0.62 ± 0.05[b]	0.49 ± 0.04[b]	0.37 ± 0.06[b]

[a] $p \leq 0.01$
[b] $p \leq 0.001$

Numbers in parentheses: normal values in our laboratory (based on 50 normal patients). CI: cardiac index; SI: stroke index; LVEDP: left ventricular end-diastolic pressure; EDV/m²: left ventricular end-diastolic volume per m²; EF: ejection fraction.

end-diastolic pressure, end-diastolic volume, and ejection fraction were mildly abnormal.

Sixteen patients (23 percent) had infarctions involving more than 20 percent of the left ventricular surface area. The infarction was anterior and superior in 10; inferior and posterior, one each; and more than one lesion in four instances. Most of these patients maintained a fairly normal resting cardiac output and stroke volume. Their hearts were, however, dilated; all of these patients had an increased end-diastolic volume and the filling pressure was abnormal in most (borderline in two cases). The ejection fraction was markedly decreased in all patients.

There were significant correlations between the size of the infarction and the left ventricular end-diastolic volume (r = 0.654), the ejection fraction (r = 0.965, Fig. 8) and the VCG estimate of infarct size (r = 0.642). A less significant correlation was found between the size of infarction and the treadmill exercise performance (r = 0.337, p < 0.01).

There was no correlation between the degree of left ventricular impairment and the number of vessels involved (r = −0.00078).

DISCUSSION

There are obvious difficulties in comparing this series with the published data on coronary arteriography, since in most studies the indication for coronary arteriography was either angina pectoris or congestive failure. In a large series of 627 patients,[15] there were 88 patients with myocardial infarction and no angina. The incidence of single-, double-, and triple-vessel disease was 47 percent,

28 percent, and 25 percent, respectively, which is significantly different from our results. The reasons for this discrepancy are not apparent. Cohen and associates[3] studied 60 patients (54 because of angina and four because of congestive failure) and found 21 with one-vessel, 14 with two-vessel, and 25 with triple-vessel disease, which is similar to our findings in asymptomatic patients.

The arteriographic score in this group of asymptomatic men post-infarction does not differ from that found by Friesinger and associates[7] in patients with typical angina pectoris.

Fifty percent of the patients in the present study have a score greater than 10. Friesinger et al have emphasized the poor prognosis in this group (score > 10) in patients with angina pec-

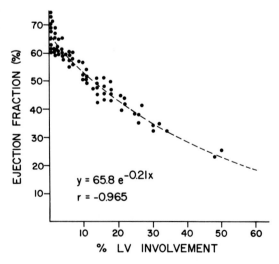

FIG. 8. Relation between ejection fraction and infarct size expressed as percent of LV involvement (see text).

tóris. These statistics may or may not apply to asymptomatic people. On the other hand, there were three deaths in our series and they each had scores of 11 or 12.

The generalized nature of this disease has also been emphasized in numerous anatomic studies—of particular interest is the study of French and Dock [5] who found significant narrowing in two arteries in 21 percent and three arteries in 35 percent of 80 cases of sudden death in young soldiers (20 to 36 years of age).

In many studies of myocardial infarction and sudden death, mention is made of cases in which coronary occlusion is not present. The possibility of myocardial infarction and subsequent normal coronary arteriograms is well known, but its frequency is debatable. In over 400 studies at our institution of patients postmyocardial infarction, we have found two with normal coronaries, both female. In this series, arteriographic evidence of obstruction was found in the appropriate location (that is, LAD for anterior infarction, circumflex for posterior, and RCA for inferior) in 100 percent of the cases. In 87 percent, the arteries were completely occluded. These results are similar to those of Proudfit, Shirey, and Sones [15] and Mitchell and Schwartz.[14]

The high incidence of patients in this study with metabolic abnormalities and other risk factors is noteworthy.[10] None of the risk factors, however, by themselves or in combinations serve as predictors of severity of the coronary artery disease. There were only seven patients in this study with completely normal cholesterol, triglycerides, and glucose tolerance tests. Of these, four had triple-vessel disease. As seen in Table 3, the cholesterol was perhaps the only significant predictor. The incidence of one-, two-, and three-vessel disease showed considerable overlapping with normal or mildly abnormal cholesterol levels. If cholesterol was in excess of 300, however, the incidence of three-vessel disease was five to one. This finding may explain the higher incidence of sudden death in patients with elevated cholesterol.[11]

The usefulness of the ECG-VCG to predict the site of the occlusion and the location of the infarction needs to be reemphasized. The high accuracy in the present study does not necessarily apply to the general population. Double-blind studies in our institution (unpublished observations) have shown that the location and size of the akinetic or hypokinetic segment can be predicted from the ECG-VCG with 86 percent accuracy.

The results of exercise testing in the present highly selected study population is in general agreement with other reports. The incidence of false negative tests (30 percent) is almost identical to that reported by Roitman et al,[17] Martin and coworkers,[12] and more recently by Bartel and colleagues.[1] The incidence of false negative tests appears related to the severity of the coronary artery lesions. Of the 17 patients in this study with single-vessel disease, 10 (59 percent) had a negative test. In contrast, a negative test was obtained in only 6 of the 39 patients with triple-vessel disease (15 percent). These findings are similar to those previously reported.[1,12,13] Stated in another way, a positive test in this population of asymptomatic postinfarction patients indicated triple vessel disease in 73 percent of the cases. If the degree of ST depression was greater than 0.3 mv, the odds for severe triple-vessel disease were overwhelming.

Cohen et al [3] and Bartel et al [1] have reached similar conclusions. The strong relationship between the exercise test and the severity of the coronary lesions may apply only to the rather homogeneous group of people selected in the present study. Froelicher and coworkers [8] studied 76 asymptomatic men with abnormal treadmill tests. Only 46 percent were found to have CAD and the incidence of one-, two-, and three-vessel disease was 49 percent, 36 percent, and 15 percent respectively. This is in sharp contrast with our findings and must be related to patient selection since they specifically excluded from their series patients with history or ECG evidence of myocardial infarction.

Ten patients had ejection fractions of less than 0.40 and in two patients the ejection fraction was 0.25. It is surprising that people with this degree of left ventricular dysfunction can be totally asymptomatic, working full-time without limitations and even be participating in an exercise program.

SUMMARY

The distribution of obstructive coronary lesions exceeding 60 percent of the normal diameter was studied in 70 asymptomatic men, 40 to 50 years of age with previous myocardial infarction.

Severe triple-vessel disease was found in 56 percent of the patients, two-vessel in 20 percent, and one-vessel in 24 percent.

Complete occlusion of an appropriate major artery was found in 65 (93 percent) of cases. The remaining five (7 percent) all had high-grade obstruction (75 percent or greater) in the appropriate proximal vessel. Eight patients, all with triple vessel disease had a left main lesion or a "left main equivalent."

The two most useful noninvasive tools to evaluate these patients were the vectorcardiogram (to predict the extent of LV dysfunction) and the treadmill exercise test (to predict the severity of the coronary arterial lesions).

Metabolic abnormalities were found in 90 percent of the patients. There was, however, no relation between these abnormalities and the severity of the coronary lesions.

References

1. Bartel A, Behar V, Peter R, Orgain E, Kong Y: Graded exercise stress tests in angiographically documented coronary artery disease. Circulation 49:348, 1974
2. Chin H, Hanashiro P, Khan A, Blankenhorn D: Glucose tolerance testing in men with myocardial infarction. Abstracts: Coronary Artery Medicine and Surgery Conf., Houston, Feb. 21–23, 1974
3. Cohen L, Elliot W, Klein M, Gorlin R: Clinical studies: coronary heart disease. Clinical, cinearteriographic and metabolic correlations. Am J Card 17:153, 1966
4. Doan A, Peterson D, Blackman J, Bruce R: Myocardial ischemia after maximal exercise in healthy men: a method for detecting potential coronary heart disease. Am Heart J 69:11, 1965
5. Dodge H, Sandler H, Ballew D, Lord J: The use of biplane angiocardiography for the measurement of left ventricular volume in man. Am Heart J 60:762, 1960
6. French A, Dock W: Fatal coronary arteriosclerosis in young soldiers. JAMA 124:1233, 1944
7. Friesinger G, Page E, Ross R: Prognostic significance of coronary arteriography. Trans Assoc Am Phys 93:78, 1970
8. Froelicher V, Yanowitz F, Thompson A, Lancaster M: The correlation of coronary angiography and the electrocardiographic response to maximal treadmill testing in 76 asymptomatic men. Circulation 48:597, 1973
9. Gensini G, Kelly A: Incidence and progression of coronary artery disease: an angiographic correlation in 1,263 patients. Arch Intern Med 129:814, 1972
10. Hanashiro P, Sanmarco M, Selvester R, Blankenhorn, D: Risk factors in males with premature atherosclerosis. Abstracts: Coronary Artery Medicine and Surgery Conf., Houston, Feb. 21–23, 1974
11. Kannel W, Dawber T, Friedman G, Glennon W, McNamara P: Risk factors in coronary heart disease. An evaluation of several serum lipids as predictors of coronary heart disease. The Framingham Study. Ann Intern Med 61:888, 1964
12. Martin C, McConahay D: Maximal treadmill exercise electrocardiography. Correlations with coronary arteriography and cardiac hemodynamics. Circulation 46:956, 1972
13. McHenry P, Phillips J, Knoebel S: Correlation of computer quantitated treadmill exercise electrocardiogram with arteriographic location of coronary artery disease. Am J Card 30:747, 1972
14. Mitchell J, Schwartz C: The relation between myocardial lesions and coronary artery disease. II. A selected group of patients with massive cardiac necrosis or scarring. Br Heart J 25:11, 1963
15. Proudfit W, Shirey E, Sones F: Distribution of arterial lesions demonstrated by selective cinecoronary arteriography. Circulation 36:54, 1967
16. Proudfit W, Shirey E, Sones F: Selective cine coronary arteriography. Correlation with clinical findings in 1,000 patients. Circulation 36:54, 1967
17. Roitman D, Jones W, Sheffield L: Comparison of submaximal exercise ECG test with coronary cineangiogram. Ann Intern Med 72:641, 1970
18. Sanmarco M, Fronek K, Phillips C, Davila J: Continuous measurement of left ventricular volume in the dog. II. Comparison of washout and radiographic technics with the external dimension method. Am J Card 18:584, 1966
19. Selvester R, Wagner J, Rubin H: Quantitation of myocardial infarct size and location by electrocardiogram and vectorcardiogram. In Quantitation in Cardiology. Snellen, Hemker, Hugenholtz, and VanBemmel, eds. Leiden University Press. 1972, pp 31–44
20. Sheffield L, Holt J, Reeves T: Exercise graded by heart rate in electrocardiographic testing for angina pectoris. Circulation 32:622, 1965

29

GLUCOSE TOLERANCE TESTING IN MEN
WITH MYOCARDIAL INFARCTION

H. P. Chin, P. K. Hanashiro, A. H. Khan,
and D. H. Blankenhorn

Transient glucose intolerance frequently occurs during the acute episode of myocardial infarction and may be confused with diabetes. Occasionally, coronary artery bypass surgery is performed on survivors of myocardial infarction or patients with ischemic heart disease. In such cases the metabolic condition of a patient must be regarded as an important determinant of the long-term effects of surgical intervention. Recent studies have suggested that glucose intolerance may indicate a predisposition to ischemic heart disease (Tzagournis et al, 1967; Heinle et al, 1969). It is generally believed that lipid and carbohydrate metabolism go hand in hand, and that a disturbance of one may lead to a change in the other (Randle et al, 1963; Gertler et al, 1972). Macdonald (1968) and Maruhama (1970) have shown that the incorporation of carbohydrates into fatty acids and triglycerides is distinctly abnormal in men with ischemic heart disease. Furthermore, a strong correlation has frequently been noted between obesity, hyperlipidemia, and diabetes (Fredrickson et al, 1967; Heinle et al, 1969; Gertler et al, 1972).

Whether or not a patient is a candidate for cardiac surgery, it is clear that knowledge of the interactions of lipid and carbohydrate metabolism in heart disease would assist the clinician in maximizing the benefits of therapy for his patient. The goal of the present study was to examine the kinetics of insulin secretion and establish relationships between glucose tolerance and circulating blood lipids in men with documented myocardial infarction.

Supported by Los Angeles County Heart Association Grant 461 and USPHS HL-14138

SUBJECTS AND METHODS

Forty men, all with histories of myocardial infarction and averaging 44 years of age (range 22 to 65 years), were tested at least two weeks after infarction. Fasting blood was drawn for determination of serum lipid levels, lipoprotein distributions, and fasting glucose with insulin levels. Then, 25 grams of glucose were injected rapidly as a 50 percent aqueous dextrose solution via an antecubital vein, and at 2.5, 5, 10, 20, 30, 40, 50, and 60 minutes after injection blood samples were obtained from the opposite arm vein for measurement of glucose and insulin levels. Glucose was analyzed by the glucose oxidase method (Saifer and Gerstenfeld, 1958) and insulin by radioimmunoassay (Hales and Randle, 1963); analyses of total cholesterol (Abell et al, 1952), free cholesterol (Chin et al, 1966), triglycerides (Chin et al, 1971), phospholipids (Chin, 1968), free fatty acids (Duncombe, 1963), and lipoprotein electrophoresis (Chin and Blankenhorn, 1968) were also performed. Rate constants for glucose utilization were derived by obtaining a least-squares fit of observed values between 20 and 60 minutes on a semilogarithmic plot of glucose concentration versus time (Hamilton and Stein, 1942; Wahlberg, 1966). The glucose rate constant (k) gives a quantitative measure of the percentage of glucose removed from the blood stream per minute. According to established criteria, k values between 0.9 and 1.1 are considered to be borderline with respect to glucose tolerance; values above 1.1 are considered normal, while those falling below 0.9 reflect chemical diabetes.

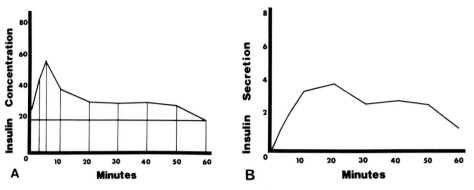

FIG. 1. Serum insulin response to intravenously administered glucose plotted in conventional manner. A. With perpendicular lines drawn from abscissa to intersect curve. B. Incremental insulin secretion (obtained from A by weighing areas above basal level for each interval) plotted against time.

Another conventional method of evaluating glucose tolerance results is to construct and examine graphs displaying temporal changes in concentrations of circulating glucose and insulin. We have extended the technique to allow examination of the dynamics of insulin response to glucose load (Fig. 1). Estimates of incremental insulin secretion and glucose stimulus above basal levels were derived in the following manner: Plots of insulin or glucose concentration versus time were divided into periods corresponding to sampling intervals, and perpendicular lines were drawn from the abscissae to intersect the curves. Incremental glucose and insulin areas (areas above basal levels) were cut and weighed for each patient tested. This procedure yielded the equivalents of integrals of the areas under the curves represented algebraically by the expression:

$$\text{Area} = C_o \int_{t_o}^{t_1} e^{-k\,t}\ dt$$

where C_o is the concentration of glucose or insulin at t_o, and k the rate constant for change in glucose or insulin between times t_o and t_1. The measurements were plotted against time to produce graphs expressing amounts of insulin secreted in response to changing serum .glucose loads. The approach is similar to that employed by others for evaluating incremental glucose and insulin responses (Lerner and Porte, 1971; Quickel et al, 1971; Genuth, 1973).

RESULTS AND DISCUSSION

Glucose k varied widely, from less than 0.3 to greater than 3.0, a tenfold difference in the rate of removal of glucose from the circulation

(Fig. 2). K values exceeded 1.1 in 18 men, fell below 0.9 in 17 men, and were within the borderline range of 0.9 to 1.1 in the remaining five. Among the subjects tested, the prevalence of reduced glucose tolerance was greater than that expected in populations of normal individuals and consistent with findings of epidemiological studies (Kannel et al, 1964; Ostrander et al, 1965).

A frequent question is whether glucose intolerance persists after myocardial infarction. In our study no significant correlation was established between k value and time since infarction, even though the patients were tested at times varying from two weeks to four years after infarction. It has previously been demonstrated that glucose k stabilizes shortly after infarction (Wahlberg, 1966). Our results are in agreement with those findings and indicate that the immediate effects of acute myocardial infarction on glucose tolerance must be of short duration; therefore, glucose tolerance can be reliably tested two or more weeks following infarction and can be included as a part of the metabolic workup at this time.

A primary goal of our study was to examine insulin secretion as a function of variations in their responses to intravenous glucose challenge. To this end, patients were placed in subgroups of low, high, and intermediate k value (Table 1). The low-k group consisted of 10 men with k values less than 0.65 (k = 0.49 ± 0.04, mean ± SEM), including three with Type II hyperlipoproteinemia, three with Type IV, and four with normal blood lipids. The high-k group consisted of nine patients with glucose k greater than 1.45 (k = 2.08 ± 0.18, mean ± SEM), including five Type II, three Type IV, and one patient with normal blood lipids. Twenty-one patients fell within the intermediate range; of these there were 2 Type II, 5 Type IV, and 13 with normal blood

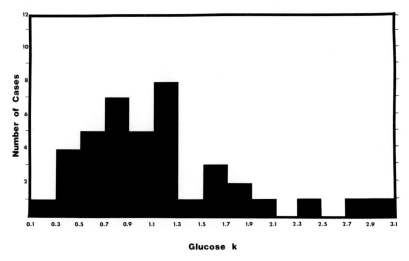

Glucose k

FIG. 2. Distribution of patients by glucose k value.

lipids and lipoprotein patterns. One patient with intermediate-k had a mixed lipoprotein disorder and exhibited simultaneous elevation of cholesterol and triglyceride levels. A total of 10 had Type II, and 11 had Type IV patterns; one patient had mixed hyperlipoproteinemia, and 18 exhibited normal lipoprotein patterns. No clear correlation was observed between lipoprotein type and glucose k value, and neither Type II nor Type IV hyperlipoproteinemia occurred with remarkably greater frequency in postinfarction patients. Serum lipid levels were variable, and subjects with high or low glucose k did not exhibit a preponderance of typical lipid values (Table 2).

As expected from differences among the subgroups in rates of glucose assimilation, the mean fasting glucose level was significantly higher in the low k group than in the high-k group (p < 0.01). Glucose concentrations after intravenous challenge rose rapidly in both groups but fell more slowly in the former than in the latter. At the same time, insulin levels rose and fell more rapidly in patients with normal glucose tolerance (Table 3). Fasting insulin levels initially appeared to be considerably higher in the low k group, but the mean value of 37.7 $\mu U/ml$ (Tables 2 and 3) included one fasting insulin of 183 $\mu U/ml$; exclu-

sion of this value from the calculation yielded a mean of 21.6 ± 2.2 (SEM) $\mu U/ml$, which did not differ significantly from values observed in men with high glucose k.

Incremental insulin secretion was more responsive to changing glucose load in high-k than in low-k patients (Fig. 3). In the former, insulin secretion rose as the size of the glucose stimulus increased and fell rapidly in company with glucose load as the need to accommodate large amounts of glucose subsided; liberation of insulin appeared closely coupled with change in glucose stimulus. In contrast, insulin secretion in patients with chemical diabetes rose slowly and continued rising even as glucose load fell, finally diminishing gradually toward the end of the experimental period. The close coupling of stimulus and response observed in patients with high glucose k was not found in low-k patients and was somewhat blunted in subjects with intermediate-k, among whom were men with normal glucose tolerance as well as some with slight-to-moderate glucose intolerance. The results suggest that two distinguishing characteristics of chemical diabetes may be faulty coupling of insulin response with glucose stimulation and reduction in the magnitude of the secretory response.

Several experimental techniques have been employed by investigators to examine patterns of insulin secretion. *In vitro* studies have demonstrated that glucose infusion causes release of insulin from isolated rat pancreas in two distinct phases (Curry et al, 1968). In man, the dynamics of insulin release are as yet not thoroughly defined; insulin response varies somewhat with the method of application of the glucose stimulus and under certain conditions may exhibit more than

TABLE 1. Patients Classified by Lipoprotein Type and Glucose k

GLUCOSE k	LIPOPROTEIN TYPE			
	Type II	Type IV	Mixed	Normal
High k	5	3	0	1
Intermediate k	2	5	1	13
Low k	3	3	0	4

TABLE 2. Mean Value for Biochemical Measurements[a]

	k	AGE (years)	% IDEAL WEIGHT	TC (mg/dl)	FC (mg/dl)	TG (mg/dl)	PL (mg/dl)	FFA (mg/dl)	α_1 (%)	α_2 (%)	β (%)	G_0 (mg/dl)	I_0 (mg/dl)
Overall	1.12	44.1	118.5	260.7	94.5	255.0	288.2	17.4	19.6	26.7	53.6	109.4	23.0
(n = 40)	±0.10	±0.9	±3.9	±10.5	±4.1	±52.8	±13.9	±1.1	±1.2	±2.7	±2.1	±8.1	±4.4
High	.2.08	43.7	109.5	280.2	97.0	191.0	304.1	16.0	21.2	20.4	58.3	82.7	19.2
(n = 9)	±0.18	±1.5	±4.4	±27.1	±7.5	±37.3	±28.1	±1.5	±2.4	±3.9	±3.5	±2.5	±4.1
Intermed.	1.02	44.2	117.9	247.3	89.3	210.8	269.3	16.1	19.8	27.1	52.9	96.2	18.4
(n = 21)	±0.04	±1.4	±3.1	±13.6	±5.5	±39.7	±13.8	±1.0	±1.4	±3.2	±2.8	±4.6	±2.1
Low	0.49	44.4	128.0	271.2	103.2	400.8	313.7	21.6	17.7	31.3	50.8	161.3	37.7
(n = 10)	±0.04	±1.8	±5.7	±19.7	±9.6	±187.2	±40.7	±3.4	±3.3	±7.7	±5.1	±25.1	±16.3

*TC: total cholesterol; FC: free cholesterol; TG: triglycerides; PL: phospholipids; FFA: free fatty acids; α_1, α_2,
β: lipoprotein distributions; G_0: fasting glucose; I_0: fasting insulin.*
[a]*mean ± SEM (standard error of the mean)*

one phase (Cerasi and Luft, 1967; Pupo and Porte, 1969; Turner et al, 1971). In our experiments a single intravenous dose of glucose was employed that resulted in biphasic release of insulin during the first hour after injection, regardless of glucose k value (Fig. 4). Both phases exhibited Gaussian distribution characteristics and similar time constants, the estimated duration of each being roughly 70 minutes. Furthermore, both components of insulin secretion could be individually quantified for a comparison of relative secretory activities. Total incremental insulin in patients with reduced glucose tolerance was estimated to be 55 percent of that in the high-k group. In patients with high-k values 80 percent of total incremental secretion occurred during the initial phase, compared with 43 percent of incremental secretion occurring in low-k patients during this phase. Moreover, insulin released during the initial phase in men with abnormal glucose tolerance was only 29 percent of that in men with normal glucose tolerance, although their second-

phase response was approximately 50 percent higher. A diminished overall insulin response to glucose stimulation in diabetes has been observed by other investigators (Cerasi and Luft, 1967; Perley and Kipnis, 1967; Bagdade et al, 1971, Quickel et al, 1971; Fraser, 1972). Cerasi and Luft (1967) have ascribed the deficient insulin response to a reduction in early insulin release as well as to an attenuation of late release. Our results confirm in part the observations cited, but demonstrate that when the intravenous challenge is administered as a single dose, glucose depression of insulin secretion in patients with impaired glucose tolerance occurs during the initial phase only, while insulin release during the second phase may be higher than normal.

In general, insulin secretion during the initial phase in the three subgroups appeared to be reflected in glucose k values. This phase comprised the major component of incremental insulin release in high-k individuals, men with unimpaired glucose tolerance who responded to glucose stimula-

TABLE 3. Serum Glucose and Insulin Concentrations during Intravenous Glucose Tolerance Tests

		TIME (minutes)								
		0	2.5	5	10	20	30	40	50	60
High k (2.08 ± 0.18)[a]										
Glucose	mean	82.7	260.8	245.8	219.3	181.0	140.3	114.9	97.2	89.0
(mg/100 ml)	SEM	2.5	18.2	11.4	7.8	11.7	10.5	10.6	11.7	8.9
Insulin	mean	19.2	87.1	105.7	82.3	66.0	51.5	40.2	37.6	30.9
(μU/ml)	SEM	4.1	20.2	16.4	17.5	15.8	9.5	5.7	6.6	4.9
Low k (0.49 ± 0.004)[a]										
Glucose	mean	161.3	330.7	321.5	284.2	268.5	257.6	246.6	231.8	226.6
(mg/100 ml)	SEM	25.1	41.1	24.8	20.8	24.7	24.7	24.1	21.6	22.9
Insulin	mean	37.7	51.1	52.2	44.9	48.4	48.1	50.9	51.6	34.7
(μU/ml)	SEM	16.3	18.5	15.4	16.0	16.4	16.5	17.7	17.0	6.7

[a]*Mean ± SEM (standard error of the mean).*

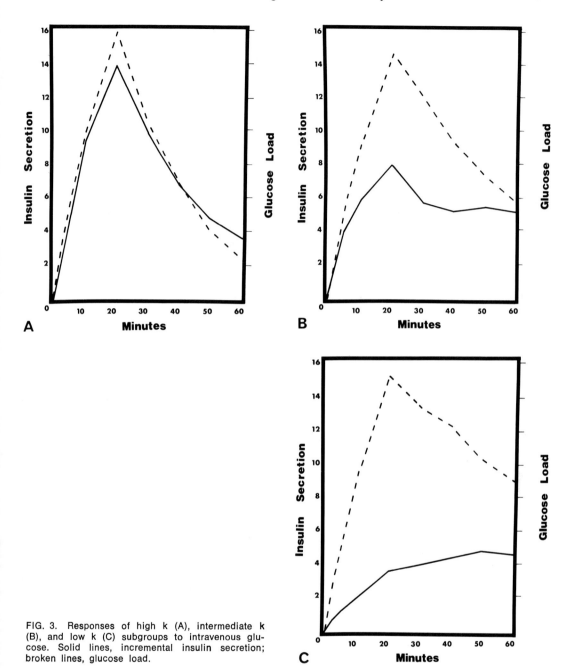

FIG. 3. Responses of high k (A), intermediate k (B), and low k (C) subgroups to intravenous glucose. Solid lines, incremental insulin secretion; broken lines, glucose load.

tion with a rapid liberation of insulin closely coupled with prevailing glucose load in time as well as magnitude of response. A drastic reduction in early secretion of insulin, because of its dominance under normal circumstances, could account for a depression of total incremental response in insulin-deficient, adult-onset diabetes. In our experiments, this may have been partly compensated by a heightened response of the second secretory phase. It is possible that biphasic insulin response stems from the existence of two pools of insulin in the pancreas that differ in latency period or sensitivity to stimulation. Alternatively, there may exist two populations in islet cells with different thresholds of response, the second response being triggered by activity of the initial phase. Both explanations would be consistent with currently available evidence (Cerasi and Luft, 1967; Curry et al, 1968; Porte and Pupo, 1969).

Extrapolation of insulin responses beyond

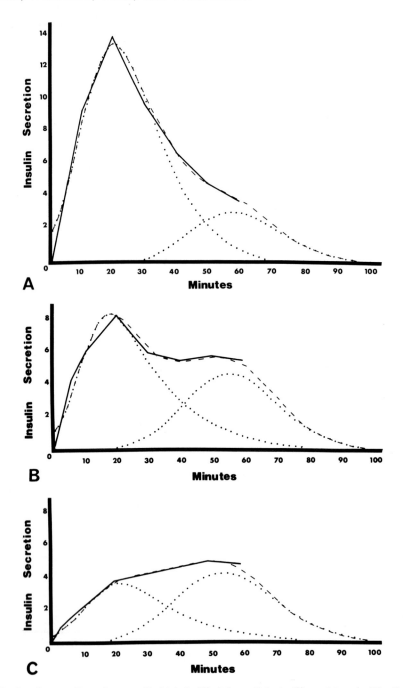

FIG. 4. Insulin secretion of men with high k (A), intermediate k (B), and low k (C) after intravenous glucose. Dotted lines, component curves constructed with DuPont 310 Curve Resolver to fit observed secretion patterns (solid line); broken line, sum of component curves.

the 60-minute sampling period resulted in intersection of the curves with the abscissae at approximately 100 minutes. This suggests that in tested patients incremental liberation of insulin would have reached completion roughly 100 minutes after glucose injection. In this regard, it is noteworthy that preliminary results of two-hour intravenous glucose tolerance tests show insulin release in the majority of cases to have returned to basal levels by two hours (Fig. 5).

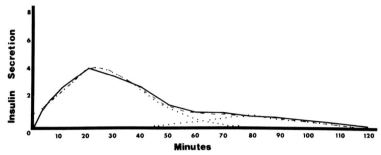

FIG. 5. Insulin secretion of an asymptomatic, noninfarcted male, age 37 years, glucose k = 1.1, followed for 120 minutes after intravenous glucose. Dotted lines, component curves constructed to fit observed secretion pattern (solid line); broken line, sum of component curves.

Hyperglycemia and hyperlipidemia frequently exist concurrently in individuals with ischemic heart disease. Our data do not show a close association of characteristic glucose k values with specific lipoprotein types and suggest that abnormal lipid metabolism need not coexist with glucose intolerance. Nevertheless, knowledge of both is relevant to an evaluation of metabolic status. Glucose tolerance may be markedly altered during an acute episode of myocardial infarction but appears stable in patients tested by intravenous glucose challenge two or more weeks after infarction.

Our study has also demonstrated that insulin secretion in postmyocardial infarction patients after a single intravenous dose of glucose is biphasic and that depression of insulin secretion is commonly found in individuals with impaired glucose tolerance. Behavior of the first secretory phase appeared to be an important determinant of the k value. In patients with reduced glucose, k secretory activity of the first phase was depressed, although secondary insulin release was somewhat higher than in men with normal glucose tolerance. Based on evidence developed thus far, it seems reasonable to suggest that therapy for diabetes should be aimed at correcting deficiencies in the first phase of insulin secretion; in this connection, various pharmacological agents have been identified that may be employed to influence the activity of this component. Knowledge concerning mechanisms controlling insulin secretion is incomplete, and it is not known whether the second phase of insulin release is affected by the kinetics of the initial phase; nonetheless it can be safely assumed that either secretory phase may be involved in lipid metabolism, which is known to be influenced by insulin action, and that therapy for diabetes is likely to affect lipid transport as well.

Epidemiological studies have shown that risk factors for coronary heart disease are additive. Glucose intolerance significantly increases coronary risk probability in every age group studied (Gordon et al, 1971) and should be treated to reduce the probability of premature death from coronary heart disease. There is every reason to believe that risk factors are also additive in postmyocardial infarction patients; in cases where arterial bypass surgery is under consideration as a therapeutic measure, presence or absence of chemical diabetes should be ascertained. Appropriate treatment of diabetes, if present, should reduce the risk of further damage to the myocardium, increase the likelihood of graft survival, and insure proper function of the arterial tree.

ACKNOWLEDGMENTS

We thank Misses Kathryn Jefcoat and Adelina SanJuan for analyses of glucose and insulin, and Mrs. Cynthia Lorion for help in preparing the manuscript.

References

Abell LL, Levy BB, Kendall FE: A simplified method for the estimation of total cholesterol in serum and demonstration of its specificity. J Biol Chem 195: 357, 1952

Bagdade JD, Bierman EL, Porte D: Basal and stimulated insulin levels: comparison of insulinogenic effects of oral glucose and intravenous tolbutamide in nondiabetic and diabetic subjects. Metabolism 20:1000, 1971

Cerasi E, Luft R: The plasma insulin response to glucose infusion in healthy subjects and in diabetes mellitus. Acta Endocrinol 55:278, 1967

Chin HP: The sphingomyelin content of human serum: a genetic study. Biochim Biophys Acta 152:346, 1968

Chin HP, Abdel-Meguid SS, Blankenhorn DH: An improved method for determination of serum and plasma triglycerides. Clin Chim Acta 31:381, 1971

Chin HP, Blankenhorn DH: Separation and quantitative

analysis of serum lipoproteins by means of electrophoresis on cellulose acetate. Clin Chim Acta 20: 305, 1968

Chin HP, Blankenhorn DH, Chin TJ: Altered partition of serum cholesterol and cholesteryl ester in a petroleum ether-ethanol-water system after incubation. Lipids 1:285, 1966

Curry DL, Bennett LL, Grodsky GM: Dynamics of insulin secretion by the perfused rat pancreas. Endocrinology 83:572, 1968

Duncombe WG: Colorimetric micro-determination of long-chain fatty acids. Biochem J 88:7, 1963

Fraser R: Metabolic disorders in diabetes. Br Med J 4:591, 1972

Fredrickson DS, Levy RI, Lees RS: Fat transport in lipoproteins—an integrated approach to mechanisms and disorders. N Engl J Med 276:34, 94, 148, 215, 273, 1967

Genuth SM: Plasma insulin and glucose profiles in normal, obese, and diabetic persons. Ann Intern Med 79:812, 1973

Gertler MM, Leetma HE, Saluste E, Rosenberger JL, Guthrie RG: Ischemic heart disease: insulin, carbohydrate, and lipid interrelationships. Circulation 46: 103, 1972

Gordon T, Sorlie P, Kannel WB: Coronary heart disease; ABI, IC—A multivariate analysis of some factors related to their incidence, Framingham study—a 16-year follow-up; Section 27, U.S. Government Printing Office, 1971

Hales CN, Randle PJ: Immunoassay of insulin with insulin-antibody precipitate. Biochem J 88:137, 1963

Hamilton B, Stein AF: The measurement of intravenous blood sugar curves. J Lab Clin Med 27:491, 1942

Heinle RA, Levy RI, Fredrickson DS, Gorlin R: Lipid and carbohydrate abnormalities in patients with angiographically documented coronary artery disease. Am J Cardiol 24:178, 1969

Kannel WB, Dawber TR, Friedman GD, Glennon WE, McNamara PM: Risk factors in coronary heart disease: An evaluation of several serum lipids as predictors of coronary heart disease: The Framingham study. Ann Intern Med 61:888, 1964

Lerner RL, Porte D: Relationships between intravenous glucose loads, insulin responses and glucose disappearance rate. J Clin Endocrinol Metab 33:409, 1971

Macdonald I: Ingested glucose and fructose in serum lipids in healthy men and after myocardial infarction. Am J Clin Nutr 21:1366, 1968

Maruhama Y: Conversion of ingested carbohydrate-14C into glycerol and fatty acids of serum triglyceride in patients with myocardial infarction. Metabolism 19:1085, 1970

Ostrander LD, Francis T, Hayner NS, Kjelsberg MO, Epstein FH: The relationship of cardiovascular disease to hyperglycemia. Ann Intern Med 62:1188, 1965

Perley M, Kipnis DM: Plasma insulin response to oral and intravenous glucose studies in normal and diabetic subjects. J Clin Invest 46:1954, 1967

Porte D, Pupo AA: Insulin responses to glucose: evidence for a two pool system in man. J Clin Invest 48:2309, 1969

Quickel KE, Feldman JM, Lebovitz HE: Enhancement of insulin in adult-onset diabetes by methysergide maleate: evidence for an endogenous biogenic monoamine mechanism as a factor in the impaired insulin secretion in diabetes mellitus. J Clin Endocrinol Metab 33:877, 1971

Randle PJ, Garland PB, Hales CN, Newsholme EA: The glucose fatty-acid cycle: its role in insulin sensitivity and the metabolic disturbances of diabetes mellitus. Lancet 1:785, 1963

Saifer A, Gerstenfeld S: The photometric microdetermination of blood glucose with glucose oxidase. J Lab Clin Med 51:448, 1958

Turner RC, Schneeloch B, Nabarro JDN: Biphasic insulin secretory response to intravenous xylitol and glucose in normal, diabetic, and obese subjects. J Clin Endocrinol Metab 33:301, 1971

Tzagournis M, Seidensticker JF, Hamwi GJ: Serum insulin, carbohydrate, and lipid abnormalities in patients with premature coronary heart disease. Ann Intern Med 67:42, 1967

Wahlberg F: Intravenous glucose tolerance in myocardial infarction, angina pectoris, and intermittent claudication. Acta Med Scand 180 (Suppl 453):1, 1966

30

A REGIONAL CARDIOVASCULAR CENTER FOR TEAM TREATMENT OF CARDIOVASCULAR DISEASE

James R. Jude, Irwin B. Boruchow,
and Ramanuja Iyengar

INTRODUCTION

With the increased incidence of cardiovascular disease, and also in the demand for diagnosis and therapy of coronary artery disease, existing facilities, generally at university hospitals, can no longer accommodate the volume of patients. Indeed, many procedures may be performed more effectively, more economically, and with better results in the clinical practice setting. Therefore, new demands for the delivery of health care have been placed on community hospitals. The specialized equipment, personnel, and technical facilities are extremely expensive unless utilized at optimal levels. Most referring physicians, especially cardiologists, wish to be involved in the diagnostic protocol and decision-making process. In order to meet the increasing demands and to offer a referring doctor the ability to participate, we have organized our resources as a team effort: initial personal physician-cardiologist-diagnostic facilities, cardiac surgical evaluation, cardiac surgery, continued home care, and long-term evaluation.

MATERIALS AND METHODS

A cardiovascular unit was created within an established 325-bed community hospital to serve as a definitive diagnostic (including stress testing, cardiac catheterization) and medical/surgical therapy center for multiple-area hospitals with over 2,000 cumulative beds. The hospital provides standard facilities for regular and vascular radiology, clinical and anatomical pathology (with a special interest in cardiovascular histology), respiratory therapy, and renal dialysis. The cardiovascular unit comprises 6,000 square feet of new space (Fig. 1) and includes offices for the surgeons, anesthesiologists, and cardiologists, two fully equipped cardiac catheterization laboratories, a biochemical laboratory, a 10-bed surgical intensive and intermediate care unit, two cardiac surgery operating rooms, conference rooms, family waiting facilities, and an extensive television communications network. One of the operating rooms is equipped with cineangiography equipment so that intraoperative coronary arteriography may be performed. The cardiovascular unit is immediately adjacent to one of the regular 48-bed hospital floors that specifically serves as a pre- and postoperative floor for cardiovascular patients. Nurses are trained in the psychological, as well as physical, needs of patients.

This facility was designed to serve a regional need. It was quite apparent that each hospital in the South Florida area could not have all of the facilities presented here, and, yet, the physicians practicing in these areas want to participate in the current effort to combat heart disease. Inpatients from the area hospitals are scheduled for diagnostic or therapeutic evaluation and returned to the referring institution (and the care of their physicians) on the same or the following day. When indicated, immediate decisions for urgent surgery have been made with the personal physician. The flow, therefore, has been from the patient's personal physician (who performs the initial evaluation and makes the decision for further diagnostic studies from his knowledge of the patient) to the medical cardiology section of the cardiovascular center. The patients are admitted to the adjacent hospital floor for appropriate diagnostic maneuvers including lipid profile, vector-

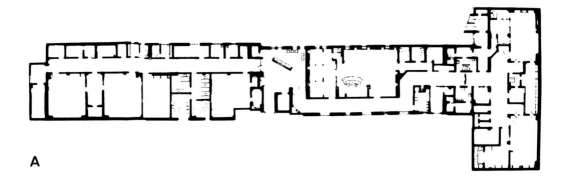

A

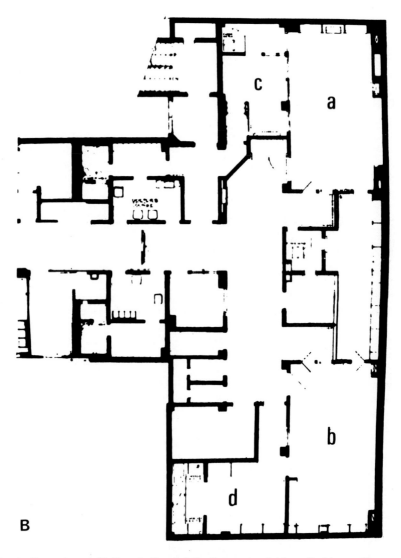

B

FIG. 1. A. Floor plan of St. Francis Hospital Cardiovascular Center. B. (a) operating room #1, (b) operating room #2, (c) gallery, (d) pump room. C. (e) surgical intensive care unit, (f) lobby and waiting area. D. (g) conference room, (h) examining rooms, (i) bathrooms, (j) chemistry laboratory. E. (k) cardiac catheterization rooms, (l) darkroom, (m) art room.

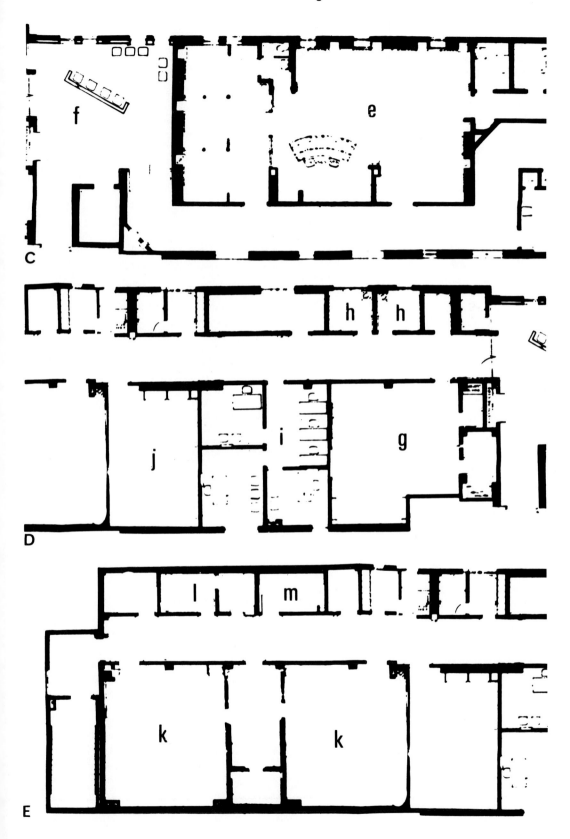

cardiography, stress testing, and full cardiac catheterization, when indicated. Surgical consultation is immediately available when the results of these studies have been completed. The information is then voice-communicated to the patient's referring doctor and a joint decision is reached as to the need for medical or surgical treatment. The patient is returned to the hospital room and may then be transferred back to his own personal physician for continued medical care or to the operating room, as the need dictates. Patients who undergo cardiac surgery are reevaluated by the cardiovascular center team, including the private physician, at specified intervals, including repeat stress testing and cardiac catheterization.

The staff of the regional cardiovascular center has participated regularly in the medical conferences of the area hospitals. By the employment of television tape cassettes, the diagnostic and therapeutic procedures used on patients referred from a particular hospital are presented. In this way, the referring physicians become active participants in the decision-making processes.

RESULTS

Using this approach and the diagnostic facilities of the regional cardiovascular center, 100 open-heart operations have been performed with an overall five percent mortality rate. A breakdown of these procedures includes coronary artery bypass grafts (54 cases), valve replacement (24 cases), combined procedures (9 cases), and other procedures (13 cases). The average patient's stay has been 10 hospital days if he undergoes surgery, at an approximate cost of $400 per day.

Intraoperative coronary angiography has yielded clinically valuable data. In one case, intraoperative coronary arteriography showed a vein bypass graft placed proximal to an obstructive lesion (Fig. 2). It was then possible to go back on cardiopulmonary bypass and correct the error. In another situation, a vein bypass was grafted to the left anterior descending coronary artery, whereas a far more severe lesion was present in a diagonal branch. This lesion was not evident on the initial cardiac catheterization but was readily apparent on the intraoperative cinecoronary arteriogram (Fig. 3). The patient was placed back on cardiopulmonary bypass, and another vein was grafted to the diagonal branch (Fig. 4). From such studies new data will become available that will help in terms of case selection and ascertaining the reasons for early and late vein graft failure.

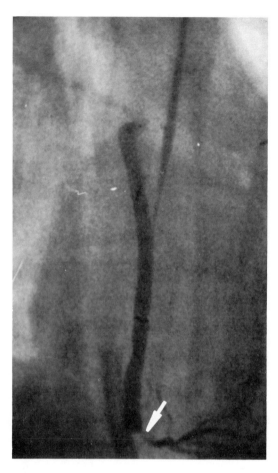

FIG. 2. Intraoperative Coronary Cineangiogram. Right coronary artery bypass graft placed proximal to obstructive lesion. Cardiopulmonary bypass reinstituted and error corrected.

DISCUSSION

Heart disease, and specifically coronary artery disease, has obviously reached epidemic proportions in the United States. It is the leading cause of death in this country and frequently affects those in the wage-earning years. Loss of productivity has been enormous. With the advent of vein bypass surgery for coronary insufficiency, the demand for open-heart facilities has burgeoned. A need, therefore, has been placed on the community hospital to perform a health-care delivery service for treatment of this national problem. Expensive and highly specialized, the service is a burden not readily accepted by hospital administrators. Conflicts result with the medical staff who

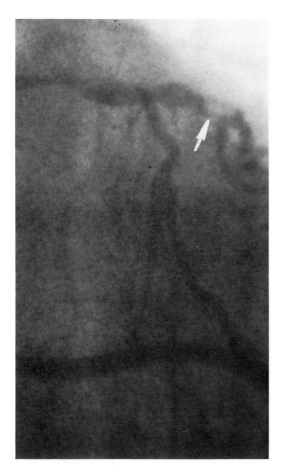

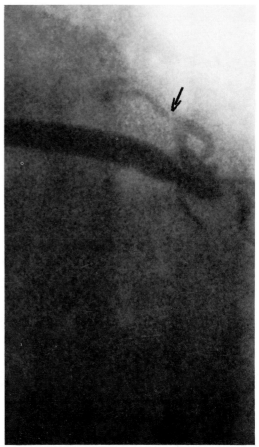

FIG. 3. Intraoperative Coronary Cineangiogram. Vein bypass to left anterior descending coronary artery. Note unsuspected severe lesion in first diagonal. Cardiopulmonary bypass reinstituted.

FIG. 4. Intraoperative Coronary Cinearteriogram. Same patient as Figure 3. Vein graft to first diagonal. Note severe proximal obstruction.

want such diagnostic and therapeutic capabilities for their patients but also wish to be a part of what has been considered academic-quality care. And, frequently, the hospital administration is not able, or even allowed, to comply with this wish because of third-party payment restrictions.

These thoughts generated the concept of the regional medical-surgical-cardiovascular center that was subsequently put into practice. It provides, by virtue of the large number of referring beds, a distribution of the cost factor and also provides quality diagnostic and therapeutic care while involving the patient's personal physician at each level, including the long-term evaluation. This facility is unique in that it is a completely consolidated patient-oriented medical-surgical unit. There are interlocking feedback communications from the patient's personal physician to center cardiologists and surgeons and back again to the

personal physician. Highly specialized and expensive capabilities have already yielded valuable results in terms of giving the quality of clinical care that is expected today. Routine intraoperative cinearteriograms provide an example of the value of these capabilities. They have been performed at the conclusion of all coronary artery bypass operations and have been particularly useful in studying the technical characteristics of the anastomoses as well as the distal coronary artery segment. If there is a technical problem with the anastomosis or if the anastomosis has been placed proximal to an obstructing lesion, correction is carried out prior to chest closure. As a research tool, it is believed that it will be possible to correlate the angiographic findings on the operating table with flow measurements of the bypass grafts in terms of prognosticating graft patency. In our recent experience, angiographically poor runoff at the time of operation is the single most important factor accounting for graft failure. Certainly, further information along these lines is needed, and we expect to obtain significant data in this regard.

SUMMARY

The concept of a regional referral center for team treatment of cardiovascular disease, especially coronary artery disease, has been presented. The establishment of regional cardiovascular centers would make academic-quality care available to all patients and their physicians as an extension of their own hospital setting.

The entire facility is directed toward efficient and economic delivery of health care.

31

CURRENT METHODS OF REDUCING THE SERUM CHOLESTEROL CONCENTRATION: RATIONALE AND AN APPROACH TO THERAPY

CARL S. APSTEIN

INTRODUCTION

Atherosclerosis probably causes more morbidity and mortality than any other pathologic process in the United States and Western Europe. The best treatment for this disease is hardly satisfactory, and, therefore, the best therapy is to prevent the atherosclerotic lesion from occurring in the first place. When this is impossible, then a "second-best" therapy is to cause regression of those lesions or, at least, to slow their rate of progression.

The purpose of this study is to review the relationship between the serum cholesterol concentration and the incidence of clinical coronary disease, to consider the evidence that the reduction of the serum cholesterol can either prevent or cause regression of coronary atherosclerotic lesions or slow their rate of progression, and to present an approach to reducing the serum cholesterol concentration.

ASSOCIATION OF CHOLESTEROL AND ATHEROSCLEROSIS

The evidence linking the serum cholesterol level with the atherosclerotic plaque is now overwhelming. This evidence comes from several sources: pathologic studies, experimental models, and epidemiologic studies. The experimental and pathologic data is based on many studies but can be summarized briefly as follows: (1) the lipid composition of atheromatous plaque shows a high content of cholesterol and cholesterol ester, (2) numerous experimental animals have been shown to develop atherosclerotic-like lesions when placed on a high-cholesterol or high-saturated-fat diet, and, (3) isotopically labeled cholesterol injected into patients ultimately can be recovered from arterial wall and atheroma at autopsy (Chobanian and Hollander, 1962), indicating that at least part of the cholesterol found in the arterial wall and the atheromatous plaque comes from the circulating cholesterol pool.

Human atherosclerosis is linked to the circulating serum cholesterol concentration by numerous careful epidemiologic studies such as those of the International Cooperative Study on Cardiovascular Epidemiology, the Framingham Study, and the Albany Study. These studies showed a very strong correlation between the serum cholesterol concentration and the risk of acquiring clinical coronary artery disease (Keys, 1971). The average data from the Framingham, Albany, and Minneapolis–St. Paul studies is shown in Figure 1. The risk of acquiring clinical coronary artery disease, relative to the average risk for the study population, is plotted against the serum cholesterol concentration. The risk of developing clinical coronary disease increases approximately as the cube, or third power, of an increase in the cholesterol concentration. Thus, the risk of developing coronary heart disease is roughly eight times as great for a patient with a cholesterol level of 360 mg percent compared to a patient with a cholesterol of 180 mg percent (Keys, 1971).

The epidemiologic data thus point out the fallacy of a so-called normal cholesterol level. The relative risk of developing coronary heart disease progressively decreases for lower cholesterol levels. Therefore, it is not meaningful to talk of a "normal" cholesterol level. Rather, the cholesterol level should be considered in terms of the associated risk of coronary heart disease. Below a level of

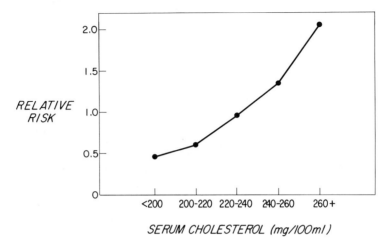

FIG. 1. Relative risk of developing coronary heart disease and the relationship to the serum cholesterol concentration (after Keys, 1971). This figure summarizes the results from the Framingham, Albany, and Minneapolis–St. Paul studies. The relative risk increases approximately as the third power of the relative increase in serum cholesterol concentration.

220 mg percent, there is not much gain from further reduction. Therefore, a level of 200 to 220 mg percent is the goal that should be sought in young middle-aged patients. In older patients it may be more difficult to achieve this goal. To consider 275 or 300 mg percent as the upper limit of normal (which is the case in many laboratories) obscures the fact that this level is associated with a relatively high risk of coronary atherosclerosis.

The incidence of coronary heart disease in four countries in age-matched populations is shown in Figure 2. There is a striking 30-fold difference between Finland and the United States and rural Yugoslavia. The average serum cholesterol levels

in these populations parallel the incidence rate. There was little difference in obesity, incidence of cigarette smoking, or hypertension in the groups studied. Although the U.S. population was more sedentary, the Finns were as active in heavy work as the Yugoslav and Greek populations. Thus, the best discriminator of the high- and low-risk coronary populations was the serum cholesterol concentration (Keys, 1971).

The Framingham Study has shown that the influence of the serum cholesterol on the risk of coronary heart disease is much greater in young men and women (Kannel et al, 1971). Figure 3 summarizes these data and shows that the risk of developing coronary heart disease in men and

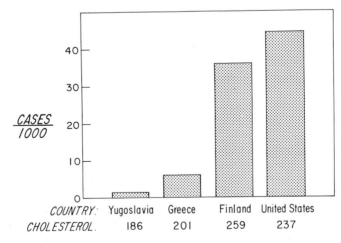

FIG. 2. Incidence of coronary heart disease in four countries, in thousands of cases (after Keys, 1971). The mean serum cholesterol concentration is shown below each country in mg/100 mi.

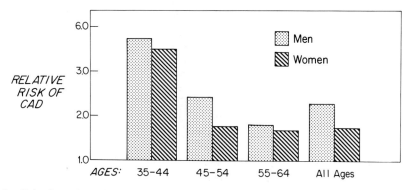

FIG. 3. Risk of an elevated serum cholesterol concentration at different ages (after Kannel et al, 1971). Each bar represents the relative risk of developing coronary heart disease in a population with a serum cholesterol concentration ≦ 220 mg percent compared to a population with a cholesterol concentration ≧ 265 mg percent. The higher serum cholesterol concentration increases the risk of coronary artery disease most strikingly in people of young middle age.

women 35 to 45 years old is five to six times as great for the group with a cholesterol level of 265 mg percent or greater compared to those of 220 mg percent or lower. In older age groups a high cholesterol still carried a high risk of coronary artery disease, but the relative risk is not as striking as in people under 45. In other words, a high serum cholesterol does not simply take years off the end of one's life; rather it increases, at a very high risk rate, the chance of developing symptomatic coronary heart disease in young middle age. This is an important practical point in terms of convincing patients to take the necessary measures to reduce their serum cholesterol level.

The Framingham Study also identified several other factors that are associated with a higher risk of coronary disease (Kannel et al, 1971). These are (1) carbohydrate intolerance as evidenced by an abnormal glucose tolerance test or frank diabetes mellitus, (2) cigarette smoking, and (3) hypertension. The relative risk of each of these factors has been summarized in tabular form and is available from the American Heart Association. In general, the cholesterol concentration is additive to or is synergistic with the other risk factors.

INFLUENCING THE NATURAL HISTORY OF ATHEROSCLEROSIS

Two studies give hope that the atherosclerotic process may be reversed or the rate of progression significantly slowed. The first is an experimental study performed in rhesus monkeys that were fed a high-cholesterol, saturated-fat diet with a resulting increase in the circulating cholesterol

from 135 to 700 mg percent (Armstrong et al, 1970). After 17 months a group of monkeys were sacrificed and revealed severe coronary atherosclerosis (Fig. 4). These lesions were not precisely analogous to the human lesion, which frequently has more fibrous tissue.

The monkeys that were not sacrificed at 17 months were placed on a low-cholesterol, high-polyunsaturated-fat diet, and the serum cholesterol decreased back to the normal range for monkeys (135 mg percent). After 40 months at the low-serum-cholesterol level the remaining monkeys were sacrificed and their coronaries examined (Fig. 5). The extent of atherosclerosis was markedly reduced compared to the coronary disease when the circulating cholesterol level was high. Thus, at least in monkeys, where coronary atherosclerosis was acutely induced with a marked elevation of the serum cholesterol concentration, there is potential for regression of these lesions.

A recent study in man (Miettinen et al, 1972) has shown that dietary modification with a resultant lowering of the serum cholesterol results in a decreased risk of coronary heart disease.

Two Finnish mental hospital populations were studied. Each was on the regular hospital diet for six years and on a cholesterol-lowering diet for six years. The dietary modifications were fairly minor; ordinary milk was replaced by an emulsion of soy bean oil in skim milk ("filled milk"), and butter and ordinary margarine were replaced by a soft margarine with a high content of polyunsaturated fatty acids. The average value of the serum cholesterol on the regular hospital diet was 275 mg percent; on the experimental diet the average cholesterol decreased to 234 mg percent. The mean age of the patients during the

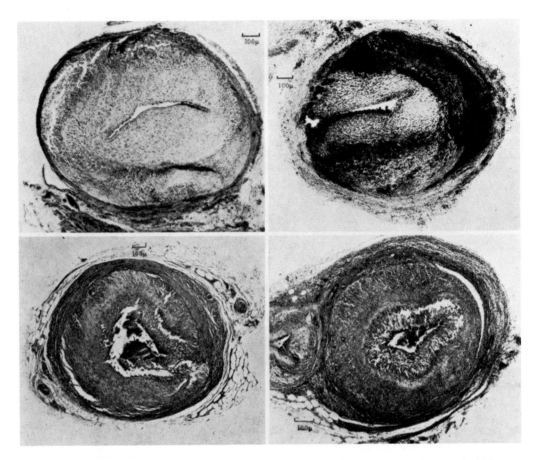

FIG. 4. Coronary atherosclerosis in rhesus monkeys maintained on a high-cholesterol, high-saturated-fat diet (from Armstrong et al, 1970).

study was 52. Thus, the intervention consisted of a modest lowering of the serum cholesterol in a middle-aged group of patients over a six-year period, with a six-year period serving as control.

The results of this study are summarized in Figure 6, and show that the incidence of coronary heart disease was significantly decreased in patients on the cholesterol-lowering diet during the period of study. The difference in death rates due to coronary heart disease in males was statistically significant. In females there was a trend toward a decreased death rate from coronary disease, but it did not achieve statistical significance during the course of the study. Deaths due to all causes were decreased by about 12 percent in males on the experimental diet; there was no change in the overall death rate for females. However, the difference in overall death rate for males was not statistically significant.

There was no increase in the incidence of malignant neoplasms on the high-polyunsaturated-fat diet; this deserves special mention since others have reported a slightly higher incidence of car-

cinoma on a high polyunsaturated fat diet (Pearce and Dayton, 1971).

On the basis of this study, therefore, it would appear that a modest decrease in the serum cholesterol over a prolonged period of time can favorably influence the death rate due to coronary heart disease in middle-aged men. Such a result does not distinguish between regression of pre-existing lesions and a decrease in the rate of progression of existing lesions, but this study does indicate that reducing the serum cholesterol concentration, even in relatively late middle age, can decrease the risk of death from coronary heart disease.

DETERMINANTS OF SERUM CHOLESTEROL

Since the incidence of coronary heart disease seems to be highly correlated with the serum cholesterol concentration, it is important to understand the determinants of the serum cholesterol level.

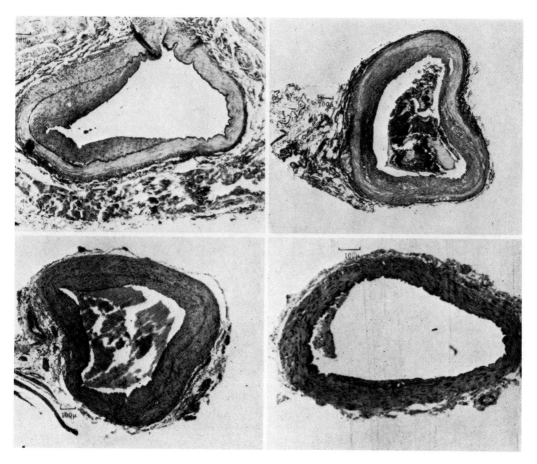

FIG. 5. Regression of coronary atherosclerosis in rhesus monkeys after 40 months on a low-cholesterol, high-polyunsaturated-fat diet (from Armstrong et al, 1970).

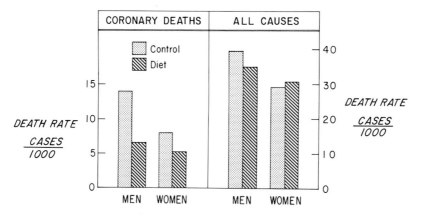

FIG. 6. Effect of cholesterol-lowering diet on deaths due to coronary heart disease in Finnish mental hospital study (death rate in thousands of cases) (after Miettinen et al, 1972).

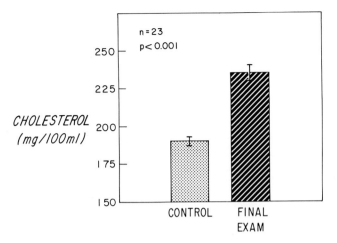

FIG. 7. Effect of mental stress on the serum cholesterol concentration (mg/100 ml) (after Grundy and Griffin, 1959).

Clearly there are a number of factors involved that can be summarized under the heading of genetic, dietary, psychological, and perhaps others of which we are unaware. The genetic aspects have recently been extensively reviewed (Goldstein et al, 1973).

As far as the dietary relationships are concerned, it has been repeatedly shown that the circulating cholesterol level bears a direct relationship to the amount of cholesterol and saturated fat in the diet (Keys, 1971). Type IV patients also increase the triglyceride and cholesterol content of the blood in relation to the amount of carbohydrate in the diet (Fredrickson and Levy, 1972).

Psychological stress has also been shown to elevate the serum cholesterol concentration (Grundy and Griffin, 1959). The serum cholesterol concentration was measured in medical students during the semester when there were no examinations, and at the end of the semester during the final examination period. There was a consistent increase in the mean serum cholesterol from 190 to 238 mg percent or an increase of 25 percent, which is greater than the increment in serum cholesterol caused by the dietary intervention in the Finnish hospital study (Fig. 7). Thus, mental stress can significantly increase the circulating cholesterol level, and this mechanism may play an important role in the pathogenesis of coronary atherosclerosis in patients who exist in psychologically stressful environments.

TREATMENT

Before an elevated serum cholesterol concentration can be treated, it must be discovered.

Thus, the first question to be considered is, *Who should have their serum cholesterol measured?*

The author's answer to this question is, *Everybody.* Measuring the serum cholesterol concentration is a benign procedure that requires only the collection of a fasting blood sample. Since the best therapy of atherosclerosis is prevention, it follows that the greatest success will be obtained the earlier that a predisposing condition (eg an elevated serum cholesterol concentration) is discovered and corrected. Thus, universal screening for hypercholesterolemia is strongly recommended.

Once an elevated serum cholesterol is discovered, there are a number of ways to approach the task of lowering it. Who should have their serum cholesterol lowered? It would seem prudent to attempt reduction of the cholesterol in those patients who are at risk. Since the risk of coronary heart disease climbs rapidly as the serum cholesterol rises above 220 mg percent and since young middle-aged patients, both male and female, have a particularly high cholesterol-associated risk of coronary artery disease, these patients should be treated aggressively in an effort to reduce the serum cholesterol below 220 mg percent.

The management of an elevated serum cholesterol and/or triglyceride level has recently been reviewed (Lees and Wilson, 1971, Levy et al, 1972). The principles to be followed in managing these conditions are as follows:

1. *The type of therapy should be individualized according to the lipoprotein phenotype of the patient.* Type II and type IV are the most common types of hyperlipoproteinemia and account for more than 90 percent of the

lipid abnormalities seen in clinical practice.

Either of these phenotypes may be associated with an elevated serum cholesterol concentration. If the triglyceride concentration is elevated out of proportion to the cholesterol concentration, then the phenotype is probably type IV. With type II, the triglyceride concentration is normal (IIa) or slightly to moderately elevated (IIb). The distinction in phenotype is important since in type II the excess cholesterol is carried in the β, or low-density lipoprotein fraction, whereas in type IV it is carried in the pre-β or very low-density lipoprotein fraction, and the optimal therapeutic regimen depends on the specific lipoprotein abnormality. Lipoprotein electrophoresis should be performed if the cholesterol or triglyceride level is abnormal in order to determine the phenotype.

2. *Dietary therapy should be the first measure taken.* Obese patients should undergo weight reduction to their optimal weight. Type IV patients are usually moderately to grossly obese, and often this type of hyperlipoproteinemia will be completely corrected with weight loss and restriction of carbohydrate intake. A low-cholesterol, low-saturated-fat, and high-polyunsaturated-fat diet is also recommended for type IV patients.

Type II patients should undergo weight reduction if obese, but often these patients are lean. This phenotype should be treated with a low-cholesterol, low-saturated-fat, and high-polyunsaturated-fat diet.

Thus, both type II and IV should be on a low-cholesterol, low-saturated-fat, high-polyunsaturated-fat diet; and type IV patients should also have a restricted carbohydrate intake.

3. *When dietary therapy is not successful in reducing the blood lipids to the desired range, pharmacological agents should be added to the regimen.* The drugs that are effective in reducing the blood lipid level can be classified by their mechanism of action. Clofibrate and nicotinic acid appear to work by inhibiting the release of lipoprotein from the liver. Other agents are effective by interrupting the enterohepatic circulation of cholesterol; these drugs are resins such as cholestyramine and colestipol, β-sitosterol (Cytellin, a naturally occurring plant sterol), and neomycin.

Clofibrate is probably the drug of choice for type IV hyperlipoproteinemia. Nicotinic acid should be tried either in combination with clofibrate, or as a substitute for it, if clofibrate fails in the treatment of type IV.

Type II hyperlipoproteinemia should be treated conservatively at first with a drug that works in the gut and is not absorbed. Cholestyramine, colestipol, β-sitosterol, or neomycin are all examples of drugs such as this, although neomycin is absorbed to a small extent.

Neomycin is not widely used despite published reports of its efficacy (Samuel et al, 1967). A recent clinical trial has substantiated the previous conclusion that neomycin is an effective and reliable agent in reducing the serum cholesterol concentration (Apstein et al, 1973). The results of this study are shown in Figure 8. The extent of reduction depends upon the pretreatment cholesterol level and the dosage. Thus, with a pretreatment level of

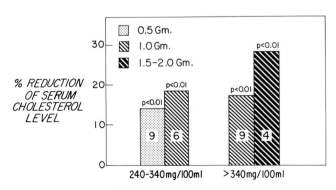

PRE-TREATMENT CHOLESTEROL LEVEL

FIG. 8. Effect of oral neomycin on the serum cholesterol concentration (after Apstein et al, 1973).

240 to 340 mg percent, there was a reduction of 15 percent and 20 percent with 0.5 and 1.0 gm/day, respectively. At higher pretreatment levels, 1.0 and 1.5 to 2.0 gm/day dosages lowered the cholesterol by 19 and 29 percent, respectively. Monthly audiograms showed no change in acoustic acuity in any of the 28 patients. Three patients had nausea or vomiting associated with taking this drug; these symptoms were relieved by taking medication with meals. Thus, low-dose neomycin appears to be an effective agent for lowering the serum cholesterol.

If treatment with a single agent that interrupts the enterohepatic circulation of cholesterol is not satisfactory, then nicotinic acid or clofibrate can be added to it.

SUMMARY

This brief review has attempted to highlight the important studies that link an elevated serum cholesterol with atherosclerosis, to suggest that there is some evidence that reduction of the circulating cholesterol can favorably influence the natural history of the disease, and to outline an approach to therapy. The therapeutic approach outlined above has successfully lowered the serum lipids in the vast majority of patients so treated. The impact of such a reduction in serum lipids on the morbidity and mortality caused by coronary artery disease has yet to be determined. However, the risk of coronary artery disease in a population with an untreated elevated cholesterol is so high that such a prudent approach to lowering the serum cholesterol appears to be warranted at this time.

References

Apstein CS, George PK, Myers GS, et al: Treatment of hypercholesterolemia with low dose oral neomycin. J Clin Invest 52:4a, 1973

Armstrong ML, Warner ED, Connor WE: Regression of coronary atheromatosis in rhesus monkeys. Circ Res 27:59, 1970

Chobanian AV, Hollander W: Body cholesterol metabolism in man. I. The equilibration of serum and tissue cholesterol. J Clin Invest 41:1732, 1962

Fredrickson DS, Levy RI: Familial hyperlipoproteinemia. In Stanbury JB, Wyngaarden JB, and Fredrickson DS (eds): The Metabolic Basis of Inherited Disease. New York, McGraw-Hill, 1972, pp 545–614

Goldstein JL, Schrott HG, Hazzard WR, Bierman EL, and Motulsky AG: Hyperlipidemia in coronary heart disease. II. Genetic analysis of lipid levels in 176 families and delineation of a new inherited disorder, combined hyperlipidemia. J Clin Invest 52:1544, 1973

Grundy SM, Griffin AC: Effects of periodic mental stress on serum cholesterol levels. Circulation 19:496, 1959

Kannel WB, Castelli WP, Gordon T, and McNamara PM: Serum cholesterol, lipoproteins and the risk of coronary heart disease. The Framingham Study. Ann Intern Med 74:1, 1971

Keys A: The diet and plasma lipids in the etiology of coronary heart disease. In Russek HI, and Zohman BL (eds): Coronary Heart Disease. Philadelphia, JB Lippincott, 1971, pp 59–76

Lees RS, Wilson DE: The treatment of hyperlipidemia. N Engl J of Med 284:186, 1971

Levy RI, Fredrickson DS, Shulman R, et al: Dietary and drug treatment of primary hyperlipoproteinemia. Ann Intern Med 77:267, 1972

Miettinen M, Turpeinen O, Karvonen MJ, Elosuo, R, and Paavilainen E: Effect of cholesterol-lowering diet on mortality from coronary heart disease and other causes. Lancet ii:835, 1972

Pearce LM, Dayton S: Incidence of cancer in men on a diet high in polyunsaturated fat. Lancet I:464, 1971

32

MEDICAL MANAGEMENT OF ANGINA PECTORIS: MULTIFACTORIAL ACTION OF PROPRANOLOL

William H. Frishman, Charles Smithen, James Christodoulou, Babette Weksler, Norman Brachfeld, and Thomas Killip

Beta-adrenergic blocking drugs have been used extensively in many countries for the treatment of a wide range of clinical disease states since their introduction by Powell and Slater (1958). Propranolol has been demonstrated by several investigators to be an effective agent in the treatment of patients with angina pectoris, causing a significant decrease in the frequency of attacks, a decline in the amount of nitroglycerin consumed and improvement in exercise tolerance (Gianelly, Goldman, et al, 1967; Hamer, Grandjean, et al, 1966; Harrison, 1972; Pitt and Ross, 1969; Prichard and Gilliam, 1971). More recently, it has been suggested that propranolol administration following acute myocardial infarction results in preservation of ischemic myocardium with limitation of infarction size. Maroko et al (1973) have shown a decrease in the area of ischemic injury of dogs with ligated coronary arteries, as measured by ST segment maps. Mueller and associates (1974) have demonstrated reversal of the ischemic metabolic response following myocardial infarction in humans with propranolol therapy.

Ischemia and angina pectoris occur when myocardial oxygen or energy demands exceed supply (Fig. 1). Myocardial requirements for oxygen rise progressively as cardiac work increases. As a consequence of autoregulatory mechanisms, arteriolar vasodilation occurs with an increase in coronary flow. In the presence of significant coronary artery disease, there are periods where sup-

ply is unable to meet demand, and thus ischemia results. Treatment may be designed to increase myocardial oxygen supply and energy availability or to reduce energy need. It is currently believed that the beneficial effects of propranolol when coronary blood flow is limited result from a reduction in myocardial oxygen requirement brought about by a decrease in heart rate, systemic blood pressure, and velocity of myocardial fiber shortening (Dwyer, Wiener, et al, 1968, Furberg and Jacobson, 1967). However, little attention has been paid to other actions of propranolol, particularly with regard to enhancement of myocardial oxygen and energy supply. Accordingly, the following studies were performed in order further to elucidate the mechanism of its action.

METHODS

Patient Studies

Nineteen patients with a history typical for ischemic heart disease were entered into a double blind controlled trial. There were 11 male and eight female patients with an average age of 54. All had definite electrocardiographic evidence of myocardial ischemia during exercise stress testing and at least three attacks of anginal chest pain per week. The patients were followed in a special angina clinic, and all initially started on placebo for a six-week period. After this period, the patients were placed at random in placebo and propranolol treatment groups. The placebo group ($n = 9$) remained on the same placebo regimen, while the drug treatment group ($n = 10$) was started on 80 mg of oral propranolol daily in four

Supported in part by USPHS Contract No. PH 43-67-11439, and in part by a grant from Ayerst Pharmaceutical Company, New York, New York

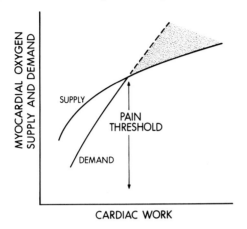

FIG. 1. Oxygen supply-demand relationship in angina pectoris. As myocardial oxygen demand increases with cardiac work, a point is reached where oxygen demand exceeds supply, resulting in ischemia (gray zone) and angina pectoris.

divided doses for two weeks followed by 160 mg daily for a further two-week period.

Exercise Testing

Bicycle ergometer exercise testing was performed by the same physician in a double blind fashion in all patients. Tests were carried out during the initial six-week placebo period and then bimonthly while on 80 and 160 mg of propranolol daily or corresponding placebo dose. A modification of the ear-ensiform system described by Arbarquez et al (1960) was used with recording of precordial leads V1, V4, V5, and modified orthogonal leads X, Y, Z, every minute throughout the study. Patients were started at a work load of 150 kpm/min and the level of work increased by 150 kpm/min every three minutes until chest pain or significant fatigue occurred. Total work performance was calculated at the summation of the products of work load and the time of pedaling at each load level. Blood pressure was recorded by the auscultatory method, and heart-rate blood pressure product, an indirect index of myocardial oxygen consumption (Robinson, 1967), was calculated at the exact end-point of exercise.

P50 MEASUREMENTS. Affinity of hemoglobin for oxygen was determined from measurement of the P50 of heparinized blood at the time of, but not preceding, exercise testing in all patients. For comparison, P50 was measured in 37 normal subjects. The partial pressure of oxygen when hemoglobin is 50 percent saturated (P50) was determined from venous blood by a modification of the mixing techniques of Edwards and

Martin (1966). Percent oxyhemoglobin saturation, hemoglobin concentration, and percent carbon monoxyhemoglobin saturation was measured on an IL-Co-Oximeter, Model 182. Appropriate radiometer electrodes were used to measure pH, PCO_2, and PO_2. The initial aliquot was divided into two parts that were exposed to nitrogen and 20 percent oxygen respectively in a tonometer incubated at 37 percent C. Five percent CO_2 was added to each gas mixture. After tonometering, equal quantities of each sample were combined to produce a mixture with 50 percent oxyhemoglobin saturation. The PO_2 observed at 50 percent saturation is reported as the P50, corrected to a pH of 7.4 using the Severinghaus nomogram.

PLATELET STUDIES. Platelet aggregation studies were performed slightly before exercise testing in all patients; and in 11, age and sex matched normal subjects.

The blood was obtained after a 12-hour fast. After an initial resting period of 30 minutes, a 19 gauge needle was inserted, without use of a tourniquet, into an antecubital vein, and a slow infusion of physiological saline was begun. After 15 minutes of rest, blood was sampled by free flow into plastic tubes containing acid citrate dextrose, $1/10$ volume acid citrate dextrose (ACD). The blood specimens were then immediately processed for analysis. The specimens were coded so that those performing the aggregation studies had no knowledge of the patient, the diagnosis, or the type of drug therapy.

Platelet aggregation studies were performed using the turbidometric method of Born (1962), as modified by Mustard et al (1964). The sample collected a few minutes earlier was placed in sterile polypropylene tubes and platelet-rich plasma (PRP) separated by immediate centrifugation for 15 minutes at room temperature at 225 g. After removal of the upper two-thirds of the PRP, the remaining PRP was recentrifuged at 4,300 g for 10 minutes at 4 C to yield platelet poor plasma (PPP). Platelet counts were performed on a Coulter Model F counter; the count of the PRP was adjusted to the range 300–400,000/mm^3, when necessary, with the autologous PPP.

Platelet aggregation studies were performed in duplicate within 90 minutes of venipuncture. The sample was kept tightly covered at room temperature until analyzed. Samples of 0.45 ml PRP were prewarmed for one minute with stirring in siliconized cuvettes placed in a Payton dual channel aggregation module (Payton Associates, Buffalo N.Y.) before aggregating agents were added. The light transmittance was recorded on a Rikin Denshi linear recorder. The blank for each study was a similarly treated sample of PPP. The aggregating agent tested was adenosine diphosphate (ADP) (Sigma, Inc. St. Louis, Mo.) maintained as a 10^{-3}M frozen stock and diluted just before use over a range of 10^{-7}M to 10^{-4}M (0.1 to 100 μM). The lowest concentration producing a full biphasic aggregation response was recorded as the threshold dose.

Animal Experiments

The effects of propranolol on myocardial metabolism have not been extensively reported. Because of the possible ability of the drug to augment myocardial glycogen stores following stress, a study was performed to evaluate this effect and to determine whether propranolol could be protective during induced acute myocardial anoxia.

BASAL STUDIES. Six rats of the Sherman strain were fed ad-lib and treated with 10 mg/kg of propranolol intraperitoneally twice daily for three days. A comparable control group received 1 cc of saline intraperitoneally for the identical period of time. Following an overnight fast, both groups were subjected to a 20-minute period of ice-water stress and then anesthetized with Nembutal prior to sacrifice. All animals were sacrificed at the same time following the last intraperitoneal injection. The hearts were rapidly removed, compressed by a Wollenberger clamp, maintained in liquid nitrogen, and subsequently assayed for glycogen, creatinine phosphate, ATP, ADP, and AMP.

PERFUSION STUDIES. Another series of 12 rats was divided into two groups of six animals each; one received saline and the other propranolol in the dosage previously noted. After 20 minutes of ice-water stress, they were anesthetized with Nembutal and then perfused aerobically (PO_2 550 mm Hg) on a modified Langendorff apparatus for 15 minutes. Hearts were paced at 300/min and contracted isovolumically following inflation of a small latex balloon catheter inserted into the left ventricle. The bubbling reservoir was set to deliver a perfusion pressure of 75 mm Hg. At the end of perfusion, left ventricular systolic pressure, dP/dt, end-diastolic pressure, and coronary flow were measured and hearts were freeze-clamped for analysis of tissue glycogen and high-energy phosphate concentration.

A third group of 12 animals was studied with an identical protocol to the above except that aerobic perfusion was followed by a five-minute paced anoxic period (PO_2, 50 mm Hg) with measurements of the same hemodynamic and metabolic parameters previously noted.

The results of all these experiments were compared in the control and propranolol treated groups.

ANALYSIS. Group means are presented with the standard error of the mean as the index of dispersion. Statistical analysis was performed using Student's t-test for independent and paired observations.

RESULTS

Patient Studies

EXERCISE TESTS. During the control period, all 19 patients in the study had positive exercise tests with typical anginal pain the endpoint. The 10 patients who received propranolol (80 mg/day) were able to increase their total mean work by 128 percent from 765 ± 125 kpm during the control period to $1,792 \pm 285$ kpm ($p < .01$) (Fig. 2). This beneficial effect on work performance was associated with a significant drop in the heart rate–blood pressure product from $16,800 \pm 1,535$ at control to $12,000 \pm 885$ after drug ($p < 0.01$) (Fig. 3). With 160 mg/day of oral propranolol, no significant change in work performance was observed when compared to the 80-mg/day dose. The placebo group demonstrated no significant changes in total work performance or heart rate–blood pressure product in the serial exercise studies done.

P50. Mean P50 data in normal subjects and in patients with angina on placebo and on oral propranolol are shown in Figure 4. The mean P50 for the 37 normal subjects was 25.81 ± 0.44 mm Hg. Patients with angina pectoris demonstrated no difference in P50 when compared to the normal subjects. Propranolol in doses of 80 or 160 mg/day did not change P50 values significantly. Mean P50 was 24.89 ± 1.10 mm Hg during control, 25.78 ± 1.36 mm Hg during 80 mg of propranolol/day, and 24.63 ± 1.10 mm Hg during 160 mg of propranolol/day.

PLATELET AGGREGATION STUDIES. All 19 patients with angina pectoris demonstrated increased in vitro platelet sensitivity to aggregating concentrations of ADP when compared to the 11 normal subjects. Mean concentration of ADP necessary for a biphasic aggregation response was 1.79 ± 0.22 μM in patients and 4.27 ± 0.75 in normals ($p < 0.001$) (Fig. 5).

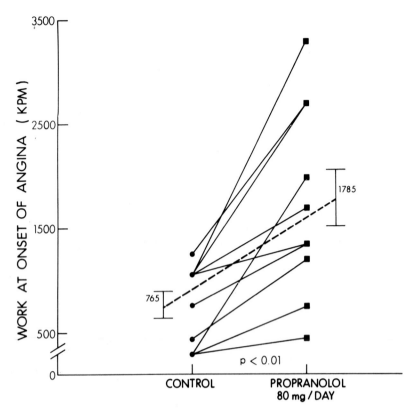

FIG. 2. Change in total work performance after propranolol treatment in patients with angina pectoris. Circles depict individual values before and squares after propranolol treatment. A significant increase in mean total work performance occurs with 80 mg/day of oral propranolol. Work is measured in kilo-pound meters (kpm).

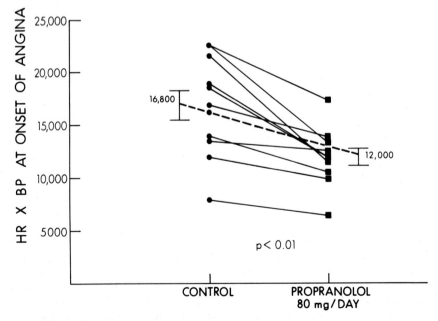

FIG. 3. Changes in heart rate–blood pressure product (HR × BP) after propranolol in patients with angina pectoris. Circles depict values before and squares after propranolol treatment. A significant mean decrease in HR × BP, an indirect measurement of myocardial oxygen consumption, is demonstrated at the end of exercise with 80 mg/day of oral propranolol.

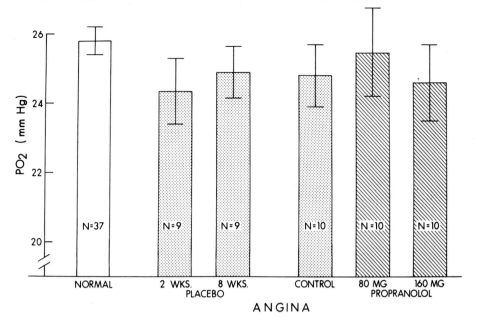

FIG. 4. P50 vs dose (placebo and propranolol) in normal subjects and patients with angina pectoris. Patients demonstrated no significant difference from normals. Neither placebo- nor propranolol-treated patients showed any change from normal.

FIG. 5. Comparison of ADP-induced platelet aggregability in normal subjects and patients with angina pectoris. Platelets of normal subjects require significantly higher concentrations of ADP to attain aggregation threshold than do platelets of normal subjects.

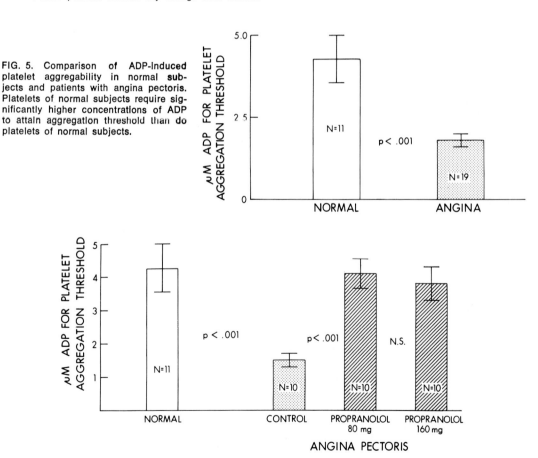

FIG. 6. Effect of oral propranolol on ADP-induced platelet aggregability in patients with angina pectoris. After propranolol, 80 mg/day, platelets of treated patients are less sensitive to ADP when compared to control. Concentration of ADP required during propranolol treatment is not significantly different from normal. Platelet responsiveness is not further changed when propranolol dose is doubled to 160 mg/day.

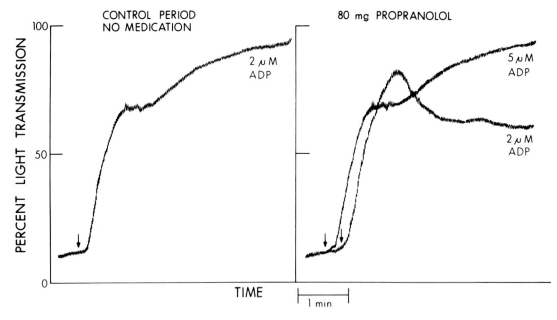

FIG. 7. Platelet aggregation with and without propranolol in a patient with angina pectoris. Degree of aggregation is related to the increase in light transmission, since clumping reduces light absorption. Arrows indicate the addition of ADP to stirred platelet-rich plasma. Left panel, during placebo therapy, 2μM ADP required for aggregation threshold. Right panel, after 80 mg/day propranolol orally, 2μM ADP is insufficient to achieve aggregation threshold. 5μM is now required and the response is within normal limits.

Serial studies while on placebo showed no change in platelet sensitivity to ADP. With propranolol, 80 mg/day, platelet aggregation response to ADP was entirely normalized, 4.10 ± 0.46 μM ADP being required to produce a biphasic aggregation response after therapy as compared with 1.50 ± 0.21 μM in these same patients before therapy ($p < 0.01$). No additional changes were noted with propranolol 160 mg/day (Fig. 6). An example of the propranolol effect on platelet aggregation in a treated patient with angina pectoris is shown in Figure 7.

Animal Experiments

Following an acute ice-water stress with liberation of catecholamines there was 44 percent higher glycogen concentration in propranolol-treated hearts (101 ± 8 μ moles/gdw in control hearts versus 146 ± 11 in propranolol hearts, $p < 0.02$). No differential effect was seen on levels of ATP (control 17.6 ± 0.9 versus treated 17.4 ± 0.8), ADP (5.10 ± 0.4 versus 44 ± 0.3), AMP (0.9 ± 0.2 versus 0.8 ± 0.1), and creatinine phosphate (18.4 ± 1.9 versus 18.7 ± 2.4). Following 15 minutes of aerobic perfusion in the second series of hearts, this difference in glycogen levels persisted (99.7 ± 4.1 μ moles/gdw for control hearts versus 126.2 ± 10.6 μ

moles/gdw for propranolol hearts, $p < 0.05$). No differential effect on high-energy phosphate levels or on myocardial hemodynamics was demonstrated.

In the third series of rats subject to the five-minute anoxic insult, cardiac function was significantly better in the propranolol treated group then in the control group (Fig. 8). Left ventricular systolic peak pressure was 15 percent higher (39.6 ± 1.3 mm Hg versus 45.6 ± 1.8 mm Hg, $p < 0.025$); dP/dt was 94 percent higher (272 ± 38 mm Hg/sec, versus 529 ± 42 mm Hg/sec $p < 0.005$), and left ventricular end-diastolic pressure was 64 percent lower (20 ± 3 mm Hg versus 7 ± 1 mm Hg, $p < 0.005$). Associated with this enhanced myocardial performance, propranolol-treated hearts showed a 32 percent increase in glycogenolytic flux during the anoxic period when compared to control (Fig. 9).

Despite improved left ventricular function, tissue ATP, ADP, and AMP levels were similar in both groups of hearts (Fig. 10).

DISCUSSION

The results of this present study suggest that the mode of action of propranolol in ischemic heart disease is more complex than a method de-

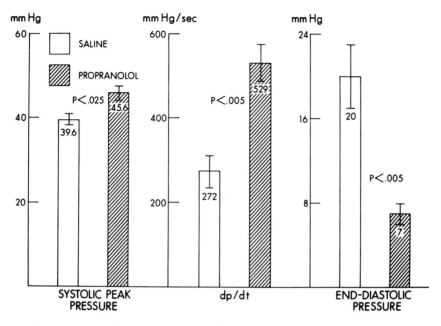

FIG. 8. Effect of propranolol pretreatment on left ventricular hemodynamics during anoxia in the isolated perfused rat heart. Propranolol-treated hearts developed higher left ventricular systolic peak pressures, higher dP/dt, and lower end-diastolic pressures than saline-treated control hearts.

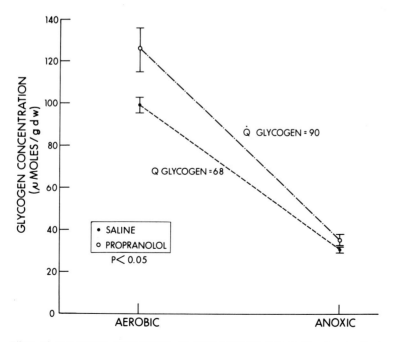

FIG. 9. Effect of propranolol pretreatment on glycogenolytic flux during anoxia. During aerobic perfusion following an acute Ice-water stress, propranolol-treated hearts have significantly higher glycogen concentrations than the heart treated with a saline. This results in enhanced glycogenolytic flux during anoxic perfusion.

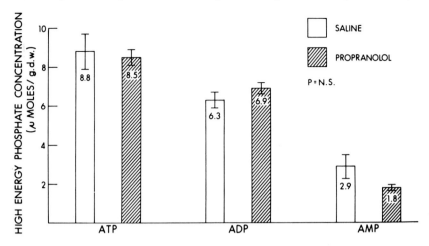

FIG. 10. Effect of propranolol pretreatment on high-energy phosphate stores during anoxia. No differential effects on myocardial ATP, ADP, or AMP levels were observed in propranolol- or saline-treated hearts.

signed solely to reduce myocardial oxygen consumption. Our studies confirm the work of others and show a significant improvement in work performance coupled with a reduction in the heart rate—blood pressure product at the end-point of exercise, suggesting a reduction in oxygen demands (Furberg and Jacobson, 1967; Harrison, 1972; Pitt and Ross, 1969; Prichard and Gilliam, 1972). However, in serial echocardiographic measurements of left ventricular end-diastolic volume reported elsewhere (Frishman, Smithen, et al, 1974), we have shown a progressive increase in this parameter with increasing propranolol dosage, an effect that would tend to increase oxygen demand. Thus, the net action of propranolol on myocardial oxygen consumption will depend on a balance between those factors that tend to decrease or increase oxygen needs.

The first suggestion that propranolol might augment myocardial oxygen or energy supply came from work by Oski and his associates (1969) on hemoglobin affinity for oxygen. It has been known for some time that reduced affinity of hemoglobin for oxygen, reflected by a rightward shift in the oxyhemoglobin dissociation curve, occurs in several clinical states characterized by chronic hypoxemia. More recently, Shappell (1969) has demonstrated the phenomenon following the acute induction of angina pectoris during atrial pacing. Also Kostuk and Sobel (1973) have described a rightward shift in the oxyhemoglobin dissociation curve during acute myocardial infarction. Oski and Miller (1972) showed that propranolol produced a similar shift *in vitro* and in normal subjects, probably by a release of membrane-bound 2, 3 diphosphoglycerate. This en-

hancement of oxygen release might be particularly important in facilitating oxygen availability to marginally perfused areas of myocardium. However, we have been unable to corroborate such an effect of propranolol in patients with angina pectoris, although Schrumph and his associates (1974) have reported an increase in the P50 in their angina patients treated with the drug.

Several observers have suggested that altered platelet function plays an important role in ischemic heart disease (Born, 1972; Mustard, 1972; Hampton and Gorlin, 1971). In the animal model, platelet aggregates have recently been demonstrated in the coronary microvasculature following catecholamine infusions and after acute severe stress (Haft, Fani, et al, 1973; Haft, Kranz, et al, 1972). The findings in this controlled study show a highly significant increase in ADP-induced platelet aggregability in patients with angina pectoris when compared to normal subjects. Although the exact mechanism for this increased aggregability in patients with angina pectoris remains unknown, the clinical implications of this observation are of interest. Infarction can occur secondarily to occlusion of a vessel by a platelet thrombus, although such platelet aggregates persist for only a few minutes. Mustard et al (1970) have produced such lesions experimentally by infusing platelet-aggregating agents into a coronary artery. Haerem (1971) reported that platelet aggregates in the epicardial coronary arteries of patients who died suddenly of cardiac causes were more numerous and larger than those found in patients without cardiac disease. The majority of patients who die suddenly and demonstrate myocardial infarction at postmortem examination are found to have incompletely obstructed coronary arteries (Haerem, 1972; Roberts, 1972). The possibility that the initial insult could be caused by an evanescent platelet thrombus in severe circumstances is attractive. The serial increase in infarction size often observed following acute myocardial infarction (Reid, Taylor, et al, 1974) could be due to formation of platelet microaggregates mediated by local release of ADP from ischemic myocardial cells, circulating platelets, and red blood cells. Agents that could alter platelet aggregability may, therefore, have a beneficial effect in management of patients with coronary artery disease, especially in the prevention of acute ischemic complications. Such possibilities are speculative and are a stimulus for further investigation.

In this study of patients with angina pectoris, there was a definite decrease in ADP-induced platelet aggregability from control, with pharmacologic doses of propranolol that increase exercise tolerance. One could speculate that an agent that protects hyperresponsive circulating platelets from the usual aggregating concentrations of ADP might well enhance myocardial oxygen delivery by preventing the formation of microaggregates during stress or ischemic states. Such a mechanism might limit the size of a myocardial infarction or improve exercise performance in patients with angina pectoris.

The preliminary animal experiments reported herein support the work of others who have emphasized the protective effect of increased glycogen stores following an acute anoxic insult. Cardiac glycogen is known to be a substrate for glycolysis during myocardial anoxia. Conn (1959) demonstrated that during anoxia, excised non-working hearts with increased glycogen content have a greater utilization of glycogen than control animals. Scheuer (1972) has shown an increased glycogen content in isolated rat hearts following physical training or depletion of catecholamines by reserpine treatment. Similar changes have been noted by Beviz (1969) using an *in vitro* system. Enhanced glycogenolysis with preservation of heart function related to the increased myocardial glycogen stores has been demonstrated by Scheuer and Stezoskil (1970). Recent studies by Hewitt et al (1973) confirmed these earlier studies and indicated a greater utilization of glycogen in animals with increased myocardial glycogen content, possibly by a mass action effect. This might also be related to a greater labile fraction of glycogen. Russell and Bloom (1955) have emphasized that myocardial glycogen, elevated by diet or drug manipulation, is not protein bound, and thus is readily available as a substrate for energy production during anoxia. Catecholamines stimulate glycogen breakdown by conversion of phosphorylase B to its active state, phosphorylase A. In our study, propranolol prevented this conversion and resulted in maintenance of myocardial glycogen stores following ice-water stress. As glycogenolysis can occur in anoxic beating mammalian hearts in the absence of humoral factors, it was anticipated that this elevated glycogen could be utilized during the anoxic period. Using the isolated rat heart model and controlling many of the variables determining oxygen consumption and propranolol action, we have shown that pretreatment with propranolol without dietary manipulation maintains cardiac glycogen stores following acute stress. This results in protection of the hearts with enhanced mechanical performance during anoxic injury. This protection appears to result from an increase in glycogenolytic flux with increased anaerobic energy production.

The possible ramifications of all these experiments to the clinical situation are still speculative, but they add new dimensions to our understanding of a complex agent with multifactorial mechanisms of action. It is now apparent that propranolol may exert its antianginal action and preserve ischemic myocardium, not only by its effect on myocardial oxygen demands but also by increasing myocardial oxygen and energy availability.

References

Albarquez RF, Freiman AH, Reichel F, La Due JS: The precordial electrocardiogram during exercise. Circulation 22:1060, 1960

Beviz A, Hjamarson A, Isaksson O: Effects of beta-adrenergic blockade, adrenaline and hypoxia on carbohydrate metabolism in the isolated working rat heart. Acta Physiol Scand 77:80, 1969

Born GVR: Aggregation of blood platelets by adenosine diphosphate and its reversal. Nature 194:927, 1962

Born GVR: Platelet pharmacology in relation to thrombosis. Adv Cardiol 4:161, 1970

Conn H, Wood J, Morales G: Rate of change in myocardial glycogen and lactic acid following arrest of coronary circulation. Circ Res 7:721, 1959

Dwyer EM, Wiener L, Cox JW: Effects of beta adrenergic blockade (propranolol) on left ventricular hemodynamics and the electrocardiogram during exercise-induced angina pectoris. Circulation 38:250, 1968

Edwards MJ, Martin R: Mixing technique for the oxygen-hemoglobin equilibrium and Bohr effect. J Appl Physiol 21:1898, 1966

Frishman W, Smithen C, Killip T: Non-invasive assessment of clinical response to oral propranolol. Am J Cardiol 33:137, 1964

Furberg C, Jacobson KA: Propranolol and angina pectoris. Acta Med Scand 181:729, 1967

Gianelly RE, Goldman RH, Treister B, et al: Propranolol in patients with angina pectoris. Ann Intern Med 67:1216, 1967

Haerem JW: Sudden coronary death: the occurrence

of platelet aggregates in the epicardial arteries of man. Atherosclerosis 14:417, 1971

Haerem JW: Platelet aggregates in intramyocardial vessels of patients dying suddenly and unexpectedly of coronary artery disease. Atherosclerosis 15:199, 1972

Haft JI, Fani K: Intravascular platelet aggregation in the heart induced by stress. Circulation 47:353, 1973

Haft JI, Kranz P, Albert F, Fani K: Intravascular platelet aggregation in the heart induced by norepinephrine: microscopic studies. Circulation 46:698, 1972

Hamer J, Grandjean T, Melendez L, Sowton E: Effect of propranolol (inderal) on exercise tolerance in angina pectoris. Br Heart J 28:414, 1966

Hampton JR, Gorlin R: Platelet studies in patients with coronary artery disease and in their relatives. Br Heart J 34:465, 1971

Harrison DC: Beta adrenergic blockade, 1972. Pharmacology and clinical use. Am J Cardiol 29:432, 1972

Hewlitt R, Lolley D, Adrouny G, Drapanas T: Protective effect of myocardial glycogen on cardiac function during anoxia. Surgery 73:444, 1973

Kostuk W, Suwa K, Bernstein E, Sobel B: Altered hemoglobin oxygen affinity in patients with acute myocardial infarction. Am J Cardiol 31:295, 1973

Maroko P, Braunwald E: Modification of myocardial infarction size after coronary occlusion. Ann Intern Med 79:720, 1973

Mueller H, Religa A, Evans R, Ayres S: Metabolic effect of propranolol on ischemic tissue in human and experimental myocardial infarction. Am J Cardiol 33:159, 1974

Mustard JF: Platelets and thrombosis in acute myocardial infarction. Hospital Practice 7:115, 1972

Mustard JF, Hegardt B, Roswell HC, MacMillan RL: Effect of adenosine nucleotides on platelet aggregation and clotting time. J Lab Clin Med 64:548, 1964

Mustard JF, Packham MA: Factors influencing platelet function: adhesion, release and aggregation. Pharmacol Rev 22:97, 1970

Oski FA, Gottlieb AJ, Deliviria-Papadopoulos M: Redcell 2,3 diphospho-glycerate levels in subjects with chronic hypoxemia. N Engl J Med 280:1165, 1969

Oski FA, Miller LD, Deliviria-Papadopoulos M: Oxygen affinity in red cells: changes induced in vivo by propranolol. Science 175:1372, 1972

Pitt B, Ross R: Beta-adrenergic blockade in cardiovascular therapy. Mod Concept Cardiovasc Dis 38: 47, 1969

Powell CE, Slater IH: Blocking of inhibitory adrenergic receptors by dichloro analog of isoproterenol. J Pharmacol Exp Ther 122:480, 1958

Prichard BNC, Gilliam PMS: Assessment of propranolol in angina pectoris: clinical dose response curve and effect on electrocardiogram at rest and on exercise. Br Heart J 33:473, 1971

Reid P, Taylor D, Kelly D, et al: Myocardial infarct extension detected by precordial ST segment mapping. N Engl J Med 290:123, 1974

Roberts WC: Coronary arteries in fatal acute myocardial infarction. Circulation 45:215, 1972

Robinson BF: Relation of heart rate and systolic blood pressure to the onset of pain in angina pectoris. Circulation 35:1073, 1967

Russell J, Bloom W: Extractable and residual glycogen in tissues of the rat. Am J Physiol 183:345, 1955

Scheuer J, Stezoski S: Effect of physical training on the mechanical and metabolic response of the rat heart to hypoxia. Circ Res 30:418, 1972

Scheuer J, Stezoski S: Protective role of increased myocardial glycogen stores in cardiac anoxia in the rat. Circ Res 27:835, 1970

Schrumpf JD, Sheps DS, Wolfson S, et al: Effects of propranolol on hemoglobin-oxygen affinity in the anginal syndrome. Am J Cardiol 33:170, 1974

Shapell SD, Murray JA, Nasser MG, et al: Acute changes in hemoglobin affinity for oxygen during angina pectoris. N Engl J Med 280:1165, 1969

33

IMPROVED MYOCARDIAL OXYGEN AVAILABILITY IN HUMAN AND EXPERIMENTAL MYOCARDIAL INFARCTION BY PROPRANOLOL

Hiltrud S. Mueller, Anna Religa, Robert G. Evans, and Stephen M. Ayres

INTRODUCTION

Clinical and experimental observations, made during the past decade, support the belief that myocardial infarction develops in a stepwise manner and that myocardial tissue may be salvaged by techniques designed to interrupt this progressive necrotic process.[26,36,58,59] Beta adrenergic blockade,[16,33,56] peripheral vasodilation,[11,13,17,22] cardiac assistance,[8,21,32,35,40,42,45] and early coronary artery surgery [1,15,28] have all been proposed as therapeutic interventions that might salvage myocardial tissue and decrease mortality from acute myocardial infarction. Our early observations that beta adrenergic stimulation produced metabolic deterioration in different stages of coronary artery disease [40,41] together with parallel studies revealing the frequent occurrence of augmented myocardial free fatty acid uptake in complicated infarction [39] suggested that beta adrenergic blockade might be useful in limiting infarct size. Further evidence supporting this are the clinical findings that beta adrenergic blockade decreases chest pain in both angina pectoris and acute myocardial infarction,[14,19,23,27,49,63,64,66] and the observation of Maroko et al [36] that beta adrenergic blockade reduces the size of experimentally produced myocardial infarcts.

We recently presented evidence that myocardial metabolic changes might be a sensitive in-

dicator of infarct size.[39] If this be the case, improvement in myocardial oxygenation with beta adrenergic blockade would be an important preliminary step in evaluating its clinical value. The present paper presents myocardial metabolic observations in 20 patients treated with propranolol during the early stages of acute transmural myocardial infarction without evidence of the left ventricular failure. These results are emphasized by the effect of propranolol on ischemic zone metabolism in experimental myocardial infarction. The studies demonstrate that beta adrenergic blockade is capable of acutely reversing the metabolic abnormalities associated with acute myocardial ischemia.

METHODS

Patients were considered for the present study if the criteria for an acute transmural myocardial infarction were met by development or presence of Q-waves, of acute elevation of ST segments, and by a history characteristic of acute myocardial infarction. Immediately after the diagnosis of acute myocardial infarction was obtained, the patients were admitted to the coronary care unit either directly from the coronary ambulance or from the emergency room.

The study was performed an average of six to eight hours after admission to the hospital. The patient was not included in the study if one or more of the following findings were observed: (1) previous history of cardiac failure; (2) symptoms of present cardiac failure such as cardiac enlargement, dyspnea, or bibasalar rales; (3) pul-

Supported in part by the John A. Hartford Foundation, Inc., and the U.S. Public Health Service National Heart and Lung Institutions Research Grants HL-12323 and HL-08074

monary venous congestion on chest radiography; (4) systolic arterial cuff pressure less than 110 mm Hg; (5) heart rate below 65 beats per minute; (6) atrioventricular or intraventricular conduction delay; and (7) history of asthma or bronchitis.

A #16 polyethylene catheter was advanced into the brachial artery via puncture of the surgically exposed radial artery. A #7 Goodale Lubin catheter was placed into the coronary sinus via cutdown of the left medial basilic vein. A #6 teflon catheter was placed into the right atrium (12 patients), a #5 Swan Ganz catheter into the pulmonary artery (8 patients) via puncture of the right femoral vein, using the Seldinger technique. Cardiac output was determined in eight patients by the direct Fick method. Coronary blood flow was measured by a modification of the method of Krasnow,[31] using I^{125} Antipyrine as the indicator. The details concerning techniques and the determination of oxygen, lactate, pyruvate, and glucose concentrations in the blood as well as plasma pH, oxygen, and carbon dioxide tension[43] and blood concentration of free fatty acids have been published previously.[12,38,62]

After control evaluation 0.1 mg/Kg propranolol was given intravenously in three divided doses at five-minute intervals. Ten minutes after the last administration of propranolol, measurements of hemodynamics, coronary blood flow, and myocardial metabolism were repeated.

Ten mongrel dogs, weighing 15 to 20 Kg, were anesthestized with sodium pentothal. Ventilation was performed through an endotracheal tube with a Harvard pump. The heart was exposed through intrasternal thoractomy and suspended in a pericardial cradle. Through the right atrium, a thin glass cannula was inserted into the coronary sinus. A small catheter was passed through the glass cannula into the vein draining the left descending artery. Acute ischemia was caused by high ligation of the left descending coronary artery. Studies were performed before, 30 minutes after ligation, and 20 minutes after propranolol (1.0 mg/Kg intravenously). Blood was sampled simultaneously from the coronary vein, the coronary sinus, and the femoral artery.

Calculation

Time-tension index per minute, TTM (mm Hg-sec/min) = mean systolic arterial pressure times systolic ejection period times heart rate. Systolic ejection rate, SER (ml/sec/M²) = stroke index divided by systolic ejection period. Coronary vascular resistance, CVR (dynes-sec-cm⁻⁵/1,000)

= mean diastolic arterial pressure minus mean right atrial pressures times diastolic filling period per minute times 1,332 divided by coronary blood flow times 0.75. Myocardial oxygen consumption, MVO_2 (ml/100g/min) = arterial-coronary sinus oxygen difference times coronary blood flow. Myocardial respiratory quotient, MRQ = coronary sinus-arterial CO_2 difference divided by arterial-coronary sinus O_2 difference. Myocardial extraction ratio, EX (percent) = arterial-coronary sinus difference divided by arterial content.

RESULTS

Twenty patients, 19 men and one woman, were studied six to eight hours following hospital admission for acute transmural myocardial infarction. The average age was 55 years and ranged from 36 to 74 years. The electrocardiogram revealed anterior wall infarction in five, anterior-lateral wall infarction in eight, and inferior wall infarction in seven patients. In three instances, the acute inferior wall infarction was associated with severe anterior-lateral wall subendocardial ischemia. Peak creatinine phosphokinase averaged 1,085 units/ml (range 146 to 2,650); initial arterial free fatty acid concentration averaged 987 $\mu M/L$ (range 100 to 1,480), of lactate 1.73 mM/L (range 0.69 to 3.44), glucose concentration averaged 184 mg percent (range 118 to 304). All 20 patients tolerated the intravenously administered propranolol well. None developed dyspnea or other clinical findings of left ventricular failure. Perfusion of skin and urine output remained adequate. Two patients complained of fatigue after propranolol. These symptoms occurred in the presence of a cardiac index of 2.70 and 2.22 L/min/M² and are probably not related to poor organ perfusion. None of the patients developed atrioventricular or intraventricular conduction delays. Anginal pain, unresponsive to meperidine or morphine therapy, disappeared in four patients after propranolol. All patients survived and left the hospital.

Initial Results of Hemodynamics and Myocardial Oxygenation in Acute Myocardial Infarction in Man

Mean values are shown in Tables 1 and 2, individual measurements in Figures 1, 2, and 3. Heart rate varied from 57 to 110 beats per minute and arterial pressures ranged from 104 to 202 mm Hg systolic, 66 to 103 mm Hg diastolic, and

TABLE 1. Effects of Propranolol on Hemodynamics and Arterial Substrate Contents

MEASUREMENT	CONTROL		PROPRANOLOL		% CHANGE	P
	Mean	±σ	Mean	±σ		
n = 20						
Heart rate (beats/min)	80	± 15	73	± 14	− 9	<0.001
Arterial systolic pressure (mm Hg)	130	± 30	107	± 23	−18	<0.001
Arterial diastolic pressure (mm Hg)	72	± 13	62	± 11	−14	<0.001
Arterial mean pressure (mm Hg)	92	± 18	76	± 16	−17	<0.001
Time-tension index (mm Hg sec/min)	2,481	±735	1,954	±531	−21	<0.001
Right atrial pressure	6.6	± 3.0	6.1	± 3.8	− 8	NS
Arterial lactate content (mM/L)	1.65	± 0.65	1.92	± 0.62	+16	0.05
Arterial free fatty acid content (μM/L)	938	±416	873	±454	− 7	NS
n = 8						
Cardiac index, L/min/M^2	2.6	± 0.46	2.0	± 0.38	−23	<0.001
Stroke index, ml/beat/M^2	32	± 6.56	28	± 5.71	−13	<0.01
Pulmonary wedge pressure (mm Hg)	12	± 4.3	14	± 2.9	+27	<0.05
Arterial-pulmonary artery O$_2$ difference (ml/100 ml)	5.0	± 1.47	5.5	± 0.96	+10	<0.01
Systemic vascular resistance (dynes-sec-cm^{-5})	1,451	±547	1,635	±578	+13	<0.001
Systolic ejection rate (ml/sec/M^2)	115	± 34	97	± 29	−16	<0.01

68 to 138 mm Hg mean (Fig. 1). Right atrial pressure varied from 2 to 10 mm Hg and pulmonary wedge pressure, measured in eight patients, ranged from 8 to 20 mm Hg. Cardiac index and arterial-pulmonary artery oxygen difference, also measured in eight of the patients, varied between 1.68 to 3.2 L/min/M² and 3.5 to 5.8 ml/100 ml respectively (Fig. 2).

Coronary blood flow averaged 77 ml/100g/min (range 56 to 96), myocardial oxygen consumption 9.20 ml/100g/min (range 7.24 to 13.8), and myocardial oxygen extraction ratios between 53 to 80 percent (Fig. 3). Coronary sinus oxygen tension varied from 20 to 37 mm Hg. Five patients revealed myocardial lactate production, and five had abnormally low myocardial lactate extraction

(below 15 percent). Lactate extraction was normal in the remaining 10 patients (Fig. 3). Free fatty acid extraction ranged from 0 percent to 50 percent; six patients had free fatty acid extractions in excess of 15 percent.

Effect of Propranolol on Systemic Hemodynamics in Man

Figure 1 shows that heart rate decreased following propranolol administration in all but three patients; the mean changed from 80 to 73 beats per minute. All indices of arterial blood pressure decreased; peak systolic pressure fell from an average of 130 to 107 mm Hg, diastolic pressure

TABLE 2. Effect of Propranolol on Coronary Blood Flow and Myocardial Metabolism

MEASUREMENT	CONTROL		PROPRANOLOL		% CHANGE	P
	Mean	±σ	Mean	±σ		
n = 20						
Coronary blood flow (ml/100g/min)	77	±11	64	± 8.5	− 17	<0.001
Coronary vascular resistance (dynes-sec-cm^{-5}/1000)	67	±14	70	±15	+ 4	NS
		±				
Myocardial O$_2$ consumption (ml/100g/min)	9.20	± 1.94	7.20	± 1.28	− 22	<0.001
Arterial-coronary sinus, O$_2$ difference (ml/100 ml)	11.93	± 1.34	11.21	± 1.68	− 6	<0.001
Coronary sinus O$_2$ tension (mm Hg)	27	± 4.9	29	± 3.9	+ 7	NS
Myocardial O$_2$ extraction (%)	65	± 5.8	62	± 7.0	− 5	NS
Myocardial lactate extraction (%)	14	±15	26	±12	+ 86	<0.001
Myocardial pyruvate extraction (%)	14	±18	14	±27	0	NS
Myocardial free fatty acid extraction (%)	14	±12	16	±10	+ 14	NS
Myocardial glucose extraction (%)	0.4	± 6.3	3.0	± 9.4	+650	NS
Myocardial respiratory quotient	0.81	± 0.09	0.91	± 0.15	+ 12	<0.01

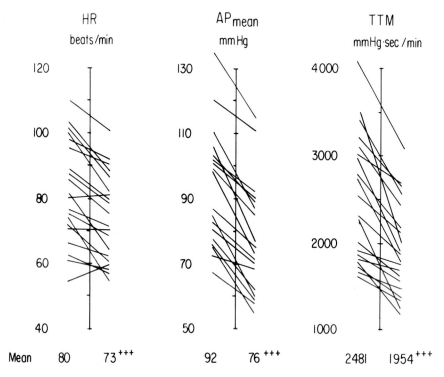

FIG. 1. Hemodynamic effects of propranolol in individual patients. Control values are shown at the left, results after propranolol at the right of the horizontal axis. Heart rate (HR), mean arterial pressure (AP_{mean}), and time-tension index per minute (TTM) uniformly decreased after propranolol. +++ $p < 0.001$

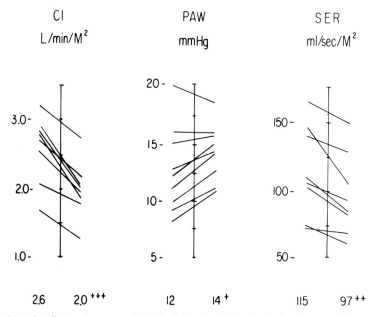

FIG. 2. Hemodynamic effects of propranolol in individual patients. Control values are shown at the left, results after propranolol at the right of the horizontal axis. Cardiac index (CI) and systolic ejection rate (SER) decreased after propranolol. Pulmonary artery wedge pressure (PAW) increased an average of 2 mm Hg. In three instances with the highest initial value, wedge pressure decreased or remained essentially unchanged. +++ $p < 0.001$; ++ $p < 0.01$; + $p < 0.05$

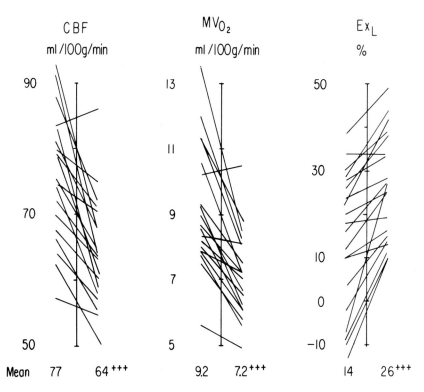

FIG. 3.   Effects of propranolol on myocardial perfusion and metabolism. Control values are shown at the left, results after propranolol at the right of the horizontal axis. Coronary blood flow (CBF) and cardial lactate utilization improved. Lactate production $(-Ex_L)$ shifted to extraction or the rate of lactate extraction increased. +++ p < 0.001

from 72 to 62 mm Hg, and mean arterial pressure from 92 to 76 mm Hg (Fig. 1, Table 1). Pulse pressure decreased from an average of 58 to 45 mm Hg. Time-tension index per minute (TTM) decreased from 2,481 to 1,954 mm Hg sec/min. Peripheral vascular resistance remained essentially unchanged or increased slightly, averaging from 1,450 to 1,645 dynes-sec-cm^{-5}.

Cardiac index decreased in all of the 8 patients in whom it was measured, averaging 2.60 L/min/M^2 before propranolol and 2.05 L/min/M^2 after the intervention (Fig. 2, Table 1). This decrease in cardiac index was associated with a widening of the arterial-pulmonary artery oxygen difference, averaging 0.45 ml/100 ml (p < 0.01). Pulmonary wedge pressure increased an average of two mm Hg. It was unchanged or decreased in three patients with the highest initial values (20, 16, and 15 mm Hg). Systolic ejection rate decreased an average of 15 percent.

Effect of Propranolol on Coronary Blood Flow and Myocardial Metabolism in Man

Coronary blood flow decreased in all but one patient (Fig. 3, Table 2). The decrease aver-

aged 17 percent and was highly significant (p < 0.001). Figure 4 shows that prior to propranolol administration, other factors in addition to arterial pressure determined coronary blood flow. The pressure-flow points were scattered (crosses). Following propranolol administration a fair relationship between mean aortic pressure and coronary blood flow developed (r = 0.43, p = 0.05); the importance of perfusion pressure for coronary blood flow became obvious.

Myocardial oxygen consumption as well as coronary blood flow decreased 22 percent after propranolol (Fig. 3). The arterial-coronary sinus oxygen difference decreased in 15 patients, remained unchanged in four, and increased in one (Fig. 5). The decrease for the entire group averaged 0.72 ml/100 (p < 0.001).

Figure 3 shows that myocardial lactate extraction increased in all but one patient, from an average of 14 percent to 26 percent (p < 0.001). All of the five patients who initially produced lactate shifted to lactate extraction after propranolol (from an average −8 percent to 14 percent). In five other patients, initial lactate extraction was below 15 percent, averaging 10 percent. Propranolol increased the rate of lactate extraction to an average of 18 percent in these patients. Lactate

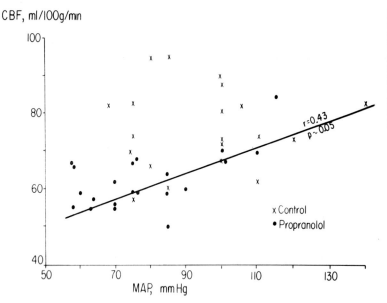

FIG. 4. Coronary pressure-flow relationship. Prior to propranolol administration, other factors in addition to mean aortic pressure (MAP) determined coronary blood flow (CBF); the pressure-flow points were scattered. Propranolol produced a certain pressure-flow relationship; flow became pressure dependent.

extraction increased or remained unchanged in the 10 patients whose initial lactate extraction was normal (above 15 percent).

Dependency of Propranolol Effect on Initial Conditions

Figure 6 shows that decrease in arterial blood pressure correlated with initial values ($p < 0.001$). The behavior of coronary blood flow and myocardial oxygen consumption was similar. Both blood flow and oxygen consumption decreased an average of 22 percent and the de-

crease was closely correlated with the initial levels ($p < 0.001$) (Fig. 7).

Effect of Propranolol on Hemodynamics and Myocardial Oxygenation in Canine Myocardial Infarction

The hemodynamic response to coronary ligation and to propranolol was characteristic (Fig. 8). Heart rate, averaging 158 beats/min during control, remained essentially unchanged after ligation, and decreased an average of 47 beats/min

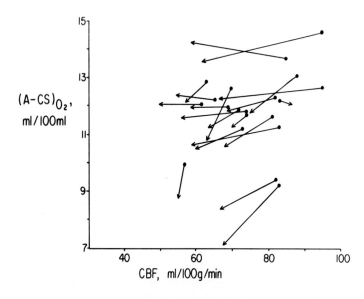

FIG. 5. Effect of propranolol on myocardial oxygen consumption. Propranolol decreased both components of myocardial oxygen consumption: coronary blood flow (CBF) *and,* in most instances, arterial-coronary sinus oxygen difference $(A-CS)_{O_2}$.

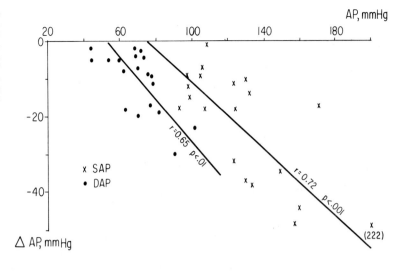

FIG. 6. Dependency of propranolol effect on initial condition. The higher the initial indices of arterial blood pressure, the greater was the decline after propranolol. SAP = systolic arterial pressure (r = 0.65; p < 0.01); DAP = diastolic arterial pressure (r = 0.72; p < 0.001).

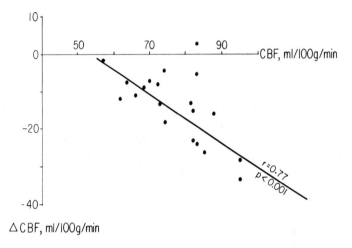

FIG. 7. Dependency of propranolol effect on initial condition. The higher the initial coronary blood flow (CBF) the greater was the decline (r = .077; p < 0.001).

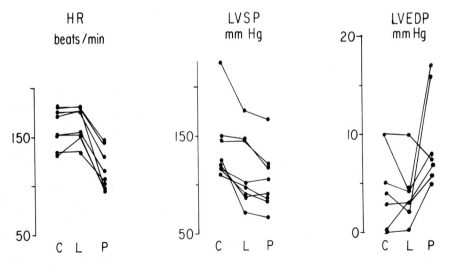

FIG. 8. Effect of propranolol in experimental myocardial infarction. Heart rate (HR), essentially unchanged after ligation (L), uniformly decreased after propranolol (P). Left ventricular systolic pressure (LVSP) fell after ligation and further after propranolol. Left ventricular end diastolic pressure (LVEDP) increased after propranolol, in average 6 mm Hg. C = control.

after propranolol (p < 0.001). Left ventricular systolic pressure, averaging 140 mm Hg during control, decreased 30 mm Hg after ligation (p < 0.01) and a further 7 mm Hg after propranolol (p < 0.05). Left ventricular end-diastolic pressure remained below 10 mm Hg in all but two animals after propranolol; the average increased from 4 to 9 mm Hg (p < 0.05).

The metabolic changes, induced by ligation and by propranolol, are summarized in Figure 9 (mean values). After ligation, myocardial oxygen extraction increased from 69 to 78 percent (p < 0.001). In all but one animal lactate was extracted by the myocardium during the control state. After ligation, lactate extraction of 35 percent shifted to production of 63 percent (p < 0.05). Myocardial glucose extraction increased after ligation from 4 to 13 percent (p < 0.05). Coronary venous pH decreased from 7.32 to 7.26 after ligation. Myocardial free fatty acid extraction ratios varied considerably during the control state, averaging 48 percent. After ligation seven of the 10 animals extracted more than 50 percent free fatty acids. Compared to control, the arterial free fatty acid content remained essentially unchanged or increased after ligation, ranging from 100 to 600 $\mu M/L$. The average free fatty acid extraction ratio increased from 48 percent at control to 63 percent after ligation (NS). Preliminary data

from our laboratory with continuous infusion of C^{14} palmitic acid indicate that only small amounts of labeled CO_2 from the palmitic acid are recovered in the coronary venous blood.

After propranolol administration myocardial lactate production of 63 percent reversed to extraction, averaging 21 percent (p < 0.05) (Fig. 9, mean value). Myocardial glucose extraction markedly decreased, from 13 to 8 percent (p < 0.05). These changes were associated with an increase in coronary venous pH from 7.26 to 7.33 (NS). Myocardial free fatty acid extraction ratios had a tendency to decrease after propranolol; the average fell from 63 to 47 percent (NS). The arterial-coronary venous differences for epinephrine and 1-norepinephrine, narrowing slightly after ligation, consistently increased after propranolol, in averages of 0.43 $\mu g/L$ for epinephrine and 1.51 $\mu g/L$ for 1-norepinephrine. These changes in the arterial-coronary venous differences of catecholamines were due mainly to changes in the coronary venous rather than in the arterial blood. Figure 10 demonstrates catecholamine levels in the coronary venous blood, the vein draining the ischemic area. After ligation, epinephrine and 1-norepinephrine levels increased in most of the experiments; epinephrine content increased from an average of 2.8 to 3.4 $\mu g/L$ (NS), 1-norepinephrine from an average of 4.1 to 4.4 $\mu g/L$ (NS).

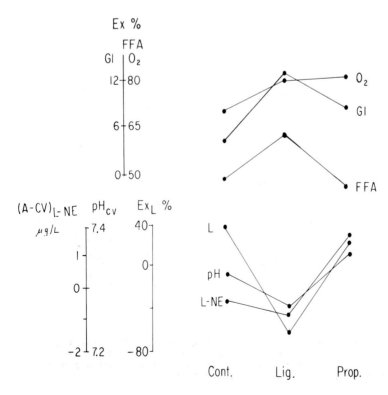

FIG. 9. Response of myocardial metabolism to ligation (Lig) and propranolol (Prop) in experimental myocardial infarction. Cont = control. After ligation, average myocardial oxygen extraction (Ex_{O_2}) increased, lactate extraction (Ex_L) shifted to production and myocardial glucose extraction (Ex_{GL}) increased. pH in the local coronary venous blood strikingly decreased. The arterial-coronary venous difference of l-norepinephrine $(A - CV)_{L-NE}$ decreased, possibly related to local catecholamine release into the circulation. These abnormalities markedly improved following propranolol.

FIG. 10. Catecholamine contents in the coronary venous blood, the effluent ischemic myocardium. After coronary ligation (Lig), epinephrine and l-norepinephrine contents increased in most experiments; following propranolol (Prop), content of both catecholamines consistently decreased, possibly related to diminished local catecholamine release by the myocardium. Cont = control.

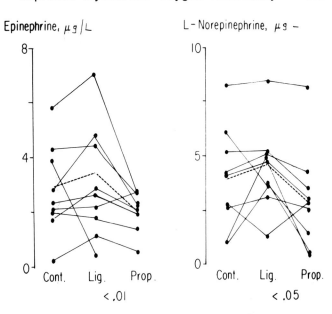

After propranolol, there was a consistent drop in the catecholamine contents. Epinephrine content in the coronary venous blood decreased from an average of 3.4 to 1.8 µg/L (p < 0.01), l-norepinephrine from an average of 4.4 to 2.2 µg/L (p < 0.05).

DISCUSSION

Salvage of jeopardized myocardial tissue is a major goal in the treatment of acute myocardial infarction. The fate of the endangered ischemic tissue, which surrounds the necrotic area following infarction, depends upon the balance between oxygen requirements and supply. The development of drugs, specifically blocking beta adrenergic stimulation, provides a method for determining whether the commonly observed increased adrenergic activity in acute myocardial infarction is a beneficial or potentially harmful adaptive response. The apparent benefits of an increase in myocardial contractility and peripheral perfusion might be overshadowed by the associated increase in myocardial oxygen requirements and by the failure of the diseased coronary bed to dilate adequately during beta adrenergic stimulation.

One of the earliest clinical uses of beta adrenergic blocking drugs was the treatment of patients with angina pectoris. After initial disappointing results with propranolol,[23,50,66] it soon became clear, that if used in high doses, it significantly improved anginal pain and reduced the amount of nitroglycerin required.[19,23,30,50,64] Sub-

sequent studies confirmed the beneficial effect of propranolol on both the patient's symptoms and his capacity to perform exercise before anginal pain occurred.[18,20,44] Robinson [52,53] demonstrated a remarkably constant relationship between development of chest pain and time-tension index per minute, a rough index of myocardial oxygen consumption. Decrease of time-tension index by nitroglycerin [52] or propranolol [34] significantly increased the exercise tolerance of the patients. Wolfson and Gorlin found a striking improvement of anginal pain by propranolol in 90 out of 104 patients, all with angiographically documented coronary artery disease.[63]

The experience with propranolol in human myocardial infarction is rather limited. In 1965, Snow [56,57] first reported a substantial reduction of mortality in acute myocardial infarction in patients who had received propranolol. These results, however, were based on a relatively small number and the studies were performed without placebo control. Several randomized double-blind studies were then initiated.[4,5,10,29] An average of 40 to 80 mg/24 hours propranolol, administered orally in about 250 patients with acute myocardial infarction, did not reveal any definite results or conclusions. Interest in the possible use of propranolol in acute myocardial infarction was revived by observations pointing to the harmful effects of isoproterenol administration in acute myocardial infarction. We demonstrated that isoproterenol produced marked deterioration of myocardial oxygenation in shock following acute myocardial infarction in man.[40] Other investigators showed that isoproterenol increased [36] while propranolol decreased infarct size [36,37] in the experimental animal. The data presented above demonstrates that acute administration of propranolol is able to improve myocardial oxygenation in patients with uncomplicated acute myocardial infarction. Data in canine myocardial infarction demonstrate that propranolol improves oxygenation of the ischemic myocardium.

The most important hemodynamic response to propranolol in our patients appeared to be a substantial decrease in myocardial contractility. This decrease was reflected by the fall in cardiac output and arterial pressure with little change in systemic vascular resistance. The fall in cardiac output was mainly due to a fall in stroke volume since heart rate changed surprisingly little, an average decrease of 7 beats per minute. Recent studies in acute myocardial infarction in man by Amsterdam et al demonstrated similar decreases in cardiac index with propranolol.[3] In both patient groups, the initial cardiac index averaged 2.6 L/min/M² and decreased after propranolol to 2.1 and 2.0 L/min/M² respectively. The mechanism of decrease, however, was different. In Amsterdam's study, cardiac index decreased mainly by fall in heart rate; and in our study, mainly by decrease in stroke volume. Much of this different behavior may be related to the difference in initial heart rate and propranolol dosage. In our patient group, initial heart rate averaged 80/min; in Amsterdam's patients it averaged 99/min. We gave 0.1 mg/Kg propranolol iv; Amsterdam gave 0.03 to 0.05 mg/Kg iv. Further evidence that propranolol reduced contractility in our patients was the increase in pulmonary wedge pressure from an average of 12 to 14 mm Hg. The reduction in contractility and increase in end-diastolic volume may have been greater than that suggested by the observed increases in wedge pressure because of associated alterations in ventricular distensibility.

Variable relationships among left ventricular pressure, volume, and compliance complicate the interpretation of changing pulmonary wedge pressure in ischemic heart disease. Ross,[54] in his Sir Thomas Lewis Lecture of 1969, reviewed the evidence indicating that sudden decreases in ventricular compliance were responsible for the appearance of prominent left ventricular "a" waves in patients with angina pectoris. Scheidt et al [55] reported similar findings in patients with angina pectoris, observing in some instances that acute elevations of left ventricular end-diastolic pressure preceded changes in heart rate and arterial pressure. Direct volume measurements made by Pepine and Wiener [47] demonstrated that end-dias-

tolic volume was unchanged while end-diastolic pressure increased during pacing-induced angina, clearly indicating that myocardial ischemia produced substantial decreases in ventricular compliance.

Our observations that propranolol produced but little change in pulmonary wedge pressure while contractility decreased might be interpreted in light of the compliance changes discussed above. Similar findings were reported by Forrester et al.[16] They noted that propranolol decreased pulmonary wedge pressure from an average of 13 to 12 mm Hg in 14 patients with acute myocardial infarction; cardiac index fell from 5.2 to 3.8 L/min/ M², and systolic blood pressure fell from 135 to 120 mm Hg. Alderman et al [2] demonstrated in patients with coronary artery disease without acute infarction that propranolol increased end-diastolic volume and compliance of the severely diseased left ventricle, but not of the ventricle with normal function. Our findings, together with those of Forrester et al and Alderman et al suggest that beta adrenergic blockade may increase left ventricular compliance in patients with myocardial ischemia, possibly by improving myocardial oxygenation.

The response of myocardial metabolism to propranolol depends upon the effect of beta adrenergic blockade on the determinants of myocardial oxygen consumption: contractility, heart rate, and wall tension. Decreasing contractility and heart rate decrease oxygen consumption. Opposing this is the observation that, in some patients, propranolol increases ventricular volume and fiber length, thus increasing wall tension and oxygen consumption. Our studies, demonstrating a 22 percent decrease in oxygen consumption per minute and a 14 percent decrease in oxygen consumption per beat, indicate that decreases in contractility and heart rate outweigh any increase in wall tension. Further evidence that these decreases in oxygen consumption represent decreased oxygen demand is the narrowing of the arterial coronary sinus oxygen difference and the striking improvement in myocardial lactate metabolism. Stated differently, in the patient group described above, the oxygen-sparing effect of decreased contractility overshadowed any oxygenwasting effect of increased cardiac size.

Direct measurements of ischemic zone metabolism in experimental myocardial infarction demonstrate that propranolol improved oxygenation of the ischemic tissue.[51] The metabolic pattern following coronary ligation, characteristic of severe myocardial hypoxia, could be reversed. After propranolol profound myocardial lactate production shifted to extraction, glucose utilization decreased, and coronary venous pH strikingly improved. Epinephrine and particularly 1-norepinephrine content in the coronary vein, increasing after ligation, consistently decreased following propranolol. These changes in catecholamine levels occurred predominantly in the coronary venous rather than in the arterial blood. It has been shown experimentally that activation of sympathetic receptors in the myocardium can occur immediately after acute myocardial ischemia. Sympathetic fibers to the myocardium are stimulated through very rapid spinal reflexes, causing release of epinephine and 1-norepinephrine from the granules into the circulation.[9] Other studies have revealed that local catecholamine release can be initiated by metabolic changes in the ischemic myocardium itself particularly by changes in myocardial pH.[65] In our experiments propranolol, improving the metabolic condition of the ischemic myocardium, might have decreased release of local catecholamines and thus diminished oxygen demand of ischemic tissue. Similar metabolic observations have been reported by Haneda, Lee, and Ganz.[25]

Coronary blood flow, the most important determinant of myocardial oxygen supply, decreased in all but one of our patients after propranolol administration. This response, previously observed in experimental myocardial infarction[46,61] might suggest propranolol to be harmful in ischemic heart disease. The overall response of the myocardium to any intervention, however, should be considered in terms of both oxygen supply and oxygen need. Our findings that myocardial lactate metabolism improved and oxygen extraction decreased indicate that reduction in myocardial oxygen demand outweighed the decrease in coronary blood flow. The fall in mean aortic pressure from 92 to 76 mm Hg certainly played an important role in the decrease of coronary blood flow from 77 to 64 ml/100g/min. While the group average for coronary vascular resistance changed little with propranolol, 12 patients increased coronary vascular resistance an average of 16 percent ($p < 0.001$). In this group both decreases in perfusion pressure and increases in resistance contributed to a decrease in coronary blood flow. Presumably, a decrease in oxygen demand improved myocardial oxygenation, evoking an autoregulatory response. Although our measurements of total coronary blood flow do not provide information relative to the distribution of blood flow within the myocardium, experimental studies demonstrate that beta adrenergic blockade does not decrease blood flow in ischemic areas. Pitt et al[48]

and Becker, Ferreira, et al[6] using different methods showed that propranolol decreased regional perfusion in nonischemic areas of the myocardium; flow in ischemic regions was essentially unchanged. Labeled microsphere studies enabled Becker, Fortuin, et al[7] to demonstrate that propranolol reversed the maldistribution of coronary blood flow, produced by coronary ligation, improving the perfusion of subendocardial regions.

Our metabolic observations in human myocardial infarction together with our animal studies and those of Haneda, Lee, et al demonstrate that beta adrenergic blockade improved oxygenation of ischemic myocardium. Although these studies present effects following acute propranolol administration, the early use of propranolol in patients with uncomplicated acute myocardial infarction may interrupt the stepwise development of myocardial necrosis, salvage potentially viable myocardium, and improve both immediate mortality and long-term ventricular function.

References

1. Adam M, Mitchel BF, Lambert CJ: Immediate revascularization of the heart. Circulation 42 (suppl II):II–73, 1970
2. Alderman EL, Coltart DJ, Robinson SC, Harrison DC: Effects of propranolol on left ventricular function and diastolic compliance in man. (Abstr) Circulation 48 (suppl IV):IV–87, 1973
3. Amsterdam EA, Hilliard G, Williams DO, et al: Hemodynamic effects of propranolol in acute myocardial infarction (Abstr). Circulation 48 (suppl IV):IV–138, 1973
4. Bay G, Lund-Larsen P, Lorensten E, Silvertssen E: Hemodynamic effects of propranolol in acute myocardial infarction. Br Med J 1:141, 1967
5. Balcon R, Jewitt DE, Davies JPH, Oram S: A controlled trial of propranolol in acute myocardial infarction. Lancet 2:917, 1966
6. Becker L, Ferreira R, Thomas M: Effect of propranolol on ST segment and regional left ventricular blood flow in experimental myocardial ischemia (Abstr). Circulation 46 (suppl II):II–129, 1972
7. Becker LC, Fortuin NJ, Pitt B: Effect of ischemia and antianginal drugs on the distribution of radioactive microspheres in the canine left ventricle. Circulation Research 28:263, 1971
8. Braunwald EJ, Covell W, Maroko PR, Ross J Jr: Effects of drugs and of counterpulsation on myocardial oxygen consumption. Observation on the ischemic heart. Circulation 39 (suppl IV):IV–220, 1969
9. Brown AM, Malliani A: Spinal sympathetic reflexes initiated by coronary receptors. Am J Physiol 212:685, 1971
10. Clausen J, Felsby M, Jorgensen FS, et al: Absence of prophylactic effect of propranolol in myocardial infarction. Lancet 2:920, 1966
11. Cohn JN: Vasodilator therapy for heart failure. The influence of impedance on left ventricular performance. Circulation 48:5, 1973
12. Dole VP: A relation between non-esterified fatty acids in plasma and the metabolism of glucose. J Clin Invest 35:150, 1956

13. Epstein SE: Hypotension, nitroglycerin, and acute myocardial infarction. Circulation 47:217, 1973
14. Epstein SE, Braunwald E: Beta-adrenergic receptor blocking drugs: Mechanisms of action and clinical applications. N Engl J Med 275:1107, 1966
15. Favaloro RG, Effler DB, Cheanvechai C, Quint RA, Sones RM Jr: Acute coronary insufficiency (impending myocardial infarction and myocardial infarction). Surgical treatment by the saphenous vein graft technique. Am J Cardiol 28:598, 1971
16. Forrester J, Chatterjee K, Parmley WW, Swan HJC: Hemodynamic profiles in acute myocardial infarction and their therapeutic implications. (Abstr) Circulation 48 (suppl IV):IV–59, 1973
17. Franciosa JA, Guiha NH, Limas CJ, Rodriguera E, Cohn JN: Improved left ventricular function during nitroprusside infusion in acute myocardial infarction. Lancet 1:650, 1972
18. Gianelly RE, Goldman RH, Treister B, Harrison DC: Propranolol in patients with angina pectoris. Ann Intern Med 67:121, 1967
19. Gilliams PMS, Prichard BNC: Propranolol in the therapy of angina pectoris. Am J Cardiol 18:366, 1966
20. Ginn WM Jr, Orgain EA: Propranolol hydrochloride in the treatment of angina pectoris. JAMA 198:1214, 1966
21. Gold HK, Leinbach RC, Mundth ED, Sanders CA, Buckley MJ: Reversal of myocardial ischemia complicating 84 acute infarction by intra-aortic balloon pumping (IABP). (Abstr) Circulation 46 (suppl II):II–22, 1972
22. Gold HK, Leinbach RC, Sanders CA: Use of sublingual nitroglycerin in congestive failure following acute myocardial infarction. Circulation 46:839, 1972
23. Grant RHE, Keelan P, Kernohan RJ, et al: Multicenter trial of propranolol in angina pectoris. Am J Cardiol 18:361, 1966
24. Hamer J, Grandjean E, Melendez L, Sowton BE: Effect of propranolol (Inderal) on exercise tolerance in angina pectoris. Br Heart J 28:414, 1966
25. Haneda T, Lee T, Ganz W: Metabolic effects of propranolol in the ischemic myocardium studied by regional sampling. (Abstr) Circulation 48 (suppl IV):IV–174, 1973
26. Harnaryan C, Bennett MA, Pentecost BL, Brewer DB: Quantitative study of infarcted myocardium in cardiogenic shock. Br Heart J 32:728, 1970
27. Harrison DC: Circulatory Effects and Clinical Uses of Beta Adrenergic Blocking Drugs. Amsterdam, Excerpta Medica, 1971
28. Hill JD, Kerth WJ, Kelly JJ, et al: Emergency aortocoronary bypass for impending or extending myocardial infarction. Circulation 43 (suppl I):I–105, 1971
29. Kahler RL, Brill SJ, Perkins WE: The role of propranolol in the management of acute myocardial infarction. In Kattus AA, Ross G, Hall VE (eds): Cardiovascular Beta Adrenergic Responses. Berkeley, Univ of Calif Press, 1970, p 213
30. Keelan P: Double-blind trial of propranolol (Inderal) in angina pectoris. Br Med J 1:897, 1965
31. Krasnow N, Rolett EL, Yuchak PM, et al: Isoproterenol and cardiovascular performance. Am J Med 37:514, 1964
32. Leinbach RC, Gold HK, Buckley MJ, Austen WG, Sanders CA: Reduction of myocardial injury during acute infarction by early application of intraaortic balloon pumping and propranolol. (Abstr) Circulation 48 (suppl IV):IV–101, 1973
33. Libby P, Maroko PR, Covell JW, et al: The effects of practolol on left ventricular function and infarct

34. Macalpin RN, Kattus AA, Winfield ME: Effect of a B-adrenergic-blocking agent (Nethalide) and nitroglycerin on the exercise tolerance in angina pectoris. Circulation 31:869, 1965
35. Maroko PR, Bernstein EF, Libby P, et al: The effects of intraaortic balloon counterpulsation on the severity of myocardial ischemic injury following acute coronary occlusion. Circulation 45:1150, 1972
36. Maroko PR, Kjekshus JK, Sobel BE, et al: Factors influencing infarct size following experimental coronary artery occlusion. Circulation 43:67, 1971
37. Maroko PR, Libby P, Braunwald E: Effects of pharmacologic interventions on left ventricular function in the severely ischemic heart. (Abstr) Circulation 46 (suppl II):II–29, 1972
38. Mosinger F: Photometric adaptation of Dole's microdetermination of free fatty acids. J Lipid Research 6:157, 1965
39. Mueller H, Ayres SM: Prognostic implications of varying myocardial fatty acid and carbohydrate metabolism in acute myocardial infarction in man. (Abstr) Circulation 46 (suppl II):II–195, 1972
40. Mueller H, Ayres SM, Giannelli S Jr, et al: Effect of isoproterenol, l-norepinephrine, and intraaortic counterpulsation on hemodynamics and myocardial metabolism in shock following acute myocardial infarction. Circulation 45:335, 1972
41. Mueller H, Ayres SM, Grace WJ: Effects of propranolol and l-norepinephrine in acute myocardial infarction in man. (Abstr) Am J Cardiol 29:282, 1972
42. Mueller H, Ayres SM, Grace WJ: Hemodynamic and myocardial metabolic response to external counterpulsation in acute myocardial infarction in man. (Abstr) Am J Cardiol 31:149, 1973
43. Mueller H, Ayres SM, Gregory JJ, Giannelli S Jr, Grace WJ: Hemodynamics, coronary blood flow and myocardial metabolism in coronary shock: response to l-norepinephrine and isoproterenol. J Clin Invest 49:1885, 1970
44. Nestel PJ: Evaluation of propranolol ("Inderal") in the treatment of angina pectoris. Med J Aust 2:1274, 1966
45. Parmley W, Chatterjee K, Michael TD, Forrester JS, Swan HJC: Systolic unloading with nitroprusside and diastolic augment with external counterpulsation (cardiassist^R): non invasive application of the principles of circulatory assist. (Abstr) Am J Cardiol 31:151, 1973
46. Parratt JR, Grayson J: Myocardial vascular reactivity after beta-adrenergic blockade. Lancet 1:338, 1966
47. Pepine CJ, Wiener L: Relationship of anginal symptoms to lung mechanics during myocardial ischemia. Circulation 46:863, 1972
48. Pitt B, Craven P: Effect of propranolol on regional myocardial blood flow in acute ischemia. Cardiovasc Res 4:176, 1970
49. Prichard BNC, Gillam PMS: Assessment of propranolol in angina pectoris: clinical dose response curve and effect on electrocardiogram at rest and on exercise. Br Heart J 33:473, 1971
50. Rabkin R, Stables DP, Levin NW, Suzman MM: The prophylactic value of propranolol in angina pectoris. Am J Cardiol 18:370, 1966
51. Religa A, Mueller H, Evans R, Ayres SM: Metabolic effect of propranolol on ischemic tissue in human and experimental myocardial infarction. (Abstr) Clin Res 21:954, 1974
52. Robinson BF: The relation of heart rate and systolic

blood pressure to the onset of pain in angina pectoris. Doctoral thesis, Univ of London, 1966

53. Robinson BF: Relation of heart rate and systolic blood pressure to the onset of pain in angina pectoris. Circulation 35:1073, 1967

54. Ross RS: Pathophysiology of coronary circulation. Br Heart J 33:173, 1971

55. Scheidt S. Wilner G, Wolk M, et al: Left ventricular dysfunction in "unstable angina pectoris." (Abstr) Circulation 46 (suppl II):II–105, 1972

56. Snow PJD: Treatment of acute myocardial infarction with propranolol. Am J Cardiol 18:458, 1966

57. Snow PJD: Effect of propranolol in myocardial infarction. Lancet 2:551, 1965

58. Sobel BE, Bresnahan GF, Shell WE, Yoder RD: Estimation of infarct size and its relation to prognosis. Circulation 46:640, 1972

59. Sobel BE, Shell WE: Jeopardized, blighted, and necrotic myocardium. Circulation 47:215, 1973

60. Srivastava SC, Dewar HA, Newell DJ: Double-blind trial of propranolol (Inderal) in angina of effort. Br Med J 2:724, 1964

61. Stein PD, Brooks HL, Matson JL, Hyland JW:

Effect of beta-adrenergic blockade on coronary blood flow. Cardiovasc Res 2:63, 1967

62. Trout DL, Estes EH Jr, Friedberg SJ: Titration of free fatty acids of plasma: a study of current methods and a new modification. J Lipid Research 1:199, 1960

63. Wolfson S, Gorlin R: Effects of propranolol in the diseased heart. In Kattus AA, Ross G, Hall VE (eds): Cardiovascular Beta Adrenergic Responses. Berkeley, Univ of Calif Press, 1970, p 151

64. Wolfson S, Heinle RA, Herman MV, et al: Propranolol and angina pectoris. Am J Cardiol 18: 345, 1966

65. Wollenberger A, Krause EG, Shabab L: Endogenous catecholamine mobilization and the shift to anaerobic energy production in the acutely ischaemic myocardium. In International Symposium on Coronary Circulation and Energetics of the Myocardium. Basel, S Karger, 1967

66. Zeft HJ, Patterson S, Orgain ES: The effect of propranolol in the long-term treatment of angina pectoris. Arch Intern Med 124:588, 1969

34

EFFECTS OF NITROGLYCERIN ON CARDIAC FUNCTION IN ACUTE MYOCARDIAL INFARCTION

David O. Williams, Jorge Otero, James Lies,
Richard R. Miller, Dean T. Mason,
and Ezra A. Amsterdam

The remarkable efficacy of nitroglycerin (NTG) in angina pectoris is well known. Equally emphasized, however, has been the traditional admonition against the use of this agent in patients with myocardial infarction because of the observed decline in systemic arterial pressure that results from the drug.

Recognition of the significance of the balance between myocardial oxygen demand and supply as the determinant of myocardial ischemia has led to interest in therapeutic interventions that may favorably affect this relation in order to preserve viable myocardium in acute myocardial infarction.[1] In addition, agents that reduce ventricular afterload or impedance to left ventricular ejection have the potential of improving left ventricular function during acute myocardial infarction without augmenting myocardial oxygen demand.[2] On the basis of these considerations, we investigated the hemodynamic effects of nitroglycerin administered sublingually to patients with acute myocardial infarction.

METHODS

The study group was composed of 16 randomly selected patients who demonstrated typical clinical, electrocardiographic, and serum enzyme manifestations of acute myocardial infarction. There were 13 men and three women in the group. The age of the patients ranged from 47 to 86 years (mean age 63.3 years). No patient was receiving diuretic agents, digitalis compounds, sympathomimetic drugs, or beta adrenergic blocking agents.

Eight patients had transmural anterior myocardial infarction, six had transmural inferior myocardial infarction and two patients had nontransmural infarctions. After informed consent was obtained, an arterial needle was inserted into a peripheral artery, and a flow-directed, balloon-tipped catheter was inserted into the pulmonary artery. Control pressures and cardiac output, determined in duplicate by the indicator dilution technique, were then obtained. Nitroglycerin, 0.4 mg, was then administered sublingually, and hemodynamic data were obtained at 5 to 10, 10 to 15, and 20 to 30 minutes. All patients were studied within 72 hours of the onset of symptoms of acute myocardial infarction.

Student's t-test for paired data analysis was used for all statistical calculations.

RESULTS

Results of hemodynamic studies are shown in Table 1. Data were analyzed after the patients were divided into two groups according to pulmonary artery wedge (PAW) pressure. Group I included those individuals whose control pulmonary artery wedge pressure (PAW) was 12 mm Hg or less (n = 6); Group II consisted of those individuals in whom PAW was over 12 mm Hg (n = 10). Fall in pulmonary artery wedge pressure was significant in both groups but of greater magnitude in those patients with initially elevated levels. In Group I, pulmonary wedge pressure declined from 7 to 4 mm Hg (p < 0.05). In Group II, reduction from 19 mm Hg to 9 mm Hg (p < 0.01) followed nitroglycerin.

A small but significant rise in heart rate, from 71 to 80 beats per minute, was seen in

TABLE 1. Mean Values

	GROUP I					GROUP II				
	Control	5–10	10–15	20–30	P	Control	5–10	10–15	20–30	P
Rate (beats/min)	71	80	77	74	<0.02	80	83	78	79	NS
PAW (mm Hg)	7	4	5	6	<0.05	19	9	12	14	<0.01
Systemic arterial pressure (mm Hg)										
Systolic	150	128	143	148	<0.01	120	110	116	120	<0.05
Diastolic	78	76	75	75	NS	71	63	66	68	<0.05
Mean	100	89	96	98	<0.02	92	78	82	85	<0.02
Cardiac index (L/min/M^2)	1.83	1.75	1.66	1.60	<0.05	1.77	1.31	1.57	1.64	<0.02
Stroke index (cc/M^2)	26	23	21	23	<0.05	24	18	21	22	<0.01
Peripheral vascular resistance (dynes-sec-cm^{-5})	2,600	2,600	2,643	2,649	NS	2,311	2,844	2,311	2,177	NS

Group I. In Group II, however, there was no significant change in heart rate.

Significant changes in mean systemic arterial pressure occurred in both groups. Group I, with an initial mean pressure of 100 mm Hg, exhibited a decline to 89 mm Hg after NTG (p < 0.02). Group II demonstrated a fall in mean arterial pressure of 92 to 78 mm Hg (p < 0.02).

In Group I patients, there was a 13 percent decrease in cardiac index from 1.83 to 1.60 L/min/m^2 (p < 0.05). Group II, however, demonstrated a decline of 26 percent from 1.77 to 1.31 L/min/m^2 (p < 0.01).

Control peripheral vascular resistance was elevated in both Groups I and II with values of 2,600 and 2,300 dynes sec cm^{-5}, respectively. Although there was a slight increase in peripheral resistance in both groups following NTG administration, neither of these changes was statistically significant.

DISCUSSION

Previous investigators have documented the hemodynamic effects of nitroglycerin in patients without coronary artery disease.[2-4] Mean systemic arterial pressure uniformly decreases, cardiac output decreases or changes minimally, and peripheral vascular resistance and venous tone, as measured in the human forearm, both decrease.[5] In addition, there is a reduction in calculated cardiac dimensions, both end systolic and end diastolic volumes diminishing. Decrease in the latter is of greater magnitude, resulting in a decrease in stroke volume.

Similar decreases in mean systemic arterial pressure, left ventricular end diastolic pressure, and pulmonary artery pressures have been noted in patients with angina pectoris consequent to coronary artery disease. Decreases in cardiac index are more consistently observed [6-9] after the nitrite

in patients with coronary artery disease than in subjects without cardiac disease.

There is only one prior report of the hemodynamic effects of nitroglycerin during myocardial infarction in man. In this study, Gold et al [11] administered nitroglycerin to patients in several stages of infarction and noted decreases in pulmonary artery wedge pressure and mean systemic arterial pressure. However, changes in cardiac output varied according to prenitroglycerin pulmonary artery wedge pressure. In those patients with elevated wedge pressure, cardiac output rose after nitroglycerin, and in those with normal wedge pressure there was a fall in cardiac output.

Our study demonstrated that nitroglycerin given during the acute phase of myocardial infarction results in a decline in pulmonary artery wedge pressure irrespective of initial pressure. Our findings differ from those of Gold, et al, however, in demonstrating a consistent decrease in cardiac output associated with the fall in pulmonary wedge, or left ventricular filling, pressure.

Thus, it appears that nitroglycerin administered during the acute phase of myocardial infarction manifests its predominant effect on left ventricular preload through its major action of systemic venodilation.[4] This decrease in left ventricular filling pressure is reflected in a fall in cardiac index and mean arterial pressure resulting in downward movement along the ascending limb of the ventricular function curve.

Reduction in left ventricular filling pressure and mean arterial pressure with little increase in pulse rate suggests a net decrease in myocardial oxygen demand, a favorable effect in terms of reducing myocardial ischemia. However, the decrease in cardiac index and perfusion pressure may counter this effect by decreasing coronary flow. Interestingly, and contrary to previous impressions, in this study nitroglycerin did not reduce ventricular afterload as reflected by changes in peripheral vascular resistance. This may be due to the vasoconstriction induced by reflex sympathetic stimulation overriding the direct vasodilating effects of the nitrite.

Thus, it is apparent that in acute myocardial infarction, nitroglycerin causes a prompt decrease in ventricular preload and decreases several major determinants of myocardial oxygen demand. These actions would confer special benefit on patients with pulmonary vascular congestion complicating acute myocardial infarction. However, these favorable effects must be weighed against a predictable, mild reduction in arterial blood pressure and cardiac output, which also result from nitroglycerin administration.

References

1. Maroko PR, Kjekshas JK, Sobel BE, Watanabe R, Covell JW, Ross J, Jr, and Braunwald E: Factors influencing infarct size following experimental coronary artery occlusions. Circulation 43:67, 1971
2. Franciosa JA, Guiha, NH, Limas CJ, et al: Improved left ventricular function during nitroprusside infusion in acute myocardial infarction. Lancet 1:650, 1972
3. Brachfeld N, Bozer J, Gorlin, R: Action of nitroglycerin on the coronary circulation in normal and mild cardiac subjects. Circulation 29:697, 1967
4. Williams, JF, Glick G, Braunwald E: Studies on cardiac dimensions in intact unanesthetized man, V effects of nitroglycerin. Circulation 32:676, 1967
5. Mason DT, Braunwald E: The effects of nitroglycerin and amyl nitrite on arteriolar and venous tone in the human forearm. Circulation 32:755, 1965
6. Gorlin R, Brachfeld N, MacLeod C, et al: Effect of nitroglycerin on the coronary circulation in patients with coronary artery disease or increased left ventricular work. Circulation 19:705, 1959
7. Chlong NA, West RO, Parker JO: Influence of nitroglycerin on myocardial metabolism and hemodynamics during angina induced by atrial pacing. Circulation 45:1044, 1972
8. Lee SJK, Surg KK, Zaragoza AJ: Effects of nitroglycerin on left ventricular volumes and wall tension in patients with ischemic heart disease. Br Heart J 32:790, 1970
9. Najmi M, Griggs DM, Kasparian H, Novack P: Effects of nitroglycerin on hemodynamics during rest and exercise in patients with coronary insufficiency. Circulation 35:46, 1967
10. Christensson B, Karietors T, Westling H: Hemodynamic effects of nitroglycerin in patients with coronary heart disease. Br Heart J 27:511, 1965
11. Gold HK, Leinback, RC, Sanders, CA: Use of sublingual nitroglycerin in congestive failure following acute myocardial infarction. Circulation 46:839, 1972

35

CORONARY ARTERIAL SPASM IN VARIANT ANGINA PRODUCED BY HYPERVENTILATION AND VALSALVA— DOCUMENTED BY CORONARY ARTERIOGRAPHY

Bertron M. Groves, Frank I. Marcus, Gordon A. Ewy, and Brendan P. Phibbs

INTRODUCTION

In 1959, Prinzmetal described a variant form of angina pectoris that was neither brought on by exertion nor relieved by rest. The pain tended to be more severe than classic angina pectoris and often recurred at about the same time each day. Approximately 50 percent of the patients had ventricular arrhythmias during the peak of their pain. Transient marked elevation of the ST-segments in the distribution of a large coronary artery was considered to be the electrocardiographic indicator of this variant form of angina. Prinzmetal suggested that the pathophysiology of this syndrome was temporary hypertonus or spasm of a large, narrowed coronary artery. His ability to reproduce ST-segment elevation in dogs by intermittently occluding a large coronary artery supported his hypothesis (Prinzmetal et al, 1959).

In 1967, MacAlpin and Kattus reported five patients with variant angina who had fixed high-grade proximal obstruction demonstrated by coronary arteriography (MacAlpin and Kattus, 1967). By 1970, MacAlpin had studied 12 patients with variant angina and found significant fixed focal lesions in each of them (MacAlpin, 1970). Between 1968 and 1973, several authors reported patients with variant angina who had either normal coronary arteriography or lesions that were only mildly stenotic (Bobba et al, 1971; Cheng et al, 1973; Gianelly et al, 1968; Kristian-Kerin et al, 1973; MacAlpin et al, 1973; Whiting et al, 1970). These cases strongly implicated the role of coronary artery spasm in the clinical syndrome of variant angina. From 1972 to 1973, coronary arterial spasm was documented angiographically in eight patients with variant angina who had normal or mildly diseased coronary arteries (Table 1). Seven of these patients had spasm of the right coronary artery (RCA) and one involved the circumflex (CMFX) branch of a single left coronary artery (LCA). The present report describes a patient with variant angina in whom spasm of the left anterior descending coronary artery (LADCA) was documented by angiography. Transient spasm was induced by hyperventilation, Valsalva maneuver, and walking.

CASE REPORT

A 40-year-old Caucasian waitress was in good health until the evening of May 10, 1973, when she experienced the onset of pain in her chest and both arms unrelated to exertion or excitement. The initial episode of pain lasted less than three minutes and was not associated with dyspnea or nausea. That night she awoke twice with similar chest pain, which subsided spontaneously. Episodes of nocturnal chest pain recurred for the three consecutive days prior to her hospitalization on May 15, 1973. The patient had a smoking history of a package a day for 15 years and had taken oral contraceptives for 12 years. Her serum cholesterol was 220 mg percent and triglycerides were 176 mg percent. Her father died at age 46 from an acute myocardial infarction. The admission electrocardiogram (ECG) revealed anterior ischemia with T-wave inversion in leads V_1 through V_4 (Fig. 1). The following day, an ECG taken during an episode of pain revealed transient anterolateral ST elevation and frequent

TABLE 1. Coronary Artery Spasm in Variant Angina

CASE REPORT	AGE/ SEX	ARTERIOGRAPHY BEFORE SPASM	ARTERIOGRAPHY DURING SPASM	ARRHYTHMIAS	TREATMENT AND COMMENTS
Guermonprez 1972	37/M	RCA 50% Proximal 1/3	RCA over 95% Proximal 1/3	– –	SVBG to distal RCA Postop–graft patent
Dhurandhar 1972	52/M	RCA less 50%	RCA over 90% Proximal 1/3	V. tach. V. fib.	SVBG to mid RCA Died six weeks postop Graft patent RCA 75% obstruction proximal 1/3
Cheng 1973	40/M	Normal	RCA over 75% Distal 1/3	–	Propranolol and isosorbide dinitrate–some improvement Repeat cath five years later Coronary arteriography normal Treadmill stress test–negative Atrial pacing– negative
Cheng 1973	43/M	Normal	RCA over 75% Proximal 1/3	–	Nitroglycerin–used as needed Atrial pacing–negative Stress test–negative
Oliva 1973	46/F	Normal	RCA 100% Multiple sites	3° AV block	Permanent pacemaker Isosorbide dinitrate– asymptomatic Bicycle stress test– negative Atrial pacing–negative
MacAlpin 1973	55/F	RCA under 60% Mid 1/3	RCA 50% Proximal	–	SVBG–distal RCA Mid 1/3 RCA spasm during surgery Intraoperative infarction Postop–graft occluded 25 months postop– asymptomatic; treadmill stress test– negative
King M 1973	42/F	RCA 50% Mid 1/3	RCA over 90% Mid 1/3	–	Isosorbide dinitrate– asymptomatic
King S 1973	58/M	Normal Single LCA	CMFX 75% Mid 1/3	3° AV block V. tach. V. fib.	SVBG–distal CMFX Postop–graft occluded Permanent pacemaker Propranolol and isosorbide dinitrate
Groves 1974 (present report)	40/F	LADCA under 60% Proximal 1/3	LADCA 100% Proximal 1/3	PVCs	Isosorbide dinitrate– improved Treadmill stress test– ST elevation

premature ventricular contractions. During the second week of hospitalization she experienced no further chest discomfort. Determinations of LDH and SGOT were normal. Serial ECGs demonstrated transient anterolateral ST elevation alternating with deep symmetric T-wave inversion (Fig. 2).

The patient was transferred to Arizona Medical Center on June 1, 1973, for evaluation of recurrent, painless episodes of ST elevation. Physical examination revealed the presence of a fourth heart sound. Right and left heart catheterization revealed that all intracardiac pressures were normal. The cardiac index was 2.4 liters/minute/

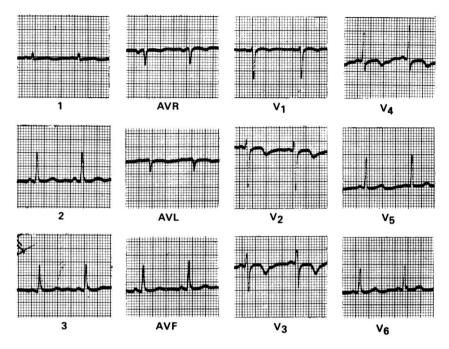

FIG. 1. Admission electrocardiogram taken on May 15, 1973. Note anterior T-wave inversion.

meter.[2] The left ventricular end-diastolic pressure at rest was four to eight mm Hg and rose to 18 to 21 mm Hg after biplane left ventricular (LV) cineangiography. Left ventricular contractility was normal. The LV ejection fraction was 0.60 in the right anterior oblique (RAO) and 0.58 in the left anterior oblique (LAO) view. There was no mitral regurgitation. Sublingual nitroglycerin was given prior to and during selective coronary arteriography performed by Judkin's technique. Coronary artery injections were recorded on 35 mm cineangiography and serial arteriograms in the LAO, lateral, and RAO views. The patient experienced no chest discomfort throughout the catheterization and no ST-segment elevation occurred.

The dominant RCA was normal (Fig. 3). The main left coronary artery was short and free of disease. The circumflex and obtuse marginal branches of the LCA were normal. The proximal left anterior descending coronary artery (LADCA) had two hour-glass-shaped lesions distal to the first septal perforator with an estimated narrowing of 50 to 60 percent (Figs. 4 and 5). The mid and distal segments of the LADCA were normal. The proximal segment of the first septal perforator was narrowed by 50 percent.

The patient's ECG was monitored for several days with no change noted in the anterolateral ischemic pattern. She remained asymptomatic on no medication. On June 6, 1973, the 12 lead ECG was recorded at rest (Fig. 6), during and after hyperventilation (Fig. 7), and during and after the Valsalva maneuver (Fig. 8). She experienced no discomfort but had ST-segment elevation as compared with the control ECG during and after these maneuvers. She was then walked on a treadmill at 1.7 mph at 0⁰ elevation for a total of three minutes. She had no pain or fatigue from this mild level of exertion but because of the development of marked anterolateral ST-segment elevation, the procedure was terminated (Fig. 9).

After it was determined that the ST-segment elevation could be produced by these maneuvers, the patient was again taken to the catheterization laboratory and selective catheterization of the LCA by Judkin's technique was performed. During this study, a vasodilator was not given. Multiple views of the LCA were recorded on both 35 mm cineangiography and serial arteriograms to reconfirm the low-grade obstructions previously described (Fig. 10). While monitoring lead V_4 the patient was asked to hyperventilate, and no ST-segment change was detected. Similarly, no change was produced by performance of a single Valsalva maneuver. However, when two Valsalva maneuvers were performed in sequence, it was noticed that the inverted T-wave in V_4 became upright and the ST-segment began to rise. A repeat cinean-

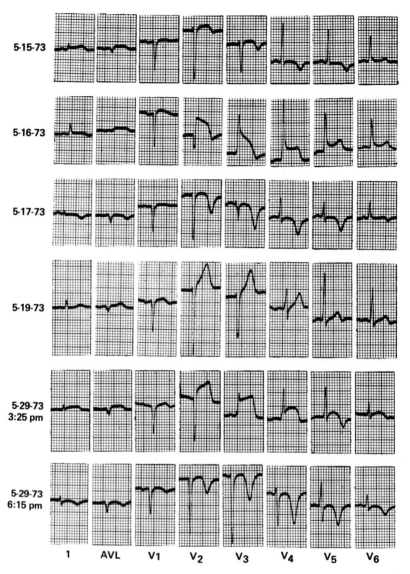

FIG. 2. Serial electrocardiograms. The ECG on May 16, 1973, was taken during chest pain. There is marked anterolateral ST-segment elevation, which was transient. Both ECGs on May 29, 1973, were taken while the patient was asymptomatic. The 6:15 P.M. tracing on May 29, 1973, demonstrates the degree of anterolateral ischemia, which persisted at the time of transfer and initial cardiac catheterization.

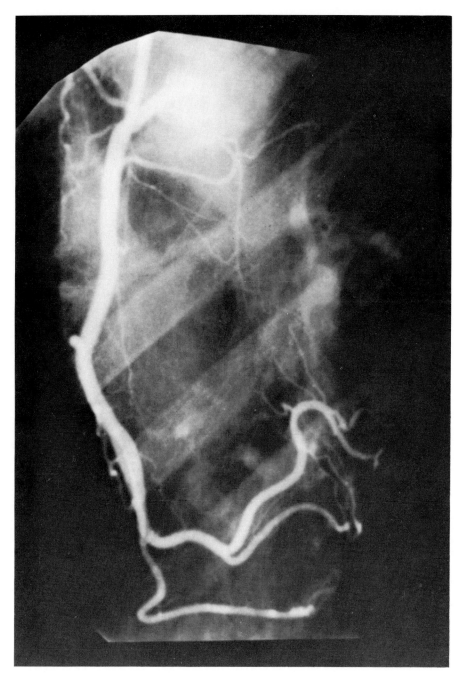

FIG. 3. Normal right coronary arteriogram, left anterior oblique view.

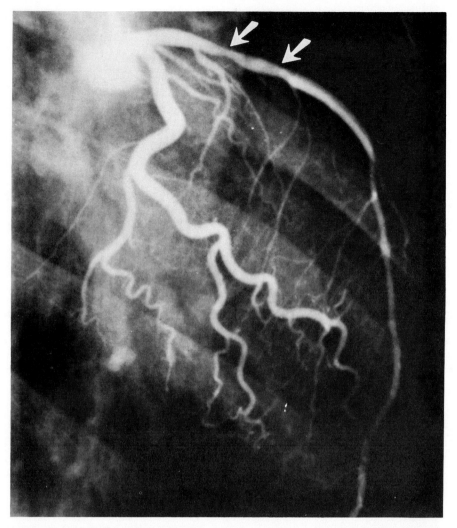

FIG. 4.   Left coronary arteriogram, right anterior oblique view. This arteriogram done on June 19, 1973, after sublingual nitroglycerin, demonstrates two proximal lesions (arrows) in the left anterior descending coronary artery with less than 60 percent obstruction.

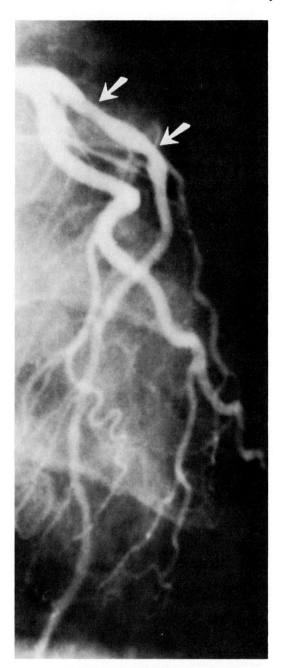

FIG. 5. Left coronary arteriogram, shallow right anterior oblique view. The arrows point to the two lesions in the proximal left anterior descending coronary artery (LADCA). Note the absence of disease in the mid and distal segments of the LADCA.

giographic injection of the LCA in the RAO view documented complete obstruction of the LADCA at the site of the most proximal lesion. The patient experienced no chest discomfort. After the ST-segment elevation resolved spontaneously within one minute, a repeat LCA injection documented resolution of the obstruction. The above sequence of events was repeated and total transient obstruction of the proximal LADCA occurred and was documented on serial arteriograms (Figs. 11 and 12).

During a 24-hour period of unrestricted activity, lead V_4 was monitored on a tape recorder. Recurrent episodes of ST-segment elevation occurred with and without the patient's awareness of chest discomfort (Fig. 13). The patient was treated with sublingual isosorbide dinitrate 10 mg every three hours while awake. Over a period of two weeks, the electrocardiographic pattern of anterolateral ischemia showed marked improvement (Fig. 14). No further episodes of chest pain or ST-segment elevation occurred. While on vasodilator therapy, a repeat 24-hour tape monitoring lead V_4 revealed no episodes of ST-segment elevation during unrestricted activity. A repeat treadmill stress test was performed. The patient exercised a total of 10 minutes before reaching her 90 percent predicted maximal heart rate. No chest discomfort, ST-segment abnormality, or arrhythmia was produced during or after exercise (Fig. 15). The patient was discharged on sublingual isosorbide dinitrate, 10 mg every three hours while awake. Eight months following discharge, she was working full time but continued to experience occasional chest discomfort.

DISCUSSION

The most common etiology of coronary arterial spasm is mechanical stimulation by an angiographic catheter (Demany et al, 1968; Gensini et al, 1962; Gorlin, 1965; and O'Reilly, 1970). The findings presented in the present case report were interpreted as episodic, transient coronary arterial spasm producing complete obstruction of the proximal LADCA. The clinical manifestations were chest pain and transient anterolateral ST-segment elevation. Several factors support the view that the coronary arterial spasm demonstrated in this patient was not induced by catheter manipulation. The area of spasm was located well beyond the depth of catheter penetration. The spasm

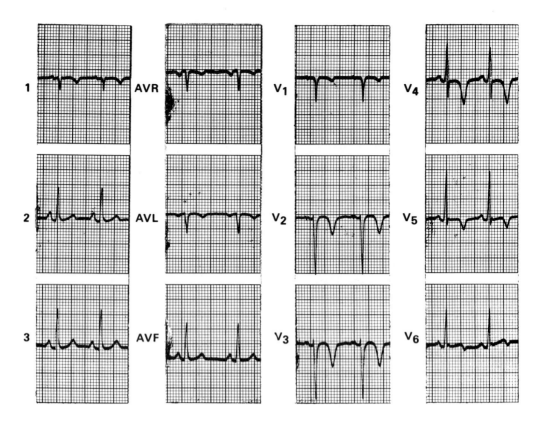

FIG. 6. Baseline electrocardiogram on June 6, 1973. The degree of anterolateral ischemia is comparable to the ECG taken at 6:15 P.M. on May 29, 1973, in Figure 2.

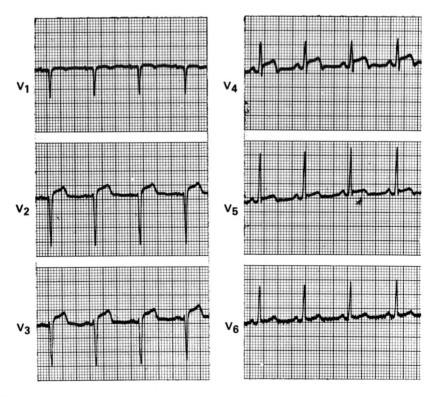

FIG. 7. Leads V_1 to V_6 of an electrocardiogram recorded immediately after hyperventilation. Note ST-segments returned to the baseline and T-waves became deeply inverted in V_2 to V_5.

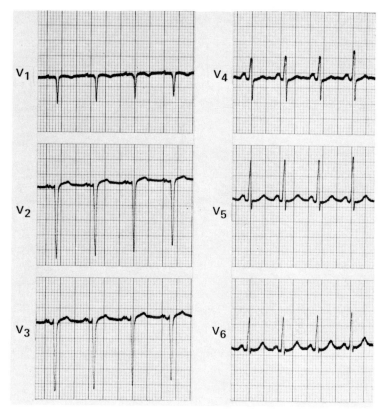

FIG. 8. Leads V_1 to V_6 of the electrocardiogram recorded immediately after Valsalva. Minor ST-segment elevation is present in V_2 to V_3 and the T-waves have become upright when compared to the control ECG in Figure 6.

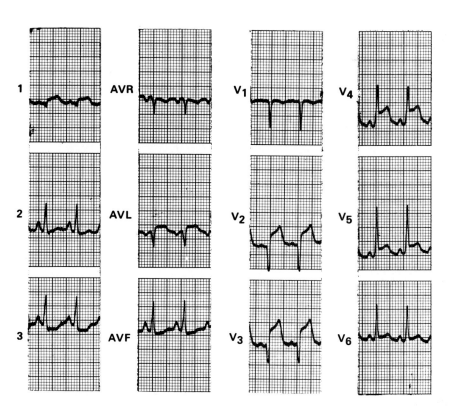

FIG. 9. Electrocardiogram recorded after three minutes of walking 1.7 miles per hour at 0 degrees elevation. Marked anterolateral ST-segment elevation is present in leads 1, AVL, and V_2 to V_6. The patient was asymptomatic.

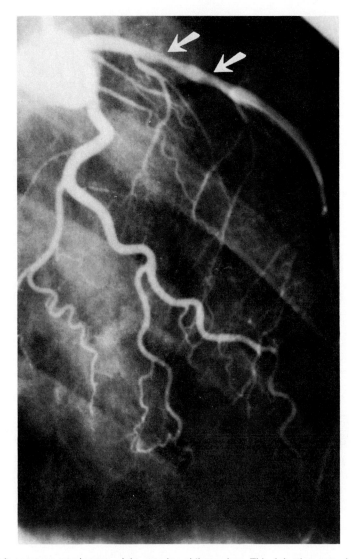

FIG. 10. Left coronary arteriogram, right anterior oblique view. This injection was done on June 6, 1973, without vasodilation. Arrows indicate the proximal lesions in the left anterior descending coronary artery, which are similar to Figure 4.

was produced and reproduced immediately after the patient performed the Valsalva maneuver while the left coronary catheter was not manipulated. Finally, the same electrocardiographic evidence for spasm had been observed during performance of the same maneuvers prior to the repeat catheterization.

The ability to produce transient spasm in this patient during coronary arteriography was based upon our observations during physiologic testing. Previous reports of patients with variant

angina have noted episodes of chest pain and ST-segment elevation in association with Valsalva maneuver, cold pressor test (Sawayama et al, 1965), drinking ice water (Hilal and Massumi, 1967), rapid eye movement sleep (King et al, 1973), and following ingestion of alcohol (Fernandez et al, 1973).

The production of coronary arterial vasoconstriction by hyperventilation was suggested by Nowlin, who monitored the electroencephalogram during sleep in patients with nocturnal angina.

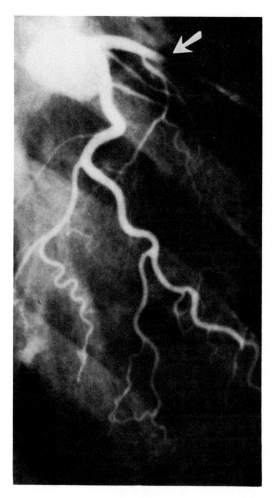

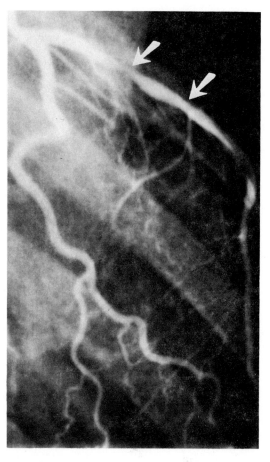

FIG. 11. Left coronary arteriogram, right anterior oblique view. This injection was done on June 6, 1973, immediately after Valsalva when the ST-segment was elevated in V_4. Note complete occlusion of the left anterior descending coronary artery at the site of proximal narrowing. The patient was asymptomatic.

FIG. 12. Left coronary arteriogram, right anterior oblique view. This injection was performed immediately after the arteriogram in Figure 11, when the ST-segment elevation had resolved within one minute. When compared to the control arteriogram in Figure 10, the proximal area of narrowing is more severe but contrast promptly filled the mid- and distal segments at the left anterior descending coronary artery. Later injections confirmed total resolution of the proximal spasm.

He reported one patient who developed ST-segment depression in response to hyperventilation that occurred shortly after the onset of rapid eye movements. He proposed that lowering of the arterial P_{CO_2} by hyperventilation might produce coronary arterial vasoconstriction (Nowlin et al, 1965).

The mechanism by which coronary arterial spasm was produced by the Valsalva maneuver in our patient is unknown. In response to the systemic hypotension produced by the increased intrathoracic pressure and reduced venous return from performance of the Valsalva maneuver, several re-

flex pressor mechanisms are stimulated. Intense vasoconstriction is part of this response (Gorlin et al, 1957; Sarnoff et al, 1948). The Valsalva maneuver was reported by Benchimol to decrease left coronary phasic arterial blood flow velocity by 45 percent as measured by a Doppler flowmeter catheter (Benchimol et al, 1972). It is possible that coronary arterial vasoconstriction is produced by the Valsalva maneuver.

Characteristically, patients with variant angina do not develop chest pain or electrocardiographic evidence of myocardial ischemia with exertion. It is important to emphasize that prior

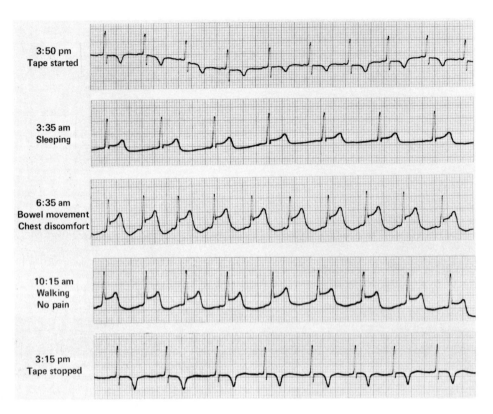

FIG. 13. 24-hour tape recording of lead V_4 prior to treatment. Transient ST-segment elevation occurred during sleep and ambulation when the patient was asymptomatic and during a bowel movement when she had chest discomfort. No arrhythmia occurred.

to treatment our patient developed marked ST-segment elevation during minimal exertion with no awareness of chest discomfort. Two weeks later, while taking sublingual isosorbide dinitrate on a regular schedule, her baseline ECG revealed resolution of the ischemic pattern. A repeat treadmill stress test at that time demonstrated that she was able to attain 90 percent of her predicted maximum heart rate with no chest discomfort or significant electrocardiographic changes.

Eight case reports in the literature have documented by angiography the existence of coronary arterial spasm in patients with variant angina (Table 1). In all of these cases, spasm involved the coronary circulation to the inferior wall of the left ventricle. Spasm of the main left coronary artery or left anterior descending coronary artery in variant angina has not been previously reported. All nine cases summarized in Table 1 had either normal coronary arteriography or less than 60 percent obstruction before spasm occurred. Four of these patients experienced significant arrhythmias.

Two required permanent transvenous pacemakers to treat recurrent complete heart block. Four patients were treated with aortocoronary saphenous vein bypass grafts. Postoperative angiograms in three patients revealed graft occlusion in two. The fourth patient treated surgically died six weeks later and was found to have a patent graft on postmortem examination. In this patient, the placement of the graft proximal to the acute marginal branch of the RCA may have been significant in view of multiple and variable areas of spasm that were demonstrated in the patient reported by Oliva. He pointed out that additional distal coronary arterial spasm could nullify the benefit of a more proximal graft (Oliva et al, 1973). It is possible that postoperative coronary arterial spasm was an adverse factor in the results of surgical therapy in variant angina reported by MacAlpin (MacAlpin et al, 1973).

Based upon experience with this patient and a review of the literature, it is our opinion that patients who present with variant angina may have

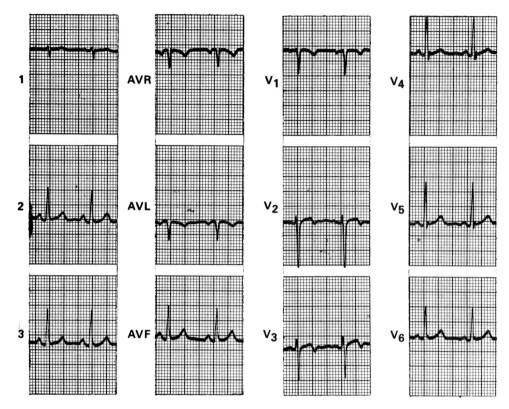

FIG. 14. Control electrocardiogram on June 20, 1973, while on sublingual isosorbide dinitrate. Minor T-wave changes are the only residual abnormality.

any one of three angiographic patterns: (1) normal coronary anatomy; (2) less than 60 percent narrowing of a large coronary artery; and (3) high-grade stenosis of a large coronary artery. Coronary arterial spasm may be superimposed upon any of the above baseline angiographic patterns. Surprisingly, angiographic documentation of coronary arterial spasm in a patient with a fixed, high-grade stenotic lesion has not been reported. When spasm occurs, its location correlates well with the distribution of ST-segment elevation.

No clinical finding has been demonstrated to predict accurately the coronary angiographic findings in patients with variant angina. Therefore, it is necessary to perform coronary angiography in all patients with variant angina for selection of appropriate therapy. When this condition is suspected, we recommended that the use of vasodilators be avoided if possible during the initial selective coronary arteriograms. If a lesion is found, repeat arteriograms should be made in multiple views after vasodilation. In cases with minimal or no coronary artery disease, it may prove helpful to have the patient perform hyperventilation and the Valsalva maneuver in an effort to produce coronary arterial spasm during catheterization. The cold pressor test may also be used.

In the absence of high-grade obstructive disease, vasodilator therapy appears to be the treatment of choice in most patients with variant angina. A pacemaker may be needed to control complete heart block. A combination of saphenous vein bypass grafting and vasodilator therapy may be required when medical therapy alone is unsuccessful.

ACKNOWLEDGMENTS

The authors wish to thank Dr. Edward Kennedy, Ganado, Arizona, for referring this patient to the Arizona Medical Center and providing the electrocardiograms used in Figures 1 and 2. We also acknowledge the secretarial assistance of Miss Deena Falkow and the services of the Audiovisual Department of the Arizona Medical Center.

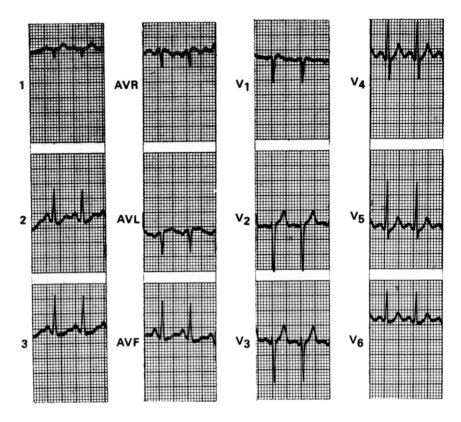

FIG. 15. Electrocardiogram taken immediately after submaximal treadmill stress test on June 20, 1973. T waves are upright in V_2 to V_6. No abnormality of the ST-segment developed.

References

Benchimol A, Wang TF, Desser KB, Gartlan JL: The Valsalva maneuver and coronary arterial blood flow velocity. Ann Intern Med 77:357, 1972

Bobba P, DiGuglielmo L, Vecchio C, Montemartini C: Coronarographic patterns in Prinzmetal's variant angina. Acta Cardiol 26:568, 1971

Cheng TO, Bashour T, Kelser GA, Weiss L, Bacos J: Variant angina of Prinzmetal with normal coronary arteriograms—a variant of the variant. Circulation 47:476, 1973

Demany MA, Tambe A, Zimmerman HA: Coronary arterial spasm. Dis Chest 53:714, 1968

Dhurandhar RW, Watt DL, Silver MD, Trimble AS, Adelman AG: Prinzmetal's variant form of angina with arteriographic evidence of coronary arterial spasm. Am J Card 30:902, 1972

Fernandez D, Rosenthal JE, Cohen LS, Hammond G, Wolfson S: Alcohol-induced Prinzmetal variant angina. Am J Card 32:238, 1973

Gensini GG, DiGiorgi S, Murad-Netto S, Black A: Arteriographic demonstration of coronary artery spasm and its release after the use of a vasodilator in a case of angina pectoris and in the experimental animal. Angiology 13:550, 1962

Gianelly R, Mugler F, Harrison DC: Prinzmetal's variant of angina pectoris with only slight coronary atherosclerosis. Calif Med 108:129, 1968

Gorlin R: Pathophysiology of cardiac pain. Circulation 32:138, 1965

Gorlin R, Knowles JH, Storey CF: The Valsalva maneuver as a test of cardiac function—pathologic physiology and clinical significance. Am J Med 22:197, 1957

Guermonprez JL, Hiltgen M, Fouchard J, et al: L'angor de Prinzmetal aspects coronarographiques et chirurgicaux. J Radiol Electrol 53:623, 1972

Hilal H, Massumi R: Variant angina pectoris. Am J Card 19:607, 1967

King MJ, Zir LM, Kaltman AJ, Fox AC: Variant angina associated with angiographically demonstrated coronary artery spasm and REM sleep. Am J Med Sci 265:419, 1973

King SB, Mansour KA, Hatcher CR, Silverman ME, Hart NC: Coronary artery spasm producing Prinzmetal's angina and myocardial infarction in the absence of coronary atherosclerosis—surgical treatment. Ann Thor Surg 16:337, 1973

Kristian-Kerin N, Davies B, Macleod CA: Nonocclusive coronary disease associated with Prinzmetal's angina pectoris. Chest 64:352, 1973

MacAlpin R: Variant angina pectoris. N Engl J Med 282:1491, 1970

MacAlpin RN, Kattus AA: Angina pectoris at rest with preservation of exercise capacity—angina inversa. Circulation 35–36 (Supp II):176, 1967

MacAlpin RN, Kattus AA, Alvaro AB: Angina pectoris at rest with preservation of exercise capacity—Prinzmetal's variant angina. Circ 47:946, 1973

Nowlin JB, Troyer WG, Collins WS, et al: The association of nocturnal angina pectoris with dreaming. Ann Intern Med 63:1040, 1965

Oliva PB, Potts DE, Pluss RG: Coronary arterial spasm in Prinzmetal angina—documentation by coronary arteriography. N Engl J Med 288:745, 1973

O'Reilly RJ, Spellberg RD, King TW: Recognition of proximal right coronary artery spasm during coronary arteriography. Radiology 95:305, 1970

Prinzmetal M, Kennamer R, Merliss R, Wada T, Bor N: Angina pectoris I. A variant form of angina pectoris. Am J Med 27:375, 1959

Sarnoff SJ, Hardenbergh E, Whittenberger JL: Mechanism of the arterial pressure response to the Valsalva test: the basis for its use as an indicator of the intactness of the sympathetic outflow. Am J Physiol 154:316, 1948

Sawayama T, Shiozu N, Niki I, Matsuura T, Ichinose S: Unusual form of impending myocardial infarction in a premenopausal woman. Jap Circ J 29:943, 1965

Whiting RB, Klein MD, VanderVeer J, Lown B: Variant angina pectoris. N Engl J Med 282:709, 1970

36

OPERATIVE TREATMENT OF PRINZMETAL ANGINA AND DYSRHYTHMIAS DUE TO SEVERE ATHEROMATOUS OBSTRUCTION OF THE RIGHT CORONARY ARTERY

Harry A. Wellons, Jr., Joel P. Schrank, and Richard S. Crampton

In the past decade, the diagnostic evaluation and management of atherosclerotic coronary artery disease has improved greatly, because of the widespread use of coronary arteriography and the introduction of surgical techniques to improve blood flow to obstructed coronary vessels. Despite these new techniques, the role of operative intervention remains controversial today, and indications for coronary surgery are not always precise, particularly in the management of variant angina pectoris. Since the report of Prinzmetal et al in 1959, over 100 cases have been reported in the literature. With the introduction of coronary arteriography, a wide spectrum of coronary artery disease in variant angina has emerged. Although most cases of variant angina occur in the presence of severe proximal atherosclerotic disease, in others atherosclerosis may be minimal or absent and attacks of severe coronary spasm have been documented. The proper management of each clinical presentation depends upon identifying the underlying pathological process. When coronary arterial spasm plays a major role and no significant fixed obstructive lesions are present, operative intervention offers little. On the other hand, if fixed obstructions are demonstrable, operation may be indicated and, in some instances, life-saving. The following cases demonstrate patients with life-threatening dysrhythmias due to severe isolated proximal atheromatous right coronary artery obstructions who were treated successfully by operative intervention.

CLINICAL EXPERIENCE

Since 1969, 12 patients have been treated at the University of Virginia Hospital with docu-mented Prinzmetal's variant angina; seven had life-threatening dysrhythmias. Of these, three with isolated proximal right coronary artery lesions are summarized below. All three had life-threatening dysrhythmias poorly controlled by medical management. Two of the patients demonstrated the difficulty of establishing the presence of a fixed obstruction in the right coronary artery by arteriography.

CASE 1: *RR, a 47-year-old male, had substernal and epigastric pain, nausea, dyspnea, sweating, and near syncope on awakening from sleep two weeks before entering the hospital. The attack subsided in a few minutes, but similar, milder episodes occurred at rest in the evening hours many times over the next two weeks. However, he was able to perform his usual heavy manual labor without symptoms. A second near-syncopal episode with vomiting prompted admission to a local hospital. There the electrocardiogram (ECG) showed sinus bradycardia with S-T segment elevation in the inferior and midprecordial leads, which persisted only during the pain. No Q-waves appeared, and cardiac enzymes did not rise. On the second night of hospitalization, near syncope and profound weakness in the absence of ischemic pain were associated with sinus bradycardia, sinus arrest, and transient S-T elevation (Fig. 1). Since treatment with atropine and isoproterenol had little effect, a temporary pacemaker was introduced, and the patient was transferred to this hospital. Examination revealed blood pressure of 120/80 mm Hg, and a prominent fourth-sound (S4) gallop. Except for transient S-T elevation in the inferior and midprecordial leads with pain, the ECG remained normal. Coronary angiography revealed a normal left coronary artery; but an isolated, long 80 percent obstruction of the proximal right coronary artery, which extended from its orifice to the point*

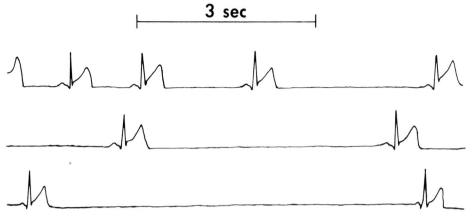

FIG. 1. Case 1. Continuous lead II during near syncope without pain. Note S-T elevation accompanied by progressive bradycardia.

of origin of the sinus node artery, persisted in spite of sublingual nitroglycerin (Fig. 2). Left ventricular contractility was normal, and left ventricular end-diastolic pressure (LVEDP) was 9 mm Hg. At operation, a long atherosclerotic plaque was found at the expected site in the right coronary artery, but the remainder of the arteries were normal to palpation. No flow came through the proximal right coronary artery. A saphenous vein bypass graft was placed from the aorta to the right coronary artery, and measured flow through the graft was 75 to 90 ml per minute. The postoperative course was uncomplicated, and no changes of infarction (Schrank et al, 1974) occurred in the ECG or vectorcardiogram (VCG). Six months after operation, the patient exercised on the treadmill for 23 minutes, completing 3 minutes at 3 miles per hour (MPH) on a 17 percent grade. The maximum heart rate was 180 per minute, and blood pressure was 160/80 mm Hg without chest pain or dysrhythmias. He refused follow-up arteriography. Twenty-five months after operation, the patient is working full-time at heavy labor without symptoms or medications.

CASE 2: JA, a 62-year-old male, experienced chest pain at rest and on exertion. Over 18 months before admission, episodes of pain were often associated with palpitation and dizziness, and he fainted twice. Treatment with isosorbide dinitrate, propranolol, and digoxin was ineffective. Three months before surgery, he had chest pain at rest, a sudden cardiac arrest, and successful resuscitation. At the time of his admission to a local hospital, the ECG showed transient elevation of the S-T segments in the inferior leads without pathologic Q-waves, but there was a serial rise and fall of cardiac enzymes. Medical management with lidocaine, propranolol, diphenylhydantoin, quinidine, hydrocortisone, and sedatives in varying doses

and combinations did not prevent frequent transient S-T elevation with salvos of ventricular tachycardia (VT) (Fig. 3). One episode of ventricular fibrillation was electrically reverted. Upon transfer to this hospital, the blood pressure was 130/80 mm Hg, and there was an S4 gallop. At cardiac catheterization, left ventricular contractility was normal, and LVEDP was 9 mm Hg. Although diffuse irregularities of the lumen were seen in many vessels, no significant coronary obstruction was detected (Fig. 4A, B). It was postulated that this ischemic pain was due to coronary spasm or small-vessel coronary disease. Transient S-T elevation, rest pain, and ventricular dysrhythmias continued to occur in spite of frequent sublingual nitroglycerin, isosorbide dinitrate, and propranolol. The right coronary arteriogram was repeated with many oblique views. An 80 percent obstruction of the middle third of the right coronary artery, which persisted after sublingual isosorbide dinitrate was appreciated only in the steep right anterior oblique view (Figure 4C). At operation, diffuse atherosclerosis was palpable only in the right coronary artery. At the site of the expected obstruction, there was marked atherosclerotic narrowing with no flow through the proximal right coronary artery. A saphenous vein bypass graft was placed from the aorta to the distal right coronary artery. The postoperative ECG and VCG did not show changes of infarction, and cardiac enzymes did not rise significantly. Three months after operation on a progressive treadmill test, he achieved a heart rate of 100 percent of predicted maximum for age on a 12 percent grade at 2 MPH without chest pain, dysrhythmias, or diagnostic ECG changes. A left ventricular angiogram revealed no abnormality of contraction, and LVEDP was 10 mm Hg. The bypass graft supplied the distal right coronary artery. The proximal right coronary artery was completely obstructed at the site of previous 80

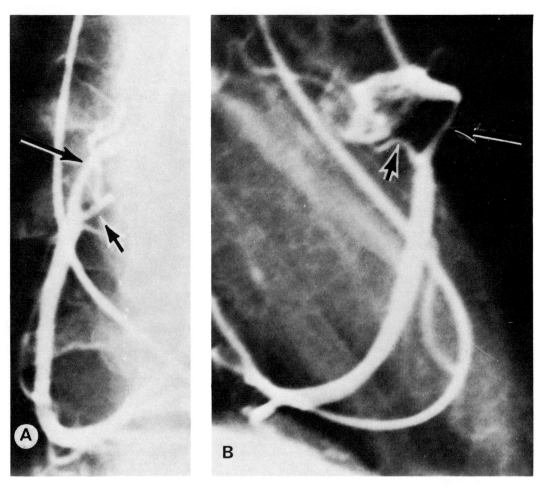

FIG. 2.   Case 1. Right coronary cut film angiogram in the AP (A) and lateral (B) views. Note long, eccentric 80 percent obstruction (large arrow) in proximal right coronary artery extending to origin of the sinus node artery (small arrow on sinus node artery).

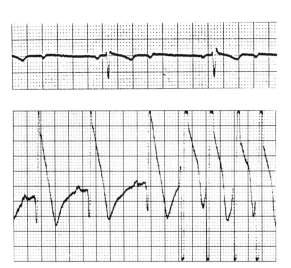

FIG. 3.   Case 2. A. Monitor lead: asymptomatic 2:1 AV block. B. Lead II: Marked S-T elevation during pain with ventricular tachycardia.

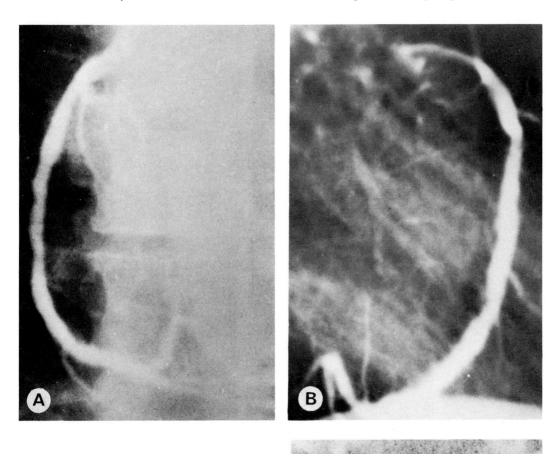

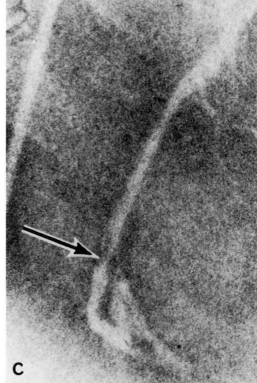

FIG. 4. Case 2. Original right coronary cut film angiogram in the AP (A) and lateral (B) views. Diffuse irregularity without significant proximal obstruction. C. Repeat coronary cine-angiogram in the 75-degree right anterior oblique view. The arrow points to an area of obstruction near the margin of the heart. The severity of obstruction is apparent only in C.

percent obstruction. Since surgery 15 months ago, he has worked and exercised actively without chest pain or syncope.

CASE 3: *FJ, a 61-year-old male, noted angina of effort five months before admission. Two months later, transient elevation of the S-T segment in the inferior leads was first documented in a local hospital. Recurrent episodes of chest pain with S-T elevation and ventricular dysrhythmias prompted investigation at another university medical center. Cinecoronary arteriography there revealed a 50 percent obstruction of the mid-right coronary artery, which was considered clinically insignificant. Left ventricular contractility was normal, and LVEDP was 11 mm Hg. The entire syndrome was attributed to spasm of the right coronary artery, and he was discharged from that center, taking sublingual and oral isosorbide dinitrate. Two weeks before admission, he again entered a local hospital, where daily episodes of pain at rest, S-T elevation, and VT unresponsive to nitrates, propranolol, procainamide, diphenylhydantoin, and lidocaine occurred. He was transferred to this hospital for reevaluation. Examination disclosed a blood pressure of 130/90 mm Hg, and a loud S4 gallop. Marked, transient S-T elevation appeared in the inferior leads during pain and frequently in the absence of pain but returned to normal within a few minutes. Sinus bradycardia, first- and second-degree AV block, and short runs of VT occurred during pain (Fig. 5.) Cardiac enzymes remained normal. Coronary arteriograms revealed minimal irregularity of the left coronary artery and an apparently insignificant mid-right coronary obstruction in all the views except the 60-degree left anterior oblique position, where an 80 percent obstructive lesion was seen in the mid-right coronary artery (Fig. 6). This lesion persisted after sublingual isosorbide dinitrate. At operation, the cause of the obstruction was found to be a long eccentric atherosclerotic plaque with minimal flow past the lesion. A saphenous vein was interposed between the aorta and the distal right coronary artery. No dysrhythmias or ischemic chest*

pain occurred postoperatively. The ECG and VCG showed no changes of infarction, and cardiac enzymes did not rise. Three months later, on a progressive treadmill exercise at 3 MPH on a 10 percent grade, he achieved a heart rate of 100 percent of predicted maximum without chest pain, dysrhythmias, or diagnostic ischemic S-T changes. Left ventricular angiography revealed no abnormalities of contraction, and LVEDP was 14 mm Hg. The saphenous vein graft to the right coronary artery was patent and filled both proximal and distal right coronary artery. The patient has returned to part-time farming and factory work and remains completely asymptomatic without nitrates one year after surgery.

DISCUSSION

These three patients represent an anatomical subset of the syndrome of variant angina pectoris described by Prinzmetal. All had severe, isolated, proximal, obstructing lesions persisting after administration of nitrates and involving one coronary artery, the distribution of which could account for the change seen on ECG during attacks. Two of the cases clearly point out the difficulty in establishing the presence of a fixed obstructing lesion. In situations where the atherosclerotic plaque is eccentrically placed, if the x-ray beam is not appropriately positioned, a false impression of patency may be given. It is, therefore, extremely important that multiple views in all of the coronary vessels be obtained, especially views of the vessel that supplies the area indicated by S-T elevation. The operative indications were felt to be well-justified by the demonstration of a fixed proximal obstruction and by the recurrent attacks associated with life-threatening dysrhythmias that responded poorly to drug therapy.

Variant angina characteristically occurs at rest or during normal activity and frequently oc-

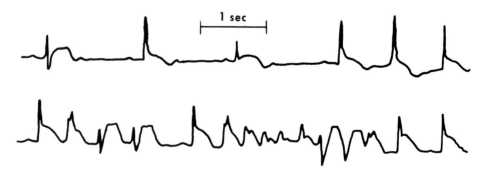

FIG. 5.　Case 3. Lead II: S-T elevation during pain with 2:1 AV block, variable AV and ventricular conduction. Bottom: S-T elevation during pain with chaotic ventricular rhythm.

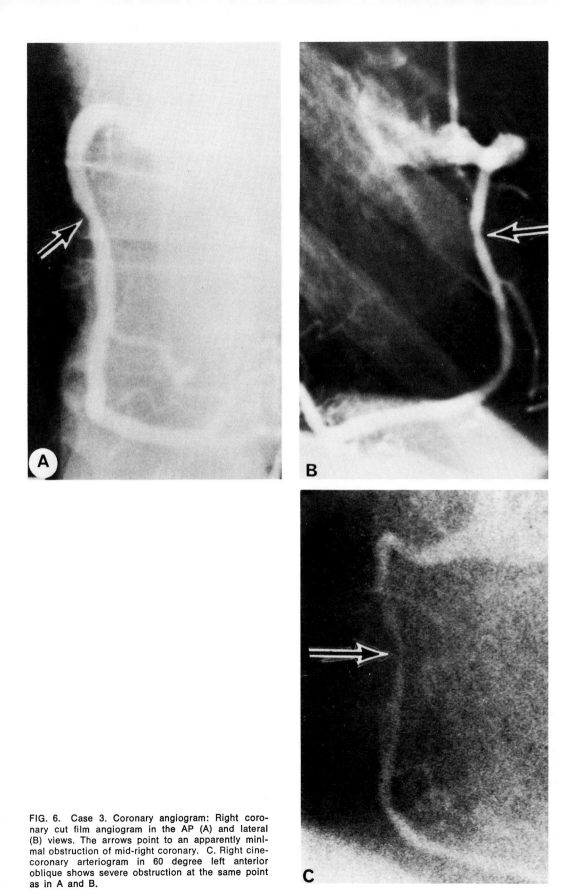

FIG. 6. Case 3. Coronary angiogram: Right coronary cut film angiogram in the AP (A) and lateral (B) views. The arrows point to an apparently minimal obstruction of mid-right coronary. C. Right cinecoronary arteriogram in 60 degree left anterior oblique shows severe obstruction at the same point as in A and B.

curs during sleep and at 24-hour intervals. The pain often is of much longer duration than that associated with classic angina and can, therefore, easily lead to the diagnosis of preinfarction angina or myocardial infarction. Interestingly, Lasser and de la Paz, 1973, have reported a case of recurrent marked S-T segment elevation without chest pain, but associated with heart block and Stokes-Adams attacks. Similar painless episodes were noted in our third case. Continuous ECG monitoring is important in establishing the diagnosis (Lunger and Shapiro, 1964; Guazzi et al, 1970). During the peak intensity of the attacks, the ECG reveals S-T segment elevation, often of a marked degree, with reciprocal S-T depression in the standard leads. Following an attack, the ECG returns to its preattack baseline. Typically, exercise testing does not precipitate attacks of variant angina but may result in S-T segment depression.

Dysrhythmias are very common during attacks and are usually ventricular in origin, although virtually every type of dysrhythmia has been recorded. First-, second-, and third-degree heart block are seen occasionally and may lead to Stokes-Adams attacks (Schwartz et al, 1966; Botti, 1966; Gillilan et al, 1969). Sinus bradycardia and arrest, more commonly a feature of patients with predominantly right coronary artery disease, was the cause of many near-syncopal attacks in our first case.

Pathophysiology

Initially Prinzmetal et al, 1959, postulated that variant angina was due to major proximal coronary artery obstructive disease with superimposed cyclic episodes of increased tone or spasm of the vessel wall resulting in the ischemic event. Pathological study of patients dying with variant angina revealed severe proximal coronary artery disease in a distribution that would account for the ECG signs of ischemia. Those patients who sustained myocardial infarctions developed them in the area of previously demonstrated ischemia, and symptoms or variant angina usually disappeared after myocardial infarction occurred (Prinzmetal et al 1959; Robinson, 1965). Variant angina in a patient who did not have severe coronary atherosclerosis was first reported by Gianelly et al, 1968. In the late 1960s, patients were more frequently studied by selective coronary arteriography, and in 1970 Whiting reported a case in which coronary arteriograms were completely normal. Cheng et al, 1973, and Oliva et al, 1973, demonstrated simultaneous elevation of the S-T segment and coronary arterial spasm and reversal of

both after administration of nitrates. Repeat contrast injections performed after the attacks had subsided revealed the coronary arteries to be normal. Dhurandhar et al, 1972, presented evidence of spasm during coronary arteriography complicated by simultaneous clinical attacks of angina. Since then, there have been several reports of patients with variant angina and normal coronary arteriograms (Christian and Botti, 1972; Kristian-Kerin et al, 1973). The experience of most observers, however, is that atheromatous occlusive disease is present in the majority of cases and in a distribution that nearly always accounts for the localized ischemic pattern of the ECG (Prinzmetal et al 1959; MacAlpin et al, 1973; Bete et al, 1973; Ruggeroli et al, 1973).

Of 23 cases of proved inferior S-T elevation associated with pain at rest and dysrhythmias, 19 underwent coronary arteriography and 17 had obstruction of right coronary blood flow (Actis Dato et al, 1972; Altieri, 1972; Cherrier et al, 1973; Cosby et al, 1972; Dhurandhar et al, 1972; Gonin et al, 1973; Gorfinkel et al, 1973; Gianelly et al, 1968; Hiltgen et al, 1973; King, Kir, et al, 1973; Lasser and de la Paz, 1973; MacAlpin et al, 1973; Nadal-Ginard and Cardenas, 1973; Oliva et al, 1973; Silverman and Flamm, 1971; Whiting et al, 1970). In five of the 17 obstructions, coronary spasm was noted, but in only one was spasm the sole cause of coronary insufficiency (Oliva et al, 1973). Of the remaining four cases with spasm, all had associated atheromatous obstruction, two seen by angiogram (Hiltgen et al, 1973; King, Kir, et al, 1973) and two missed by angiogram, but subsequently identified at autopsy (Cosby et al, 1972; Dhurandhar et al, 1972). Thus, 16 of 19 had proximal atheromatous right coronary stenosis.

S-T segment elevation similar to that seen in man has been demonstrated experimentally in dogs by temporary occlusion of a major coronary trunk (Ekmekci et al, 1961). S-T segment elevation is associated with a more severe and widespread area of epicardial ischemia than ischemia resulting in S-T segment depression. These observations confirm the clinical impression that variant angina is due to intermittent occlusion of a major coronary trunk, perhaps in part on a basis of increased vasomotor tone of the coronary vessels. Why this phenomenon occurs at rest is as yet unexplained. The fact that both painful and painless attacks occur more frequently at rest without change of heart rate or blood pressure rules out increased heart work and oxygen demand as the cause. More likely there are cyclic increases in arterial tone, which, when superimposed at the site of a stenotic lesion, especially if it is eccentrically placed, will then produce profound coronary narrowing and ischemia.

Spasm in normal coronary arteries, especially in the right coronary near the catheter tip, was demonstrated by Demany et al, 1968, in seven of 750 coronary arteriograms. The demonstration of the absence of recent thrombosis in cases of fatal myocardial infarction further implicates increased vasomotor tone in ischemic episodes (Roberts, 1972).

In summary, it is now clear that a wide spectrum of anatomical findings may occur in patients with variant angina. Most cases are still noted to have discrete proximal obstructive lesions in one or more coronary arteries, but in certain cases arterial spasm assumes a much greater role for reasons at present unclear.

Natural History and Prognosis

Unfortunately, the natural history of variant angina is not well known. Many of the reported cases do not have sufficiently long or detailed follow-up. Prinzmetal et al, 1959, found that of 35 cases, 11 went on to have myocardial infarction, and three died as a result of their disease. Almost all patients who had myocardial infarction and survived were completely relieved of their symptoms. In a later review, Silverman and Flamm in 1971 suggested a rather grim outlook, reporting that 50 percent of patients developed myocardial infarction or died within one year of the onset of symptoms. Review of the current literature suggests that the prognosis is not quite so grave. Variability in prognosis occurs because patients with variant angina have different pathological findings. Series that include a large proportion of patients with normal coronary arteriograms and presumed arterial spasm report good overall prognosis on medical therapy, although myocardial infarction or death still does occur in patients with only spasm (Gianelly et al, 1968; Cheng et al, 1973; Christian and Botti, 1972). Medical treatment, therefore, must be aggressive and patients carefully followed.

These different pathophysiological mechanisms must be identified by coronary arteriograms with multiple oblique views, with and without sublingual nitrates, before a rational basis for therapy can be established. Significant disease is easy to overlook. Indeed, it has been shown by pathological study that a high percentage of coronary arteriograms may be interpreted falsely as negative (Vlodaver et al, 1973). Factors that contribute to a false negative evaluation include technique, an eccentric, slitlike lumen adjacent to the atheroma, insufficient number of oblique views, and comparison of a narrowed segment with an already diseased vessel. The difficulty of interpreting arteriograms of the right coronary artery is emphasized by our second and third cases and three fatal cases of variant angina. Cosby et al, 1972, interpreted two cases as having normal arteriograms but at autopsy found significant stenosis of the right coronary artery ostia. In the case of Dhurandhar et al, 1972, right coronary obstruction was attributed solely to spasm, but after death a few weeks later, a 75 percent obstruction by an eccentric right coronary plaque was found in the same area. These five cases very aptly demonstrate that severe fixed obstructions due to eccentrically placed plaques or ostial lesions may not be readily apparent on conventional views. Not only are eccentric lesions missed more frequently, but flow characteristics also indicate that a small change in cross-sectional area or perfusion pressure cause a greater reduction in flow in eccentric lesions than in those centrally placed (Logan et al, 1974). In addition, the site of an eccentrically placed atheroma may be more responsive to local vasomotor changes because the portion of the wall free of disease retains its ability to contract. Conversely, if severe spasm occurs during coronary arteriography, one may falsely interpret this as representing a fixed obstruction. These pitfalls of arteriography emphasize the necessity of obtaining multiple views during the procedure and of demonstrating the persistence of fixed obstruction after administration of potent coronary vasodilators.

Management: Medical and Permanent Pacing

The objectives in the treatment of variant angina include prevention of recurrent attacks of pain, control of associated dysrhythmias, and hopefully the prevention of myocardial infarction and death. Early cases were treated with a variety of agents, with varying degrees of success. Prinzmetal et al, 1959, found administration of nylidrin hydrochloride useful in addition to nitroglycerin. The importance of antidysrhythmic drugs was also emphasized. Although Guazzi et al, 1971, found propranolol useful, King, Kir, et al, 1973, found propranolol treatment associated with increase in pain in a patient with spasm demonstrating a minimally diseased coronary vessel. Isosorbide dinitrate, however, resulted in symptomatic relief. Basically, the medical management of this problem differs little from that of severe classical angina pectoris.

Sinus bradycardia, complete heart block, and

Stokes-Adams attacks occur not infrequently with variant angina and may be fatal (Schwartz et al, 1966; Cosby et al, 1972). Six patients with episodic inferior S-T elevation have been treated with permanent cardiac pacemakers (Oliva et al, 1973; Nadal-Ginard and Cardenas, 1973; Whiting et al, 1970; Cherrier et al, 1973; Lasser and de la Paz, 1973; Gianelly et al, 1968). Before pacing, all had episodes of complete heart block during S-T elevation, and five had syncopal attacks. Three did not undergo coronary angiography (Nadal-Ginard and Cardenas, 1973; Cherrier et al, 1973; Lasser and de la Paz, 1973), and, of these, one died suddenly after six months without syncope (Cherrier et al, 1973). Of the three examined angiographically, two had no atheromas (Oliva et al, 1973; Whiting et al, 1970), and one had insignificant atheromas (Gianelly et al, 1968). The latter patient died suddenly eight months after initiation of pacing. The four surviving patients were alive and improved from six to 12 months after initiation of pacing. Although offering some protection from syncope, pacing seems to have little influence on control of recurrent attacks of angina, and the death rate of two out of six patients is high.

Management: Surgical

Surgical intervention in the management of this syndrome was first reported by Silverman and Flamm, 1971, who obtained good results in two of the three patients treated. In 34 surgically treated cases, including our three, there has been a variable degree of success (Silverman and Flamm, 1971; Kahn and Landry, 1970; MacAlpin et al, 1973; King et al, 1973; Bete et al, 1973; Linhart et al, 1972). Although follow-up information is limited, two-thirds of the patients have done well and are improved after operation. There have been only two deaths reported in the surgical group, and two cases of myocardial infarction. In only rare instances of follow-up have coronary arteriograms been obtained, but in one series, three of eight coronary artery bypass grafts were found to be occluded (MacAlpin et al, 1973).

Surgical results in angiographically identified, isolated right coronary obstruction with episodic S-T elevation, including our three cases, indicate that 10 of 13 patients, aged 40 to 62 years, have done very well for two to 27 months postoperatively. Twelve of the 13 had single saphenous vein bypass grafts of the right coronary obstruction; one had a patch graft (Hultgren et al, 1967). A 39-year-old man died five days after operation (Silverman and Flamm, 1971). A 55-

year-old woman with marked spasm at operation had an infarction three days later due to occlusion of the graft and became asymptomatic thereafter (MacAlpin et al, 1973). A 52-year-old man with spasm died six weeks after operation (Dhurandhar et al, 1972). This latter patient had a patent graft at autopsy in addition to a severe proximal atheromatous right coronary obstruction missed at preoperative angiography. Of the 10 asymptomatic patients, four have had postoperative angiograms showing a patent graft at three months (present cases) and six months (Actis-Dato et al, 1972; Gorfinkel et al, 1973). In three of these cases, the narrowed right coronary artery had become totally occluded.

In contrast, four patients, aged 42 to 73 years, without coronary surgery and without cardiac pacing fared poorly, with isolated right coronary obstruction. Three died, one, two, and 21 months after diagnosis (Altieri, 1972; Hiltgen et al, 1973; Cosby et al, 1972). Three underwent coronary angiography (Hiltgen et al, 1973; King, Kir, et al, 1973; Cosby et al, 1972). In a 42-year-old woman, a right ostial obstruction was not detected until autopsy after sudden death 21 months later (Cosby et al, 1972). A 73-year-old man without angiography died after a month of observation with acute posterolateral myocardial infarction, rupture of the left ventricle at the area of infarction, hemopericardium, and right coronary obstruction (Altieri, 1972). A 41-year-old man (Hiltgen et al, 1973) was not autopsied after sudden death. A 42-year-old female did well during four months of observation after angiography (King et al, 1973). Two of the three who died suddenly had experienced episodes of complete heart block during attacks (Altieri, 1972; Cosby et al, 1972).

Thus, on balance, it appears that bypassing the right coronary obstruction surgically is superior to pacing and to medical therapy when second- and third-degree AV block and ventricular tachycardia and fibrillation complicate Prinzmetal angina due to right coronary obstruction.

The selection of treatment in each case depends basically on the nature of the lesions involved. Those patients who fall clearly in the realm of medical therapy are those in whom no significant fixed obstructive disease can be found or no clearly demonstrable coronary artery spasm is seen on arteriography. Also to be included in this group are patients with single isolated lesions and minimal clinical symptoms easily controlled by drug therapy and uncomplicated by life-threatening arrhythmias. Operative intervention should be considered in those patients refractory to medical therapy in the face of demonstrable fixed obstructive disease of one or more vessels.

Isolated right coronary obstructive disease is unique in the spectrum of variant angina, due to its frequent association with life-threatening dysrhythmias and because severe fixed obstructive lesions may be easily overlooked during arteriography in this vessel. Our experience supports the belief that operative intervention is indicated and beneficial in patients selected according to the above criteria.

SUMMARY

Three cases of Prinzmetal's variant angina pectoris with life-threatening dysrhythmias associated with isolated atheromatous obstruction of the right coronary artery are presented, and the recent literature is reviewed. Variant angina occurs in a spectrum of pathophysiological settings, ranging from severe coronary artery spasm in presumably normal vessels to severe atherosclerotic occlusive disease involving all three major vessels. The value of coronary arteriography in evaluation of patients with variant angina and the selection of operative versus nonoperative management are discussed.

References

Actis-Dato A, Baldrighi G, Passoni F, et al. Angina di Prinzmetal: quadro coronarografica e terapia chirurgica. Minerva Med (Supplemento) 1:4901, 1972

Altieri S: La forma variante di angina pectoris: ressegna della letteratura contributo casistico—inquadramento nosologico—prospettive fisiopathegenetiche. Minerva Cardioang 20:239, 1972

Bete JM, Shubrooks SJ, Block PC, Hutter, AM: Prinzmetal's angina pectoris, clinical and anatomical spectrum and results of coronary artery bypass surgery (abstract). Circulation (Suppl IV) 48:145, 1973

Botti RE: A variant form of angina pectoris with recurrent transient complete heart block. Am J Cardiol 17:443, 1966

Cheng TO, Bashour T, Kelser GA, Weiss L, Bacos J: Variant angina of Prinzmetal with normal coronary arteriograms: a variant of the variant. Circulation 47:476, 1973

Cherrier F, Cuilliere M, Dodinot B, Hua G: Angor de Prinzmetal: aspects coronarographiques; considerations therapeutiques. A propos de 7 observations. Arch Mal Coeur 66:579, 1973

Christian N, Botti RE: Prinzmetal's variant angina pectoris with prolonged electrocardiographic changes in the absence of obstructive coronary disease. Am J Med Sci 263:225, 1972

Cosby RS, Giddings JA, See JR, Mayo M: Variant angina: case reports and critique. Am J Med 53:739, 1972

Demany MA, Tombe A, Zimmerman HA: Coronary artery spasm. Dis Chest 53:714, 1968

Dhurandhar RW, Watt DL, Silver MD, Trimble AS, Adelman AG: Prinzmetal's variant form of angina with arterial spasm. Am J Cardiol 30:902, 1972

Ekmekci A, Toyoshima H, Kwoczynski JK, Nogaya T, Prinzmetal M: Angina pectoris IV: Clinical and experimental differences between ischemia with S-T elevation and ischemia with S-T depression. Am J Cardiol 7:412, 1961

Gianelly R, Mugler F, Harrison DC: Prinzmetal's variant of angina pectoris with only slight coronary atherosclerosis. Calif Med 108:129, 1968

Gillilan RE, Hawley RR, Warbasse JR: Second degree heart block occurring in a patient with Prinzmetal's variant angina. Am Heart J 77:380, 1969

Gonin A, Berthou JD, Delaye J, et al. Angor de Prinzmetal: apports de la coronarographie et discussion de la chirurgie de revascularisation: a propos de 13 cas comportant 10 coronarographies selectives et 9 pontages aorta-coronariens. Arch Mal Coeur 66:571, 1973

Gorfinkel H, Inglesby T, Lansing A, Goodin R: S-T segment elevation, transient left posterior hemiblock, and recurrent ventricular arrhythmias unassociated with pain: a variant of Prinzmetal's anginal syndrome. Ann Intern Med 79:795, 1973

Grubbay ER: Prinzmetal's variant angina. Can Med Assoc J 83:164, 1960

Guazzi M, Fiorentini C, Polese A, Magrini F: Continuous electrocardiographic recording in Prinzmetal's variant angina pectoria: report of four cases. Br Heart J 32:611, 1970

Guazzi M, Magrini F, Fiorentini C, Polese A: Clinical electrocardiographic and hemodynamic effects of long term use of propranolol in Prinzmetal's variant angina pectoris. Br Heart J 33:889, 1971

Hiltgen M, Guermonprez J, Sellier P, et al: Angor de Prinzmetal: a propos de 16 cineangiographies coronaries selectives et 13 interventions (Pontages aorto-coronaries). Arch Mal Coeur 66:553, 1973

Hultgren H, Calciano A, Platt F, Abrams H: A clinical evaluation of coronary arteriography. Ann J Med 42:228, 1967

Khan AH, Landry AB: Variant angina: letter to editor. Ann Intern Med 76:335, 1970

King MJ, Kir LM, Kaltman AJ, Fox AC: Variant angina associated with angiographically demonstrated coronary artery spasm and REM sleep. Am J Sci 265:419, 1973

King SB, Mansour KA, Hatcher CR, Silvermann ME, Hart NC: Coronary artery spasm producing Prinzmetal's angina and myocardial infarction in the absence of coronary atherosclerosis. Am Thorac Surg 16:337, 1973

Kristian-Kerin N, Davies B, MacLeon CA: Nonocclusive coronary disease associated with Prinzmetal's angina pectoris. Chest 64:352, 1973

Lasser RP, de la Paz NS: Repetitive transient myocardial ischemia, Prinzmetal type, without angina pectoris, presenting with Stokes-Adams attacks. Chest 64:350, 1973

Linhart JW, Beller EM, Talley RC: Preinfarction angina: clinical hemodynamic and angiographic evaluation. Chest 61:312, 1972

Logan SE, Tyberg JV, Parmley WW, Swan HJC: The relationship between coronary perfusion pressure flow, and resistance in stenosed human coronary arteries: the critical importance of small changes in percentage stenosis (abstract). Am J Cardiol 33:153, 1974

Lunger M, Shapiro A: Continuous electrocardiographic monitoring in nocturnal angina. Am J Cardiol 13:119, 1964

MacAlpin RN, Kattus AA, Alvaro AB: Angina pectoris at rest with preservation of exercise capacity: Prinzmetal's variant angina. Circulation 47:946, 1973

Oliva PB, Potts DE, Pluss RG: Coronary arterial spasm in Prinzmetal's angina; documentation by coronary arteriography. N Engl J Med 288:745, 1973

Nadal-Ginard B, Cardenas M: Prinzmetal's angina with

recurrent and transitory atrio-ventricular block. Acta Cardiol 28:214, 1973

Prinzmetal M, Kennamer R, Merliss R, Wada T, Bor N: Angina pectoris: I. A variant form of angina pectoris. Am J Med 27:375, 1959

Roberts WC: Coronary arteries in fatal acute myocardial infarction. Circulation 45:215, 1972

Robinson JS: Prinzmetal's variant angina pectoris: report of a case. Am Heart J 70:797, 1965

Ruggeroli CW, Cohn K, Langston M: Prinzmetal's variant angina: a pathophysiological and clinical kaleidoscope (abstract). Circulation (Suppl IV) 48:211, 1973

Schrank JP, Slabaugh TK, Beckwith JR: The incidence and clinical significance of ECG-VCG changes of myocardial infarction following aortocoronary saphenous vein bypass surgery. Am Heart J 87:46, 1974

Silverman ME, Flamm ME: Variant angina pectoris: Anatomic findings and prognostic implications. Ann Intern Med 75:339, 1971

Vlodaver Z, Frech R, Van Tassel RA, Edwards JE: Correlation of the antemortem coronary arteriogram and the post mortem specimen. Circulation 47:162, 1973

Whiting RB, Klein MD, VanderVeer J, Lown B: Variant angina pectoris. N Engl J Med 282:709, 1970

37

PRINZMETAL'S VARIANT ANGINA: SURGICAL MANAGEMENT AND PHYSIOLOGIC ASPECTS

WILLIAM H. GAASCH, ROBERTO LUFSCHANOWSKI,
MIGUEL A. QUINONES, ROBERT D. LEACHMAN,
and JAMES K. ALEXANDER

Variant, or Prinzmetal's, angina pectoris may be defined as a clinical syndrome characterized by development of chest pain at rest with concomitant transient ST segment elevation in the electrocardiogram. In Table 1, some of the characteristic features of variant angina are summarized and compared with those of classic angina pectoris. Of particular note are the observations that variant angina is not precipitated by exercise, that arrhythmias and heart block are frequently noted during pain, and that the hemodynamic alterations associated with variant angina suggest a reduction in myocardial oxygen supply during pain, in contrast to increased myocardial oxygen demands in classic angina (MacAlpin et al, 1973; Prinzmetal et al, 1960; Gaasch et al, 1974; Guzaai et al, 1971; Whiting et al, 1970). While localized stenoses of the coronary arteries are frequently demonstrated in variant as well as classic angina, the additional occurrence of coronary artery spasm has been documented in variant angina (Dhurandhar et al, 1972). Likewise, coronary artery spasm has been documented during pain in patients with angiographically normal coronary arteries (Cheng et al, 1973; Oliva et al, 1973).

Since proximal localized stenosis can be easily identified by arteriography in patients with variant angina and the caliber and appearance of the distal vessel frequently suggests that saphenous vein bypass would be an easy technical procedure, surgical therapy for this condition has seemed a promising approach (Silverman and Flamm, 1971). However, experience with saphenous vein aortocoronary bypass surgery (SVACBS) in the treatment of variant angina has resulted in variable degrees of success, and thus the role of surgery in this syndrome has remained controversial. In this presentation, we propose to describe our experience with six patients having variant angina and undergoing bypass surgery, and to review 18 other surgically treated cases gathered from the literature (Gaasch et al, 1974). Additionally, we will summarize some hemodynamic and anatomical observations relating to variant angina that have implications regarding the therapeutic approach to this condition.

SURGICAL MANAGEMENT OF VARIANT ANGINA

Six patients with variant angina were treated by SVACBS. Information on locations of the stenotic lesions, whether they were spastic or occlusive in nature (on arteriography), and the results of surgery is summarized in Figure 1. Of the six patients, two developed myocardial infarction postoperatively, one had continued pain, and one died; only two had relief of pain without postoperative infarction.

Figure 2 summarizes the results of surgical treatment in a total of 24 cases of variant angina, six of our own, and 18 surveyed from the literature, with 21 of the total 24 treated by SVACBS. In this figure the designation *successful* indicates that patients were pain-free postoperatively without myocardial infarction or known graft occlusion. A *qualified success* indicates that the patient was pain-free postoperatively but experienced myocardial infarction and/or documented graft occlusion. *Lack of improvement* indicates continued

**TABLE 1. Summary and Comparison of the Characteristic Features of
Variant Angina and Classic Angina**

	VARIANT ANGINA	CLASSIC ANGINA
Pain	At rest, sometimes cyclic	Exertional
EKG	ST elevation Arrhythmias and heart block frequent Negative exercise test	ST depression Arrhytmias and heart block infrequent Positive exercise test
Pathophysiology	Reduced myocardial O_2 supply Extensive coronary artery spasm	Increased myocardial O_2 demand Localized atherosclerotic coronary artery occlusive lesions

pain irrespective of graft patency. *Mortality* figures include deaths up to 30 days after surgery. Successful surgical results were achieved in only 38 percent of the entire group. Of the nine patients in the successful category, four had patent grafts, and the graft status was unknown in the remaining five. These results are in striking contrast to those reported postoperatively with classic angina (Morris et al, 1972; Hall et al, 1973; Sheldon et al, 1973). Significant symptomatic improvement occurs in about 90 percent and complete relief of pain is achieved in two-thirds of patients with classic angina treated by SVACBS. The mortality figure of 12.5 percent for variant angina again contrasts with that found in patients with classic angina; in the latter group mortality is of the order of two to six percent in patients with good left ventricular function. Myocardial infarction occurred intra- or postoperatively in five of the 24 variant angina cases, to give an incidence of approximately 20 percent. Of the 12 patients with variant angina having postoperative studies, the grafts were occluded in seven, or over 50 percent. Graft patency at one year in patients with classic angina usually has been reported in the range of 75 to 85 percent. Of four patients with

variant angina and documented coronary spasm, none showed postoperative improvement. Analysis of the surgical results in terms of single-vessel versus multiple-vessel involvement yields figures comparable to those for the overall group.

At present the natural history of variant angina is not well known, and the risks of medical and surgical management are not clearly defined; additionally, the evaluation of these therapeutic approaches is complicated by the similarity of variant angina to the intermediate coronary artery syndrome (unstable angina). Nevertheless, it is clear that the results of bypass surgery with variant angina are by no means as favorable as those with classic angina, and importantly surgery has been uniformly unsuccessful in those patients with documented coronary spasm. If the pain of variant angina is related to reduced myocardial oxygen supply produced by coronary artery spasm, saphenous vein aortocoronary bypass surgery would appear to be an inadequate approach. Coronary artery denervation by adventitial stripping in combination with bypass might provide a more satisfactory therapeutic result.

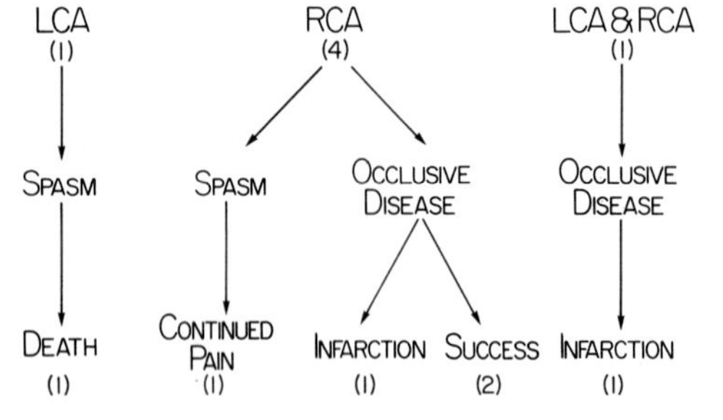

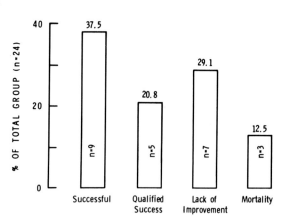

FIG. 1. Information on the locations of the stenotic lesions, whether they were spastic or occlusive in nature, and the results of saphenous vein aortocoronary bypass (SVACBS) surgery in 6 patients with variant angina.

FIG. 2. Summary of the results of surgical treatment in a total of 24 cases of variant angina (6 of our own, and 18 cases surveyed from the literature).

HEMODYNAMIC AND ANGIOGRAPHIC ASPECTS OF VARIANT ANGINA

In the remainder of this discussion certain hemodynamic and anatomical observations with therapeutic implications in patients with variant angina will be presented, some of which have been interpreted as indicating that (1) angina in these patients is associated with a reduction in myocardial oxygen *supply* rather than increased myocardial *demand,* and (2) major coronary artery spasm does play a role in variant angina, but not always.

The electrocardiogram and left ventricular (LV) pressure recordings from a patient with variant angina are shown in Figure 3. The patient spontaneously developed pain during cardiac catheterization; there was little change in heart rate or LV systolic pressure during pain, while the LV

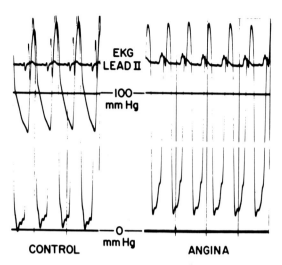

FIG. 3.   Electrocardiogram and left ventricular pressure from a patient with variant angina. Note the impressive rise in left ventricular end-diastolic pressure. There was no significant change in the heart rate or blood pressure during angina.

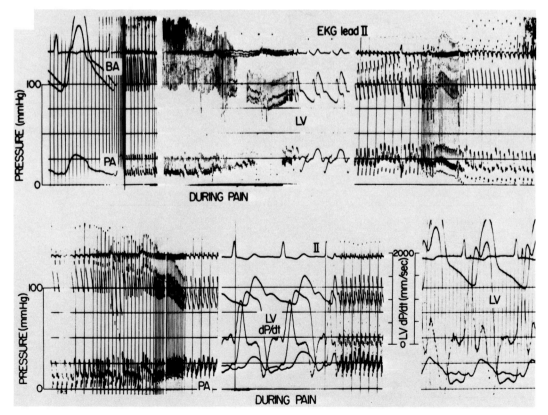

FIG. 4.   Brachial artery, pulmonary artery, and left ventricular pressures prior to and during two episodes of spontaneous angina in a patient with variant angina.

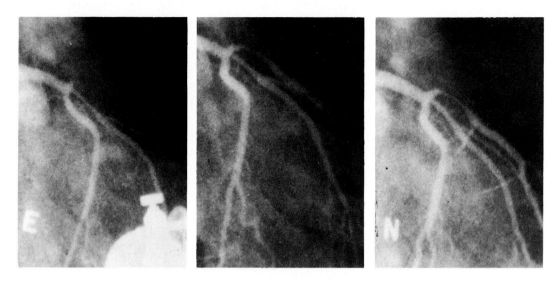

FIG. 5. Left coronary arteriogram from a patient with variant angina. In the panel on the left, there is extensive spasm of the left anterior descending artery associated with pain and ST elevation in EKG lead V_1. One minute after sublingual nitroglycerin (middle panel), the vessel begins to opacify and two minutes later (panel on the right) the distal vessel remained unchanged when compared to other films taken prior to the spasm The nitroglycerin was also associated with prompt relief of pain and reversal of the EKG changes.

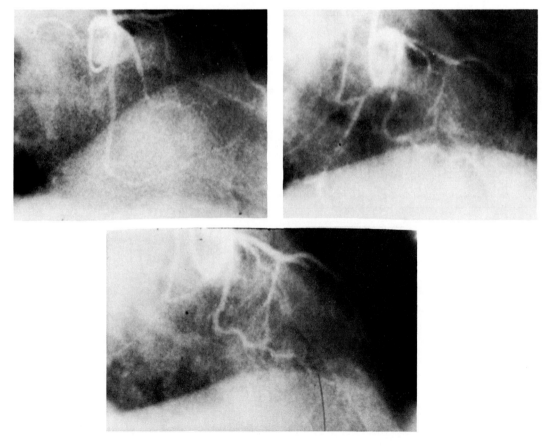

FIG. 6. Left coronary arteriogram in a patient with variant angina showing variable spasm of the left circumflex artery.

end-diastolic pressure increased from 7 to 34 mm Hg. Note the ST elevation in EKG lead II. LV volume angiography in this patient (prior to and during angina) revealed that reductions in the systolic ejection fraction, the stroke volume and the mean and peak rate of ejection, and hypokinesis of the apex and the diaphragmatic wall of the LV wall developed. The LV end-diastolic volume did not change significantly (3 cc/m² increase) during pain. This data can be interpreted as suggesting (1) there were no circulatory changes prior to or during pain that might result in an increase in the myocardial oxygen demands, (2) severe impairment of LV systolic performance was present during angina, and (3) a marked reduction in LV diastolic compliance occurred during pain.

Figure 4 shows a simultaneous recording of brachial artery, pulmonary artery, and LV pressure from another patient with variant angina experiencing spontaneous pain during heart catheterization. During both attacks of angina there was a distinct fall in systemic arterial pressure and an increase in the LV end-diastolic (and pulmonary artery) pressure; LV peak dP/dt fell during pain. As in the previous case, there were no circulatory changes prior to or during angina that might result in an increase in the myocardial oxygen demands.

An increase in the triple product (pressure-time index) of LV systolic pressure, heart rate, and systolic ejection period is generally recorded prior to and during pain in patients with classic angina and in those with unstable angina (Cohn and Gorlin 1972; Cannom et al, 1974). The increased myocardial oxygen demands thought to parallel a rise in the pressure-time index results in a supply-demand imbalance and leads to myocardial ischemia. In contrast, data from patients with variant angina suggest that there is no increase in myocardial oxygen demands to account for myocardial ischemia and that factors other than increased demand must be implicated.

Arteriographic evidence of coronary artery spasm in patients with variant angina has been reported by several authors. To our knowledge, the first report of major coronary artery spasm documented under direct vision at operation was made by MacAlpin and associates (1973). They observed elevation of ST segments in the inferior leads and spasm of the right coronary artery in a patient with variant angina at operation when the heart was exposed prior to coronary bypass surgery. In 1968, Ross and Gorlin reported angiographic evidence of coronary artery spasm associ-

ated with hypotension and ST elevation as a complication of cardiac catheterization. Recently Cheng and associates (1973) and others (Oliva et al, 1973) have reported coronary artery spasm during pain in patients with variant angina.

In Figure 5, the left coronary arteriogram from a patient with variant angina is shown. The panel on the left shows the vessel shortly after the intravenous infusion of 0.35 mg ergotamine tartrate. At this time, the anterior descending branch of the left coronary artery was not opacified, the patient was experiencing substernal pain, and elevation of ST segments was recorded in V_1. Sublingual administration of nitroglycerin (NTG) produced relief of the pain and reversal of the EKG changes within two minutes. In the middle panel the anterior descending branch of the vessel is just beginning to opacify with injection of contrast material (one minute after NTG) and in the panel on the right, obtained after the pain had subsided, the anterior descending branch opacifies well distally with some persistent proximal segmental narrowing. This segmental lesion was present prior to the ergotamine infusion and did not change with repeated use of NTG. We have interpreted this as extensive coronary artery spasm during an attack of variant angina induced by ergotamine. As in the cases discussed above, the pressure-time index did not increase during pain in this patient.*

Left coronary arteriograms obtained during cyclic pain in another patient with variant angina are shown in Figure 6. Spasm of the posterior descending branch of the circumflex vessel is seen during spontaneous pain. The vessel is widely patent in the panel on the upper left; a segmental obstruction appears (just above the diaphragm) in the panel on the upper right; in the lower panel the vessel is completely obliterated. This patient experienced repeated attacks of chest pain associated with ST segment elevation and ventricular tachycardia, during successive obliterations of several major coronary arteries. Each attack was associated with hypotension.

Angiographic studies of another patient with the clinical syndrome of variant angina are shown

---

* This patient was initially treated with isosorbide dinitrate (5 mg every four hours) and reserpine (1.0 mg per day) with a good clinical response. Two additional patients (one with normal coronary arteriograms and one with a single lesion of the right coronary artery) have been successfully treated with reserpine (RDL, unpublished observations).

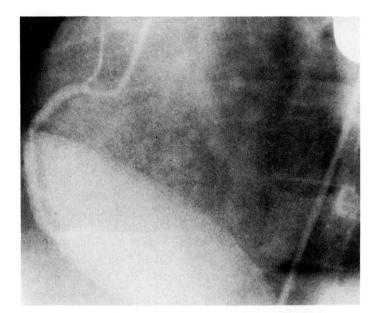

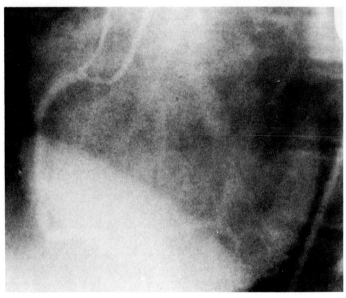

FIG. 7. Right coronary arteriogram from a patient with variant angina. The upper panel was obtained prior to pain, and the lower panel was taken during an attack of pain and ST elevations. There was no change of appearance in the vessel during pain.

in Figures 7 and 8. This patient had a six-week history of recurrent substernal chest pain that occurred at rest; the treadmill exercise test was negative. ST segment elevation was recorded in EKG leads 2, 3, and AVF during pain, but in contrast to other patients with variant angina a rise in arterial blood pressure and heart rate was consistently recorded during the attacks of pain. At the time of coronary arteriography, the left coronary artery was entirely normal. The right coronary arteriogram shown in Figure 7 (upper panel) was obtained at a time when the patient was pain-free. There was a high-grade proximal lesion of

the right coronary artery. Three minutes after this arteriogram was obtained, the patient developed an elevation of the systemic arterial pressure to 180/100 mm Hg, (from a previous level of 120/70) and an increase in heart rate from 70 to 120 beats/min; this was associated with chest pain and ST elevation in lead II. A second right coronary arteriogram (Fig. 7, lower panel) was obtained during this attack of pain and the vessel appeared unchanged when compared to the previous film. The pain persisted in spite of sublingual NTG, but later responded to morphine administration. Figure 8 shows the appearance of the right coro-

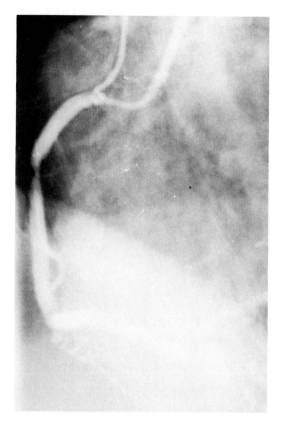

FIG. 8. Right coronary arteriogram (spot film) taken from the same patient as is shown in Figure 7. This film was taken after the administration of nitroglycerin. The vessel remains unchanged when compared to both panels in Figure 7.

nary artery five minutes after NTG was administered; no change in the appearance of the vessel can be appreciated. Minimal T-wave inversion in the inferior leads persisted for one month, but no definite evidence of infarction was uncovered. Although this patient had the typical clinical syndrome of Prinzmetal's variant angina, coronary artery spasm could not be demonstrated during pain; and importantly an increase in the pressure-time index was measured during pain. Thus, a reduction in coronary blood flow or myocardial oxygen supply may be implicated in some, but not all, cases of variant angina.

COMMENT

An analysis of our data in conjunction with those in the literature indicate that the results of SVACBS in patients with variant angina are not as favorable as those currently being obtained in patients with classic angina pectoris. In contrast to classic angina, hemodynamic observations suggest no change or reduction in myocardial oxygen demands during attacks in most patients with variant angina. The role of major coronary artery spasm in variant angina appears well documented, but this mechanism may not be implicated in all cases. Unfortunately the natural history of this syndrome remains undefined and thus, evaluation of the various forms of therapy in variant angina is difficult.

References

1. Cannom DS, Harrison DC, Schroeder JS: Hemodynamic observations in patients with unstable angina pectoris. Am J Cardiol 33:17, 1974
2. Cheng TO, Bashour T, Kelser GA, et al: Variant angina of Prinzmetal with normal coronary arteriograms: a variant of the variant. Circulation 47:476, 1973
3. Cohn PF, Gorlin R: Abnormalities of left ventricular function associated with the anginal state. Circulation 46:1065, 1972
4. Dhurandhar RW, Watt DL, Silver MD, et al: Prinzmetal's variant form of angina with arteriographic evidence of coronary arterial spasm. Am J Cardiol 30:902, 1972
5. Gaasch WH, Adyanthaya AV, Wang VH, et al: Prinzmetal's variant angina: hemodynamic and angiographic observations during pain. Am J Cardiol 35:683, 1975
6. Gaasch WH, Lufschanowski R, Leachman RD, Alexander JK: Surgical management of Prinzmetal's variant angina. Chest 66:614, 1974
7. Guazzi M, Polese A, Fiorentini C, et al: Left ventricular performance and related hemodynamic changes in Prinzmetal's variant angina pectoris. Br Heart J 33:84, 1971
8. Hall RJ, Dawson JT, Cooley DA, et al: Coronary artery bypass. Circulation (Suppl III) 48:146, 1973
9. MacAlpin RN, Kattus AA, Alvaro AB: Angina pectoris at rest with preservation of exercise capacity: Prinzmetal's variant angina. Circulation 47:946, 1973
10. Morris GC, Reul GJ, Howell JF, et al: Follow-up results of distal coronary artery bypass for ischemic heart disease. Am J Cardiol 29:180, 1972
11. Oliva PB, Potts DE, Pluss RG: Coronary arterial spasm in Prinzmetal angina: Documentation by coronary arteriography. N Engl J Med 288:745, 1973
12. Prinzmetal M, Ekmekci A, Kennamer R, et al: Variant form of angina: previously undelineated syndrome. JAMA 174:102, 1960
13. Ross RS, Gorlin R: Coronary arteriography. In Braunwald E, Swan HJC (eds): Cooperative study on cardiac catheterization. American Heart Association monograph #20, New York. III–67, 1968
14. Sheldon WC, Rincon G, Effler DB, Proudfit WL, Sones FM Jr: Vein graft surgery for coronary artery disease. Circulation (Suppl III) 48:184, 1973
15. Silverman ME, Flamm MD: Variant angina pectoris: Anatomic findings and prognostic implications. Ann Intern Med 75:339, 1971
16. Whiting RB, Klein MD, Vander Veer J, et al: Variant angina pectoris. N Engl J Med 282:709, 1970

38

PREINFARCTION ANGINA—WHAT IS IT?

William G. Williams, Harold Aldridge,
Malcolm D. Silver, and Alan S. Trimble

A number of clinical syndromes characterized by rapid progression of angina or a change in a stable pattern of angina have been recognized. These have been previously termed acute coronary insufficiency, the intermediate syndrome, acute myocardial ischemia, preinfarction angina, impending infarction, status anginosus, unstable angina, accelerated angina, and crescendo angina. All are characterized by the above-mentioned pain patterns and do not progress to immediate myocardial infarction. They do not have electrocardiographic evidence of infarction and have normal serum enzymes.

The first 400 patients with aortocoronary bypass grafting done at the Toronto General Hospital have been reviewed. The in-hospital mortality in patients with stable angina was 2 percent. However, there was a small group of patients who had unstable or "preinfarction" angina. The in-hospital mortality in this group of patients was unacceptably high.

Thirty-two patients with unstable angina were reviewed: Two distinct groups could be identified, which we termed crescendo angina and acute coronary insufficiency.

CRESCENDO ANGINA

In crescendo angina, there is an increased frequency in pain with or without lesser provocation, a duration of less than 15 minutes, and prompt relief by coronary vasodilators. Some patients show transient ECG changes of ischemia during pain but not of infarction.

Supported by the Ontario Heart Foundation.

ACUTE CORONARY INSUFFICIENCY

In acute coronary insufficiency there is characteristic anginal pain lasting more than 20 minutes with incomplete or no relief with coronary vasodilators, transient ECG changes of ischemia but not of infarction, and normal serum enzyme studies.

All 32 patients had recurrent angina up to the time of operation and had been unresponsive to vigorous medical management with coronary vasodilators, beta adrenergic blockers, diuretics, and hospitalization.

CLINICAL INFORMATION

The patients with unstable or "preinfarction angina" were classified as crescendo angina (16 patients) or acute coronary insufficiency (16 patients). The baseline data are listed in Table 1. Apart from the angina pattern, there were no significant differences in the clinical background of these patients.

TABLE 1. Clinical Information

	CRESCENDO	ACI
Male	14	12
Female	2	4
Mean age	49	54
Age range	39–64	41–65
Previous MI	12	10
Duration of symptoms (mos)	13	9

Hemodynamic Data

Complete catheter data were available in all but one of the patients. A summary of the mean values is presented in Table 2. The only finding of statistical significance was the ratio diastolic perfusion time index over tension time index (DPTI/TTI). This was calculated from the (post-angiographic) left ventricular and aortic pressure tracings as described by Buckberg in 1972. The values of DPTI/TTI are illustrated in Figure 1.

ANGIOGRAPHY

Left Ventricular Contractility

Contractility was assessed using the criteria of Lansdown in 1968 and is illustrated in Table 3. The ACI group has slightly better contractility, though the difference was not significant.

TABLE 2. Hemodynamic Data

	CRESCENDO	ACI
Cardiac index (L/min/m^2)	3.15	2.72
Stroke vol. index (ml/m^2)	40.4	32.5
Cardiac work (g – m)	4,020	3,295
LVEDP (mm Hg)	13.4	13.8
DPTI/TTI	0.86 ± 0.06	0.65 ± 0.05

TABLE 3. LV Contractility

ANGIOGRAPHY	CRESCENDO	ACI
Grade I	2	4
Grade II	7	10
Grade III	5	2
Grade IV	2	0

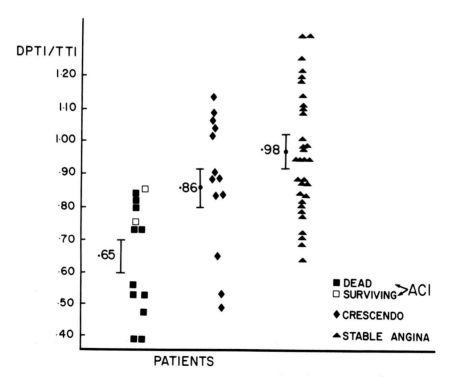

FIG. 1. The calculated values for the Diastolic Perfusion Time Index over Tension Time Index (DPTI/TTI) are illustrated graphically for these groups of patients. The mean value for the acute coronary insufficiency group (0.65) is in a critical range and is significantly different (P < 0.01) than either the crescendo angina patients or a control group of 32 patients with stable angina.

Coronary Arteriography

Stenotic lesions of 75 percent or greater were present in all three coronary arteries in nine of the crescendo group patients and 12 of the acute coronary insufficiency patients. There were no patients in either group with single coronary artery disease. The distribution of significant lesions is shown in Table 4.

TABLE 4. Distribution of Coronary Artery Disease[a]

	CRESCENDO	ACI
RCA	14 pts.	14 pts.
LAD	14 pts.	15 pts.
Circumflex	11 pts.	15 pts.

[a]*Stenotic lesions of 75 percent or greater.*

SURGICAL MANAGEMENT

Our policy from the outset has been to delay operation in the "preinfarction patient." Subsequent operation for "stable" angina carries a low (2 percent) in-hospital mortality. In the 32 patients under consideration, the "preinfarction" or unstable angina pattern persisted in spite of complete in-hospital medical treatment.

Our operative technique has included full-flow normothermic cardiopulmonary bypass with moderate hemodilution. The heart has been electrically fibrillated with alternating current, and anoxic arrest has been limited to less than 20 minutes at any one time.

TABLE 5. Distribution of Aortocoronary Grafts

	CRESCENDO	ACI
RCA	12	12
LAD	15	12
Circumflex	1	4
Total	28	28

The distribution of aortocoronary grafts is shown in Table 5. Two patients in the crescendo group and one in the acute coronary insufficiency group underwent internal mammary artery implantation at the time of their vein bypass graft. In addition, one patient with acute coronary insufficiency underwent resection of a left ventricular aneurysm at the time of vein grafting.

OPERATIVE RESULTS

Patient Survival

There were no deaths in the 16 patients with crescendo angina. In marked contrast to this, there were 12 deaths in the 16 patients with acute coronary insufficiency. Nine of these 12 deaths occurred within 12 hours of operation, either as a result of failure to wean from bypass, or as a result of progressive low-output syndrome. The three other deaths in the acute coronary insufficiency group were preceded by a lesser degree of low output syndrome leading to myocardial infarction in two and pulmonary embolism in the third.

Graft Patency

Postoperative information regarding graft patency is available for nine of the patients in the crescendo group and 13 patients in the acute coronary insufficiency group. The graft patency rates were 87 percent and 82 percent, respectively.

AUTOPSY MATERIAL

Autopsy was performed in nine of the 12 patients who died; all of the deaths were in the acute coronary insufficiency group. These nine patients had received a total of 15 aortocoronary bypass grafts and 11 (73 percent) were patent.

The relative infrequency of classical myocardial infarction was surprising. In spite of a history of 13 previous myocardial infarctions in these nine patients, only four classical infarctions could be identified histologically. Two of these infarcts had occurred relatively recently and were associated with a single occluded aortocoronary bypass graft. All of these four hearts with classical infarcts also had extensive areas of subendocardial fibrosis.

The typical lesions found in these hearts are illustrated in Figure 2. The subendocardial muscle showed extensive ischemic injury of varying age. This consists of extensive focal myofibrillary degeneration or myocytolysis in the earlier stages and subsequent organization and replacement by fibrous tissue in the chronic stage. These lesions are not localized to the distribution of a single coronary artery but are distributed throughout the entire subendocardial layer of the ventricular wall. Subendocardial ischemic damage was

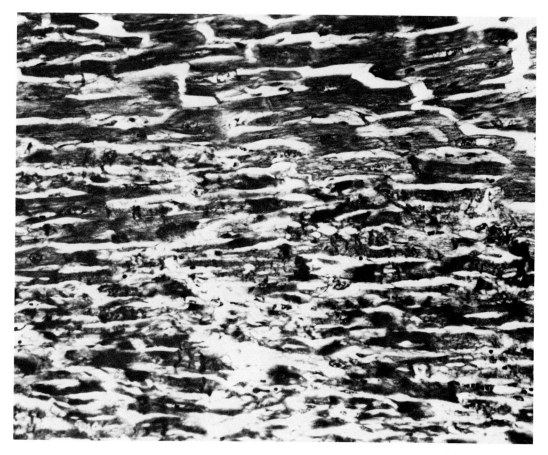

FIG. 2. Extensive myofibrillary degeneration is seen in the subendocardium. The myocardial fibers in the upper third of the photograph are normal. (Hematoxalin and Eosin × 50)

extensive even in hearts with patent grafts, including one patient with a triple graft. In effect, these hearts all showed evidence of ongoing myocardial necrosis in the subendocardial region.

DISCUSSION

Aortocoronary bypass grafting in patients with stable angina is a very safe procedure. In our initial experience with 400 patients, there were only eight hospital deaths. In marked contrast however, we had 12 hospital deaths in a group of 32 patients who underwent operation with a clinical diagnosis of "preinfarction" angina. When these patients were reviewed carefully, they could be classified into two distinct groups: crescendo angina and acute coronary insufficiency (ACI) angina. All of the deaths occurred in the ACI subgroup. The criteria used in isolating the ACI subgroup were those of Fischl in 1973. It must be stressed that these patients were having recurrent

bouts of ACI, unresponsive to medical management, up to the time of operation. Single bouts of ACI are common. Paul Wood in 1968 stated that 10 percent of patients with coronary artery disease present with ACI. Almost all patients with a single bout of acute coronary insufficiency become clinically stable. Our surgical results in patients with a history of one previous bout of acute coronary insufficiency are identical to those patients with stable angina. The problem group in our series has been the 16 patients (4 percent of the total surgical series) in whom the bouts of acute coronary insufficiency were recurrent up to the time of operation in spite of medical treatment.

The high-risk group of patients (ACIs) could not be isolated on the basis of standard hemodynamic or angiographic assessment. They could be isolated by calculating myocardial blood flow distribution on the basis of Buckberg's supply/demand ratio. The mean value of DPTI/TTI for the ACI group was in the critical range for subendocardial ischemia. This value was significantly different (p < 0.01) from the crescendo group of patients. A random group of 32 patients undergoing bypass surgery for stable angina were also measured and the ratios are included in Figure 1.

The low DPTI/TTI ratio in the ACI group suggests that these patients had significant subendocardial ischemia prior to operation. All nine of the autopsied hearts showed extensive areas of subendocardial ischemia, necrosis, and fibrosis. It seems likely to us that the prolonged pain of acute coronary insufficiency is due to subendocardial ischemia. Recurrent bouts of ACI lead to subendocardial cell death in spite of absent ECG and enzyme changes. Because of our high surgical mortality, we do not feel justified in operating on this small group of patients with the same techniques that we have used in the past. Specifically, subendocardial blood flow must be increased to allow these patients to survive operation.

Other authors have not had difficulty with the "preinfarction" group of patients. In Thomas's collective review of 16 authors' work, the operative mortality in 420 patients was only 4.3 percent. The questions we must ask are, "What are *we* doing wrong?" "Are we talking about the same group of patients?" "What is 'preinfarction' angina?" "What must we change in our operative technique to lower hospital mortality in this group of ACI patients?"

SUMMARY

A review of our initial experience with aortocoronary bypass vein grafts in 400 patients uncovered a small number of patients in whom the operative mortality was unacceptably high. This group of 32 patients had a clinical picture described as "preinfarction" or unstable angina. In half of these patients the unstable angina followed a crescendo pattern; the other half were classified as recurrent acute coronary insufficiency. Operative results in the crescendo group were excellent and did not differ from patients with stable angina.

In contrast, the operative mortality in the ACI group was 75 percent. The myocardial blood-flow distribution at catheterization, calculated by the Buckberg formula, showed that these patients had a critical circulation in their subendocardium. At autopsy, all of the hearts examined had extensive subendocardial necrosis of varying ages. This necrosis occurred in spite of absent ECG and enzyme changes. Salvage of this small group of patients will require some means of improving subendocardial blood flow so that they can tolerate surgery.

References

Buckberg GD, Fixler DE, Archie JP, Hoffman JIE: Experimental subendocardial ischemia in dogs with normal coronary arteries. Circ Res 30:67, 1972

Editorial. Intermediate coronary syndrome. Br Med J 3:601, 1973

Fischl SJ, Herman MV, Gorlin R: The intermediate coronary syndrome. N Engl J Med 288:1193, 1973

Fowler NO: "Preinfarctional" angina: a need for an objective definition and for a controlled clinical trial of its management. Circulation 44:755, 1971

Gazes PC, Mobley EM, Faris HM, Duncan RC, Humphries GB: Preinfarctional (unstable) angina—a prospective study—ten year follow-up. Circulation 48:331, 1973

Lansdown EL, Aldridge HE, Spratt EH: Angiographic assessment of the ischemic left ventricle: a preliminary report. Can Med Assoc J 99:1171, 1968

Najafi H, Henson D, Dye WS, et al: Left ventricular hemorrhagic necrosis. Ann Thorac Surg 7:550, 1969

Reichenbach DD, Benditt EP: Catecholamines and cardiomyopathy: the pathogenesis and potential importance of myofibrillar degeneration. Hum Pathol 1:125, 1970

Schlesinger MJ, Reiner L: Focal myocytolysis of the heart. Am J Pathol 31:443, 1955

Spencer FC, Glassman E: Preinfarction angina: current therapeutic considerations. Am J Cardiol 32:382, 1973

Thomas CS, Alford WC, Burrus GR, Stoney WS: Aorta-to-coronary artery bypass grafting: Indications and contraindications—an interim review. Ann Thorac Surg 16:201, 1973

Wood, P: Diseases of the Heart and Circulation, 3d ed. London, Eyre & Spottiswoode, 1968

39

PREINFARCTIONAL (UNSTABLE) ANGINA: A PROSPECTIVE STUDY—TEN-YEAR FOLLOW-UP
Prognostic Significance of Electrocardiographic Changes

PETER C. GAZES, E. MIMS MOBLEY, JR., HENRY M. FARIS, JR.,
ROBERT C. DUNCAN, G. BADGER HUMPHRIES,
and JAMES A. L. GLENN

INTRODUCTION

The terms "impending coronary occlusion," "acute coronary insufficiency," "intermediate coronary syndrome," "coronary failure," "status anginosus," "preinfarction angina," and "unstable angina," among others, have been used for patients who experience a sudden increase in frequency of angina, or more severe and prolonged cardiac pain than the usual angina. The pain often occurs at rest.

In our study, 140 patients with preinfarctional angina were followed for 10 years. The objective of this study was to determine the survival rate of this group and to discover whether it was possible to predict the patient's prognosis on the basis of electrocardiographic findings. Now that saphenous vein graft bypass techniques for direct myocardial revascularization have been developed, recording the natural history of preinfarctional angina has become even more important. At present, there are no specific criteria for selection of surgical candidates. The ubiquitous nature of angina makes it very difficult to pick out the patients with this syndrome who would probably die without surgical intervention. It would be helpful if types of angina pectoris could be defined and distinguished by their natural history.

MATERIALS AND METHODS

The 140 consecutive patients from a private practice (PCG) who satisfied our criteria for pre-infarctional angina were included in this study prior to 1961. The criteria were as follows:

Type 1. Initial onset of progressive, crescendo (increase in frequency, severity, and duration) angina and pain at rest in a patient previously free of symptoms.
Type 2. Same as in Type 1, *occurring suddenly* in a patient with known stable angina.
Type 3. Episodes of prolonged pain at rest, of more than 15 minutes, not related to obvious precipitating factors such as anemia or arrhythmias.

The 140 patients were admitted to the hospital, usually within 48 hours but not later than two weeks after the onset of their preinfarctional symptoms. Patients were excluded from the study if, during the first 48 hours, electrocardiographic changes indicated the development of an acute myocardial infarction or if enzyme levels rose significantly. They were also excluded when first examined if significant cardiomegaly was present, or if there was evidence of congestive heart failure. Whenever there was an associated disease that could shorten a patient's life, that patient was not included in the study. The 140 patients meeting selection criteria were divided into groups according to the electrocardiographic findings noted at rest or occurring transiently during or just after an episode of pain. The transient findings included ischemic ST and/or T-wave changes. Patients with known previous myocardial infarction or bundle branch block had old tracings documenting these findings.

Seven groups were noted with different electrocardiographic recordings:

Group 1. Ischemic ST depression of the horizontal type of at least 1 mm (0.1 mV) or greater, with T-wave inversion (17 patients)

Group 2. Ischemic ST depression without T-wave inversion (26 patients)

Group 3. Old myocardial infarction pattern with or without transient ST or T-wave changes (25 patients)

Group 4. ST elevation (five patients)

Group 5. Previous bundle branch block with or without transient ST or T-wave changes (11 patients)

Group 6. T-wave inversion only (32 patients)

Group 7. Normal (24 patients)

Each patient was included in only one group. Twelve patients in Group 3 and one patient in Group 5 had superimposed transient ST depression during pain. In addition, seven patients in Group 3 and two in Group 5 had transient T-wave inversion. These patients were not included in Groups 1, 2, or 6.

The 140 patients were a uniform group in that they fulfilled our criteria for preinfarctional angina and their illness was incapacitating. Fifty-four patients continued to have typical angina or prolonged ischemic pain after 48 hours of bed rest despite maximum therapeutic measures. These patients began to respond poorly to nitroglycerin and required frequent doses of opiates for relief. A daily record of pain and the use of nitroglycerin was kept during the hospital period so that at the end of the 10 years these 54 patients were separated and distinguished as an early high-risk subgroup.

During the 10-year period, data were compiled by personal follow-up examinations, telephone calls to family physicians, patients, or their families. In certain instances death certificates and autopsy reports were reviewed. The data included the following: age, sex, body build, family history, occupation, pre-existing conditions (hypertension, diabetes, myocardial infarction), pain characteristics, physical findings, laboratory findings, and patient's course. The patients were treated with periods of rest, nitrites (long-acting and sublingual nitroglycerin), sedatives, analgesia, and low calorie–low fat diets. The beta-blocker drugs were not available until the later part of this study. Ninety-one patients received warfarin and/or heparin.

Follow-up life table analysis was employed

TABLE 1. Sex Distribution of 140 Patients in Seven Electrocardiographic Groups

SEX	GROUP							TOTAL
	I	II	III	IV	V	VI	VII	
Male	14	22	20	4	8	26	19	113
Female	3	4	5	1	3	6	5	27

Reproduced from Gazes PC et al: Preinfarctional (unstable) angina—a prospective study—ten year follow-up. Circulation 48:331, 1973, by permission of the authors, publisher, and the American Heart Association, Inc.

to determine survival by using the method described by Remington and Schork, 1970.[23] We followed 113 patients either to the time of death or for 120 months. Twenty-seven patients were lost to follow-up prior to 120 months. Comparisons of the yearly survival rates were made for the electrocardiographic groups using the standard normal z-test.

RESULTS

Of the 140 patients in this study, 113 were male and 27 female, a ratio of 4:1 (Table 1). Tables 2 and 3 compare the clinical features of the total group and the high-risk subgroup with respect to age, electrocardiographic groups, and preinfarction criteria. The ages ranged from 35 years to 72 years. The average age was 56 years for the total group and 57 years for the high-risk subgroup. Patients with Type-2 pain had prior stable angina for an average of 2.8 years. In addition, 25 of these Type-2 patients had suffered a myocardial infarction that occurred on the average of 3.3 years earlier. Table 4 summarizes the main features of the high-risk subgroup.

TABLE 2. Patient Population According to Age and Electrocardiographic Groups

AGE	GROUP													
	I		II		III		IV		V		VI		VII	
	T	S	T	S	T	S	T	S	T	S	T	S	T	S
35–44	1		4		2	2	0		0		4		2	
45–54	0		7	3	4	3	1	1	0		9		5	2
55–59	9	6	7	2	11	3	1	1	5	3	9	2	8	2
60–72	7	6	8	5	8	4	3	2	6	3	10	3	9	1

T = total group of 140 pts. S = high-risk subgroup of 54 pts.

Reproduced from Gazes PC et al: Preinfarctional (unstable) angina—a prospective study—ten year follow-up. Circulation 48:331, 1973 by permission of the authors, publisher, and the American Heart Association, Inc.

TABLE 3. Clinical Presentation of Preinfarction Angina According to Criteria (three types)

TYPE	TOTAL GROUP (no. pts.)	HIGH-RISK SUBGROUP (no. pts.)
1	27	3
2	109	51
	(Prior to MI-25)	(Prior to MI-12)
3	4	
1 and 3	5	
2 and 3	27	15

Reproduced from Gazes PC et al: Preinfarctional (unstable) angina—a prospective study—ten year follow-up. Circulation 48:331, 1973 by permission of the authors, publisher, and the American Heart Association, Inc.

TABLE 4. Features of High-Risk Preinfarction Subgroup

FEATURE	NO. PTS.[a]
Frequent in-hospital pain	54 (100)
ST change during pain	33 (61)
Normal ECG during pain	5 (9)
Prior stable angina	51 (94)

Reproduced from Gazes PC et al: Preinfarctional (unstable) angina—a prospective study—ten year follow-up. Circulation 48:331, 1973 by permission of the authors, publisher, and the American Heart Association, Inc.
[a]*Percent of patients in parentheses.*

Seventy-seven of the 140 patients expired. Fifty-five percent (63 of 114) of the males died, and 51 percent (14 of 27) of the females died. Seventy-three of these deaths were the result of coronary events such as sudden death, sudden death with angina, heart failure, or myocardial in-farction. The other four patients died from non-coronary events: two had cerebrovascular accidents, one had carcinoma of the stomach, and one had an automobile accident.

Figure 1 depicts the probability of survival for the total group, the high-risk subgroup, and

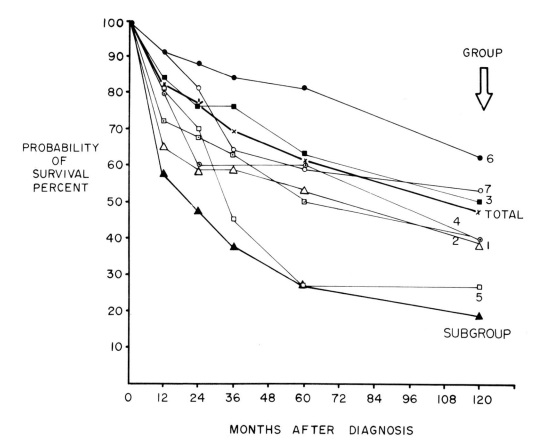

FIG. 1. Survival curves (determined by life table analysis) of patients in the total group, high-risk subgroup, and in the 7 electrocardiographic groups. Reproduced from Gazes PC et al: Preinfarctional (unstable) angina—A prospective study—ten year follow-up Circulation 48:331, 1973, by permission of the authors, publisher, and the American Heart Association, Inc.

for each of the seven electrocardiographic groups. Patients in electrocardiographic Groups 6 and 7 had a higher survival rate during the first two years when compared to patients of groups 1 and 2 (p < 0.05). Patients in Group 5 had the worst prognosis after the first two years.

The seven electrocardiographic groups are neither mutually exclusive nor based on comparable types of descriptors; patients with ST and T changes may also have an old myocardial infarction and/or bundle branch block. The descriptors of ST and T changes relate to acute coronary insufficiency (the patient's problem at the time of observation), while old myocardial infarction and bundle branch block relate to remote events that may not have similar effects upon short-term prognosis. Therefore, the data was analyzed for patient survival according to whether they had ST, T, or no changes during rest or transiently during, or just after, pain. Figure 2 depicts the probability of survival for the total group, high-risk subgroup, and total group minus the high-risk subgroup according to these three electrocardiographic groups. In the total group, the survival for patients with ST changes differs from those with T-wave changes (P < 0.05) throughout all periods, but only for the first year when compared with patients with no changes. There was no difference statistically among the three electrocardiographic groups for the high-risk subgroup and for the total group minus the high-risk subgroup.

If the high-risk subgroup is subtracted from the total group, the remaining 86 patients have better prognoses. Figure 3 compares the cumulative survival rate of these three groups.

Figure 4 compares the number of deaths and myocardial infarctions that occurred within three months of the onset of preinfarctional angina for the total group and the high-risk subgroup. Two of these patients had severe chest pain for over 30 minutes and died suddenly on the way to the hospital. The other patients with infarctions were diagnosed in the hospital. Twenty-nine of the 140 (20.7 percent) patients developed an acute myocardial infarction and the mortality rate associated with this complication was 41.4 percent (12 of 29 patients) for this three-month period. The total mortality during this period was 10 percent (14 of 140 patients). Fifteen of the 29 patients who developed an infarction were on anticoagulants. There were seven deaths in this group and five deaths in the 14 patients who were not on anticoagulants.

Nineteen of the 54 high-risk subgroup patients (35 percent) developed an acute myocardial infarction during the three-month period with an associated mortality of 63 percent (12 of 19 patients). The total mortality during this period was 26 percent (14 of 54 patients). In fact, all of the deaths in the first 12 weeks were entirely in this high-risk subgroup. Table 5 compares the number of infarctions that developed prior to three months

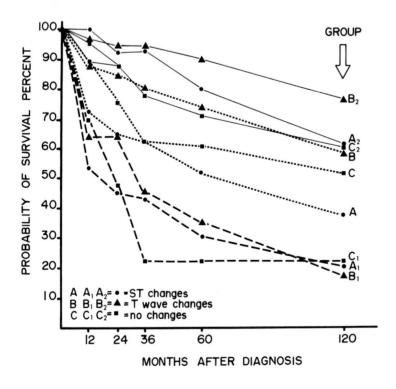

A $A_1 A_2 = $ •-• ST changes
B $B_1 B_2 = $ ▲-▲ T wave changes
C $C_1 C_2 = $ ■-■ no changes

FIG. 2. Survival curve (determined by life table analysis) of patients in the total group (A, B, C), high-risk subgroup (A_1, B_1, C_1), and total group minus high-risk subgroup (A_2, B_2, C_2) for the 3 electrocardiographic groups.

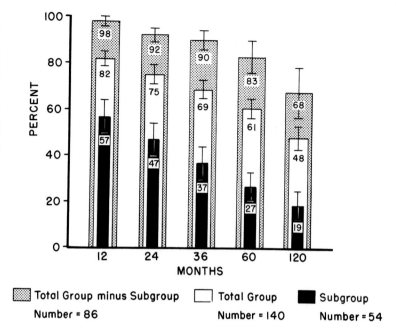

FIG. 3. Comparison of the cumulative proportion of patients surviving in the total group (n = 140), high-risk subgroup, (n = 154), and in the total group minus the subgroup (n = 86). Reproduced from Gazes PC et al: Preinfarctional (unstable) angina—a prospective study—ten year follow-up. Circulation 48: 331, 1973, by permission of the authors, publisher, and the American Heart Association, Inc.

in both the total group and the high-risk subgroup with associated deaths broken down into each of the seven electrocardiographic groups. In Table 6 the number of patients who developed infarctions are compared according to the three types of our preinfarctional criteria.

Table 7 compares the incidence of hyper-

tension, diabetes, and hypercholesterolemia in the total and in the high-risk subgroup. Hypertension was considered present if the blood pressure was 140/90 or greater, and hypercholesterolemia if the cholesterol was over 240 mg percent. Hypertension was present prior to the onset of angina. The incidence of diabetes is low for such patients.

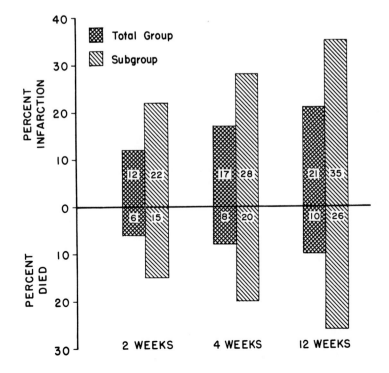

FIG. 4. Myocardial infarctions and deaths that occurred prior to 3 months in the total group and in the high-risk subgroup. Reproduced from Gazes PC et al: Preinfarctional (unstable) angina—a prospective study—ten year follow-up. Circulation 48: 331, 1973, by permission of the authors, publisher, and the American Heart Association, Inc.

TABLE 5. Number of Patients That Developed Infarction and Associated Death in Each of the Seven Electrocardiographic Groups

	GROUP												
	I		II		III		IV		V		VI		VII	
	T	S	T	S	T	S	T	S	T	S	T	S	T	S
Pts.	17	12	26	10	25	12	5	4	11	6	32	5	24	5
Infarcted	5	5	6	5	6	5	1	1	1	1	5	1	5	1
	(29.7)	(41.7)	(23)	(50)	(24)	(41.7)	(20)	(25)	(9)	(16.6)	(15.6)	(20)	(20.8)	(20)
Died from infarct	5	5	3	3	3	3	0	0	0	0	1	1	0	0
	(100)	(100)	(50)	(60)	(50)	(60)					(20)	(20)		

T = total group; S = high-risk subgroup. Percent of patients in parentheses.
Reproduced from Gazes, PC et cl: Preinfarctional (unstable) angina—a prospective study—ten year follow-up.
Circulation 48:331, 1973, by permission of the authors, publisher, and the American Heart Association, Inc.

However, glucose tolerance tests were not performed on all patients, and all of those designated had been diagnosed as diabetic prior to this study.

During the first year after onset of preinfarctional angina, 18 percent (25 of 140) of the patients died. Seventy-four percent (104 of 140) had less angina, and the anginal pattern of the remaining 8 percent (11 of 140) remained unchanged. It is difficult to evaluate change in the quality of these patients' lives since many adjusted their exertion in order to reduce the anginal attacks. Approximately 50 percent of these patients resumed normal activity.

DISCUSSION

The distinction between preinfarctional angina and more chronic varieties of angina may be difficult since they may overlap. In the present series, all patients demonstrated a clear change in their clinical status and satisfied the usual criteria for the preinfarction syndrome. As others have noted, many of these patients will not develop myocardial infarctions. For this reason, the term "preinfarctional angina" is misleading, and this syndrome should be referred to as "unstable angina." High-risk patients, with frequent and prolonged attacks of angina continuing after 48 hours of bed rest without significant response to therapy, should be recognized, since they have a very poor prognosis. In addition, 94 percent (51 patients) in our high-risk subgroup also had prior stable angina, and all except five had electrocardiographic changes during an attack. Ischemic ST depression occurred in 29 of these patients (seven with prior myocardial infarcts) and ST elevation in four patients. These ST changes accounted for 61 percent (33 of 54) of the electrocardiographic changes in this high-risk subgroup. Twelve of the 54 high-risk patients died during the first month (average, eight days after admission). The earliest deaths in this high-risk subgroup occurred in two patients: one at 48 hours after hospitalization and the other at 72 hours.

Patients with prior bundle branch block, especially after the second year in the study, had the worst prognosis. This may be accounted for

TABLE 6. Number of Patients That Developed Infarction with Associated Death Prior to Three Months According to the Preinfarction Criteria (3 Types)

TYPE	TOTAL GROUP		HIGH-RISK SUBGROUP	
	Infarcts	Deaths	Infarcts	Deaths
1	1	–	–	–
2	22	9	14	9
2 with prior infarct	6	3	5	3
3	–	–	–	–

Reproduced from Gazes, PC et al: Preinfarctional (unstable) angina—a prospective study—ten year follow-up. Circulation 48:331, 1973, by permission of the authors, publisher, and the American Heart Association, Inc.

TABLE 7. Incidence of Hypertension, Diabetes, and Hypercholesterolemia

	TOTAL: 140 PTS.	HIGH-RISK GROUP: 54 PTS.
Hypertension	46 (32)	29 (54)
Diabetes	13 (9)	7 (13)
Hypercholesterolemia	69 (49)	17 (31)

Percent of patients in parentheses.
Reproduced from Gazes, PC et al: Prefarctional (unstable) angina—a prospective study—ten year follow-up. Circulation 48:331, 1973, by permission of the authors, publisher, and the American Heart Association, Inc.

by the fact that five of the patients in this group were between 55 and 60 years of age, and six were over 60 years of age. In addition, the six deaths in the group were sudden, with coronary occlusions, suggesting, in view of the bundle branch block, that trifascicular block may have developed. The deaths were distributed equally between the two types of bundle branch block.

In the high-risk subgroup, those with electrocardiographic changes of ischemic ST depression (Groups 1 and 2) or prior myocardial infarction (Group 3), or those with prior stable angina had the highest incidence of acute infarction and associated death prior to three months (Tables 5 and 6). Vakil (1964)[31] reported an overall incidence of 40.6 percent for acute myocardial infarctions within this same period in 360 cases with preinfarctional angina. Infarctions in that study occurred in 36 percent of the 190 patients treated with anticoagulant therapy, and this complication developed in 49 percent of 156 patients treated conservatively, with associated mortalities of 26 percent and 37 percent respectively. Fulton et al (1972)[10] reported an incidence of 14 percent of patients developing myocardial infarctions who had preinfarctional angina, with an 11 percent mortality due to this complication. The high mortality of the patients in our group with acute myocardial infarctions, superimposed on the preinfarctional syndrome, was probably due to the fact that all except one of these patients had prior stable angina. In addition, six of the patients with stable angina had also experienced a prior infarction. Furthermore, our patients were referred to a medical center, whereas Fulton's cases were collected from the records of general practitioners and probably were seen much earlier in the evolution of their disease.

In another study, of 100 patients with acute coronary insufficiency who were medically treated, six developed an acute myocardial infarction and survived; the one-year survival rate was 85 percent. A follow-up study of 47 patients with unstable angina revealed 8 percent in-hospital deaths and 17 percent late deaths (within 14 months). The survival rates of these two studies are approximately the same as that found in our total group for the same follow-up periods. The Framingham study[14] could predict that almost 30 percent of patients with angina (stable or complicated) over the age of 55 would die within eight years, or an average of 3.7 percent annually. The cases of preinfarctional angina were not separately analyzed in that study. The mortality rate for our 140 patients over the 10-year period averaged approximately five percent per year, and for the

54 high-risk subgroup patients, eight percent annually. After subtracting the high-risk subgroup from the total, the remaining 86 patients had an annual mortality rate of 3.2 percent. The five-year mortalities for these three groups were 8, 14.5, and 3.4 percent, respectively. These figures are much higher than those representing the 10-year period for the total and high-risk subgroups, since most of the deaths in these two groups occurred during the first five years. The average annual mortality for an average age of 56 years (similar to our total group), for a 10-year period involving the general population is 1.7 percent for the United States and 2.2 percent for South Carolina.

Our study is the first reported long-term follow-up study on preinfarctional angina. The immediate effectiveness of saphenous vein bypass grafts for coronary artery disease is recognized. In the literature to the present time,[1-9,11-22,24-26,28-30,32] there have been approximately 361 patients reported that have had saphenous vein bypass graft surgery for preinfarctional angina, with an average mortality of seven percent. These patients were not compared with similar groups treated medically. In addition, the lack of uniformity of criteria in these studies for preinfarctional angina (these groups of patients were not homogeneous) and paucity of information regarding long-term myocardial function and patient survival makes it very difficult to compare these surgical results with our medically treated groups. Recently, several short-term follow-up studies were reported comparing surgically and medically treated groups. Scanlon et al[27] reported on 70 patients with accelerated angina. Forty-eight of these patients were treated surgically, with a mortality of 12.5 percent; 22 patients treated without surgery had a mortality of 27 percent. The follow-up period for this study was not clearly stated. Another study, comparing 38 patients with preinfarctional angina treated with conventional medical therapy to 21 patients having aortocoronary graft, with a mean follow-up of 6.4 months, revealed a mortality of 20 percent and 14 percent, respectively.

Coronary arteriography was not performed on our patients since this study began prior to 1961. However, all of the patients had an unequivocal history of angina, and 83 percent had electrocardiographic changes at rest or during an episode of pain. Symptomatic coronary artery disease has been found to be accompanied by arteriographic evidence of moderate or severe obstruction of one or more major coronary vessels. Normal electrocardiograms can be found in patients in whom severe coronary artery disease could be demonstrated by coronary arteriograms.

A recent study reported the natural history of severe proximal coronary disease as defined by cineangiography in 200 patients with a seven-year follow-up. It was found that single-vessel anterior descending disease has a four percent yearly attrition rate, or 30.5 percent seven-year mortality; single right coronary or circumflex lesions, 1.8 percent yearly death, or 12.5 percent in seven years; two-vessel disease, 44 percent; and three-vessel disease 70 percent mortality in seven years. Our total group mortality compares with that of the two-vessel disease group and our high-risk subgroup with that of three-vessel disease.

SUMMARY

A total of 140 patients with preinfarctional (unstable) angina were followed for 10 years for the purpose of determining the natural history and the prognostic significance of electrocardiographic findings. The cumulative survival rate for the 140 patients was as follows: 12 months: 82 percent; 24 months: 75 percent; 36 months: 69 percent; 60 months: 61 percent; and 120 months: 48 percent. Twenty-one percent (29 of 140) of the patients developed an acute myocardial infarction within three months of onset of the diagnosis of preinfarctional angina with an associated mortality of 41.4 percent (12 of 29). A combination of high-risk factors in a patient, eg, frequent angina in the hospital, prior stable angina, and ischemic ST change during pain, identified his as a high-risk case. The high-risk subgroup (54) had a cumulative survival rate as follows: 12 months: 57 percent; 24 months: 47 percent; 36 months: 37 percent; 60 months: 27 percent; and 120 months: 19 percent. Thirty-five percent (19 of 54 patients) of this subgroup developed a myocardial infarction within three months of the onset of preinfarctional angina, with an associated mortality rate of 63 percent (12 of 19 patients). The total deaths in the first three months were entirely in this high-risk subgroup. At the first-year follow-up, 18 percent (25 of 140) of the patients died; 74 percent (104 of 140) had less angina; and 8 percent (11 of 140) did not show a change in their anginal pattern.

Patients with coronary artery disease with unstable angina who do not respond to in-hospital medical management within 48 hours (usually in a setting of preexisting angina pectoris) have a 12-week mortality of 26 percent and should be considered for urgent coronary artery bypass surgery. These data can be used as a basis for evaluation of surgical results.

References

1. Bolooki H, Vargas A, Ghahramani A, et al: Aorto-coronary bypass graft for preinfarction angina. Chest 61:247, 1972
2. Cheanvechai C, Effler DB, Loop FD, et al: Emergency myocardial revascularization. Am J Cardiol 32:901, 1973
3. Cohn LH, Fogarty TJ, Daily PO, Shumway NE: Emergency coronary artery bypass. Surgery 70:821, 1971
4. Dumesnil JG, Gau G, Callahan J, et al: Emergency myocardial revascularization with saphenous vein bypass graft (abstr). Am J Cardiol 29:269, 1972
5. Favaloro RG, Effler DB, Groves LK, Sheldon WC, Jones JM Jr: Direct myocardial revascularization by saphenous vein graft. Ann Thorac Surg 10:97, 1970
6. Favaloro RG, Effler DB, Cheanvechai C, Quint RA, Sones FM Jr: Acute coronary insufficiency (impending myocardial infarction) and myocardial infarction. Surgical treatment by the saphenous vein graft technique. Am J Cardiol 28:598, 1971
7. Flemma RJ, Johnson D, Tector AJ, Lepley D Jr, Blitz J: Surgical treatment of preinfarction angina. Arch Intern Med 129:828, 1972
8. Fowler NO: "Preinfarctional" angina. Circulation 44:755, 1971
9. Freedberg AS, Blumgart HL, Zoll PM, Schlesinger MJ: Coronary failure: the clinical syndrome of cardiac pain intermediate between angina pectoris and acute myocardial infarction. JAMA 138:107, 1948
10. Fulton M, Lutz W, Donald KW, et al: Natural history of unstable angina. Lancet 1:860, 1972
11. Graybiel A: The intermediate coronary syndrome. US Armed Forces Med J 6:1, 1955
12. Hill JD, Kerth WJ, Kelly JJ, et al: Emergency aortocoronary bypass for impending or extending myocardial infarction. Circulation 43, 44 (suppl I): I-1, 105, 1971
13. Johnson WD, Lepley D: An aggressive surgical approach to coronary disease. J Thorac Cardiovasc Surg 59:128, 1970
14. Kannel WB, Feinleib M: Natural history of angina pectoris in the Framingham Study. Am J Cardiol 29:154, 1972
15. Krauss KR, Hutter AM, DeSanctis RW: Acute coronary insufficiency: Course and follow-up. Circulation 45,46 (suppl I):I-1, 66, 1972
16. Lambert CJ, Adam M, Geisler GF, et al: Emergency myocardial revascularization for impending infarctions and arrhythmias. J Thorac Cardiovasc Surg 62:522, 1971
17. Martinez-Rios MA, Bruto DaCosta BC, Cecena-Seldner FA, Gensini GG: Normal electrocardiogram in the presence of severe coronary artery disease. Am J Cardiol 25:320, 1970
18. Master AM, Jaffe HL, Field LE, Donoso E: Acute coronary insufficiency: its differential diagnosis and treatment. Ann Intern Med 45:561, 1956
19. Moberg CH, Webster JS, Sones FM, Jr: Natural history of severe proximal coronary disease as defined by cineangiography (200 patients, 7 year follow-up). (Abstr) Am J Cardiol 29:282, 1972
20. Papp C, Smith KS: Status anginosus. Br Heart J 22:259, 1960
21. Proudfit WL, Shirey EK, Sones FM Jr: Selective cine coronary arteriography: correlation with clinical findings in 1000 patients. Circulation 33:901, 1966

22. Public Health Service Life Table. In Vital Statistics of the United States. US Dept of HEW. Vol II, Sec 5, 1969

23. Remington RD, Schork MA: Statistics with application to the Biological and Health Sciences. Englewood Cliffs, NJ, Prentice-Hall, 1970, p 344

24. Resnik WH: Preinfarction angina. I. The transaminase test—A diagnostic aid. II. An interpretation. Mod Concepts Cardiovasc Dis 31:751, 1962. Ibid, 31:757, 1962

25. Robinson WA, Smith RF, Stevens TW, Perry JM, Friesinger GC: Preinfarction syndrome: evaluation and treatment. Circulation 46 (suppl II): II–212, 1972

26. Sampson JJ, Eliaser M Jr: Diagnosis of impending acute coronary artery occlusion. Am Heart J 13:675, 1937

27. Scanlon PJ, Nemickas R, Moran JF, et al: Accelerated angina pectoris. Clinical hemodynamic, arteriographic and therapeutic experience in 85 patients. Circulation 47:19, 1973

28. Segal BL, Likoff W, van den Broek H, et al: Saphenous vein bypass surgery for impending myocardial infarction. Critical evaluation and current concepts. JAMA 223:767, 1973

29. South Carolina State Life Table, vol 2, no 41, US Dept of HEW, Public Health Service, 1959–61

30. Spencer FC: Bypass grafting for preinfarction angina. Circulation 45:1314, 1972

31. Vakil RJ: Preinfarction syndrome—management and follow-up. Am J Cardiol 14:55, 1964

32. Watkins JC, Russel RO, Rackley CE: Follow-up of unstable angina in a myocardial infarction research unit. Circulation 46 (suppl II): II–23, 1972

40

EMERGENCY SURGERY FOR HIGH-RISK PREINFARCTION ANGINA

Peter Hairston, William H. Lee, Jr.,
and James E. May

Coronary artery bypass for the treatment of coronary arterial occlusive disease has gained wide acceptance and application since it was initially envisioned by Alexis Carrel in 1910. The procedure generally consists of autogenous vein or internal mammary bypass grafting of critical obstructions in the coronary artery. The objective is to establish immediate restoration of blood flow to ischemic heart muscle in order to effect relief of angina pectoris, improve ventricular function (Chatterjee, Swan, et al, 1972; Hairston, Newman, et al, 1973), and prevent subsequent myocardial damage. Applied on an elective basis, the procedure appears to have accomplished this objective successfully (Cooley, Dawson, et al, 1973; Favaloro, 1969; Hutchinson, Green, et al, 1974; Sampson, Eliaser, 1937).

Naturally interest has now turned to applying these revascularization techniques to emergency intervention in patients with preinfarction angina (Favaloro, Effler, et al, 1971; Harrison, Shumway, 1972; Sheldon, Rincon, et al, 1973), a syndrome variously described as impending coronary occlusion (Sampson, Eliaser, 1937), acute coronary insufficiency (Master, Jaffe, et al, 1956), intermediate coronary syndrome (Graybiel, 1955), coronary failure (Freedberg, Blumgart, et al, 1948), status angiosus (Papp, Smith, 1960), and unstable angina (Fowler, 1971). Fundamental to this approach is the premise that there is a recognizable stage in the evolution of ischemic heart disease when clinical signs suggest that infarction of the myocardium is impending. The controversy associated with this aggressive approach stems from the potential hazards associated with operating on such gravely ill patients, as well as the difficulties inherent in predicting the course of patients with preinfarction syndrome.

Gazes (Gazes, Mobley, et al, 1973) has recently reported a long-term follow-up study in which the prognostic significance of preinfarction unstable angina in patients managed on a medical regimen has been assessed. A "high-risk" subgroup was defined on the basis of several factors, including frequent angina in the hospital, prior stable angina, and ischemic ST change during anginal pain, which appeared to indicate a highly lethal potential. This report is a critical analysis of a similar group of patients, categorized as high risk, in whom direct immediate myocardial revascularization was performed on an emergency basis.

MATERIAL AND METHODS

Patient Selection

Forty-four patients with preinfarction syndrome, characterized by a combination of "high-risk" factors, were incapacitated by their illness and referred by the Cardiology Service at the Medical University Hospital for consideration of emergency coronary bypass surgery (Table 1). These patients were considered "high risk" on the basis of one or more of the following factors:

1. the presence of typical angina or prolonged ischemic pain despite maximum therapeutic measures
2. crescendo angina in a patient previously free of symptoms
3. crescendo angina in a patient with prior stable angina
4. ischemic ST change during anginal episodes

TABLE 1. Patient Profile

PTS.	NO.
Age (yrs)	
30–40	7
40–50	16
50–60	10
>60	11
(Avg. age: 50)	
Male	34
Female	10
White	43
Black	1

The patients were monitored in the Coronary Care Unit while undergoing a medical regimen consisting of bed rest, sedatives, narcotics, nasal oxygen, and coronary vasodilators. Anticoagulants were not employed routinely since, generally, surgery was performed within 48 hours of the patient's admission. Left heart catheterization, including cineangiography by the Sones technique, was performed with results as noted in Table 2. A 70 percent or greater obstruction of the coronary lumen was considered significant. Only six patients had a single-vessel obstruction; 15 had two obstructed vessels; and 23 had three vessels involved. Ventricular dysfunction as manifested by segmental or diffuse dyskinesis, paradoxical wall motion, or elevated left ventricular end-diastolic pressure was encountered in 34 patients. Aortic or mitral valve dysfunction with hemodynamic impact sufficient to require replacement was detected in two patients. All patients were considered to be in Functional Class IV of the New York Heart

TABLE 2. Catheterization/Angiography Data

	NO.
Coronary occlusion[a]	
One vessel	6
Two vessels	15
Three vessels	23
Ventricular dysfunction	
Dyskinesis	
Segmental	26
Diffuse	8
Aneurysm	2
LVed >12	33
Valve dysfunction	
Aortic	1
Mitral	1

[a]Considered significant if narrowing greater than 70 percent in either oblique projection.

TABLE 3. Factors Compounding Operative Risk in 44 Patients—Functional Class IV[a]

	NO. PTS.
Diabetes	8
Cardiac enlargement	5
Hypertension	7
Previous infarction	21

[a]New York Heart Association Functional Classification.

Association Classification. Factors considered significant in compounding the operative risks in these 44 patients are listed in Table 3. None of the patients were in clinical congestive failure, but five manifested significant cardiac enlargement, and 21 had documented evidence of previous myocardial infarction.

Operative Technique

Suitable lengths of autogenous vein, generally the saphenous, were obtained, with meticulous care in handling, through multiple incisions in the medial thigh and lower leg. The veins were irrigated with heparinized blood and gently distended to check for leaks. The proximal vein-to-aorta anastomosis was performed first, generally, utilizing a partial aortic occlusion clamp to create an elliptical aortotomy incision. Total cardiopulmonary bypass was employed utilizing a Bentley oxygenator, moderate body hypothermia, intermittent ischemic cardiac arrest with topical application of iced Ringer's lactate, and left ventricular decompression through a catheter inserted via the right superior pulmonary vein. The distal vein to artery anastomosis was performed by isolated occlusion of the vessel avoiding total myocardial ischemia whenever possible. All anastomoses were created with monofilament nylon in a continuous fashion.

Operative Procedures (Table 4)

A total of 104 saphenous vein grafts were inserted in the 44 patients, with the majority of patients requiring more than a single graft. The internal mammary artery was utilized in two patients, one of whom had developed recurrence of angina attributed to occlusion of a vein graft previously placed to the left anterior descending coronary artery. Coronary endarterectomy was requisite to adequate vessel reconstruction in 10 patients. Aortic or mitral valve replacement was required in two patients. Resection of a sizable ventricular

TABLE 4. Operation Performed: 44 Patients

OPERATION	NO.	NO. PTS.
Saphenous vein graft	104	
Single		5
Double		15
Triple		23
Internal mammary bypass	2	
Endarterectomy	10	
Valve replacement	2	
Aortic		1
Mitral		1
Ventricular reconstruction	1	

aneurysm containing thrombus was necessary in one patient.

Results (Tables 5 and 6)

A single intraoperative death occurred presumably secondary to a massive myocardial infarction; this was a female patient with severe diffuse occlusive disease who required a three-vessel revascularization. She suffered cardiac arrest in the Intensive Care Unit two hours following the initial operative procedure and, therefore, was returned immediately to surgery. The graft to the dominant right coronary artery was found to be occluded with thrombus. Patency was reestablished, but the myocardium became progressively unresponsive to cardiotonic agents, and intractable arrest ensued.

TABLE 5. Results—44 Patients

	NO.	%
Hospital deaths	4	9
Late deaths (15 mo)	1	5
(25 mo)	1	
Living (7–27 mo)	38	86
Total	44	

On the fourth day following surgery, one patient died of a massive intracerebral hemorrhage attributed to a head injury suffered in a fall three days prior to the operation. The intracerebral bleeding was probably exacerbated by the heparin required during the surgery. One patient died of myocardial insufficiency on the eighth day following a three-vessel revascularization and coincident mitral valve replacement. The fourth hospital death was due to aortic aneurysm rupture in a patient in whom an aortic valve had been implanted and a three-vessel revascularization had been performed.

TABLE 6. Death Analysis—Six Patients

	TIME	NO.
Myocardial infarction	(OR)	1
Massive CVA	4 days	1
Myocardial insufficiency	8 days	1
Aortic aneurysm rupture	18 days	1
Arrhythmia—(etiology?)	15 mo	1
Unknown and sudden	25 mo	1

There have been two late deaths, one at 15 months and the other at 25 months, both in active asymptomatic patients gainfully employed at the time of their deaths. Autopsies were not obtained in either case.

Thirty-eight patients (86 percent) are living seven to 27 months following surgery (Table 7). Twenty-six patients are free of angina and have discontinued all cardiac medications except digitalis. Eight patients express significant improvement of their angina with coincident reduction in the required medication and would be placed in New York Heart Association Functional Class II. Twenty-five patients are gainfully employed, and nine patients are either retired and living active lives or else functioning in a capacity that they consider normal without financial gain. Therefore, 89 percent of the living patients are symptomatically and functionally improved following the operative procedure.

TABLE 7. Life Analysis[a] 38 Patients

	NO.	SUBTOTAL	%
Angina free	26	34	89
Angina improved	8		
Gainfully employed	25	34	89
Activity normal	9		

[a]*Two patients were angina free and gainfully employed at time of late sudden death but are not included. See Table 6.*

Two patients required second operative procedures as a result of recurrent angina and angiographic demonstration of vein graft occlusion. Both patients improved following the second procedure, and one is gainfully employed.

Myocardial infarction was documented by electrocardiography in six patients all within the perioperative period. Four of these patients manifested no symptoms, and five are included in the group of survivors who are gainfully employed.

Postoperative Catheterization (Table 8)

Ten patients have been restudied, one patient twice, for varying degrees of symptom recurrence. A total of 25 grafts were studied and 17 (68 percent) found to be patent. In nine of the patients at least one graft was noted to be patent. One patient with a single graft to the left anterior descending coronary, a middle-aged female with severe diabetes, was studied 12 days following surgery due to recurrence of severe anterior chest pain. She was found to have occluded the graft and developed moderate ventricular dyskinesis over the left anterior ventricular surface. A second operative procedure was not performed, and the patient is presently controlled on medication and is gainfully employed.

TABLE 8. Postop Catheterization—11 Patients

GRAFTS		OPEN	CLOSED
LAD	9	6	3
RCA	7	5	2
CCA[a]	7	5	2
LIMA[b]	2	1	1
Total	25	17	8

[a] Circumflex coronary artery.
[b] Left internal mammary artery.

DISCUSSION

The myocardium deprived of adequate oxygen supply, as occurs with coronary artery occlusion, evokes recognizable premonitory signs that herald impending and frequently inevitable myocardial damage. On the basis of these signs standardized criteria are developing for definition of the clinical state foreshadowing imminent infarction, commonly referred to as the preinfarction syndrome (Harrison, Shumway, 1972). Coincidentally there is increasing awareness of the high morbidity (myocardial infarction), and mortality that characterizes the natural history of unstable or preinfarction angina (Fulton, Luntz, et al, 1972; Hochberg, 1971; Soloman, Edwards, et al 1969). Coronary artery bypass applied as emergency intervention in patients manifesting the prodromal signs of myocardial infarction is gaining enthusiasm. The results of direct immediate myocardial revascularization in these patients, although

variable, have been significantly better than those obtained in similar patients treated by medical regimen (Lambert, Adam, et al, 1971). However, a valid comparison awaits analysis of the treatment methods when they are applied to patients in whom there is uniformity of recognizable premonitory signs heralding impending myocardial damage.

The present study utilized the criteria described by Gazes (Gazes, Mobley, et al, 1973) in his 10-year follow-up of 140 nonoperated patients with unstable angina. Gazes identified a high-risk subgroup that manifested a combination of factors: frequent angina in the hospital, prior stable angina, and ischemic ST change during pain. The 12-month mortality of this subgroup was 43 percent. Thirty-five percent developed a myocardial infarction within three months of the unstable angina with an associated mortality of 63 percent.

The 44 patients selected for the present study comprise a similar high-risk subgroup who continued to have typical angina or prolonged ischemic pain after 48 hours of bed rest despite maximum therapeutic measures. Efforts were made to exclude the possibility of acute myocardial infarction, and coronary angiography was performed followed by coronary bypass surgery as an emergency procedure. A 9 percent hospital mortality and a 4.5 percent late mortality reflect a considerable improvement in the prognosis of unstable angina with surgical management.

The hospital mortality was encountered solely in patients with triple-vessel disease. This might be anticipated from the data of Friesinger (Friesinger, Page, et al, 1970), Moberg (Moberg, Webster, et al 1972) and more recently Webster (Webster, Moberg, et al, 1974), who reports an extremely high natural attrition in patients with severe proximal coronary disease involving three vessels.

Myocardial infarction was encountered in six patients (13 percent, resulting in one death, all in the perioperative period. Gazes reported a much higher infarction rate (28 percent at one month) in his comparable subgroup. The frequency of electrocardiographic changes compatible with myocardial infarction after coronary bypass ranges from 8 to 35 percent. The absence of symptomatology in the majority of these patients suggests that the presence of new Q-waves may reflect the unmasking of preexisting infarction rather than development of new infarction (Bassan, Oatfield, et al, 1974).

Graft patency of 68 percent was found in 11 patients studied following surgery, all of whom had recurring symptomatology. Hopefully, this does not reflect the status of the remaining asymptomatic patients. Coronary endarterectomy and the liberal use of bifurcation grafts in the early part of the series have been shown to enhance early graft occlusion (Cooley, Dawson, et al, 1973; Tradd, Larsen, et al, 1973). Avoidance of these techniques as well as the more liberal use of the internal mammary artery (Green, 1972) is anticipated to result in a prolongation of graft patency.

Thirty-eight patients are living, and of the survivors 89 percent are either free of angina or significantly improved. In addition, these patients are either gainfully employed or pursuing an active life. It is concluded that immediate direct coronary artery bypass for the relief of myocardial ischemia in the selected patient whose preinfarction syndrome is characterized by a combination of high-risk factors affords considerable promise, especially when compared to a similar group in whom surgery was not performed.

References

Bassan MM, Oatfield R, Hoffman I, Matloff J, Swan HJC: New Q waves after aortocoronary bypass surgery. N Engl J Med 290:349–53, 1974

Carrel A: On the experimental surgery of the thoracic aorta and the heart. Ann Surg 52:93, 1910

Chatterjee K, Swan HJC, Parmley WW, et al. Depression of left ventricular function due to acute myocardial ischemia and its reversal after aortocoronary saphenous vein bypass. N Engl J Med 286:1117–22, 1972

Cooley DA, Dawson JT, Hallman GL, et al. Aortocoronary saphenous vein bypass. Ann Thorac Surg 16:380–90

Favaloro RG: Saphenous vein graft in the surgical treatment of coronary artery disease. J Thorac Cardiovasc Surg 58:178, 1969

Favaloro RG, Effler DB, Cheanvechai C, Quint RA, Sones FM Jr: Acute coronary insufficiency (impending myocardial infarction and myocardial infarction): Surgical treatment by the saphenous vein graft technique. Am J Cardiol 28:598, 1971

Fowler NO: "Preinfarctional" angina. Circulation 44:755, 1971

Freedberg AS, Blumgart HL, Zoll PM, Schlesinger MJ: Coronary failure: the clinical syndrome of cardiac pain intermediate between angina pectoris and acute myocardial infarction. JAMA 136:107, 1948

Friesinger GC, Page EE, Ross RS: Prognostic significance of coronary arteriography. Trans Assoc Am Physicians 83:78–92, 1970

Fulton M, Lutz W, Donald KW, et al. Natural history of unstable angina. Lancet 1:860, 1972

Gazes P, Mobley EM Jr, Farris HM Jr, Duncan RD, Humphries GB: Preinfarction angina (unstable)—a prospective study—10-year follow-up. Circulation 48:331–37, 1973

Graybiel A: The intermediate coronary syndrome. US Armed Forces Med J 6:1, 1955

Green GE: Internal mammary artery-to-coronary artery anastomosis: Three year experience with 165 patients. Ann Thorac Surg 14:260, 1972

Hairston P, Newman WH, Daniell HB: Myocardial contractile force as influenced by direct coronary surgery. Ann Thorac Surg 15:364–70, 1973

Harrison DC, Shumway N: Evaluation and surgery for impending myocardial infarction. Hosp Practice 7:49–58, 1972

Hochberg HM: Characteristics and significance of prodromes of coronary care unit patients. Chest 59:10, 1971

Hutchinson JE III, Green GE, Mekhjian HA, Kemp HG: Coronary bypass grafting in 376 consecutive patients, with three operative deaths. J Thorac Cardiovasc Surg 67:7–16, 1974

Lambert CH, Adam M, Geisler GF, et al. Emergency myocardial revascularization for impending infarctions and arrhythmias. J Thorac Cardiovasc Surg 62:522, 1971

Master AM, Jaffe HL, Field LE, Donoso E: Acute coronary insufficiency: its differential diagnosis and treatment. Ann Intern Med 45:561, 1956

Moberg CH, Webster JS, Sones FM Jr: Natural history of severe proximal coronary disease as defined by cineangiography (200 patients, 7 year follow-up). (Abstr) Am J Cardiol 29:282, 1972

Papp C, Smith KS: Status angiosus. Br Heart J 22:259, 1960

Sampson JJ, Eliaser M Jr: Diagnosis of impending acute coronary artery occlusion. Am Heart J 13:675, 1937

Sheldon WC, Rincon G, Effler DB, et al. Vein graft surgery for coronary artery disease. Circulation 48: suppl III:III-184–III-189, 1973

Soloman HA, Edwards AL, Killip T: Prodromata in acute myocardial infarction. Circulation 40:463, 1969

Traad EA, Larsen PB, Gentsch TO, Gosselin AJ, Swaye PS: Surgical management of the preinfarction syndrome. Ann Thorac Surg 16:261–71, 1973

Webster JS, Moberg C, Rincon G: Natural history of severe proximal coronary artery disease as documented by coronary cineangiography. Am J Cardiol 33:195–200, 1974

41

PREINFARCTION ANGINA: SURGICAL AND MEDICAL MANAGEMENT

George E. Berk, Stephen J. Gulotta, John B. Morrison,
Martin J. Kaplitt, Stephen L. Frantz,
and Vellore T. Padmanabhan

There are few terms in the medical literature more surrounded with ambiguity and confusion than "preinfarction angina." There are a variety of terms used by various investigators to describe this entity, eg, "unstable angina" (Fowler, 1971), "intermediate coronary syndrome" (Graybiel, 1955), "impending coronary occlusion" (Sampson and Eliaser, 1937), "impending myocardial infarction" (Lawrence, 1971), "coronary failure" (Freedberg, Blumgart, et al, 1971), and "accelerated angina pectoris" (Scanlon, Nemickas, et al, 1973).

These terms, used interchangeably, have in common an attempt to delineate a group of patients with angina who have a high risk of developing myocardial infarction with its attendant morbidity and mortality.

Over the past few years the advent of direct saphenous vein coronary artery bypass has made surgical intervention in this group of patients feasible. Although it has been enthusiastically advocated by some investigators, the loose definitions used have made it difficult to assess surgical therapy on an objective basis. The principal difficulty lies in the fact that the syndrome of preinfarction angina has been defined by very subjective clinical criteria, which, over the years, have varied from "new or altered ischemic cardiac pain" (Scanlon, Nemickas, et al, 1973) to relatively complex, multifactoral definitions (Conti, Brawley, et al, 1973). Moreover, the immediate and remote natural history of the syndrome is not known, and the risks of diagnostic intervention and major surgery in patients with severely compromised myocardial vascular supply are uncertain.

With the above considerations in mind, this study was undertaken to (1) define precisely a subgroup of patients with rigorous criteria for preinfarction angina; (2) assess the short-term prognosis of such a group managed medically; and (3) gauge the risk and efficacy of aggressive surgical intervention in such patients.

MATERIALS AND METHODS

All admissions with the diagnosis of ischemic heart disease to the ICU or CCU of North Shore University Hospital from January 1973 to August 1973 were considered for inclusion in the study (850 patients). Of these, all patients with electrocardiographic and/or enzymatic evidence of acute myocardial infarction on admission were excluded, as were those with evidence of acute MI in the first 48 hours of hospitalization. Criteria for acute MI were (1) new Q-waves on ECG, or (2) ST segment and T-wave changes with transient elevation of cardiac enzymes (SGOT > 55, CPK > 200, LDH > 200) and compatible clinical picture. Also excluded were patients without convincing evidence of coronary arterial disease by ECG or careful history, those with preexisting bundle branch block or liver disease in whom the diagnosis of MI was difficult to ascertain, and those patients with significant disease of other organ systems. Of the remaining group, the following criteria were said to constitute preinfarction angina: (1) change in preexisting anginal pattern or new onset of classical symptoms of angina pectoris; (2) severe chest pain occurring at complete bed rest; (3) electrocardiographic changes occurring at the precise moment of chest pain reverting completely to a preexisting pattern no longer than 30 minutes after cessation of pain; the changes included significant ST segment elevation, ST segment depression of 2 mm or more, heart block, or transient bundle branch block; and (4) no electrocardiographic or enzymatic evidence of myocardial infarction.

During the first four months of the study, all patients who fulfilled the above criteria (13 patients) were treated medically—ie, oxygen, complete bed rest under constant monitoring in the CCU, sedation, long-acting sublingual nitrates, and propranolol in varying doses and regimens as determined by their private cardiologists. Cardiac catheterization and coronary angiograms were not done in this group, being considered part of aggressive management.

During the latter four months of the study, all patients with preinfarction angina were studied with cardiac catheterization and coronary angiography after careful examination of serial ECGs and enzymes to exclude acute infarction. The mean time for diagnosis to catheterization was five days, during which time medical management (as determined by the patient's private physician) was utilized.

Right and left heart catheterization, left ventriculography and selective coronary angiography were performed in the postabsorptive state under mild pentobarbital sedation. The right heart was entered via the left femoral vein approached percutaneously. A platinum-tipped end hole catheter was used for pressure measurements. This also served as an electrode catheter in the event pacing became necessary during the procedure. Left heart catheterization, left ventriculography, and coronary angiography were performed by the Seldinger technique utilizing the left femoral artery. Intracardiac and intravascular pressures were measured using P23 db Statham strain gauges and recorded with a DR-12 Electronics for Medicine recorder. Cardiac output was determined by the indicator dilution technique using indocyanine green dye and a Gilford densitometer.

Cine studies were performed with a Phillips C-arm fluoroscopic unit at 60 frames per second, using 35 mm SF-2 Dupont film. Left ventriculography was performed in a single-plane 30-degree right anterior oblique projection. Selective coronary arteriography was done in the AP, RAO, and LAO projections, using the Judkins technique.

Measurements of cardiac output, left ventricular end-diastolic pressure, and ventriculography were used to assess left ventricular function. The left ventriculogram provided information relating to contractility and helped define areas of abnormal wall motion.

The above studies were done in the operating room with the entire cardiac team on standby. The cardiopulmonary bypass apparatus was in the room and primed with saline. Twelve units of cross-matched whole blood were available. All patients with high-grade occlusive lesions deemed amenable to bypass surgery (defined as greater than 85 percent stenosis of a proximal vessel as gauged by at least three observers) were then treated with one, two, or three saphenous vein grafts. Surgery was done immediately following angiography in each case.

Surgically and medically treated patients were compared as to age, sex, prior MI, and risk factors (diabetes, hypertension, family history of coronary artery disease, lipid abnormalities, smoking, and cardiomegaly). Diabetes was defined as abnormal glucose tolerance test (peak blood glucose greater than 160 mg percent after 60 minutes) with or without glycosuria. Hypertension was defined as consistent elevations in systolic blood pressure over 140 and/or diastolic blood pressure over 90. Lipid abnormalities included serum cholesterol greater than 250 mg percent. Smoking of a significant degree was defined as more than one pack a day for over 10 years. Cardiomegaly meant a cardiothoracic ratio of greater than 0.5.

The results of medical and surgical therapy were compared in terms of types of ECG change, incidence of myocardial infarction, occurrence of complications such as congestive heart failure, shock, and ventricular fibrillation in short-term follow-up (three months). Congestive heart failure was defined as the occurrence of two or more of the following: pulmonary vascular congestion on chest x-ray, basilar râles without evidence of infection, and ventricular gallop. Shock consisted of systolic blood pressure less than 85 for at least three consecutive hours, oliguria (less than 15 cc of urine per hour) for the same period of time, peripheral vasoconstriction, and altered state of higher integrative function. In addition to the above, surgical patients were evaluated for postpericardotomy syndrome, defined as typical pericarditic chest pain with friction rub, fever, and elevated sedimentation rate.

RESULTS

Table 1 shows a comparison between risk factors in medically and surgically managed patients. The medically managed group had a mean

TABLE 1. Risk Factors

	MEDICAL[a]	SURGICAL[a]
Number	13	11
Age	60	51
Male	13	–
Female	9	2
Diabetes	4	4
Hypertension	4	4
Family history	6	7
Lipid abnormality	1	0
Smoking	7	6
Cardiomegaly	1	0
Prior MI	4	3

[a]*One patient had two discrete preinfarction episodes eight months apart and was included in both groups.*

age of 60 as compared with a mean age of 51 in the surgically managed group. There was a marked male preponderance in both groups with all 13 of the medical group and 9/11 of the surgical group being male. The most commonly encountered risk factors in both groups were smoking and positive family history of ASHD. In each group these occurred in more than 50 percent of cases. Diabetes, hypertension, and prior infarction were intermediate in occurrence, being present in about a third of both groups. Lipid abnormality and cardiomegaly were unusual, each occurring in one case of the medically managed group.

Table 2 summarizes the results of medical therapy in the initial group of 13 patients. Preinfarction ECG changes were extremely variable, consisting of ST segment depressions and/or T-wave inversions in six cases; in the anterolateral leads (I, AVL, V4-6) in two cases, in the anterior leads (V1-3) in three cases, and in the inferior leads (II, III, AVF) in one case. In the remaining seven cases, ST elevations occurred, in the inferior leads in five cases, and in the anterior leads in three cases (one case had elevations in both areas at different times). There was no correlation between presence of ST segment elevation versus depression and subsequent development of infarction or complications, and there was no significant relationship between areas of ST segment changes and subsequent course. Nine of 13 patients treated medically evolved acute infarctions as documented by Q-waves and enzyme elevations; two of these were anterolateral wall infarctions, three were anterior wall, and four were inferior wall. As might be expected, the area of infarction correlated in all cases with the area of ST segment change in the preinfarction state.

The time from preinfarction to infarction varied from one to 13 days in this group. In terms of complications, seven of nine patients who evolved acute infarctions also developed heart failure significant enough to require therapy with digitalis and/or diuretics. Three of the nine de-

TABLE 2. Results of Medical Therapy

PT.	AGE	PREINFARCT ECG CHANGE	MI	DAYS FROM PREINFARCT TO MI	CHF	SHOCK	VF/VT	SEQUELLAE (3 mos.)
LB	72	ST depression I, AVL, V5–6	ALMI	3	No	No	No	Pain-free
PG	47	ST depression V1–3	No	–	No	No	No	Preinfarction treated surgically 8 months later
BH	76	T inversion V1–4	AMI	8	No	No	No	Pain-free
TL	49	ST elevation 2, 3, AVF	No	–	No	No	No	Lost to follow
MG	59	ST depression V1–3	ASMI	2	Yes	No	No	Sudden death after discharge (1 week)
MB	63	ST elevation 2, 3 AVF	DMI	3	Yes	No	No	Persistent CHF
IW	57	ST elevation 2, 3 AVF	DMI	3	Yes	No	No	Pain-free
FB	66	ST elevation	No	–	No	No	No	Pain-free
ES	59	ST elevation V1–3	No	–	No	No	No	Persistent pain without MI
JJ	69	ST depression V2–6	ALMI	4	Yes	No	No	Intermittent pain persists
WH	67	ST elevation 2, 3 AVF	DMI	13	Yes	Yes	Yes	Died day 15 of acute MI
WN	62	ST elevation V1–3 & 2, 3, AVF	AMI	3	Yes	Yes	Yes	Intermittent pain persists
JP	47	ST depression 2, 3, AVF, V5–6	DMI	1	Yes	Yes	Yes	Died acute DMI day 3

TABLE 3. Results of Surgical Therapy

PT.	AGE	PREINFARCT ECG CHANGES	CATH FINDINGS	GRAFTS DONE	MI	CHF	ARRHYTHMIA	POST PERICARDOTOMY	PAIN ON FOLLOW-UP
JB	63	3 degree heart block	90% prox. LAD	LAD	–	–	–	–	No
RF	53	LBBB	90% LMCA, 90% prox. LAD	LAD	–	–	–	–	No
BG	44	ST elevation 2, 3, AVF	100% prox. LAD, 90% prox. RCA	RCA	DMI	–	–	–	No
DR	46	ST elevation 2, 3, AVF	90–100% prox. RCA	RCA	–	–	–	–	No
MT	53	ST depression I, AVL, V5–6	95% prox. LAD, 80% prox. CIRC	LAD, CIRC	–	–	–	–	No
EF	55	T-wave inversion V2–6	85% prox. RCA, 70% prox. LAD, 100% mid-LAD	RCA, LAD	–	–	AF	Yes	No
GN	40	ST depression 2, 3, AVF, V5–6	Diffuse disease RCA; 90% prox. LAD, CIRC	LAD, CIRC	–	–	–	–	No
MD[a]	53	ST elevation V1–4	Diffuse triple-vessel disease		No surgery done, no evidence MI				
AN	59	ST depression 2, 3, AVF, V5–6	90% LMCA, 90% prox. LAD; 2 90% lesions RCA	RCA, LAD (with gas endarterectomy)	–	–	–	–	No
TD	48	T inversion V1–6	90% prox. LAD; 80% RCA	LAD RCA	–	–	–	–	No
PG	47	ST depression V1–6	100% RCA, 90% prox. LAD, 90% obtuse marginal	RCA, LAD CIRC	–	–	–	–	No
BK	37	ST depression 1, AVL, V4–6	95% lg. 1st diagonal	1st diagonal	–	–	–	Yes	No

[a]Excluded from study.

TABLE 4. Summary

	MEDICAL	SURGICAL
Number	13	11
Mortality	3	0
Acute MI	9	1
CHF	7	0
Shock	3	0
Ventricular fibrillation	3	0

veloped ventricular tachycardia or fibrillation requiring DC countershock. Three suffered cardiogenic shock, and two of the three died. A third patient died suddenly one week after hospital discharge, presumably of a cardiovascular event. Of the 10 survivors, three continued to have pain during the period of follow-up, and one patient again presented with preinfarction angina eight months later.

The results in the surgically treated group are summarized in Table 3. In this group of 11 patients receiving 18 grafts, aggressive cardiac catheterization and immediate surgery was associated with no mortality. All patients studied had high-grade stenosis of one or more proximal vessels; eight of the 11 had double- or triple-vessel disease. Only one patient, who had severe three-vessel disease with poor runoff, was considered inoperable. In terms of morbidity one patient was felt to have sustained an acute MI during the operative period, and two patients had postpericardotomy syndromes manifested by pleuritic chest pain, fever, new rubs, and transient arrhythmia in one case. None of these patients demonstrated significant heart failure or ventricular arrhythmias. On three-month follow-up, all surgically managed patients were free of anginal pain. Of note was a high incidence of transient ventricular fibrillation during catheterization (four of 11 patients), demonstrating the marked cardiac irritability of this group.

Table 4 summarizes the surgical and medical results in our group of patients with preinfarction angina, including the period of hospitalization and three months after discharge.

DISCUSSION

It has been a subject of great controversy in the literature as to the prognosis of "preinfarction angina" in terms of morbidity and mortality. Indeed, a recent article (Conti, Brawley, et al, 1973) asserts that "mortality rates for patients with unstable angina treated medically range from

3 to 40 percent." The great divergence in these figures is obviously due in great measure to the rigor with which one defines the preinfarction state. Thus, Kraus, Hutter, et al (1972) report an 86 percent survival rate of "preinfarction" patients treated medically over a year's time but define preinfarction angina as "pain lasting over 30 minutes" without evidence of MI. Fulton, Lutz, et al (1972) reported only a 14 percent infarction rate over an 18-month period in patients with unstable angina but again included in their group all patients with altered chest pain. Chalmers (1972) summarized the results of medical therapy in nearly 1,000 patients, from five papers utilizing varying definitions, and found a mortality rate varying from 0 to 27.7 percent (average 20.8 percent). When one becomes much more specific in defining the preinfarction state, however, the natural history of this entity appears much more grim. Scanlon, Nemickas, et al (1973) took a group of patients with "accelerated angina pectoris" (increasing frequency and severity of anginal attacks, rest or nocturnal angina, often ischemic ST and T-wave changes with pain) and defined a selected high-risk subgroup on the basis of significant lesions on coronary angiography. When followed on medical therapy, 59 percent suffered acute myocardial infarction with 27 percent mortality in this group, and an additional nine of the 57 patients considered for surgery had an acute MI preoperatively. Gazes, Mobley, et al (1973), in a recent retrospective study over 10 years, compared a group with preinfarction angina defined as "progressive crescendo angina and pain at rest" with a "high-risk subgroup" that, in addition to progressive angina, had transient ECG changes occurring during episodes of pain. In the less rigorously defined group 21 percent developed an acute MI in the initial eight months after diagnosis, with an associated mortality of 41.4 percent; the 12-month survival in the group was 82 percent. In contrast, the high-risk subgroup had a 35 percent incidence of acute MI in the three months following diagnosis with an associated mortality of 63 percent and a 12-month survival of only 57 percent.

Our experience with a high-risk subgroup closely parallels that of Gazes. Fully 70 percent of our group treated medically sustained an acute infarction during their hospitalization, and the mortality after follow-up for three months was 23 percent. It might be argued that "optimal" medical therapy was not given, but there is currently much active debate as to what constitutes optimal therapy for impending infarction. Our patients received propranolol in varying dosages, round-the-clock sublingual vasodilators, morphine sulfate, and other therapy deemed appropriate.

When one examines the surgical experience in preinfarction angina, the definition is again critical. For example, Flemma, Johnson, et al (1972) report only a 2.5 percent operative mortality with 78/80 patients "improved" but define the preinfarction state as simply "increased angina at rest . . . poorly responsive to medical therapy." Auer, Johnson, et al (1971), utilizing a similar definition, report no infarctions or mortality in 41 consecutive patients. These groups are obviously quite distinct from patients in a high-risk subgroup with rigorous criteria such as those reported here. The experience with such groups in the literature is somewhat limited. Miller, Cannom, et al (1973) reported a well-selected group of 67 patients who underwent saphenous vein bypass, with a mortality rate of 10.4 percent and a late death rate of 3.3 percent. A recent review by Conti, Brawley, et al (1973) on a rigorously selected subgroup indicated an operative mortality of 22 percent. Our initial experience, as summarized previously, shows no mortality and minimal morbidity in 11 consecutive patients treated with aggressive surgical management. On this basis we feel that surgical therapy in the preinfarction state is, at this time, associated with significantly lower morbidity than medical management. The variance of these results from those of Conti are somewhat difficult to explain but may be due in part to the presence of unrecognized myocardial infarction in this group of patients. It is noteworthy that the period between angiography and surgery in Conti's patients averaged 6.3 days. In our group the angiography was considered to be the first step in aggressive management and was done in the majority of cases in the operating room with pump standby. Most patients underwent surgery immediately following angiography, thereby minimizing the number of patients suffering small infarctions during or subsequent to the catheterization and decreasing the early surgical mortality.

CONCLUSIONS

Aggressive cardiac catheterization and coronary angiography immediately followed by saphenous vein bypass was successfully utilized in 11 consecutive cases of rigorously defined preinfarction angina. These results were contrasted with a similar group treated medically in which there was a high incidence of acute infarction and mortality. It is concluded that aggressive angiography and surgical management may offer significant therapeutic advantages over medical management in the preinfarction state.

References

Auer JE, Johnson WD, Flemma RJ, Tector AJ, and Lepley D: Direct coronary artery surgery for impending myocardial infarction (abstr). Circulation 44 (Suppl II):II 102, 1971

Bolooki H, Vargas A, Ghahramani A, et al: Aorto-coronary bypass graft for preinfarction angina. Chest 61:247, 1972

Chalmers T: Randomization and coronary artery surgery. Ann Thorac Surgery 14:323, 1972

Cohen LH, Fogarty TJ, Daily PO, and Shumway NE: Emergency coronary artery bypass. Surgery 70:821, 1971

Conti RC, Brawley RK, Griffith LS, et al: Unstable angina pectoris: morbidity and mortality in 57 consecutive patients evaluated angiographically. Am J Cardiology 32:745, 1973

Dumesnil JG, Gau G, Callahan J, et al: Emergency revascularization with saphenous vein graft. Am J Cardiology 29:260, 1972

Favaloro RG, Effler DB, Cheanvechai C, Quint RA, and Sones FM Jr: Acute coronary insufficiency: impending myocardial infarction and myocardial infarction. Am J Cardiology 28:598, 1971

Flemma RJ, Johnson WD, Tector AJ, Lepley D Jr, and Blitz J: Surgical treatment of preinfarction angina. Arch Intern Med 129:828, 1972

Fowler NO: "Preinfarctional" angina: a need for an objective definition and for a controlled clinical trial of its management. Circulation 44:755, 1971

Freedberg AS, Blumgart HL, Zoll PM, and Schlesinger MJ: Coronary failure: the clinical syndrome of cardiac pain intermediate between angina pectoris and acute myocardial infarction. JAMA 138:107, 1948

Fulton M, Lutz W, Donald KW, et al: Natural history of unstable angina. Lancet 1:860, 1972

Gazes PC, Mobley EM Jr, Faris HM Jr, Duncan RC, and Humphries GB: Preinfarctional (unstable) angina—a prospective study—ten year follow up. Circulation 48:331, 1973

Graybiel A: The intermediate coronary syndrome. US Armed Forces Med J 6:1, 1955

Krauss KR, Hutter AM Jr, and DeSanctis RW: Acute coronary insufficiency: course and follow up. Arch Intern Med 129:808, 1072

Lambert CJ, Mitchel BF, Adam M, and Geisler GF: Emergency myocardial revascularization for impending myocardial infarctions. Chest 61:479, 1972

Lawrence GH: Coronary revascularization for impending myocardial infarction (abstr). Circulation 44 (Suppl II):190, 1971

Linhart JW, Beller BM, and Talley RC: Preinfarction angina: clinical, hemodynamic and angiographic evaluation. Chest 61:312, 1972

Miller DC, Cannom DS, Fogarty TJ, et al: Saphenous vein coronary artery bypass in patients with "preinfarction angina." Circulation 47:234, 1973

Pfeifer J, Hultgren H, Alderman E, Angell W, and Shumway N: Surgical intervention in impending myocardial infarction (abstr) Circulation 44 (Suppl II): 211, 1971

Robinson WA, Smith RF, Stevens TW, Perry JM, and Friesinger GC: Preinfarction syndrome: evaluation and treatment. Circulation 46 (Suppl II):II-212, 1972

Sampson JJ, Eliaser M Jr: Diagnosis of impending acute coronary artery occlusion. Am Heart J 13:675, 1937

Scanlon PJ, Nemickas R, Moran JF, et al: Accelerated angina pectoris: clinical, hemodynamic, arteriographic and therapeutic experience in 85 patients. Circulation 47:19, 1973

Spencer FC: Bypass grafting for preinfarction angina. Circulation 45:1314, 1972

Sustaita H, Chatterjee K, Matloff JM, et al: Emergency bypass surgery in impending and complicated acute myocardial infarction. Arch Surg 105:30, 1972

Vogel JH, McFadden RB, Love JW, and Jahnke EJ: Emergency vein bypass for the preinfarction syndrome. Chest 59:606, 1971

42

CLINICAL, ARTERIOGRAPHIC, AND SURGICAL EXPERIENCE WITH THE IMPENDING MYOCARDIAL INFARCTION SYNDROME

James F. Pfeifer, Herbert N. Hultgren, Martin Lipton, William W. Angell, and William R. Brody

Many recent published reports of the impending myocardial infarction syndrome (IMIS) have clearly demonstrated an association with a high risk of death or nonfatal infarction within three months to three years after the onset of symptoms.[1-4] The risk is higher in patients who have ECG evidence of prior myocardial infarction, who have prior stable angina, and who have continued chest pain and ST-T changes during their hospital stay. Studies have also demonstrated that coronary arteriography and surgical intervention can be carried out with an acceptably low mortality and will result in relief of chest pain in a substantial number of patients over a one-to-two-year follow-up period.[5-16]

Fewer reports are available where clear diagnostic criteria for the diagnosis of the IMIS have been employed and described in a consecutive series of patients with subsequent arteriography and surgery.[17-20] Further data are needed on this problem to facilitate the selection of patients who have a high incidence of arteriographically demonstrated coronary disease, who are at high risk of death or infarction, and who would be suitable for coronary surgery. The purpose here is to describe the clinical and arteriographic features of a group of patients who fulfilled acceptable diagnostic criteria for the IMIS and who subsequently had coronary surgery performed with a low mortality and an excellent postoperative result.

MATERIALS AND METHODS

Patients referred to the CCU with chest pain were selected for angiography and possible surgery if they exhibited any of the following symptoms:

1. Stable angina with a recent increase in severity.
2. Recent onset of angina without clinically evident infarction.
3. Episodes of acute coronary insufficiency or rest angina of at least 15 minutes duration.
4. Symptomatic ventricular arrhythmias of recent onset.

Patients with any of the above symptoms of longer than three months' duration were not included in this study.

An increase in severity of established angina was diagnosed when episodes of angina became more frequent, more prolonged, or appeared at rest or at night, without other evident causes such as increased physical activity, mental stress, or changes in medical therapy. Usually angina appeared with less physical effort and required an increase in nitroglycerin consumption. Established angina was defined as stable angina of six months or more in duration. Acute coronary insufficiency was diagnosed when anginal chest pain occurred at rest without evident cause, lasted more than 15 minutes, and was not relieved by nitroglycerin. Such episodes were frequently accompanied by systemic symptoms such as dyspnea, sweating, weakness, palpitations, nausea, or vomiting, and Demerol or opiates were frequently required for pain relief. Symptomatic ventricular arrhythmias consisted of episodes of ventricular tachycardia or fibrillation that produced symptoms of palpitation or disturbances of consciousness.

In addition to the above features, objective

evidence of coronary disease was required in the form of either ECG signs of prior myocardial infarction or acute changes in the T-waves or ST segments during episodes of chest pain.

Patients were observed for several days in the CCU with continuous ECG monitoring, daily 12-lead ECG's, daily determination of serum enzymes (SGOT-LDH-CPK) as well as daily clinical examinations.

Patients with ECG or serum enzyme evidence of acute myocardial infarction were excluded from the study. On the basis of prior experience in this hospital, two successive serum enzyme levels exceeding the following values were considered to be evidence of acute infarction: CPK > 200 units, SGOT > 90 units, LDH > 800 units, when the upper normal limit of these values was 60, 40, and 350 units, respectively.[24]

Selective coronary arteriography was performed using the Judkin's technique. Left ventricular angiograms were performed after coronary arteriography via retrograde passage of a loop catheter into the LV. If surgically suitable lesions were present, saphenous vein bypass graft surgery (SVBGS) was performed within 72 hours of the arteriogram. Informed consent was obtained prior to arteriography.

RESULTS

Forty patients were studied and had selective coronary arteriography; 37 had surgery; 38 were males; and the mean age was 53 years (range 35 to 72).

Clinical Presentation

1. Stable angina of over six months had been present prior to the onset of the IMIS in 27 patients (68 percent). The mean duration was 66 months (range 6 months to 16 years).

2. Increased severity of angina occurred in all of the above 27 patients or 100 percent of the total number of patients. The mean duration was 31 days (range 1 to 180 days).

3. Recent onset of angina occurred in 13 patients. The mean duration was 37 days (range 3 to 150 days).

4. Acute coronary insufficiency or angina at rest occurred in 29 patients (75 percent). In nine patients (23 percent) acute coronary insufficiency was the only presenting complaint. In all patients with symptoms of acute coronary insufficiency these attacks preceded hospital entry from one day to 12 weeks (mean 4.8 weeks).

5. Two patients had chest pain at rest and experienced episodes of syncope due to ventricular tachycardia and short periods of ventricular fibrillation reverting spontaneously to sinus rhythm.

These data are summarized in Table 1.

Associated Risk Factors

1. In 14 of 30 (47 percent) ECG evidence of prior myocardial infarction was present in the resting ECG.

2. In 15 of 33 patients (45 percent) a history of prior infarction was obtained, but the resting ECG did not show evidence of infarction in five of 15 (33 percent).

3. A family history of coronary disease was obtained in 20 of 32 patients (63 percent).

4. A history of prior hypertension was present in nine of 25 patients (36 percent), and a diastolic pressure exceeding 89 mm Hg was present in eight of 38 patients (39 percent).

5. Serum cholesterol levels exceeding 300 mg percent were present in five of 35 patients (14 percent), and serum tri-

TABLE 1. Clinical Presentations of Impending Myocardial Infarction Syndrome

TYPE OF CHEST PAIN	NO. PTS.	%	DURATION-MEAN	RANGE
Stable angina > 6 mos	27	67.5	66 Mos	6 mos to 16 yrs
Accelerated angina	27	100.0	31 Days	1 to 180 days
Recent onset of angina	13	32.0	37 Days	3 days to 5 mos
Acute coronary insufficiency	29	75.0[a]	4.8 Wks	1 day to 12 wks
Ventricular arrhythmia	2	5.0	2 Mos	1 mo to 3 mos

[a]*23 percent presented with coronary insufficiency as the sole complaint.*

glyceride levels exceeding 250 mg percent were present in four of 23 patients (17 percent). A history of diabetes was present in four of 25 patients (16 percent). Twelve of 24 patients (50 percent) had fasting blood sugars in excess of 100 mg percent.

6. A positive smoking history was present in 27 of 28 patients (96 percent).

TABLE 2. Associated Risk Factors in Patients with Impending Myocardial Infarction Syndrome

FACTOR	NO. OBS.	NO. POSITIVE	%
EGG Prior MI	30	14	47
History only MI	33	15	45
Family history CAD	32	20	63
HBP history	25	9	36
DP > 89 mm	38	8	39
Chol > 300	35	5	14
Trig > 250 or 200	23	4	17
Smoking	28	27	96
Fasting blood sugar > 100	24	12	50

Risk factors are summarized in Table 2.

Electrocardiographic Changes

The following general types of acute ECG changes were observed either during symptoms or in the CCU.

1. Prominent inversion of T-waves of greater than 5 mm below the baseline (giant T-wave inversion). This was observed in 19 of 40 patients (48 percent). The T-waves exhibited terminal inversion, a "cove plane" contour, and the QT interval was usually prolonged (Fig. 1). These changes were most frequently seen in the anterior lateral or inferior lateral leads and less frequently in only the inferior or anterior leads. (These changes often persisted for many days even in the absence of continuing chest pain.)

2. T-wave inversion of lesser magnitude.

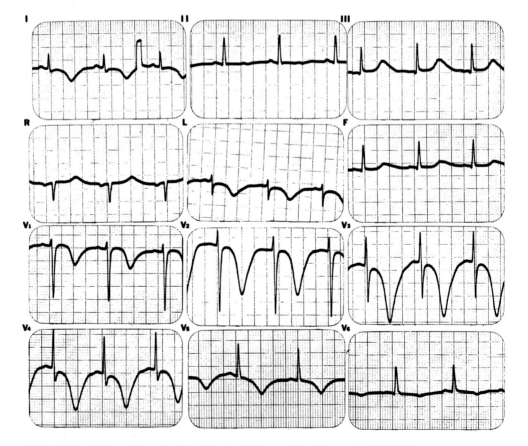

FIG. 1. Deep T-wave inversion in a 53-year-old housewife with recurrent episodes of acute coronary insufficiency of three weeks' duration. A severe proximal stenosis of the LAD was present. She has had no symptoms two years after a single bypass graft, which was shown to be patent 15 months after surgery.

These changes were observed in five of 40 patients (13 percent) and frequently accompanied or followed ST segment depression. Both of the above types of T-wave inversion often persisted for several days following the occurrence of chest pain.

3. ST segment depression. These changes occurred in 13 of 40 patients (36 percent) and were frequently transient occurring only during chest pain. The changes were observed in both anterior and inferior leads (Fig. 2).

4. ST segment elevation. This change was observed in nine of 40 patients (23 percent) and was usually transient occurring during chest pain (Fig. 3A–B). Subsequent T-wave inversion or the appearance of Q-waves was not observed.

5. Two patients had recurrent episodes of syncope associated with the onset of ventricular tachycardia at a rate of 180/min. This reverted to ventricular fibrillation lasting 10 to 30 seconds with the spontaneous resumption of a slow sinus rhythm with incomplete AV block. The episodes were preceded by chest pain at rest and elevation of ST segments in inferior leads.

6. Ventricular premature beats occurred in 17 of 32 (53 percent) patients and atrial arrhythmias occurred in 16 of 24 patients (66 percent). Sinus bradycardia was observed in 5 of 35 patients (14 percent). All five had acute ST-T-wave changes in inferior leads. ECG changes in all patients are summarized in Table 3.

Serum Enzyme Changes

CPK levels exceeded 60 units in 11 patients ($11/31 = 35$ percent), SGOT levels exceeded 40 units in 13 patients ($13/34 = 38$ percent), and LDH levels exceeded 350 units in 12 patients ($12/33 = 36$ percent). Highest serum enzymes were 481 (CPK), 151 (SGOT), and 1,044 (LDH). None of these patients had clinical

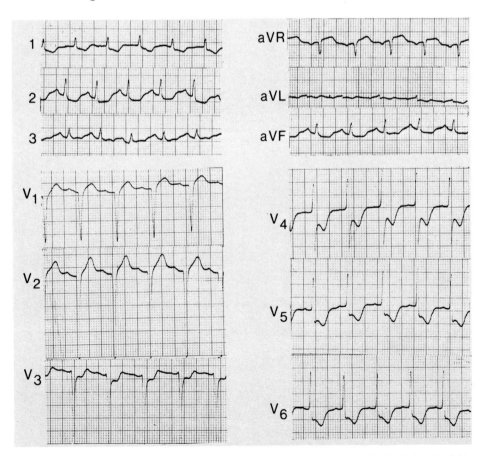

FIG. 2. Ischemic ST depression during chest pain in a 72-year-old veteran who had chronic stable angina with 24 hours of crescendo angina. Triple coronary disease was demonstrated. ST segments became isoelectric when pain was relieved.

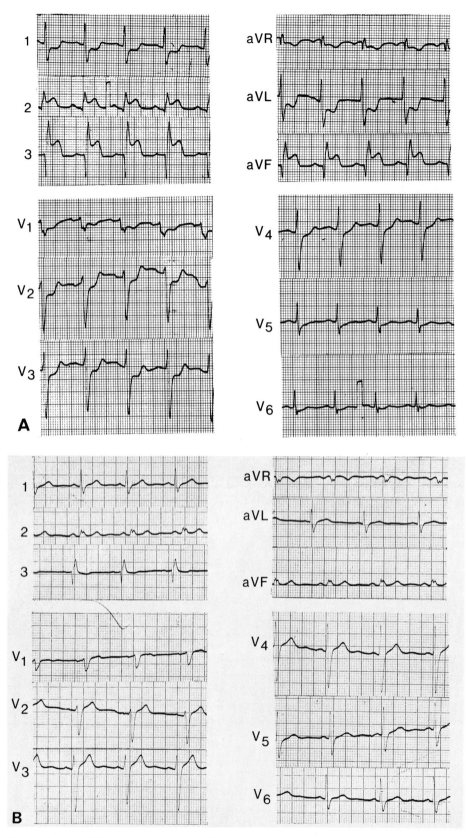

FIG. 3. A. Acute ST segment elevation during chest pain in a 55-year-old man with increasingly severe angina and rest pain over a 30-day period. An inferior myocardial infarction had occurred one year previously. Triple coronary disease was present. B. Same patient after relief of pain.

TABLE 3. Electrocardiographic Changes
Occurring during Hospital Observation of
Impending Myocardial Infarction Syndrome

	NO. PTS.	%
Giant T ↓	19/40	48
Lesser T ↓	5/40	13
ST ↓	13/40	36
ST ↑	9/40	23
Ventricular tachy or fib	2/40	5
Ventricular PMBs	17/32	53
Atrial arrhythmia	16/24	66
Sinus bradycardia	5/35	14

TABLE 4. Coronary Arteriographic Findings
in 40 Patients with Impending Myocardial
Infarction Syndrome. Lesions Listed Are
Those Resulting in > 50% Narrowing
of the Artery

	NO.	%
Left Main	4	10
LAD	33	82
Left Circumflex	17	42
Right Main	24	60
Posterior Descending	10/32	31
Contraction Abnormality	25/37	67
Ejection Fraction <60%	5/23	21
Collateral Vessels	24/38	63

or electrocardiographic evidence of myocardial infarction. The data are shown in Figure 4.

Clinical Observations

None of the patients had clinical evidence of shock or acute left ventricular failure. Clinical signs of arteriosclerosis or left ventricular dysfunction (S_4 gallop, precordial systolic bulging, apical systolic murmurs) were observed in several patients, but systematic studies were not made.

Heart Rate and Blood Pressure

Systematic observations of heart rate and blood pressure during attacks of pain were not made. In 40 patients the heart rate ranged from 55 to 122 beats/min (mean 75). In 12 patients (30 percent) the heart rate exceeded 80 beats/min. In 14 patients (37 percent) the diastolic blood pressure was 90 mm or more. Hypotension (< 100/70) was not observed in any patient. The mean systolic pressure in 37 patients was 135 mm, and the mean diastolic pressure was 84 mm.

Coronary Arteriography

Coronary arteriography was performed in all patients without serious complications. All patients had severe disease of two or more major coronary arteries. In 23 patients (58 percent) severe disease of the three major coronary arteries was present. Four patients had severe narrowing of the left main coronary artery. Left ventricular

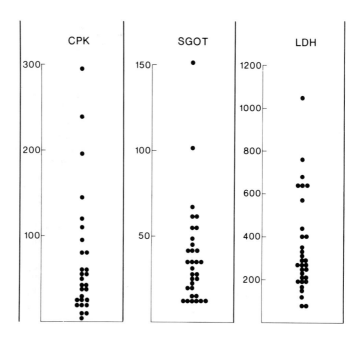

FIG. 4. Serum enzyme levels in patients with impending myocardial infarction. Each point represents the highest value observed for each patient during the period of hospital observation.

TABLE 5. Operative Details in Patients with Impending Myocardial Infarction Syndrome

OPERATION	NO.	R.C.	POST. DESC.	LAD	L. CIRC.	MARG.	OBLIQUE
Single SVBG	9	3		6			
Double SVBG	19	12	3	16	2	4	1
Triple SVBG	7	5	1	7	3	3	2
Other	2	2	0	2	1	2[a]	1

[a]Both grafts in same patient.

angiography revealed moderate abnormalities of LV contraction in 24 of 37 patients (65 percent). Mean ejection fraction calculated in 20 patients was 69 percent (range 33 to 88). These data are summarized in Table 4.

Surgical Intervention

Saphenous vein bypass graft surgery was employed in 37 patients (93 percent). Three patients were not operated on. Two had diffuse disease not amenable to bypass surgery and one elected to receive medical therapy. The operative details are summarized in Table 5. One operative death occurred in a 59-year-old patient with stable angina of eight years' duration and a history of diabetes. Increasingly severe angina had been present for two weeks prior to admission. Pain was associated with ST depression in lateral leads, and prominent deep T-wave inversion was present in inferior leads. The highest preoperative enzyme levels recorded were as follows: SGOT, 43 units; LDH, 400 units; and CPK, 60 units. Coronary arteriography revealed severe disease of the LAD, circumflex, circumflex marginal, and right main arteries. No LV angiogram was done. Bypass grafts were placed to the RCA and LAD, but at the conclusion of the procedure the LV became hypodynamic and the patient could not be brought off bypass. No autopsy was obtained.

Acute myocardial infarction was noted in the immediate postoperative period in three patients (12.3 percent).

Follow-up Studies

Follow-up observations are available on all patients from 2 to 36 months (mean 13 months). Eight of 35 (23 percent) have been followed for less than five months. No late cardiac deaths occurred. There was one operative death and one late death from leukemia.

Complete relief of chest pain was noted in 21/35 (60 percent), substantial improvement in 9/35 (26 percent), and little change in 5/35

(14 percent). Chest pain other than angina was reported in 3/35 (8.6 percent).

No patient had an increase in symptoms following surgery. Two patients were reoperated, one of whom is presently pain free, the other has mild angina, and his grafts were occluded at angiography one month after a second bypass graft operation.

Angiographic graft visualization was performed in 25/35 (71 percent) operated patients. At least one graft was patent in 21/25 patients (84 percent). Of 51 grafts studied 42 (83 percent) remain patent.

Subsequent to surgery, late myocardial infarction occurred in 2/35 (5.7 percent) of operated patients. Four of 35 (11 percent) have moderate symptoms of left ventricular heart failure.

Of the two nonoperated patients, one sustained an acute myocardial infarction while hospitalized with his preinfarction angina and has subsequently been pain free. The other patient continues to have moderate angina but is able to carry out moderate activity on medical management.

DISCUSSION

An important aspect of the selection of patients for angiography and possible surgery are the diagnostic criteria employed. In the present report the following clinical presentations were identified: (1) Stable angina with a recent increase in severity, (2) episodes of acute coronary insufficiency or rest angina, (3) recent onset of angina, and (4) symptomatic serious ventricular arrhythmias. Four published reports contain similar diagnostic criteria.[17-20]

Patients with symptoms of greater than three months' duration were not included in the present study. Only 10 percent of patients had symptoms of greater than two months' duration prior to hospital entry. The upper limit of duration of symptoms for the diagnosis of the IMIS is clearly arbitrary and various intervals from 30 days to several weeks have been employed. Many reports do not provide this information. An upper time limit of two to three months appears reasonable. Soloman and other workers have studied prodromal symptoms of patients with acute myocardial infarction and have reported that such symptoms may occur as long as two months prior to infarction.[22]

An important additional diagnostic criterion is ECG evidence of acute myocardial ischemia or serious ventricular arrhythmia occurring during symptoms. All of the patients in the present study exhibited such changes at least once during symptoms. This is a necessary criterion since in the absence of diagnostic ECG changes many patients with chest pain syndromes not related to coronary artery disease might be subjected to the risk of coronary arteriography. However, this criterion may be too strict and thus may exclude patients with coronary disease from arteriography. For example, a patient may have a severe episode of acute coronary insufficiency at home without ECG monitoring, be placed on nitrites and Inderal, be admitted to the hospital, and demonstrate no ECG changes during further episodes of pain. In a controlled evaluation of the role of surgery, such patients should probably not be included. Patients who do not exhibit acute ECG changes during symptoms but who have ECG evidence of an old myocardial infarct or who have had a positive ECG exercise test in the past would be accepted for evaluation by some workers.

Acute myocardial infarction should be excluded by appropriate ECG and serum enzyme studies as well as clinical evaluation since the object of surgical intervention in the IMIS is to prevent infarction, and surgery in the presence of acute infarction is more hazardous than when an acute infarct is not present. It is clear that some degree of focal, disseminated infarction or minor subendocardial infarction is present in many patients with the IMIS.[26] This is evidenced by prolonged ischemic ECG changes (deep T-wave inversion or ST depression) and minor rises in serum enzymes. In the present study such enzyme elevations occurred in 65 percent of patients. These changes should not exclude a patient from consideration for surgery. It is evident from the present study that despite modest, transient enzyme elevations in a majority of patients the operative mortality and the incidence of intraoperative myocardial infarction were low—2 percent and 12 percent, respectively.

The term "impending myocardial infarction syndrome" was employed in the present study to include the various clinical presentations that carry a high risk of immediate or late myocardial infarction. This term has some disadvantages, the most obvious one being that myocardial infarction is not clearly imminent in a majority of patients with this syndrome. This is evident by the relatively long duration of symptoms—ie, up to three months—and the relatively low incidence of acute infarction observed by others during the hospital stay. Unstable angina is used by some workers to describe this syndrome. It has the advantage of describing the symptoms experienced by most patients if one includes rest angina or acute coronary insufficiency under the general term of "angina." The term also places less emphasis upon the possibility of acute myocardial infarction as a sequel to the pain syndrome. Other terms have also been employed, such as preinfarction angina, accelerated angina, and the intermediate coronary syndrome.

Conventional medical therapy of the IMIS consists of measures that reduce cardiac work, dilate coronary vessels, and control cardiac arrhythmias. In the present study, prior to the institution of medical therapy, 12 patients had heart rates exceeding 80 beats per minute (31 percent), 14 patients had diastolic blood pressures of 90 mm or more (34 percent), and ventricular premature beats occurred in 51 percent. Thus, one-third to one-half of the patients were suitable for medical therapy including propranolol, hypotensive drugs, and antiarrhythmic agents.

The diagnostic criteria presented in this paper will select patients who are very likely to have severe, operable coronary disease revealed by arteriography. Only two of the 40 patients in the present study were unsuitable for surgery because of severe, diffuse disease. None had a normal arteriogram. Fischl and his workers described 23 patients who were selected by similar diagnostic criteria.[20] One patient had a normal arteriogram. A comparison of Fischl's data and data from the present study is shown in Table 6. The clinical features are similar. Conti presented data on 57 patients with unstable angina who were selected using similar criteria.[21] One patient had a normal arteriogram. Ernst observed five normal arteriograms in 65 patients.[23]

Results of medical management in patients with the IMIS who fulfill the diagnostic criteria used in the present paper and who have had coronary arteriography should be examined. Four such reports are available describing 42 patients.[17-20] The 14-month mortality was 14 percent and the incidence of nonfatal infarction was 16 percent. Data on the quality of life are not available. Randomization was not performed.

TABLE 6. Comparison of Data from Patients with Intermediate Coronary Syndrome Reported by Fischl et al[20] with Data Obtained in Present Study

	FISCHL	PRESENT STUDY	GAZES
Number	23	40	140
Mean age	49	53	56
Prior infarction (%)	50	47	18
Stable angina	78	68	78
ST depression (%)	91	36	31
T inversion (%)	87	61	35
ST elevation (%)	22	23	3.5
Minor enzyme elev.			
CPK (%)	26	35	
SGOT (%)	35	38	
LDH (%)	57	36	
Ejection fraction	0.54	0.69	

Other reports describe the course of similar patients with the IMIS who have not had coronary arteriography. Such reports contain some patients who probably would have normal coronary arteriograms. Gazes noted a 25 percent mortality in three years in 140 patients. Twenty-six (18.5 percent) developed an acute myocardial infarct within 12 months, and 25 patients (18 percent) died.[3] Krauss studied 100 patients and noted an 8 percent incidence of acute infarction in 20 months and a 22 percent mortality.[2] The risk of infarction and death was higher in patients who presented with a deterioration of chronic angina compared to patients with new ischemic pain. Watkins reported a follow-up study of 46 patients with unstable angina and observed a 6.5 percent incidence of infarction and a 24 percent incidence of death within 14 months.[4] Robinson noted a 32 percent infarction incidence and an 18 percent mortality in 6.4 months in 38 patients.[5] Beamish and Storrie have presented similar data.[1] Analysis of the four reports above indicate that over an 11-month period in 324 patients there was a 14 percent incidence of nonfatal infarction and a 20 percent mortality.

It is difficult to evaluate the current results of surgical therapy since in most surgical reports the diagnostic criteria employed are not described and the incidence of intraoperative infarction is not stated. A review of eight reports indicates an immediate operative mortality of 9.1 percent and an incidence of intraoperative infarction of 12.4 percent. The 30-day operative mortality will be slightly higher and an unknown incidence of late deaths and nonfatal infarction during the first year should be considered. These are estimated at 2 percent and 4 percent. Thus, at one year after surgery the mortality will be approximately 11 percent and the incidence of nonfatal infarction (intraoperative and late) will be approximately 16 percent. Viewed in this perspective surgery might appear to offer little advantage over medical treatment except for the relief of chest pain and angina, which was reported to be complete or substantial in 74 percent of the surgical reports cited.

The group of patients presented in this study appeared to have been improved by surgery since at 10 months the mortality was 2.5 percent (one operative death), the incidence of infarction was 12 percent (all intraoperative infarctions), and 61 percent were either free of angina or substantially improved. Final proof of the value of surgery in the IMIS can only be obtained from a large-scale, prospective randomized study in which surgical therapy is compared with medical management.

References

1. Beamish R, Storrie V: Impending myocardial infarction: recognition and management. Circulation 21:1107–15, 1960
2. Krauss K, Hutter A Jr, DeSanctis R: Acute coronary insufficiency: course and follow-up. Arch Intern Med 129:808–13, 1973
3. Gazes P, Mobley E, Faris H, Duncan R, and Humphries G: Preinfarctional (unstable) angina —a prospective study—ten year follow-up. Circulation 48:331, 1973
4. Watkins J, Russell R and Rackley C: Follow-up of stable angina in a myocardial infarction research unit. Circulation, Supp II:23, 1972
5. Robinson W, Smith R, Stevens T, Perry J, Friesinger G: Preinfarction syndrome: evaluation and treatment. Circulation 46: Supp II:212, 1972
6. Lambert C, Adam M, Geisler G, et al: Emergency myocardial revascularization for impending infarctions and arrhythmias. J Thorac Cardiovasc Surg 62:522–28, 1971
7. Pifarre R, Spinazzola A, Nemickas R, et al: Emergency aortocoronary bypass for acute myocardial infarction. Arch Surg 103:525–28, 1971
8. Favaloro R, Effler D, Cheanvechai C, et al: Acute coronary insufficiency (impending myocardial infarction). Am J. Cardiol 28:598–607, 1971
9. Bolooki H, Sommer L, Ghahramani A, et al: Cardiovascular hemodynamics in the course of impending myocardial infarction: the effects of emergency revascularization. Circulation 44:Supp II: 143, 1971
10. Linhart J, Beller B, and Talley R: Preinfarction angina: clinical, hemodynamic and angiographic evaluation. Chest 61:312–16, 1972
11. Harrison D and Shumway N: Evaluation and surgery for impending myocardial infarction. Hospital Practice 49–58, Dec 1972
12. Flemma R, Johnson W, Tector A, et al: Surgical treatment of preinfarction angina. Arch Intern Med 129:828–30, 1972
13. Scanlon P, Nemickas R, Moran J, et al: Accelerated angina pectoris: clinical, hemodynamic, arteriographic and therapeutic experience in 85 patients. Circulation 47:19–26, 1973
14. Segal B et al: Saphenous vein bypass surgery for

impending myocardial infarction: critical evaluation and current concepts. JAMA 223:767, 1973

15. Miller D, Cannom D, Fogarty T: Saphenous vein coronary artery bypass in patients with "pre-infarction angina." Circulation 47:234–41, 1973

16. Schroeder J, Berndt T, Cannom D, et al: Long-term results of surgery for unstable angina pectoris. Circulation 48:Supp IV:216, 1973

17. Rahimtoola S, Bonchek L, Starr A, Anderson R, Bristow, J: Late results after emergency aorto-coronary bypass surgery for unstable angina. Circulation 48:Supp IV:205, 1973

18. Cheanvechai C, Effler D, Loop F, et al: Emergency myocardial revascularization. Am J Cardiol 32:901–8, Dec 1973

19. Traad E, Larsen P, Gentsch T, Gosselin A, and Swaye P: Surgical management of the pre-infarction syndrome. Ann Thorac Surg 16:261–72, Sept 1973

20. Fischl S, Herman M and Gorlin R: The intermediate coronary syndrome: clinical, angiographic and therapeutic aspects. N Engl J Med 288:1193–98, 1973

21. Conti C et al: Unstable angina pectoris: morbidity and mortality in 57 consecutive patients evaluated angiographically. Am. J. Cardiol 32:745–50, 1973

22. Selden R, Anderson R, Ritzmann L, Neill W: A prospective randomized study of medical vs. surgical therapy for acute coronary insufficiency. Circulation 48:Supp IV:217, 1973

23. Ernst S, VanHarpen G, Vermuelen F, Bruschke A: Impending first myocardial infarction: medical vs. surgical management. Circulation 48:Supp IV:161, 1973

24. Hultgren H, Miyagawa M, Buch W, Angell W: Ischemic myocardial injury during coronary artery surgery. Am Heart J 82:624, 1971

25. Soloman H, Edwards A and Killip T: Prodomata in acute myocardial infarction. Circulation 40:463, 1969

26. Snow PJD, Jones AM, Duber KS: A clinico-pathological study of coronary disease. Br Heart J 18:435, 1956

43

UNSTABLE MYOCARDIAL INFARCTION

Samuel A. Kinard, Edward B. Diethrich, Robert M. Payne,
David Goldfarb, Vincent E. Friedewald,
and Joel E. Futral

Aortocoronary bypass has been used in the treatment of patients with "preinfarction syndrome" with an operative mortality similar to or slightly higher than that for patients with stable angina pectoris (Scanlon et al, 1973; Favaloro et al, 1971; Bolooki et al, 1971, 1972; Auer et al, 1971; Conti et al, 1971; Lawrence, 1971). Because preinfarction syndrome does not invariably lead to myocardial infarction, Fowler (1971) has suggested that this condition be termed "unstable angina pectoris." Preinfarction syndrome, as defined by Gazes et al (1973), is classified into three types:

Type I. Initial onset of progressive crescendo angina (increase in severity, frequency and duration) and pain at rest in a patient previously free of symptoms.

Type II. Same as Type I, but occurring in a patient with known stable angina.

Type III. Episodes of prolonged pain at rest, lasting more than 15 minutes and not related to such obvious precipitating causes as anemia and arrhythmias.

Vakil et al (1964) presented a similar definition of preinfarction syndrome. Table 1 lists the incidence of myocardial infarction and death within three months of the onset of preinfarction symptoms in these two series of 140 (Gazes) and 346 (Vakil) patients. Myocardial infarction occurred within the first three months in 20.7 percent of all patients reported by Gazes and in 36.3 percent of Vakil's anticoagulated patients, with mortality rates of 10 percent and 9.5 percent, respectively. Gazes's high-risk group included those patients who continued to have chest pain 48 hours following hospitalization in spite of maximum medical therapy. Myocardial infarction

occurred in 35 percent of these cases, with a mortality factor of 63 percent among those who had myocardial infarctions. Overall, the death rate in the high-risk group was 26 percent over the three-month period.

A small number of patients with unstable angina pectoris have transient ST segment elevation associated with chest pain. This condition was originally described by Prinzmetal et al (1959, 1960) and is known as Prinzmetal's angina. The incidence of infarction and death in such patients, particularly from arrhythmias, is somewhat higher than in the unstable angina group as a whole, particularly if coronary artery spasm is excluded as a cause of the syndrome. Pfeifer et al (1971) operated on eight patients with transient ST segment elevation with no operative mortality.

ST segment elevation associated with the hyperacute stage of myocardial infarction may persist for a number of hours before the development of the classical QRS changes indicative of myocardial infarction. In patients with Prinzmetal's angina, as well as in those with transient ST segment elevation without QRS changes, a small area of myocardial necrosis may occur. Myocardial infarction in certain areas of the myocardium may not produce any abnormalities of the electrocardiogram. These patients, then, are in an intermediate stage between ischemia and infarction of the myocardium, and it is likely that small areas of necrosis have been produced in the myocardium.

Myocardial infarction may be either an all-or-none event or a slowly progressing phenomenon. In dogs, because of constant extensive collateral circulation, infarction has been shown to progress for periods as long as 12 to 18 hours (Cox et al, 1968). Likewise, a patient with good collateral circulation may have a small area of necrosis

TABLE 1. Comparison of Preinfarction Syndrome Morbidity and
Mortality for Patient Series Reported by
Gazes (1973) and Vakil (1964)

	NO. PTS.	DEATH RATE— 3 mos (%)	INFARCTION RATE—3 mos (%)	DEATH RATE FROM INFARCTION (%)
Gazes 1973				
All patients	140	10	20.7	41.4
High risk	54	26	35.0	63.0
Vakil 1964				
No anticoagulant	156	23.7	49.4	48.1
Anticoagulant	190	9.5	36.3	26.1

bordered by a much larger area of ischemia, which will deteriorate progressively over several hours until total infarction of the ischemic area has occurred. Operative intervention for the treatment of acute myocardial infarction has been used in patients with associated cardiogenic shock with, as expected, a very high operative mortality (Keon et al, 1973; Leinbach et al, 1973; Mundth et al, 1970; Reul et al, 1973). This mortality rate is, however, somewhat lower than that reported by Leinbach et al (1973) for a series of patients undergoing medical treatment for cardiogenic shock. Intraaortic balloon pumping with infarctectomy and vein bypasses were combined, resulting in an operative mortality rate of 63 percent. In the series reported by Reul et al (1973), the occurrence of cardiac arrest prior to surgery significantly increased the incidence of mortality in the absence of cardiogenic shock. Two of their three patients with preoperative cardiac arrest expired.

In those patients with recent myocardial infarction without the complications of cardiogenic shock or cardiac arrest, operative mortality has varied considerably. Seven of eight patients with acute myocardial infarction reported by Scanlon et al (1971) survived operative therapy. Two of eight patients with large transmural infarctions reported by Anderson et al (1972) expired. Three of eight patients with myocardial infarction and persistent chest pain reported by Reul et al (1973) expired. Dawson et al (1973) related operative mortality to the timing of the operation following acute infarction. The mortality for their series was 50 percent (nine of 18 patients) in those undergoing operation within one week of myocardial infarction and 6.3 percent when the operation was performed 31 to 60 days after the infarction. Four of their five patients (80 percent) operated on within 24 hours of infarction died.

MATERIALS AND METHODS

In the two years from October 1971 to October 1973, a total of 16 patients with unstable myocardial infarction underwent operation at the Arizona Heart Institute. Two of the 16 had Prinzmetal's angina with transient ST segment elevation associated with chest pain; two had an intermediate syndrome of chest pain with persistent ST segment elevation without QRS change; and 12 had myocardial infarction followed by episodes of angina pectoris.

Of the two patients with Prinzmetal's angina, both had anterior descending coronary arterial lesions causing ST segment changes (Table 2), and one also had a right coronary arterial lesion. Of the two patients with intermediate syndrome, both had right coronary arterial lesions, and one had a left anterior descending coronary arterial lesion causing ST segment elevation (Table 2).

TABLE 2. Coronary Arterial Disease Distribution
for Patients with Prinzmetal's Angina and
Intermediate Syndrome

	NO. PTS.	LVed ELEV.	TOTAL
Prinzmetal's angina			
Single vessel (*LAD*)	1		
Double vessel (*LAD* + RCA)	1	1	2
Intermediate syndrome			
Single vessel (*RCA*)	1	0	
Double vessel (*LAD* + RCA)	1		2

Electrocardiogram results included ST elevation without QRS change during angina. In each case the italicized vessel was responsible for the ST segment elevation.

TABLE 3. Coronary Arterial Disease Distribution for Patients Experiencing Persistent Angina Pectoris Following Acute Myocardial Infarction

	NO. PTS.	LVed ELEV.	TOTAL
Single vessel			
LAD	3		
RCA	1	2	4
Double vessel			
LAD + RCA	2		
LAD + LCC	2	3	
LCC + LAD	1		5
Triple vessel			
LAD + RCA + LCC	1	0	2
RCA + LAD + LCC	1		
Quadruple vessel			
LAD + LM + LCC + RCA	0		1
Total			12

The vessel responsible for the area of necrosis is italicized. LCC: left circumflex coronary artery; LM: left main coronary artery.

Of the 12 patients with postinfarction angina pectoris, four had single-vessel disease, five had double-vessel involvement; two triples; and one quadruple (Table 3). Of these 12 patients, nine had myocardial infarction caused by stenosis or occlusion of the anterior descending coronary artery; two, of the right coronary artery; and one, of the circumflex coronary artery.

OPERATIVE TREATMENT

Aortocoronary bypass was accomplished within the first seven days after acute infarction in five patients, from eight to 14 days in three patients, and from 15 to 29 days in four patients (Table 4). Six of these patients underwent single aortocoronary bypass to the left anterior descending coronary artery, and three had right coronary artery bypass. Four had double bypass to the left anteior descending and right coronary arteries, and two had bypass to the left anterior descending and circumflex coronary arteries. One patient underwent triple coronary bypass (Table 5).

TABLE 4. Time from Myocardial Infarction to Performance of Aortocoronary Bypass for Series of 12 Postinfarction Patients

DAYS	NO. PTS.
0– 7	5
8–14	3
15–29	4

TABLE 5. Breakdown by Number of Patients of Types of Aortocoronary Bypass Performed in Series of 16 Patients

	NO. PTS.
Single vessel	
LAD	6
RCA	3
Double vessel	
LAD + RCA	4
LAD + LCC	2
Triple vessel	
LAD + LCC + RCA	1

RESULTS

The operative mortality for this series of 16 patients was zero. In all cases, the electrocardiogram taken in the postoperative period showed evolutionary changes of the infarction zone without new QRS changes.

CONCLUSIONS

The zero mortality rate appears to be related to the selection of patients who had relatively small areas of necrosis. This was presumed after observation of low serum enzyme levels, limited distribution of Q-wave abnormalities on the electrocardiogram, and a limited area of abnormally contracting ventricle. Furthermore, because the vessel involved (usually the left anterior descending coronary artery) supplied a large area of the myocardium, continued chest pain indicated the presence of a large area of ischemia adjacent to the smaller necrotic zone. The timing of the operation relative to the initial episode of myocardial infarction apparently had no effect on operative mortality in this selected group of patients. None of these patients had cardiogenic shock, and none had developed cardiac arrest prior to the operation.

References

1. Anderson R, Hodam R, Wood J, Starr A: Direct revascularization of the heart—early clinical experience with 200 patients. J Thorac Cardiovasc Surg 63:353–59, 1972
2. Auer JE, Johnson WD, Flemma HL, Tector AJ, Lepley D Jr: Direct coronary artery surgery for impending myocardial infarction. Circulation 44 (Suppl II):102, 1971
3. Bolooki H, Sommer L, Ghahrumani A, Concha D, Slavin D, Semberg L: Cardiovascular hemodynamics in the course of impending myocardial in-

farction: the effects of emergency revascularization. Circulation 44 (Suppl II):143, 1971

4. Bolooki H, Vargas A, Ghahrumani A, Sommer LS, Orvald T, Jude JR: Aortocoronary bypass graft for preinfarction angina. Chest 61:247–52, 1972

5. Conti CR, Greene B, Pitt B, Griffith L, Humphries O, Brawley R, Taylor D, Bender H, Gott V, Ross RS: Coronary surgery in unstable angina pectoris. Circulation 44 (Suppl II):154, 1971

6. Cox JL, McLaughlin VW, Flowers NC, Horan LG: The ischemic zone surrounding acute myocardial infarction: its morphology as detected by dehydrogenase staining. Am Heart J 76:650–59, 1968

7. Dawson JR, Fall RJ, Hallman GL, Cooley DA: Mortality of coronary artery bypass after previous myocardial infarction. Am J Cardiol 31:128, 1973

8. Favaloro RG, Effler DB, Cheanvechai D, Quint RA, Sones FM Jr: Acute coronary insufficiency (impending myocardial infarction) and myocardial infarction: surgical treatment by the saphenous vein graft technique. Am J Cardiol 28:598, 1971

9. Fowler NO: "Preinfarctional" angina. Circulation 44:755, 1971

10. Gazes PC, Mobley EM Jr, Faris HM Jr, Duncan RC, Humphries GB: Preinfarctional (unstable) angina—a prospective study—ten year follow-up: prognostic significance of electrocardiographic changes. Circulation 48:331–37, 1973

11. Keon WJ, Bedard P, Shankar KR, Akyrekli Y, Nino A, Berkman F: Experience with emergency aortocoronary bypass grafts in the presence of acute myocardial infarction. Circulation 47-48 (Suppl III):151, 1973

12. Lawrence GH: Coronary revascularization for impending myocardial infarction. Circulation 44 (Suppl II):190, 1971

13. Leinbach RC, Gold HK, Dinsmore RE, Mundth ED, Buckley MJ, Austen WG, Sanders CA: The role of angiography in cardiogenic shock. Circulation 47–48 (Suppl III):95, 1973

14. Mundth ED, Yurchak PM, Buckley MJ, Leinbach RC, Kantrowitz AR, Austen WG: Circulatory assistance and emergency direct coronary artery surgery. N Engl J Med 283:1382, 1970

15. Pfeifer J, Hultgren H, Alinheman E, Angell W, Shumway N: Surgical intervention in impending myocardial infarction. Circulation 44 (Suppl II): 211, 1971

16. Prinzmetal M, Kennamer R, Merliss R, Wada T, Boor N: Angina pectoris: 1. a variant form of angina pectoris: preliminary report. Am J Med 27:375, 1959

17. Prinzmetal M, Ekmekci A, Kennamer T, Kwoczynski JK, Shulin H, Toyoshima H: Variant form of angina pectoris: previously undelineated syndrome. JAMA 175:1794, 1960

18. Reul GJ, Morris GC Jr, Howell JF, Crawford ES, Stelter WJ: Emergency coronary artery bypass grafts in the treatment of myocardial infarction. Circulation 47–48 (Suppl III):177, 1973

19. Scanlon PJ, Nemickas R, Tobin JR Jr, Anderson W, Montoya A, Pifarre R: Myocardial revascularization during acute phase of myocardial infarction. JAMA 218:207–12, 1971

20. Scanlon PJ, Nemickas R, Morgan JF, Talano JV, Amirparviz F, Pifarre R: Accelerated angina pectoris: clinical, hemodynamic, and therapeutic experience in 85 patients. Circulation 47:19–26, 1973

21. Vakil RJ: Preinfarction syndrome—management and follow-up. Am J Cardiol 14:55, 1964

CARDIOGENIC SHOCK AND COUNTERPULSATION

44

THERAPEUTIC ALTERATIONS OF PRELOAD, AFTERLOAD, AND CONTRACTILE STATE IN PATIENTS WITH POWER FAILURE FOLLOWING ACUTE MYOCARDIAL INFARCTION

William W. Parmley, Kanu Chatterjee,
James S. Forrester, and H. J. C. Swan

Preload, afterload, and contractile state are the three major determinants of the mechanical performance of the heart. In simplified terms the preload can be considered as the level of left ventricular filling pressure and is important because it affects diastolic fiber length. In the absence of mitral valve stenosis there is a close relationship between mean left ventricular diastolic pressure, mean left atrial pressure, and pulmonary capillary wedge pressure, With the recent introduction of balloon flotation catheterization of the pulmonary artery, pulmonary capillary wedge pressure can be easily and safely measured in acutely ill patients.[6] Such measurements provide an indirect measurement of the left ventricular filling pressure and can be of vital clinical significance in the therapy of patients with acute myocardial infarction. If the left ventricular filling pressure is low, then cardiac output may be inadequate because the ventricle is operating at a reduced level on its ventricular function curve. If left ventricular filling pressure is too high, then pulmonary congestion and edema result in increased respiratory and cardiac work. Thus, in patients with power failure following an acute myocardial infarction, optimization of left ventricular filling pressure is an important goal so that pulmonary congestion is minimized but cardiac performance maximized.

The relationship of left ventricular filling pressure to cardiac performance can be measured with a triple lumen balloon-tipped catheter.[3] With the use of this catheter, cardiac output can be obtained with the thermodilution technique; in addition to measurements of pulmonary artery and pulmonary capillary wedge pressure. Figure 1 demonstrates the relationship between the left ventricular stroke work index and pulmonary capillary wedge pressure in 21 patients admitted with the confirmed diagnosis of acute myocardial infarction. In each patient a teflon needle was also placed in the radial or brachial artery to monitor systemic arterial blood pressure and thus calculate stroke work index. Left ventricular function curves were described in each patients by either volume infusion or diuresis. In patients with a pulmonary capillary wedge pressure greater than 18 mm Hg, preload was reduced by diuretic therapy with furosemide. In patients with filling pressures below 14 mm Hg, volume infusion was given to raise pulmonary capillary wedge pressure. Thus, over a given range, a left ventricular function curve could be described for each patient. The solid rectangle encompasses pulmonary capillary wedge pressures of 15 to 18 mm Hg. With pressures below this level it is apparent that reduction in filling pressure also reduced stroke work index in accord with the Frank-Starling mechanism. For pressures above this level, increasing pulmonary capillary wedge pressure did not appreciably change left ventricular stroke work index. Therefore, above this level, patients were working on the flat portion of their ventricular function curve. Thus, in this group of patients with acute myocardial infarction the optimal level of left ventricular filling pressure was 15 to 18 mm Hg. It should be remembered, of course, that because of the dis-

Supported in part by General Research Support Grant, USPHS # 5 SO1 RR 05468. This work was done by Dr. Parmley during the tenure of an Established Investigatorship of the American Heart Association.

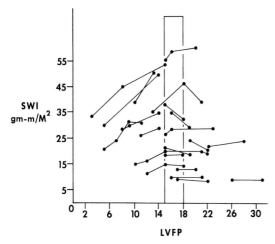

FIG. 1. Ventricular function curves in 21 patients with acute myocardial infarction. Left ventricular filling pressure was altered either by volume infusion or diuresis. The rectangle identifies the optimal level of left ventricular function in these patients.

parity that exists between central venous pressure and pulmonary capillary wedge pressure, one cannot use central venous pressure as an index of volume infusion in acute myocardial infarction.[2]

Following the optimization of preload, it is common practice to consider the administration of a variety of inotropic and/or pressor drugs. In general, however, the use of such agents has been disappointing in that they have not altered the prognosis in cardiogenic shock. More importantly, they may precipitate serious arrhythmias or aggravate the imbalance between oxygen supply and demand in ischemic myocardium. These effects are illustrated for two drugs commonly employed in the acute therapy of cardiogenic shock, namely digitalis and norepinephrine. For purposes of comparison patients were divided into three groups: nine patients with uncomplicated infarction, five with left ventricular failure, and five in cardiogenic shock. Figure 2 illustrates the response of these patients to the intravenous administration of an average dose of 1 mg digoxin. Note that those patients without left ventricular failure had the greatest increase in cardiac output and left ventricular stroke work index. On the other hand, the patients with left ventricular failure and shock showed a decreasing beneficial response. Thus, the patients who needed the drug most responded least, while those patients who did not need the drug responded in a beneficial manner.

A similar type of response is seen following the administration of norepinephrine. Figure 3 plots the response of two groups of patients with acute myocardial infarction. Fifteen surviving pa-

tients with mild to moderate ventricular failure, most of whom did not need the drug, had the greater increase in stroke volume and stroke work. The patients with severe power failure, who subsequently died, averaged very little response. The lack of a substantial effect, together with a potential increase in ventricular irritability and oxygen consumption, suggest that positive inotropic agents do not have a major beneficial role in the therapy of power failure following acute myocardial infarction. Experimental evidence has also suggested that such positive inotropic drugs can actually increase the surrounding ischemic area and subsequently increase infarct size.[4]

A lack of substantial response of the heart in power failure to positive inotropic agents appears to be related to several factors. First of all these hearts have the largest infarcts, and therefore the largest areas of nonresponsive myocardium. Secondly, the remaining normal myocardium is already maximally stimulated by intrinsic cathecholamines, making it difficult, if not impossible, to stimulate it any more. For all of these reasons it appears unlikely that positive inotropic agents will make a major impact on the mortality associated with power failure following myocardial infarction. It should be pointed out, however, that a few patients will individually respond in a beneficial manner (Fig. 3). This underscores the importance of monitoring hemodynamic changes in individual patients following any form of therapy. This allows the physician to choose forms that appear to be beneficial in each patient, rather than assuming that any individual will always respond as the average of a larger group.

Even though inotropic agents have not been

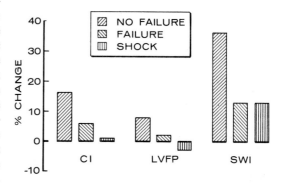

FIG. 2. Hemodynamic effects of intravenous digoxin in 19 patients with acute myocardial infarction. Nine patients had no evidence of left ventricular failure, five had mild to moderate left ventricular failure, and five were in cardiogenic shock. The percentage changes in cardiac index, left ventricular filling pressure, and stroke work index are indicated for the three groups of patients.

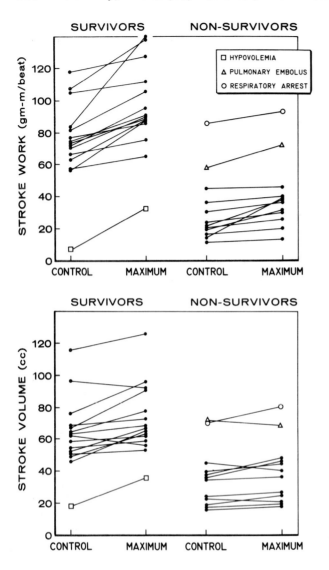

FIG. 3. Hemodynamic responses to infusions of norepinephrine in 25 patients following acute myocardial infarction. Also included are one patient with a pulmonary embolus and another with a respiratory arrest. Individual changes in stroke work and stroke volume are shown for each patient. Most of the 15 surviving patients had only mild or moderate left ventricular failure and did not require the drug for therapy. The 12 nonsurvivors had severe power failure, for which norepinephrine was given as a therapeutic agent.

very beneficial in the setting of cardiogenic shock, recent studies have suggested that afterload reduction with vasodilator drugs may produce substantial hemodynamic benefit and also reduce mortality. By reducing aortic impedance to ejection, cardiac output can be increased with no change in contractile state. To evaluate such therapy we have recently studied 38 patients with acute myocardial infarction.[1] Phentolamine was used intravenously by a constant infusion pump in 11 patients. Five mg of phentolamine was administered in the first minute followed by an infusion rate of 0.1 to 2 mg per minute. Nitroprusside was infused in the remaining 27 patients at a rate of 16 to 200 mcg per minute with the use of an infusion flow controller. The infusion rate of either drug was gradually increased until mean arterial pressure decreased by not more than 20 mm Hg or

until there was a significant decrease in pulmonary capillary wedge pressure. The infusion rate was then kept constant, and hemodynamic and metabolic measurements were repeated. For the evaluation of therapy, patients were divided into three groups on the basis of their filling pressure and stroke work index. Group I included patients with filling pressures less than 15 mm Hg (9 patients). Group II included patients with left ventricular filling pressures greater than 15 mm Hg and a stroke work index greater than 20 g-m/m² (14 patients). Group III included patients with left ventricular filling pressures greater than 15 mm Hg and a stroke work index less than 20 g-m/m² (15 patients).

The majority of patients in Group I were free of signs and symptoms of left ventricular failure. Twelve of 14 patients in Group II had clinical and radiologic signs of left ventricular failure. Ten had clinical and radiologic evidence of frank pulmonary edema. All patients in Group III had clinical evidence of left ventricular failure, and 14 of the 15 patients had frank pulmonary edema. Furthermore the majority of the patients in the latter group were hypotensive, and eight patients had clinical features of cardiogenic shock.

Generally, a beneficial hemodynamic response (increase in cardiac output and reduction in pulmonary capillary wedge pressure) occurred only after a reduction in arterial pressure. In a few patients, however, these beneficial effects occurred without any substantial change in arterial pressure. An example of this latter type of patient response is shown in Figure 4. During the administration of nitroprusside, mean arterial pressure was essentially unchanged, pulmonary capillary wedge pressure fell from 24 to 13 mm Hg, and cardiac index increased from 2.6 to 3.2 L/min/m². Coronary sinus blood flow and myocardial oxygen consumption were reduced slightly, presumably because of the reduction in preload and heart size. The fact that cardiac output can go up despite little or no change in arterial pressure reflects the fact that the increase in cardiac output counterbalances the decrease in systemic vascular resistance and thus maintains arterial blood pressure. Since there always appears to be a reduction in aortic impedance (pressure divided by flow), it is preferable to refer to these effects as due to a reduction in aortic impedance, since blood pressure will not change in some patients.

The usual hemodynamic response in each group, was decreased systemic and pulmonary vascular resistance, decreased pulmonary, right atrial and left ventricular filling pressures, together with a slight to moderate decrease in mean arterial pressure (Table 1). Cardiac index increased consistently in Group II and III patients but not in Group I patients. Individual changes in stroke volume index and left ventricular filling pressure are illustrated in Figure 5. In Group I patients with an initial left ventricular filling pressure of less than 15 mm Hg, the fall in left ventricular filling pressure during vasodilator therapy was usually accompanied by a fall in stroke volume index and a slight tachycardia. In Group II and III patients, however, a reduction in left ventricular filling pressure was usually accompanied by an increase in stroke volume index and cardiac index. It appears therefore that cardiac performance may not improve in patients with a normal left ventricular filling pressure, but significant improvement may be expected in patients with elevated left ventricular filling pressures and depressed cardiac performance (Table 1).

These changes are better illustrated in Figure 6, where percentage changes in left ventricular filling pressure, stroke volume index, and cardiac index are indicated for the three groups. Despite the same percentage reduction in left ventricular filling pressure there was little change in stroke volume index or cardiac index in Group I. However, in the sicker patients (Group II and III), there were significant increases in stroke volume index and cardiac index with no change in heart rate.

The effects of such therapy on metabolic parameters are listed in Table 2. In general, coronary sinus flow was reduced in Groups II and III patients with no significant change in the arterial-coronary sinus oxygen difference. Myocardial oxygen consumption was reduced in all

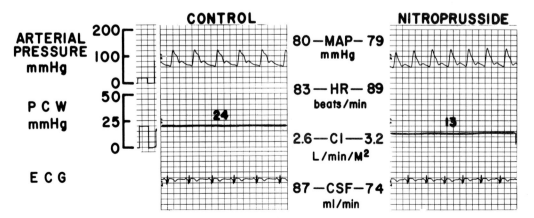

FIG. 4. Effects of nitroprusside infusion in a representative patient with acute myocardial infarction. Control tracings are on the left while those during nitroprusside infusion are on the right. The numbers in the middle represent hemodynamic values before and during nitroprusside administration.

TABLE 1. Hemodynamic Effects of Nitroprusside in Patients with Acute Myocardial Infarction

	HR/min	$\overline{BP}$ (mm Hg)	$\overline{RA}$ (mm Hg)	$\overline{PCW}$ (mm Hg)	CI (L/min/M^2)	LVSWI (g–M/M^2)	SVR (dynes sec cm^{-5})
GROUP I (n = 9)							
C	88±7 (SEM)	92±2	6±1	11±1	2.7±.2	36±5	1,520±120
NP	99±7[a]	83±3[a]	4±1[a]	7±1[a]	2.8±.3	30±5[a]	1,320±100[a]
GROUP II (n = 14)							
C	93±3	101±4	10±1	22±1	2.5±.2	34±2	1,740±160
NP	95±2	85±4[a]	6±1[a]	14±1[a]	3.1±.3[a]	35±2	1,270±140[a]
GROUP III (n = 15)							
C	100±3	83±2	13±1	27±3	1.7±.1	14±1	1,770±170
NP	100±4	74±2[a]	9±1[a]	18±2[a]	2.2±.2[a]	18±1[a]	1,290±100[a]

C: control; NP: nitroprusside.
[a]*P < 0.05, NP vs. c.*

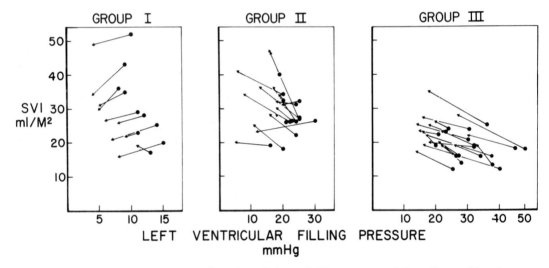

FIG. 5. Individual changes in stroke volume index and filling pressure during nitroprusside administration in the three groups of patients defined in the text. The dot end of each line represents the control measurements while the arrow tip indicates measurements made during nitroprusside administration in each patient.

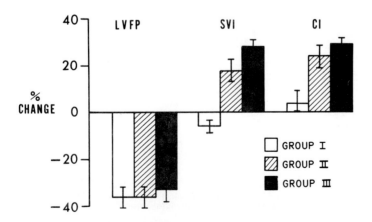

FIG. 6. Percentage changes in left ventricular filling pressure, stroke volume index, and cardiac index during nitroprusside administration, in the three groups of patients defined in the text.

TABLE 2. Effects of Nitroprusside on Myocardial Metabolism

	CSF (ml/min)	ART.–CS O_2 DIFF. (vol%)	MVO_2 (ml/min)	LACTATE EXTRACTION (%)
GROUP I (n = 6)				
C	117±11 (SEM)	13.2±1.1	16.1±3.0	20±4
NP	121±8	11.9± .9	14.4±1.6	19±4
GROUP II (n = 6)				
C	135±15	10.7± .9	14.5±2.2	21±4
NP	120±20	10.2± .8	12.0±1.9	16±8
GROUP III (n = 7)				
C	136±12	11.0± .7	15.7±1.1	10±5
NP	120±7	10.6± .8	12.6±1.2[a]	13±4

C: control; NP: nitroprusside.
[a]$P < 0.05$, NP vs. C.

three groups although this reached a level of significance only in Group III patients, who presumably had the greatest reduction in heart size. There was no significant change in lactate extraction, Thus, the hemodynamic benefits produced by vasodilator therapy were accompanied by a reduction in myocardial oxygen demand, which should favorably influence the balance between oxygen supply and demand in the ischemic myocardium.

A potentially deleterious effect of afterload reduction, however, is a reduction in arterial pressure. In particular, a reduction in diastolic pressure will reduce the perfusing pressure of the coronary arteries and might therefore reduce oxygen delivery to the ischemic myocardium. In order to maintain diastolic perfusing pressure, a few

patients have undergone simultaneous augmentation of diastolic pressure with a noninvasive external counterpulsation device (Cardiassist®). Figure 7 shows the representative effects of this combined therapy in a patient with acute myocardial infarction. The left-hand panel shows control values of arterial pressure and pulmonary capillary wedge pressure together with the ECG and cardiac index. Following the administration of nitroprusside there was a slight fall in arterial pressure together with a fall in pulmonary capillary wedge pressure from 28 to 18 mm Hg. This was accompanied by an increase in cardiac index from 1.76 to 2.39 L/min/m². The addition of external counterpulsation (right-hand panel) restored diastolic pressures to control values and produced a slight further increase in cardiac index. These

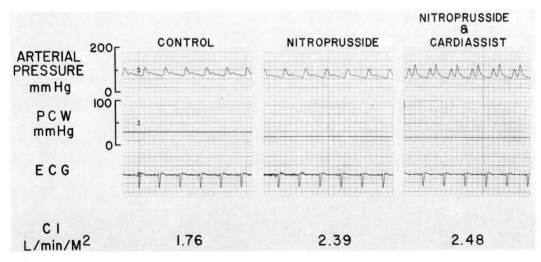

FIG. 7. Tracings from a representative patient who received nitroprusside administration, followed by the combination of external counterpulsation and nitroprusside. The diastolic augmentation in arterial pressure with external counterpulsation is seen in the upper right-hand trace. Pulmonary capillary wedge pressure was 28 mm Hg control, 18 mm Hg during nitroprusside therapy, and 17 mm Hg with the addition of external counterpulsation.

findings are representative of results in nine patients who have undergone combined therapy with nitroprusside and external counterpulsation.[5]

Although the results with inotropic agents have been disappointing relative to the mortality of power failure accompanying acute myocardial infarction, recent experience suggests that vasodilator therapy may not only improve cardiac performance but may reduce mortality.[1] Thus of the 15 patients in Group III, 9 (60 percent) survived. In the present study, 19 patients, nine of whom had clinical cardiogenic shock, had a cardiac index less than 2.3 L/min/m² and an elevated left ventricular filling pressure. Of these, 12 patients (63 percent) including four with cardiogenic shock, survived. Similarly, of 16 patients with a left ventricular stroke work index less than 25 g-m/m² and an elevated left ventricular pressure, nine (54 percent) survived. While these numbers are admittedly small, results in our unit prior to impedance reduction therapy suggest that the mortality of this group of patients was approximately 85 percent with conventional therapy, including optimization of preload and the use of various inotropic agents.

In summary, it is apparent that alterations of preload and afterload can have substantial effects on the hemodynamic performance of patients with acute myocardial infarction. Alterations of contractility with conventional inotropic agents appear to produce effects primarily in those patients who need them least, and to have little effect in the patients with more severe power failure. Optimization of left ventricular filling pressure is important in those patients with very low or very high filling pressures. Elevation of low filling pressures to an appropriate level will increase ventricular

performance. Reduction of high filling pressures will reduce the signs and symptoms of pulmonary congestion. In addition, reduction of impedance or afterload in patients with high filling pressures can produce a substantial reduction in filling pressure together with an increase in cardiac index and may favorably influence the mortality of cardiogenic shock. Potentially deleterious effects of lowering diastolic coronary perfusing pressure can be offset by the simultaneous application of external counterpulsation. The application of these therapeutic techniques to the management of patients with acute power failure appears to offer promise in optimizing hemodynamic status and reducing mortality.

References

1. Chatterjee K, Parmley WW, Ganz W, et al: Hemodynamic and metabolic responses to vasodilator therapy in acute myocardial infarction. Circulation 48:1183, 1973
2. Forrester J, Diamond G, HcHugh T, Swan HJC: Filling pressures in the right and left sides of the heart in acute myocardial infarction: a reappraisal of central-venous-pressure monitoring. N Engl J Med 285:190, 1971
3. Forrester J, Diamond G, Swan HJC: Pulmonary artery catheterization: a new technique in treatment of acute myocardial infarction. Geriatrics (October): 65, 1971
4. Maroko PR and Braunwald E: Modification of myocardial infarction size after coronary occlusion. Ann Intern Med 79:720, 1973
5. Parmley WW, Chatterjee K, Charuzi Y, Swan HJC: Hemodynamic effects of non-invasive systolic unloading (Nitroprusside) and diastolic augmentation (External counterpulsation) in patients with acute myocardial infarction. Am J. Cardiol 33:819, 1974
6. Swan HJC, Ganz W, Forrester J, et al: Catheterization of the heart in man with use of a flow-directed balloon-tipped catheter. N Engl J Med 288:477, 1970

45

THE INTRAAORTIC BALLOON PUMP IN CARDIOGENIC SHOCK, AND AS A PREOPERATIVE ADJUNCT IN HIGH-RISK MYOCARDIAL REVASCULARIZATION

George N. Cooper, Jr., Karl E. Karlson, Dov Jaron,
Arun K. Singh, Charles D. Price,
and Robert Capone

Before 1961, support of the acutely ischemic or acutely failing myocardium consisted mainly of oxygen, pharmacologic agents, water restriction, and bed rest. Epinephrine, L-norepinephrine, and isoproterenol have been mainstays of blood pressure support but have come under scrutiny because of the metabolic deficits they induce. Epinephrine infusion has been associated with increased pulmonary shunting (Nomoto et al, 1974). In small doses, it may be less dangerous to the heart than norepinephrine in treatment of low-output states (Sullivan and Forlin, 1967), but myocardial injury from large doses has been noted (Piscatelli and Fox, 1968).

Isoproterenol enhances myocardial contractility, but the concomitant augmentation of myocardial oxygen demand exceeds the oxygen delivery. L-norepinephrine improves lactate metabolism, but myocardial oxygen extraction remains abnormally high (Mueller et al, 1972). The beneficial hemodynamic effects of in-series counterpulsation have been seen experimentally (Jaron et al, 1968; Shilt et al, 1967; Tomecek et al, 1969; Brown et al, 1967; Powell et al, 1970; Corday et al, 1970; Tyberg et al, 1970; Feola et al, 1969). Because intraaortic balloon counterpulsation appears to offer the unique combination of decreasing myocardial oxygen demand while improving oxygen availability (Mueller et al, 1972), this modality has become clinically attractive. We have seen varying results from balloon pumping in acute myocardial infarction and post cardiopulmonary bypass. We have been impressed, however, with the benefits of elective preoperative counterpulsation in high-risk patients requiring myocardial revascularization procedures.

METHOD OF COUNTERPULSATION

The patients are taken to the operating room where local anesthesia is supplemented with small doses of Innovar. Controlled respiratory support via an endotracheal tube is obtained, if necessary, in unstable cardiogenic shock patients. Intraaortic balloon pumping is accomplished with the AVCO three-chambered balloon.* Insertion of the balloon is usually via the common femoral artery. The balloon is advanced up the aorta until the left radial artery pressure wave is altered, signifying that the balloon is at the subclavian artery takeoff. It is then withdrawn 2 to 3 cm. A chest x-ray taken immediately has shown satisfactory balloon position in each case with this method. After the balloon is in position, a segment of beveled 10-mm dacron graft, placed over the balloon before insertion, is sutured with 4-0 prolene double-armed sutures end to side onto the incision in the common femoral artery. To secure a dry field for suturing an umbilical tape is doubly looped around the artery proximally, tightening it on the balloon catheter, and a vascular clamp is placed distally. To prevent clotting at the suture line, 5,000 to 7,500 units of heparin are given intravenously just before balloon insertion, and weak heparin solution is injected proximally and distally before tightening tape and clamp. Heavy silk ties around the graft secure the balloon catheter in place.

* AVCO Corp., Everett, Mass.

After securing the catheter, the graft is trimmed, leaving 3 to 4 cm remaining in the wound. The wound is copiously irrigated with kanamycin solution and closed with chromic catgut and nylon. At the time of balloon removal, the graft is exposed and permitted to bleed momentarily after the balloon is withdrawn, to flush out debris. The base of the graft is then carefully sutured and the excess graft removed. The wound is again irrigated with kanamycin and closed as before. Fibrin accumulation in the graft segment has been appreciable despite heparinization for the duration of balloon pumping. Routine passage of Fogarty catheters has not been practiced, but this is done if the pedal pulse has not been good or if there is a large buildup of clot in the arteriotomy site. Appropriate balloon timing is determined by setting inflation on the dicrotic notch, while deflation is set so that diastolic augmentation ends immediately prior to the upstroke of the systolic pressure curve.

RESULTS

Intraaortic balloon counterpulsation was used in 23 patients (Table 1). Eight patients had acute myocardial infarction with shock. Five were assisted because of acute left ventricular failure after cardiopulmonary bypass. Three were counterpulsed for preinfarction angina just prior to urgent operation. Seven had counterpulsation on an elective basis before, during, and after revascularization. Three of these had left main coronary stenosis and three had poor ventricular function with

**TABLE 1. Counterpulsation Experience
(23 Patients): 12/72–2/74**

1. Acute ischemia
   (a) Acute myocardial infarction with shock   (8)
   (b) Impending infarction or preinfarction
       angina   (3)
2. Postcardiopulmonary bypass
   Low output in postbypass period   (5)
3. Preoperatively
   a. Critical stenosis of left main coronary
      proximal left anterior descending with
      proximal circumflex   (3)
   b. Poor ventricles with questionable distal
      coronaries and severe angina   (3)
   c. Severe unstable angina with tight LAD
      and circumflex plus severe aortic stenosis
      with ventricular hypertrophy   (1)

Total   23

questionable distal coronaries. One of the elective cases had coronary stenoses, severe aortic stenosis, and left ventricular hypertrophy.

Acute Myocardial Infarction with Shock

These eight cases (Table 2) represent our initial experience with balloon counterpulsation. Although our logistics with intraaortic balloon pumping in shock are better in 1974 than in late 1972, none of the patients in this category survived. Four were operated upon, and two of these survived postoperatively for two and 13 days, respectively. Three of the four patients who were not offered operation had very poor ventriculograms, poor general status with significant secondary organ deterioration, or unacceptable distal coronary vessels. The fourth patient died before he could be studied.

Acute Postperfusion Cardiac Failure

Critical left main coronary stenosis was present in three of these patients whose hemodynamics abruptly deteriorated upon induction of anesthesia or before bypass. Only one of these patients survived operation, responding to three days of balloon pump support. One other postbypass was a 27-year-old girl with type II hyperlipidemia who had been on propranolol preoperatively and who was weaned very quickly from the balloon. In the fifth case, severe iliofemoral disease precluded passage of the balloon. We dissected a plaque from the iliac artery with the balloon, necessitating reoperation and iliac endarterectomy with a Fogarty balloon catheter and vein patch graft of the common femoral artery.

Urgent Preoperative Counterpulsation for Preinfarction Angina

There were three patients in this group. One had persistent severe angina and recurrent ventricular tachycardia before transfer to our hospital. He had a balloon inserted on arrival, was rendered pain-free, and underwent uneventful cardiac catheterization and surgery for critical stenosis of the left anterior descending coronary artery. The second patient had persistent anginal pain and ST segment changes after coronary angiography. A balloon was inserted, and he became asymptomatic and underwent uneventful myo-

TABLE 2. Balloon Pumping for Myocardial Infarction with Shock

PT.	AGE	DIAGNOSIS	TIME FROM ADM. TO INSERTION OF BALLOON	TYPE OF SURGERY	OUTCOME
LP	53	AMI, shock, ventri-ular aneurysm	23 days	Aneurysmectomy, 1 vein graft	Died immed. after sur-gery—V tach.
JS	56	AMI, shock	21 days	None	Poor vessels, bad ventri-cle, no surgical candi-date, died
AB	49	AMI, shock	9 days	None	Expired preangiogram
JLaC	61	AMI, failure, ruptured papillary muscle	8 days	Vein graft and mitral valve replacement	Reoperation—delayed homopericardium, in-anition, sepsis, died on 13th day.
MT	70	AMI shock	24 hrs	Vein graft and aneurysmectomy	Finally operated upon on 19th day. Died 2d po day
LF	54	AMI, shock, acute VSD	14 hrs	Vein graft, repair of VSD	System infarcted, died at at operation
EF	56	AMI, shock	10 hrs	None	Inadequate augmentation incorrect volume set-ting, died preangiogram
IW	56	AMI, shock	12 hrs	None	Obese diabetic with poor vessels, no surgical candidate

cardial revascularization the next day. The third patient had preinfarction angina after catheteriza-tion. When ST segment changes appeared, she had a balloon inserted with complete relief of pain and underwent successful coronary bypass the next day.

Elective Preoperative Counterpulsation

Seven patients had elective preoperative counterpulsation. Four of these patients had criti-cal lesions in the left main coronary artery or proximal left anterior descending coronary with unstable symptoms. One of these patients had, in addition, tight aortic stenosis with left ventricular hypertrophy. Three others had marked angina with very poor ventricular function. All of these patients had counterpulsation beginning on the afternoon before the day of coronary bypass sur-gery. These patients comprised a high-risk group, but they all survived with a minimum of intra-or postoperative difficulty. This was in marked contrast to the group with left main stenosis in whom we did not use this elective balloon con-cept. There were several noticeable advantages of elective preoperative counterpulsation. Stabiliza-tion of anesthesia induction with maintenance of good systemic and coronary perfusion despite tran-sient lowering of systolic pressure was seen in

each case. In addition, there was very little need for inotropic support in the immediate postperfu-sion setting or postoperatively. Counterpulsation was continued for an average of 2.5 days after surgery. Twenty-four hours before balloon re-moval, weaning is usually begun: assisting only one of two beats for 6 to twelve hours, then one of four beats for 6 to twelve hours, then removing the balloon in the operating room.

COMPLICATIONS

Femoral Arterial Insufficiency (Three Patients)

Two patients had clots in the femoral ar-tery or at the graft site, requiring Fogarty catheter thrombectomy either during the period of counter-pulsation or at the time of balloon removal. These patients had lapses in heparin administration, but others with adequate heparinization had fibrin buildup in the graft site at the time of balloon removal.

In only one patient did a leg actually be-come irretrievably compromised but this was in one of our postoperative shock patients who also had diabetes. Passage of a Fogarty catheter into the distal posterior tibial artery did not produce a clot. A very low flow state was present at this time, which may have accounted for both the limb ischemia and the patient's death.

Femoral Wound Problems (Three Patients)

One patient had transient serious drainage from the groin wound. In another patient who developed a wound hematoma during the night before surgery, and had a superficial wound separation, which healed secondarily. In the third patient, technical difficulty with the artery at the time of insertion followed by two balloon repositioning led to a distorted femoral artery, which was repaired at time of removal. Two weeks after discharge the patient bled from his arteriotomy site, necessitating further repair, which was followed by complete recovery.

Mechanical Difficulty (Four Patients)

In one instance, there was a high leak from the system due to a cracked condensation collection chamber, which was easily replaced. On another occasion, ineffectual balloon pumping was caused by a defective fuse. In one patient the balloon catheter broke because of undue twisting just on the balloon side of the device connecting the small diameter to the clear plastic tube.

DISCUSSION

Acute Myocardial Infarction with Shock

At the end of 1972, we instituted counterpulsation in selected cases of acute myocardial infarction with shock (AMIS). It became apparent that with counterpulsation, cardiogenic shock would be relieved, at least temporarily. Attempts at weaning from the balloon pump without the benefits of myocardial revascularization were not successful.

Some success in cardiogenic shock with counterpulsation alone was seen in 1968 by Kantrowitz, who noted a 43 percent survival without further surgical intervention. Our experience does not allow us this degree of optimism. We now proceed with coronary angiography soon after balloon insertion, and an operative decision is made promptly.

Some impressions can be gained from our experience with counterpulsation in the AMIS situation. We have seen that delay in angiography

or surgery is fruitless. The catabolic effects of prolonged bed rest alone are sizable (Randall, 1970; Howard et al, 1946). The additional catabolic effects of surgery will tend to weigh against a patient already depleted by the time a delayed surgical decision is finally made. This point is illustrated by a patient who had rupture of a posterior papillary muscle due to a posterior infarction. Counterpulsation was instituted on the eighth day, and she had an uneventful mitral valve replacement and saphenous vein bypass. Inanition, poor healing, (despite attempts at hyperalimentation), thrombocytopenia, and a late hemopericardium requiring reoperation one week later, were not well tolerated. She died with sepsis. This patient would possibly have had more reserve if she had had counterpulsation and operation had been instituted soon after admission to the hospital, rather than on the eighth day after entry.

In any case of cardiogenic shock there may be necrosis of 40 percent of the left ventricular myocardium (Dunkman et al, 1972). We therefore assume that in these acute operative attempts we may have to resect a portion of ventricle. We have not had difficulty closing a ventriculotomy in the early postinfarction period, so that if a patient is balloon dependent and anatomically a candidate for surgery one should not delay operation hoping for a stronger or more recoverable ventricle in a few days.

The judgment of whether or not to counterpulse a marginal patient is not easily answered. Things such as age, ultimate survival chances, and general operability must be considered, and combined medical-surgical judgment is desirable upon admission. We are impressed with the improvement in hemodynamics with balloon counterpulsation and will continue to use this modality in cardiogenic shock.

Limitation of the extent of myocardial infarction by counterpulsation is an interesting concept (Mundth et al, 1973; Caulfield et al, 1972; Maroko et al, 1972). This may lead to earlier use of balloon pumping in infarction as an attempt to limit infarct extension and consequent shock.

Early revascularization for acute myocardial infarction is an emerging concept that we are examining closely. Several workers have shown very respectable survival with early operation (Keon et al, 1973; Pifarre et al, 1971). Cheanvechai et al, in 1973, reported survival of 27 of 30 acute myocardial infarction patients after operation within the first four to 10 hours post infarction. Applicability of this early operation concept, however valid, is in large part a function of adequacy of hospital logistics, and because these vary widely, there will be varying degrees of aggressiveness in acute infarction.

Balloon Pump Immediately after Cardiopulmonary Bypass

Three of these patients had critical stenosis of the left main coronary artery, and they all did poorly before bypass, with hypotension, and acute heart failure and concomitant ECG changes. The two nonsurvivors were young men with good distal vessels on angiography, both having rather routine coronary bypass procedures. Neither of these hearts beat effectively after bypass, and in neither was counterpulsation particularly effective in restoring hemodynamics. The left ventricles dilated and did not contract effectively, as if they had sustained infarction intraoperatively. This was ultimately corroborated by our pathologist.

Buckley et al in 1973 used counterpulsation after bypass in 26 patients with 10 long-term survivors. Berger et al in 1973, reported six survivors out of 14 patients with postcardiotomy cardiogenic shock. Although counterpulsation can indeed be used after cardiopulmonary bypass, our feeling is that if possible one should try to avoid the postperfusion power failure situation by selective application of balloon pumping preoperatively.

Preoperative Counterpulsation

Reports by others (Sharma et al, 1973; Kisslo et al, 1973), have indicated a relatively high surgical risk in patients with left main coronary stenosis. Because of these, and our own initial surgical mortality in patients with severe left main coronary stenosis, we now use preoperative intraaortic balloon pumping in this entity. We have extended the concept to some cases of very proximal severe stenosis of both the left anterior descending and circumflex, cases of poor ventricular contraction with questionable distal coronary anatomy, and severe aortic stenosis with marked left ventricular hypertrophy.

This policy has yielded gratifying results in 10 patients (Table 3), whose surgical risk was judged to be unusually high, in that all survived with a minimum of intra- or postoperative difficulty.

Although blood volume has been restored preoperatively, there is very frequently a blood pressure drop on anesthesia induction, even when done with caution and expertise. Critical left main coronary stenosis will not allow adequate myocardial perfusion with reduced pressure, but our impression is that balloon counterpulsation

will supply the needed perfusion pressure and at the same time unload the ventricle, making the induction and pre-bypass period less likely to produce myocardial ischemia.

In addition to a smooth anesthesia induction period with balloon pumping, one has the advantage of continuing the pulsatile intraaortic pressure augmentation during cardiopulmonary bypass (Fig. 1), using an ECG simulator * or one of the operating room personnel to provide an ECG signal to trigger the balloon. This provides pulsatile flow throughout the entire pump run. We have not yet quantitated any definite benefit from pulsatile as opposed to nonpulsatile flow, but there is experimental evidence to indicate that pulsatile flow during cardiopulmonary bypass may be more physiologic and offer better tissue perfusion than nonpulsatile flow (Mukherjee et al, 1973; Shepard and Kirklin, 1969; Jacobs et al, 1969). In 1972, Berger described the feasibility and benefits of intraaortic-balloon-pump-induced pulsatile flow during cardiopulmonary bypass.

In the three patients with severe unstable preinfarction angina, the balloon was inserted before catheterization in one, and after catheterization in two. In each, the anginal pain subsided immediately, and coronary bypass was accomplished uneventfully within 24 to 48 hours, whenever optimum operating room circumstances became available. Application of balloon pumping in preinfarction angina renders the patient asymptomatic and decreases his immediate jeopardy. Therefore, surgical timing in this situation becomes somewhat less critical, and unplanned early morning or late night revascularization procedures have been replaced with a more orderly approach during daylight hours.

Three patients had severe angina with questionable distal coronary anatomy and ventricles that were marginal at best. One of these had recurrent heart failure as a prominent symptom. With preoperative balloon pumping, each had very routine triple coronary bypass surgery with stable hemodynamics postoperatively.

One patient in the preoperative group had left ventricular hypertrophy with aortic stenosis in addition to stenosis in the proximal left coronary system. He was especially stable in the immediate postoperative period, unlike our most recent patient with aortic stenosis and ventricular hypertrophy, who was a strapping 41-year-old man who was not counterpulsed. Bilateral coronary per-

---

* Heart Simulator—HS-1, Paradise Electronics Development Corp., Randolph, Mass.

TABLE 3. Preoperative Balloon Pumping

PT./AGE	BALLOON INDICATION	OPERATION	COMMENT
GL/57	Severe preinfarction angina—unstable—V Tach. on Inderal	Vein bypass to LAD	Adm'd—cath'd & operated; balloon rendered case elective
WA/53	Severe angina—unstable—rest pain	Triple coronary bypass	Uneventful perioperative course
FO'S/62	Preinfarction angina—3, very tight stenoses	Double bypass, acute inferior infarction intraoperatively	Atrial pacing and balloon supported patient. Recovered nicely
AM/50	Angina—left main coronary stenosis	Triple bypass with IMA to LAD	Smooth induction and perioperative course
JL/46	Severe angina—LAD occl. flush with main	IMA to LAD, R. gas endart	Uneventful perioperative course
HR/56	L Main stenosis, diabetes, poor vessels, preinfarction episode	Double bypass—terrible mid-LAD but good distal flow with graft	Perioperative course uneventful
JP/53	Severe angina with failure, poor ventricle	Triple coronary bypass	Uneventful perioperative course, no failure postop
HV/41	Severe angina poor ventricle	Triple coronary bypass	Uneventful perioperative course
AR/53	Severe unstable angina with very poor ventricle	Double bypass	Uneventful perioperative course
RJ/56	Severe angina—tight LAD & Circ. with AS	AV Repl, veins to LAD & Circ	Uneventful perioperative course

fusion was carried out at 32 C with the heart beating, and valve replacement was uneventful. Although he ultimately did well, he sustained a subendocardial myocardial infarction postoperatively, significantly prolonging his convalescence. Hottenrott et al, in 1973, have shown that the subendocardium in hypertrophied hearts becomes ischemic during cardiopulmonary bypass, especially during ventricular fibrillation. Subendocardial ischemia has also been produced by lowering coronary diastolic blood pressure, raising left ventricular diastolic pressure, and shortening diastole (Buckberg et al, 1972). It is possible that even though preoperative counterpulsation may not diminish afterload in a ventricle with aortic stenosis, it may increase the coronary perfusion gradient through the hypertrophied ventricle, thus decreasing subendocardial ischemia. Counterpulsation after aortic valve replacement should then help to unload the ventricle, as well as augment coronary perfusion, and subendocardial ischemia should again be minimized.

Balloon Timing

Jaron et al, in 1970, showed by experimental measurements of the afterload phase angle, that the hemodynamic benefits of in-series intraaortic balloon assistance are highly dependent on precise timing of the diastolic pulse. Maximum benefits in left ventricular mechanical work, tension time index, and coronary flow occurred when this phase angle was 180 degrees, ie, balloon systole 180 degrees out of phase with ventricular systole.

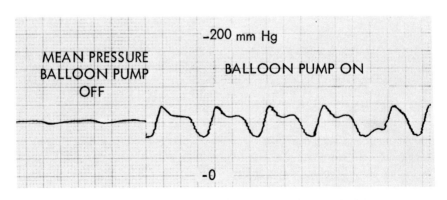

FIG. 1. Pulsatile flow induced by balloon pump while on total bypass.

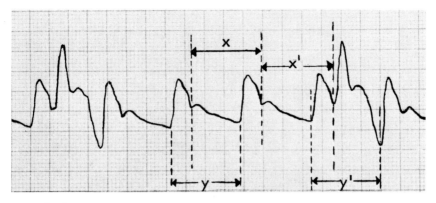

FIG. 2. Calibration of balloon pump timing should have assisted and unassisted cardiac cycles of equal duration (see text).

Deviations from this phase angle were associated with less than optimal cardiovascular hemodynamics. Other recent work also indicates that the hemodynamics efficiency of in-series assistance is highly dependent on the timing of the device within the cardiac cycle (Weber et al, 1972; Jelinek et al, 1972). Using a radial artery catheter, a pressure tracing was obtained (Fig. 2) showing an example of the calibration of balloon timing. The driving unit was set at a ratio of one assisted beat to three unassisted beats. Time from one unassisted dicrotic notch to another (x) should be equal to the time from the dicrotic notch of an unassisted beat to that of the following assisted beat (x'). Similarly, the time between beginning of systole in two adjacent unassisted beats (y) should be the same as the time between onset of systole in an assisted beat and the following unassisted beat (y').

If one uses only ECG as a timing guide without concomitant scrutiny of the arterial pressure curve, one can inadvertently impose excessive afterload by inflating too early or insufficient diastolic augmentation by inflating too late. Deflating too late would increase afterload. It is possible that deflating too early could cause a diminution in central aortic pressure, the abruptness of which could cause retrograde blood flow from the periphery or the coronary arteries into the aorta. Figure 3 shows deflation too far ahead of the opening of the aortic valve. The very short segment between the end of aortic runoff and the beginning of systole (t-t') represents the time in which this flow reversal phenomenon could take place. The dotted line demonstrates more appropriate deflation at the end of diastole. Figure 4 shows spontaneous rhythm (A) followed by early inflation (B) in a postoperative patient. With the inflation too early, the patient's ventricular ejection is diminished, because the ventricle now ejects against an increased aortic pressure. With the correct inflation setting (C), diastolic augmentation is maximal and does not occur until the aortic valve is closed.

Need for balloon timing adjustment when changing the pacing site is seen in Figure 5A, B, and C, showing sequential switching from atrial pacing to spontaneous rhythm, then to ventricular pacing. In Figure 5B and C the augmentation is quite late and must be moved leftward toward the

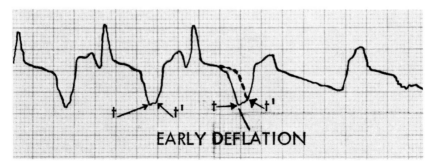

EARLY DEFLATION

FIG. 3. Early balloon deflation may cause momentary retrograde flow from systemic periphery toward aorta. Transient increase in aortic pressure before systole represented by t = t'.

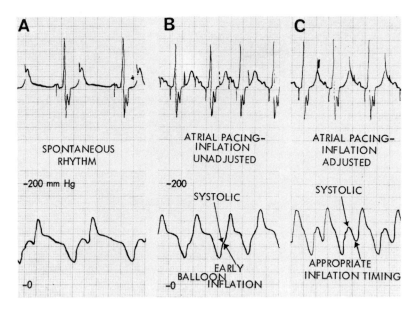

FIG. 4. Early inflation of balloon retards ventricular ejection (B), whereas inflation after aortic valve closure causes better augmentation (C).

dicrotic notch. Figure 5D shows resumption of atrial pacing with restoration of satisfactory systolic and diastolic pressures.

Buckley noted in 1973 that balloon assist has been successful in patients who sustain intraoperative ischemic injuries and noted that with stable rhythm survival rates have been high.

Benefits of combined atrial pacing and balloon pumping were seen in one of our preinfarction angina patients. She sustained an intraoperative inferior myocardial infarction with heart block. Spontaneous systolic pressure without coun-

terpulsation immediately post-bypass was 60 mm Hg. With diastolic augmentation on ventricular pacing she needed minimal to moderate inotropic support. Several hours after surgery it was found that her heart block was no longer present and her heart could be paced via the atrial wire placed at surgery. Figure 6 shows a tracing taken during ventricular pacing. The systolic pressure is 60 mm Hg and the diastolic 80 mm Hg. The second part of the tracing, taken after several hours, showed the systolic pressure augmented by atrial pacing, and the increase in diastolic augmentation

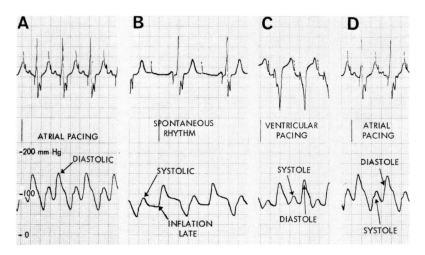

FIG. 5. Rapid sequential switching from one pacing site to another shows need to adjust balloon timing each time (see text).

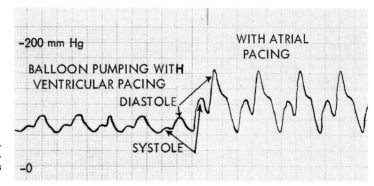

FIG. 6. Systolic pressure is augmented by atrial pacing and diastolic balloon augmentation is increased.

by the balloon. Subsequent to this she was hemodynamically greatly improved, and she went on to recover uneventfully.

SUMMARY

1. Intraaortic balloon counterpulsation has been used in 23 patients. It temporarily restores acceptable hemodynamics in cardiogenic shock. Counterpulsation with or without surgical treatment has resulted in no survival in eight cardiogenic shock patients.

2. Salvage with counterpulsation used after cardiopulmonary bypass was achieved in only one of three patients with main left coronary stenosis with acute post-perfusion heart failure.

3. Elective preoperative counterpulsation was used in seven high-risk revascularization patients with survival and smooth perioperative courses in all seven. Anesthesia induction with left main coronary stenosis was especially uneventful.

4. Counterpulsation in three preinfarction angina patients provided elective operative circumstances with uneventful recovery.

5. Preoperative counterpulsation in aortic stenosis with severe ventricular hypertrophy may diminish subendocardial ischemia immediately before and after valve replacement.

6. Proper balloon timing is important for optimum diastolic pressure augmentation.

References

Berger R, Saine V: Conversion of non-pulsatile cardiopulmonary bypass to pulsatile flow by intraaortic balloon pumping during revascularization for cardiogenic shock (Abstr). Circulation 45:46, 1972 (suppl)

Berger RL, Virender K, Ryan T, Sokol D, Keefe J: Intraaortic balloon assist for post cardiotomy cardiogenic shock. J Thorac Cardiovasc Surg 66:906, 1973

Brown BG, Goldfarb D, Topaz SR, Gott VL: Diastolic augmentation by intraaortic balloon: circulatory hemodynamics and treatment of severe acute left ventricular failure in dogs. J Thorac Cardiovasc Surg 53:789–804, 1967

Buckberg GD, Fixler DE, Archie JC, Hoffman JIE: Experimental subendocardial ischemia in dogs with normal coronary arteries. Circ Res 30:67, 1972

Buckberg GD, Towers B, Paglia DE, Mulder DG, Maloney JV: Subendocardial ischemia after cardiopulmonary bypass. J Thorac Cardiovasc Surg 64:669, 1972

Buckley M, Craver J, Gold H, et al: Intraaortic balloon pump assist for cardiogenic shock after cardiopulmonary bypass. Circulation 47 and 48:90, 1973

Buckley M: Discussion of Berger et al. J Thorac Cardiovasc Surg 66:914, 1973

Caulfield JB, Dunkman WB, Feinberg RC: Cardiogenic shock: myocardial morphology with and without artificial left ventricular counterpulsation. Arch Pathol 93:532, 1972

Cheanvechai C, Effler D, Loop FD, et al: Aorto coronary artery graft during early and late phases of acute myocardial infarction. Ann Thorac Surg 16:249, 1973

Corday E, Swan JC, Lang TW, et al: Physiologic principles and application of circulatory assistance for the failing heart: intraaortic balloon circulatory assist in venoarterial phase partial bypass. Am J Cardiol 26:595–602, 1970

Dunkman WB, Leinbach RC, Buckley, et al: Clinical and hemodynamic results of intraaortic balloon pumping and surgery for cardiogenic shock. Circulation 46:465, 1972

Feola M, Norman NA, Haiderer O, Kennedy JH: Assisted circulation: experimental intraaortic balloon pumping. In Artif Heart Prog Conf Proc Washington DC, 1969, pp 637–57

Harvard JE, Bigham ES Jr, Eisenberg H, Wagner D, Bailey E: Nitrogen and mineral balances during starvation and graduated feeding in healthy young males at bed rest. Bull Johns Hopkins Hosp 78:282, 1946

Jacobs L, Klopp E, Seamone W, Topaz S, Gott V: Improved organ function during cardiac bypass with a roller pump modified to deliver pulsatile flow. J Thorac Cardiovasc Surg 58:703, 1969

Jaron D, Yahr W, Tomecek J, et al: Hemodynamic changes during intracorporeal circulatory assistance by means of phase-shift balloon pumping in experimental cardiogenic shock. Proc 21st Ann Conf Engl Med Biol 10:20.2, 1968

Jaron D, Tomecek J, Freed PS, et al: Measurement of ventricular load phase angle as an operating criteria for in-series assist devices: hemodynamic studies utilizing intraaortic balloon pumping. Trans Am Soc Artif Intern Organs 16:466–71, 1970

Kantrowitz A, Tjonneland S, et al: Mechanical intra-aortic cardiac assistance in cardiogenic shock. Arch Surg 97:1000, 1968

Keon WJ, Bedard P, Akyurekli Y: Experience with emergency myocardial revascularization. Circulation 48 (Suppl IV):54, 1973

Kisslo RP, Behar V, Bartel A, Kong Y: Left main coronary artery stenosis. Circulation 48 (Suppl IV):57, 1973

Maroko PR, Bernstein EF, Libby P, et al: Effects of intraaortic balloon counterpulsation on the severity of myocardial ischemic injury following acute coronary occlusion: counterpulsation and myocardial injury. Circulation 45:1150, 1972

Mueller H, Ayres SM, Giannelli, et al: Cardiac performance and metabolism in shock due to acute myocardial infarction in man: response to catecholamines and mechanical cardiac assist. Trans NY Acad Sci 34:309–33, 1972

Mukherjee N, Beran A, Hirai J, et al: In vivo determination of renal tissue oxygenation during pulsatile and non-pulsatile heart bypass. Ann Thorac Surg 15:354, 1973

Mundth ED, Buckley MJ, Geinbach RC, et al: Surgical intervention for the complications of acute myocardial ischemia. Ann Surg 178:379, 1973

Nomoto S, Berk JL, Hager JF, Koo R: Pulmonary anatomic arterio-venous shunting caused by epinephrine. Arch Surg 108:201, 1974

Pifarre R, Spinazzola A, Nemickas R, et al: Emergency aorto coronary bypass for acute myocardial infarction. Arch Surg 103:525, 1971

Piscatelli R, Fox L: Myocardial injury in epinephrine overdosage. Am J Cardiol 21:735–37, 1968

Powell WJ, Daggett WM, Magro AE, et al: Effects of intraaortic balloon counterpulsation on cardiac performance, oxygen consumption and coronary blood flow. Am J Cardiol 25:122, 1970

Randall HT: Nutrition in surgical patients. Am J Surg 119:530, 1970

Sharma S, Khaja F, Heinke R, Goldstein S, Easley R: Left main coronary artery lesions: risk of catheterization, exercise test and surgery. Circulation 48 (Suppl IV):53, 1973

Shepard RB, Kirklin JW: Relation of pulsatile flow to oxygen consumption and other variables during cardio pulmonary bypass. J Thorac Cardiovasc Surg 58:694, 1969

Shilt W, Freed PS, Khalil G, Kantrowitz A: Temporary non-surgical intra-arterial cardiac assistance. Trans Am Soc Artif Intern Organs 13:322–28, 1967

Sullivan JM, Gorlin R: Effect of L-epinephrine on the coronary circulation in human subjects with and without coronary artery disease. Circ Res XXI:919, 1967

Tomecek J, Jaron D, Tjønneland S, Kantrowitz A: Phase-shift cardiac assistance with a valve balloon: experimental results. Trans Am Soc Artif Intern Organs 15:406–11, 1969

Tyberg JV, Keon WJ, Sonnenblick EH, Urschel CW: Effectiveness of intraaortic balloon counterpulsation in the experimental low output state. Am Heart J 80:89, 1970

Weber KT, Janicki JS, Walker AA: Intraaortic balloon pumping; an analysis of several variables affecting balloon performance. Trans Am Soc Artif Intern Organs 18:486–91, 1972

Weber KT, Janicki JS, Walker AA, Kirklin JW: An assessment of intraaortic balloon pumping in hypovolemic and ischemic heart preparations. J Thorac Cardiovasc Surg 64:869–77, 1972

46

THE USE OF AVCO INTRAAORTIC BALLOON CIRCULATORY ASSISTANCE FOR PATIENTS WITH CARDIOGENIC SHOCK, SEVERE LEFT VENTRICULAR FAILURE, AND REFRACTORY, RECURRENT VENTRICULAR TACHYCARDIA

Melvin R. Platt, James T. Willerson, John T. Watson, Stephen J. Leshin, George Curry, R. R. Ecker, Stephen P. Londe, and Winifred L. Sugg

Left ventricular assist devices of various types have been successfully used to support the failing circulation. The most extensive experience has been with the use of intraaortic balloon counterpulsation to improve hemodynamics and support patients in cardiogenic shock. The present report summarizes our own experience with this mode of therapy, using the device developed by AVCO laboratories.* Most of the 29 patients studied had cardiogenic shock as a primary problem, but a smaller group representing patients with medically refractory left ventricular failure or refractoy ventricular tachycardia will also be discussed (Table 1).

CLINICAL MATERIAL

These patients were all treated at Parkland Memorial Hospital in Dallas, Texas, over a two-year period (1971–73). The 29 patients included 24 males and 5 females, with an age range of 37 to 71 (mean 52.1) years. The duration of balloon support ranged from two hours to 21 days (mean 4.6 days). Five patients were supported for eight hours or less; counterpulsation was ineffective in these five patients, and all died within the eight hours. Nine patients were weaned from balloon support, including eight in shock and one

* Furnished by the Southwestern Medical Foundation.

with ventricular tachycardia. In these patients, the duration of support averaged 5.9 days.

Cardiogenic shock was defined as a systolic blood pressure less than 85 mm Hg associated with signs of decreased organ and tissue perfusion (mental confusion, urine output less than 20 cc/hr, cold, clammy extremities, etc). All other causes for shock were ruled out, including sepsis, hypovolemia, drug-induced hypotension, and rhythm disturbances, though the latter commonly accompanied the shock syndrome, as noted in Table 2. If hypotension *only* occurred at times of serious rhythm abnormalities, then the patient was not included as a shock patient.

Patients in cardiogenic shock were all monitored in our intensive care unit, and continuous monitoring was obtained of arterial pressure, urine output (Foley catheter inserted), pulmonary artery pressure (Swan-Ganz catheter inserted), and a single-lead ECG. Periodic monitoring of pulmonary wedge pressure, cardiac output (green dye method), chest x-ray, complete ECG, temperature, and laboratory data (blood gases, renal function, cardiac enzymes, and hematologic parameters) was also obtained. A trial of volume expansion was used in those patients with initial wedge pressures below 12 to 14 mm Hg, but if an increase to 18 to 20 mm Hg did not reverse the shock state, then vasopressors were given, usually norepinephrine. Patients with mean wedge pressures above 20 to 22 mm Hg were given diuretics and digitalis in addition to vasopressors. Acid-base

TABLE 1. Balloon-Supported Patients

NAME	AGE/ SEX	DIAGNOSIS	LENGTH OF SUPPORT	OUTCOME
RLS[a]	58/M	Cardiogenic shock, cardiomyopathy	65 hrs[b]	Died; pneumonia 7 days after balloon removed
WH	45/M	Cardiogenic shock, alcoholism	56 hrs[b]	Died; neurologic complications 7 days after balloon removed
IR	71/F	Cardiogenic shock, acute inferior MI	21 hrs	Died; no benefit from support
WJ[a]	62/M	Cardiogenic shock (10 days after antero-lateral MI; recurrent arrhythmias, failure	29 hrs	Died; cardiac cath., deemed inoperable
LC[a]	43/M	Severe refractory failure, coronary artery disease	9 days	Operated upon, discharged; died 2 mos later of choledocholithiasis
GL[a]	45/M	Cardiogenic shock, acute inferior MI	6 days[b]	Discharged; alive 26 months later
WSR	57/M	Cardiogenic shock, acute anteroseptal MI	10 days[b]	Weaned from balloon, died 3 wks later (arrhythmia)
JA[a]	51/M	Cardiogenic shock, acute anterior MI	2 hrs	Died; no benefit from balloon
EF[a]	45/M	Cardiogenic shock, acute anterior MI	3 days	Operated; died in low output
WT	61/M	Cardiogenic shock, acute anterolateral MI, recurrent ventricular tachycardia	24 hrs	Died on balloon support
PL[a]	50/M	Cardiogenic shock, acute anterior MI, recurrent ventricular tachycardia	2 days	Operated; died in low output
WP[a]	62/M	Cardiogenic shock, acute anteroseptal MI	3 days	Operated; died in low output
FS	56/M	Cardiogenic shock, acute anterolateral MI	4 hrs	Died; no benefit from balloon
VC[a]	57/M	Cardiogenic shock, acute inferior MI	4 days[b]	Discharged; had bypass 9 months later
JF[a]	57/F	Cardiogenic shock, acute anteroseptal MI, recurrent ventricular tachycardia	9 days[b]	Operated; died of recurrent ventricular tachycardia
SS[a]	53/F	Cardiogenic shock, acute anteroseptal MI, recurrent ventricular tachycardia	5 days	Died of refractory ventricular tachycardia
PM	44/F	Intraoperative acute anterolateral MI; severe left ventricular failure	8 days	Died of refractory ventricular tachycardia
WR	49/M	Cardiogenic shock, severe left ventricular failure	4 days	Died; no benefit from balloon
NL	37/M	Cardiogenic shock, acute anterior MI	24 hrs	Died; no benefit from balloon
RA[a]	44/M	Cardiogenic shock, acute anteroseptal MI, severe left ventricular failure, recurrent ventricular tachycardia	2 days	Died; refractory ventricular tachycardia
JH	45/M	Acute anteroseptal MI, refractory ventricular tachycardia	2 hrs	Died; no benefit from support
EH[a]	70/M	Cardiogenic shock, acute anterior MI	17 days	Died; cardiac cath., deemed inoperable
RS	48/F	Cardioversion followed by recurrent ventricular tachycardia	3 days[b]	Discharged
ER	55/M	Cardiogenic shock after mitral valve replacement	9 days[b]	Weaned; 2 wks later died of pulmonary disease
LE	50/M	Cardiogenic shock (? cause), refractory ventricular tachycardia	6 days[b]	Weaned; 2 days later died of arrhythmia
JS	40/M	Cardiogenic shock, acute anterior MI	8 hrs	Died; no benefit from balloon
GA	45/M	Cardiogenic shock, acute inferior MI, severe left ventricular failure	2 hrs	Died; no benefit from balloon
KK[a]	69/M	Cardiogenic shock, acute anterior MI	21 days	Died on balloon support
JW[a]	45/M	Cardiogenic shock, acute anterolateral MI, severe ventricular failure	5 days	Operated; died in low output

[a] *Cardiac catheterization data available.*
[b] *Weaned from balloon support.*

TABLE 2. Hemodynamic Status for 29 Patients

	NO. PTS.
Cardiogenic shock	25
Acute MI	21
Anterior MI	17
Inferior MI	4
Other[a]	4
No shock	4
Acute MI	2
Other[b]	2

[a] Cardiomyopathy: 2 patients, MVR, probable AMI.
[b] Cardioversion, chronic LV failure

TABLE 3. Technical Problems with the Intraaortic Balloons

	NO. PTS.
Inability to insert device	1[a]
Retrograde dissection	1[b]
Bilateral groin exploration required	2
Crack in plastic condensation trap, making balloon unworkable	1

[a] Not in series.
[b] Balloon functioned.

and electrolyte abnormalities were corrected, and if all the above measures failed to correct the hemodynamic abnormalities, then counterpulsation was considered appropriate. A decision regarding the use of intraaortic counterpulsation was made as soon as it became clear that the patient did require at least a few hours of pressor support. Those patients supported for refractory left ventricular failure and ventricular tachycardia had similarly failed to respond to vigorous attempts at medical management.

TECHNIQUES

The balloon catheter was inserted under sterile conditions in the groin with the better femoral pulse, and its position was checked fluoroscopically. A woven Dacron graft was sutured to the common femoral artery at the site of balloon insertion. In the present series, only one patient was encountered in whom all manipulations to provide correct balloon placement were unsuccessful, and the other groin was subsequently successfully utilized. Another patient required bilateral groin exploration; she was a diabetic with bilateral superficial femoral artery obstruction, and she developed distal ischemia in her extremity two days after the balloon was inserted. It was successfully changed to the other femoral artery, and though this patient was balloon-dependent and eventually died of recurrent arrhythmias, postmortem exam revealed no obstruction in either lower extremity other than that from chronic atherosclerosis. Another patient (JW) with severe atherosclerosis had the balloon inserted into an extraintimal plane with retrograde dissection of the balloon at the level of the proximal common iliac artery. The dissection involved the entire length of the thoracic and abdominal aorta, but not the aortic arch. Counterpulsation was only partially effective, but this patient was catheterized and operated upon, eventually dying after a total of five days of balloon assist. Autopsy showed the adventitia of the aorta to be intact with no obvious compromise of any of the branch vessels of the aorta.

In one patient, not in the series, we were unable to insert the balloon device in either groin, and the patient died in cardiogenic shock without benefit of counterpulsation. She was a small woman with weak femoral pulses due to severe bilateral aortoiliac disease. While it is recognized that weak lower extremity pulses are at least a relative contraindication to the use of intraaortic counterpulsation, it is often difficult to be sure that altered femoral artery pulse characteristics are not due to the shock state itself; even the usual bruits may be absent when the two situations coexist.

All patients were heparinized during the period of counterpulsation with two exceptions; these two patients had previous clotting abnormalities, and neither developed complications from balloon insertion or later, during the several days of circulatory assistance.

In only one instance did a mechanical malfunction prevent satisfactory counterpulsation, and in that case a crack in a plastic condensation trap allowed leakage of helium and prevented proper balloon function. (Table 3). The patient died in shock before this could be remedied, and he is not included in the present series. In all patients in whom counterpulsation was successfully employed, the three-segmented AVCO balloon reliably produced the well-documented counterpulsation effects of lowering systemic arterial systolic pressure, decreasing mean pulmonary capillary wedge pressure, and increasing systemic arterial diastolic pressure. Cardiac output increased moderately in all patients in whom it was measured.

Weaning from the balloon was done by

omitting counterpulsation every other beat, and if tolerated it was decreased to every fourth beat over a period of several days. If no hemodynamic deterioration occurred 24 hours after supporting a patient one out of four beats, then it was considered safe to remove the balloon. At the time of removal the previously placed graft was simply trimmed and sutured closed. No long-term morbidity resulted; one patient (VC) developed a superficial wound infection, which did not prolong his hospitalization and healed satisfactorily. Another wound infection, however, precluded reinsertion of the balloon 10 days after its removal; this patient's course (JF) is described in the results section. It is unlikely that the infection influenced her course.

RESULTS

Cardiogenic Shock

Twenty-five patients in cardiogenic shock were treated with the intraaortic balloon (Table 4). Twenty-one (84 percent) had an acute myocardial infarction as the etiology; in 17 of these, the infarct was anterolateral or anteroseptal, and in four it was inferior (Table 2). Two of the latter four were the only long-term survivors in the shock group. Among the four patients with shock but without acute infarction were two patients with cardiomyopathy (alcoholism in WH, idiopathic in RLS), one with possible but unproven myocardial infarction (LE), and one patient who had had a double coronary bypass graft four months before and was undergoing mitral valve replacement for papillary muscle dysfunction when he developed cardiogenic shock, requiring support (ER).

TABLE 4. Shock Patients Benefited by Balloon Support, 18 Patients

WEANED (8)		DEPENDENT (10)		
Living (2)	Died (6)	Cath. on Support (9)		Died (1)
		Inoperable (5)	Operated (4)	WT[a]
GL	RLS	SS[a]	PL[a]	
VC	WH	WJ[a]	EF	
	WSR	RA[a]	JW	
	JF[a] (op)	EH	WP	
	LE	KK		
	ER (post op)			

op: operation performed
[a]*These patients also had recurrent ventricular tachycardia (7). Italicized patient had shock reversed; 10 days later required catheterization and operation for refractory ventricular tachycardia.*

TABLE 5. Cause of Death after Weaning from Balloon, 6 Patients

	PT.
Refractory ventricular tachycardia	JF
Pneumonia	RLS[a]
Neurologic complications	WH[b]
Acute development of complete heart block	WSR, LE
Chronic pulmonary insufficiency, right heart failure	ER

[a]*Cardiomyopathy.*
[b]*Seven days after balloon removed.*

In the group of patients in shock, 18 (72 percent) showed hemodynamic improvement from counterpulsation, with consequent increased urine output, improved sensorium, and decreased dependence on vasopressors. However, only eight patients could be weaned from the support device, and six of these went on to die of further complications but without recurrent shock (Table 5). The remaining 10 patients improved with counterpulsation but could not be weaned; nine of these underwent cardiac catheterization on balloon support for consideration of operative intervention. Regarding the catheterization findings (Tables 6 and 7), the left anterior descending (LAD) coronary artery was significantly involved in all patients with cardiogenic shock, as has been noted before (Leinbach, Dinsmore, et al, 1972). With one exception (SS = 41 percent) the ejection fractions of all patients catheterized in shock were 25 percent or less. Three-vessel disease was noted in 5/9, two-vessel involvement in 3/9, and single-vessel involvement in one patient (WP). The two long-term survivors (GL—alive 26 months and asymptomatic; VC—alive 12 months after shock and 3 months after double coronary bypass done for persistent angina) were not catheterized during shock, but both had studies about nine months after the acute episode and both demonstrated three-vessel disease at that time and ejection fractions of 40 percent and 37 percent respectively.

Four patients were operated upon while on balloon support (Table 8). Interestingly, one of the patients (PL) had a complete reversal of the shock state prior to surgery, but urgent surgery was dictated by refractory ventricular tachycardia, which was not controlled by counterpulsation and antiarrhythmic agents. A bypass was placed to the right coronary artery (RCA) with a mean flow of 60/min, and an anterior infarct was resected, but he died 11 hours later in a low-output state. Patient EF also had a RCA bypass (mean flow 75 cc/min) and resection of an apical aneurysm but also died five hours after operation. Patient WP,

TABLE 6. Catheterization Data–Nonoperated Patients

PT.	LVEDP	CO	VENTRICULOGRAM	EF	EDV	ESV	CORONARY ANATOMY
WJ	35	4.5	Diffuse hypokinesis, akinetic distal AL wall & apex	22	273	212	T–LAD 4+–RCA, CCA
SS	20	3.7	Slight paradox distal AL wall & apex	41	175	104	T–LAD, CCA
RA	20	3.5	Not done (dye reaction)	–	–	–	4+–LAD, RCA, CCA
RLS	14	2.2	Diffuse hypokinesis	23	371	246	Normal
EH	28	–	Diffuse hypokinesis with slight paradox distal AL wall	22	276	216	T–RCA 4+–LAD 3+–main left
KK	24	–	Hypokinetic AL wall & apex	16	314	262	T–LAD, RCA 3+–CCA
JA[a]	16	4.8	Hypokinetic AL wall & apex	54	159	73	T–main left
GL[b]	18	4.6	Diffuse hypokinesis, akinetic distal inferior wall	40	134	80	T–RCA 4+–LAD, CCA

CO = cardiac output; EF = ejection fraction; EDV = end diastolic volume; ESV = end systolic volume; T = total occlusion; 4+ = 90% obstruction or more; 3+ = 70% obstruction or more; AL = anterolateral.
[a]*Study was done before cardiogenic shock developed.*
[b]*Study was done approximately nine months after balloon assist.*

TABLE 7. Catheterization Data–Operated Patients

PT.	LVEDP	CO	VENTRICULOGRAM	EF	EDV	ESV	CORONARY ANATOMY
LC	32	5.0	Diffuse hypokinesis, akinetic distal AL wall & apex	20	596	476	T–LAD, RCA, CCA
PL	20	5.7	Diffuse hypokinesis, slight paradox distal AL wall	23	214	164	T–RCA 4+–LAD
EF	18	8.4	Diffuse hypokinesis, slight paradox distal AL wall and apex	16	165	139	T–LAD 4+–RCA
JF	19	–	Diffuse hypokinesis, slight paradox distal AL wall and apex	21	166	131	T–LAD 4+–RCA
WP	20	–	Same as above	22	170	132	T–LAD
JW	45	–	Hypokinetic AL wall & apex, slight paradox of apex	25	154	115	T–main left 3+–RCA
VC[a]	5	3.9	Slight diffuse hypokinesis, slight paradox of apex	37	246	131	T–RCA 4+–LAD 3+–CCA

[a]*Preoperative study done nine months after balloon assist.*
Italicized patients were in cardiogenic shock when studied.

with a total occlusion of the LAD but no other significant disease, underwent resection of the area of infarction only, but he would not tolerate weaning from bypass. Patient JW had a massive anterior, lateral, and septal infarct, which was too extensive to resect. The RCA was bypassed with a mean flow of 45 cc/min, but the graft placed to the LAD had a flow of less than 10 cc/min; the latter graft was attempted because retrograde filling was seen on angiogram, and indeed the LAD was a 2-mm smooth vessel from its upper third to the apex. The patient survived for four days but never really improved, and postmortem exam revealed both grafts to be patent and a massive infarct (six to eight days old) involving approximately 75 percent of the left ventricular muscle. The main left coronary artery was totally occluded by thrombus overlying a severe stenosis.

Severe Left Ventricular Failure (Table 9)

Two patients were supported for severe left ventricular failure that was refractory to the usual medical agents.

Patient LC was a 43-year-old man with a previous myocardial infarction followed by severe symptoms of congestive heart failure. He was admitted with massive anasarca, and after all usual measures were exhausted he was placed on peritoneal dialysis with only partial control. Balloon support was tried, and he had gratifying improvement, with increased

TABLE 8. Operative Results

PT.	BALLOON SUPPORT	PROCEDURE	RESULT
LC	9 days	SVG to RCA, infarctectomy	Discharged
PL	2 days	SVG to RCA, infarctectomy	Died
EF	3 days	SVG to RCA, infarctectomy	Died
WP	3 days	Infarctectomy	Died
JW	5 days	SVG to RCA, LAD	Died
JF	8 days	Plication of infarct, SVG to LAD	Died
VC[a]	4 days	SVG to RCA, LAD	Discharged

SVG: saphenous vein graft.
[a]*Weaned from balloon support after four days, discharged but returned with severe angina and underwent elective revascularization.*

diuresis and improved strength, but he remained markedly dependent upon balloon support. At cardiac catheterization left ventricular pressures were alternately taken on and off the balloon, going from 100/22 to 28 mm Hg off to 85/16 to 18 mm Hg on balloon support. A left ventriculogram showed a huge heart with some apical paradox; coronary ateriograms demonstrated a high total LAD occlusion, total circumflex coronary artery occlusion 2 cm from its origin, and total RCA occlusion in its distal third! (These findings were confirmed at autopsy two months later). At operation a right coronary bypass achieved a flow of 70 cc/min, and a very small apical aneurysm was resected. The postoperative course was prolonged, but he recovered and was discharged. He remained limited at home but was improved compared to his previous status. However, about a month after discharge he was admitted with another acute episode of what was interpreted as severe failure, associated with abdominal pain but no fever. He rapidly became hypotensive and died. Autopsy revealed an impacted common duct stone with evidence of cholangitis. The vein graft was patent and no acute cardiac injury was found.

Patient PM was 44 years old, with hypercholesterolemia, severe angina, and left ventricular failure. He was operated upon at another hospital after angiograms revealed severe three-vessel disease and a posterior aneurysm. Three vein by-passes were done, and the aneurysm was plicated, but he had an intraoperative anteroseptal myocardial infarction and had a very stormy postoperative course, mostly due to severe left-sided failure. After nine days with only minimal improvement he was transferred to our unit for balloon support. Soon after counterpulsation was begun, he started to diurese and the pulmonary wedge pressure fell from the 18 to 20 mm Hg range to 10 to 12. Though he was able to maintain this improvement for several days, he never made further gains and could not be weaned. He survived for 8 days on balloon support, with the major problem in the last few days being recurrent ventricular tachycardia, and he finally succumbed to an uncontrollable rhythm disturbance. Autopsy was refused.

Recurrent, Refractory Ventricular Tachycardia (Table 6)

Our single success in this category is patient RS, who had long-standing mitral stenosis treated by a successful closed commissurotomy in 1962. She was admitted with the recent onset of atrial fibrillation, for cardioversion. During the procedure she converted to normal sinus rhythm, but she developed recurrent ventricular tachycardia, which could not be controlled medically. Counterpulsation was begun, and she very rapidly became stable, with occasional premature ventricular contractions but no further serious arrhythmias. She was weaned from the balloon after three days but still had some ventricular irritability, which by this time responded to the usual antiarrhythmic drugs. She was discharged and subsequently admitted for cardiac catheterization, which revealed normal coronary arteries with a small mitral valve gradient. She is currently doing well and remains in sinus rhythm.

Balloon support was tried in patient JH, a 45-year-old man who arrived at the hospital in ventricular fibrillation and was converted; ECG showed an acute anteroseptal infarct. He had recurrent ventricular tachycardia (VT) over the next few days but responded to a standard medical regimen and slowly improved. However, 29 days after admission he developed recurrent VT requiring multiple drugs and frequent D/C shocks. The intraaortic balloon was inserted, but the same course of refractory intermittent VT persisted, and after two hours of counterpulsation he could no longer be resuscitated.

Two other patients in this category were operated upon; both patients had cardiogenic shock controlled by counterpulsation, but the VT was not controlled.

PL was a 50-year-old man with an anterior infarction, initially in left heart failure, but he re-

TABLE 9. Balloon Support in Severe Refractory Left Ventricle Failure

LC	Improved by balloon support (9 days), operation performed successfully, late death (noncardiac)
PM	Postop myocardial infarction after triple bypass grafting, severe failure improved by balloon but could not be weaned (8 days)

sponded to standard therapy and improved until his fourth hospital day, when he developed recurrent VT. This was finally controlled by a combination of antiarrhythmic drugs, but on the eighth day of hospitalization, these episodes recurred and were associated with cardiogenic shock. Counterpulsation reversed the shock state but provided no improvement with regard to the VT, and he required multiple defibrillations; this obviously made catheterization difficult, but it was completed and showed severe three-vessel disease and an anterior paradoxical segment. Operation included a RCA graft with a mean flow of 60 cc/min and resection of the infarct. After this he had no further ventricular tachycardia but died 11 hours postoperatively in a low-output state despite balloon support.

The other operative case was JF, a 57-year-old hypertensive diabetic with two previous infarcts who presented with an acute anteroseptal infarct with pulmonary edema. Her edema could be medically controlled, but on her fourth hospital day she went into cardiogenic shock. Balloon support was started, and within a few hours all vasopressors were stopped. She was supported for eight days and was successfully weaned from support. However, though the shock state was reversed, she continued to have ventricular irritability throughout balloon support and after removal of the balloon. Ten days after the balloon had been removed (22 days of hospitalization) she developed more frequent episodes of VT; the balloon was not reinserted because it had not controlled her arrhythmias before. There was also a superficial wound infection where the balloon had been inserted. This was considered to be a contraindication to reinsertion on that side, and the other femoral artery was potentially to be used for perfusion during operation. She was catheterized and found to have a totally occluded LAD and severe, diffuse obstruction in the RCA; an apical area was noted to have slight paradoxical movement. Operation was performed and included a vein bypass to the LAD (flow of only 10 cc/min; technically satisfactory but involving a severely diseased vessel) and plication of the apical infarct. Infarctectomy was not done because of the small size of the left ventricle. Postoperatively, she initially did very well, requiring vasopressors but with much less irritability. However, she developed recurrent VT and died 48 hours after operation.

DISCUSSION

Intraaortic balloon counterpulsation using the AVCO device has been utilized clinically by our group for the past two years. The majority of the patients (21/29) supported were those with cardiogenic shock due to acute myocardial infarction. Whereas approximately a third of the patients in shock (8/25) survived their episode of pump failure and could be weaned from the balloon, only two patients were actually discharged from the hospital, simply an indication of the multiple organs adversely affected by the shock process.

Cardiac catheterization can be carried out safely in this group of gravely ill patients and provides essential guides for planning therapy. Ten patients in shock were dependent upon balloon support; nine were catheterized and four subsequently were operated upon. Thus, less than half the patients studied were considered operable, though we were relatively aggressive in accepting patients for operation, excluding those with no acceptable runoff beyond obstructed vessels and those with more than 50 percent of the ventricular volume involved unless there was a significant paradoxical segment. It is obvious from analyzing the surgical cases, however, that even these criteria were not strictly adhered to, especially in the younger patients. Cardiac outputs appeared to be an insensitive guide in this group of patients, but the ejection fractions were consistently depressed to 25 percent or less; the exception was one of 41 percent (patient SS), probably the result of an undiseased dominant RCA (confirmed at autopsy), which allowed vigorous contraction of the posterior left ventricle.

Autopsy results have confirmed the catheterization data, with the exception that we have seen some widely patent vessels that did not fill by collateral on coronary angiograms (always a left-coronary branch); the significance of this situation is uncertain, but it may represent the destruction of the collateral bed by the infarct process or obstruction to flow by cellular swelling and suggests that the outflow bed is irreversibly damaged. This may explain the very low flow in the LAD graft of JW, since this flow was otherwise unexpected in a 2-mm artery with no distal obstructions, and autopsy confirmed that the graft was technically adequate. In our small surgical group with shock (four patients) we were unsuccessful in reversing their downhill courses. Other series have shown more optimistic results (Sanders, Buckley, et al, 1972), and thus an aggressive approach still seems reasonable in carefully selected patients.

Of particular importance is the experience we had with cardiogenic shock associated with an acute inferior myocardial infarction. Two of four such patients survived with counterpulsation alone, and though this is a small group, others have tended to show similar trends (Leinbach, Buckley, et al, 1971). Of the two patients who died, one was the oldest patient in the study (71 years old —IR—21 hours on support) and the other (GA) was only supported for two hours with no benefit. There is obviously a stage of cardiogenic shock when balloon support is not enough; we had seven patients in shock who showed no improvement at all, but a review of this group revealed no obvious differences in age, location of infarcts, or duration of shock prior to starting assist. Autopsy results were not available in most of these patients.

The two patients with primarily left ventricular failure both showed prompt improvement on balloon support, and our only survivor of those operated on while on support (LC) falls into this category. The other patient (PM) also responded well but after eight days succumbed to ventricular tachycardia. It is unlikely that many patients supported for left ventricular failure will survive unless remedial surgery can be performed, as in the first case. The second patient had already undergone an apparently satisfactory revascularization nine days before, and it was hoped that with balloon support he could recover from the intraoperative infarction.

Ventricular tachycardia proved to be a particularly difficult problem (Table 10). It should be noted that many of the patients with cardiogenic shock who improved on balloon support also had runs of VT early in their course, and at this stage the irritability was often decreased by support. However, it was the recurrence of irritability seven or more days after the acute infarct that seemed to show little improvement with ballon support. The patient (RS) with VT cardioversion was definitely improved by counterpulsation, but this is an unusual case and subsequent coronary studies were normal. The two patients operated upon died, and both survived for too short a time for us to

make any definite conclusions about the effect of operation on their arrhythmias.

Regarding the two patients with cardiogenic shock due to cardiomyopathy, it should be recognized that these patients were originally thought to represent coronary artery disease, and they were supported for that reason. It is of some interest, however, that both patients responded favorably and could be weaned from support, though both went on to die of other complications. Unless the myopathy has some reversible etiology (alcoholism?), it would be difficult to justify such extraordinary efforts to support the majority of patients with this diagnosis.

We have not included pure mechanical problems, such as ventricular septal defect or mitral insufficiency associated with acute infarction, though some may argue that an akinetic or paradoxically moving area of myocardium is also a mechanical problem. We also have not included patients supported in low-output states after valve or other open-heart surgery, with the exception of patient ER, and this seemed appropriate since his entire problem (coronary insufficiency requiring previous double coronary bypass, mitral insufficiency due to papillary muscle dysfunction, and postoperative cardiogenic shock) was on the basis of coronary artery disease. His case demonstrates the value of counterpulsation even in the end stage of this disease, though heart transplantation or mechanical hearts may offer the only hope of a near normal existence for such patients.

SUMMARY

Twenty-nine patients supported with the AVCO intraaortic balloon have been analyzed; most were supported for cardiogenic shock, but the problems of left ventricular failure and ventricular tachycardia have also been discussed. Approximately one-third of the patients in shock could be weaned from support, but most (6/8) eventually died in the hospital. Another 10 patients were dependent on balloon support, and nine underwent cardiac catheterization, with the consistent findings of significant LAD obstruction in all patients (except one cardiomyopathy), ejection fractions of 25 percent or less (with one exception—41 percent), and apical wall motion abnormalities in all patients, with slight paradox in 6/8 studied during shock. An improved prognosis in inferior infarcts associated with shock is suggested.

Ventricular tachycardia (VT) was poorly controlled, especially if it occurred after the first

TABLE 10. Balloon Support in
Ventricular Tachycardia

PT.

JH	Acute anteroseptal MI without shock but with refractory ventricular tachycardia, unimproved by two hours of balloon support
RS	Cardioversion for atrial fibrillation resulted in refractory ventricular tachycardia, which responded to balloon support over three days; normal coronary anatomy
JF	Cardiogenic shock reversed by balloon support, but recurrent ventricular tachycardia persisted; operation unsuccessful
PL	Same as above, with shock responding but tachycardia still recurring; operation unsuccessful

four days of hospitalization for an acute infarct. Four patients were operated on during balloon support for cardiogenic shock, but none survived; in one of these the urgency of operation was because of VT. Another patient was operated upon because of refractory VT occurring 10 days after removal of balloon support for cardiogenic shock; she did not survive. The only patient operated on for refractory left ventricular failure survived, but later died of an unrelated problem.

Intraaortic balloon support can be rapidly, safely, and effectively utilized in the situations described, both as "primary" therapy and as support to accomplish cardiac catheterization and possibly operation. Salvage in this group of patients remains low, and selection of criteria for operability remains difficult.

References

1. Dunkman WB, Leinbach RC, Buckley MJ, et al: Clinical and hemodynamic results of intra-aortic balloon pumping and surgery for cardiogenic shock. Circulation 46:465, 1972
2. Kantrowitz A, Tjønneland S, Freed PS, et al: Initial clinical experience with intra-aortic balloon pumping in cardiogenic shock. JAMA 203:113, 1968
3. Kantrowitz A, Krakauer JS, Rosenbaum A, et al: Phase-shift balloon pumping in medically refractory cardiogenic shock. Arch Surg 99:739, 1969
4. Kasser IS, Kennedy JW: Measurement of left ventricular volumes in man by single-plane cineangiocardiography. Invest Radiol 4:83, 1969
5. Leinbach RC, Buckley MJ, Austen WG, et al: Effects of intraaortic balloon pumping on coronary flow and metabolism in man. Circulation 43: Suppl 1: 71, 1971
6. Leinbach RC, Dinsmore RE, Mundth ED, et al: Selective coronary and left ventricular cineangiography during intraaortic balloon pumping for cardiogenic shock. Circulation 45:845, 1972
7. Maroko PR, Bernstein EF, Libby P, et al: Effect of intraaortic balloon counterpulsation on the severity of myocardial ischemic injury following acute coronary occlusion; counterpulsation and myocardial injury. Circulation 45:1150, 1972
8. Mundth ED, Buckley MJ, Leinbach RC, et al: Myocardial revascularization for the treatment of cardiogenic shock complicating acute myocardial infarction. Surgery 70:78, 1971
9. Powell WJ, Daggett WM, Magro AE, et al: Effects of intraaortic balloon counterpulsation on cardiac performance, oxygen consumption, and coronary blood flow in dogs. Circ Res 26:753, 1970
10. Sanders CA, Buckley MJ, Leinbach RC, Mundth ED, Austen WG: Mechanical circulatory assistance; current status and experience with combining circulatory assistance, emergency coronary angiography, and acute myocardial revascularization. Circulation 45:1292, 1972
11. Scheidt S, Aschein R, Killip T III: Shock after acute myocardial infarction: a clinical and hemodynamic profile. Am J Cardiol 26:556, 1970
12. Scheidt S, Wilner G, Mueller H, et al: Intra-aortic balloon counterpulsation in cardiogenic shock; report of a cooperative clinical trial. N Engl J Med 288:979, 1973
13. Sugg WL, Webb WR, Ecker RR: Reduction of extent of myocardial infarction by counterpulsation. Ann Thorac Surg 7:310, 1969
14. Watson JT, Willerson JT, Fixler DE, Browning RM, Sugg WL: Changes in collateral coronary blood flow (CCBF) distal to a coronary occlusion during intra-aortic balloon pumping (IABP). Trans Am Soc Artif Intern Organs 19:402, 1973

47

INTRAAORTIC BALLOON COUNTERPULSATION AND CARDIAC SURGERY

John F. Neville, Jr., Frederick B. Parker, Jr., E. Lawrence Hanson, and Watts R. Webb

INTRODUCTION

We have used intraaortic balloon pumping (IABP) for the management of acute left ventricular failure in three categories of patient treatment: (1) treatment of the postbypass patient who is unable to maintain an adequate peripheral circulation even with the aid of blood volume replacement and positive inotropic agents; (2) preoperative stabilization of patients with surgically correctable complications of acute myocardial infarction; and (3) management of patients with acute myocardial infarction who did not have surgically remedial lesions or did not require emergency surgical intervention. This report is concerned with the first two categories.

IABP does not pump blood from the left ventricle to the aorta. It can improve left ventricular function only in proportion to its ability to improve ventricular emptying during systole. This improvement is primarily mechanical by reducing the pressure the left ventricle must generate to store a given stroke volume in the central aorta, thereby permitting a more efficient emptying of the ventricle. The reduction in pressure permits more of the ventricle's limited work capacity to be spent in moving volume rather than generating pressure. The higher diastolic pressure increases coronary blood flow when this parameter is pressure limited. Increased oxygen availability may further aid contractility. To be successful, IABP requires that acute left ventricular failure be reversible to the point where the patient can eventually provide an acceptable unassisted cardiac output. By interrupting the vicious cycle of the low cardiac output syndrome, this becomes possible.

METHOD

Before using IABP in postbypass patients we determine that cardiac output is clinically inadequate despite (1) volume replacement to a left atrial or left ventricular diastolic pressure of 25 mm Hg; (2) repeated periods of partial or total bypass; and (3) a variety of positive inotropic agents. With increasing experience, the length of time wasted in testing these adjuncts has decreased. The positive inotropic agents are not usually discontinued in the operating room. In the recovery room, we try to wean the patient off these agents while receiving maximum balloon assist. After a period of observation, balloon assistance is slowly decreased while monitoring left atrial pressure and clinical signs of cardiac output. If either shows evidence of an unfavorable hemodynamic response, full assistance is reinstituted. This titration of response and degree of assistance is continued until it is obvious that the patient can support his own circulation. The balloon is then removed.

The preoperative use of IABP has followed a somewhat similar pattern in that various modes of medical therapy (volume therapy, inotropic agents, and rhythm stabilization) have failed to restore adequate left ventricular function. Patients are now being seen earlier in their time course as the ability of IABP to improve hemodynamics has become accepted. After a maximum period of 24 to 48 hours on IABP, the necessary diagnostic cardiac catheterization procedures are performed during IABP. If a surgically correctable lesion is found, surgery is performed. IABP is usually required in the postbypass period.

Our study has not included patients seen

early enough within the optimum time for salvage of myocardium through the use of emergency revascularization. The use of revascularization has been only as an important adjunct to the basic treatment indicated for complications of myocardial infarction.

MATERIAL

There have been 22 patients in whom IABP has been used postoperatively (Group I). The procedures have been: seven aortic valve replacements, two mitral valve replacements, two double valve replacements, five aortocoronary bypass grafts, and six resections of chronic left ventricular aneurysms. In the latter group, four had additional procedures including mitral valve replacement or bypass vein grafts.

There have been 11 patients requiring preoperative IABP for complications of acute myocardial infarction (Group II). The major indications for surgery were acute left ventricular aneurysms (13 to 42 days) in four patients, acute mitral insufficiency in four patients including one with a posterior aneurysm requiring simultaneous aneurysmectomy, a chronic aneurysm complicated by recent total occlusion of another coronary artery in two patients, and one acute VSD.

RESULTS

In Group I, eleven patients were successfully weaned from IABP and these were able to maintain an adequate circulation with only conventional medical management. There were nine patients whose left ventricular failure was progressive, and the use of IABP could not prevent death. There were four late hospital deaths due primarily to the complications of sepsis and/or renal failure. The overall salvage rate has been 40 percent.

In Group II, seven patients were successfully weaned off IABP postoperatively. The IABP was used for up to 14 days postoperatively with successful weaning. These patients had the same problems postweaning as were seen in Group I. A total of four were unable to improve left ventricular function sufficiently to permit weaning. One patient developed intractable ventricular fibrillation postbypass despite IABP. One with an acute VSD, extensive septal infarction, and an acute anterior aneurysm did not have sufficient functioning of the left ventricle to support an adequate circulation even with IABP. There were

three late deaths, leaving an overall salvage rate of 36 percent.

The high incidence of late deaths masks the ability of IABP to sustain life until the left ventricle can regain sufficient function to maintain an adequate circulation. In both Groups I and II, 60 percent of the patients were successfully weaned from IABP. The remaining 40 percent either died in the operating room or early postoperatively with intractable arrhythmias or low cardiac output. The late deaths reduced the survival to 40 percent and reflect the complications that result from either pre- or intraoperative periods of low cardiac output.

COMPLICATIONS

One patient who had been on IABP for several days preoperatively had the opposite femoral artery used for arterial return during bypass. Autopsy confirmed the presence of cerebral fibrin emboli, possibly washed off the balloon. We now routinely use aortic cannulation for perfusion. One patient with known peripheral vascular insufficiency and severe diabetes developed gram-negative myositis on the side of the IABP catheter and ultimately required amputation. Following death from both renal and congestive heart failure, autopsy revealed thrombotic occlusions of the hepatic and renal arteries, which were thought to be emboli from thrombi on the left ventricular infarction. In three other patients there have been local or distal thrombi. This problem seems to have been solved by the technique of catheter insertion described previously,[1] full heparinization, and routine passage of a Fogarty catheter antegrade and retrograde at decannulation.

DISCUSSION

IABP is not a panacea since it cannot pump more blood than the left ventricle can put into the aorta. Even though we have used it successfully for a three-week period, it cannot be used indefinitely and requires a reversible state of acute left ventricular failure. Within these constraints, IABP is clearly a valuable adjunct to conventional medical management. The mechanisms by which it achieves improvement in myocardial function have clear advantages when compared to the conflicting physiologic effects of positive inotropic agents.

The presently available equipment for IABP is reliable and basically easy to use. It can be safely used for relatively long periods of time without requiring the constant attendance of a physician or special technician. It will permit survival of surgical patients who otherwise would die of the vicious circle established by low cardiac output. It will provide the same benefit to patients with acute myocardial infarction and its complications, increasing the safety of the diagnostic procedures necessary to select patients for surgical intervention.

IABP has developed from the work of Kantrowitz.[2,3] It has a role in the management of acute myocardial infarction [3,4,5,6] including emergency revascularization. This report reaffirms [1] that the use of IABP will permit a significant salvage rate in patients undergoing surgical correction of the complications of myocardial infarction. Similarly it permits survival in the acute left ventricular failure that occasionally follows cardiac surgery.[1,8] It has developed into a valuable clinical tool that should receive increasing application.

References

1. Parker FB Jr, Neville JF Jr, Hanson EL, Webb WR: Intraaortic balloon counterpulsation and cardiac surgery. Ann Thorac Surg 17:2, 1974

2. Kantrowitz A, Kantrowitz A: Experimental augmentation of coronary flow by retardation of the arterial pressure pulse. Surgery 34:678, 1953

3. Kantrowitz A, Tjonneland S, Freed PS, Phillips SJ, Butner AP, Sherman JL Jr: Initial clinical experience with intraaortic balloon pumping in cardiogenic shock. JAMA 203:113, 1968

4. Mundth ED, Turchak PM, Buckley MJ, Leinbach RC, Kantrowitz A, Austen WG: Temporary mechanical circulatory assistance and emergency direct coronary artery surgery for the treatment of cardiogenic shock complicating acute myocardial infarction. N Engl J Med 283:1382, 1970

5. Mundth ED, Buckley MJ, Leinbach RC, DeSanctis RW, Sanders CA, Kantrowitz A, Austen WG: Myocardial revascularization for the treatment of cardiogenic shock complicating acute myocardial infarction. Surgery 70:78, 1971

6. Sanders CA, Buckley MJ, Leinbach RC, Mundth ED, Austen WG: Mechanical circulatory assistance: current status and experience with combining circulatory assistance, emergency coronary angiography, and acute myocardial revascularization. Circulation 45:1292, 1972

7. Bregman D, Goetz RH: Clinical experience with a new cardiac assist device—the dual chambered intra-aortic balloon assist. J Thorac Cardiovasc Surg 62:577, 1971

8. Buckley MF, Craver JM, Gold HK, Mundth ED, Daggett WM, Austen WG: Intra-aortic balloon pump assist for cardiogenic shock after cardiopulmonary bypass. Circulation 47–48 (Suppl III):90, 1973

48

ADVANCES IN CLINICAL INTRAAORTIC BALLOON PUMPING

David Bregman, Eduardo N. Parodi, Keith Reemtsma, and James R. Malm

Intraaortic balloon pumping (IABP) is currently the supportive temporary mechanical treatment of choice for the management of refractory left ventricular power failure.[4,6-10]

It is the purpose of this chapter to outline those clinical and technical advances in IABP that have increased patient survival and have facilitated the application of IABP, especially in the operating room.

METHODS AND MATERIALS

Clinical experience at our institution has been with the unidirectional dual-chambered intraaortic balloon in conjunction with the Datascope System 80.*[4,6-10] The dual-chambered balloon is constructed from polyurethane and has a spherical distal chamber which inflates initially during diastole, thereby gently occluding the aorta (Fig. 1). This is immediately followed, in the same diastolic interval, by the inflation of a narrower, cylindrical proximal chamber, which pumps the intraaortic blood unidirectionally toward the aortic root. The result is a phasic occlusion of the descending thoracic aorta during diastole. The usual clinical balloon employed is 30 cc with an 18-mm distal occluding balloon and a 14-mm proximal pumping balloon.

The Datascope System 80 is a fail-safe, mobile, cardiac assist console that is completely self-sufficient and needs no other ancillary support to

* Manufactured by the Datascope Corporation, Paramus, N.J.

Supported in part by National Institutes of Health Research Grant #HL 12738.

function.[6] The unit synchronizes IABP with the R-wave of the EKG, but it can also trigger from the arterial pressure wave. Arrhythmia tracking is a built-in feature. Carbon dioxide is the driving gas, and a safety chamber is utilized in a closed system to minimize the potential hazard of balloon rupture. An electrically isolated monitor provides digital readouts of hemodynamic parameters and of body temperature. Built-in batteries facilitate transport of a patient undergoing balloon assist.

TECHNICAL ADVANCES

Balloon Management

A 10-mm side-arm woven Dacron graft is sutured end-to-side to the common femoral artery (Fig. 2). The graft stump should be about 2.5 to 3 cm long.

If, after the arteriotomy has been negotiated, the balloon cannot be advanced, do not exert excessive force on the balloon catheter. Remove the balloon and insert a Fogarty[R] catheter to assess patency of the vessel. If the vessel appears patent, try inserting the balloon again on the same side. If this is unsuccessful, remove the balloon and manually bend the balloon catheter, 0.5 to 1 cm distal to the lucite tip to a 45 degree angle (Fig. 3).[5] The flexible stainless steel wire strut within the proximal pumping balloon will maintain this angulated position. Now, reinsert the balloon and when the obstruction is reached, rotate the balloon and catheter. This maneuver will frequently allow the balloon to pass a tortuous or arteriosclerotic juncture or an angulated aortoiliac bifurcation. By the advent of this technique, we have now treated

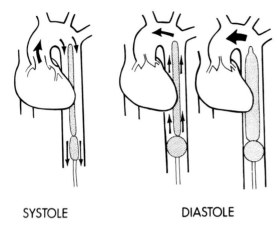

SYSTOLE   DIASTOLE

FIG. 1. Action mechanism of the unidirectional dual-chambered intraaortic balloon. The distal spherical balloon inflates slightly earlier in diastole and phasically obstructs aortic flow. The larger cylindrical proximal balloon then pumps the blood unidirectionally toward the aortic root. Both balloons are then completely deflated by an active vacuum just prior to ventricular ejection.

several patients in whom difficulty was initially encountered but, nevertheless, in whom the balloon was easily inserted in the ipsilateral extremity, thereby sparing the patient additional surgery while at the same time enabling the earlier application of cardiac assistance. In our earlier experience, such a patient would have required a contralateral femoral arteriotomy, often with the same unsuccessful attempt.

The wound is irrigated thoroughly and is closed in layers. No sutures should be placed around the balloon catheter, either subcutaneously or at the skin level, since these may saw through the catheter over a period of time. Instead, the balloon catheter is taped to the skin, similarly to taping a chest tube. These dressings are changed every 48 hours, even after the balloon has been removed. Usually 12 to 24 hours after surgery, one of the many weaning techniques is utilized.[4] The balloon is not left in the patient in the nonpulsating state for more than one hour since this may predispose to platelet build-up.[2] In fact, if a bal-

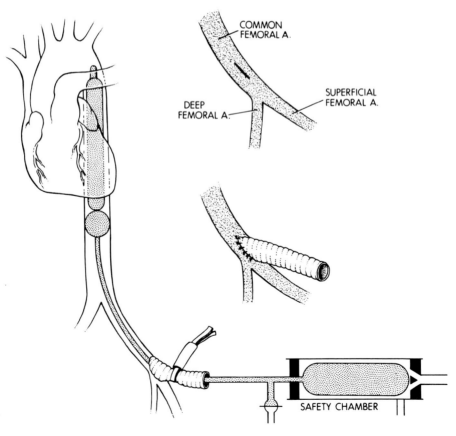

COMMON FEMORAL A.

SUPERFICIAL FEMORAL A.

DEEP FEMORAL A.

SAFETY CHAMBER

FIG. 2. Usual technique of dual-chambered intraaortic balloon insertion.

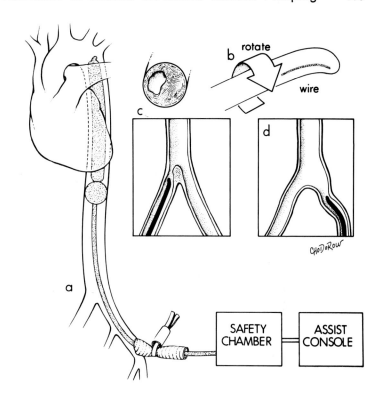

FIG. 3. Simple method to facilitate difficult intraaortic balloon insertion. A. Proper position of dual-chambered intraaortic balloon just distal to left subclavian artery. Note that the balloon is inserted through a Dacron prosthesis, which is snared, permitting perfusion of the distal extremity during the period of cardiac assistance. B. Technique of bending and rotating distal balloon catheter during insertion. C. Balloon negotiating eccentric arteriosclerotic stenosis. D. Balloon passing through an arterial tortuosity.

loon is *in situ* during cardiopulmonary bypass, the balloon is partly inflated every 15 seconds to prevent this complication. After removing the balloon, one has the choice of leaving a short segment of graft and oversewing it, removing the graft completely and repairing the artery primarily, or using a vein patch. The first is our preferred technique since it is easily accomplished at the bedside. A

Fogarty[R] catheter is frequently passed down the ipsilateral extremity at the time of balloon removal to extract any peripheral debris.[24]

Pressure Triggering

Another feasibility with a System 80 equipped with an "A" model monitor (850A,

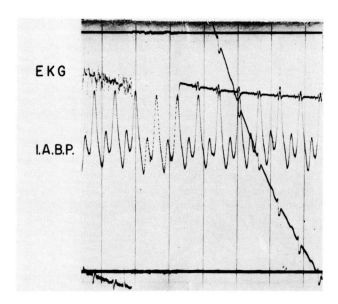

FIG. 4. Tracing demonstrating IABP utilizing a pressure trigger. In this instance, although an electrocautery distorted the EKG, IABP nevertheless remained smooth and synchronous.

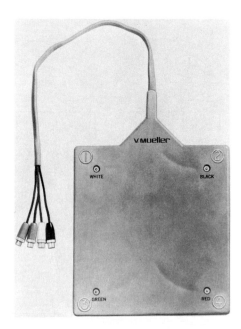

FIG. 5. V. Mueller's EKG pad for rapid acquisition of the electrocardiogram in the operating room. After placing the pad beneath the patient's back, it is rapidly connected to the System 80.

860A, 865A) is the ability to trigger cardiac assistance from the arterial pressure wave alone. This can be utilized in the cardiac arrest situation in conjunction with either closed or open chest cardiac massage, or when a situation arises where electrical interference becomes excessive, such as in the operating room when an electrocautery is used (Fig. 4). With this mode of synchronous cardiac assistance, one can rapidly begin IABP in the operating room by simply acquiring aortic pressure with a needle under emergency circumstances.

EKG Pad

Since one cannot predict with great accuracy which patients in the operating room will need IABP, an early difficulty encountered was the securing of standard limb leads on these patients while they were covered with the sterile operative drapes. To circumvent this problem, an EKG pad * (Fig. 5) has been acquired, which can simply be placed under the patient's back by the anesthesiologist. There is a rapid connection to the System 80, and a crisp EKG is uniformly obtained. When the chest is closed, the standard

EKG leads are then applied and the EKG pad is disconnected prior to transporting the patient to the recovery room.

RECENT ADVANCES IN MANAGEMENT DURING CLINICAL IABP

The measurement of left atrial pressure in the operating room during IABP is mandatory, since these patients are initially extremely volume sensitive. During IABP, fluids should be administered to maintain a mean left atrial pressure of 20 to 25 mm Hg. The peak augmented blood pressure should be maintained at 100 to 110 mm Hg. If this peak pressure cannot be obtained, and an inotropic agent is required, Levophed® (norepinephrine) is the agent of choice in coronary patients, and frequently this agent can be discontinued after a short period of initial response. IABP can be continued in postoperative patients after the endotracheal tube is removed and is well tolerated. Balloon support is usually continued for 12 hours, even if the patient appears stable shortly after his arrival in the recovery room. A chest x-ray is taken promptly in the recovery room to ascertain balloon position. A proximal arterial pressure line (ie above the balloon) is necessary, and it is usually connected to a Sorenson Intraflow® * to facilitate patency. The radial artery is usually preferred for pressure monitoring.

In the operating room, our routine for postoperative patients requiring IABP is to reverse the patients' heparinization with protamine. No anticoagulants are utilized for the first 48 hours.[4] If IABP must be continued longer than this, 10 to 15 cc per hour of low molecular weight dextran (Rheomacrodex®) is utilized.

It is extremely important to wash all powder off the surgeon's gloves prior to initially handling the balloon, since powder granules can act as a nidus for platelet aggregations and emboli. In our experience, we have not encountered any emboli with this regimen.

As an additional note, it should be mentioned that a balloon used clinically should *never* be used again for several reasons. After usage, the balloon membrane may retain small deposits of foreign protein, which may not be eliminated even with thorough washing. This foreign protein may serve as a nidus for the deposition of platelets and other formed elements of the blood, which may

---

* V. Mueller, Chicago, Illinois.

* Sorenson Research Company, Salt Lake City, Utah.

result in eventual thrombosis. In addition, the risk of serum hepatitis transferred from one patient to another is a reality. Finally, during balloon removal, it is possible that the balloon membrane may become damaged due to scratching as the balloon exits through the graft in the groin. With additional clinical usage, this defect in the membrane could weaken its structural integrity and thereby encourage the risk of balloon rupture.[4]

CLINICAL OBSERVATIONS ON CORONARY BLOOD FLOW DURING IABP

During the past year, we have encountered five high-risk adult male patients undergoing coronary revascularization procedures who required intraoperative balloon support to wean them from cardiopulmonary bypass after the usual methods were unsuccessful. The clinical data relating to this group of patients can be seen in Table 1. Three patients had associated left ventricular aneurysms, and two of these were resected. A total of nine coronary arteries were revascularized. Four patients were long-term survivors assisted for an average of 17 hours and were discharged from the hospital, while one patient expired in the operating room after an initial hemodynamic response to IABP.

The coronary graft blood flows in these patients, as measured with a square-wave electromagnetic flowmeter,* can be seen in Table 2. There was a uniform increase in coronary blood flow (CBF) in all patients when the balloon was initially turned on, as compared to the graft flows measured during cardiopulmonary bypass (average increase = 117 percent). Although patient #2 also increased his graft flow during IABP, he had diffuse arteriosclerotic coronary artery disease, which precluded the development of adequate CBF in either of his grafts at any time.

One hour after the initial graft flows were measured during IABP, repeat measurements were performed on and off the balloon, just prior to chest closure (Table 2). The changes in CBF that can be attributed to the balloon (measurements on and off IABP just prior to chest closure) demonstrated an average increase of 80 percent (range 50 to 100 percent: median = 83 percent). Specific patient tracings illustrating the improvement in CBF seen with unidirectional IABP can be seen in Figures 6 and 7.

* Carolina Medical Electronics, Winston-Salem, N.C.

NEW BALLOONS

Pediatric IABP

A pediatric single-chambered balloon has been developed (volume: 10 cc; OD: 9 mm) on a special catheter. Its clinical uses have not yet been defined, but it may play a role in the management of an infant with myocarditis and congestive heart failure, or in the management of a postoperative infant with a low output state.

Left Ventricular Balloon Pumping (LVBP)

In the experimental low output state, IABP may be hemodynamically ineffective, and a more direct left ventricular assist device may be required. A left ventricular balloon has been shown to be an extremely effective cardiac assist device in the experimental low output setting by its ability to cause a rapid fall in left atrial pressure and in left ventricular end diastolic pressure with concomitant improvement in aortic pressure, aortic flow, and coronary blood flow.[11,14,22] In its present form, it is introduced directly into the left ventricular cavity via the apex of the left ventricle, and, after circulatory hemodynamics improve, a transition can readily be made to IABP and the left ventricular balloon removed. A pear-shaped model for clinical use is available.[11]

DISCUSSION

A greater understanding regarding the role of IABP in conjunction with managing a cardiogenic shock patient or a patient undergoing open-heart surgery has evolved recently and has markedly improved patient survival.

Initially, it was felt that IABP would be the significant definitive therapeutic modality in the management of a patient with cardiogenic shock.[64] However, clinical experience has shown that this is not the case, and a survival of only 15 to 17 percent [18,26] can be expected with IABP alone, although, to some extent, this figure will vary with the temporal sequence of the initiation of IABP. Clearly, the earlier IABP is initiated during the course of management of a cardiogenic shock patient, the higher will be the survival rates from this intervention alone.[4,8,9] A significant number of these balloon dependent patients can now safely undergo angiography while on con-

TABLE 1. Intraoperative Unidirectional Intraaortic Balloon Pumping (IABP) in Conjunction with Coronary Revascularization–Clinical Data, Columbia-Presbyterian Medical Center (1973–1974)

PT.	AGE/ SEX	DIAGNOSIS	OPERATION PERFORMED	DURATION OF IABP (hrs)	OUTCOME
GB	41/M	ASHD + LV aneurysm	Aneurysm resection + bypass grafts to LAD and CIRC	1	Long-term survivor
JC	62/M	ASHD	Bypass grafts to RCA and LAD	1	Expired in OR
NN	58/M	ASHD + LV aneurysm	Aneurysm resection + bypass graft to RCA	6	Long-term survivor
WZ	54/M	ASHD + LV aneurysm	Bypass graft to CIRC	45	Long-term survivor
ES	49/M	ASHD	Bypass grafts to RCA, LAD, and CIRC	15	Long-term survivor

ASHD: Arteriosclerotic heart disease; CIRC: circumflex coronary artery; OR: operating room.

tinuous intraaortic balloon support and can then undergo definitive open-heart surgery based on their individual pathologic anatomy.[25]

In addition, a uniform survival in excess of 50 percent has been achieved in those patients who require IABP to wean them from cardiopulmonary bypass.[1,12,15,20,21,23,25,28]

Of the clinical advances discussed, perhaps the most significant is the documentation of the increase in CBF with unidirectional balloon support.[4] Previous reports in the literature have been conflicting regarding the changes in CBF during intraaortic balloon support in man. Reports of single-chambered IABP have demonstrated clinical increases of up to 36 percent.[19] Previous reports with the three-segment modification of the single-chambered balloon showed that the trend during balloon assist was toward a diminished net coronary flow:[13] The flow fell in seven studies, was unchanged in three, and rose in only four.[17] A more recent clinical three-segment balloon report showed an average increase in CBF of 38 percent (in open-chest patients)[1] as compared to the 80 percent increase seen with the unidirectional

TABLE 2. Intraoperative Unidirectional IABP-Coronary Graft Blood Flow, Columbia-Presbyterian Medical Center, 1973–74 (cc/min)

PT.	PRE-IABP (on bypass)			IMMEDIATELY AFTER START OF IABP			FLOW PRIOR TO CLOSURE OF CHEST					
							On IABP			Off IABP		
	RCA	LAD	CIRC	RCA	LAD	CIRC	RCA	LAD	CIRC	RCA	LAD	CIRC
GB		35	5		50 (AP = 50)	30		80 (AP = 90)	50		50	30
JC	5	0		10	0 (AP = 30)		20	15 (AP = 50)		ND	ND	
NN	20			35	(AP = 50)		80	(AP = 90)		40		
WZ			40		(AP = 70)	60		(AP = 100)	90			60
ES	15	25	20	25	60 (AP = 60)	35	50	150 (AP = 100)	55	25	75	30

AP: mean arterial pressure (mm Hg); ND: not determined.

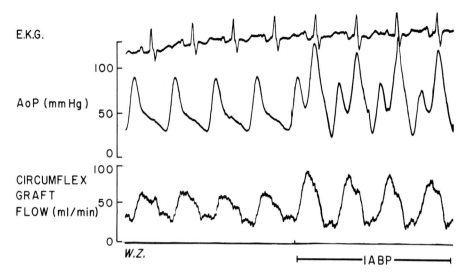

FIG. 6.   Dual-chambered IABP in a patient assisted after aortocoronary bypass graft surgery. Note the doubling of the circumflex coronary graft blood flow when IABP was instituted. Tracing speed 25 mm/sec. EKG: electrocardiogram; AoP: aortic pressure.

dual-chambered balloon reported herein. This confirms the previously reported increase in coronary blood flow, which had been documented in the experimental low output state.[27] It is the combination of increasing myocardial oxygen supply and decreasing myocardial oxygen demand that accounts for the improved physiology seen with IABP.[3]

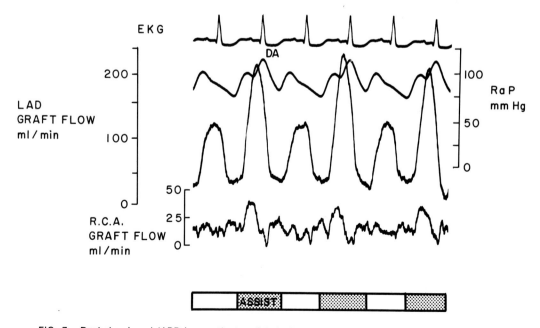

FIG. 7.   Dual-chambered IABP in a patient assisted after aorto-coronary bypass graft surgery. Note 100 percent increase in both LAD and RCA graft flows during assist on every other beat. Tracing speed 25 mm/sec. DA: diastolic augmentation; LAD: left anterior descending; RCA: right coronary artery; RaP: radial artery pressure; Assist: IABP period.

The initial clinical use of LVBP will undoubtedly occur in the operating room when a postsurgical patient in a profound low cardiac output state cannot benefit from IABP. Perhaps with further advances in balloon materials and in catheter designs, an indwelling left ventricular balloon will be designed for prolonged support.

The recent technical advances in IABP that were discussed have greatly facilitated the application of IABP in the operating room. Perhaps the advance facilitating difficult balloon insertions[5] by utilizing a bend in the proximal balloon catheter is most timely, since an incidence of up to 15 percent of difficulty or inability to insert intraaortic balloons has been reported.

At the present time, more than 750 patients have been assisted worldwide with unidirectional dual-chambered IABP. It is hoped that the recent clinical and technical advances reported herein will help to continue the trend of improved patient survival with this encouraging form of temporary mechanical cardiac assistance.

References

1. Berger RL, Saini VK, Ryan TJ, Sokol DM, Keefe JF: Intraaortic balloon assist for postcardiotomy cardiogenic shock. J Thorac Cardiovasc Surg 66:906, 1973
2. Bernstein EF, Murphy AE: The importance of pulsation in preventing thrombosis from intraaortic balloons. A note of caution. J Thorac Cardiovasc Surg 62:950, 1971
3. Braunwald E, Covell JW, Maroko PR, Ross JR Jr: Effects of drugs and of counterpulsation on myocardial oxygen consumption. Circulation 40:220 (Suppl 4), 1969
4. Bregman D: Dual-chambered Intraaortic balloon counterpulsation. In Ionescu MI, Wooler GH (eds): Current Techniques in Extracorporeal Circulation. London, Butterworths, 1974 (in press)
5. Bregman D, Bolooki H, Malm JR: A simple method to facilitate difficult intraaortic balloon insertions. An Thorac Surg 15:636, 1973
6. Bregman D, Goetz RH: A failsafe cardiac assist system for intraaortic balloon pumping. Trans Am Soc for Artif Int Organs 18:505, 1972
7. Bregman D, Goetz RH: A new concept in circulatory assistance—the dual-chambered intraaortic balloon. Mount Sinai J Med 39:123, 1972
8. Bregman D, Goetz RH: Clinical experience with a new cardiac assist device—the dual-chambered intraaortic balloon assist. J Thorac Cardiovasc Surg 62:577, 1971
9. Bregman D, Kripke DC, Cohen MN, Laniado S, Goetz RH: Clinical experience with the unidirectional dual-chambered intraaortic balloon assist. Circulation 43,44:82 (Suppl 1), 1971
10. Bregman D, Kripke DC, Goetz RH: The effect of synchronous unidirectional intraaortic balloon pumping on hemodynamics and coronary blood flow in cardiogenic shock. Trans Am Soc for Artif Int Organs 16:439, 1970
11. Bregman D, Parodi EN, Malm JR: Left ventricular and unidirectional intraaortic balloon pumping: effects on hemodynamics in canine cardiogenic shock. J Thorac Cardiovasc Surg 67:553, 1974
12. Buckley MJ, Craver JM, Gold HK, et al: Intraaortic balloon pump assist for cardiogenic shock after cardiopulmonary bypass. Circulation 47,48:90 (Suppl 3), 1973
13. Buckley MJ, Leinbach RC, Kastor JA, et al: Hemodynamic evaluation of intraaortic balloon pumping in man. Circulation 41,42:130 (Suppl 2), 1970
14. Donald DE, McGoon DC: Circulatory support by a ventricular balloon pump. Circulation 43,44:96 (Suppl 1), 1971
15. Housman LV, Bernstein EF, Braunwald NS, Dilley RB: Counterpulsation for intraoperative cardiogenic shock. Successful use of intraaortic balloon. JAMA 224:1131, 1973
16. Kantrowitz A, Tjonneland S, Freed PS, et al: Initial clinical experience with intraaortic balloon pumping in cardiogenic shock. JAMA 203:135, 1968
17. Leinbach RC, Buckley MJ, Austen WG, et al: Effects of intraaortic balloon pumping on coronary flow and metabolism in man. Circulation 43,44:77 (Suppl 1), 1971
18. Malm JR: What's new in cardiothoracic surgery. Surg Gynecol Obstet 136:191, 1973
19. Mueller H, Ayres SM, Conklin EF, et al: The effects of intraaortic counterpulsation on cardiac performance and metabolism in shock associated with acute myocardial infarction. J Clin Invest 50:1885, 1971
20. Mundth ED, Yurchak PM, Buckley MJ, et al: Circulatory assistance and emergency direct coronary artery surgery for shock complicating acute myocardial infarction. N Engl J Med 283:1382, 1970
21. Parker FB Jr, Neville JF, Hanson EL, Webb WR: Intraaortic balloon counterpulsation and cardiac surgery. Ann Thorac Surg 17:602, 1974
22. Petrovsky BV, Shumakov VI: Artificial heart implanted into the organism. Kardiologia 8:14, 1967
23. Philips PA, Marty AT, Miyamoto AM: A clinical method for detecting subendocardial ischemia following cardiopulmonary bypass. J Thorac Cardiovasc Surg 69:30, 1974, 1975
24. Saini VK, Berger RL: Technique of aortic balloon catheter deployment with the use of a Fogarty catheter. Ann Thorac Surg 14:440, 1972
25. Sanders CA, Buckley MJ, Leinbach RC, Mundth ED, Austen WG: Mechanical circulatory assistance—current status and experience combining circulatory assistance, emergency coronary angiography, and acute myocardial revascularization. Circulation 45:1292, 1972
26. Scheidt S, Wilner G, Mueller H, et al: Intraaortic balloon counterpulsation in cardiogenic shock. Report of a co-operative clinical trial. N Engl J Med 288:979, 1973
27. Talpins NL, Kripke DC, Yellin E, Goetz RH: Hemodynamics and coronary blood flow during intraaortic balloon pumping. Surg Forum 19:122, 1968
28. Webb WR, Parker FB, Jr, Neville JF Jr, Hanson EL: Coronary artery disease: surgical management of acute emergencies. NY State J Med 73:2572, 1973

49

CLINICAL EVALUATION OF SYNCHRONOUS EXTERNAL CIRCULATORY ASSISTANCE IN CARDIOGENIC SHOCK

Harry S. Soroff, William C. Birtwell, Robert L. Norton,
Charles T. Cloutier, Linda A. Begley,
and Joseph V. Messer

In the late 1950s Birtwell developed the idea of assisting a failing circulation by "counterpulsation." This entailed withdrawing blood from the arterial system during cardiac systole (to lessen the afterload against which the heart contracts) and returning the blood during cardiac diastole (to augment the coronary perfusion pressure).

The first experiments with counterpulsation, published by Clauss et al in 1961, documented the hemodynamic effects in animals. The same year Jacobey et al (1961) published experiments showing that counterpulsation could stimulate the development of coronary collateral circulation. In 1966 we reported our first attempts to use counterpulsation as a treatment for patients in profound shock following myocardial infarction (Birtwell et al, 1966). The results were not successful, mainly because of the technical difficulties involved in aspirating blood during cardiac systole from a severely diseased arterial system.

A more promising approach to synchronous assisted circulation is external counterpulsation (ECP), a noninvasive method conceived by our group (Birtwell et al, 1963) and at the same time, by Dennis et al (1963) and Osborne et al (1963). Over the past dozen years we have conducted many ECP studies with healthy animals, with

experimental cardiogenic shock preparations, and with normal persons (Soroff et al, 1964; Giron et al, 1966; Ruiz et al, 1968; Nishimura et al, 1970; Antebi et al, 1970; Cloutier et al, 1971; Soroff et al, 1971).

The hemodynamic effects of ECP are similar to those of counterpulsation as it was originally conceived. However, the external method does not require arterial cannulation or extracorporeal handling of blood. Experiments have shown that application of positive pressure to the lower extremities during cardiac diastole can increase the diastolic pressure by 40 to 50 percent, while the release of pressure or the application of negative pressure during cardiac systole can lower the systolic pressure by about 30 percent. Studies have indicated that ECP increases the venous return to the heart because of the unidirectional valves in the peripheral venous bed.

With a patient in shock, the effect of ECP on systolic pressure may be obscured by the status of the cardiovascular system and its control mechanisms, because the tendency of ECP to reduce the systolic pressure is somewhat offset by the potential of the left ventricle to eject a larger stroke volume against the reduced effective vascular resistance. Nevertheless, in cardiogenic shock accompanied by myocardial ischemia, the increased coronary flow that ECP provides may improve cardiac function and thus indirectly affect the hemodynamic response to counterpulsation.

In this report we describe a cooperative clinical study, conducted over a period of a year and a half, in which 25 patients suffering from cardiogenic shock following myocardial infarction were treated with external counterpulsation.

Supported in part by grants from the General Clinical Research Centers Program of the Division of Research Resources, National Institutes of Health (FR-54), the National Heart and Lung Institute (HE-08164-06A1, HE-08613, HL-14902-02), the John A. Hartford Foundation Inc., Medical Innovations, Inc., and the Upjohn Company

METHODS

Patients were treated at 10 different hospitals in or near metropolitan Boston.

Our ECP team consisted of two physicians, a nurse, a biochemistry technician, and an engineer. Alerted by a paging system, we were usually able to assemble at a patient's bedside in less than an hour, but in some cases we took as long as two hours. The assisted circulation equipment was transported to the patient in a small truck. Calls for the team were originated by referring physicians, who had agreed to participate in the study.

Patient Selection

We did not exclude any patient whose physician felt that a trial of ECP was warranted. The diagnosis of cardiogenic shock, made by the referring physician, was based solely on conventional clinical criteria: recent myocardial infarction, low systolic blood pressure (80 mm Hg or less), oliguria (urine output of 30 cc/hour or less), cold and clammy skin, and mental lethargy or confusion. (Measurements of variables such as cardiac index would have been very useful but, except for rare instances, were simply not available to us.) We included patients who, despite fluid-loading, required vasopressors for more than four hours to maintain a systolic pressure of 80 to 100 mm Hg; and we included those whose arterial pressure remained low even though diuretics increased the urine output.

Treatment Protocol

When the ECP team was called, the medical personnel in immediate charge of the patient began to carry out the following procedures.

If necessary, a transvenous pacemaker was inserted for control of heart-block. Digitalis (Digoxin) was given if needed. Assisted ventilation through an endotracheal tube was provided if oxygenation by mask or nasal catheter proved inadequate. A Foley catheter was inserted if it had not already been done.

A catheter was inserted for measurements of central venous pressure. (In a few cases a Swan-Ganz catheter was used to measure pulmonary artery wedge pressure.) If the central venous pressure was below 10 cm H_2O, the patient was challenged with 150-cc aliquots of fluid over a one-hour period in an attempt to increase the preload of the left ventricle. For monitoring of arterial pressure, a polyethylene catheter (ga. 14-19) was inserted into a radial artery through an incision in the skin.

Arterial lactate, pH, PCO_2, and PO_2 values were determined frequently. Metabolic acidosis was corrected with sodium bicarbonate; and urine volume was measured hourly.

When the ECP team arrived, the assist system was placed around the patient's lower limbs, and ECP was applied for up to two hours. Vasopressors were discontinued as soon as possible—in most cases within 15 to 30 minutes. If the hemodynamic response during ECP was less than optimal, several measures could be taken. Fluid (5 percent glucose in water or lactated Ringer's solution) was administered until the venous pressure rose to about 15 cm H_2O. Methylprednisolone sodium succinate (Solu-Medrol) or other steroid drugs were given to increase the vasodilatation, and if steroids were ineffective, chlorpromazine (Thorazine) was given. In most patients, mephentermine (Wyamine) (500 mg per 500 cc) was slowly infused during the last 15 to 30 minutes of assisted circulation to ensure an adequate peripheral vasomotor tone following ECP.

If a systolic blood pressure of at least 90 mm Hg could not be maintained without vasopressors, ECP was applied for additional two-hour periods until the blood pressure was stable or the patient died.

Mode of Circulatory Assistance

The counterpulsation equipment * used in this study consisted of a self-contained, portable console with a hydraulic power supply, a vacuum pump, a water supply, a synchronous electronic control unit, and monitoring for pressure and EKG (Fig. 1). The only requirement was a standard 110-V electrical outlet.

Rigid, cone-shaped casings with hinged covers were easily and quickly placed around the patient's lower extremities without moving the patient from bed. An inelastic, waterproof fabric lines the metal leg housings. The fabric was sealed around the patient's waist with a belt. Water was pumped into and out of the space between the metal casing and the fabric by a large piston with Bellofram seals, driven by a high pressure hy-

---

* The circulatory assist system, developed in our laboratory, was manufactured by Medical Innovations, Inc., Waltham, Mass.

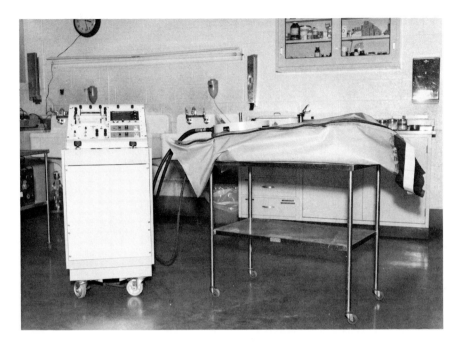

FIG. 1. Console and actuator for external counterpulsation.

draulic cylinder and controlled by a servovalve. The pumping equipment allowed application of positive pressure up to 250 mm Hg and negative pressure to −50 mm Hg over the surface of the limbs. The hydraulic coupling provided good frequency response and permitted accurate control of the shape and phase of the external pressure pulse.

Initially, only the positive pressure pulse was used. The positive pressure was slowly increased until there was a maximum increase in the diastolic blood pressure. This was usually achieved with the machine operating at a phasic pressure of 0 during cardiac systole and 200 mm Hg during cardiac diastole.

Once the vascular bed was actively dilated, and an adequate intravascular volume was ensured, a positive-negative mode of assist was begun. With the machine operating at pressures varying from −30 mm Hg during cardiac systole to +200 mm Hg during cardiac diastole, the hemodynamic response may be markedly improved, as illustrated in Figure 2.

Of crucial importance is the synchronization of the counterpulsation pump with the action of the heart (Soroff et al, 1963). In a previous report (Soroff et al, 1969), we showed an example of the undesirable arterial pulse pattern resulting from overlap of pump systole and cardiac

systole. Such improper phasing may be associated with increased myocardial oxygen consumption, increased hemolysis, and damage to the aortic valve and endocardium.

RESULTS

Pertinent data on the first 20 patients in this series were tabulated and analyzed in detail. The condition of each of these patients before, during, and after assisted circulation is summarized in Tables 1 through 4. Case numbers indicate the order in which the patients were admitted to the study—beginning with Patient #1 in February of 1971 and going through to Patient #20 in January of 1972. These patients, 16 men and four women, ranged in age from 47 to 78, with an average of 63 years.

Categorization of Outcome

NONSURVIVORS.   Six patients died during ECP, and five patients showed some response but died soon after.

SHORT-TERM SURVIVORS.   Two patients had a normal blood pressure without vasopressors and showed adequate tissue perfusion

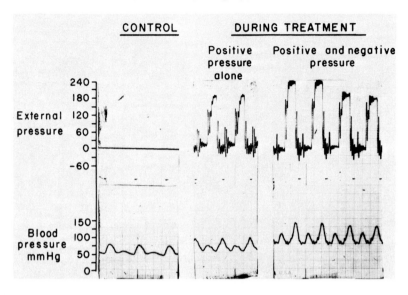

FIG. 2.   Improvement in hemodynamic effects of external counterpulsation with positive-negative pressure mode as compared with positive pressure alone.

(as reflected in urine output and clinical appearance) following ECP. However, one died three days later, and the other died three weeks later. In both cases the cause of death was noncardiac in nature and was unrelated to counterpulsation.

LONG-TERM SURVIVORS. Seven patients responded well and were eventually discharged from the hospital.

Comparison of Survivors and Nonsurvivors

As can be seen in Table 1, the order in which patients were admitted to the study was not related to mortality, nor were the results a function of the hospital in which the patient was treated.

To determine whether the nine survivors had been at less risk than the 11 nonsurvivors *before* ECP, we calculated each patient's Peel Index (Table 1). This index (Peel et al, 1962), a prognostic tool for grading the severity of an infarct, takes into account a variety of factors that affect mortality—age, sex, history of heart disease, and immediate problems such as shock, congestive heart failure, EKG abnormalities, and arrhythmias. Normally a person with an index of 20 or over has less than a 25 percent chance of surviving. The average Peel Index of our survivors was 20; the average of those who died was 21.

The average age of the survivors was 64. The average age of the patients who died was 62. There was little difference between survivors and nonsurvivors with respect to either the loca-

tion of infarct or associated factors such as previous infarction. Four of the 11 patients who died and three of the nine survivors had had previous infarctions. Eight of the patients who died and five of the survivors were in deep coma when ECP was begun. X-rays showed that almost all of the patients had pulmonary edema, congestion, or areas of pneumonitis.

Arrhythmias and Heart-Block (Table 1)

Eight of the patients who died and eight of the patients who survived had various forms of arrhythmias before ECP. There were four instances of *partial* heart block in the deaths as compared with two in the survivors, and three instances of *complete* heart-block in the deaths as compared with one in the survivors. Five of the patients who died and four of the survivors needed pacemakers before ECP was begun.

Onset of Shock and Timing of Treatment (Table 2)

Two patients, one who lived (#7) and one who died (#10), had sustained their infarctions 108 hours before the onset of shock. With these patients included, the average time between infarction and development of shock was 30 hours in the patients who died and 22 hours in the survivors. Not including these patients, the averages were 17 hours and 10 hours, respectively.

The interval from the time that the diag-

TABLE 1. Patients' Condition Prior to External Counterpulsation

CASE NO.[a]	HOSP.[b]	PT.	SEX/AGE	YRS SINCE PREVIOUS MI[c]	EKG DIAG.[c]	PEEL INDEX	ARRHYTHMIAS AND/OR HEART BLOCK[d]	PACE-MAKER	COMA 1+ to 4+	PULMONARY DISEASE CLIN. AND X-RAY DIAG.
Death during assist										
4	StE	MP	M/57	—	Apical	17	PVC's	—	1+	Pulmonary edema
10	NWH	RL	F/69	2 IMI	AMI	28	Atrial tach.	Yes	4+	Vasc. engorgement, pulmonary edema
11	BCH	FK	M/67	old IMI	AMI	28	Vent. tach., sinus tach., bradycardia, arrest. bifas.[e] block, c.h.b.	Yes	4+	Cong. heart failure, rt.l.l. pneumonia
14	JH	TL	M/63	—	Ant Sep	21	Vent. fib, arrest, v.p.b.	—	4+	Unilateral pulmonary edema
16	BCH	HF	F/67	—	Ant-lat Inf	18	Rt. b. br. block, lt. ant. hemiblock	—	2+	Rt. l. l. infiltrate, edema
20	PBBH	WL	M/47	—	Ant Sep Lat	19	Atrial & nodal tach., c.h.b.	Yes		Edema
Death after temporary hemodynamic response										
1	BCH	HF	M/60	6 AMI	IMI	27	Vent. fib., vent. tach., atrial fib., bilat. b. br. block	—	4+	Pulmonary congestion
2	StE	JT	M/73	—	IMI	22	Bradycardia, atrial fib, PVC, nodal rhythm	Yes	1+	Pulmonary edema
9	MH	LC	M/66	—	IMI	11	Complete heart-block	Yes		Pulmonary congestion
13	BCH	DT	F/56	—	Ant-lat	17		—		Pulmonary edema
17	CCGH	SS	M/59	6 IMI	AMI	23	PAC, PVC, sinus tach., atrial tach.	—	2+	Pulmonary edema
Short-term survivors										
5	MH	MR	M/71	old AMI	Apical	27	Sinus tach.		4+	Pulmonary edema
19	BCH	AM	M/78	—	Ant-lat	22	PVC, vent tach., arrest, bifas.[e] rhythm	Yes	4+	Pulmonary edema
Long-term survivors										
3	MH	FO	M/51		AMI	7	Sinus bradycardia		1+	Pulmonary edema, vascular engorgement
6	FUH	IK	M/54		Ant Sep	19	PVC, sinus tach.			
7	BCH	WW	M/65		AMI	22	PVC, AV block, c.h.b., AV dissoc.	Yes	1+	Bibasilar rales
8	MH	BC	M/48		IMI	14	PVC with bigeminy, cardiac arrests		4+	Rales, pulmonary
12	BCH	TC	M/78		Ant-lat Sep	22	Nodal, PVC, vent tach., rt. & lt. b. br. block	Yes		Pulmonary edema
15	BCH	BH	F/60	10,9, 1/2 AMI	Ant-lat	27	PVC, lt. b. br. block, transient bifasicular	Yes		Bibasilar rales, chronic obstructive lung disease, pulmonary edema
18	NEMCH	BS	M/72	11 MI	PMI	20				

[a] Numbered in order of admission to study.

[b] StE: St. Elizabeth's; NWH: Newton-Wellesley; BCH: Boston City; JH: Jordan; PBBH: Peter Bent Brigham; MH: Milford; CCGH: Cardinal Cushing General; FUH: Framingham Union; NEMCH: New England Medical Center.

[c] MI: Myocardial infarction; IMI: inferior MI; AMI: anterior MI; PMI: posterior MI.

[d] PVC: premature ventricular contraction; PAC: premature atrial contraction.

[e] bifascicular.

TABLE 2. Clinical Status of Patients before External Counterpulsation

CASE NO.	INFARCT TO SHOCK (hr)	TIME IN SHOCK BEFORE ECP (hr)	BP (mm Hg) WITH PRESSORS	PRESSORS Drug	PRESSORS Hrs.	FLUID INTAKE (cc)	URINE OUTPUT[a] V_0	V_1	pH	PO_2	PCO_2	CVP (cm H_2O)	ARTERIAL LACTATE[b] (mg%)
Death during assist													
4	32	13	60/40	Lev[c]	13	1,345 (8 hr)	19	4	7.37	48	24	20	32
10	108	2	70/40	Iso[c], Met[c]	2	2,040 (8 hr)	7	30[d]	7.44	63	24	28	—
11	24	9	70/58	Iso, Met, Lev	3.5, 2.5, 1.5	800 (8 hr)	40	0[d]	7.45	48	41	26	48
14	5	6	75/50	Met, Lev	4	1,000 (8 hr)	0	0[d]	7.44	35	30	—	45
16	Admitted in shock	12	66/40	Iso, Lev	10, 1	2,600 (8 hr)	0	7	7.42	80	28	14	90
20	24	20	64/44	Lev	20	600 (8 hr)	0	60[d]	7.44	58	22	10[f]	21
Death after temporary response													
1	Admitted in shock	5.75	70/54	Lev	5	500 (5 hr)	14	0	7.42	110	40	11	—
2	12	10	60/40	Met, Iso	2, 10	1,150 (8 hr)	19	5[d]	7.40	86	45	15	30
9	75	13	60/40	Met	13	200 (8 hr)	12	4[d]	7.40	114	22	18	26
13	6	7	85/65	Lev	4	475 (6 hr)	0	50[d]	—	—	—	28[e]	34
17	36	24	75/45	Met	11	870 (8 hr)	2	10[d]	7.30	38	33	14[e]	—
Short-term survivors													
5	1	4.5	80/60	Met	2.5	2,652 (8 hr)	0	40[d]	7.20	58	42	3	44
19	3	4	100/50	Lev	4	250 (8 hr)	0	46[d]	7.36	57	59	20	198
Long-term survivors													
3	36	24	92/70	Met	23.5	1,360 (10 hr)	30	10	7.38	84	38	0	13
6	7-10	14	80/60	Lev, Iso	5, 9	930 (8 hr)	30	117[d]	7.41	66	35	14	12
7	108	6.5	80/50	Iso	6.5	1,520 (9 hr)	10[d]	0	7.42	65	28	20	16
8	4	6	80/50	Met	5.5	560 (7 hr)	0	40	7.50	55	30	10	19
12	24	6	90/60	Lev	6	645 (5 hr)	0	50[d]	7.33	78	40	19	15
15	5	7	80/60	Lev	7	1,425 (8 hr)	0	290[d]	7.42	79	47	13	49
18	6	5	80/55	Met	4	1,850 (16 hr)	10	12[d]	7.25	91	38	12	26

[a] V_0: urine output (cc/hr) at time of diagnosis of shock; V_1: urine output (cc/hr) immediately preceding assist.
[b] Normal value for arterial lactate is 6.75 ± 0.81 mg%.
[c] Lev: Levarterenol; Iso: Isoproterenol; Met: Metaraminol.
[d] Patient was given a diuretic (mannitol, furosemide, or ethacrynic acid).
[e] Pulmonary capillary wedge pressure (mm Hg).
[f] Pulmonary artery mean pressure (mm Hg).

FIG. 3. Arterial blood pressure, central venous pressure, and blood gas values of 9 survivors and 11 nonsurvivors.

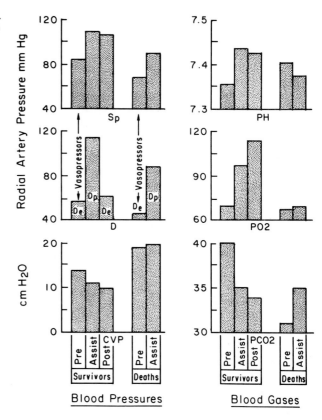

nosis of shock was made to the start of ECP averaged 10 hours for the nonsurvivors and 8.5 hours for the survivors. All of the patients were given vasopressors when shock was diagnosed and were on vasopressors at the time that assisted circulation was begun.

Physiological Measurements (Fig. 3)

The *arterial blood pressure* at the time of the diagnosis of cardiogenic shock was taken by sphygmomanometer. The average for the nonsurvivors was 69/47 and for the survivors 85/57. The average systolic pressure of the survivors was significantly higher ($p < 0.001$) than that of the patients who died both before and during ECP. Both survivors and nonsurvivors showed similar increases in systolic pressure during the assist, but at the time that ECP was begun, the patients who died were in more profound shock than the survivors. The average diastolic pressure of the survivors was also significantly higher ($p < 0.01$) than that of the nonsurvivors, both before and during ECP.

The average *central venous pressure* was 19 cm H_2O in those who died and 14 cm H_2O in the survivors. The difference was not statistically significant. As might be expected, however, the central venous pressure of the survivors fell to 11 cm H_2O during the assist, while the average in the nonsurvivors was 20 cm H_2O ($p < 0.05$).

At the time that shock was diagnosed, the urine output (V_0 in Table 2) averaged 10 cc/hour for the patients who died and 16 cc/hour for the patients who survived. Fluid therapy was intensified at that time, and 15 of the patients who were oliguric were given diuretics. Nine responded, and by the time ECP was begun, the average urine output (V_1) was 15 cc/hour in the patients who died and 67 cc/hour in the survivors.

Biochemical Measurements (Fig. 3)

At the time of diagnosis of shock the average *arterial lactate concentration* of the patients who died was 32 mg percent while that of the survivors was 15 mg percent. During assist, as the clinical condition of the survivors improved, the lactate levels fell slightly, but in the nonsurvivors the level rose to 38 mg percent ($p < 0.05$).

The *pH and PO₂* of the arterial blood were similar in nonsurvivors and survivors at the time shock was diagnosed. The average PO_2 of the survivors increased during assist to 95 mm Hg while in those who died it remained unchanged, but the difference was not statistically significant because of a wide scatter of the data. The PCO_2, however, was significantly lower in the nonsurvivors than in the survivors before ECP ($p < 0.05$) —perhaps reflecting a compensatory mechanism for metabolic acidosis, since the pH of the blood was similar in both groups.

Quality of Counterpulsation

Our criteria for judging the effectiveness of ECP are given in a footnote to Table 3. In general, the hemodynamic response to counterpulsation was good even in patients who died. The augmentation of their diastolic pressure during assist was comparable to that of the survivors (Table 3).

The poorest hemodynamic response to counterpulsation was observed, not surprisingly, in the patients who died during the assist. Of the five patients whose response to ECP was transient, two showed a substantial increase in mean pressure as well as an increase in diastolic pressure to a level above the systolic pressure.

In the nonsurvivors the average diastolic pressure was raised only to the level of the systolic pressure (90/89 mm Hg). In the survivors, the average blood pressure was 109/114 mm Hg during ECP.

Counterpulsation was carried out for an average of 4.4 hours in the patients who died and an average of three hours in the survivors. Three patients who died (#14, #16, and #20) were counterpulsated repeatedly; in one case for a total of nearly 19 hours (Table 3). Among the survivors, the longest total period of ECP was five hours.

Effect of Vasodilators

Eight of the patients who died and five of the patients who survived were given steroids or chlorpromazine in an attempt to produce vasodilatation and thus to improve tissue perfusion. The vasodilatation and the concomitant administration of fluids were well tolerated during ECP.

Course of Patients after ECP (Table 4)

Patients #2, #13, and #17 responded well initially the ECP, and vasopressors were discontinued. However, they became hypotensive several hours later, and when ECP was reapplied it was not effective. They all died during, or soon after, the second period of ECP.

The two short-term survivors (#5 and #19) and one long-term survivor (#6) are worthy of mention. Patient #5 was operated on for a polyp of the stomach. A limited wedge resection was carried out. During the operation the patient suffered a myocardial infarction and went into shock. ECP was begun 330 minutes later. Hemodynamic values stabilized after 142 minutes of ECP, and vasopressors were no longer required. However, the patient developed acute pancreatitis and peritonitis and died three days later.

Patient #19 suffered cardiac arrest about 3.5 hours after a myocardial infarction. He was resuscitated and placed on vasopressors but remained in coma. Although he responded well to five hours of ECP in that his hemodynamic status improved, he did not regain consciousness. He was transferred from the coronary care unit to a general medical ward, where he required continuous assisted ventilation. He died three weeks later of respiratory complications.

Patient #6 was discharged from the hospital and did well until eight months later, when he developed severe left heart failure associated with a ventricular aneurysm. Coronary angiography revealed severe three-vessel disease involving the proximal circumflex and left anterior descending arteries, both of which were completely occluded, and the right coronary artery, which was diffusely diseased. The left ventricular ejection fraction was diminished to 33 percent. Several days later the patient died suddenly at home.

Details of One Survivor's Course

Patient #12, a 78-year-old man, was admitted with severe chest pain, the third occurrence in three days. An EKG showed a complete right bundle branch block with left axis deviation and S-T segment elevation over $V_2 - V_5$. The problem was diagnosed as an acute anteroseptal myocardial infarction. There was nothing in the patient's medical history of particular relevance except for the occurrence of "two-pillow" orthop-

TABLE 3. Patients' Clinical Condition and Requirement for Medications during External Counterpulsation

AVERAGE VALUES DURING EXTERNAL COUNTERPULSATION

CASE NO.	Peak Syst/Peak Diast BP (mm Hg)	Urine Output (cc/hr)	CVP (cm H_2O)	Arterial Lactate (mg%)	pH	PO_2	PCO_2	QUALITY OF ECP[a]	MEAN % INCR. DIAST. PRESS.[b]	PRESSOR DRUGS, STEROIDS, CHLORPRO.[a]	SERIOUS ARRHYTHMIAS	ECP (min)
Death during assist												
4	60/64	9	20	36	7.38	52	27	Fair	50	Met, Iso, Mep, Lev, Metp (2 gm) Chl (10 gm)	Atrial tach.	33
10	84/84	23	16	–	–	–	–	Fair	100			
11	72/64	10	30	93	7.36	57	35	Poor	5	Lev, Iso, Chl (10 gm)	Complete electrical dissociation, arrest	180
14	91/99	0	–	58	7.33	80	40	Good	100	Lev, Mep (2 gm)		480
16	85/90	15	14	63	7.41	133	30	Good	125	Lev, Mep, Metp, (1.5 gm)		480
20	98/99	95	32[d]	30	7.53	40	29	Good	125	Dex (4 cc)	Vent. tach. to asystole	
Death after temporary hemodynamic response												
1	90/110	8	–	–	7.41	87	38	Excel.	100	Metp (2 gm)	Atrial premature beats	120
2	68/68	12	20	20	7.47	54	44	Fair	70	Iso, Metp (1.5 gm)		76
9	118/122	17	18	25	–	–	–	Excel.	300			75
13	97/98	80	28[e]	37	7.27	86	41	Good	50	Metp (1.5 gm)		120
17	95/80	17	–	–	7.27	38	33	Good	77		Atrial tach., atrial premature beats	120
Short-term survivors												
5	90/95 at end of ECP	68	3	54	7.39	50	32	Good	50	Hyd (3 gm)		142
19	130/155 at end of ECP	83	17	90	7.50	105	48	Excel.	300	Lev, Metp (2 gm)		300
Long-term survivors												
3	112/106	32	2	13	7.39	91	38	Good	50			111
6	112/128	76	11	12	7.43	67	34	Excel.	100			159
7	115/122	55	–	14	7.38	217	36	Excel.	140			130
8	104/107	35	15	14	7.32	85	35	Good	100	Met, Mep, Lev, Dex (12 gm)	Vent fib., arrest	270
12	105/106	50	15	22	–	–	–	Good	76	Metp (2.5 gm)		204
15	92/91	35	13	–	7.59	66	36	Good	50	Lev (10 min), Metp (2 gm)		205
18	122/119	11	18	24	7.47	107	24	Good	116	Met		120

[a] Poor: little or no increase in diastolic pressure. Fair: diastolic pressure equal to systolic but no significant increase in diastolic pressure. Good: diastolic pressure equal to systolic plus significant increase in systolic pressure. Excellent: increase in systolic pressure and diastolic pressure greater than systolic pressure.

[b] As compared with preassist values.

[c] Met: Metaraminol; Iso: Isoproterenol; Mep: Mephentermine; Metp: Methylprednisolone sodium succinate; Chl: Chlorpromazine; Dex: Dexamethasone; Lev: Levarterenol; Hyd: Hydrocortisone sodium succinate.

[d] Pulmonary artery mean pressure (mm Hg).

[e] Pulmonary capillary mean pressure (mm Hg).

TABLE 4. Clinical Status of

CASE NO.	CONDITION AFTER ECP	VASOPRESSORS GIVEN AFTER ECP
Death during assist		
4	Could not maintain BP without assist; cardiac arrest during intubation	Levarterenol
10	Arrest following intravenous MS	–
11	BP not maintained when ECP discontinued	–
14	Cardiopulmonary arrest	–
16	BP not maintained without ECP	Levarterenol
20	Arrest immediately following ECP	Levarterenol, Phenylephrine, Mephentermine
Death after temporary hemodynamic response		
1	Ventricular tachycardia; cardiac arrest in 45 min	Isoproterenol
2[a]	Hemodynamically stable (with isoproterenol and glucagon) for 2 hr	Isoproterenol
9	Stable for 2 hr. Hypotension and arrest following morphine.	None for 2 hr, then metaraminol
13[a]	Stable for 20 hr	Mephentermine for 2 hr
17[a]	Stable for 20 hr	–
Short-term survivors		
5	BP stable at 100/70	–
19	Stable BP	–
Long-term survivors		
3	Stable	–
6	Stable	Mephentermine
7	Stable	Mephentermine
8	Stable	Metaraminol
12	Stable	–
15	Stable	Mephentermine
18	Stable	Mephentermine

[a]*Required ECP 24 hr after first period of assist; course of second treatment described in Results Section.*

Patients after External Counterpulsation

LONG-TERM FOLLOW-UP	POSTMORTEM FINDINGS
–	Occlusion of LAD and CIRC. Congestive heart failure with pulmonary congestion and edema
–	No autopsy
–	No autopsy
–	Thrombosis of LAD. Acute myocardial infarction involving anterolateral walls. Atelectasis, acute pulmonary edema
–	No autopsy
–	Old and recent occlusions of right coronary artery with myocardial infarction involving all the septum and anterior third of left ventricular wall and apex. Pulmonary edema
–	No autopsy
–	Severe atherosclerosis of all 3 coronary arteries. Myocardial infarction involving all the walls of the left ventricle including the interventricular septum. Acute pulmonary congestion and edema
–	No autopsy
–	No autopsy
–	Severe narrowing of all vessels with old occlusion of anterior descending arteries. Old, healed posterior left ventricular infarct. Recent myocardial infarction involving 2/3 of septum, anterior wall, apex, and lower posterior left ventricular wall. Bilateral pulmonary edema
Died 3 days later of peritonitis	Peritonitis, acute pancreatitis. Acute anteroseptal infarction. Right and left coronaries slightly narrowed but patent
Remained in coma and died in 3 wk of pulmonary edema and congestion	No autopsy
Alive 12 mo	–
Died 8 mo later of myocardial infarction	–
Alive 8 mo	–
Alive 8 mo	–
Alive 6 mo	–
Alive 5 mo	–
Alive 2 mo	–

nea and nocturia several weeks before admission.

He was given 5 mg morphine on admission and an additional 11 mg over the next two hours. At that point he developed periods of nodal rhythm and had ventricular tachycardia at rates of 100 to 110, alternating with NSR at a rate of 100. A chest X-ray showed pulmonary venous congestion, and the examining physician noted that there were bilateral basilar rales. The patient was given lidocaine (Xylocaine) for tachycardia, plus 40 mg furosemide (Lasix) intravenously. He was then transferred to the coronary care unit where a transvenous pacemaker was inserted. Arrhythmias continued to occur, and over a period of five hours he required a lidocaine drip of 4 mg/minute plus several 100-mg bolus injections of lidocaine. His central venous pressure at that time was 19 cm H_2O. He was given another 40 mg furosemide and 0.25 mg digitalis (Digoxin). His vital signs remained stable.

On admission to the coronary care unit, his blood pressure was 150/70, his pulse was 110 and irregular, and his respirations were 18. His temperature was normal. Physical examination revealed: *Neck*—external veins distended 3 to 4 cm above the angle of Louis. *Chest*—bilateral basilar rales, more prominent on the right. *Heart*—no palpable PMI; distant heart sounds; a soft S_4 gallop at the apex; no murmurs or audible rubs. Over the next few hours his blood pressure gradually fell to 90/60, and his urine output dropped

to zero. A levarterenol (Levophed) drip (8 mg in 500 cc of 5 percent glucose in water) was begun.

Six hours after the diagnosis of cardiogenic shock was made, a Swan-Ganz catheter and a radial artery catheter were inserted and external counterpulsation was begun. At that time the patient's urine output was 50 cc/hour, and his blood pressure with vasopressors was 115/65 mm Hg.

Figure 4 shows the patient's response to ECP. The levarterenol drip was discontinued after 17 minutes of assist. The first of three periods of ECP was 52 minutes long. There was a marked increase in diastolic peak pressure and a modest initial decrease in systolic peak pressure during each period of assist. Similarly, the systolic mean decreased slightly and the diastolic mean rose markedly. The mean radial artery pressure rose somewhat during the course of treatment. Since the central venous pressure remained fairly constant, the increase in mean pulmonary capillary wedge pressure when methylprednisolone (solu-Medrol) was given during the third period of ECP, suggests that the left ventricle was unable to accommodate itself to the increased fluid load although the right ventricle remained competent. The systemic vascular resistance decreased at the end of the third period of ECP (Fig. 5), probably as a result of the steroid therapy. During the second and third periods, the systolic ejection period became shorter while the diastolic coronary filling period became longer (Fig. 6).

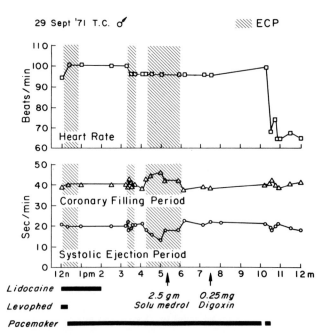

FIG. 4. Hemodynamic effects of external counterpulsation in one survivor. Blood pressure changes in one survivor during 6-hour period from noon (12n) to 6 P.M. when external counterpulsation was applied intermittently, and during the subsequent 6 hours. Lidocaine (Xylocaine) and levarterenol (Levophed) were given continuously during the periods marked by horizontal bars. Methylprednisolone sodium succinate (Solu-Medrol) and digitalis (Digoxin) were each given once, at the times marked by the arrows. A pacemaker was used, as indicated by the lowest horizontal bar, until about 10 P.M.

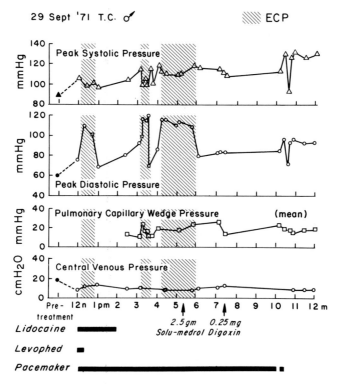

FIG. 5. Hemodynamic effects of external counterpulsation in one survivor. Systemic vascular resistance was calculated as

$$\frac{\text{arterial mean pressure } - \text{ right atrial mean pressure (or central venous pressure)}}{\text{cardiac output}} \times 80$$

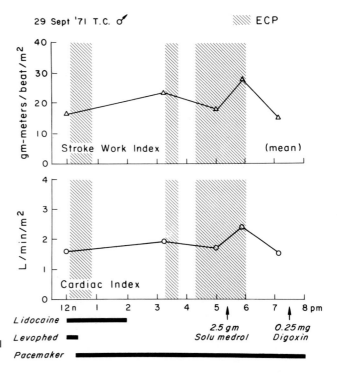

FIG. 6. Hemodynamic effects of external counterpulsation in one survivor.

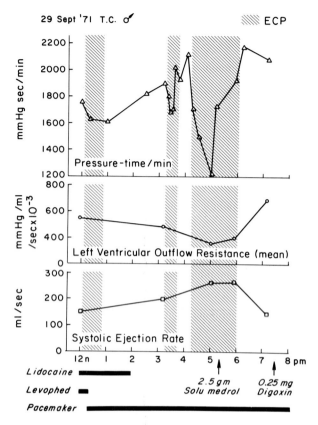

FIG. 7. Hemodynamic effects of external counterpulsation in one survivor. The stroke work index was calculated as

$$\frac{13.6 \times (\text{arterial systolic mean} - \text{pulmonary capillary wedge pressure}) \times \text{cardiac index}}{\text{heart rate}}$$

Arterial blood gases did not change significantly. Both the cardiac index and the stroke work index increased somewhat, especially after the administration of steroids in the third period (Fig. 7). This was probably because of an increase in left ventricular preload and reduced peripheral resistance resulting from the fluid-loading and vasodilatory effects of the steroids. Since the mean systolic pressure did not rise at the time, the increased work of the heart was related primarily to the increased flow.

The PTM values, which are closely correlated with myocardial oxygen consumption (Levine and Wagman, 1962), were reduced during the three periods of ECP (Fig. 8). Although the left ventricular outflow resistance fell only slightly during the first two periods of ECP, a marked decrease occurred at the end of the third period (Fig. 8). The systolic ejection rate went up most dramatically when steroids were given during the third period (Fig. 8). It appears that for this

patient steroids markedly enhanced the hemodynamic effects of counterpulsation.

The patient was discharged from the hospital and has remained well.

Sequential Analysis of Mortality Statistics

To determine if ECP could be considered a significantly better treatment than current approaches to cardiogenic shock, we used a sequential design—a useful technique when the number of subjects is limited and studies must be done in a clinical setting where there is no practical possibility of having adequate controls or where the referring physicians consider a paired control design unacceptable. A detailed explanation of sequential analysis is given in a classic book by Wald (1947) and in other statistical texts.

For our sequential analysis, we needed four

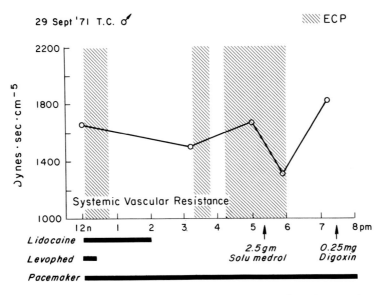

FIG. 8. Hemodynamic effects of external counterpulsation in one survivor. Pressure time per minute was calculated as the systolic mean pressure multiplied by the systolic ejection period per minute. Left ventricular outflow resistance was calculated as the systolic mean pressure multiplied by the systolic ejection period per beat, divided by the stroke volume. The systolic ejection rate was calculated as the stroke volume divided by the systolic ejection period per beat (or as the cardiac output divided by the systolic ejection period per minute).

values: P_0, the present estimated rate of survival from cardiogenic shock; P_1, the survival rate that we were willing to consider, on clinical grounds, to be a worthwhile improvement over the current rate; alpha, which—as in any statistical test—represents the probability of erroneously rejecting ECP as a beneficial treatment; and beta, which represents the probability of erroneously accepting ECP as a beneficial treatment. These values were set at P_0: 15 percent, P_1: 45 percent, α: 0.001, β: 0.001.

On the basis of these values, a graph was drawn as in Figure 9. The lower slanted line, H_0, marks the points at which the unfavorable hypothesis should be accepted (that is, there is no significant improvement in survival rate when ECP is used). The upper slanted line, H_1, represents the points at which the unfavorable hypothesis should be rejected (that is, ECP could be considered an improvement over standard therapeutic techniques).

The slope of both H_0 and H_1 were calculated as follows:

$$S = \frac{\log \left[\frac{1 - P_0}{1 - P_1} \right]}{\log (P_1/P_0) - \log \left[\frac{1 - P_1}{1 - P_0} \right]}$$

The intercept of H_0 is given by h_0, which is calculated as follows:

$$h_0 = \frac{\log \left[\frac{\beta}{1 - \alpha} \right]}{\log (P_1/P_0) - \log \left[\frac{1 - P_1}{1 - P_0} \right]}$$

The intercept of H_1 is given by h_1, which is calculated as follows:

$$h_1 = \frac{\log \left[\frac{1 - \beta}{\alpha} \right]}{\log (P_1/P_0) - \log \left[\frac{1 - P_1}{1 - P_0} \right]}$$

As we treated each consecutive patient with ECP, we plotted an appropriate point on the graph to show whether the patient had lived or died; and at each point we decided, on the basis of the cumulative record, whether or not to continue our study.

Of our total group of 25 patients, 12 survived. On the basis of the sequential analysis, we can consider this 48 percent survival rate a significant improvement over the current survival rate in cases of cardiogenic shock.

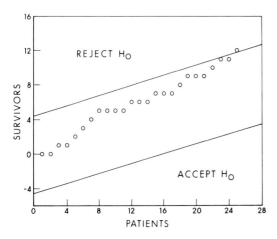

FIG. 9. Sequential analysis of clinical experience in the management of patients in cardiogenic shock. $P_0 = 0.15$; $P_1 = 0.45$; $\alpha = 0.001$; $\beta = 0.001$.

DISCUSSION

Selection of Patients

As far as we know, there were no important differences between the survivors and nonsurvivors that resulted from unwitting biases in patient selection or variations in initial treatment. Both groups were of about the same age range; their chances for survival, based upon the Peel Index, were virtually identical; and they had similar types of infarctions (Table 1). The order in which patients were admitted into the study had no apparent effect on the outcome, nor did it seem to matter in which of the hospitals a patient was treated.

The hospitals included both university-affiliated and community-based institutions, some without house staff. Further, since the hospitals are widely scattered, they serve different types of patient populations in terms of socioeconomic strata and racial and ethnic origins. Some might feel that the resulting demographic heterogeneity of our subject group, plus the variability in initial treatment, cast doubt on the validity of our conclusions. In our opinion, however, these are strengthening factors since they minimized the possibility of our patients, as a group, being either unusually resistant or unusually vulnerable to the sequelae of a myocardial infarction.

Nevertheless, there were some differences between the patients who survived and those who did not—differences that might be important in the future in choosing candidates for assisted cir-

culation. At the time of the diagnosis of cardiogenic shock, the peak systolic pressure was significantly higher in those who survived than in those who died, and the central venous pressure was significantly lower. Although there was little difference in the urine output at the time of diagnosis, the patients who died did not respond to fluids or diuretics and their urine output became significantly lower at the time ECP was begun. Neither arterial lactate concentrations nor arterial blood gases were significantly different statistically in the two groups at the time of diagnosis. During ECP, the increase in both systolic and diastolic pressures was significantly greater in the survivors. Central venous pressure dropped in the survivors but remained high in the patients who died. Arterial lactate levels rose to an even higher level in those who died, whereas the levels fell in those who survived.

Diagnosis of Cardiogenic Shock

Tables 1 and 2 show that all our patients had met the usual clinical criteria of cardiogenic shock and that every effort was made to treat them by standard procedures. Still, the diagnosis of cardiogenic shock or "pump failure" covers degrees of severity ranging from mild to terminal. Although the diagnosis was made in each case according to the same general criteria, it is clear from the data that, for the most part, the patients who did not survive were in deeper shock than those who did. (In future studies, in a controlled environment, we would obviously want to include routine measurements of cardiac output and pulmonary capillary wedge pressures as criteria for application of assisted circulation.)

Even though the Myocardial Infarction Research Units have now established precise, quantitative criteria for diagnosing cardiogenic shock, most hospitals are not equipped to make the necessary measurements. As a rule, physicians must base their diagnoses on clinical judgment. For example, urine volume is generally considered a good indicator of renal perfusion pressure. In our patients, urine output at the time of diagnosis of shock was 30 cc/hour or less; but many of the patients responded to diuretics and fluid-loading, so that by the time ECP was begun nine of the patients had a urine output of over 30 cc/hour. All of them, however, were still suffering from cardiogenic shock as evidenced by low blood pressure, need for vasopressors, clammy skin, and mental confusion.

One patient who survived (#3) was in only mild pump failure and had the lowest Peel Index of all our patients. However, the fact that he required vasopressors for 23.5 hours indicated a poor prognosis. Similarly, Patients #6 and #12 required prolonged treatment with vasopressors to maintain a normal blood pressure. Before vasopressors were administered, their pressures had been 80/60 and 90/60, respectively. Patient #6 was observed for six hours and Patient #12 for 14 hours before ECP. During that time, whenever vasopressors were discontinued their systolic pressures dropped to 80 mm Hg or below.

Timing of Application

A major problem in planning the management of patients in cardiogenic shock is the difficulty of quickly determining the underlying pathologic lesion. However, Don Michael et al (1972), in a retrospective study of 100 patients dying of cardiogenic shock secondary to myocardial infarction, was able to identify three subgroups whose clinical courses reflected fairly distinct pathology. The first subgroup (57 percent) had cardiac ischemia with loss of function in a major portion of the myocardium. The second subgroup (15 percent) had a specific mechanical lesion provoking shock in an infarcted ventricle. The third subgroup (28 percent) gave a history of a previous infarction, had cardiomegaly, and had a limited but critical infarction in an already grossly damaged ventricle.

We think that early application of ECP might help to preserve myocardial function in the first and third groups by decreasing myocardial oxygen requirements and increasing the coronary collateral circulation. Experiments have shown that coronary vascular resistance is somewhat reduced during counterpulsation (Soroff et al, 1963)—an indication that dormant collateral channels may be opened during the procedure. Other experiments in our laboratory (Nishimura et al, 1970) have confirmed that the function of an ischemic portion of the left ventricle could be preserved and protected by early application of counterpulsation. In a control group, a 45-minute period of ischemia irreversibly damaged 85 percent of the ischemic tissue. When counterpulsation was applied during the ischemic period, only 23 percent of the tissue was irreversibly damaged; and when a 45-minute period of counterpulsation preceded the 45-minute occlusion, only 48 percent of the involved tissue was irreversibly damaged. In another series (Kataoka et al, 1973), when ECP was applied throughout a 45-minute period of ischemia, only 31 percent of the involved tissue was irreversibly damaged, compared

with 71 percent in a control group; yet similar EKG changes occurred in both groups during and after the period of coronary artery occlusion.

We feel, on the basis of our experimental data (Nishimura et al, 1970) that the *sooner* counterpulsation is applied after the onset of a myocardial infarction the more effective it will be in protecting the viability of the myocardium. In both the survivors and the nonsurvivors in our clinical series, the average delay from the time that shock was diagnosed to the time that ECP was begun was about nine hours. Ideally, ECP should be instituted within two hours.

There is also some evidence that ECP could eventually become an important tool in the prevention of myocardial infarction. In one animal experiment (Antebi et al, 1970) we produced diffuse coronary occlusions by injecting microspheres into the coronary arteries. When ECP was applied before or immediately after the injection, 50 percent of the animals survived, compared with only 27 percent in a control group. The difference was most marked and was statistically significant at higher doses of microspheres. Postmortem coronary angiograms suggested that the lower mortality in the counterpulsated groups was associated with the opening of collateral coronary channels.

This concept has been extended to the study and treatment of patients with angina. Banas et al (1972) have found that ECP can help relieve anginal symptoms. They have also shown that in angina patients ECP enhances the development of coronary collaterals, providing one or two coronary vessels are partly open.

Response of Patients to ECP

Sequential analysis of mortality statistics indicated that the survival rate we obtained was a statistically significant improvement over the current 10 to 20 percent survival rate in cases of cardiogenic shock (Shubin and Weil, 1967). Although figures on mortality vary somewhat, 85 percent appears to be a reasonable estimate of the actual death rate from cardiogenic shock following myocardial infarction. Based on that estimate, a 48 percent survival rate could have occurred by chance alone less than once in 1,000 similar groups of patients. Still, the sequential analysis was not designed to quantify the effectiveness of our treatment. We need to do—and hope others will do—more carefully controlled studies to characterize further the types of patients for whom ECP would be most beneficial and to determine if patients who respond to ECP might survive cardiogenic shock without circulatory assist.

Nonetheless, from experience gained to date, it is usually possible to foresee the ultimate outcome of a given patient early in the course of ECP. If a patient does not respond hemodynamically to counterpulsation despite adequate fluid-loading and the use of vasodilators, the prognosis is usually grave. A response should be noticeable within 45 minutes after the use of positive-negative pressure assist and appropriate adjunctive therapy. Patients who show a dramatic response to counterpulsation within 45 minutes—that is, elevation of diastolic pressure above the systolic level and a gradual rise of mean and peak systolic pressures—usually survive the period of pump failure. With patients who show a good but not excellent response (elevation of diastolic pressure to the level of systolic pressure and a small rise in systolic pressure), it is difficult to assess their chances for survival until several hours have elapsed. As can be seen from Table 3, some patients in the latter category survived, while some did not.

In two patients (#16 and #20) ECP was prolonged to no avail. It appears to us on the basis of our current data that if a patient has not responded to external counterpulsation by six or, at most, eight hours, assisted circulation will not be adequate therapy. The only reasonable alternative, at that point, may be corrective coronary artery surgery, an approach that we believe should be reserved until assisted circulation has been tried.

In patients who recover and are discharged from the hospital, long-term follow-up studies are needed to assess both their residual cardiac function and possible sequelae such as mitral insufficiency or ventricular aneurysm that are amenable to corrective surgery.

ACKNOWLEDGMENTS

Studies were carried out in cooperation with Boston City Hospital, Peter Brent Brigham Hospital, Cardinal Cushing General Hospital, Framingham Union Hospital, Jordan Hospital, Milford Hospital, New England Medical Center, Newton-Wellesley Hospital, St. Elizabeth's Hospital, and Symmes Hospital.

The following physicians participated in these studies: John S. Banas, Oscar H. L. Bing, David Borkenhagen, Alfred Brilla, Robert J. Carey, Gerald L. Evans, Athanasios Flessas, Richard Gorlin, William B. Hood, Michael Lesch, Charles Lutton, James W. McDowell, Robert E. Olson, Burton Polansky, Richard M. Regnante, Thomas J. Ryan, Gordon A. Saunders, James J. Sidd, Samuel Stewart, and Theodore Waltuch.

Phyllis Childs, John Coleman, Frank Graham, Nubar Hagopian, Jerry L. Jones, Sheila O'Connell, Harold S. Sauer, Elaine C. Trivus, and Gail Woodhead provided technical and nursing assistance.

Judith Linn edited this report.

References

Antebi E, Giron F, Zawahry MD, Birtwell WC, Soroff HS: Experimental evaluation of external circulatory assist as a treatment for coronary occlusion. Surg Forum 21:154, 1970

Banas JS, Brilla A, Soroff HS, Levine H: Evaluation of external counterpulsation for the treatment of severe angina pectoris. Circulation 45 & 46 (Supplement 2):74, 1972 (abstract)

Birtwell WC, Soroff HS, Giron F, et al: Synchronous assisted circulation. Can Med Assoc J 95:652, 1966

Birtwell WC, Soroff HS, Sachs BF, Levine HJ, Deterling RA Jr: Assisted circulation: V. The use of the lungs as a pump; a method for assisting pulmonary blood flow by varying airway pressure synchronously with the EKG. Trans Am Soc Artif Intern Organs 9:192, 1963

Clauss RH, Birtwell WC, Albertal G, et al: Assisted circulation: I. The arterial counterpulsator. J Thorac Cardiovasc Surg 41:447, 1961

Cloutier CT, Soroff HS, Giron F, et al: The physiologic effects of synchronous external circulatory assistance in patients in cardiogenic shock. Surg Forum 22:187, 1971

Dennis C, Moreno JR, Hall DP, et al: Studies on external counterpulsation as a potential measure for acute left heart failure. Trans Am Soc Artif Intern Organs 9:186, 1963

Don Michael TA, Forrester JS, Allen HN, et al: Identification of clinical subsets in cardiogenic shock. Am J Cardiol 29:280, 1972

Giron F, Birtwell WC, Soroff HS, et al: Assisted circulation by synchronous pulsation of extramural pressure. Surgery 60:894, 1966

Jacobey JA, Taylor WJ, Smith GT, Gorlin R, Harken DE: A new therapeutic approach to acute coronary occlusion: II. Opening dormant coronary collateral channels by counterpulsation. Surg Forum 12:225, 1961

Kataoka K, Birtwell WC, Norton RL, Soroff HS: Experimental evaluation of coronary collateral enhancement by external counterpulsation. Trans Am Soc Artif Intern Organs 19:408, 1973

Nishimura A, Giron F, Birtwell WC, Soroff HS: Evaluation of collateral blood supply by direct measurement of the performance of ischemic myocardial muscle. Trans Am Soc Artif Intern Organs 16:450, 1970

Osborn JJ, Main FB, Gerbode FL: Circulatory support by leg or airway pulses in experimental mitral insufficiency. Circulation 28:781, 1963

Peel AAF, Semple T, Wang I, et al: A coronary prognostic index for grading the severity of infarction. Br Heart J 24:745, 1962

Ruiz U, Soroff HS, Birtwell WC, et al: Assisted circulation by synchronous pulsation of extramural pressure. J Thorac Cardiovasc Surg 56:832, 1968

Shubin H, Weil MH: Treatment of shock complicating acute myocardial infarction. Prog Cardiovasc Dis 10:30, 1967

Soroff HS, Birtwell WC, Norton RL, et al: Experimental and clinical studies in assisted circulation. Transplantation Proc 3:1483, 1971

Soroff HS, Giron F, Ruiz U, et al: Physiologic support of heart action. N Engl Med J 280:693, 1969

Soroff HS, Levine HJ, Sachs BF, Birtwell WC, Deterling RA Jr: Assisted circulation: II. Effects of counterpulsation on left ventricular oxygen consumption and hemodynamics. Circulation 27:722, 1963

Soroff HS, Ruiz U, Birtwell WC, Deterling RA Jr, Collins JA: Synchronous external circulatory assist. Trans Am Soc Artif Intern Organs 10:79, 1964

Wald A: Sequential Analysis. NY, Wiley Publishers, 1947

50

STABILIZATION OF THE ACUTE MYOCARDIAL INFARCTION PATIENT BY BALLOON COUNTERPULSATION

Jacob Rosensweig and Shekhar Chatterjee

Circulatory support by balloon counterpulsation has been applied clinically in a variety of conditions. These conditions are characterized by low cardiac output and central and peripheral hypoperfusion.[1,2,5,9,10,11,15] Evidence is accumulating that indicates the relative safety and potential effectiveness of balloon counterpulsation. In acute myocardial infarction, counterpulsation was originally restricted to cases of cardiogenic shock,[16] but more recently, the indications were extended to include a variety of circumstances theoretically capable of responding to assisted circulation.[15] This report summarizes our experience with 19 such patients in whom balloon pumping was utilized to improve their clinical status and facilitate recovery.

CLINICAL MATERIAL

Patients with acute myocardial infarction diagnosed by electrocardiographic findings and elevated serum enzyme levels, not responding to conventional therapy, were accepted for mechan-

ical circulatory support. The indications for counterpulsation related to symptoms or signs of cardiogenic shock or persistent acute myocardial ischemia (Table 1).

The majority of shock patients were over 60 years of age (mean 61 years). Most were male, and all except one had documented previ-

TABLE 1. Indications for Intraaortic Balloon Counterpulsation for Acute Myocardial Infarction

Cardiogenic shock: Refractory to medical therapy
Clinical signs
Cardiac index ($<$ L/m^2/min)
Hypotension ($<$ 90 mm Hg)
Oliguria, anuria ($<$ 10 cc/30 min)

Persistent acute myocardial ischemia
Pain
Electrocardiogram
Extension of infarct
Ventricular arrhythmia
LV failure (PAW $>$ 20 mm Hg)

TABLE 2. Clinical Summary: Cardiogenic Shock, Nine Patients

Age	42–75 (mean 61)
Sex	
Male	6
Female	3
Previous myocardial infarction	
0	1
+	4
++	2
+++	2
Time interval between infarction and shock (hrs)	1–72 (mean 23)
Duration in shock (hrs)	3–30 (mean 16)
Clinical status	
Rhythm	
Tachyarrhythmia	7
Multiple PVC	2
Cerebral	
Obtunded	7
Comatose	2
Renal	
Oliguric	5
Anuric	4
Pulmonary congestion/edema	9
CVP (cm H$_2$O)	16–24 (mean 20)
Specific therapy	
Vasopressors	8
Diuretics	4
Digitalis	6
Antiarrhythmic drugs	4

ous myocardial infarction. The mean interval between acute infarction and shock was 24 hours, and the mean duration of shock prior to counterpulsation was 16 hours. The patients were congested, confused, or comatose, severely oliguric or anuric, and demonstrated tachycardia or multiple ventricular extrasystoles. The right ventricular filling pressure was normal or elevated in each instance, and the patients were considered refractory to pharmacologic therapy (Table 2).

In the ischemic group, nine of the 10 patients were male. The average age was 56 years. Only two of the 10 had a previous history of myocardial infarction. Eight of the patients complained of persistent chest pain, and two devel-

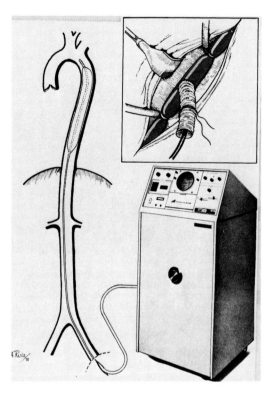

FIG. 1. Sketch illustrating passage of the intraaortic balloon catheter through an end-to-side femoral artery graft (insert), proper positioning of the balloon in the thoracic aorta, and the ACVO pump. (Reproduced by permission of Conn Med, February 1974)

TABLE 3. Clinical Summary: Persistent Acute Myocardial Ischemia, Ten Patients

Age	36–75 (mean 56)
Sex	
Male	9
Female	1
Previous myocardial infarction	
0	8
+	2
Recent MI	
Initial	
Anteroseptal	6
Anterior	4
Extension	
Lateral wall	3
Inferior wall	4
Angina	
Persistent	8
Recurrent	2
Time interval: of symptoms to assist	
<2 days	5
>2 days	5
Clinical status	
Rhythm	
Tachyarrhythmia	7
Multiple PVC	8
V. fibrillation	1
Cerebral	
Obtunded	10
Comatose	0
Renal	
Oliguric	10
Anuric	0
Pulmonary congestion/edema	10
CVP (cm H_2O)	18–20 (mean 19)
Specific therapy	
Vasopressors	1
Diuretics	8
Digitalis	8
Antiarrhythmic drugs	2

oped acute recurrent angina. Six patients showed evidence of infarct extension. Although not in frank shock, the patients were mentally obtunded, were oliguric, and demonstrated ventricular irritability. In this group, prior treatment had not included the use of vasopressors. The central venous pressure before counterpulsation averaged 19 cm of water (Table 3).

TECHNIQUE

The AVCO * triple segment intraortic balloon catheter and pump system was used (Fig. 1). Volume displacement of the balloon was 30 cc. A catheter was inserted under local anesthesia through a femoral arteriotomy. The distance from the arteriotomy to the sternal notch was measured, which usually resulted in placement of the tip of the catheter, just distal to the origin of the left subclavian artery. The position was confirmed

* AVCO Everett Research Laboratory, 2385 Revere Beach Parkway, Everett, Mass. 02149.

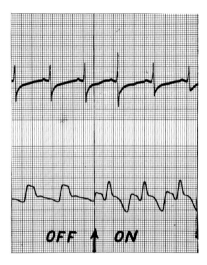

FIG. 2. Traces showing the effects of balloon counter-pulsation on arterial pressure. Systolic pressure is reduced, ejection period is shortened, diastolic pressure augmented, and end diastolic pressure lowered.

by roentgenogram of the chest and counterpulsation was instituted. A woven dacron graft was then sutured to the arteriotomy and tied about the catheter. The catheter was allowed to exit at the lower end of the wound. Aortic pressure was monitored by a catheter inserted through a right ulnar or radial arteriotomy and pulmonary wedge pressure by a Swan-Ganz catheter.* Once counterpulsation was instituted, vasopressor was discon-

* Edwards Laboratories, 1721 Red Hill Avenue, Santa Ana, Calif. 92705.

tinued. Accurate synchronization was always readily achieved. Optimal hemodynamic effects were evident when the balloon was inflated at aortic valve closure and deflated so as to produce maximal lowering of end-diastolic aortic pressure (Fig. 2). Systolic pressure was decreased 13 percent (6 to 19 percent) in cardiogenic shock patients and 13 percent (4 to 28 percent) in the ischemic group. The diastolic pressure was augmented 39 percent (25 to 64 percent) in the former group and 26 percent (13 to 40 percent) in the latter. Weaning from the pump was carried out over a 3 to 4 hour period by sequentially reducing the ratio of augmented heart beats from 1:1 to 1:8. On termination of counterpulsation, the catheter was removed and the graft trimmed and suture ligated. Passage of a Fogarty catheter into the distal superficial femoral and profunda femoral arteries was carried out when deemed appropriate. Systemic anticoagulation during counterpulsation was maintained at minimal levels using a heparin dose of 40 mg every six hours, intravenously.

RESULTS

Patients in shock were supported for 20 to 201 hours (mean 63 hours). All were hemodynamically improved. Mentation cleared, heart rate slowed, pulmonary congestion diminished, color improved, and urine output increased (Figs. 3 and 4). One patient developed fatal ventricular

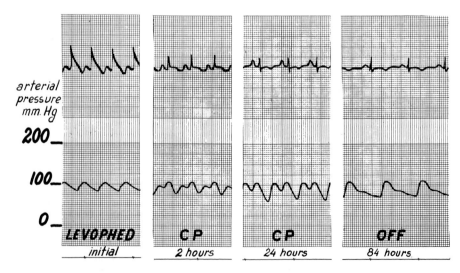

FIG. 3. Arterial pressure and electrocardiographic traces following institution of counterpulsation in a shock patient. Norepinephrine infusion was discontinued when circulatory support was begun. Note progressive slowing of heart rate and lessened injury pattern during pumping with maintenance of a satisfactory arterial pressure following termination of support.

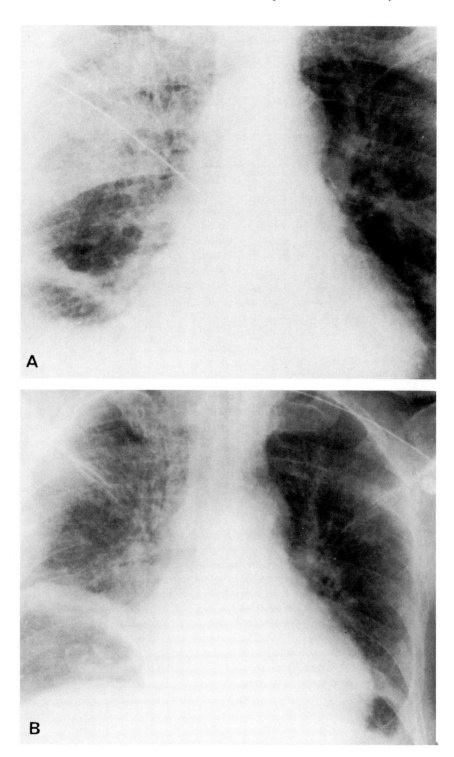

FIG. 4. Roentgenogram of the chest prior to (A) and after 24 hours of balloon counterpulsation (B) showing clearing of extensive pulmonary edema in the right lung.

fibrillation while on circulatory support, and another, a 73-year-old male, who showed no sustained improvement after 24 hours (cardiac output while supported 3.2 liters per minute; with pump off, 0.9 liters per minute) died shortly after elective termination of counterpulsation. Seven patients were weaned from the pump, but, three subsequently died of intractable heart failure. Review of the five deaths indicated that each patient had sustained multiple previous infarctions and that autopsy showed extensive involvement of left ventricular myocardium either by fibrosis or acute infarction, with rupture of the interventricular septum in one case. However, improved cardiovascular status persisted in four patients following cessation of pumping and they recovered uneventfully (Table 4).

Ischemic patients were assisted for an average of 52 hours (9 to 94 hours). All showed rapid clinical improvement. Chest pain quickly abated, heart rate slowed, arrhythmias disappeared,

TABLE 4. Results: Counterpulsation for Cardiogenic Shock, Nine Patients

Duration of assist (hrs)	20–201 (mean 63)
Immediate result	
Improved	9
No improvement	0
Off assist	8
Died	
During assist	1
Post assist	4
Discharged	4

and urine output increased (Fig. 5). Lessened myocardial ischemia was generally apparent electrocardiographically within 24 hours and in four of six cases there was complete disappearance of evidence of recent infarct extension (Figs. 6 and 7). Diminution of cardiac silhouette was frequently observed (Fig. 8). Every patient was successfully weaned from the pump. Nine of the 10 cases made a progressive recovery and were discharged (Table 5).

COMPLICATIONS

The balloon catheter could not be inserted in two patients because of bilateral iliac artery occlusion or tortuosity. In one instance, despite

TABLE 5. Results: Counterpulsion for Persistent Acute Myocardial Ischemia, Ten Patients

Duration of assist (hrs)	9–94 (mean 52)
Immediate result	
Improved	10
No improvement	0
Off assist	10
Discharged	9
Died	(1 intractable heart failure)

proper positioning of the catheter in the thoracic aorta, marked iliac tortuosity produced obstructive kinking preventing rhythmic inflation of the balloon (Fig. 9). Dissection of an atherosclerotic aorta opposite the balloon was discovered at autopsy in a patient, who had been assisted for nine days. In one case, transient foot drop developed after 24 hours, in a patient with antecedent superficial femoral artery occlusion. Embolic or thrombotic phenomenon was not observed. Hemolysis was minimal, and plasma hemoglobin never rose above 10 mg percent. Platelet counts decreased initially in some patients but returned to normal within 48 hours. Superficial wound infection developed in two cases, which responded to drainage and local therapy.

FOLLOW-UP

Two patients in the shock group are well and active at 16 and 32 months. However, two patients died suddenly at five and six months; both revealing, at postmortem examination, localized proximal occlusion with patent distal runoff in the affected coronary artery. On the basis of this early experience, routine angiographic assessment has been recommended in all patients following recovery and four have since undergone elective aortocoronary bypass and three, ventricular aneurysmectomy.

DISCUSSION

The clinical observations tend to substantiate previous experimental findings that counterpulsation increases cardiac output and lessens myocardial ischemia while effectively maintaining peripheral and visceral blood flow.[6] Positive effects on ventricular function were observed, and, as

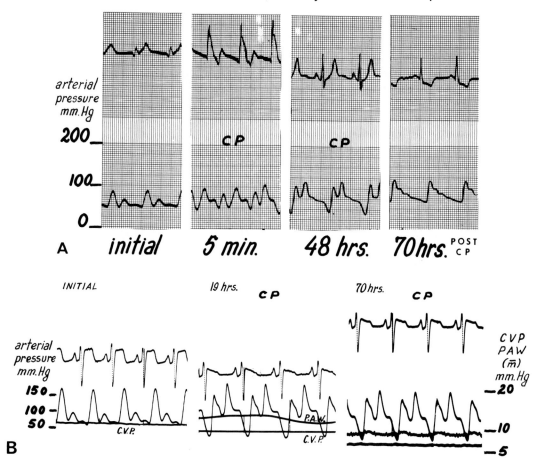

FIG. 5. Serial electrocardiographic and arterial pressure tracings of a hypotensive patient with intractable angina treated by counterpulsation for 70 hours. Abolition of chest pain correlated with effective diastolic augmentation and sustained increased arterial pressure. B. Hemodynamic studies in a patient with extensive acute anterolateral myocardial infarction and persistent angina. Marked diastolic augmentation was achieved. Heart rate slowed, and there was progressive decline in pulmonary artery wedge and central venous pressures associated with improved cardiac output.

others reported, the extent of infarcted myocardium was significantly reduced in some cases.[12,17]

Technical simplicity and minimal blood and tissue trauma make balloon pumping an attractive modality for circulatory support in acute myocardial infarction. Its potential value was indicated in our series by hospital recovery of four of nine patients in cardiogenic shock (49 percent) and nine of 10 patients manifesting unstable persistent or recurrent ischemia (90 percent).

The recovery index in cardiogenic shock was half that observed in the ischemic group, nevertheless, it is impressive when compared to the poor prognosis of patients treated medically.[8] Survival of shock patients in this series was twice

that observed by other investigators and was probably related to earlier institution of circulatory support.[16] Since maximal hemodynamic benefit is achieved within 48 hours, when left ventricular function curves reach optimal levels, continued pump dependency may indicate myocardial infarction of more than 60 percent of left ventricular wall, a condition incompatible with recovery.[3] We agree with those who recommend angiographic assessment of all pump dependent patients but question whether emergency surgery will increase overall salvage.[17] Early surgery of pump-supported patients should be considered, however, if there is evidence of ruptured interventricular septum or papillary muscle.[4]

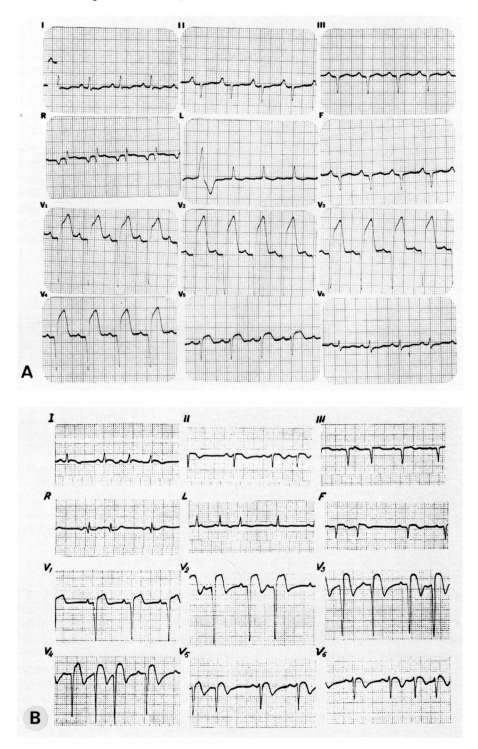

FIG. 6. Electrocardiograms of a patient admitted with acute anteroseptal myocardial infarction (A) showing evidence of extension and increased ischemia on the following day (B). Marked improvement and resolution of current injury was obvious after 12 hours (C) and 36 hours (D) of balloon counterpulsation.

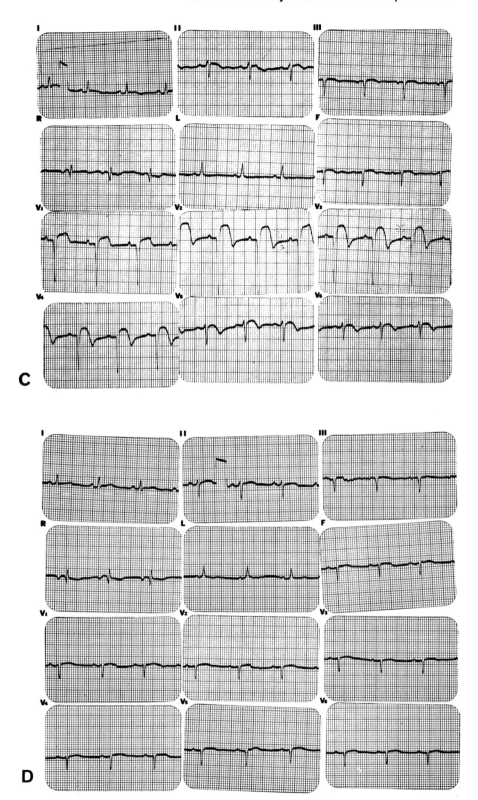

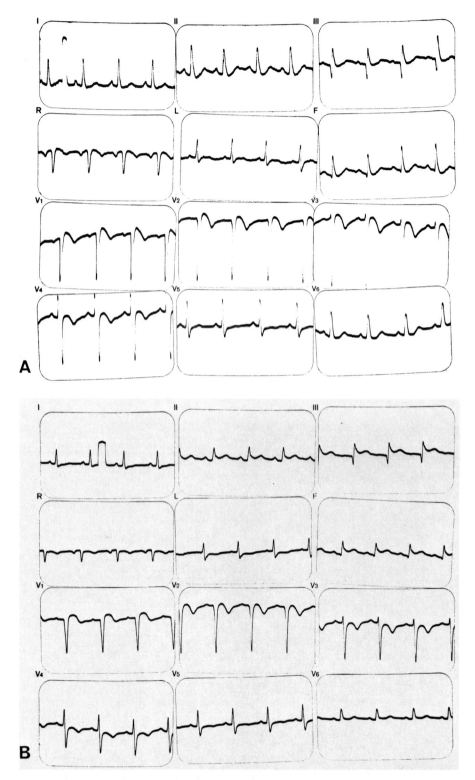

FIG. 7. Electrocardiograms of a patient admitted with acute anteroseptal myocardial infarction (A). Forty-eight hours later, recurrent chest pain was associated with current of injury involving the inferior wall (B). After 24 hours (C) and 48 hours (D) of balloon counterpulsation, evidence of inferior wall extension was no longer apparent with lessened ischemia anteriorly.

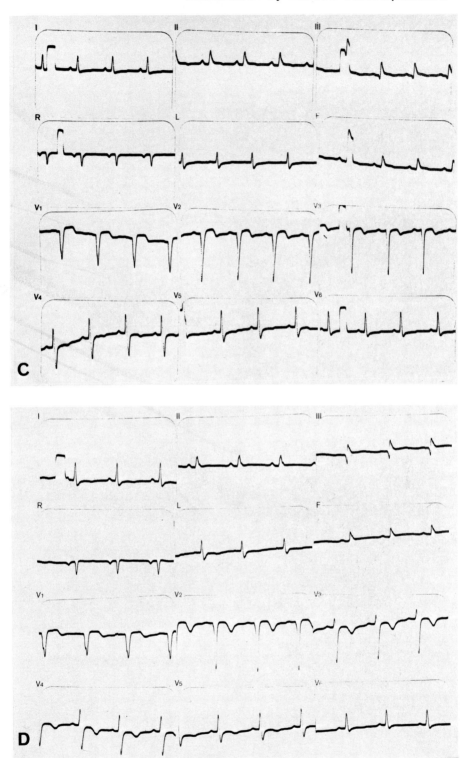

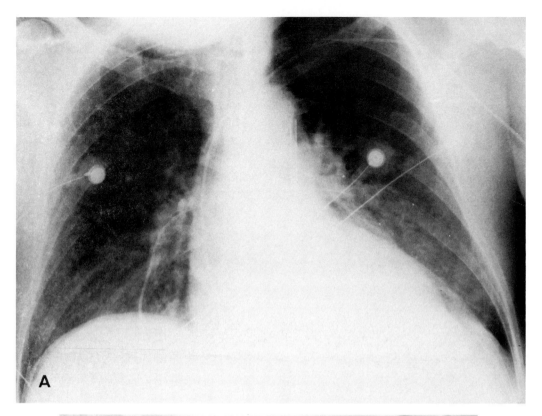

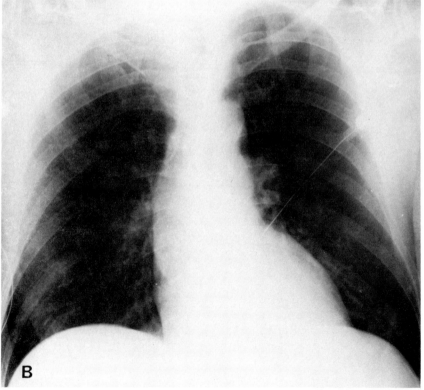

FIG. 8. Chest roentgenogram of a patient with extensive acute anterolateral myocardial infarction showing cardiomegaly (A). Despite the development of an anterior wall left ventricular aneurysm, balloon pumping resulted in diminution of heart size (B), which maintained throughout the subsequent hospital stay (C).

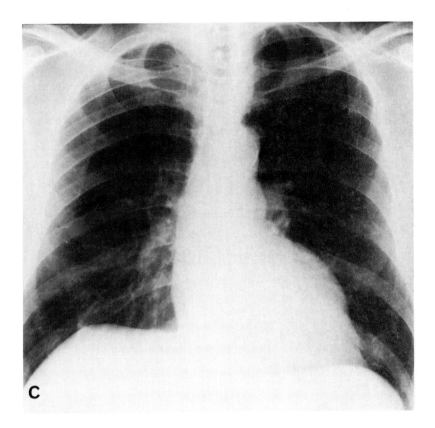

C

In the ischemic group, counterpulsation apparently prevented further deterioration of myocardial function, acute pump failure, or fatal arrhythmia. It also permitted deferral of angiographic studies and emergency surgery to more elective lesser risk circumstances.[7,14] Although some have advocated emergency catheterization and surgery once counterpulsation is instituted,[13] we feel that if circulatory dynamics are improved and the clinical condition of the patient is stabilized, it may be wiser not to intervene and to allow primary recovery to proceed. Only one patient, with an occlusion of the left main coronary artery, may have been salvaged by emergency revascularization, but the extent of left ventricular infarction would have precluded a good result. Persistent or recurrent anginal pain is an ominous symptom reflecting continuing critical myocardial ischemia. In our opinion, it should be considered a primary indication for circulatory support. We have been very impressed with its rapid resolution following institution of counterpulsation. This remarkable observation, manifest by most patients, suggests that counterpulsation should also be worthwhile in preinfarction syndrome.

CONCLUSIONS

In acute myocardial infarction, counterpulsation should be used when it offers the greatest likelihood of helping the patient. Efforts should be directed to restricting irreversible loss of ischemic myocardium by increasing coronary collateral flow and by reducing left ventricular work and myocardial oxygen requirements in all unstable patients early in the course of acute infarction. The aim of treatment should be avoidance of catastrophic arrhythmia and shock. Finally, it must be noted that whenever counterpulsation is utilized, it is imperative that following recovery, sites of coronary occlusion and the extent of myocardial damage be ascertained to determine candidacy for revascularization or reparative surgery. The sudden death of operable patients after discharge from hospital suggests that elective revascularization and/or aneurysmectomy following initial stabilization by counterpulsation may increase long-term survival.

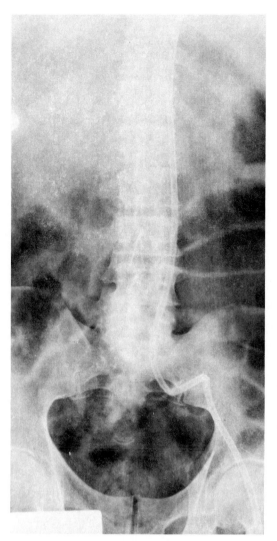

FIG. 9. Roentgenogram revealing obstructive kinking of the balloon catheter in a tortuous iliac artery, which prevented rhythmic inflation.

References

1. Berger RL, Saini VK, Long W, Hechtman H, Hood W: The use of diastolic augmentation with the intra-aortic balloon in human septic shock with associated coronary artery disease. Surgery 74: 601, 1973

2. Berger RL, Saini VK, Ryan TJ, Sokol DM, Keefe JF: Intraaortic balloon assist for post cardiotomy cardiogenic shock. J Thorac Cardiovasc Surg 66: 906, 1973

3. Braunwald E, Covell JW, Manoko PR, Ross J: Effects of drugs and of counterpulsation on myocardial oxygen consumption—observation on the ischemic heart. Circulation 39 Supplement 4:220, 1969

4. Buckley MJ, Mundth ED, Daggett WM, Austin WG: Surgical therapy for early complication of myocardial infarction. Surgery 70:814, 1971

5. Buckley MJ, Craver MJ, Gold HK, Mundth ED, Daggett WM, Austin WG: Intra-aortic balloon pump assist for cardiogenic shock after cardiopulmonary bypass. Circulation 48 Supplement III:III–90, 1973

6. Chatterjee S, Rosensweig J: An evaluation of intraaortic balloon counterpulsation. J Thorac Cardiovasc Surg 61:405, 1971

7. Cohn LH, Gorlin R, Herman M, Collins JJ: Indications and results of surgery for acute syndromes of coronary heart disease. Circulation 45 Supplement II:III–140, 1972

8. Cronin RFP, Moore S, Marpole DG: Shock following myocardial infarction: a clinical survey of 140 cases. Can Med Assoc J 93:57, 1965

9. Dilley RB, Ross J, Bernstein EF: Serial hemodynamics during intra-aortic balloon counterpulsation in cardiogenic shock. Circulation 48 Supplement III:III–99, 1973

10. Lamberti J, Cohn LH, Lesch M, Collins JJ: Intra-aortic balloon counterpulsation for post-operative left ventricular power failure. Circulation 48 Supplement IV:IV–188, 1973.

11. Leinback RC, Gold HK, Dinsmore RE, Mundth ED, Buckley MJ, Austin WG, Sanders CA: The role of angiography in cardiogenic shock. Circulation 48 (Supplement II):III–95, 1973

12. Manoko PR, Bernstein EF, Libby P, Delania GA, Covell JW, Ross J, Braunwald E: Effects of intra-aortic balloon counterpulsation on the severity of myocardial ischemic injury following acute coronary occlusion. Circulation 45:1150, 1972

13. Mundth ED, Yurchak PM, Buckley MJ, Leinbach RC, Kantrowitz AR, Austin WG: Circulatory assistance and emergency direct coronary artery surgery for shock complicating acute myocardial infarction. N Engl J Med 283:1382, 1970

14. Reul GJ, Morris GE, Howell JF, Crawford ES, Stelter W: Emergency coronary artery bypass grafts in the treatment of acute myocardial infarction. Circulation 45 (Supplement II):II–110, 1972

15. Rosensweig J, Chatterjee S, Czarnecki S, Bernstein S: Role of balloon counterpulsation in the "acute coronary" patient. Conn Med 38:54, 1974

16. Scheidt S, Wilner G, Mueller H, Summers D, Lesch M, Wolf G, Krakauer J, Rubenfine M, Fleming P, Noon G, Oldhem N, Killip T, Kantrowitz A: Intraaortic balloon counterpulsation in cardiogenic shock. N Engl J Med 288: 979, 1973

17. Sugg WL, Webb WR, Ecker RR: Reduction of extent of myocardial infarction by counterpulsation. Ann Thorac Surg 7:310, 1969

51

THE SURGICAL MANAGEMENT OF VENTRICULAR FAILURE WITH LOW EJECTION FRACTIONS
The Prophylactic Use of Intraaortic Balloon Counterpulsation

Armand A. Lefemine, Hyung S. Moon, Athanasios Flessas, Thomas J. Ryan, and K. Ramaswamy

Coronary artery disease produces a variety of surgical problems. The indications for surgical intervention beyond the treatment of intractable angina are not clearly defined and remain controversial. Congestive heart failure secondary to postinfarction scars or fibrosis responds poorly or not at all to revascularization and is associated with a greatly increased hospital and late mortality.[1,2,3,4] It is difficult to compare series and results because of differences in selection of patients. The clinical state usually manifests dyspnea on exertion and fatigue. Angina may or may not be present. Additional findings such as edema, ascites, rales, and pleural effusion add to the seriousness of the condition. Cardiac catheterization offers a means for a more precise definition of ventricular failure and its cause. If saccular ventricular aneurysm is excluded, as a cause of left ventricular failure, there remain a group of patients who demonstrate large, dilated, poorly contracting ventricles with large systolic and diastolic volumes and low ejection fractions by ventriculography. Localized ventricular wall dysfunction in the form of akinesis and dyskinesis is often apparent usually anteriorly and apically. If the contractile area is large enough, compensation by the Frank-Starling mechanism results in overstretching the remaining myocardium and failure that cannot respond to revascularization alone. The law of LaPlace $(T = PXR)$, which relates tension and myocardial oxygen consumption[5] to the radius of the ventricle, indicates that if the radius or size of the ventricle is reduced by resection of a localized scar or noncontractile area, tension would be reduced and the remaining functional muscle fibers would be returned to a more favorable position on the Frank-Starling curve. There is general agreement that ejection fractions below 40 percent represent severe impairment of ventricular function often regarded as a contraindication for bypass operations. Left ventricular end-diastolic pressures and stroke volume index while helpful are more variable and less reliable indicators of failure. Thus patients with congestive failure should benefit more if a reconstruction of the ventricle is added to revascularization and valve replacement. This report presents the results of 20 patients treated by resection of akinetic and dyskinetic segments and revascularization by vein or internal mammary artery bypasses.

PATIENTS

Patients varied in age from 40 to 62 years with 16 males and four females. All were selected for operation because of disability resulting from dyspnea on exertion, fatiguability, and disabling angina (10 patients). All had ejection fractions of 40 percent or less. Calculations of end-diastolic and end-systolic volumes are available in 17 patients. Comparable postoperative studies are available in 10 patients at intervals of three to four weeks (four patients), three months (one patient), six months (three patients), and eight months (two patients) following operation. All patients had large areas of akinesis with minor dyskinesis in anterior and apical segments exceeding 25 percent of ventricular wall area. Coronary arteriorgraphy revealed three patients with one-vessel disease, eight patients with two-vessel disease, and nine patients with three or more severely diseased coronary arteries. Five patients had some degree of mitral insufficiency. Classified according to the New York Heart Association criteria: two were in functional class II, 10 were in functional class III, and eight patients were in functional class IV.

TECHNIQUES

Cardiopulmonary bypass utilized hemodilution with hematocrit of 20 percent, frozen red cells, albumin, mannitol, and hypothermia of 30 C. Anoxic arrest is never used. Induced ventricular fibrillation with apical decompression of the left ventricle is standard. The saphenous vein, flushed with heparinized oxygenated blood, was used to construct bypasses in 19 patients and the internal mammary artery in one. All coronary anastamoses were performed with a running 7–0 or 6–0 Prolene suture and two-power magnification.

Excision and exclusion of nonfunctional ventricular wall was judged by ventriculogram and by careful observation of the beating heart before induction of ventricular fibrillation. It is also helpful to palpate the wall between two fingers because a definite demarcation is usually clear at the transition to normal myocardium. Observation of the interior of the ventricle will demonstrate a transition from smoother wall to more trabeculated and glistening endocardium. The excision has not included septum or the area of LAD coronary artery. An elliptical full thickness specimen is taken from the length of the incision. The endocardium is cleared of all thrombi or cholesterol material, and the incision is closed by mattress sutures of O Tevdek through strips of thick Teflon felt placed on either side of the closure.

The Avco intraaortic balloon was inserted through one femoral artery either at the same time as cannulation for cardiopulmonary bypass or later through the femoral arteriotomy used for bypass. The balloon was positioned by palpation of the descending thoracic aorta. Balloon pulsation was started as soon as the balloon was placed and continued during cardiopulmonary bypass if it was in place. The early placements were for patients in whom we anticipated difficulty removing pump-oxygenator support because of a severe degree of failure. A portable battery operated Avco pump allowed us to continue counterpulsation while patient was in transit to the intensive care area. Intraaortic balloon counterpulsation was continued for one to five days depending on blood pressure and urine output. Vasopressors were used as needed. Defibrillation is usually no problem. Removal of pump support often requires the use of adrenalin, 1:10,000, in intermittent doses. If the intraaortic balloon is in position, this is used as part of the weaning process. Anticoagulation was not used for the first 48 hours; following this a heparin infusion was given continuously by Harvard pump at a rate of 1,000 units per hour. Postoperatively the most sensitive indicator of adequate cardiac output is the urine output. Left atrial pressure is essential to determine volume replacement during the first 48 hours. Gross observation of the first derivative or upstroke of the aortic pressure curve also helps to judge left ventricular contractility. Cardiac catheterization and retrograde aortic catheterization of the coronary arteries and left ventricle were performed in standard fashion. End-diastolic and end-systolic volumes and ejection fraction were calculated from single plane left ventriculography in the 30-degree right anterior oblique position.[6]

RESULTS

Twenty patients with ejection fractions of 40 percent or less underwent resection of noncontractile ventricular wall and revascularization by vein bypass or internal mammary artery anastomosis (Fig. 1). The mitral valve was replaced in one. The preoperative hemodynamic profile of the group is found in Table 1. Ejection fraction averaged 27 percent with an end-diastolic volume index of 136 cc/m² and an end systolic volume index of 100 cc/m². Left ventricular end-diastolic pressure averaged 24 mm Hg with a cardiac index that was low normal. The operations and results are presented on Table 2. The operative mortality was 5 percent, or one patient who died of an air

TABLE 1. Preoperative Hemodynamics, Twenty Patients

	MEAN	SD	N
EF	28.1	8.7	20
EDV	244.4	52.4	17
ESV	178.1	54.7	17
EDVI	134.2	33.5	17
ESVI	98.3	33.1	17
CI	2.5	.68	20
LVEDP	23.9	8.4	20
SVI	29	8.8	20

EF: ejection fraction; EDV: end-diastolic volume; ESV: end-systolic volume; EDVI: end-diastolic volume index; ESVI: end-systolic volume index; CI: cardiac index; LVEDP: left ventricular end-diastolic pressure; and SVI: stroke volume index.

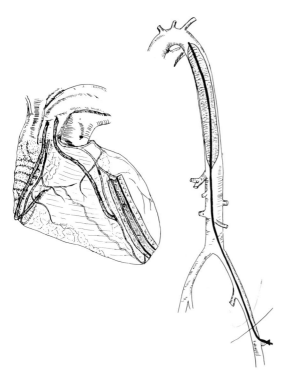

FIG. 1. Double coronary bypass and ventricular resection with intraaortic balloon.

pump. This 54-year-old man was admitted because of chronic and progressive congestive heart failure, functional classification IV D (New York Heart Association). Chronic edema, pleural effusions, hyperbilirubinemia, ascites, hepatomegaly, and rales, where characteristic. The electrocradiogram revealed old anterior and posterior myocardial infarctions. Coronary and ventricular angiography demonstrated a large dilated left ventricle with anterior akinesis, occlusion of the right coronary artery, and 80 percent stenosis of the LAD coronary artery. His cardiac index was 1.7 L/min/m², and the ejection fraction was 25 percent. Postoperatively, counterpulsation was continued for 48 hours (Fig. 3). His recovery was smooth and uncomplicated though prolonged by weakness and fatigue. A postoperative catheterization revealed no change in the ejection fraction. One other patient is a definite failure of therapy, though she is still alive 30 months after her operation. This 53-year-old woman underwent resection of an anterior-apical segment and a triple coronary bypass for occlusion of the right and LAD artery and stenosis of the circumflex artery. A myocardial infarction three weeks after operation resulted in chronic heart failure and angina.

The remainder of the group, 15 patients, have demonstrated varying clinical and hemodynamic improvement when followed for an average of 17.5 months (three to 37 months). Postoperative hemodynamic studies are available in 10 of the survivors, three weeks to eight months after operation. Figure 4 shows the individual preoperative and postoperative comparisons. Only one patient was returned to normal hemodynamics; however, even a small improvement of left ventricular function as judged by ejection fraction and volumes was associated with marked clinical improvement. Figures 5, 6, and 7 illustrate the varying degrees of improvement in patients who had excellent clinical results. One patient (Fig. 5), a 44-year-old man was an invalid because of dyspnea and fatigue. Angina was an occasional symptom. Postoperatively he was able to return to work

embolus. Late mortality was 15 percent, or three patients, all of whom succumbed to low cardiac output and failure. The late deaths are important since they are related to left ventricular failure and represent possible improvement in the operative approach. In two patients, mitral insufficiency of relatively minor degree was left uncorrected and is considered a cause of persistent failure and low output in one and late failure (six months) in the other. The third late death was due to an inadequate amount of functional myocardium because of extensive fibrosis and atrophy (Fig. 2). This last patient is an interesting case study because he is the first in whom we planned and carried out the prophylactic use of the intraaortic balloon

TABLE 2. Clinical Results

OPERATIONS	NUMBER OF PATIENTS	HOSPITAL MORTALITY	LATE MORTALITY	GOOD RESULTS
Resection	2	0	0	2
Resection, single bypass	4	0	0	3
Resection, double bypass	11	0	3	8
Resection, triple bypass	2	0	0	1
Resection, double bypass, mitral valve	1	1	0	0
Total	20	1	3	14
(Percent)		(5)	(15)	(70)

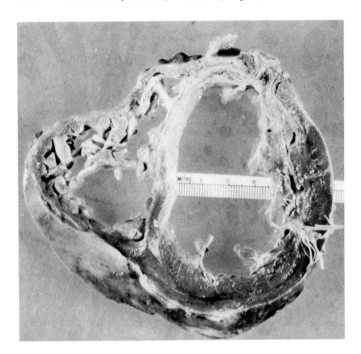

FIG. 2. A patient who died three months after double bypass and resection from chronic low output state. Note the dilated ventricular cavities, the extensive scar anteriorly and septally, and the thin myocardium.

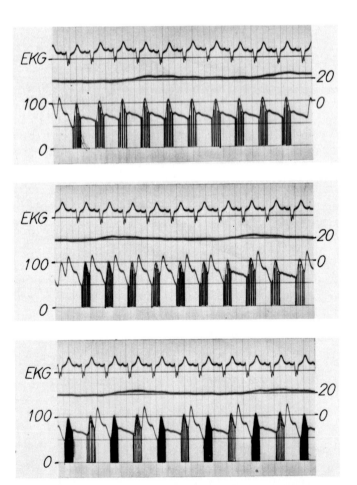

FIG. 3. Counterpulsation postoperatively in a patient (CS) with advanced congestive failure. Postoperative course was uncomplicated in spite of the advanced and irreversible cardiac changes. Scale on left: AP; scale on right: left atrial.

FIG. 4. Failure group, pre- and post-operative hemodynamics. Note the consistent changes in ejection fractions (EF), end-diastolic volume (EDV), and end-systolic volumes (ESV). Cardiac index (CI), stroke volume index (SVI), and left ventricular end-diastolic pressures (LVEDP) were more variable.

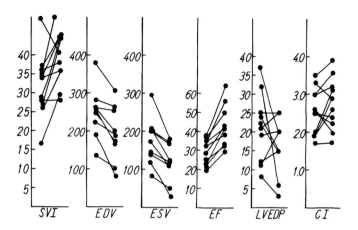

as a Department of Public Works employee doing moderate physical labor outdoors. His improvement has been maintained for three years. Noteworthy in his studies is that the ejection fraction increased from 22 percent to 33 percent, and end-systolic volume decreased 202 cc to 170 cc. Cardiac index and stroke volume were both significantly increased, though LVEDP remained unchanged. Another patient (Fig. 6) was able to double his

ejection fraction from 21 percent to 42 percent with corresponding improvements in other parameters. Though the EF and ESV and EDV are not normal, he has returned to his job and a normal life style without restrictions or medications two years later. Figure 7 illustrates the changes in a patient whose circulatory and ventricular dynamics returned to normal. This 43-year-old man was operated upon because of crescendo angina and

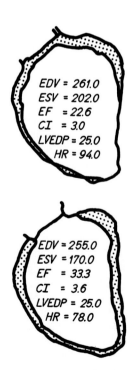

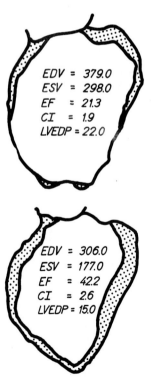

FIG. 5. A contraction diagram of patient CA, who achieved a good clinical result with small improvements in ejection fraction (EF), end-systolic volume (ESV), cardiac index (CI), and stroke volume index (SVI) without change in left ventricular end-diastolic pressure (LVEDP). Top: preoperative; bottom: postoperative.

FIG. 6. A contraction diagram of patient JM with a good clinical result. Ejection fraction (EF) was doubled, though not to normal levels. This was associated with significant reduction of EDV, ESV, and LVEDP. Cardiac index (CI) was significantly better. Top: preoperative; bottom: postoperative.

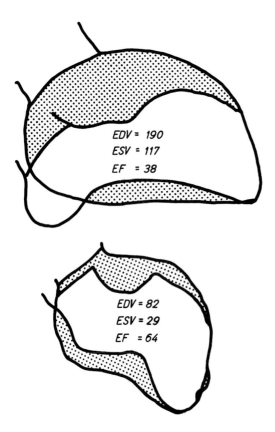

FIG. 7. Contraction diagram of the patient WM, whose hemodynamics were returned to normal following resection and bypass procedure. Top: preoperative; bottom: postoperative.

an acute myocardial infarction of 10 days' duration. The anterior and apical wall were akinetic. Ejection fraction was 38 percent, and EDV and ESV were significantly elevated. LVEDP was 24 mm Hg. The intraaortic balloon was inserted 48 hours before operation and continued for 72 hours after operation. His postoperative course was un-

TABLE 3. Postoperative Hemodynamics

	PREOP MEAN	POSTOP MEAN	P	SIGNIFICANCE OF DIFFERENCE
EF	29.4	42.9	0.001	S
EDV	247.7	192.6	0.001	S
ESV	177.6	117.3	0.001	S
CI	2.48	2.88	0.05	S
SVI	31.8	41.1	0.02	S
LVEDP	21.1	16.4	0.1	NS

EF: ejection fraction; EDV: end-diastolic volume; ESV: end-systolic volume; CI: cardiac index; SVI: stroke volume index; and LVEDP: left ventricular end diastolic pressure.

complicated except for reconstruction of the femoral artery. Table 3 analyzes the pre- and postoperative changes for significance. The ejection fraction was increased and the end-diastolic and end-systolic volumes were significantly decreased to the P 0.001 level in spite of the fact that two patients in the group were not improved. Ejection fraction rose from a mean of 29 percent to 42 percent. End-diastolic volume decreased from 246 cc to 191 cc. End-systolic volume decreased from 177 cc to 117 cc. The changes in cardiac index, stroke volume index, and LVEDP were more variable. The change of LVEDP was not statistically significant. The variation in LVEDP, a common criterion for left ventricular failure, may be explained by the changes of compliance, which may vary with the degree of dyskinesia. The compliance of the left ventricular wall may be decreased by the resection and buttressing of the wall with a corresponding rise in the LVEDP in spite of improvement of other parameters. We find the LVEDP a poor index of improvement.

Four patients were managed by the elective and prophylactic use of intraaortic balloon counterpulsation. One patient required preoperative counterpulsation because of crescendo angina and acute myocardial infarction. In the other three patients the balloon was placed either before or after the extracorporeal bypass through the unused femoral artery because of congestive failure and ejection fractions of 29 percent, 25 percent, and 16 percent. The last two patients were in advanced stages of failure with peripheral edema, ascites, and pleural effusions. Only one patient required vasopressors postoperatively (EF 16 percent) in addition to balloon counterpulsation (Fig. 8). All had stable hemodynamics and urine output and uncomplicated postoperative courses. The indications for use of the balloon prophylactically evolved from our initial experience with the first 12 patients, 10 of whom required vasopressors immediately following the operation for unstable blood pressures, and two of whom developed anuria and acidosis. Ejection fractions of 30 percent or less were all unstable postoperatively for about 48 hours and required constant attention to blood volume, inotropic agents, fluids, diuretics, and pH. The intraaortic balloon was planned in one additional patient but was not accomplished because of aortoiliac disease. Removal of pump support was difficult, and she was managed with isoproterenol and aramine for 48 hours. Because aortoiliac disease is common in this group we now resort to preoperative aortography if the intraaortic balloon is felt to be essential to survival (Figs. 9 and 10).

The pathology of the diseased segments re-

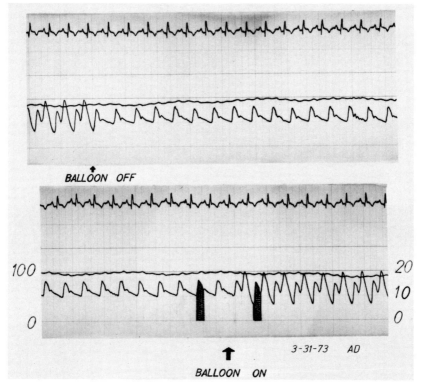

BALLOON OFF

100   20
                                       10
0   0

3-31-73   AD

BALLOON ON

FIG. 8. Postoperative intraaortic balloon counterpulsation in patient AD whose ejection fraction was 16 percent. Note the reduction of left atrial (scale at right) pressure and increase of aortic (scale at left) pressure when balloon pump is on.

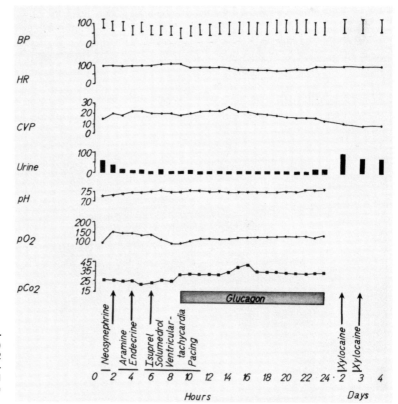

FIG. 9. Hemodynamics post-operatively in a patient (CA) with ejection fraction of 22 percent without balloon assistance. Note the oliguria and anuria as well as multiple use of drugs.

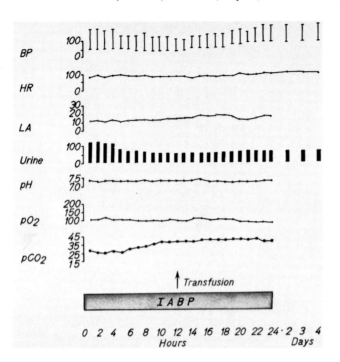

FIG. 10. Hemodynamics postoperatively in a patient (EH) with ejection fraction of 29 percent with balloon assistance. Note the absence of vasopressors and inotropic agents, normal urine input, and stable blood pressure.

veals a wide variety of fibrosis mixed with normal muscle. These segments are always thicker than the classic ventricular aneurysm, though there may be a thinned-out area at the apex. Generally one can identify the diseased segment by palpating a distinct difference between a thinned-out adynamic segment and the thicker normal segment. The same area can be identified by observing lack of contraction. Fibrosis is not always evident on the surface, and except for the lack of contraction the surface may appear as normal myocardium (Fig. 11). The usual finding is a mixture of muscle and fibrosis (Fig. 12). The endocardial and myocardial

fibrosis usually involve septum and usually extend up the posterior wall to the base of the papillary muscles. The resection usually involves the apex of the heart to the papillary muscles as well as the anterior segment often including the diagonal branch of the anterior descending coronary artery. No attempt was made to include the LAD coronary artery or the septum in the resection. The LAD artery was usually patent, and a bypass proceedure, either vein or internal mammary artery, was performed in all but two cases. The extent of the resection has not been a serious limitation when these boundaries are observed.

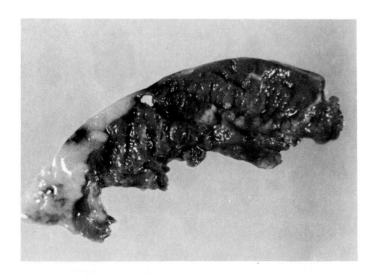

Fig. 11. A gross specimen showing full thickness of resected specimen. There is very little subendocardial fibrosis though the segment was non-contractile.

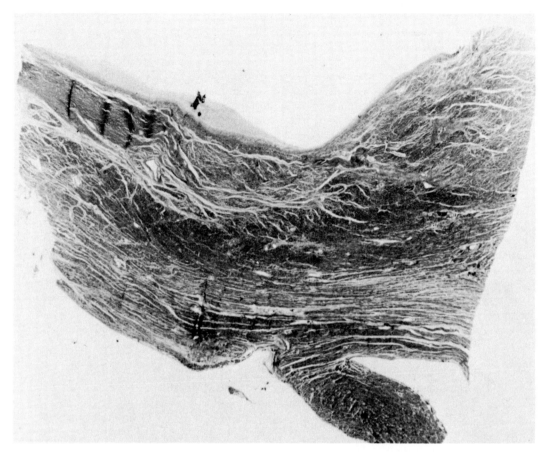

FIG. 12. Microscopic section of an akinetic segment. Note the large amount of normal muscle with scattered areas of fibrosis.

DISCUSSION

The large hypodynamic heart resulting from left ventricular failure and coronary artery disease has been indentified with poor functional results and increased operative mortality. The large saccular aneurysm with paradoxing wall has been excluded from this discussion because it is clearly established that resection is the treatment of choice and is effective in rehabilitating most of the patients. The patients under consideration are characterized clinically by symptoms of dyspnea and fatigue, some have angina, and some have obvious congestive failure. Angiography demonstrates a symmetrically dilated left ventricular cavity with large systolic and diastolic volumes and a generally reduced contraction of the ventricular wall except for the base. Segmental akinesis and dyskinesis can usually be identified though this may be difficult at times because of high wall tension.

There has been a tendency to reject patients as candidates for revascularization if their ejection fractions are less than 40 percent because of the increased risk and poor results. Our own experience agrees with the findings of Spencer et al[1] that vein bypass is not an adequate solution for congestive heart failure resulting from advanced coronary artery disease. Kouchoukos et al[7] found that resection plus a single bypass in a group with severe congestive failure did not offer hope of salvage since a third died from the operation, a third died within months after the operation, and the remainder were not improved. Mundth et al[2] reported 40 patients with congestive failure undergoing vein bypass, some with resection of ventricular aneurysm, with an operative mortality of 15 percent, and a late mortality of 7 percent. This last group was not defined by volumes and ejection fractions. Eighty percent were classified as good or excellent results on clinical grounds. On the other hand Schimert[8] and Kitamara et al[9] have produced evidence that resection of the adynamic segments of coronary artery disease is a valid approach for improving ventricular function with or without vein bypass and mitral valve replacement. Our initial studies [10] with postoperative clinical and hemodynamic evaluations for periods up to 36 months convince us that combined resection of segmental akinesis and dyskinesis combined with indicated vein bypasses and mitral valve replacements can improve the left ventricle to compensation and restore the patient to a normal life.

There are good theoretical reasons for adding resection of large akinetic areas to revascularization and valve replacement for the ventricle in failure. The mechanism of failure is probably a functional or absolute loss of contractile myocardium due to fibrosis exceeding the ability of the remaining functional units to compensate by the Frank-Starling mechanism. This results in enlargement of the ventricle and overstretching of the fibers as decompensation increases. This is reflected by the rise in LVEDP, the increase of end-diastolic and end-systolic volumes, and a reduction of cardiac index, and the ejection fraction. Wall tension, myocardial oxygen consumption, and functional radius of the left ventricle are all directly related to each other and this relationship is expressed by the law of LaPlace: $T = P \times R$.[11] In heart failure a greater ventricular end-diastolic pressure and volume are required to deliver a normal or reduced stroke volume.[12] Thus the heart with coronary artery disease and a large localized scar or noncontractile area has two causes of pump failure that can be corrected. The most direct approach to improving ventricular function would be to reconstruct the ventricle with a smaller functional radius by resection or exclusion of the noncontracting area. A reduction of radius automatically produces a reduction of wall tension and myocardial oxygen consumption and improves the strength and speed of fiber contraction by reducing the stretch to a more favorable portion of the Frank-Starling curve. The value of vein bypass alone for producing these same effects in advanced stages of ventricular failure must be questioned, though there is some evidence that hypokineses can be improved or restored to normal by revascularization.[13]

Another aspect of vein bypass in the poor-risk, ventricular-failure group is the possibility of patients being functionally worse because of the operation. Siderys and colleagues [3] found that one-third of those with severe left ventricular impairment showed elevation of left ventricular end-diastolic pressures, and 17 percent showed deterioration of their ventriculograms in the postoperative period.

The operative mortality associated with vein bypass alone in the poor-risk group with severe left ventricular impairment varies widely in reported series from 15 percent to 56 percent.[1,2,3,4,7] This is obviously related to variation in the composition of the groups as well as the inherent risk of performing a major operation that does not improve ventricular function in most of the patients. Even with procedures expected to improve ventricular function, the first 48 hours postoperatively are a period of critical hemodynamic instability. Elective intraaortic balloon counterpulsation has added a measure of support and stability that we feel has been instrumental in the survival of patients who otherwise could not be considered for surgery. Our experience indicates that this poor-risk group can be operated upon for revascularization with safety and good functional results if the operation includes procedures to improve the functional status of the left ventricle such as resection of adynamic segments and replacement of an insufficient mitral valve. The safety of the operation in part depends on the availability of circulatory support in the immediate postoperative period.

SUMMARY

Twenty patients with coronary artery disease and left ventricular failure characterized by ejection fractions of 40 percent or less have been treated by resection of akinetic segments and coronary artery bypasses. In one patient the mitral valve was also replaced. Operative mortality was five percent, or one patient who died of air embolus. Late mortality was 15 percent, or three patients who died of low cardiac output states within six months of the operation. Uncorrected mitral insufficiency was a significant factor in two of these, while the third revealed inadequate remaining myocardium. The remainder have been followed for three to 36 months and demonstrate significant improvement in 14 patients (70 percent). Only one of the survivors is in chronic failure, the result of a postoperative myocardial infarction. We feel that reconstruction of the ventricle to reduce the functional radius by resection of the noncontractile segments anteriorly and apically is an important part of the surgical treatment of ventricular failure secondary to coronary artery disease. Revascularization and mitral valve replacement should be carried out as indicated by the arteriography.

References

1. Spencer FC, Green GE, Tice DH, Walsh E, Mills NL, Glassman E: Coronary artery bypass grafts for

congestive heart failure. J Thorac Cardiovasc Surg. 62:4, 1971

2. Mundth E, Hawthorne JW, Buckley MJ, Dinsmore R, Austen WG: Direct coronary artery revascularization in the treatment of cardiac failure. Arch Surg 103:529–34, 1971

3. Siderys H, Pittman JN, Herod G: Coronary artery surgery in patients with impaired left ventricular function. Chest 61:482, 1972

4. Sewell WH: Lifetable analysis of the results of coronary surgery. Chest 61:481 1972

5. Shaffer AB, Katz LN: Hemodynamic alterations in congestive heart failure. N Engl J Med 276:853, 1967

6. Kasser IS, Kennedy JW: Measurement of left ventricular volume in man by single plane cineangiography. J Invest Radiol 4:83, 1963

7. Kouchoukos NT, Doty DB, Buettner LE, Kirklin JW: Treatment of post-infarction cardiac failure by myocardial excision and revascularization. Circulation 45–56:I–72, 1972

8. Schimert G, Lajos TZ, Bunnell IL, Green DG, Falsetti HI, Gage AA, Dean DC, Bernstein M: Operation for cardiac complication following the assessment of myocardial performance in man by hemo-dynamic and cineangiographic techniques. Am J Cardiol 23:511, 1969

9. Kitamara S, Echevarria M, Kay JH, Krohn BG, Redington JV, Mendez A, Zubiate P, Dunne EF: Left ventricular performance before and after removal of the noncontractile area of the left ventricle and revascularization of the myocardium. Circulation 45:1005, 1972

10. Lefemine AA, Moon HS, Flessas A, Ryan TJ, Ramaswamy K: Myocardial resection and coronary artery bypass for left ventricular failure following myocardial infarction. Results in patients with 40 percent or less ejection fraction. Ann Thorac Surg 17:1, 1974

11. Braunwald E, Ross J, Gault JH, Mason DT, Millo C, Gave IT, Epstein SE: Assessment of cardiac function. Ann Intern Med 70:369, 1969

12. Ross J: The assessment of myocardial performance in man by hemodynamic and cineangiographic techniques. Am J Cardiol 23:511, 1969

13. Saltiel J, Lesperance J, Bourassa MG, Castonguay Y, Compeau L, Grondin P: Reversibility of left ventricular dysfunction following aorto-coronary bypass grafts. Am J Roentgen 110:739, 1970

52

IMPROVED CARDIOPULMONARY BYPASS TECHNIQUES FOR MYOCARDIAL REVASCULARIZATION

G. Doyne Williams and Raymond C. Read

The precise suturing required in myocardial revascularization is best achieved with a motionless and bloodless heart. Commonly this ideal is approached using total cardiopulmonary bypass and aortic cross-clamping above the coronary arteries to provide ischemic arrest. Unfortunately, this otherwise satisfactory technique interrupts for extended periods of time coronary perfusion in hearts with established ischemic disease. This results in significant deterioration of myocardial function.

Technical advances in cardiac surgery now permit repair of most congenital and acquired lesions, and investigative and clinical interest is shifting to the successful management of patients with severely compromised myocardial function. Thus, techniques of total cardiopulmonary bypass that provide optimum operating conditions and yet injure the myocardium least must be sought.

Three major conditions affecting the myocardium during total cardiopulmonary bypass must be considered: temperature, coronary artery perfusion, and cardiac mechanism (ie arrest, fibrillation, or normal beat). Investigators are also currently seeking myocardial protection by providing increased energy substrate to the heart during periods of compromised perfusion. These techniques, however, have not yet developed clinical stature (Hewitt et al, 1974 and Iyengar et al, 1973).

TEMPERATURE

Myocardial protection by reduced temperature was experimentally demonstrated by Fuhrman et al in 1950, who lowered the metabolic rate of rat heart slices 90 percent when the temperature was lowered from 37 C to 10 C. The feasibility of whole-organ cardiac preservation by reduced temperature was supported by successful canine cardiac transplantation several hours after harvesting of the donor heart (Lower et al, 1962).

Impressive clinical results with the use of local cardiac hypothermia were initially reported by Hurley et al in 1964. Tetralogy of Fallot, ventricular septal defect, and left ventricular outflow obstruction in 120 patients were repaired under hypothermic cardiac arrest with an operative mortality of only 3.3 percent. This group has recently reported upon a series of 283 patients receiving aortic, mitral, or multiple valve replacements or coronary artery bypass grafts under local cardiac hypothermia with an overall mortality of only 4.7 percent. This achievement is underlined by the Class III and IV status of many of the patients in the series (Griepp et al, 1973).

Cold saline pericardial lavage produced epicardial temperatures of 10 to 15 C and intramyocardial temperatures of 15 to 20 C. No detectable differences were reported between the patients receiving intermittent coronary perfusion during hypothermia and those who received no coronary perfusion. Myocardial damage, however, has been demonstrated under conditions of ischemia at a myocardial temperature of 30 C, so cooling of the myocardium to the 15 to 20 C range would seem desirable if coronary artery perfusion is not provided (Isom et al, 1973).

CORONARY ARTERY PERFUSION

Artificial perfusion of the coronary arteries even when accomplished with well-oxygenated undamaged blood at flows, temperatures, and pressures equal to those normally encountered in the patient is not an entirely physiologic situation (Bloodwell et al, 1969). Early support for continuous coronary artery perfusion during cardiac surgical procedures was provided by the favorable reports of Littlefield et al, 1960; Bahnson et al, 1960; and Kay et al, 1958. The reasonableness of this approach to myocardial protection during bypass, as well as the favorable clinical results, led to its widespread adoption. Histological proof of myocardial protection by coronary artery perfusion was provided by Kottmeier and Wheat in 1966, serving further to support the technique. Complications of coronary artery perfusion have included ostial and intimal tears due to poorly fitting or forcefully manipulated coronary cannulae, inadequate circulation because of unrecognized coronary artery anomalies (Lillehei et al, 1964), sinus of Valsalva perforation (Bjork, 1964), and dissection of the coronary artery with hemorrhage (Heilbrunn and Zimmerman, 1965). Air embolism and occlusion of small coronary arteries were added to this list of complications by Bloodwell et al in 1969. In spite of these shortcomings normothermic artery perfusion has contributed significantly to patient survival. However, one must recognize its limitations, and situations do occur in which effective myocardial protection cannot be achieved with coronary artery perfusion alone due to extensive coronary artery disease, forcible retraction of the heart, ventricular hypertrophy, or combinations of the three. In these instances additional measures must be employed, and these will be discussed later.

myocardium have been recognized both experimentally and clinically as a result of normothermic anoxic arrest (Burnett and Ashford, 1965; Stemmer et al, 1973; Ebert et al, 1962; Cooley et al, 1972; and Griepp et al, 1973).

"Stone Heart" or left ventricular rigor, unresponsive to resuscitation and defibrillation, has been found to occur after approximately 90 minutes of ischemic normothermic arrest in dogs. Interestingly, the *right ventricle* in these preparations remained flaccid and could be defibrillated. Damage was found in the mitochondria by ultrastructural studies. Left ventricular mitochondria were destroyed as rigor developed, but those in the right ventricle remained preserved after two hours of normothermic ischemic arrest (Armstrong et al, 1973). We also find that even limited periods of normothermic total cardiac ischemia (15 minutes) may introduce abnormalities in lactate metabolism and oxygen consumption that no degree of subsequent myocardial perfusion can correct (Isom et al, 1973, and Lajos et al, 1974). In contrast, experimental studies, as well as clinical experience, have shown that local cardiac hypothermia (15 to 20C) in conjunction with total ischemia provide some degree of myocardial protection for periods averaging up to 1.5 hours (Stemmer et al, 1974, and Griepp et al, 1973). Additionally, the use of intermittent periods of coronary perfusion as an adjunct to normothermic ischemic arrest is found to improve the histological appearance of the hearts so treated in contrast to those subjected to continuous ischemic arrest (Lajos et al, 1974; Stemmer et al, 1973; and Benzing et al, 1973).

ANOXIC NORMOTHERMIC CARDIAC ARREST

Anoxic normothermic cardiac arrest is held by some to be tolerated by the myocardium for limited periods of time (Bloodwell et al, 1969). Perhaps support for this thesis accumulated because postoperative survival of the patient has served in the past as our primary index for judging the adequacy of an operative procedure and its attendant perfusion. Patient survival figures have now stabilized at an acceptable level for most experienced cardiac surgery teams and the postoperative status of the myocardium itself is emerging as a very important index of operative success. Patients have undergone "successful" cardiac procedures only to become cardiac cripples due to a damaged myocardium (Iyengar et al, 1973). Serious structural and functional changes in the

CARDIAC MECHANISMS

Previously, some myocardial protection during cardiopulmonary bypass was felt to be afforded by induced fibrillation. Less myocardial oxygen consumption has been demonstrated during ventricular fibrillation in contrast to the beating, working heart, and an increased myocardial oxygen consumption during ventricular fibrillation has been found secondary to vasodilatation (McKeever et al, 1958; and Read et al, 1956).

Impairment of myocardial metabolism and function has been demonstrated experimentally during continuous ventricular fibrillation (Reis et al, 1967). Other studies have suggested that induced fibrillation diverts blood away from the subendocardial muscle layer. (Hottenrott et al, 1973). Further, this latter effect has been demonstrated to be of most significance when ventricular hypertrophy is present, a point of obvious clinical significance.

Blood flow to the subendocardial region is found to increase when the normal ventricle fibrillates spontaneously. In contrast, coronary artery blood is diverted away from the subendocardial layer of hypertrophied hearts during fibrillation and these hypertrophied hearts do not increase their oxygen consumption during fibrillation. (Isom et al, 1973). The vulnerability of the subendocardial myocardium of hypertrophied canine hearts to hypoxia was demonstrated by Iyengar in 1973.

Optimum myocardial perfusion of all layers is found when the heart is beating normally with empty ventricles, and coronary artery perfusion from the aortic root is uninterrupted.

PERFUSION TECHNIQUES FOR MYOCARDIAL PROTECTION

The foregoing suggests that several potentially adequate techniques of myocardial protection during cardiopulmonary bypass are available and that combinations may be even more beneficial. We have evolved three basic techniques for myocardial perfusion and protection during various bypass procedures as described below. These perfusion techniques are applicable to a variety of open cardiac procedures. However, their application to myocardial revascularization is emphasized here.

With these techniques, we maintain high normothermic corporeal flows and establish coronary artery perfusion either by individual cannulation of the coronary arteries or via selective perfusion of the aortic root. Selective cardiac hypothermia is suggested for those cases exhibiting compromised coronary arteries, ventricular hypertrophy, or procedures requiring forcible cadiac retraction that may impair coronary flow. Ventricular fibrillation is avoided except in those cases requiring unusually precise suturing that would be compromised by normal cardiac activity.

The basic perfusion is conducted with a Temptrol oxygenator and roller-type arterial pump. Flow rates of approximately 70 cc per kilogram per minute are maintained with a perfusate temperature of 37 C. The hemodilution prime is adjusted with dextrose 5 percent in one-half normal saline so that the hematocrit during perfusion is approximately 23 to 30 percent. (The average

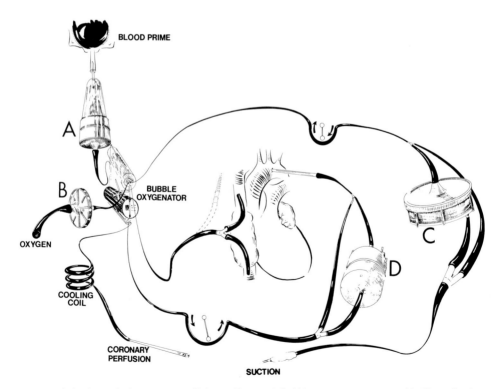

FIG. 1. A basic perfusion system utilizing a Temptrol bubble type oxygenator with filters in the arterial, coronary suction, oxygen, and blood prime lines. A. SWANK Transfusion Filter #IL-200, Pioneer Filters Inc., 4650 S.W. Pacific Avenue, Beaverton, Oregon, 97005. B. Pall Oxygen Filter, #ORDIH, Pall Corporation, Biomedical Products Division, Glen Cove, Long Island, New York, 11542. C. SWANK Coronary Suction Filter #CA-100. D. Barrier Arterial Filter #1320, Johnson and Johnson, New Brunswick, New Jersey, 08903.

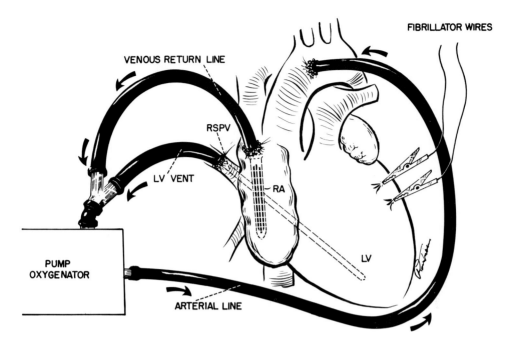

FIG. 2. System for normothermic perfusion of normal-sized hearts with good ventricular function.

preoperative hematocrit was 40 percent for the entire group, and it was 25 percent during the perfusion.)

Appropriate filters are used in the arterial line, the oxygen line, and the coronary suction line. The blood prime is filtered as it is introduced into the oxygenator (Fig. 1).

We have noted that our patients wake more quickly and have had virtually no postperfusion sensorial dullness since the introduction of a fully filtered, high-flow, hemodilution perfusion system. Additionally, less postperfusion pulmonary venoarterial shunting has followed the introduction of these systems.

For purposes of myocardial protection, the patients are divided into three categories.

1. Patients with normal-sized left ventricles of good function whose surgical procedure does not require opening the aortic root.
2. Patients with hypertrophied ventricles and/or compromised function whose surgical procedure does not require opening the aortic root.
3. Patients requiring opening of the aortic root.

We used the perfusion system as outlined in Figure 2 for patients in category 1. The venous return is obtained from the right atrium with a specially designed single multiple opening cannula (Figure 3), which leads to a 0.5-inch Mayon tubing venous return line. The 0.5-inch

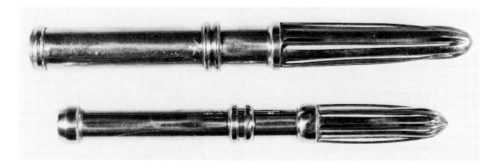

FIG. 3. Specially constructed right atrial cannulae for collection of venous return. The upper (adult) cannula is 14 cm long and is used with a half-inch venous return line. The lower (pediatric) cannula is 12 cm long and accepts three-eighths-inch venous return line.

diameter line provides a much more efficient siphon effect than the ⅜-inch line that we used previously and must be used if flows of 70 cc per kilogram are to be consistently obtained. The cannula is inserted via a purse-string suture in the right atrial appendage so that its tip lies just within the orifice of the inferior vena cava. A similar single right atrial catheter venous return collection system has also been used extensively by Sewell.

The left ventricle is vented with an L-shaped, size-20 French, Bardic catheter,* which is bent as shown in Figure 4 by autoclaving while taped to a strip of firm cardboard. The shape facilitates the insertion of the catheter with minimal displacement of the heart. This catheter is inserted through a purse string suture in the anterior surface of the right superior pulmonary vein and is then manipulated across the left atrium through the mitral valve to the tip of the left ventricle. The catheter is attached to a side arm of the 0.5-inch venous return line so that the siphon effect of this system is applied to the left ventricular chamber.

The highly efficient siphon effect of this system can almost totally remove the blood from the right atrium and only negligible amounts pass through the pulmonary circuit to be picked up by the left ventricular vent catheter. For example, in one group of 36 patients with an average systemic flow of 5,400 cc per minute, at a mean arterial pressure of 80 mm of mercury, the flow through the left ventricular vent catheter (as measured with the electromagnetic flowmeter) averaged only 175 cc per minute. Forcible retraction of the ventricles in a cephalad direction may compromise the position of the right atrial cannula so that increased blood flows through the pulmonary circuit to the left ventricle. We have measured up to 350 cc per minute through the vent under these conditions, and while not particularly harmful the increased flow can be ablated by slight repositioning of the retracted ventricles.

The properly positioned right atrial and left ventricular vent catheters in conjunction with strong siphonage from the 0.5-inch venous return line empty the heart almost completely, and the chambers often reveal the intracardiac vacuum by inversion of their walls. The cardiac mechanism becomes very gentle and relaxed, and one can perform anastomoses to the proximal right coronary artery and left anterior descending coro-

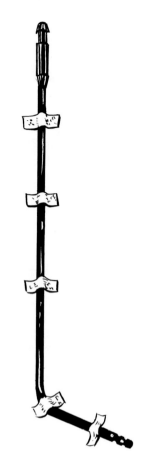

FIG. 4. The left ventricular vent catheter is shaped as shown by autoclaving while taped to a strip of firm cardboard.

nary artery without induced ventricular fibrillation although we often fibrillate normal-sized hearts that have good function. The surprising ease with which the empty and finely fibrillating heart can be moved about within the pericardium to provide exposure of the circumflex and posterior descending coronary arteries deserves special emphasis.

The heart is defibrillated following completion of the saphenous vein to coronary artery distal anastomoses, and the left ventricular vent is clamped when adequate cardiac activity has resumed. The patient is then, if possible, taken off cardiopulmonary bypass and the proximal saphenous vein anastomosed to an isolated segment of the anterior ascending aorta using a Beck clamp. The pump time is thus usually confined to that required for the saphenous vein coronary artery anastomoses. Should adequate

* C. R. Bard, Inc., Murray Hill, N.J.

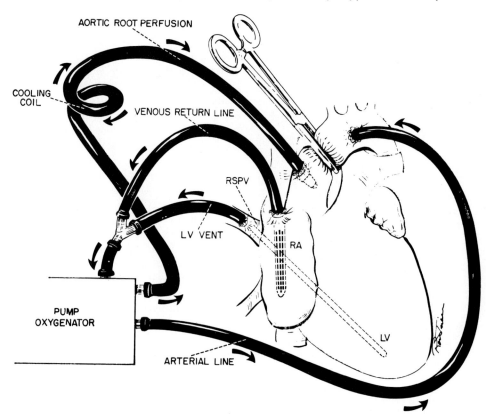

FIG. 5. Hypothermic perfusion system for enlarged hearts or those with compromised coronary circulation and/or impaired ventricular function. Cooled blood is introduced via the aortic root as indicated.

cardiac activity not immediately resume, the patient can remain on CPBP while the proximal anastomoses are completed and the left ventricular vent is unclamped to provide less load for the recovering ventricle. The aorta is never cross-clamped in this group, and normothermic perfusion of the coronary arteries remains undisturbed throughout the procedure. We have commonly used this technique in patients with normal-sized hearts and good ventricular function requiring myocardial revascularization and/or left ventricular aneurysmectomy.

Similar procedures are performed on patients with hypertrophied ventricles and/or compromised ventricular function with the technique depicted in Figure 5. This differs from the previous technique only in the addition of aortic root coronary artery perfusion with cooled blood. Cardiopulmonary bypass is instituted exactly as described previously and the aorta is then cross-clamped just proximal to the corporeal perfusion cannula as shown. A size-12 French Bardic catheter is then inserted through a small stab wound in the proxi-

mal aortic root and held in place with a single mattress suture. Care is taken to insert the catheter only far enough to cover the last side hole so that it does not cause aortic valvular insufficiency. The catheter is then perfused with cooled blood using a separate Sarns pump with flow adjusted to 300 cc per minute. We commonly cool to 28 to 30 C and the temperature is regulated by the num-

TABLE 1. Temperature of Aortic Root or Coronary Artery Perfusate as Related to Length of Tubing Immersed in Ice Slush and Flow Rate

INCHES OF 1/4" MAYON TUBING IN ICE	FLOW RATE (CC/MINUTE)					
	50	100	150	200	250	300
125	10C	17C	21C	23C	25C	26C
100	12C	19C	23C	25C	26C	28C
75	15C	22C	25C	26C	28C	30C

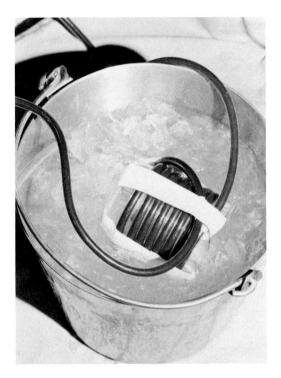

FIG. 6. The cooling coil is formed by wrapping a pre-selected length of one-fourth-inch Mayon tubing around a glass cylinder and immersing in ice slush.

ber of inches of ¼-inch Mayon tubing immersed in ice slush (Table 1, Figure 6). The perfusion pressure of the aortic root is constantly measured and averages 70 to 80 mm Hg at a flow of 300 cc per minute and a myocardial temperature of 28 C. The corporeal perfusion remains at 37 C. Should the aortic root be forcefully manipulated during perfusion, the aortic valve may become incompetent with loss of perfusion pressure, and the 300 cc flow may not be sufficient to immediately "seat" the aortic valve. This is easily corrected by slightly opening the aortic cross-clamp until the aortic root becomes "firm" and then reapplying it. The heart becomes cool within two to three minutes following cold perfusion and usually reaches the desired temperature in less than five minutes.

Myocardial activity diminishes markedly due to the lowered temperature in combination with the empty cardiac chambers and if fibrillation does not spontaneously occur it is possible to do many saphenous vein to coronary artery anastomoses without intentionally fibrillating the heart. This is, of course, preferred because of the undesirable effects of ventricular fibrillation in the presence of ventricular hypertrophy under perfusion conditions. The aortic cross-clamp is removed when the distal saphenous vein coronary artery

anastomoses are completed and the aortic root perfusion catheter is removed from the aorta. The Beck clamp can be placed as the catheter is withdrawn, and the catheter entry hole can be enlarged and used as a point of anastomosis for one of the saphenous vein grafts. Cardiac rewarming occurs rapidly when aortic root perfusion with normothermic corporeal blood ensues and defibrillation, if necessary, is performed when the cardiac temperature reaches 27 C. Bypass is discontinued when cardiac activity recovers adequately and the proximal aortic saphenous vein anastomoses are completed as previously described.

Patients whose procedure requires opening of the aortic root (aortic valve replacement in combination with coronary artery revascularization) are perfused with the system shown in Figure 7. Right atrial blood is collected as before with the special right atrial cannula in conjunction with a 0.5-inch diameter venous return line. The siphon-type left ventricular vent is not used, however, as air can enter the left ventricular cavity by way of the open aorta and might "air-lock" the venous return line. Left ventricular blood is therefore aspirated as shown with a separate sump type catheter introduced by way of the right superior pulmonary vein and attached coronary suction. The coronary artery orifices are cannulated separately, and each cannula * is perfused with a separate pump and monitored with an individual pressure gauge. Coronary perfusion blood passes through an appropriate length of 0.25-inch tubing immersed in ice slush to achieve the desired temperature, as indicated in Table 1. We try not to exceed a myocardial perfusion pressure of 100 mm of mercury. Coronary artery vascular resistance decreases during the procedure allowing adequate perfusion at lower pressures and flows. Lower coronary artery flows will produce still lower perfusate temperatures, as shown in Table 1, and myocardial protection remains adequate. Failure to diminish coronary artery perfusion flow as the resistance decreases in the hypothermic heart may result in overperfusion and intramyocardial hemorrhage. Precise, constant monitoring of the flows and pressures is essential.

Careful preoperative inspection of the coronary cineangiograms is mandatory if maximum myocardial perfusion and protection is to be provided. The left anterior descending coronary artery may arise very close to the origin of the main left coronary artery and be occluded by the normally

* Spencer-Malette Coronary Artery Perfusion Cannula, V. Mueller Co., 6600 W. Touhy Ave., Chicago, Ill.

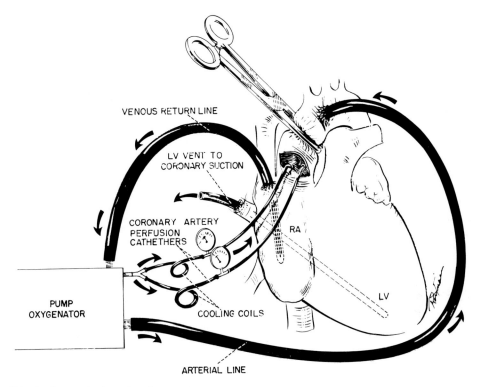

FIG. 7. System for hypothermic perfusion of the coronary arteries in procedures requiring an open aortic root.

placed coronary *perfusion* catheter.* Knowledge of this anatomy preoperatively has allowed us to perfuse both the circumflex and left anterior descending coronary arteries with separate catheters introduced through the same aortic ostium.

Should coronary artery disease or anatomy seem to obviate adequate perfusion even with the use of hypothermic blood, then one must consider the use of topical ice water lavage to prevent myocardial deterioration. Regardless, we feel that coronary artery perfusion, if possible, should be used in conjunction with the topical cooling. Griepp et al (1973) have, however, demonstrated what they feel is adequate myocardial protection with the use of topical hypothermia alone in both pediatric and adult patients.

Mitral valve replacement requires separate superior and inferior vena caval catheters due to the forcible anterior retraction of the right atrium utilized for mitral valve exposure via the midline sternotomy incision. This particular type of retraction can compromise the right atrial cannula and impair venous return to the pump oxygenator, and this is the only instance in which we have

encountered difficulty with the single metallic right atrial cannula. Myocardial cooling can, of course, be carried out with the previously described techniques regardless of the type of venous return collection system employed.

Valve replacement (aortic or mitral) is always completed prior to the revascularization procedure. We commonly come off bypass following the valve replacement to confirm good valve function and then go on partial bypass with left ventricular venting for the skip graft anastomoses using selective cardiac hypothermia when indicated.

We have used these techniques in over 100 cases of coronary artery revascularization, some in combination with ventricular aneurysmectomy, aortic valve replacement, or mitral valve replacement. There were three operative deaths in the series.

Only one patient has failed to come off bypass. This patient was in progressive, terminal left heart failure and was operated upon as a last effort at salvage. Severe triple-vessel disease was surgically repaired, but the postperfusion cardiac output was inadequate. Postmortem examination of the heart revealed extensive small-vessel disease. The other two patients had good cardiac output following bypass but succumbed to severe ven-

* Spencer-Malette Coronary Artery Perfusion Cannula, V. Mueller Co., 6600 W. Touhy Ave., Chicago, Ill.

tricular arrhythmias at three and five days post-operatively.

We have been most favorably impressed with the ease of coming off bypass and the absence of postperfusion cerebral and pulmonary morbidity experienced since these techniques of myocardial protection in combination with high-flow, hemodilution perfusion have been utilized.

ACKNOWLEDGMENTS

The assistance of Certified Perfusion Technicians Jane Calloway, Joe Womble, and Elvis Wright in the preparation of material for the manuscript is gratefully acknowledged by the authors.

References

1. Allardyce DB, Yoshida SH, Ashmore PG: The importance of microembolism in the pathogenesis of organ dysfunction caused by prolonged use of the pump oxygenator. J Thorac Cardiovasc Surg 52:706, 1966
2. Armstrong RG, Stanford W, Cline RE, Guillebeau J: The stone heart. Ann Thorac Surg 16:480, 1973
3. Bahnson HT, Spencer FC, Busse EFG, Davis FW: Cusp replacement and coronary artery perfusion in open operations on the aortic valve. Ann Surg 152:494, 1960
4. Benzing G, Stockert J, Nave E, Kaplan S: Intermittent myocardial ischemia during cardiopulmonary bypass. J Thorac Cardiovasc Surg 65:108, 1973
5. Bjock VO: Aortic valve replacement. Thorax 19:369, 1964
6. Bloodwell RD, Kidd JN, Hallman GL, et al: Cardiac valve replacement without coronary perfusion: clinical and laboratory observations. In Brewer LA (ed): Prosthetic Heart Valves. Springfield, Thomas, 1969, p 397
7. Braimbridge MV, Darracott S, Clement AJ, Bitensky L, Chayen, J: Myocardial deterioration during aortic valve replacement assessed by cellular biological tests. J Thorac Cardiovasc Surg 66:241, 1973
8. Burdette WJ, Ashford TP: Structural changes in the human myocardium following hypoxia. J Thorac Cardiovasc Surg 50:210, 1965
9. Cooley DA, Reul GL, Wukasch DC: Ischemic contracture of the heart: "stone heart." Am J Cardiol 29:575, 1972
10. Ebert PA, Greenfield LJ, Austin WG, Morrow AG: Experimental comparison of methods for protecting the heart during aortic occlusion. Ann Surg 155:25, 1962
11. Fuhrman GJ, Fuhrman FA, Field J: Metabolism of rat heart slices, with special reference to effects of temperature and anoxia. Am J Physiol 163:642, 1950
12. Gervin AS, McNeer JF, Wolfe WG, Puckett CL, Silver D: Ultrapore hemofiltration during extracorporeal circulation. J Thorac Cardiovasc Surg 67:237, 1974
13. Griepp RB, Stinson EB, Shumway NE: Profound local hypothermia for myocardial protection during open heart surgery. J Thorac Cardiovasc Surg 66:731, 1973
14. Heilbrunn A, Zimmerman JM: Coronary artery dissection: a complication of cannulation. J Thorac Cardiovasc Surg 49:767, 1965
15. Hewitt RL, Lolley DM, Adrouny GN, Drapanas T: Protective effect of glycogen and glucose on the anoxic arrested heart. Surgery 75:1, 1974
16. Hottenrott CE, Towers B, Kurkji HJ, Maloney JV, Buckberg G: Hazard of ventricular fibrillation In hypertrophied ventricles during cardiopulmonary bypass. J Thorac Cardiovasc Surg 66:742, 1973
17. Hurley EJ, Lower RR, Dong E, Pillsbury RC, Shumway, NE: Clinical experience with local hypothermia in elective cardiac arrest. J Thorac Cardiovasc Surg 47:50, 1964
18. Isom OW, Kuten ND, Falk EA, Spencer FC: Patterns of myocardial metabolism during cardiopulmonary bypass and coronary perfusion. J Thorac Cardiovasc Surg 66:705, 1973
19. Iyengar SRK, Ramchand S, Charrette EJP, Iyengar CKS, Lynn RB: Anoxic cardiac arrest: an experimental and clinical study of its effects. Part I. J Thorac Cardiovasc Surg 66:722, 1973
20. Kay E, Head LR, Nagueira C: Direct coronary artery perfusion for aortic valve surgery. JAMA 168:1767, 1958
21. Kessler J, Patterson R: The production of microemboli by various blood oxygenators. Ann Thorac Surg 9:221, 1970
22. Kottmeier CA, Wheat MW: Ultrastructural evaluation of myocardial preservation during cardiopulmonary bypass: the mitochondrion. J Thorac Cardiovasc Surg 52:786, 1966
23. Lajos TF, Cerra FB, Montes M, Seigel, JH: A permanent experimental model for reversible myocardial anoxia. Ann Thorac Surg 17:20, 1974
24. Lillehei CW, Bonnabeau RC Jr, Levy MJ: Surgical correction of aortic and mitral valve disease by total valve replacement. Geriatrics 19:240, 1964
25. Littlefield JB, Lowicki EM, Muller WH Jr: Experimental left coronary artery perfusion through an aortotomy during cardiopulmonary bypass. J Thorac Cardiovasc Surg 40:685, 1960
26. Lower RR, Stofer RC, Hurley EJ, et al: Successful homotransplantation of the canine heart after anoxic preservation for seven hours. Am J Surg 104:302, 1962
27. McKeever LP, Gregg DE, Canney PC: Oxygen uptake of the nonworking left ventricle. Circ Res 6:612, 1958
28. Ramsey HW, de la Torre A, Linhart JW, Wheat MW: Complications of coronary artery perfusion. J Thorac Cardiovasc Surg 54:714, 1967
29. Read RC, Johnson JA, Lillehei CW: Coronary flow and resistance in the dog during total body perfusion. Surg Forum 7:286, 1956
30. Reis RL, Cohn LH, Morrow AG: Effects of induced ventricular fibrillation on ventricular performance and cardiac metabolism. J Thorac Cardiovasc Surg (Suppl I) 35:I–234, 1967
31. Robisek F, Tam W, Daugherty HK, Mullen DC: Myocardial protection during open heart surgery. Ann Thorac Surg 10:340, 1970
32. Sewell WH: Personal Communication
33. Stemmer EA, McCart P, Stanton WW Jr, et al: Functional and structural alterations in the myocardium during aortic cross-clamping. J Thorac Cardiovasc Surg 66:754, 1973

53

PERFUSION DURING AORTOCORONARY BYPASS GRAFT SURGERY

Charles C. Reed, Robert M. Keenan, Diane K. Clark, Denton A. Cooley, and Arthur S. Keats

The question of what constitutes adequate perfusion has been debated since the Azygos flow principle was described by Andreasen and Watson in 1951.[1] Twenty years of experience has not resolved such basic questions as optimal perfusion rates or pressures,[2,3,4,5,6] the need for general or local hypothermia,[7,8] the need for coronary perfusion,[9] or the degree of acceptable hemodilution.[10,11,2,12] In addition, advancing technology presents new questions such as the need for in-line filters and the merit of pulsatile flow. In an attempt to assess the critical nature of some of these questions, a review of the perfusion characteristics of patients undergoing coronary artery bypass graft surgery during a 22-month period was undertaken.

MATERIALS AND METHODS

Between January 1, 1972, and October 31, 1973, a total of 1,809 patients underwent coronary artery bypass graft surgery. Altogether, these patients had 4,132 saphenous vein bypass grafts from the ascending aorta to the distal coronary arteries. The group included patients who had valve replacement or resection of left ventricular aneurysm in addition to coronary artery bypass. All patients were perfused through the ascending aorta or femoral artery using a roller pump and a disposable bubble oxygenator. Carbon dioxide in oxygen was the oxygenating gas, and no volatile anesthetic was administered during cardiopulmonary bypass. Extracorporeal filtration was utilized only in the cardiotomy return line. Five percent dextrose in lactated Ringer's (20 ml/kg) was the only solution used to prime the perfusion circuit. Heparin 25 mg/l was added to the prime, and 3 mg/kg was administered to the patients.

Flow rates were maintained optimally between 40 and 60 ml/kg/min with 35 ml/kg/min as the minimum acceptable perfusion rate. Decompression of the left ventricle was accomplished by a left atrial vent. Moderate (30 to 32 C esophageal) systemic hypothermia was induced by extracorporeal cooling at the onset of bypass, and the myocardium was cooled topically with saline slush. Ischemic arrest was then instituted by clamping the ascending aorta. Perfusion was terminated as early as possible after the aortic clamp was released after surgical repair, and heparin was reversed with protamine sulfate as soon as venous and aortic cannulae were removed.

RESULTS

Deaths within 30 days after operation of these 1,809 consecutive patients was 5.8 percent (Table 1). There was so significant difference in mortality in any of the subgroups by number of

TABLE 1. Coronary Artery Saphenous Vein Bypass Operations (1/1/72 to 10/31/73)

NO. SAPHENOUS GRAFTS	NO. PTS.	EARLY DEATHS*	% MORTALITY
1	287	20	6.9
2	772	39	5.1
3	701	43	6.1
4	47	3	6.3
5	2	0	0
Total	1,809	105	5.8

*Death within thirty days.

saphenous grafts, nor was the mortality different in the subgroup of 144 patients who had coronary endarterectomy in addition to coronary artery bypass (5.6 percent mortality). We were unable to relate any perfusion characteristics to mortality. Survivor and nonsurvivor groups were similar in mean and range values of perfusion rate (Table 2), urine output, degree of hemodilution (Table 3), and ischemic arrest time (Table 4) (p > 0.05).

DISCUSSION

Perfusion Pressure

For most of the bypass period in all patients, perfusion flow ranged between 40 and 60 ml/kg/min, and at this flow rate, arterial pressures measured in the radial artery ranged between 40 and 60 mm Hg. Not rarely, perfusion pressure approached and at times exceeded 100 mm Hg without apparent cause especially toward the end of the bypass period. When approaching 90 mm Hg, treatment was instituted to avoid excessive back bleeding into the heart and additional blood trauma by a high flow through the coronary return system. Hypertensive perfusion always responded transiently to trimetaphan (Arfonad) or isoproterenol (Isuprel) and less reliably to phentolamine (Regitine). For a longer effect, chlorpromazine (Thorazine) was usually effective.

Excessively low perfusion pressure was usually associated with low perfusion rate and most commonly occurred at the onset of bypass. The commonest cause of low perfusion rates was inadequate venous return from malposition of the caval catheters. If adjustment of caval catheters and lowering the blood reservoir level in the oxygenator failed to provide adequate flow, additional lactated Ringer's was added to the oxygenator and the volume translocated to the intravascular compartment to provide increased venous return. At times 5 to 6 liters of electrolyte solution representing the sum of prime volume, administered by intravenous solution, and added prime were required to achieve satisfactory flow rates.

High perfusion rates per se obviously do not necessarily indicate high tissue perfusion. Rates in excess of 80 to 100 ml/kg/min may simply represent arterial-venous shunting as in tetralogy of Fallot. Even in the absence of such obvious shunting, there is no assurance that high pump flow rates lead to high perfusion of organs requiring high flow by virtue of sensitivity to oxygen lack. Indeed the converse is possible. We have been

TABLE 2. Comparison of Perfusion Rate in Survivors and Nonsurvivors of Coronary Bypass Operations

	SURVIVORS	NONSURVIVORS*
Perfusion rate (ml/Kg/min)	47.2	46.9
Range	30–112	30–67
SEM	±0.22	±1.0
Number of patients	1,707	102

Within 30 days of operation.

TABLE 3. Comparison of Hematocrit Values and Urine Output in Survivors and Nonsurvivors of Coronary Bypass Operation (Mean and Range)

	SURVIVORS	NONSURVIVORS
Preoperative Hematocrit	43.7 (33.3–54.6)	42.3 (22.2–51.6)
Hematocrit during bypass	24.5 (15–36.9)	23.7 (15.6–35.7)
Urine output during bypass	264 ml (0–1270)	286 ml (0–1600)

TABLE 4. Comparison of Ischemic Arrest Time in Survivors and Nonsurvivors of Coronary Bypass Operation

	SURVIVORS	NONSURVIVORS
Ischemic time (minutes)	48.6	60.9
Range	16–122	17–122
SEM	±0.39	±1.9

unable to correlate postoperative neurological defects (slow awakening, delirium, or neurological deficit) with low perfusion flows or pressures except in a few exceptional circumstances. Shumway's group [8] reported excellent results with perfusion rates of 35 ml/kg/min, as have Zudhi and associates [13] with perfusion rates not exceeding 20 ml/kg/min; both used moderate systemic hypothermia. At the flow rates used in our patients, the output of urine was steady during bypass without the addition of mannitol or diuretics, but only in response to the large water load provided before and during bypass. Urine production was approximately 250 ml during one hour of perfusion (Table 3).

Hemodilution

With the increasing shortage of stored blood and the rising incidence of hepatitis after blood transfusion, in one report, with as high as 51 percent of patients undergoing open-heart surgery,[14] hemodilution as a means of blood conservation assumes an even more appealing aspect. Added advantages include the lower resistance to flow of low hematocrit blood, suggesting better capillary and tissue perfusion and the capability of operating upon patients whose religious beliefs preclude blood transfusion. Hematocrit values as low as 15 were observed during bypass in our patients, and this value was considered our lowest acceptable degree of hemodilution. This dilution to less than half normal was not associated with postoperative coagulation problems, water intoxication, or congestive failure from excessive electrolyte solution. The excess water was rapidly diuresed early in the postbypass period particularly if furosemide (Lasix) in 20 to 40 mg doses was given at the end of operation. The mean hematocrit during bypass in our patients was 24.5 percent which represented a 56.1 percent reduction from preoperative values.

Ischemic Arrest

Ischemic arrest was achieved by clamping the ascending aorta after core cooling to 30 C esophageal and topical cooling the myocardium with saline slush. Although mean ischemia time was 12 minutes longer in the nonsurvivor group (Table 4), this difference was not significant (p < 0.05). Ischemic arrest for up to 122 minutes was tolerated by these patients, as indicated by postoperative mortality (Table 4). Griepp and Shumway[8] however reported aortic cross-clamp times from 21 to 138 minutes in a similar group of patients and could not relate cross-clamp time to mortality, requirement for postoperative inotropic support, duration of postoperative ventilation, duration of intensive care, or hospital stay. Reul et al[15] in a study of 493 coronary bypass patients concluded that fatal myocardial complications were related to preexisting disease rather than duration of aortic occlusion or ischemic arrest. Coronary perfusion was not used in our patients because of its attendant complications including myocardial hemorrhage, coronary artery dissection, dislodgement of arteriosclerotic material, and myocardial infarction. Similarly, continuous prolonged electrical fibrillation was not used because of possible subendocardial hemorrhagic necrosis.[16] Ischemic contracture of the heart ("Stone Heart")[17] was not observed in this group of patients.

Hypothermia

Rapid cooling was begun as soon as bypass was instituted by a venous line heat exchanger and a 4 C cooling reservoir.[18] Cooling to an esophageal temperature of 30 C required about 5 to 15 minutes, and neither serious arrhythmias nor hypotension appeared during this relatively rapid cooling. Cooling rates seldom exceeded 1 C per minute. On rewarming, the water temperature in the reservoir was never allowed to exceed 42 C, with a resulting blood-water temperature gradient of not more than 12 C, and in most instances the gradient was less than 8 C owing to the cooling effect of the blood on the water in the warming reservoir.

Filters

A depth-type dacron wool filter* was employed in the cardiotomy return line. Since the major portion of blood trauma occurred in the coronary suction system, which also returns most of the biological debris to the circuit, filtration in this subsystem was considered mandatory. We selected the depth-type filter because it is more effective in removing this biological debris than is the grid-type filter.[19]

We have not used arterial line filtration because of our concern for further blood trauma by passing fragile erythrocytes at high velocities through small apertures. Plasma hemoglobin determinations do not reflect sublethal damage and subsequent short life spans of those injured, but still viable, erythrocytes.[20]

Oxygenators

Six different bubble oxygenators were used in this group of patients: Travenol, Rygg, an experimental bag type, Bentley, Harvey, and Galen. Mortality in our patients was not related in any way to the type of oxygenator used. Each oxygenator was satisfactory when employed in a manner that recognized its individual operating

---

* Pioneer Filters, Incorporated, Beaverton, Ore.

characteristics and limitations. For example, one was extremely efficient in CO_2 removal while another tended to retain CO_2 and still another was slower in rewarming capacity. One oxygenator may well appear to be inferior in performance when operated under conditions most suitable for another oxygenator. For example, we found that the optimal blood to gas flow ratio was higher when using the Bentley oxygenator, lower in the Travenol, and lowest in the Harvey when maintaining an arterial PO_2 between 100 and 200 mm Hg as the criterion. The Bentley would certainly appear to be grossly unsatisfactory in oxygenating capacity if it were operated with the Harvey blood to gas flow ratio.

Some of the problems encountered at times during this study apart from the specific individual operating characteristics include the following: inadequate oxygenating capacity (even at blood flow rates less than 5 liters/min) of all the oxygenators used, inadequate defoaming capability in all except the Rygg and Travenol, blood-to-air leaks in all oxygenators, fibrin and frank clot formation despite adequate heparinization in all oxygenators, and inadequate rewarming capacity in the Bentley. Floating particulate matter in several of the oxygenators prompted our investigation of particulate contamination. Average particulate contamination as high as 130,000 particles larger than 20 micron per oxygenator was demonstrated in oxygenators as received from the manufacturer. As a result of these findings, each oxygenator is now rinsed and the prime filtered through a 5 micron filter * prior to use.

Although we found no correlation between mortality from operation and any perfusion characteristics reviewed, we recognize the limitations of such data. A careful review of morbidity, more detailed analysis of the course of perfusion, as well as details of surgical technique and postoperative care, might enable us to identify complications ascribable to perfusion alone. In the absence of such detailed information and from the absence of gross correlations in this study, we believe the perfusion systems and techniques described are safe and effective.

SUMMARY

We have reviewed the perfusion characteristics of 1,809 consecutive patients undergoing cardiopulmonary bypass for aortocoronary bypass graft surgery. We could not correlate mortality in

* Millipore Corporation, Bedford, Mass.

this group with duration of ischemic arrest, degree of hemodilution, urine output, perfusion rates, perfusion pressures, or oxygenators used. Based on this experience our criteria for adequate perfusion of these patients include perfusion rates of 40 to 60 ml/kg/min, perfusion pressure between 40 and 60 mm Hg, acceptable arterial and venous blood gas values, some urinary output, and the presence of EEG activity.

References

1. Andreasen, AT, Watson F: Experimental cardiovascular surgery. Br J Surg 39:548, 1951–52
2. Wilson HE, Dalton ML, Kiphart RJ, Allison WM: Increased safety of aorto-coronary bypass surgery with induced ventricular fibrillation to avoid anoxia. J Thorac Cardiovasc Surg vol 64 2:193, 1972
3. Kilman JW, Williams TE Jr, Kakos GS, Craenan J, Hosier DM: Surgical correction of the transposition complex in infancy. J Thorac Cardiovasc Surg vol 66 3:387, 1973
4. DeWall RA, Lillehei RC, Sellers RD: Hemodilution perfusions for open-heart surgery: use of five percent dextrose in water for the priming volume. N Engl J Med vol 266 21:1078, 1962
5. Zuhdi N, McCollough B, Carey J, Krieger C, Greer A: Hypothermic Perfusion for Open-Heart Surgical Procedures. J Int Coll Surg vol 35 3:319, 1961
6. Cooley DA, Beall AC Jr, Grondin P: Open-heart operations with disposable oxygenators: five percent dextrose prime and normothermia. Surgery 52:713, 1962
7. Stemmer EA, McCart P, Stanton WW Jr, Thibault W, Dearden LS, Connolly JC: Functional and structural alterations in the myocardium during aortic crossclamping. J Thorac Cardiovasc Surg vol 66 5:754, 1973
8. Griepp RB, Stinson EB, Shumway NE: Profound local hypothermia for myocardial protection during open-heart surgery. J Thorac Cardiovasc Surg vol 66 5:731, 1973
9. Isom OW, Kutin ND, Falk EA, Spencer FC: Patterns of myocardial metabolism during cardiopulmonary bypass and coronary perfusion. J Thorac Cardiovasc Surg vol 66 5:705, 1973
10. Hirsch DM, Hadidian C, Neville WE: Oxygen consumption during cardiopulmonary bypass with large volume hemodilution. J Thorac Cardiovasc Surg vol 56 2:197, 1968
11. Cruz AB Jr, Callaghan JC: Hemodilution in extracorporeal circulation: large or small non-blood prime? J Thorac Cardiovasc Surg vol 52 5:690, 1966
12. Miyauchi Y, Inoue T, Paton BC: Comparative study of priming fluids for two-hour hemodilution perfusion. J Thorac Cardiovasc Surg vol 52 3:413, 1966
13. Zuhdi N, Carey J, Greer A: Hemodilution for body perfusion. J Okla Med Assn 56:88, 1963
14. Walsh JH, Purcell RH, Morrow AG, Chanock RM, Schmidt PJ: Posttransfusion hepatitis after open-heart operations. JAMA 211:261, 1970
15. Reul GJ, Morris GC Jr, Howell JF, Crawford ES, Sandiford FM, Wukasch DC: The safety of ischemic cardiac arrest in distal coronary artery bypass. J Thorac Cardiovasc Surg vol 62 4:511, 1971
16. Najafi H, Henson D, Dye WS, Javid H, Hunter JA, Callaghan R, Eisenstein R, Julian OC: Left ventricular hemorrhagic necrosis. Ann Thorac Surg vol 7 6:550, 1969

17. Cooley DA, Reul GJ, Wukasch DC: Ischemic contracture of the heart: "stone heart." Am J Cardiol 29:575, 1972

18. Reed CC, Phillips PA, Coleman PA, Clark DK, Cooley DA: A disposable heat exchanger for normothermia and hypothermia: initial evaluation and utilization in avoiding ischemic contracture of the heart (stone heart). The Le J vol 1 1:4, 1972

19. Reed CC, Milam JD, Clark D, Wukasch DC, Sandiford FM, Hallman GL, Cooley DA: A comparative hematological study of the barrier and swank extracorporeal blood filter. AmSECT Proceedings 1:36–40, 1973

20. Bernstein EF, Indeglia RA, Shea MA, Varco RL: Sublethal damage to the red blood cell from pumping. Cardiovasc Surg 35–36:226, 1967

54

A SIMPLE METHOD OF PRODUCING PULSATILE FLOW DURING CLINICAL CARDIOPULMONARY BYPASS USING INTRAAORTIC BALLOON PUMPING

George Pappas, Peter P. Steele,
and Bruce C. Paton

The advantages of pulsatile over nonpulsatile flow for isolated organ and total body perfusion have been documented (Dalton et al, 1965; German et al, 1972; Jacobs et al, 1969; Mandelbaum and Burns, 1965; Many et al, 1968; Mukherjee et al, 1973; Nakayama et al, 1963; Ogata et al, 1960; Paquet, 1969; Shepard and Kirklin, 1969; Trinkle et al, 1970). Current pulsatile pumps have had little clinical use during cardiopulmonary bypass (CPB) because of complexity, unreliability, hazards, low output, high line pressures, and hemolysis (Trinkle et al, 1969). The standard roller pump, which produces a nonpulsatile flow, has provided an acceptable form of pumping as attested by its wide clinical applicability. Adverse effects have been described with its use, however, especially after prolonged procedures (Hultgren et al, 1973). Because of the multiple advantages of pulsatile over nonpulsatile flow, a continued search for a simple and reliable method of pulsatile flow during cardiopulmonary bypass is needed.

Intraaortic balloon pumping (IABP) is used with increasing frequency in patients with cardiogenic shock (Kantrowitz et al, 1968; Scheidt et al, 1973) and following cardiopulmonary bypass (Buckley et al, 1973). Clinical use of IABP during CPB to convert a nonpulsatile roller pump flow to a pulsatile flow is described. The details of clinical and biochemical results and changes as well as a comparison between nonpulsatile and pulsatile flow forms the basis of this report.

METHODS AND MATERIALS

On May 8, 1973, a patient who had an acute myocardial infarction, in cardiogenic shock, required IAPB and mitral valve replacement. It was decided at the time to continue balloon pumping while on CPB. The arterial pressure tracing demonstrated a pulsatile wave produced by balloon pumping (Fig. 1). Since then a total of 33 patients were subjected to this form of pusatile flow during CPB.

Balloon Insertion

The AVCO * intraaortic balloon pump was used in all patients. The balloon can be inserted into the common femoral artery or distal ascending aorta. The latter approach is simple and can avoid injury to the abdominal aorta or its branches, especially in the presence of aneurysmal or obliterative disease of these vessels. The balloon can be activated at any time in fragile patients, without the need of supportive drugs, with their potential hazards. Standard cannulation for cardiopulmonary bypass can be accomplished even with the balloon inserted into the ascending aorta. The area required on the ascending aorta for inserting the balloon is relatively small. For coronary artery surgery requiring multiple vein grafts with a short ascending aorta, the balloon can then be inserted via a femoral artery. Intraarterial pressure monitoring from the left radial artery is preferred. The desired position of the balloon is in the descending thoracic aorta. Monitoring the left radial artery will insure the position of the balloon. With mechanical interference in the radial arterial trace, the balloon should be advanced down the descending thoracic aorta until a clean arterial tracing is obtained. Prior to cardiopulmonary bypass, the balloon volume is reduced to one half

* Hoffman-LaRoche, Inc., Cranbury, N.J.

FIG. 1. Radial artery pressure tracing with pulsatile and nonpulsatile flows during cardiopulmonary bypass and intraaortic balloon support.

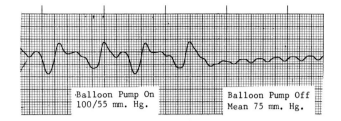

to allow adequate flow around the balloon. It is conceivable that a fully inflated balloon may produce undue obstruction at the balloon site resulting in high line pressure, hemolysis, and trauma to the aorta. To ensure that undue obstruction is not present, arterial pump line pressure should be measured. With excessively high pressures, the balloon volume should be reduced further. Balloon inflation and deflation controls on the AVCO pump can be adjusted to produce a normal-appearing arterial pulse tracing.

BALLOON PUMP ACTIVATION.   Triggering of the balloon pump can be achieved in two ways: (1) The patient's ECG can provide diastolic augmentation while on CPB. This can be done in instances when the heart rate and rhythm is reasonable to allow proper synchronous balloon pumping. (2) External fixed pacing is provided by attaching two additional limb electrodes to a pacemaker pack (Fig. 2). Fixed pacing at any predetermined rate can be used in the event of arrhythmias or bradycardia or during

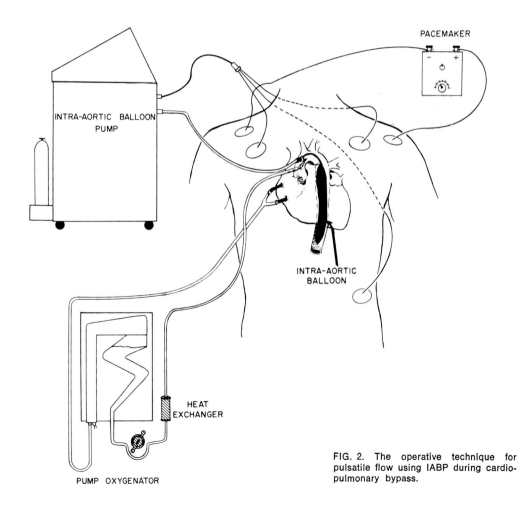

FIG. 2. The operative technique for pulsatile flow using IABP during cardiopulmonary bypass.

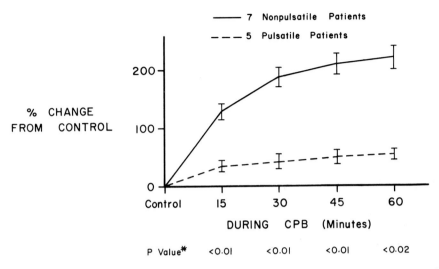

FIG. 3. Changes in coronary sinus lactates in patients having nonpulsatile and pulsatile flow during cardiopulmonary bypass.
* Student's t-test comparing nonpulsatile to pulsatile flow values.

ventricular fibrillation (often desired in coronary artery surgery). The conversion of diastolic augmentation to and from fixed pacing can be done with ease, depending upon the particular circumstance. Diastolic augmentation is preferred while the heart is beating since coronary perfusion is most physiologic at this time.

Weaning from CPB. After completion of the cardiac procedure, diastolic augmentation is used to support the heart and other vital organs while weaning the patient from CPB. During cessation of CPB this technique has provided an

important form of mechanical assist without the need of supportive drugs with their potential hazards: arrhythmia, possible myocardial necrosis (Leszkovszky and Gal, 1967), and local platelet aggregation (Mustard and Packham, 1972). Whenever hemodynamics become stable, the balloon can be removed following decannulation. If hemodynamics are unstable or the patient is in cardiogenic shock, mechanical support with return of the balloon to its full volume can be continued. Continued support via a femoral artery is preferred. If peripheral routes are impossible or haz-

TABLE 1. Changes in Total LDH in Patients Having Nonpulsatile and Pulsatile Flow during Cardiopulmonary Bypass (CPB)

	BEFORE CPB control	1 HR on CPB	1 HR off CPB	4 HR off CPB	1 DAY po	4 DAYS po	7 DAYS po
Nonpulsatile flow (10 patients)							
Mean[a]	70	121	166	203	228	194	103
SEM	6	19	18	22	45	44	14
Percent change from control	–	+87	+137	+190	+229	+177	+48
Pulsatile flow (16 patients)							
Mean[a]	69	87	113	142	121	121	136
SEM	13	24	10	11	14	21	29
Percent change from control	–	+26	+65	+107	+75	+75	+97
P values[b]	–	<0.05	<0.02	<0.05	<0.05	–	–

[a] Total LDH (IU/L).
[b] Student's t-test comparing patients with nonpulsatile and pulsatile flow.

TABLE 2. Changes in SGOT in Patients Having Nonpulsatile and Pulsatile Flow during Cardiopulmonary Bypass (CPB)

	BEFORE CPB (Control)	FOLLOWING CPB			
		4 hr	1 day	4 days	7 days
Nonpulsatile flow (7 patients)					
Mean[a]	11.7	72.5	132.7	88.0	29.6
SEM	2.1	66.1	190.1	156.5	18.4
Percent change from control	–	–38	+1,034	+652	+154
Pulsatile flow (16 patients)					
Mean[a]	20.2	36.1	31.5	23.0	19.8
SEM	18.1	18.2	16.3	11.9	7.6
Percent change from control	–	+80	+60	+15	–5
P values[b]	–	–	–	<0.01	–

[a] SGOT (IU/L).
[b] Student's t-test comparing patients with nonpulsatile and pulsatile flow.

ardous, however, support via the ascending aorta is conceivable and the balloon can be removed at a later date when the patient is stable. If such a route is the only source available, a woven 10-mm dacron graft can be sewn to the ascending aorta. The balloon catheter inside the graft can be tunneled subcutaneously and hemostasis controlled at this area by ligating the graft over the catheter. Subsequent removal can be achieved under local anesthesia with ligation of the graft.

Biochemical Studies. CORONARY SINUS LACTATE STUDIES. A coronary sinus catheter was inserted prior to instituting CPB. Samples were drawn before CPB (control) and at 15, 30, 45, and 60 minutes during CPB. Lactate determinations were made according to the method of SIGMA Chemical Co., St. Louis, Mo. Determinations were made in five pulsatile flow patients and seven nonpulsatile flow patients (Fig. 3).

TOTAL LDH. Total lactic dehydrogenase was determined before, during (one hour on), and following CPB (one hour, four hours, one day, four days, and seven days). Sixteen pulsatile flow patients were compared with 10 nonpulsatile patients (Table 1).

LIVER FUNCTION STUDIES. SGOT (Serum glutamic oxalic transaminase), alkaline phosphatase, and serum bilirubin determinations were drawn before CPB (control), four hours off CPB and at one, four, and seven days postoperatively. Seven nonpulsatile flow patients were compared to 16 pulsatile flow patients (Table 2).

MISCELLANEOUS STUDIES. Plasma hemoglobins were determined before and immediately following CPB.

Patient Material. LOW-RISK PATIENTS. There were 11 low-risk patients requiring single-vein bypass (six patients), double coronary artery bypass (four), and mitral valve replacement (one).

HIGH-RISK PATIENTS. Twenty-two high-risk patients are listed in Table 3. Some in this category may be questioned as high risks. How-

TABLE 3. "High-Risk" Patients Having Pulsatile Flow during CPB Using IABP

CARDIAC DISEASE TREATED	NO. PTS.
Acute MI, CGS, VSD	1
Acute MI, CGS, mitral insufficiency	2
Left main coronary disease	
Triple CAB	2
Triple CAB with LVEF 36 percent	1
Double CAB	1
LV aneurysmectomy (failure, no angina)	3
Preinfarction angina	
Double CAB	2
Prinzmetal's angina	
Double CAB	1
Triple CAB	3
Double CAB with severe LV failure	2
Prolonged CPB	
AVR, MVR (X2)	1
MVR (X2)	1
AVR, acute renal failure	1
MVR, giant LA	1
Total	22

MI: myocardial infarction; CGS: cardiogenic shock; VSD: ventricular septal defect: CAB: coronary artery bypass: AVR: aortic valve replacement: MVR: mitral valve replacement; LV: left ventricle; CPB: cardiopulmonary bypass; LA: left atrium.

TABLE 4. Changes in LV Ejection Fractions in Coronary Artery Bypass Patients with Nonpulsatile and Pulsatile Flow during CPB

	LEFT VENTRICULAR EJECTION FRACTION (%)			
	Preop Control[a]		Postop (Radioisotope)	
	LV Cine	Radioisotope	1 day	10 days $\pm$ 2
Nonpulsatile flow (20 patients)				
Mean $\pm$ SEM	46.1 $\pm$ 4.2	52.2 $\pm$ 2.9	38.7 $\pm$ 3.2	43.0 $\pm$ 3.4
P values[b]	–	–	$<$0.05	NS
Percent change from control	–	0	–26	–18
Pulsatile flow (19 patients)				
Mean $\pm$ SEM	52.2	51.2 $\pm$ 3.1	61.8 $\pm$ 3.5	66 $\pm$ 3.1
P value[b]	–	–	$<$0.05	$<$0.01
Percent change from control	–	–	+21	+29
P value[c]	–	–	$<$0.001	$<$0.001

[a] $r = 0.86$; $P < 0.001$ for correlation LVEF from cineangiography with LVEF from radioisotope (N = 26). Regression equation is $Y = 0.77x + 13$.
[b] Student's t-test, P value comparing with control radioisotope technique.
[c] Student's t-test, P value comparing radioisotope technique between pulsatile and nonpulsatile flow patients.

ever, we and our cardiologists felt that these patients had a potentially high operative mortality rate. Two patients requiring valve replacement had unusually long cardiopulmonary bypass. One required an aortic valve replacement (stented homograft) and a Yacoub mitral homograft (which appeared malfunctional), and the latter was removed and replaced with a prosthetic valve. The total CPB time was nearly six hours. A similar problem in the mitral region was encountered in another patient requiring three hours of CPB. Another aortic valve patient had an inadvertently contaminated fresh homograft (Candida albicans) inserted. The patient was treated with Amphotericin-B for two weeks with secondary acute renal failure. It was elected to use pulsatile flow during reoperation on the aortic valve in an effort to protect the kidneys from further injury during CPB.

Hemodynamic Studies. Left ventricular ejection fractions (LVEF percent) were measured in coronary artery bypass procedures in 19 patients by radioactive Indium (In[113m]) and precordial counting before operation and at one and 10 $\pm$ two days postoperatively (Table 4). Determining LVEF using this radioisotope technique and a single scintillation probe correlates well (r: 0.90; p < 0.001; n: 67) with values obtained by cineangiography (Steele et al). A comparable group of pulsatile flow (PF) and nonpulsatile flow (NPF) coronary artery surgical patients were studied (Table 5).

TABLE 5. Left Ventricular Ejection Fraction Patient Data

	NONPULSATILE	PULSATILE
Number of patients	20	19
Number of grafts		
Single	3	6
Double	13	9
Triple	4	4
Total	41	36
Preop MI	14	12
Preinfarction angina	3	3
Left main disease	3	3
Preop arrhythmia and angina	1	1
Deaths	1[a]	0

[a] Died three days postop from an arrhythmia whose surgery was for arrhythmia and angina.

RESULTS

Clinical Results

Of the 33 patients having pulsatile flow, only one early death (3 percent) occurred. This patient was treated for acute myocardial infarction, cardiogenic shock, and mitral insufficiency. IABP was required before and continued during cardiac catheterization. The patient had severe mitral valve insufficiency secondary to acute papillary muscle dysfunction that required mitral replacement. IABP was discontinued three days postoperatively. The patient was ambulating and died of an arrhythmia 16 days postoperatively. The remaining patients left the hospital and have been clinically improved. One patient who required aortic and two mitral valve replacements (mechanical failure occurred in the first mitral) had an unusually long period of CPB and IABP (six hours). The patient had an uneventful postoperative period without impairment of cerebral, hepatic, or renal function. Serial determinations of BUN, creatinine, SGOT, alkaline phosphatase, LDH, and LDH isoenzymes were within normal limits.

No supportive drugs were needed in our patients during or following operation. Temporary IABP (two to three days) was required in two patients postoperatively. Both of these patients were treated for acute myocardial infarction (papillary muscle dysfunction), cardiogenic shock, and severe mitral insufficiency. Except for these two, postoperative low cardiac output syndrome was not observed. During the first 24 hours postoperative, urinary output did not fall below 30 cc/hr and diuretics were not needed. Prior to use of the IABP and CPB, 20 to 30 percent of a comparable group of patients did develop various levels of low cardiac output syndrome requiring diuretics and/or supportive drugs.

Pulsatile flow was used in another patient with acute renal failure (BUN 120 mg. percent, creatinine 6.0 mg percent) secondary to a two-week course of Amphotericin-B therapy. Intraoperative cultures of a directly sewn aortic homograft grew Candida albicans. Following antibiotic therapy, the homograft was removed in the face of acute renal failure. Pulsatile flow was used to avoid further jeopardizing renal function. During and following operation, the patient had a brisk diuresis, and renal function returned to normal within 10 days.

HEMODYNAMIC STUDIES. *Arterial pressure measurements* were made during CPB with and without pulsatile flow (Fig. 1). IABP produced pressures from 75/50 to 130/70 during CPB. All saphenous vein grafts were attached to the aorta prior to instituting CPB. Coronary artery anastamoses were then performed on CPB with induced fibrillation. After completion of the anastamoses, all vein grafts demonstrated excellent palpable pulsations during pulsatile flow. The pulsations disappeared with cessation of IABP. This apparent drop in pressure was substantiated by arterial pressure measurements of saphenous vein grafts (Fig. 4).

Peripheral vascular resistance and a rising mean arterial pressure, using the standard roller pump without IABP, tend to increase during CPB with passage of time. This phenomenon did not occur in our pulsatile patients, and perfusion pressures were well within normal levels even up to six hours.

Left ventricular ejection fractions (percent) using the radioisotope Indium were determined in two groups having coronary bypass procedures. Both were comparable in regards to the extent of their coronary disease, their preoperative LVEF, the procedures performed (Table 5), the operative technique, and the anesthesia used. All determinations of LVEF (percent) were made in the awake patient. In 20 nonpulsatile patients, there was a significant depression of LVEF the day following operation (preoperative control 52.2 percent to 38.7 percent) (Table 2). At $10 \pm two$ days, the ejection fraction had returned toward preoperative values although it was still depressed (43 percent). However, in the group of pulsatile patients, the ejection fraction significantly increased the day following operation (preoperative 51.3 percent to 61.8 percent). At $10 \pm two$ days after operation, the LVEF continued to be significantly increased to 66 percent. When these two groups of patients with coronary artery surgery are compared, postoperative left ventricular function is significantly better in the pulsatile group ($p < 0.001$).

BIOCHEMICAL STUDIES. *Coronary Sinus Lactates* were determined before and during CPB at 15, 30, 45, and 60 minutes. In seven nonpulsatile patients there was an increase above control (+128 percent, +183 percent, +213 percent, and +221 percent) at the various time intervals. The respective values in a group of five pulsatile patients were +38 percent, +40 percent, +50 percent, and + 53 percent. There was a significant difference ($p < 0.01$) between the two groups (Fig. 3).

Total Serum Lactic Dehydrogenase was determined serially before, during, and following CPB (Table 1). In those receiving continuous roller pump flow (10 patients), the percent increase was much higher than in 16 pulsatile patients. The difference between the two groups was significant ($p < 0.05$).

SGOT levels were serially determined before and after CPB in seven patients having nonpulsatile flow and 16 having pulsatile flow. Elevations were much lower in the pulsatile group ($p < 0.01$)

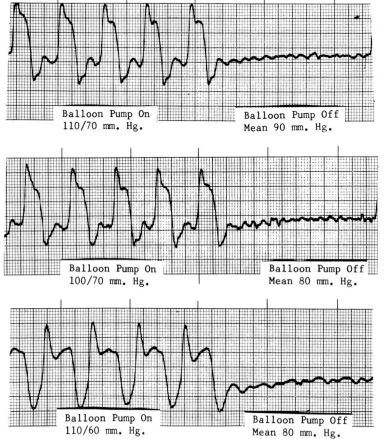

FIG. 4. Arterial pressure tracings with pulsatile and nonpulsatile flow using IABP and CPB. Top: right coronary bypass graft; middle: LAD coronary bypass graft; bottom: radial artery. Mean arterial line pressure, balloon pump on: 150/140 mm Hg; balloon pump off: mean 145 mm Hg.

especially at four days postoperative, when the two groups were compared (Table 2).

Serum Bilirubin and Alkaline Phosphatase were slightly elevated postoperatively. These elevations were similar in both groups.

Erythrocyte Hemolysis as determined by plasma hemoglobin taken immediately after CPB (45 minutes to 3 hours) averaged 77 mg percent in 11 pulsatile patients, as compared to 58 mg percent in 11 nonpulsatile patients.

Renal Function was not impaired postoperatively as measured by hourly urine output, urea nitrogen, and creatinine.

DISCUSSION

It is not the purpose of this chapter to review in detail the literature contrasting pulsatile and nonpulsatile flow. The physiologic and hemodynamic importance of pulsatile blood flow has been described by several groups (Mandelbaum and Burns, 1965; Many et al, 1968; Wilkens et al, 1962). Several reports have documented the superiority of pulsatile flow during CPB over continuous roller pump flow. These advantages include better tissue capillary perfusion (Ogata et al, 1960), less metabolic acidosis (Jacobs et al, 1969), increased oxygen consumption (Shepard and Kirklin, 1969), and excellent venous return with little tendency to internal pooling of blood (Nakayama et al, 1962). Studies using left heart bypass with pulsatile flow resulted in better renal tissue perfusion as evident by less renal tissue hypoxia and metabolic acidosis when compared with nonpulsatile flow (German et al, 1972; Mukherjee et al, 1973). In addition, Wright and Sanderson, 1972, studied the morphologic effects of pulsatile and continuous blood flow in the brain. They observed that less diffuse nerve cell changes were present in the pulsatile group and that focal changes were present in both groups. The focal lesions were probably due to circulating gas microbubbles and/or blood cell aggregates. Wakabayashi et al, 1972, studied the heart in dogs. Their studies demonstrated that coronary artery perfusion and myocardial oxygen consumption were more stable with pulsatile coronary perfusion.

The pulse contour produced with IABP during CPB resembles a normal pulse contour and appears much superior to that of the roller pump. The unique feature with the AVCO balloon is that it is trisegmented. The middle segment inflates first, with the end segments following. This feature allows dispersion of the pulse in both directions as it lies in the descending thoracic aorta. It would appear that with the unidirectional balloon (Bregman et al, 1971), ie pulsations toward the coronary arteries, pulsatile flow distal to the balloon would be less apparent. The attractive feature with IABP is synchronous diastolic augmentation. In the beating heart during CPB this is an important feature in coronary perfusion since flow to the vulnerable subendocardial muscle is primarily diastolic. In situations where there is bradycardia, erratic cardiac rhythm, and desired ventricular fibrillation (as in coronary artery surgery), an external pacing source can be used to activate the balloon. The empty, beating heart during CPB requires less O_2 than the fibrillating heart. Even in the fibrillating heart, we noted in our patients that pulsatile flow has resulted in less coronary sinus lactate production secondary to better myocardial perfusion and less anaerobic metabolism. In addition, improved postoperative myocardial function (LVEF) occurred in patients having pulsatile flow. This supports the experimental work of Wakabayashi et al, 1972. With pulsatile coronary perfusion, ischemic injuries frequently encountered (especially after prolonged perfusions) may be avoided. Hultgren et al, 1973, stressed the degree of myocardial injury encountered during surgery. Their incidence of perioperative infarction was 7 percent, with ischemic changes (ECG) of up to 30 percent. The long-term effects of this have not yet been determined. Better coronary perfusion may avoid the low cardiac output syndrome, varying degrees of subclinical subendocardial necrosis, or lethal frank circumferential left ventricular necrosis (Hultgren et al, 1973; Taber et al, 1967). In a recent experimental study, Allard et al, 1973, using radioisotope microspheres in young pigs, found that during ventricular fibrillation and with left ventricular hypertrophy, there is a redistribution of blood flow with deprivation to the subendocardial muscle. They suggested that this finding may account for the clinical setting of diffuse subendocardial necrosis. It is conceivable that PF may provide better myocardial perfusion in patients with hypertrophied ventricles. In a series of experiments

reported by Buckberg et al, 1972, the normal endoepicardial flow ratios per gram of tissue (1:1), as measured by radioactive microspheres, fell to 0.1:1 when the diastolic flow fraction fell. Pulsatile flow may improve the endoepicardial flow ratios, thereby improving subendocardial perfusion. The majority of patients who develop diffuse subendocardial necrosis most often have aortic valve disease and LVH. Unfortunately, our system of balloon pulsatile flow is not applicable during aortic valve replacement because of the necessity of cross-clamping the ascending aorta. However, the syndrome of LV necrosis has been encountered in some of our patients receiving nonpulsatile flow, as well as others (Najafi et al, 1967; Taber et al, 1967) not having aortic valve replacement. Under these circumstances, balloon pulsatile flow may play an important role in the prevention of this lesion in nonaortic valve patients. Pulsatile coronary perfusion might also prevent the problem of the "stone heart" (Cooley et al, 1972). Although the latter syndrome has been described in patients having ischemic cardiac arrest, we have observed the phenomenon in patients having coronary perfusion. Our data suggest that nonpulsatile coronary blood flow to an already jeopardized myocardium (coronary disease) results in some degree of injury to the myocardium. This injury outweighed the beneficial effects of the bypass procedures resulting in a significant depression in left ventricular performance postoperatively. However, the dual benefit of pulsatile coronary perfusion and coronary bypass procedures results in an overall improvement in cardiac function. The long-term effects of pulsatile versus nonpulsatile flow on the myocardium is not known.

The disadvantage with our system is that it cannot be used during aortic valve replacement when the aorta is clamped. In addition, aortic valve insufficiency is also a contraindication to IABP and CPB because of the increased load on the left ventricle that would occur during balloon pumping. However, when multiple valve replacement is required following aortic valve replacement, the remaining procedure(s) can be performed using pulsatile flow, especially for prolonged perfusion. In one of our patients, this technique was used during and following the initial aortic valve replacement.

The use of pulsatile flow to other vital organs during bypass would appear superior to that of continuous flow. This difference is probably not significant for short perfusion periods. When perfusions are in excess of two hours, some degree of impairment of renal, hepatic, and CNS as well as cardiac function probably exists with continuous flow. With prolonged perfusions, pulsatile flow may prove beneficial in protecting vital organ function. In other studies, less hepatocellular injury (rise in SGOT) was present in pulsatile patients. Renal dysfunction is not an infrequent occurrence following open-heart operations. Recently, Abel et al, 1974, noted that 39 percent of 507 adult patients developed renal failure of some degree (BUN > 50 mg percent or creatinine > 2.0 mg percent) postoperatively. We did not note any evidence of postoperative renal dysfunction in the patients receiving pulsatile flow. One of our patients requiring an unusually long bypass (nearly six hours) had pulsatile flow during the entire procedure. Postoperatively he did not develop any depression of vital organ function. Certainly a single case does not attest to the superiority of pulsatile flow; however, past experience with unusually prolonged perfusion has resulted in either death or often depressed vital organ function postoperatively. Overall, better tissue perfusion occurred in our pulsatile patients as evidenced by lower elevations of total LDH when compared with continuous flow.

Another advantage of pulsatile flow occurs during the cessation of bypass. No supportive drugs were needed in our patients. In critically ill patients, supportive drugs such as epinephrine, isoproterenol, and aramine have on occasion resulted in serious arrhythmias. Isoproterenol has also been known to produce ischemic injuries to the myocardium (Leszkovszky and Gal, 1967). Also, platelet aggregation and thrombosis have been attributed to these agents (Mustard and Packham, 1972). The use of mechanical support can avoid the use of these drugs, and perhaps more important, it provides better coronary flow in the face of poor LV performance while weaning the patient off bypass. Injury to the myocardium and other vital organs probably exists in those patients having low perfusion pressures after bypass. In only two of our patients was postoperative balloon pumping required (both had preoperative cardiogenic shock). The lack of necessity for supportive drugs and diuretics during the postoperative period would support the hypothesis that less myocardial damage occurs in those patients receiving pulsatile flow. This is further substantiated by our studies of improved LVEF following coronary artery surgery and PF.

Hemodynamically, the pressure gradient across the current available arterial cannulae is still significant. With the use of other pulsatile pumps, this gradient is greatly intensified. Excessively high line pressures do not occur with the use of IABP since the balloon is beyond the arterial cannulation site. Balloon pumping that augments the arterial pressure produces an increase in line pressure depending upon the degree of obstruction at the site of the balloon. The volume can be adjusted to minimize high-line pressures. Erythrocyte destruction is slightly greater during pulsatile flow when compared with the roller pump alone. Gross hemoglobinuria, when it occurs, is transient and clears within a few hours postoperatively. Similar observations have been noted in nonpulsatile CPB.

The ease of insertion and removal of the balloon into the femoral artery or ascending aorta makes this form of pulsatile flow attractive. No complications secondary to the balloon have been noted in any of our patients.

CONCLUSION

A simple method of producing pulsatile flow during cardiopulmonary bypass using intraaortic balloon pumping in 33 patients is described. The procedure is simple, safe, and effective in producing a physiologic pulsatile flow. In a comparable group of coronary bypass patients, left ventricular performance (LVEF) during the postoperative period was statistically better in the pulsatile versus the nonpulsatile group. Low cardiac output syndrome was not noted during the postoperative period, and no supportive drugs were needed during or following operation. Less hepatocellular injury and no renal failure was noted in the pulsatile group. Excessively high line pressure and hemolysis was not significantly different from continuous roller pump perfusion. No complications were associated with IABP. Only one death (preoperative cardiogenic shock) occurred in 33 patients (3 percent). This method of pulsatile flow may prove to be superior to other types.

ACKNOWLEDGMENTS

We gratefully acknowledge the technical assistance of Clyde Jordan, Terry Jackson, and Judith Stoughton.

References

Abel RM, Wick J, Beck CH, Buckley MJ, Austen WG: Renal dysfunction following open-heart operations. Arch Surg 108:175, 1974

Allard JR, Shizgal HM, Dobell ARC: Distribution of myocardial blood flow during cardiopulmonary bypass in normal and hypertrophied left ventricles. Surg Forum 24:178, 1973

Bregman D, Kripke DC, Cohen MN, Laniado S, Goetz

RH: Clinical experience with the unidirectional dual-chambered intraaortic balloon assist. Circulation 43 (Suppl I):I–82, 1971

Buckberg GD, Fixler DE, Archie JP, Hoffman JIE: Experimental subendocardial ischemia in dogs with normal coronary arteries. Circ Res 39:67, 1972

Buckley MJ, Craver JM, Gold HK, Mundth ED, Daggett WM, et al: Intraaortic balloon pump assist for cardiogenic shock after cardiopulmonary bypass. Circulation 48 (Suppl III):III–90, 1973

Cooley DA, Reul GJ, Wukasch DC: Ischemic contracture of the heart "stone heart." Am J Cardiol 29:575, 1972

Dalton ML, McCarty RT, Woodward KE, Barila TG: The army artificial heart pump. II. Comparison of pulsatile and nonpulsatile flow. Surgery 58:810, 1965

German JC, Chalmers GS, Hirai J, Mukherjee ND, Wakabayashi A, Connolly JE: Comparison of nonpulsatile and pulsatile extracorporeal circulation in renal tissue perfusion. Chest 61:65, 1972

Hultgren HN, Miyagawa M, Buch W, Angell WW: Ischemic myocardial injury during cardiopulmonary bypass surgery. Am Heart J 85:167, 1973

Jacobs LA, Klopp EH, Seamone W, Topaz SR, Gott VL: Improved organ function during cardiac bypass with a roller pump modified to deliver pulsatile flow. J Thorac Cardiovasc Surg 58:703, 1969

Kantrowitz A, Tjonneland S, Freed PS, Phillips SJ, Butner AN, et al: Initial clinical experience with intraaortic balloon pumping in cardiogenic shock. JAMA 203:113, 1968

Leszkovszky GP, Gal G: Observations in isoprenaline-induced myocardial necrosis. J Pharm Pharmac 19:226, 1967

Mandelbaum I, Burns WH: Pulsatile and nonpulsatile blood flow. JAMA 191:121, 1965

Many M, Soroff HS, Birtwell WC, Wise HM, Deterling RA: The physiologic role of pulsatile and nonpulsatile blood flow. Arch Surg 97:917, 1968

Mukherjee ND, Beran AV, Hirai J, Wakabayashi A, Sperling DR, et al: In vivo determination of renal tissue oxygenation during pulsatile and nonpulsatile left heart bypass. Ann Thorac Surg 15:354, 1973

Mustard JF, Packham MA: Factors influencing platelet function; adhesion release and aggregation. Pharmac Reviews 22:97, 1972

Najafi H, Henson D, Dye WS, Javid H, Hunter JA, et al:

Left ventricular hemorrhagic necrosis. Ann Thorac Surg 7:550, 1967

Nakayama K, Tamiya T, Yamamoto K, Izumi T, Akimoto S, et al: High-amplitude pulsatile pump in extracorporeal circulation with particular reference to hemodynamics. Surgery 54:798, 1963

Ogata T, Ida Y, Nonoyama A, Takeda J, Sasaki HA: Comparative study of the effectiveness of pulsatile and nonpulsatile blood flow in extracorporeal circulation. Arch Jap Chir 26:29, 1960

Paquet KJ: Hemodynamic studies in normothermic perfusion of the isolated pig kidney with pulsatile and nonpulsatile flows. J Cardiovasc Surg 1:45, 1969

Scheidt S, Wilner G, Mueller H, Summers D, Lesch M, et al: Intraaortic balloon counterpulsation in cardiogenic shock: report of a co-operative clinical trial. N Engl J Med 288:979, 1973

Shepard RB, Kirklin JW: Relationship of pulsatile flow to oxygen consumption and other variables during cardiopulmonary bypass. J Thorac Cardiovasc Surg 58:694, 1969

Steele PP, VanDyke D, Trow RS, Anger HO, Davies H: A simple and safe bed-side method for serial measurement of left ventricular ejection fraction, cardiac output and pulmonary blood volume. Br Heart J 36:122, 1974

Taber RE, Morales AR, Fine G: Myocardial necrosis and postoperative low-cardiac-output syndrome. Ann Thorac Surg 4:12, 1967

Trinkle JK, Helton NE, Bryant LR, Griffen WO: Pulsatile cardiopulmonary bypass: clinical evaluation. Surgery 68:1074, 1970

Trinkle JK, Helton NE, Wood RE, Bryant LR: Metabolic comparison of a new pulsatile pump and a roller pump for cardiopulmonary bypass. J Thorac Cardiovasc Surg 58:562, 1969

Wakabayashi A, Kubo T, Gilman P, Zuber WF, Connolly JE: Pulsatile pressure-regulated coronary perfusion during ventricular fibrillation. Arch Surg 105:36, 1972

Wilkens H, Regelson W, Hoffmeister FS: The physiologic importance of pulsatile blood flow. N Engl J Med 267:443, 1962

Wright G, Sanderson, JM: Brain damage and mortality in dogs following pulsatile and nonpulsatile blood flows in extracorporeal circulation. Thorax 27:738, 1972

55

AUTOMATED CIRCULATORY SUPPORT SYSTEMS

Richard E. Clark, Thomas B. Ferguson, Ronald W. Hagen, Phillip S. Berger, and Clarence S. Weldon

A high-flow, low-volume perfusion device was sought, specifically designed for membrane oxygenators and which obviated marginal flow capacity with gravity drainage, shunting with recirculation lines, and poor volume control between two occlusive pumps. Inexpensive volume displacement and pressure LVDT transducers and newly devised circuits have been used to control an arterial pump and venous roller pump, respectively. The venous system is sensitive to changes as little as 0.1 cm of negative water pressure and automatically controls the pump to any preset venous pressure. Occlusion of the venous line causes the venous pump to stop ≤ 1 sec depending on the flow rate. The system has been tested with the Travenol 0.25-6.0 M^2 and the GE 1-4 M^2 membrane oxygenators. The systems have been applied to a Sarns modular (high and low flow), Sarns console, and Med-Science heart lung machines. Eleven 24-hour partial bypass perfusions were performed on puppies weighing 1,300-6,400 gms with 91 percent (10/11) surviving. Total bypass has now been performed on 26 adult mongrel dogs 8 to 28 kg for 1 to 4 hrs and seven patients for 1.73, 2.65, 3.12, 3.37, 4.08, 4.48, and 4.53 hrs. Hemodilution without blood prime has been used in all the clinical perfusions. It is concluded that a high-flow, low-prime twin-pump occlusive perfusion system has been developed for membrane oxygenators that gives a high degree of safety and ease of perfusion without open reservoirs, recirculation lines, and other undesirable features.

Supported in part by NIH Division of Research Resources Grant RR 00 396 and HISMA 5 TO1 HS 00074 Technology in Health Care Training Grant

INTRODUCTION

The advent of practical membrane oxygenators has imposed new requirements for perfusion systems. Early experimental models of membrane oxygenators had high resistances to blood flow and low mass transfer coefficients.[2] These deficiencies have been markedly improved although most units still impose a 20 to 100 mm pressure gradient at 5 liters of flow. Consequently, several solutions have been sought since gravity drainage may be insufficient to overcome resistance to blood flow through the oxygenator and the remainder of the system. One solution was to design a membrane oxygenator that would withstand the negative pressure from an arterial pump so that blood could be aspirated through the device without breakage of the membranes.[3] Such an approach with the thin sheet membranes of copolymer, silicone rubber, or polytetrafluoroethylene still imposes the hazard of membrane fracture. Should the membrane break, gas is sucked into the blood, and the system must be stopped immediately.

A second approach has been the use of a two-pump system in which the venous pump overcomes the resistance within the oxygenator circuit by pushing blood through the oxygenator, thus establishing a positive transmembrane pressure gradient of blood with respect to oxygen. Most users have utilized a recirculation line between the output of the oxygenator and the venous pump.[4,5] However, this requires that the venous pump maintain a blood flow that is 5 to 10 percent greater than the arterial blood flow. This requirement is extremely limiting when such a membrane oxygenator system is applied to total bypass because of the frequent changes of venous return secondary to movement of the heart and the cannulae and an unexpected loss of volume. Should the venous pump become slower in its output than the arterial pump, then direct shunting of unoxygenated blood across the recirculation line to the arterial line occurs. Our aim was to develop a closed high-flow, low-prime complete membrane oxygenation system that (1) had no open reservoirs, (2) did not require a recirculation line, (3) placed minimal back pressure on the outlet side of the membrane oxygenator, and (4) utilized a venous pump to overcome the resistance of small venous cannulae, ie for use in infants. These requirements made obvious the need for maintenance of a constant blood volume between the two occlusive pumps and the need for some method to overcome the extremely little human reaction time required to avoid cavitation of blood caused by an excess vacuum from the venous pump. This report outlines our four-year development of automated controls for a twin-pump, membrane oxygenator system.

MATERIALS AND METHODS

The first effort was directed toward the problem of maintenance of a constant volume between the two occlusive pumps. A small 75 ml silicone rubber-polyester tricot reinforced bag was fabricated * (Fig. 1). A holder for this bag was fabricated in our shops (Fig. 2). An LVDT displacement transducer † was purchased and assembled into the holder. Appropriate circuitry (Fig. 3) was designed and fabricated for the Sarns high- and low-flow modular pumps and for the Med-Science console with minor modification. The output of the control circuit was directed to the SCR controller of the pump. If the venous pump output was greater than the arterial pump, the closed reservoir bag increased in size displacing the plunger of the LVDT transducer, which in turn caused an increase in the output of the arteral pump. Similarly, when the output of the arterial pump was greater than the venous pump, the bag tended to collapse, the plunger extended, and the arterial pump slowed. Bench testing and modifications were required to select appropriate time constants in order to prevent ex-

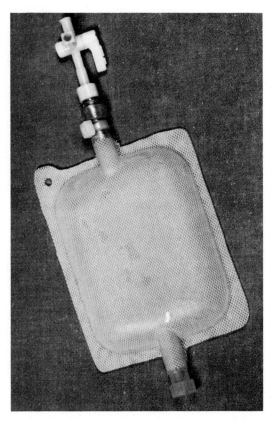

FIG. 1. Reinforced silicone rubber reservoir used for arterial pump control. The reservoir was placed between the outlet of the membrane oxygenator and the arterial pump.

cessive sawing of the arterial pump and obtain a smooth linear decrease or increase of pump speed with changes in blood volume.

The venous pump controller consisted of an LVDT pressure transducer,* amplifier, and controlling circuit. The flow resistance of the venous cannulae are offset by a voltage dialed into the controller box (Fig. 4), so that alterations in the *in vivo* central venous pressure govern the speed of the venous pump. Should sudden occlusion occur, a negative pressure develops in the transducer, which in turn rapidly slows the venous pump or completely turns it off. Similarly, the venous pump will run at greater speeds when the central venous pressure becomes increased. Consequently, both venous and arterial pumps are autocontrolled by independent sensing devices.

Animal testing used 38 adult mongrel dogs and 11 puppies. Thirty-two adult dogs were util-

---

* Travenol Laboratories, Morton Grove, Ill. 60053.
† Schaevitz Engineering Company, Pennsauken, N.J. 08110.

* Biotronex, Silver Spring, Md. 20910.

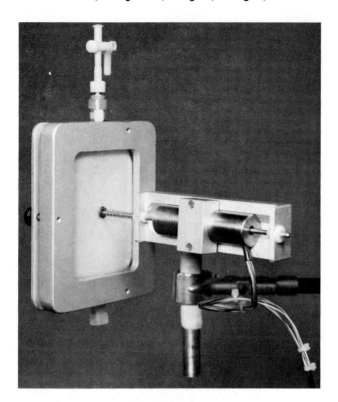

FIG. 2. The bag and transducer have been assembled into the holder.

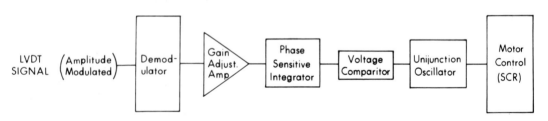

FIG. 3. Schematic circuit diagram for autocontroller for the arterial pump.

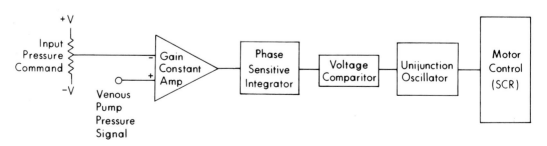

FIG. 4. Schematic circuit diagram for autocontroller for the venous pump.

ized for acute studies of component testing, 12 of which had partial bypass using the veno-venous method without entering the chest or abdomen. The purpose of these experiments was to test the oxygenation capabilities of the GE and Travenol membrane oxygenators at the 0.5 and 1.0 M^2 and 0.25 and 0.75 M^2 sizes, respectively. Additionally, these studies permitted rapid evaluation of the volume displacement system for the arterial pump. Pressure measurements * were made across the membrane oxygenator and the volume displacement system to ascertain its alterations with respect to flow. Sixteen adult mongrel dogs weighing 8 to 28 kilograms were anesthetized with sodium Nembutal and placed on a Harvard ventilator. Total cardiopulmonary bypass was instituted through the ascending aorta or in retrograde manner through the femoral artery.

The purposes of these experiments were to test the following:

1. The influence of various sized venous cannulae on the venous controller.
2. The influence of a recirculation line on oxygenation and line pressures under simulated clinical situations and errors.
3. The problems encountered with gravity flow through the two membrane systems, should this method be found necessary because of equipment failure.

Heat exchange was accomplished with the disposable Travenol unit or a Mayo tube-in-shell heat exchanger. Additionally, various bubble traps, both of the Sarns and Mayo configurations, were utilized as well as 40-micron polyester † screen mesh filters and packed polyester-wool filters.‡ The final system chosen consisted of the venous pump and its controlling subsystem, the Travenol membrane oxygenator, which was sized according to the calculated maximal oxygen consumption of the animal, a Travenol disposable heat exchanger, the LVDT volume displacement transducer system, the arterial pump, and a packed polyester-wool filter. Water to the heat exchanger was controlled by a pressure regulating device.§ Maximal flows were utilized as judged by a central venous pressure of zero to minus one cm of water. Perfusions were performed for two hours at 38 C. Finally,

six total bypass survival experiments were performed.

Continuous 24-hour partial bypass studies were done on 11 puppies, weighing 1,300 to 6,400 grams, which were anesthetized with Innovar, intubated, and placed on a Harvard ventilator. Cutdowns were performed in each groin, and catheters passed for measurement of the arterial and distal inferior vena caval pressures, and a venous cannula was inserted via the opposite femoral vein to the right atrium. Inflow was through the femoral artery. Alternative procedures involved cutdowns in the neck to utilize the external jugular vein for withdrawal and the carotid artery for inflow. Innovar was given intramuscularly as required to keep the animal sedated, and after the first two hours of perfusion the animal usually did not require the ventilator. The system was primed the afternoon before surgery with approximately 200 to 400 cc of Ringer's Lactate without dextrose and with a concentration of heparin at 10 unit/ml. Prior to perfusion, this initial priming solution was discarded and the system was reprimed with buffered Ringer's Lactate containing a concentration of heparin of 1 unit/ml and 5 percent dextrose. The purpose of this prepriming regimen was to thoroughly wet the membranes and permit absorption of heparin onto the silicone rubber surfaces. During the perfusion complete blood counts, chemistries, and blood gases were performed, and weights obtained before and after perfusion. Three puppies were perfused in the veno-venous mode and the remainder by the veno-arterial route.

Seven patients have been perfused using a Travenol 6 M^2 membrane and the components described above. The duration of operations and perfusions are listed in Table 1. In addition to the frequent study of the blood cellular components, ionic concentrations, pH, and gas tensions, special diffusion immuno-assays were performed for IgA, IgC, IgM, C'2, and C'3 protein fractions.

* Hewlett-Packard, Waltham, Mass. 02154. Transducers 267 BC and 268 BC, 350 preamplifier and recording system.
† Johnson and Johnson, Chicago, Ill. 60638.
‡ Pioneer Filters, Inc., Beaverton, Ore. 97005
§ Bentley Laboratories, Inc., Irvine, Calif. 92705.

TABLE 1. Clinical Experience with Automated Membrane Perfusion System

CASE NO.	OPERATION	PERFUSION TIME
1	Triple valve replacement	4 hr 53 min
2	Triple coronary bypass	4 hr 29 min
3	Emergency AVR	1 hr 44 min
4	AVR and MVR	2 hr 39 min
5	AVR and double coronary bypass	4 hr 5 min
6	Quadruple coronary bypass	5 hr 16 min
7	AVR and MVR	3 hr 22 min

RESULTS

Testing of the arterial controller revealed the device to be sensitive to maximal volume displacements of 6.5 ml and minimal displacements of 3.8 ml. Reaction time was a function of rotational roller speed, but initial changes for a 10 percent change in rotational speed took place within 0.5 sec or less. The venous system sensitivity was dependent upon the offset voltage and the time constant used in the circuit. In all cases, the system can be made sensitive to changes as little as 0.1 cm of water negative pressure, and occlusion of the venous line will cause the venous pump to stop in less than one second. The system was tested with the Sarns high-flow modular pumps and console for total body perfusion of dogs and humans and the Sarns low-flow pumps for the partial bypass perfusions in puppies. Additionally, the Med-Science console was used for five total body perfusions in dogs.

Six dogs underwent two hours of maximal flow perfusion at 38 C and four survived. The two deaths were iatrogenic. One was a result of an unrecognized disconnection of the ventilator six hours after perfusion was terminated, and the second death occurred when an overdose of Digoxin was given.

The eleven 24-hour partial perfusions performed on puppies were successful (Table 2).

TABLE 2. Characteristics of 24-Hour Puppy Perfusions

	BEFORE BP	DURING BP	AFTER BP
Arterial P_{O_2}	72	90	67
Buffer base	−2.2	−0.8	−2.3
Inlet P_{O_2}	−	42	−
Outlet P_{O_2}	−	175	−
Hematocrit	−	27%	−
Plasma Hgb	−	−	17 mg%

One animal succumbed 11 hr after the start of bypass from an arrhythmia, the etiology of which was not determined. Ten animals were long-term survivors. A summary of data is shown in Tables 3 and 4, and the clinical course of one animal is shown in Figure 5.

Seven patients have undergone membrane perfusions ranging in time from 1 hr 44 min to 5 hr 16 min using the 6 M^2 system. The perfusion systems have worked well and closely followed changes in blood volume and volume between pumps. With a decrease in perfusate tem-

perature to 28 C, only three to four 0.75 M^2 units were required to maintain a P_aO_2 at 28 C of 100 mm Hg. Minimal gas flows of 0.5 to 1.0 L/min are required at this temperature. The heat exchanger was judged to be efficient with an average rewarming time of 17 min for a temperature change of 8 C.

DISCUSSION

The path of progress for membrane oxygenators has been a tortuous and difficult one. Industrial technology has brought the membrane oxygenator to a point where it is small, disposable, sterile, pyrogen-free, and reasonably efficient in terms of mass transfer.[1] With this development, special problems have arisen. First is the need for design of the pumping systems around the pressure limitations of the particular membrane oxygenator. Both membrane units utilized in these experiments required positive pressure on the arterial side of the oxygenator. Neither oxygenator could withstand high vacuums, which could occur if the venous return lines were inadvertently clamped or kinked. Secondly, venous pump systems are required where high cannulae resistance must be overcome; for example, in partial bypass in infants. Finally, the need for a two-pump system has required use of a volume displacement transducer between two occlusive pumps, if no recirculation line is used. It is believed that a recirculation line between the arterial and venous

TABLE 3. Summary of 24-Hour Puppy Perfusions

Number of puppies	11
Weight range	1,320–6,400 gm
Average initial weight	3,426 gm
Blood infused	60 cc/kg
Crystalloid infused	60 cc/kg
Average weight gain	17%
Number of long-term survivals	10

TABLE 4. Experimental Experience Automated Membrane Perfusion System

MODE	NO.	DURATION (hr)	PERCENT SURVIVAL
Partial bypass	12 dogs	4–8	100
	11 puppies	24	91
Total bypass			
Acute	20 dogs	2–6	0
Survival	6 dogs	2	67

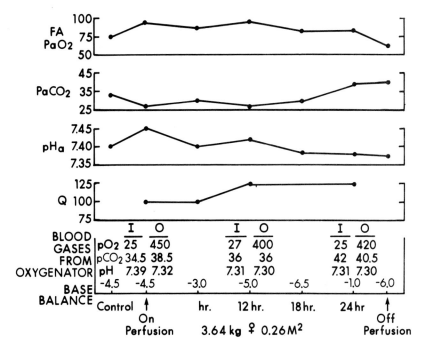

FIG. 5. Variable versus time plot for one 24-hour perfusion in a puppy.

pumps severely limits the application of membrane oxygenators to total bypass, requiring frequent alterations of the venous pump during the average clinical perfusion. The human reaction time permitted is extremely short, and consequently recirculation lines frequently permit shunting and do not prevent implosions.

The devices described in this report are neither a panacea nor usable in every application. We believe that the Travenol system may be used on gravity drainage if the volume displacement reservoir is set at the level of the exit of the oxygenator outlet and adjusted so that there is minimal back pressure, ie 0 to 10 mm Hg. Increasing the height of the reservoir linearly diminishes flow. The venous controlling device becomes of much more importance where small cannulae are to be used, either for total bypass or at the bedside for extracorporeal ventilatory assistance. This device permits an almost maintenance-free perfusion, which is automated and sensitive to venous blood volume and to any mechanical obstruction of venous inflow to the pump. As the venous pressure decreases, the venous pump automatically decreases and will shut off in the face of a negative pressure of greater than 5 cm of water. The arterial pump, on an independent controlling system, will automatically follow the venous pump. The purpose of these experiments was to develop, test, and evaluate automated devices that could be applied to a variety of commercially available

roller pumps and demonstrate their efficacy in use under a variety of requirements for extracorporeal perfusion. The systems have been tested on puppies, adult dogs, and patients in both partial venovenous and venoarterial modes, as well as total bypass in the venoarterial manner. The oxygenators utilized adequately transferred oxygen and carbon dioxide under all experimental and clinical conditions. The heat exchangers and other components have performed satisfactorily as reported by others. It is our opinion that automated devices have a role in high-flow, low-prime extracorporeal perfusion systems involving membrane oxygenators where no blood gas interface or open reservoir exists, and these elements provide degrees of safety and effectiveness for long-term perfusions where minimal human reaction time is permitted and little maintenance is required.

ACKNOWLEDGMENTS

We gratefully acknowledge the technical assistance of William B. Petty, Andrew L. Bodicky, Richard A. Beauchamp, and Phillip K. Spohn.

References

1. Boyd JC, Moran JF, Clark RE: An analysis of the operating characteristics of the 0.25 M² Travenol infant membrane oxygenator. Surgery 71:262, 1972

2. Clowes GHA Jr, Hopkins AL, Neville WE: An artificial lung dependent upon diffusion of oxygen and carbon dioxide through plastic membranes. J Thorac Surg 32:630, 1956

3. Kolobow T, Bowman RL: Construction and evaluation of an alveolar membrane artificial heart-lung. Trans Am Soc Artif Intern Organs 9:238, 1963

4. Pierce EC II: The membrane lung: its excuse, present status, and promise. J Mt Sinai Hosp. NY 34: 437, 1967

5. Pierce EC II: Extracorporeal Circulation for Open-Heart Surgery. Springfield, Ill, CC Thomas, 1969, p 41

56

MYOCARDIAL PROTECTION DURING ANOXIC CARDIAC ARREST IN AORTOCORONARY BYPASS SURGERY

S. R. K. Iyengar, E. J. P. Charrette,
C. K. S. Iyengar, and R. B. Lynn

Intermittent or continuous aortic cross-clamping is used in aortocoronary bypass surgery. Myocardial damage incidental to such anoxic conditions can be a significant factor in the incidence of arrhythmias, myocardial infarction, and low output failure, which are the major complications after direct revascularization.

Anoxic tolerance of the myocardium is primarily dependent upon the extent to which anaerobic energy is available. Preservation of the structural and functional integrity of the mammalian myocardium by providing adequate substrate for glycolysis in the perfusate and elimination of stasis of acid metabolites under anaerobic conditions has been well documented. [69,99] Our experimental and clinical observations support this.[41,42] However, this aspect of myocardial protection during anoxic arrest in cardiac surgery has not been fully explored and provides a promising area for further clinical and experimental evaluation. Our principal aim is to present pertinent data relevant to the pathophysiology of anoxic cardiac arrest and discuss the rationale of BEKS hypothermic coronary flush for myocardial protection during interruption of coronary circulation.

METHODS AND MATERIAL

Experimental Data

CONTROL GROUP. Our initial investigation was directed toward studying the effects of anoxic cardiac arrest on first the normal and then

Supported by the Ontario Heart Foundation Grant No. 2–4.

the hypertrophied canine left ventricle.[41,42] With 60 to 75 minutes of anoxic arrest, five normal dogs in the control group developed subendocardial hemorrhagic necrosis (Fig. 1) and low output failure and died intraoperatively (Tables 1, 2). Six dogs in the control group with left ventricular hypertrophy produced by subcoronary aortic stenosis [43] developed much more extensive subendocardial lesions (Fig. 2), four of six dogs failed to come off bypass, and all died intraoperatively (Tables 3, 4).

BEKS HYPOTHERMIC CORONARY FLUSH. In a group of five normal dogs and four dogs with left ventricular hypertrophy produced by subcoronary aortic stenosis, the coronary bed was intermittently flushed with 500 ml of BEKS solution during 60 to 75 minutes of anoxic arrest. The solution was made up of 400 ml of plain Ringers solution, 100 ml of low molecular weight dextran in 10 percent dextrose, 4 mEq KCl, 10 mEq $NaHCO_3$, and 1,000 units of heparin. The temperature was 20 to 25 C and the pH 7.5 to 7.7. The solution was run in under gravity flow into the aortic root or by direct cannulation of the coronary arteries.

After 60 to 75 minutes anoxic arrest, none of the five normal dogs showed evidence of subendocardial hemorrhagic necrosis at autopsy (Fig. 3) or low output failure (Tables 1, 2). Four of them survived for one to four days, and the fifth dog was alive and well at 14 months when it was electively sacrificed after cardiac catheterization. Normal hemodynamics and histology of the myocardium was present. The four dogs with left ventricular hypertrophy came off bypass and maintained a stable blood pressure in contrast to the control dogs (Tables 3, 4). The subendocardial lesions were superficial and patchy (Fig. 4).

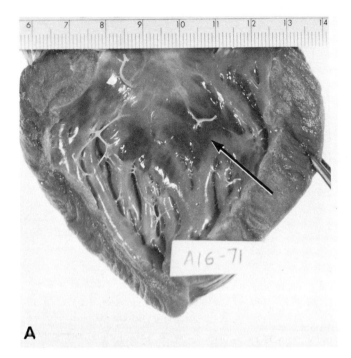

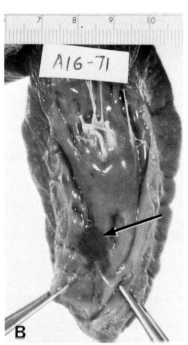

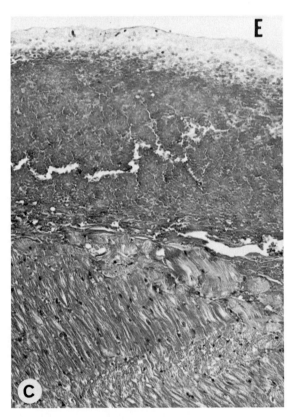

FIG. 1. Left ventricle of normal heart subjected to 65 minutes of anoxic arrest and showing subendothelial hemorrhage (arrows). A. Septal surface. B. Base of papillary muscle and adjoining ventricular wall. C. Microscopic section showing subendocardial hemorrhagic necrosis. E: endocardial surface. Hematoxylin-phloxine-saffron × 125 (From Iyengar et al, Ann Thorac Surg, 1972. Courtesy of Little Brown and Company, 1972).

TABLE 1. Extent and Distribution of Left Ventricular Lesions in Ten Normal Dogs Subjected to Anoxic Cardiac Arrest

DOG NO.	ANOXIC ARREST (min)	ACUTE HEMORRHAGIC NECROSIS		
		Endocardium	Inner Third	Middle Third
Control (5 dogs)				
C1	60	Patchy, widespread	0	0
C2	60	Patchy	0	0
C3	65	Patchy, widespread	0	0
C4	75	Patchy, widespread	minimal	0
C5	65	Patchy, widespread	0	0
BEKS coronary flush				
E1	70	0	0	0
E2	60	0	0	0
E3	65	0	0	0
E4	65	Patchy, hemorrhage only		
E5	75	0	0	0

Adapted from Iyengar et al, Ann Thorac Surg, 1972. Courtesy of Little, Brown and Company, 1972.

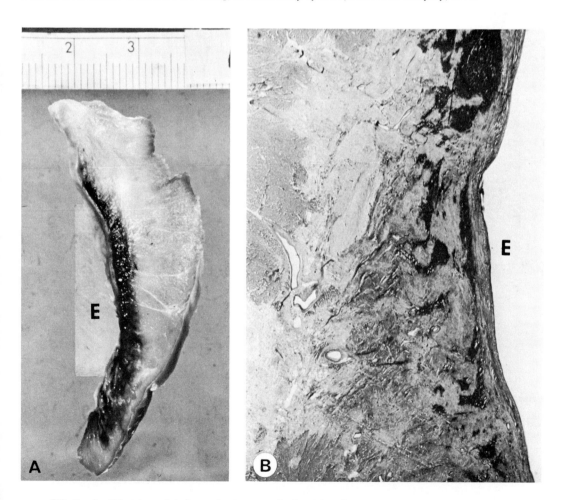

FIG. 2. A. Subendocardial hemorrhagic necrosis involving inner one-third to one-half of the hypertrophied left ventricle after 60 minutes of anoxic arrest. (E: endocardial surface.) B. Microscopic section that shows chronic ischemic changes involving the inner half of the hypertrophied left ventricle with superimposed hemorrhagic necrosis after anoxic arrest. Hematoxylin-phloxine-saffron stain. × 12.5 (From Iyengar et al, J Thorac Cardiovasc Surg, 1973. Courtesy of CV Mosby Company, 1973).

TABLE 2. Hemodynamic and Survival Data in Ten Dogs Subjected to Experimental Anoxic Cardiac Arrest

GROUP AND DOG NO.	WEIGHT	ANOXIC ARREST (min)	BYPASS TIME (min)	BEFORE THORACOTOMY				AFTER BYPASS				SURVIVAL AFTER BYPASS
				CO	HR	AP Systolic	AP Diastolic	CO	HR	AP Systolic	AP Diastolic	
Control (5 animals)												
C1	28	60	100	—a	145	190	94		150	70	30	2 hr
C2	27	60	100	3.71	150	163	90	2.32	100	94	45	2 hr
C3	27	65	110	4.78	220	189	95	—	155	65	35	15 min
C4	26	75	110	4.49	190	190	100	—	145	60	30	15 min
C5	32	60	105	—a	140	170	90		145	50	35	50 min
Experimental (5 animals) BEKS coronary flush												
E1	25	75	115	3.87	160	169	93	1.85	115	120	80	Alive and active at 14 mos
E2	27	70	110	5.10	170	171	94	2.36	150	100	60	18 hr
E3	33	60	130	2.24	125	168	88	3.42	140	130	75	16 hr
E4	26	65	100	4.45	190	190	100	1.84	130	129	74	4 days
E5	26	65	95	3.95	150	205	110	1.71	150	165	85	12 hr

aNot measured.
C2 was normotensive for 90 minutes after bypass.

CO: cardiac output; HR: heart rate; AP: arterial pressure.
Adapted from Iyengar et al, Ann Thorac Surg, 1972. Courtesy of Little Brown and Company, 1972.

TABLE 3. Extent and Distribution of Left Ventricular Lesions in Ten Dogs with Subcoronary Aortic Stenosis Subjected to Anoxic Cardiac Arrest

GROUP AND DOG NO.	LVH (percent)	ANOXIC ARREST (mins)	CHRONIC CHANGES			ACUTE HEMORRHAGIC NECROSIS			COMMENTS
			Microinfarcts	Fibrosis	Ischemic Changes	Endocardium	Ventricular Wall Inner Third	Ventricular Wall Middle Third	
Control (6 dogs)									
C1	11	60	+	+	+	Extensive	+	+	Failed to come off bypass
C2	27	67	+	+	+	Extensive	+	0	Died at 6 hrs postop; hemothorax and atelectasis
C3	13	60	0	0	+	Extensive	+	0	Failed to come off bypass
C4	24	66	+	+	+	Extensive	+	0	Failed to come off bypass
C5	18	60	+	+	+	Extensive	+	0	Failed to come off bypass
C6	24	60	0	0	+	Extensive	+	0	Died at 50 mins from VF
BEKS coronary flush (4 dogs)									
B1	17	60	+	0	+	Patchy	0	0	Died at 75 mins from hemorrhage
B2	14	60	0	+	+	0	0	0	Died at 10 hrs post-op hemothorax
B3	20	60	0	+	+	Patchy	0	0	Died at 2 hrs, hemothorax
B4	24	60	+	+	+	Patchy	0	0	Died at 5 hrs postop hemothorax and atelectasis

LVH: left ventricular hypertrophy; +: present; 0: absent; VF: ventricular fibrillation.   From Iyengar et al, J Thorac Cardiovasc Surg, 1973. Courtesy of CV Mosby Company, 1973.

TABLE 4. Hemodynamic and Survival Data in Ten Dogs with Subcoronary Aortic Stenosis Subjected to Anoxic Cardiac Arrest

GROUP AND DOG NO.	ANOXIC ARREST (min)	BYPASS TIME (min)	BEFORE THORACOTOMY CO	HR	AP Systolic	AP Diastolic	AFTER BYPASS CO	HR	AP Systolic	AP Diastolic	SURVIVAL AFTER BYPASS
Control (6 dogs)											
C1	60	100	2.46L	110	175	95	—	VF	—	—	Failed to come off bypass
C2	67	113	4.5L	105	227	105	1.62L	110	128	75	6 hrs
C3	60	135	3.75L	115	174	100	—	VF	—	—	Failed to come off bypass
C4	66	140	3.5L	116	190	95	—	VF	—	—	Failed to come off bypass
C5	60	160	—	120	136	88	—	VF	—	—	Failed to come off bypass
C6	60	125	—	140	170	90	—	145	50	35	50 mins
BEKS coronary flush (4 dogs)											
B1	60	85	4.0L	175	148	117	—	130	90	50	75 mins
B2	60	101	2.8L	155	160	136	—	115	97	55	12 hrs
B3	60	90	3.0L	130	110	88	1.6L	110	86	42	2 hrs
B4	60	91	6.0L	160	235	185	2.8L	135	142	73	5 hrs

CO: cardiac output; HR: heart rate; AP: arterial blood pressure; VF: ventricular fibrillation; L: Liter. From Iyengar et al, J Thorac Cardiovasc Surg, 1973. Courtesy of CV Mosby Company, 1973.

TABLE 5. Clinical Data on Five Patients with "Stone Heart" after Anoxic Cardiac Arrest

PT.	AGE/SEX	DIAGNOSIS	GRADIENT (mm Hg)	NYHA CLASSIFICATION	ANOXIC ARREST (mins)	COMMENTS
AS	60/M	AS	60	Class 3	50	AVR, failed to come off bypass
LK	56/M	AS	50	Class 3	55	AVR, failed to come off bypass
OF	61/M	AS	70	Class 3	60	AVR, failed to come off bypass
GM	51/M	AS and AI	65	Class 4	55	AVR, failed to come off bypass
AG	54/M	AS, LADC block	100	Class 3–4	50	AVR, LADC bypass, failed to come off bypass

AS: aortic stenosis; AI: aortic insufficiency; LADC: left anterior descending coronary; NYHA: New York Heart Association. From Iyengar et al, J Thorac Cardiovasc Surg, 1973. Courtesy of CV Mosby Company, 1973.

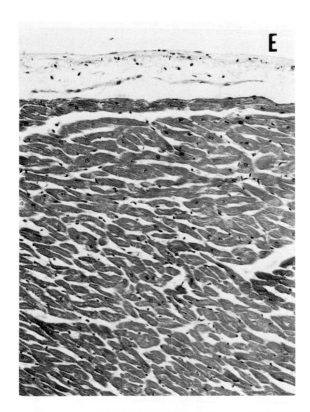

FIG. 3. Normal myocardium with perfusion of left coronary artery with a physiologic solution during 65 minutes of anoxic arrest. E: endocardial surface. Hematoxylin-phloxine-saffron. × 125 (From Iyengar et al, Ann Thorac Surg, 1972. Courtesy of Little Brown and Company, 1972).

FIG. 4. A. Superficial patchy subendocardial hemorrhage (arrow) in a hypertrophied canine left ventricle that has BEKS coronary flush during 60 minutes of anoxic arrest. (E: endothelial surface.) B. Superficial subendocardial hemorrhagic necrosis in hypertrophied canine left ventricle with BEKS coronary flush during 60 minutes' anoxic arrest. E: endocardial surface. Hematoxylin-phloxine-saffron. × 50. (From Iyengar et al, J Thorac Cardiovasc Surg, 1973. Courtesy of CV Mosby Company, 1973.)

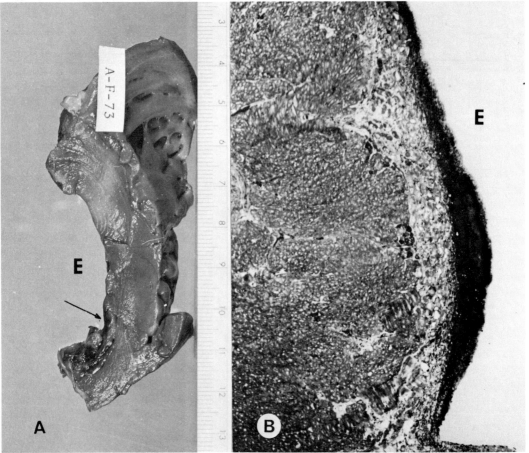

Clinical Data

We reviewed our experience with aortic valve replacement under anoxic arrest in relation to the incidence of ischemic contracture of the heart or "stone heart." Five patients could not be weaned from bypass in spite of all efforts to reverse the firm tetanic contraction of the left ventricle. All five cases were operated on under general body hypothermia of 30 to 32 C and topical cooling of the heart with ice-cold Ringers solution.

Impressed by the protective action of the BEKS solution on the myocardium during anoxic arrest that we observed in our experimental work, we started flushing the coronary bed intermittently with the BEKS solution during aortic valve replacement. None of the 12 patients in whom the coronary bed had been flushed developed ischemic contracture of the heart. All of them came off the bypass and were stable hemodynamically. The hemodynamic and clinical data of these two groups of patients are summarized in Tables 5 and 6, respectively.

Subendocardial ischemic damage has been reported in hypertrophied right ventricle associated with congenital heart disease.[11] We have used aortic root flush with the BEKS solution in total correction of tetralogy of Fallot. Apart from the likely benefit on the hypertrophied right ventricle, the solution fills the aortic cusps, thus making them clearly visible, and helps to avoid damage by aiding in the correct placement of sutures to close the ventricular septal defect.

Aortic root flush is carried out by inserting a Cooley needle into the ascending aorta in aortocoronary bypass surgery (Fig. 5). During each period of aortic cross-clamping 100 to 150 ml of the BEKS solution is run in under gravity flow. The intermittent flushing is controlled by the use of a pinch cock.

We have encountered subendocardial hemorrhage in one patient who had aortocoronary bypass for preinfarction angina (Fig. 6). All the anastomoses of the bypass graft had been done without aortic cross clamping. The patient developed arrhythmias and low output failure; he died on the first postoperative day.

PATHOPHYSIOLOGY OF ANOXIC ARREST

Subendocardial hemorrhagic necrosis, low output failure, and conduction abnormalities have been observed by us clinically and experimentally after anoxic cardiac arrest.[41,42] They represent a combination of the effects of anoxic damage on the myocardial cell, the conduction system, and the coronary microcirculation. The following discussion based on a review of the literature reveals the complex nature of the pathogenesis of anoxic damage.

Myocardial Cell

ENERGY REQUIREMENT DURING ARREST. An arrested heart requires energy for

TABLE 6. Clinical Data on Twelve Patients with BEKS Coronary Flush during Cardiac Arrest

PT.	AGE (yrs)	SEX	DIAGNOSIS	GRADIENT (mm Hg)	NYHA CLASSIFICATION	ANOXIC ARREST (mins)	COMMENTS
CK	52	M	AI, RCA Stenosis	0	Class 3	60	AVR, RCA bypass
DW	28	M	AS and AI	35	Class 3	50	AVR
BW	57	F	AS	110	Class 3	70	AVR, RCA bypass
MR	56	F	AS and AI	125	Class 3	60	AVR
RD	60	M	AS	75	Class 3	50	AVR
RM	67	M	AS	60	Class 4	75	AVR[a]
JE	62	M	AS	70	Class 3	55	AVR
BC	71	M	AS	115	Class 3	60	AVR
DB	27	F	MS, MI AS, AI	—	Class 4	85	MVR and AVR
GC	67	M	AS	125	Class 4	60	AVR
AM	26	M	AI	—	Class 3	50	AVR
EY	60	F	AS	120	Class 4	60	AVR

[a] Bjork-Shiley valve ring came apart after placing all sutures requiring resuturing a second one in position.
AS: aortic stenosis; AI: aortic insufficiency; RCA: right coronary artery; LADC: left anterior descending coronary; AVR: aortic valve replacement; NYHA: New York Heart Association.
Adapted from Iyengar et al, J Thorac Cardiovasc Surg, 1973. Courtesy of CV Mosby Company, 1973.

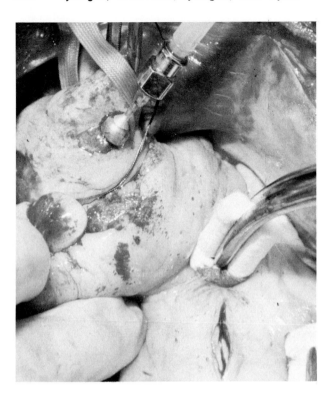

FIG. 5. Cooley needle in aortic root for BEKS hypothermic coronary flush. Arteriotomy in left anterior descending coronary artery is seen. Insert shows the needle.

chemical work to maintain the various energy-dependent subcellular systems. The sodium-potassium pump in the cell membrane, the calcium pump of the sarcoplasmic reticulum, and the mitochondria are the major components of the fine structure of the myocardial cell, which require energy for preservation of function and structure.

The extracellular fluid has a high sodium and a low potassium concentration (Fig. 7). The intracellular fluid has a high potassium and low sodium content. There is a transmembrane resting potential of −80 mv, which is generated by the separation of charges resulting from differential ion movements through the membrane.[103] There is

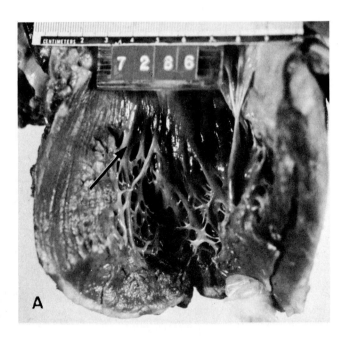

FIG. 6. A. Subendocardial hemorrhage (arrow) in a patient who had aortocoronary bypass for preinfarction angina. B. Microscopic section showing subendocardial hemorrhage (arrow). C. Microscopic section from an area adjacent to (B) showing conduction bundle (arrow) (Hematoxylin-phloxine-saffron; × 50).

A

FIG. 7. A model showing the fine structure of the myocardial cell, the sodium and calcium pump.

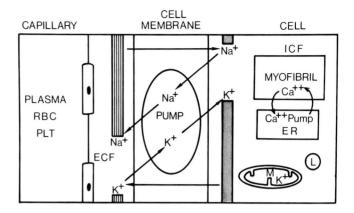

passive efflux of K^+ and influx of Na^+ along this electrochemical gradient. In order to maintain a steady state, active transport of K^+ to the interior and Na^+ to the exterior of the cell against this electrochemical gradient is necessary and requires metabolic energy.[103] In the highly specialized cardiac tissue with rhythmic activity, the fluxes of sodium and potassium assume great importance [2] and continuous expenditure of energy is required for their maintenance.[103] Irreversible injury to the Na^+ pump can be a crucial factor in the recovery of function after anoxia. Ten to 20 percent of the resting metabolism is required for the sodium pump.[103]

Several studies have been made to determine the oxygen requirement of the arrested mammalian heart.[4,5,25,29,59,68,87] The heart arrested by potassium citrate consumes 1.4 to 2.5 ml of oxygen per 100 g of tissue; whereas, a fibrillating heart requires 3.7 to 14.6 ml of oxygen for 100 g of tissue. The arrested heart uses 25 to 30 percent of the oxygen consumption of a working heart.[29]

ENERGY RESERVE DURING ARREST. The capacity of the human coronary bed estimated from postmortem specimens is 2 to 6 ml/100 g of tissue.[27] Assuming the total water content of the heart to be 60 percent of the weight, the hemoglobin concentration to be 15 g percent with 100 percent O_2 saturation, the total amount of oxygen available in a 300-g heart at the time of aortic cross-clamping is about 3 to 5 ml, which would approximately meet the oxygen requirements of an arrested heart for less than five minutes. The myocardial oxygen tension falls to its lowest levels within minutes.[9] The minimum pO_2 tension of the cytochrome oxidase, the terminal electron trans-

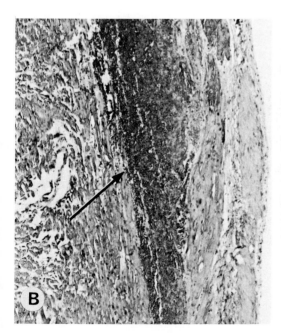

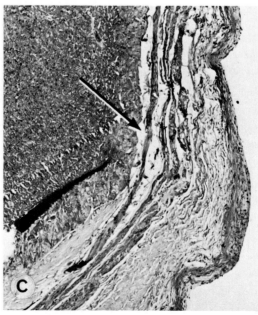

port enzyme of the mitochondria is 5 mm Hg. Energy stored by cardiac myoglobin would suffice to sustain only six additional beats at rest, in the absence of oxygen and glycolytic energy sources.[66]

Glycogen is the primary substrate for anaerobic glycolysis. There is a close correlation between the cardiac carbohydrate concentration and the survival time during anoxia.[60,63] With an initial glycogen content of 600 mg percent the energy requirements of the heart can be sustained for 4.2 minutes at resting metabolic rates.[68] The glycogen content of the adult human heart is about 200 mg percent.[8] During anaerobiosis there is depletion of cardiac glycogen,[26] and also the rate of glycolysis is considerably slower.[68,87] Anaerobic glycolysis totally stops below a pH of 6.[76]

Thus, it would appear that the myocardium has a meager reserve of substrates during anoxic arrest. In addition several important changes occur with the transition from aerobic to anaerobic metabolism that could hinder the efficient utilization of the limited energy resources, cause rapid dissipation of substrates, and inhibit glycolysis. Under anaerobic conditions breakdown of glucose proceeds via the Embden-Meyerhof glycolytic pathway up to the stage of lactic acid. Glycolysis liberates only 9 percent of the energy available in the glucose molecule.[67]

CATECHOLAMINES. There is release of endogenous myocardial catecholamines during anoxia.[102] Increased noradrenaline release and a corresponding increase in lactate production has been shown to occur in isolated rabbit hearts perfused anaerobically and in anoxic canine myocardium [88] (Fig. 8). During anoxic arrest the autonomic innervation of the heart is intact. Any sympathoadrenal stimulation secondary to cardiopulmonary bypass could also exert its influence on the cardiac sympathetic nerves and cause catecholamine release. Apart from anoxia, an increase in PCO_2 and a fall in pH stimulate release of sympathomimetic agents.[24]

Catecholamines increase myocardial oxygen consumption [30,100] and accelerate glycolysis,[58,68] both of which are wasteful in an arrested heart.

It takes several minutes before the onset of total arrest after aortic cross-clamping. The duration, rate, and intensity of myocardial contractility during this interval can be a significant factor in the early depletion of energy reserves. The His-Purkinje fibers are electrophysiologically very sensitive to adrenaline and noradrenaline.[32] Excessive release of endogenous catecholamines can result in enhanced automaticity of the His-Purkinje fibers [32] and contribute to increased activity and energy consumption preceding the onset of com-

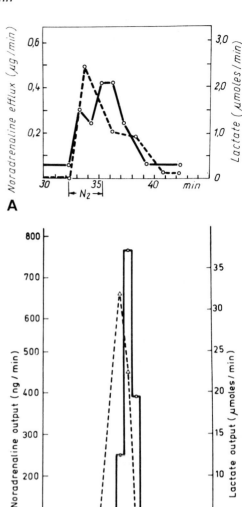

FIG. 8. A. Release of noradrenaline (solid line) and lactate (broken line) from an isolated perfused rabbit heart following anoxia by switch to anaerobic perfusion (from Shahab et al, 1972). B. Net output of noradrenaline and lactate from a portion of the dog's heart. The oblique bars on the abscissa denote the period of occlusion of the left anterior descending coronary artery. Noradrenaline output is represented by the solid line, lactate by the broken line. (From Shahab, Wollenberger, et al, courtesy of Churchill Livingstone, London, 1972.[88])

plete arrest. Increased serum levels of myocardial enzymes and extensive myocardial damage can be produced by the administration of catecholamines in intact hearts.[37,85,86]

Eosinophilia, swelling, and ultimately massive necrosis have been observed in hearts exposed to increasing amounts of catecholamines.[36] Electronmicroscopic and histoenzymatic abnormalities were shown to be the early consequences of catecholamine excess before any lesions detectable by classical histological methods appeared.[36]

CATION SHIFTS. Normally a relatively constant intracellular composition of electrolytes is maintained. Massive intramyocardial shifts of electrolytes can be induced by ischemia.[44] K^+, Na^+, Ca^{++}, and Mg^{++} are the principal cations that are subject to shifts during anoxia. Their altered distribution has an effect on the cellular metabolism, sodium pump, electrophysiology, mitochondrial function, and contractility of the myofilaments.[1,2,15,16,19,21,35,44,46,48,51,57,79,90,92,98,103,104,105]

Interruption of coronary circulation during bypass surgery results in a loss of intracellular potassium and again in intracellular sodium as shown by myocardial biopsies.[92] Depletion of intramyocardial potassium would be favorable to increased myocardial vulnerability to arrhythmias.[92] There is efflux of potassium from acidotic myocardial cells and influx of Ca^{++} into the cell.[19] Large changes in contraction can result from very small changes in intracellular ion content.[51] Na^+ efflux and K^+ influx are temperature sensitive.[103] At 3 C there is a progressive loss of intracellular K^+ in rat diaphragm muscle reaching 50 percent of the intracellular content.[57] During rewarming, active transport of the potassium into the cell takes place at the expense of metabolic energy. There is a tremendous loss of myocardial potassium during fibrillation.[90] A local impairment of cellular metabolism may lead to local accumulation of potassium, thus lowering the threshold and shortening the fiber action potential.[82] Perhaps an augmented sodium permeability of the damaged membrane may cause an extra excitation. Alterations in the normal concentrations of the cations in the extracellular water produce changes in the glycolytic rate of tissue cells.[22,79] There is an interdependence between energy-coupled reactions and mitochondrial potassium.[15] There is an increase in mitochondrial calcium and decrease in potassium, magnesium, and nitrogen content after ischemic injury.[46] As serum potassium levels do not reflect the intracellular potassium content, it is difficult to know the role of myocardial potassium shifts in the genesis of arrhythmias and low output failure after anoxic arrest.

pH AND PCO_2 CHANGES. A rising PCO_2[9,24,95] and accumulation of lactic acid from anaerobic metabolism lead to a fall in myocardial pH. The coronary sinus blood pH after 30 minutes of anoxic arrest in dogs was in the markedly acidotic range of 6.8 to 6.99. The average peak PCO_2 reading observed during 30 minutes of cardiac anoxia in dogs was 147 mm Hg in the subepicardial region while the deep myocardial readings averaged 223 mm Hg.[9] The significance of this variation is not clear.

ULTRASTRUCTURE. Nowhere is the relationship of fine structure to function better illustrated than in the myocardium.[13] Biochemical and electron microscopic studies of the fine structure of the human and mammalian cardiac tissue,[13,14,45,46,47,61,99] subjected to anoxia suggest that one of the earliest features of irreversible injury in myocardial cells may be alterations in membrane permeability. Myocardial cells are almost completely dependent upon aerobic mitochondrial metabolism for their energy requirements. Irreversible anoxic damage is associated with margination of nuclear chromatin, virtual absence of glycogen, marked relaxation of myofibrils, and characteristic mitochondrial abnormalities, which include swelling, loss of matrix density, and appearance of amorphous matrix densities. Cells irreversibly injured by ischemia and then reperfused with arterial blood show striking cellular swelling, severe contraction bands, and the appearance of granular mitochondrial densities.[47]

Lysosomes are subcellular organelles that contain hydrolytic enzymes. Normally the release of these enzymes is regulated to meet the catabolic needs of the cell. Loss of integrity of lysosomal membrane under the influence of anoxia and acidosis can lead to escape of the hydrolytic enzymes and disintegration of the intracellular structures.[97]

Coronary Microcirculation

About half of the heart's weight is made of noncontractile material, and the coronary microvasculature forms an important component of this tissue.[10] In the newborn there is one capillary for four myocardial fibers corresponding to 4,000 capillaries per mm^2 of tissue. In the adult there is one capillary per muscle fiber with a density of 3,000 to 4,000 capillaries per mm^2. The capillary diffusing area per cm^3 of tissue is 1,145 cm^2 in children, and 1,184 cm^2 in adults. The maximum diffusing distance is 8μ.[27]

Not all myocardial capillaries are functional at all times. The presence of connections between arterioles, metarterioles, precapillaries, and venules in both men and dogs suggests arteriovenous shunting to be an integral component of the coronary microcirculation accounting for a dynamic changing state of capillary patency and function.[27] Autoregulation of flow and maintenance of homeostasis by regulating the exchange of metabolites and substrates across the capillary wall are the vital functions of the microcirculation.[28]

The effects of anoxia on the coronary microvasculature is, therefore, of great importance in determining the recovery of function after anoxic cardiac arrest. The following changes have been observed in the myocardial capillaries after cardiac arrest in dogs.[77] There is weakening of the connective tissue elements. Rouleaux formation and swelling of erythrocytes occur. Upon reperfusion after arrest of the circulation, focal areas of capillary rupture with tissue hemorrhage are seen. There is a diminution in myocardial oxygen consumption on reperfusion, which varies directly with the duration of anoxia. There is believed to be arteriovenous shunting in the post anoxic period.[9]

The following changes in the ultrastructure of the capillaries of rats under the influence of serotonin, a normal constituent of platelets, have been observed.[71] Discontinuity of endothelial lining permits escape of chylomicrons, plasma proteins, platelets, erythrocytes, and leucocytes. In the course of time, large deposits of these particles accumulate within the wall of the vessel and start to dissect its layers.

A discussion of the pathogenesis of vascular damage in relation to our earlier experimental work on anoxic cardiac arrest has been reported.[41] Stasis of blood in the coronary microcirculation results in sludging of red cells and release of vasoactive substances. Alterations in the metabolism of anoxic myocardial cells result in leakage of acid metabolites and vasoactive substances. The normal electrical charges of the formed elements of the blood and of the capillary endothelium are reversed. The net result of the biophysical and biochemical changes is damage to the capillary endothelium.

Conduction System

The conduction system has a unique structure and function.[10,83,84] There is reason to believe that anoxic damage to the conduction system can result in an alteration in the normal sequence of depolarization, which could result in asynchronous ventricular contraction. The cells of the conduction system have a small number of myofibrils.[10] It may be that their contraction serves only the purpose of diminishing the shear forces that would develop between myocardial and Purkinje cells if the latter remained purely passive.

Their involvement in subendocardial ischemic damage could cause stretching of the conduction elements, which is said to be one of the factors favoring the genesis of arrhythmias.

In the longitudinal direction, the Purkinje cells are joined to the intermediate cells that connect them to myocardial cells. Increasingly large numbers of myofibrils are present in the intermediate cells as they approach the true myocardial cells. They must contribute to some extent to the overall contractile force, judging from morphological evidence.[10] This is likely to be compromised by subendocardial damage.

The entire subendocardial surface on the left side is richly lined by Purkinje fibers,[84] and the subendocardium also happens to be the area most vulnerable to subendocardial hemorrhagic necrosis.[41,42] This morphologic coincidence of the distribution of the conduction fibers and the pathological lesions (Figs. 5, 9) is likely to result in electrophysiologic alterations, which play a potential role in the low-output state in the postanoxic period. The peripheral Purkinje system appears to have a suitable anatomic arrangement to set up a well-defined circus movement and, thus, predispose to increased vulnerability to conduction abnormalities.[33]

Furthermore the His-Purkinje system is liable to damage and altered electrophysiology by the metabolic alterations, catecholamine release, fall in pH, rise in PCO_2, anoxia, cation shifts, and vascular stasis during anoxic cardiac arrest.[20,32,55,75,83]

Recovery of Function

The detrimental effects of cardiac arrest have been pointed out by several studies.[12,26,41,42,]

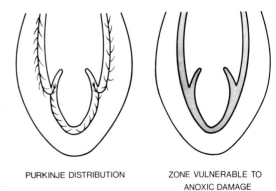

PURKINJE DISTRIBUTION   ZONE VULNERABLE TO
                                    ANOXIC DAMAGE

FIG. 9. Diagrammatic representation of left ventricular wall showing subendocardial distribution of Purkinje system (left) and zone vulnerable to anoxic damage (right).

[52,80,96] Myocardial failure can occur in the presence of normal oxidative metabolism.[68] Mechanical response to hypoxia appears related to a large extent to alterations in the coupling of excitation and contraction.[94] Even when the myocardial injury is in a reversible state, it can still have adverse effects in the postanoxic period in two ways. Reoxygenation of areas of myocardium that are in varying stages of recovery may induce disparities in the times at which contraction and relaxation occur. The overall effect on the course of contraction will be dyssynchrony between normal regions and those rendered hypoxic and then reperfused. This may occur despite the fact that peak force development may be little altered, and functional aneurysm or asynergic contraction in areas of ischemia may thus ensue despite local force production.[94] Localized areas of ischemic damage, particularly in the subendocardial region after anoxic arrest as seen in our experimental work, would favor such a situation.

It would thus appear that there is no one common denominator present in the pathogenesis of anoxic myocardial damage. Several factors play a role, and the early irreversible changes involve biochemical alterations, the ultrastructure, and membrane permeability.

METHODS TO IMPROVE ANOXIC TOLERANCE

Hypothermia has been found to be useful both experimentally and clinically.[6,7,14,23,31,40,49,63,87,91] Cold exerts its beneficial influence by reducing the metabolic needs.[23] However, it is not the ideal solution for the following reasons. The method is cumbersome, and rewarming wastes valuable perfusion time.[53] Cooling the arrested heart to between 21.5 and 25 C decreased the oxygen consumption to 7 percent of the oxygen consumption of the initial working heart.[5] Therefore moderate hypothermia does not totally abolish chemical work. The factor of intramyocardial acidosis still exists from accumulation of acid metabolites, although at a slower rate.[19,20] Stasis of blood and its associated ill effects on the microvasculature are not eliminated. Some obscure mechanism results in depletion of glycogen content of the heart during hypothermia.[68] There is progressive loss of K^+ from the cell during cooling, which needs to be pumped back during rewarming.[57,91,103] Hearts of dogs subjected to one to four hours of moderate or deep hypothermia have shown foci of necrotic muscle fibers with occasional cellular reaction in the myocardium.[81] Similar changes were observed

in the long-term canine survivors after hypothermia. After hypothermic arrest there is damage to the oxygen consuming capacity of the myocardium.[87]

In a comparative study of three techniques of hypothermia, recovery of myocardial function was 40 to 60 percent of normal with topical cooling, 80 percent of normal with selective cooling, and 90 percent of normal with cold aortic root perfusion.[89] It would thus appear that core cooling with provision of energy substrates and elimination of stasis of acid metabolites is superior to surface cooling alone.

The five cases of stone heart seen in our experience (Table 5) occurred in spite of total body cooling to 30 to 32 C and topical cooling of the heart with ice-cold Ringer's solution. This prompted us to investigate the myocardial potential for extended anaerobic metabolism in the presence of adequate substrate. We observed structural and functional myocardial protection [41,42] in the normal and hypertrophied canine left ventricle when the coronary bed was intermittently flushed with the BEKS solution (Tables 1 to 4, Figs. 3, 4). Impressed with the experimental findings, we have used this technique for the past three years in clinical practice, and we have not encountered any "stone heart" during this period in a group of patients comparable to those in whom ischemic contracture occurred in our earlier experience (Tables 5, 6).

Hypothermic BEKS coronary flush combines the advantages of core cooling, provision of energy substrate, elimination of acid metabolites, and vasoactive substances. The solution we are currently using is made up of 400 ml of plain Ringers solution, 100 ml low molecular weight dextran in 10 percent dextrose, 10 mEq $NaHCO_3$, 4 mEq KCl, 1,000 units heparin, 1 unit regular insulin, and 10 mg solucortef. The temperature of the solution is 20 to 25 C and the pH 7.5 to 7.7. In cases of aortic valve replacement, the coronary arteries are directly flushed intermittently; in aortocoronary bypass, correction of tetralogy of Fallot and ventricular septal defect, a Cooley needle is inserted into the ascending aorta (Fig. 5) and the solution is run in under gravity flow whenever the aorta is cross clamped.

Mechanical flushing alone of the coronary bed under anaerobic conditions in the absence of glucose did not preserve function and fine structure of isolated rat hearts [99] (Fig. 10). At a temperature of 20 to 25 C, chemical work is not totally abolished, and hence there is need for adequate substrate for anaerobic energy production. Therefore, we have included several pharma-

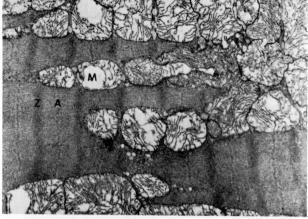

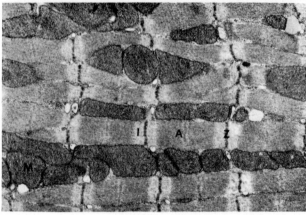

FIG. 10. (Top) After 60 minutes of aerobic perfusion and 30 minutes' anaerobic perfusion in the absence of glucose. The mitochondria appear enlarged and show decreased electron opacity of the matrix and displacement and separation of cristae. The intramitochondrial microbodies are not seen. Transverse tubules are difficult to recognize. The myofibrils are contracted and demonstrate wide Z areas and absence of I bands. (Bottom) After 60 minutes of aerobic perfusion and 30 minutes anaerobic perfusion in the presence of glucose. The mitochondria, myofibrils, and transverse tubules are well preserved. The intramitochondrial microbodies are diminished in size and number. Longitudinal tubules are not dilated. (From Weissler et al: J Clin Invest, 1968.)

cologic agents in the BEKS solution. The protective action of these agents on anoxic myocardium is supported by several experimental studies.[3,15,17,18,34,62,65,68,69,70,73,78,99] They are also intended to prevent or minimize the detrimental effects of the various metabolic and histochemical alterations associated with myocardial ischemia discussed in the preceding section on the pathophysiology of anoxic cardiac arrest.

Administration of glucose was noted to increase the content of glycogen and creatine phosphate by increasing the ATP formation beyond the needs of the heart for ATP utilization.[7] During 30 minutes of anoxia, inclusion of glucose in the perfusate resulted in marked improvement in electrical and mechanical performance of the heart as well as enhanced recovery during the subsequent period of reoxygenation. Lactic acid production was five times greater in the glucose-supported heart than in an anoxic heart without glucose. Electron microscopy revealed that pathologic alterations in the mitochondria and dilatation of the longitudinal tubules were averted with glucose[99] (Fig. 10).

Another interesting facet of the action of glucose is the experimental evidence, which shows that glucose in adequate concentrations in the perfusate stimulates mitochondria to produce energy through extraglycolytic pathways in the absence of oxygen.[72] This can be of importance in an anoxic heart. Extraglycolytic energy production by the mitochondria was further increased by the combination of tricarboxylic acid metabolites and glucose in the perfusate of the anoxic heart. Of further interest is the increased survival of rabbits during hemorrhagic shock when tricarboxylic acid metabolites were introduced into the animal.[18] It does appear that mitochondrial reactions can be stimulated to generate substantial amounts of energy through extraglycolitic pathways. Formation of high-energy phosphate bonds has been shown to occur in mammalian tissue by the utilization of α-acetoglutarate and oxalacetate under anaerobic conditions.[38]

Insulin lowers the threshold for myocardial glucose extraction and thus facilitates intracellular transfer of glucose.[34,62,68] Isolated mitochondria from anoxic cardiac tissue appeared to have a defect in the phosphorylative reactions followed by a blockage of the respiratory chain, which was prevented by insulin-glucose-potassium solution.[15]

Insulin, glucose, and potassium infusion prevents the loss of potassium from ischemic myocardial cells.[15,17,66,69] In experimental coronary artery ligation, the size of the infarction has been shown to be significantly reduced by insulin-glucose-potassium infusion.[56]

Theoretically the cessation of all contractile activity by the addition of potassium to the perfusion medium could reduce the oxygen demand to a level that could be satisfied by the maximum observed rate of anaerobic glycolysis during total anoxia.[69] Perfusate containing glucose plus 11.6 mEq KCl/L was found to produce a cardiac output on cessation of anoxia comparable to that in hearts that had not been anoxic at all.[69]

The protective action of hydrocortisone on the myocardium has been shown.[64,93] It appears to reduce the incidence of myocardial necrosis in rats with potassium depletion.[93] Acidotic myocardial failure in isolated heart preparations was mitigated by the administration of hydrocortisone.[64] Hydrocortisone also has a stabilizing action on the lysosomal and cell membranes.[97,101]

Low-molecular-weight dextran prevents intravascular aggregation of red cells by preventing the development of adhesive properties on surfaces of corpuscles.[54] The cells do not adhere to each other or the walls of the blood vessels.

Future research in this area should be directed toward the development of pharmacologic agents that will preserve structural, functional, and metabolic integrity of the myocardium for a sufficient period of time to allow total operative repair while the aorta is cross-clamped.[53]

The technique of BEKS coronary flush also provides an experimental model to evaluate methods that will achieve better myocardial protection during anoxic arrest by further pharmacological manipulation.

We are currently engaged in the evaluation of several other pharmacologic agents, addition of which to the BEKS solution may enhance its protective action.

SUMMARY

Our investigations revealed that normal dogs subjected to 60 minutes of anoxic cardiac arrest developed subendocardial hemorrhagic necrosis, low output failure, and died intraoperatively. The hypertrophied canine left ventricle was found to be much more vulnerable to anoxic damage than the normal canine heart. Both experimentally and clinically, flushing the coronary bed with BEKS solution (20 to 25 C) during anoxic arrest appears to provide structural and functional myocardial protection.

A complex series of ultrastructural, metabolic, electrophysiologic, and vascular changes take place during anoxic arrest. Their exact nature and role in the pathogenesis of myocardial damage is still not completely understood. The earliest irreversible changes occur at the level of membrane permeability and ultrastructure.

There is fairly conclusive evidence to show that provision of adequate substrate and prevention of stasis of vasoactive and acid metabolites during anoxia can preserve the glycogen content, high-energy phosphate bonds, ultrastructure, and recovery of function of the myocardium after anoxic cardiac arrest.

Myocardial protection to prevent anoxic damage incidental to aortic cross-clamping in cardiac surgery is important. We have found hypothermic BEKS coronary flush a convenient and practical method. It has the following advantages: (1) simple technique; (2) rapid core cooling to any desired level; (3) prevention of stasis of blood, vasoactive, and acid metabolites; (4) provision of substrate and optimal conditions for anaerobic energy production; (5) protection of the vascular and cellular membranes; and (6) research model to evaluate pharmacologic agents to improve even further the safe limit of anoxic arrest.

ACKNOWLEDGMENTS

We gratefully acknowledge the assistance of Dr. S. Ramchand, Dr. S. M. Wassan, and Dr. H. J. Manz for review of pathology, Medical Photography division of Queen's University; Mr. Winston Offord for technical assistance; and Mrs. Wendy Gollogly for secretarial help.

References

1. Angelakos ET, Deutsch S, Williams SL: Sensitivity of the hypothermic myocardium to calcium. Circ Res 5:196, 1957
2. Armitage AK, Burn JH, Gunning AJ: Ventricular fibrillation and ion transport. Circ Res 5:98, 1957
3. Bajusz E, Selye H: The chemical prevention of cardiac necrosis following occlusion of coronary vessels. Can Med Assoc J 82:212, 1960
4. Berglund E, Monroe RG, Schreiner GL: Myocardial oxygen consumption and coronary blood-flow during potassium induced cardiac arrest and during ventricular fibrillation. Acta Physiol Scand 41:261, 1957

5. Berne RM, Jones RD, Cross FS: Oxygen consumption of the hypothermic potassium arrested heart. Proc Soc Exp Biol Med 99:84, 1958

6. Bernhard WF, Gross RE: The rationale of hypothermic cardioplegia in the management of congenital anamolies affecting the aortic valve, coronary arteries and proximal aortic arch. Ann Surg 156:161, 1962

7. Bernhard WF, Schwartz HF, Mallick NP: Intermittent cold coronary perfusion as an adjunct to open heart surgery. Surg Gynec Obstet 111:744, 1960

8. Boyd W: Pathology for the physician. Philadelphia, Lea Febiger, 1965, p 33

9. Brantigan JW, Perna AM, Gardner TJ, Gott VL: Intramyocardial gas tensions in the canine heart during anoxic cardiac arrest. Surg Gynec Obstet 134:67, 1972

10. Brecher GA, Galletti PM: Functional anatomy of cardiac pumping. In Hamilton WF (ed): Handbook of Physiology, section 2: Circulation, vol 2, Washington, DC, American Physiological Society, 1963, pp 762–71

11. Buckburg GD, Towers B, Pagia DE, Mulder DG, Maloney JV: Subendocardial ischemia after cardiopulmonary bypass. J Thorac Cardiovasc Surg 64:669, 1972

12. Buja LM, Levitsky S, Ferrans VJ, et al: Acute and chronic effects of normothermic anoxia on canine hearts. Circulation 43:44, 1971

13. Burdette WJ, Ashford TP: Structural changes in the human myocardium following hypoxia. J Thorac Cardiovasc Surg 50:210, 1965

14. Burdette WJ, Ashford TP: Response of myocardial fine structure to cardiac arrest and hypothermia. Ann Surg 158:513, 1963

15. Calva E, Mujica A, Nunez R, et al: Mitochondrial biochemical changes and glucose-KCl-insulin solution in cardiac infarct. Am J Physiol 211:71, 1966

16. Carden NL, Steinhaus JE: Role of magnesium ion in the initiation of ventricular fibrillation produced by acute coronary occlusion. Circ Res 5:405, 1957

17. Cherbakoff A, Toyama S, Hamilton WF: Relation between coronary sinus plasma potassium and cardiac arrhythmia. Circ Res 5:517, 1957

18. Chick WL, Weiner R, Cascarano J, Zweifach BW: Influence of Kreb-cycle intermediates on survival in hemorrhagic shock. Am J Physiol 215:1107, 1968

19. Covino BG, Hegnauer AH: Electroylytes and pH changes in relation to hypothermic ventricular fibrillation. Circ Res 3:575, 1955

20. Covino BG, Hegnauer AH: Hypothermic ventricular fibrillation and its control. Surgery 40:475, 1956

21. Dennis J, Moore RM: Potassium changes in the functioning heart under conditions of ischemia and of congestion. Am J Physiol 123:443, 1938

22. Drummond GI, Duncan L, Fricsen AJD: Some properties of cardiac phosphorylase b kinase. J Biol Chem 240:2778, 1965

23. Edwards WS, Tuluy S, Reber WE, Siegel A, Bing RJ: Coronary bloodflow and myocardial metabolism in hypothermia. Ann Surg 139:275, 1954

24. Feinberg H, Gerola A, Katz LN: Effect of changes in blood CO_2 level on coronary flow and myocardial oxygen consumption. Am J Physiol 199:349, 1960

25. Fuhrman FA, Fuhrman GJ, Field J: Oxygen consumption of excised rat tissues following acute anoxic anoxia. Am J Physiol 144:87, 1945

26. Goldman BS, Trimble AS, Sheverini MA, et al: Functional and metabolic effects of anoxic cardiac arrest. Ann Thorac Surg 11:122, 1971

27. Gregg DE, Fisher LC: Blood supply to the heart. In Hamilton WF (ed): Handbook of Physiology, section 2: Circulation vol 2. Washington, DC, American Physiological Society, 1963, p 1521

28. Gregg DE, Fisher LC: Blood supply to the heart. In Hamilton WF (ed): Handbook of Physiology, section 2: Circulation, vol 2, Washington, DC, American Physiological Society, 1963, p 1528

29. Gregg DE, Fisher LC: Blood supply to the heart. In Hamilton WF (ed): Handbook of Physiology, section 2: Circulation, vol 2, Washington, DC, American Physiological Society, 1963, pp 1537–41

30. Gregg DE, Fisher LC: Blood supply to the heart. In Hamilton WF (ed): Handbook of Physiology, section 2: Circulation, vol 2, Washington, DC, American Physiological Society, 1963, p 1549

31. Gregg DE, Fisher LC: Blood supply to the heart. In Hamilton WF (ed): Handbook of Physiology, section 2: Circulation, vol. 2, Washington, DC, American Physiological Society, 1963, p 1559

32. Han J: Ventricular vulnerability in myocardial ischaemia. In Oliver MF, Julian DG, Donald KW (eds): Effect of Acute Ischaemia on Myocardial Function. London, Churchill Livingston, 1972, pp 141–56

33. Han J: The concepts of re-entrant activity responsible for ectopic rhythms. Am J Cardiol 28:253, 1971

34. Hackel DB: Effect of insulin on cardiac metabolism of intact normal dogs. Am J Physiol 199:1135, 1960

35. Harris AS, Bisteni A, Russel RA, Brigham JC, Firestone JE: Excitatory factors in ventricular tachycardia resulting from myocardial ischemia: potassium a major excitant. Science 119:200, 1956

36. Herbaczynska-Cedro K: Loss of myocardial enzymes in relation to enhanced adrenaline secretion in an early stage of experimental infarction. In Oliver MD, Julian DG, Donald KW (eds): Effect of Acute Ischaemia on Myocardial Function. London, Churchill Livingston, 1972, p 109

37. Highman B, Maling HM, Thompson EC: Serum transaminase and alkaline phosphatase levels after large doses of norepinephrine and epinephrine in dogs. Am J Physiol 196:436, 1959

38. Hunter FE Jr: Anaerobic Phosphorylation due to a coupled oxidation reduction between α-Ketoglutaric acid and oxalacetic acid. J Biol Chem 177:361, 1949

39. Hufnagel CA, Conrad PW, Schanno J, Pifarre R: Profound cardiac hypothermia. Ann Surg 153:790, 1961

40. Hurley EJ, Dong E, Stoffer RC, Shumway NE: Isotopic replacement of the totally excised canine heart. J Surg Res 2:90, 1962

41. Iyengar SRK, Ramchand S, Charrette EJP, Lynn RB: An experimental study of subendocardial hemorrhagic necrosis after anoxic cardiac arrest. Ann Thorac Surg 13:214, 1972

42. Iyengar SRK, Ramchand S, Charrette EJP, Iyengar CKS, Lynn RB: Anoxic cardiac arrest: an experimental and clinical study of its effects, part I. J Thorac Cardiovasc Surg 6:722, 1973

43. Ieyngar SRK, Charrette EJP, Iyengar CKS, Lynn RB: An experimental model with left ventricular hypertrophy caused by subcoronary aortic stenosis in dogs. J Thorac Cardiovasc Surg 66:823, 1973

44. Jennings RB, Sommers HM, Kaltenbach JP, West JJ: Electrolyte alterations in acute myocardial ischemic injury. Circ Res 14:260, 1964

45. Jennings RB, Herdson PB, Sommers HM: Structural and functional abnormalities in mitochondria isolated from ischemic dog myocardium. Lab Invest 20:548, 1969

46. Jennings RB, Moore CB, Shen AC, Herdson PB:

Electroylytes of damaged myocardial mitochondria. Proc Soc Exp Biol Med 135:515, 1970

47. Jennings RB, Ganote CE: Ultrastructural changes in acute myocardial ischemia. In Oliver MF, Julian DG, Donald KW (eds): Effect of Acute Ischaemia on Myocardial function. London, Churchill Livingstone, 1972, pp 50–74

48. Keating RE, Weichselbaum TE, Alanis M, et al: The movement of potassium during experimental acidosis and alkalosis in the nephrectomixed dog. Surg Gynec Obstet 96:323, 1953

49. Kusunoki T, Cheng H, McGuire HH Jr, Bosher LH: Myocardial dysfunction after cardioplegia. J Thorac Cardiovasc Surg 40:813, 1960

50. Lambert PB, Frank HA, Bellman S, Williams JA: Electrical excitability of ventricular myocardium in relation to graded changes in coronary inflow. J Surg Res 1:251, 1961

51. Leonard E, Hajdu S: Action of electrolytes and drugs on the contractile mechanism of the cardiac muscle cell. In Hamilton WF (ed): Handbook of Physiology, section 2: Circulation, vol 1, Washington, DC, American Physiological Society, 1962, pp 155–75

52. Levitsky S, Sloane RE, Mullin EM, McIntosh CL, Morrow AG: Normothermic myocardial anoxia. Ann Thorac Surg 11:228, 1971

53. Levitsky S: Discussion of paper: functional and structural alterations in the myocardium during aortic cross clamping. J Thorac Cardiovasc Surg 66:768, 1973

54. Long DM, Sanchez L, Varco RL, Lillehel CW: The use of low molecular weight dextran and serum albumin as plasma expanders in extracorporeal circulation. Surgery 50:12, 1961

55. Maling HM, Moran NC: Ventricular arrhythmias induced by sympathomimetic amines in unanesthetized dogs following coronary artery occlusion. Circ Res 5:409, 1957

56. Maroko PR, Libby P, Sobel BE, et al: Effect of glucose-insulin-potassium infusion on myocardial infarction following experimental coronary artery occlusion. Circulation 45:1160, 1972

57. May G, Barnes BA: Comparison of magnesium and potassium efflux from incubated rat diaphragms. Am J Physiol 199:246, 1960

58. Mayer SE, Williams BJ, Smith JM: Adrenergic mechanisms in cardiac glycogen metabolism. Ann NY Acad Sci 139:686, 1966

59. McKeever WP, Gregg DE, Canney PC: Oxygen uptake of the nonworking left ventricle. Circ Res 6:612, 1958

60. Merrick AW, Meyer DK: Glycogen fractions of cardiac muscle in the normal and anoxic heart. Am J Physiol 177:441, 1954

61. Miller DR, Rasmussen P, Klionsky B: Reversibility of morphologic changes following elective cardiac arrest. Ann Surg 159:208, 1964

62. Morgan HE, Henderson MJ, Regen DM, Park CR: Regulation of glucose uptake in muscle. I. The effects of insulin and anoxia on glucose transport and phosphorylation in the isolated perfused heart of normal rats. J Biol Chem 236:253, 1961

63. Mott JC: The ability of young mammals to withstand total oxygen lack. Br Med Bull 17:144, 1961

64. Nahas GG: Effect of hydrocortisone on acidotic failure of the isolated heart. Circ Res 5:489, 1957

65. Newsholme EA, Randle PJ: Regulation of glucose uptake by muscle. 5. Effects of anoxia, insulin, adrenaline and prolonged starving on concentrations of hexose phosphates in isolated rat diaphragm and perfused isolated rat heart. Biochem J 80:655, 1961

66. Olsen RE: Physiology of cardiac muscle. In Hamilton WF (ed): Handbook of Physiology, sec-

67. Olsen RE: Physiology of cardiac muscle. In Hamilton WR (ed): Handbook of Physiology, section 2: Circulation, vol 1, Washington, DC, American Physiological Society, 1962, p 205

68. Olsen RE: Physiology of cardiac muscle. In Hamilton WF (ed): Handbook of Physiology, section 2: Circulation, vol 1, Washington, DC, American Physiological Society, 1962, pp 210–26

69. Opie LH, Lochner A, Owen P, et al: Substrate uptake in experimental myocardial ischaemia. Evaluation of role of glucose, fatty acids and glucose-insulin-potassium therapy. In Oliver MF, Julian DG, Donald KW (eds): Effect of Acute Ischaemia on Myocardial Function. London, Churchill Livingstone, 1972, p 184

70. Opie LH, Lochner A, Owen P, et al: Substrate uptake in experimental myocardial ischaemia. Evaluation of role of glucose, fatty acids and glucose-insulin-potassium therapy. In Oliver MF, Julian DG, Donald KW (eds): Effect of acute ischaemia on myocardial function. London, Churchill Livingstone, 1972, p 196

71. Palade GE: Blood capillaries of the heart and other organs. Circulation 24:368, 1961

72. Penny DG, Cascarano J: Anaerobic rat heart: effects of glucose and tricarboxylic acid-cycle metabolites on metabolism and physiological performance. Biochem J 118:221, 1970

73. Regan TJ, Harman MA, Lehan PH, Burke WM, Oldewurtel HA: Ventricular arrhythmias and K^+ transfer during myocardial ischemia and intervention with procainamide, insulin or glucose solution. J Clin Invest 46:1657, 1967

74. Reeves RB: Metabolism and efficiency of a working turtle heart. Fed Proc 18:498, 1959 (abstract)

75. Reuter H, Gettes LS, Katzung BG: Cation movements during excitation of the heart. In Oliver MF, Julian DG, Donald KW (eds): Effect of Acute Ischaemia on Myocardial Function. London, Churchill Livingstone, 1972, pp 157–63

76. Relman AS: Metabolic consequences of acid-base disorders. In Robison RR (ed): Kidney International. New York-Heidelberg-Berlin, Springer-Verlag, 1972, p 347

77. Reynolds SRM, Kirsch M, Bing RJ: Functional capillary beds in the beating KCl arrested and KCl arrested perfused myocardium of the dog. Circ Res 6:600, 1958

78. Robb JS: Maintenance of perfused mammalian hearts. Circ Res 11:184, 1953

79. Rogen DM, Young DAB, David WW, Jack J Jr, Park CR: Adjustment of glycolysis to energy utilization in the perfused rat heart—the effect of changes in the ionic composition of the medium of phosphofructokinase activity. J Biol Chem 239:381, 1961

80. Sarin CL, Harr RW, Ross DN: Effects of extracorporeal circulation on left ventricular function with and without anoxic arrest. J Thorac Cardiovasc Surg 56:395, 1968

81. Samuli Sarajas HS: Evidence of heart damage in association with systemic hypothermia in dogs. Am Heart J 51:298, 1956

82. Schaefer H, Haas HG: Electrocardiography. In Hamilton WF (ed): Handbook of Physiology, section 2: Circulation, vol 1, Washington, DC, American Physiological Society, 1962, pp 389–96

83. Scher AM, Young AC, Malmgren AL, Erickson RV: Activation of interventricular septum. Circ Res 3:56, 1955

84. Scher AM: Excitation of the heart. In Hamilton WF, (ed): Handbook of Physiology, section 2: Circulation, vol 1, Washington, DC, American Physiological Society, 1962, pp 287–316

85. Schenk EA, Moss AJ: Cardiovascular effects of

sustained norepinephrine infusions. II Morphology. Circ Res 18:605, 1966

86. Schenk EA, Galbreath R, Moss AJ: Cardiovascular effects of sustained norepinephrine infusion. III Lactic dehydrogenase isoenzyme release. Circ Res 18:616, 1966

87. Sealy WC, Young WG, Lasage AM, Brown IW: Observations on heart action during hypothermia induced & controlled by a pump oxygenator. Ann Surg 153:797, 1961

88. Shahab L, Wollenberger A, Krause EG, Genz S: The effect of acute ischaemia on catecholamines and cyclic AMP levels in normal and hypertrophied myocardium. In Oliver MF, Julian DG, Donald KW (eds): Effect of Acute Ischaemia on Myocardial Function. London, Churchill Livingston, 1972, p 98

89. Stemmer EA, Aronon WS, Connolly JE: Selective deep hypothermia of the heart during aortocoronary surgery. Abstract (149) Coronary Artery, Medicine and Surgery Conference, Houston, Tex, 1974

90. Swan H: Discussion of paper by Young WG, Harris JS: The role of intracellular & extracellular electrolytes in the cardiac arrhythmias produced by prolonged hypercapnia. Surg 36:636, 1954

91. Swan H, Zeavin I, Holmes JH, Montgomery V: Cessation of circulation in general hypothermia. I. Physiological changes and their control. Ann Surg 138:360, 1953

92. Taggart PI, Slater JDH: Cation gradients in ischaemic human myocardium with observations on tissue and plasma catecholamines. In Oliver MF, Julian DG, Donald KW (eds): Effect of Acute Ischaemia on Myocardial Function. London, Churchill Livingston, 1972, pp 164–80

93. Tucker VL, Hanna H, Kaiser CJ, Darrow DC: Cardiac necrosis accompanying K^+ deficiency and administration of corticosteroids. Circ Res 13:420, 1963

94. Tyberg JV, Yeatman LA, Parmley WM, Urschel CW, Sonnenblick EH: Effects of hypoxia on mechanics of cardiac contraction. Am J Physiol 218:1780, 1970

95. Waddell WJ, Butler TC: Calculation of Intracellular pH from the distribution of 5,5-Dimethyl-2, 4-oxazoladinedione (DMO). Application to skeletal muscle of the dog. J Clin Invest 38: 730, 1959

96. Waldausen JA, Braunwald NS, Bloodwell RD, Cornell WP, Morrow AG: Left ventricular function following elective cardiac arrest. J Thorac Cardiovasc Surg 39:799, 1960

97. Walter JB, Isreal MS: General Pathology. London, JA Churchill, 1970, pp 37–40

98. Weber A: The role of calcium In the regulation of muscle activity. In Briller SA and Conn HL (eds): Myocardial Cell, Philadelphia, Univ of Penn Press, 1969, pp 140–41

99. Weissler AM, Kruger FA, Nobuhisa Baba, et al: Role of anaerobic metabolism in the preservation of functional capacity and structure of anoxic myocardium. J Clin Invest 47:403, 1968

100. Whalen WJ: Oxygen consumption and tension of isolated heart muscle during rest and acivlty using a new technique. Circ Res 5:556, 1957

101. Wilson JW: Cellular stabilization with synthetic steroid compounds on cardiopulmonary bypass, abstract (140), Coronary Artery Medicine and Surgery Conference, Houston, Tex, 1974

102. Wollenberger A, Krause E, Heier G: Stimulation of 3′, 5′—cyclic AMP formation in dog myocardium following arrest of blood flow. Biochem and Biophys Res Comm 36:664, 1969

103. Woodbury W: Cellular electrophysiology of the heart. In Hamilton WF (ed): Handbook of Physiology, section 2: Circulation vol 1, Washington, DC, American Physiological Society, 1962, pp 239–44

104. Woodbury W: Cellular electrophysiology of the heart. In Hamilton WF (ed): Handbook of Physiology, section 2: Circulation vol 1, Washington, DC, American Physiological Society, 1962, p 276

105. Young WG, Sealy WC, Harris JS: The role of intracellular and extracellular electrolytes in the cardiac arrhythmias produced by prolonged hypercapnia. Surgery 36:636, 1954

57

INCREASE IN MYOCARDIAL CREATINE PHOSPHATE FOLLOWING AORTIC CROSS-CLAMPING AND REPERFUSION

Sidney Levitsky, Harold Feinberg, Frederick J. Merchant, and Edward L. Nirdlinger II

Normothermic anoxic arrest by aortic cross-clamping during open-heart surgery is associated with myocardial metabolic alterations. The effects on function are incompletely understood, but empirical clinical experience indicates that the maximum safe ischemic time should be limited to 20 to 40 minutes. Previous canine experiments show that normothermic arrest exceeding 30 minutes is associated with delayed development of myocardial fibrosis and measurable depression of cardiac contractility.[1] Nevertheless, the technique of normothermic anoxic arrest is widespread, despite the lack of quantitative studies to elucidate the metabolic effects of this procedure.

In our laboratory, we have previously demonstrated, sequentially, the effects of altered myocardial metabolism induced by normothermic arrest and reperfusion.[13] The purpose of this report is to focus on the increases in myocardial creatine phosphate observed following the reperfusion period and to attempt to alter levels of this substance in a salutary manner by other pharmacologic agents in order to preserve myocardial metabolic integrity.

METHODS

Studies in the Intact Animal

CONCTRACTILITY MEASUREMENT. Ten mongrel dogs weighing 18 to 22 Kg were anesthetized with sodium pentobarbital (30 mg/

Supported in part by the American Heart Association Grant-in-Aid #72-925 and intramural research funds provided by the West Side Veterans Administration Hospital, Chicago, Ill.

Kg.) A right heart bypass preparation that permitted the regulation of coronary and systemic arterial perfusion pressures was used (Fig. 1). A large cannula placed into the right atrium and right ventricle diverted all blood returning to the heart into a graduated cylinder and subsequently the effluent was returned to the pump oxygenator. The details of this system have been described previously.[11,12]

After extracorporeal bypass was initiated, the main pulmonary artery was ligated and the left atrium opened widely. The mitral valve leaflets and chordae tendineae were excised. A soft latex balloon mounted on a perforated Teflon plug was inserted into the left ventricle and held in place by a purse-string suture encompassing the mitral annulus. A 3-mm metal cannula in direct continuity with the balloon emerged from the plug and was connected by suitable rigid couplings to two pressure transducers (Statham P23DB) for simultaneous measurement of left ventricular end-diastolic pressure (LVEDP). The analog signals were fed into a Brush 440 direct writing recorder, and the first derivative of the left ventricular pressure signal (LV dP/dt max) was obtained with an analog differentiating circuit. In addition, a stiff vinyl catheter connected to a calibrated syringe was used to vary balloon volume. Another catheter was placed in the thoracic aorta for recording aortic pressure. Mean aortic pressure was maintained at 75 mm Hg throughout the experiment by varying flow through the femoral artery cannula. Heart block was obtained by ligation of the atrioventricular node after the initiation of bypass. A constant heart rate of 120 to 150 beats/min was maintained for each animal by electrical stimulation of the right ventricle. Body and myocardial tem-

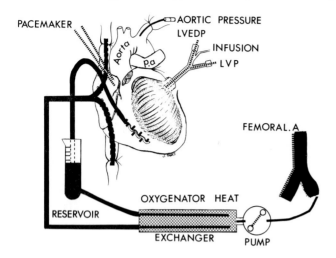

FIG. 1. Bypass preparation used to evaluate myocardial contractility. The intraventricular balloon volume is varied to length-tension curves but remains constant when inscribing force-velocity curves.

peratures were monitored and maintained between 36.5 C and 37.5 C with a heat exchanger in the perfusion circuit. In addition, during the period when the aorta was cross-clamped, the chest cavity was closed to maintain the heart at body temperature and prevent surface cooling of the heart by convective air currents.

After the mitral valve plug was in place, the balloon was inflated in 5 ml increments with 20 to 50 ml of saline solution until the LVEDP rose to 20 to 25 mm Hg. Recordings of LVEDP were obtained at each volume increment after a stable response was observed, and a diastolic compliance curve was inscribed. The balloon was deflated and then reinflated with 20 to 35 ml of saline until the LVEDP was in the range of 5 to 15 mm Hg. The exact volume was recorded, and high-speed tracings of LVEDP, LVP, and LV dP/dt max were obtained.

Force-velocity relationships were determined using the following formulas:

$$\text{Velocity} = \frac{dP/dt}{28P} \quad \text{and} \quad \text{Force} = \frac{1.36\ P\ r_i^2}{r_o^2 - r_i^2}$$

where P equals LVP, r_i and r_o equal the internal and external ventricular wall radii, respectively, and the series elastic modulus is assumed to equal 28. These calculations have been presented in detail by others.[5] At the conclusion of each experiment, the weight of the left ventricle, including the intraventricular septum, was determined after the right ventricle and both atria had been excised. Coronary blood flow was measured by the timed collection of the right heart drainage after the balloon was deflated. The oxygen content of coronary arterial blood and of blood drained from the right heart was measured manometrically and

used to calculate myocardial oxygen consumption (MVO_2).[6]

The aorta was then cross-clamped for one hour. The coronary arteries were reperfused for 30 minutes after the aortic clamp was removed before repeating the contractility studies initially performed during the control period. The heart was defibrillated by a single electric shock 15 minutes after the resumption of coronary perfusion. Statistical analysis was performed on a computer programmed to compare grouped data with unequal variance. Individual groups were compared using a two-tailed Student's t-test.

BIOCHEMICAL STUDIES. Nineteen mongrel dogs weighing 18 to 22 kg were anesthetized and placed on cardiopulmonary bypass in the manner described above. After stabilization of the preparation, full-thickness biopsies were obtained from the right ventricle by utilizing the stop-freeze technique as described by Wollenberger;[19] the biopsy site was then closed with sutures. After venting the left ventricle with an apical cannula, the aorta was cross-clamped for 60 minutes. Additional biopsies were obtained at the end of 60 minutes and again after 30 minutes of reperfusion. The specimens, weighing between 350 to 370 mg, were stored in liquid nitrogen and assayed for adenosine triphosphate (ATP), adenosine diphosphate (ADP), adenosine monophosphate (AMP), creatine phosphate (CP), creatine phosphokinase (CPK), glycogen, and lactate by methods previously described.[13]

Isolated Heart Experiments

After receiving intravenous heparin, 300 mg/Kg, 22 adult male albino rabbits weighing 1.5 to 2.5 Kg were sacrificed by a blow to the head. The chest was opened and the heart rapidly excised and cooled in 0 C Krebs-Ringers bicarbonate solution. The heart was then perfused through an aortic arch cannula using a modification of Langendorff's method at a rate of 30 to 40 ml/min.[4] The perfusate, oxygenated with 95 percent oxygen–5 percent carbon dioxide and maintained at a temperature of 37 C, contained the following: sodium chloride 100 mM/1; potassium chloride 4.7 mL/1; potassium dihydrophosphate 1.18 mM/1; magnesium sulfate 1.16 mM/1; sodium biocarbonate 25 mM/1; calcium chloride 1.09 mM/1; sodium pyruvate 4.9 mM/1; sodium fumarate 6.2 mM/1; and glucose 11.6 mM/1. After 70 minutes of perfusion the experiments were terminated; the beating hearts were quick-frozen with liquid-nitrogen-cooled biopsy tongs and analyzed for CP and ATP.

The animals were divided into seven groups and perfused as outlined in Table 1. Myocardial anoxia was achieved by cross-clamping the ascending aorta. Creatine * (0.14 mM/1) and regular insulin † (40 units/1) were added to the perfusate as indicated in the protocol.

TABLE 1. Isolated Rabbit Heart Perfusions

GROUP	N	20 MIN	30 MIN	20 MIN
I	4	Perf	Perf	Perf
II	3	Perf+Cr	Perf+Cr	Perf+Cr
III	3	Perf	Anox	Perf
IV	3	Perf+Cr	Anox	Perf+Cr
V	3	Perf	Anox	Perf+Cr
VI	3	Perf+Cr+Ins	Perf+Cr+Ins	Perf+Cr+Ins
VII	3	Perf+Cr+Ins	Anox	Perf+Cr+Ins

Perf: perfusion with oxygenated Krebs solution. Cr: 0.14 m M/1 creatine added to perfusate; Anox: ascending aorta cross-clamped; Ins: 40 units/1 regular insulin added to perfusate.

RESULTS

Intact Animal

CONTRACTILITY STUDIES. Following one hour of normothermic arrest, mean LV dP/dt max decreased 63 percent from 1050 ± 177 to 363 ± 56 mm Hg/sec (p < 0.001). Using maximum measured velocity as an index of con-

* Creatine · H_2O obtained from Sigma Chemical Co., St. Louis, Mo.
† Regular insulin (Iletin ®) manufactured by Lilly, Indianapolis, Ind.

tractility free of pre- and after-load factors, there was a significant decrease of 29 percent or 0.36 ± 0.03 to 0.26 ± 05 circumference/sec (p < 0.05) during the anoxic and reperfusion periods (Table 2). In addition, length-tension curves used to assess diastolic compliance were decreased in all of the animals following the anoxic period.

After the anoxic period and 30 minutes of reperfusion, coronary blood flow increased 28 percent (not statistically significant). However, despite the apparent increase in flow, myocardial oxygen consumption ($M\dot{V}O_2$) decreased 35 percent (Table 2).

METABOLIC STUDIES. Following 60 minutes of normothermic anoxia, the total high-energy phosphate moieties (ATP + ADP + AMP) decreased from 6.22 ± 0.16 to 2.34 ± 0.35 μmoles/g. Reperfusion demonstrated only a minimal increase to 2.83 ± 0.12 μmoles/g indicating continued myocardial metabolic impairment. Similarly, glycogen declined 62.5 percent during the anoxic period. However, following reperfusion there was a significant return toward normal (Table 2). CPK was mildly elevated following the anoxic interval and returned to normal after reperfusion. CP underwent a marked decline from 4.2 ± 0.37 to 0.49 ± 0.03 μg/g during anoxia and then exceeded control values, ie: 5.5 ± 0.82 μg/g, following reperfusion.

Isolated Heart Studies

There were no significant differences in CP levels in any of the seven groups (Table 1). The CP levels in the rabbit heart preparation (of this small series) in group III did not appear to be significantly different, although lower from control group I (Table 3).

On the other hand, if the anoxic heart is taken as the control for anoxic hearts treated with insulin and/or creatine, it is seen that CP values exceed anoxia alone and approach the nonanoxic hearts (group I). These changes are not significant in this small series, and further experiments are needed.

ATP levels fell 49 percent following the 30-minute anoxic period and reperfusion (groups I and III). Creatine infusion during reperfusion (group V) and/or preceding the anoxic period (group IV) resulted in an apparent increase in ATP levels as compared to the anoxic noncreatine-perfused group III (Table 3). The combination of creatine and insulin before and after the anoxic period (group VII) appeared to result in

TABLE 2. Metabolic and Contractility Studies in Intact Dog

	CONTROL	60-MIN ANOXIC ARREST	30-MIN REPERFUSION
ATP+ADP+AMP (μ moles/g)	6.22 ± 0.16	2.34 ± 0.35	2.83 ± 0.12
Glycogen (μ g/g)	$6,463 \pm 441$	$2,420 \pm 125$	$3,641 \pm 520$
Creat. Phos. (μ g/g)	4.20 ± 0.37	0.49 ± 0.03	5.50 ± 0.82
CPK (IU)	9.7 ± 0.76	12.3 ± 1.2	10.3 ± 1.1
LV dp/dt max (mm Hg/sec)	$1,050 \pm 177$	–	363 ± 56
Max meas vel (Circum/sec)	0.39 ± 0.03	–	0.26 ± 0.05
CBF (ml/min)	123 ± 71	–	158 ± 100
M$\dot{V}O_2$ (ml/min)	3.85 ± 1	–	2.5 ± 0.79

ATP: adenosine triphosphate; ADP: adenosine diphosphate; AMP: adenosine monophosphate; Creat. phos: creatine phosphate; LV dp/dt max: first derivative of left ventricular pressure; Max meas vel: maximum measured velocity; CBF: coronary blood flow; M$\dot{V}O_2$: myocardial oxygen consumption per 100 g of left ventricle.

the greatest enhancement of ATP levels. Since these studies are preliminary and small numbers of animals are involved, it is premature to attach great significance to the apparent differences between groups.

DISCUSSION

Short periods of normothermic anoxic arrest are in widespread clinical use and appear to be safe. Nevertheless, there has been some concern that deteriorating myocardial function and concomitant injury associated with any arrest period may be associated with chronic damage to the heart that may not be appreciated in the immediate postoperative period.[1] The marked depression in postanoxic contractility and the persistence of myocardial metabolic abnormalities observed in this study attest to the requirement of better measures to prevent permanent cardiac injury.

Following 60 minutes of arrest, high-energy phosphate levels appeared to reach a point of irreversibility. Total adenine nucleotides were lost as a result of ATP breakdown to ADP and AMP followed by dephosphorylation to adenosine.[2] This was further broken down to inosine, hypoxanthine, and xanthine.[7] Anaerobic glycolysis, evidenced by depressed glycogen levels following the anoxic period, contributed to further depression of ATP levels below that necessary to maintain contractile function. Further glycolysis during ischemia was stimulated by endogenous release of myocardial catecholamines resulting in activation of phosphorylase via cyclic AMP.[18]

CP rose immediately after reperfusion and exceeded control levels while ATP values experienced only a minimal increase. The rise in CP was probably the result of the fact that free creatine levels are maintained even in the ischemic state.[6] Thus, return of oxidative phosphorylation, the high level of phosphate in the ischemic heart, and restored CPK activity could result in rapid

TABLE 3. Isolated Heart Metabolic Studies

GROUP	STATE	ATP	p	CP	p
I	Control	1.65 ± 0.36	–	3.38 ± 0.47	NS
II	Cr	1.72 ± 0.19	NS	2.94 ± 0.64	NS
III	Anox	0.85 ± 0.13	<0.01	2.42 ± 0.29	NS
IV	Cr–Cr	1.00 ± 0.25	<0.01	3.30 ± 0.23	NS
V	Per–Cr	0.98 ± 0.09	<0.01	3.28 ± 0.48	NS
VI	Cr+Ins	1.60 ± 0.07	NS	3.34 ± 0.35	NS
VII	Cr+Ins–Cr+Ins	1.12 ± 0.10	<0.05	2.98 ± 0.26	NS

restoration of CP. Studies corroborating the rapid return to normal and overshoot of CP have been reported by Ellis and coworkers.[3]

If the heart could be loaded with creatine during the pre- or postanoxic period, then the capacity to phosphorylate the creatine may induce high CP levels that maximally convert ADP and thus may enhance the formation of ATP. Since ATP is not a substrate for adenosine production, the inexorable breakdown of APD to AMP and to adenosine could be halted or perhaps reversed; thus, postanoxic contractility might also be preserved as a result of maintaining the adenyl moieties as ATP.

Others have reported increases in myocardial creatine in rat and rabbit hearts following perfusion with creatine.[10,14] In addition, insulin has been shown to increase creatine uptake by skeletal muscle.[8] Perfusion of the isolated heart preparations with creatine at five times normal plasma levels showed no evidence of increasing cardiac creatine levels. These observations are in disagreement with those reported by Olivo and coworkers.[14] In addition, the levels of CP in the isolated perfused hearts are lower than those observed by other workers. These discrepancies may be related to the method used in sacrificing the rabbit. Lee and associates have shown variations in cardiac CP in animals killed by potassium arrest, acetylcholine arrest, and a blow on the head. The decrease in the latter group is related to the outpouring of catecholamines following the blow on the head and was duplicated with epinephrine infusions.[9] The addition of 40 units/1 insulin to the creatine-Ringers perfusate also failed to increase myocardial CP. Nevertheless, there appeared to be a progressive increase in ATP. It has been suggested that treatment with insulin may increase cardiac glycogen stores and, therefore, anaerobic production of ATP during myocardial anoxia. This mechanism may be involved in the observed elevated postanoxic ATP levels and is being investigated.

Creatine is thought to cross skeletal muscle membranes against a concentration gradient via a saturable transport mechanism, which requires oxygen and is inhibited by 2-4 dinitrophenol and cooling.[5] This creatine uptake seems to be enhanced in the presence of insulin *in vivo*.[8] The fact that in the present experiments no increased cardiac creatine levels were observed following creatine perfusion suggests that the amount of myocardial creatine is regulated at a fixed level. The failure of insulin to increase cardiac creatine concentrations may be due to delay in the action of insulin beyond the period of our experiment

or to the fact that insulin either has no effect on cardiac creatine (in contradiction to skeletal muscle) or that its effect is exerted on creatine uptake through some mechanism not present in the isolated heart preparation. Nevertheless, the apparent enhancement of ATP in these pilot experiments warrants further studies in the intact animal and additional determinations as to whether the increases in ATP have a functional equivalent.

SUMMARY

Normothermic anoxic arrest induced by aortic cross-clamping during open-heart surgery is associated with myocardial metabolic alterations whose effects on function are incompletely understood. In 29 dogs supported by cardiopulmonary bypass and subjected to 60 minutes of normothermic arrest followed by 30 minutes of reperfusion, contractility (isovolumetric balloon) and metabolites ("stop-freeze biopsy") were studied. Despite reperfusion, total nucleotides ($p < 0.001$) and contractility ($p < 0.001$) were depressed. However, creatine phosphate (CP) increased ($p < 0.01$), and creatine phosphokinase returned toward normal. These data suggest that normothermic anoxic arrest causes an efflux of adenine nucleotides from the cell and extensive glycogenolysis while, at the same time, preserving creatine for energy pools. Nevertheless, the increase in CP does not appear to be sufficient to sustain a normal level of contractility following the anoxic insult.

References

1. Buja LM, Levitsky S, Souther SG, Ferrans VJ, Roberts WC, Morrow AG: Acute and chronic effects of normothermic anoxia on canine hearts: light and electronmicroscopic evaluation. Circulation (Suppl 1) 43:44, 1971
2. Deuticke B, Gerlack E: Abban freier nucleotide in hert, skeletmuskel, gehirn and leber der ratte bei sauerstoffmangel. Pfluegers Arch 292:239, 1966
3. Ellis SB, Evans GT, Hallaway BE, Phibbs C, Freier EF: Myocardial creatine phosphate and nucleotides in anoxic cardiac arrest and recovery. Am J Physiol 201:687, 1961
4. Feinberg H, Boyd E, Tanzini G: Mechanical performance and oxygen utilization of the isovolumic rabbit heart. Am J Physiol 215:132, 1968
5. Fitch CG, Shields RP: Creatine metabolism in skeletal muscle. J Biol Chem 241:3611, 1966
6. Isselhard W, Mauer W, Stremmel W, et al: Stoffwechsel des kanichenherzens in situ wahrend asphyxie und in der post-asphyktischhen erholung. Pfluegers Arch 316:164, 1970
7. Katori M, Berne RM: Release of adenosine from anoxic hearts: relationship to coronary flow. Circ Res 19:420, 1966

8. Koszalka TR, Andrew CL: Effect of insulin on the uptake of creatine-1-C14 by skeletal muscle in normal and x-irradiated rats. Proc Soc Exp Biol Med 139:1265, 1972

9. Lee YCP, DeWall RA, Visscher MB: State of creatine in mammalian heart muscle. Am J Physiol 198:855, 1960

10. Lee YCP, Visscher MB: On the state of creatine in heart muscle. Proc Nat Acad Sci 47:1510, 1961

11. Levitsky S, Mullin EM, Sloane RE, Morrow AG: Experimental evaluation of pentazocine: effects on myocardial contractility and peripheral vascular resistance. Am Heart J 81:381, 1971

12. Levitsky S, Sloane RE, Mullin EM, McIntosh CL, Morrow AG: Normothermic myocardial anoxia: effects on canine heart and left ventricular outflow obstruction. Ann Thorac Surg 11:229, 1971

13. Merchant FJ, Feinberg H, Levitsky S: Sequential analysis of altered myocardial metabolism and contractility induced by normothermic arrest and reperfusion. J Surg Res 16:153, 1974

14. Olivo F, Vianello A, Baroni P, D'Alberton A: Glycocyamine and isonine as precursors of creatine phosphate and adenosine triphosphate in muscle fibers. Ital J Biochem 12:216, 1964

15. Taylor RR, Ross J, Covell JW, Sonnenblick EH: A quantitative analysis of left ventricular myocardial function in the intact, sedated dog. Circ Res 21:99, 1967

16. Van Slyke DD, Neill JM: The determination of gases in blood and other solutions by vacuum extraction and manometric measurement. J Biol Chem 61:523, 1924

17. Weissler AM, Altshuld RA, Gibb LE, Pollack ME, Kruger SA: Effect of insulin on the performance and metabolism of the anoxic, isolated perfused rat heart. Circ Res 32:108, 1973

18. Wollenberger A, Krause EG, Heier G: Stimulation of 3', 5'-cyclic AMP formation in dog myocardium following arrest of blood flow. Biochem Biophys Res Commun 36:664, 1969

19. Wollenberger A, Ristau O, Schoffa G: Eine einfache Technik der extrem schnellen Abkuhlung grosserer Gewebsstucke. Pfluegers Arch 27:339, 1960

58

CARDIOVASCULAR TOXIC FACTOR (CVT) IN PATIENTS UNDERGOING CARDIOPULMONARY BYPASS

R. W. M. Frater, Rita McConn, Yasu Oka, E. Yellin, and Arnold Nagler

Nagler and Levenson, 1972, described a passively transferrable lethal factor (PTLF) in the plasma of animals in irreversible shock that causes death when transfused into animals in mild reversible shock. In summary, the current information on PTLF is as follows (Nagler and Levenson 1974):

1. PTLF is found in the plasma of normal and germ-free rats subjected to irreversible shock.

2. On column chromatography on DEAE cellulose PTLF activity resides in a fraction eluted with 0.02M phosphatase buffer, pH 5.3. Ultracentrifugation and immune electrophoresis produced data consistent with the PTLF activity residing in an aggregated gamma globulin.

3. PTLF is heat stable and nondialysable and appears to be a polypeptide with a molecular weight greater than 10,000.

4. Injection of PTLF intraventricularly into the heart of the frog, Rana pipiens, produced no change in ventricular activity; nor did it produce any effect on a Langendorff rabbit heart preparation.

5. Incubation of PTLF with a white blood cell lysate (prepared from acid lysis of white cells) produced material that caused depression or cessation of frog heart ventricular contractility. Incubation of plasma from animals in irreversible shock with WBC lysate also produced cardiotoxic activity. Lysate by itself had no effect on ventricular activity, and incubation with plasma or plasma fractions from normal animals or animals in mild shock similarly produced no cardiotoxin.

6. Incubation of PTLF with acid phosphatase produced the same effect as incubation with WBC lysate.

7. Direct injection of endotoxin (E coli 011B4) had no effect on the frog heart preparation by itself or after incubation with PTLF.

8. PTLF may also be designated as a cardiotoxin precursor. It is hypothesized that it may be a white cell Leukokininogen, which is activated by a white cell derived protease in a system such as that described by Greenbaum, 1969.

9. Injection into intact anesthetized dogs of plasma that is positive for cardiotoxin by the frog bioassay produces an immediate fall in ventricular pressure and dP/dt, a rise and then a fall in coronary blood flow, and a probable fall in peripheral vascular resistance (Fig. 1). The effect on ventricular pressure lasts approximately 1.5 minutes, suggesting inactivation or consumption of the toxin. Because of the effect on vasculature evident in these experiments, the term cardiovascular toxic factor (CVTF) has been used instead of cardiotoxic factor (Yellin et al, 1973).

10. PTLF was not found in the blood of 24 normal donors. Of 35 patients in our ICU, 12 who had no shock and only minimal bleeding had weak or negative titers of toxic factor or PTLF. Twelve had moderately high titers on one or two occasions. Some of these latter patients had bled significantly but had not been in shock. A fall in

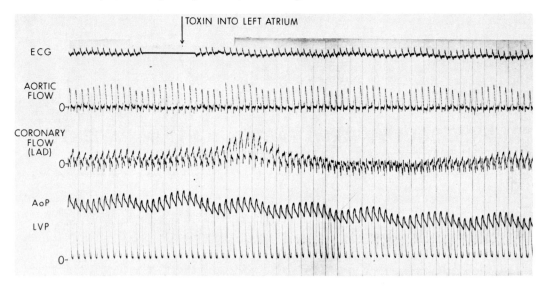

FIG. 1. Effect of injection of CVTF into an intact, unshocked, anesthetized dog. Electrocardiogram: ↓ – injection of 5 cc of human plasma with ++++ CVTF activity into left atrium. Note the modest fall in aortic flow, the immediate rise and then fall in coronary flow, and the fall in left ventricular and aortic pressures.

titers to normal coincided with clinical recovery. In patients with shock due to various causes, ++++ levels of toxic factor were seen. All were dead within 24 hours of the development of ++++ levels. The plasma of these patients on further analysis appeared to contain the same factor that had been present in the animal experiments (Nagler and Levenson, 1973).

With this body of preliminary information available, it was decided to look for PTLF and CVTF in patients undergoing open-heart surgery.

METHODS

Blood was collected according to the following schedule:

1. after premedication, before induction
2. from the bypass machine after priming (one unit of 'fresh" CPD blood, less than 72 hours old, and 3,000 ml of "Normosol-R" * with, in addition, albumin, calcium, chloride, sodium bicarbonate, and heparin)
3. five minutes after the start of bypass
4. at the end of bypass
5. at the end of the operation
6. in some cases 24 hours later

---

* McGan Laboratories balanced electrolyte infusion.

The plasma was tested for CVTF by the frog bioassay and then incubated with white cell lysate to convert PTLF or toxic factor precursor to active CVTF in order to assess the presence of PTLF, again by the frog heart bioassay.

Twenty-four patients were studied. In 13, cardiac outputs and pulmonary arteriovenous shunting were measured before and after cardiopulmonary bypass as well as white cell lysosomal enzymes and oxygen dissociation curves. By a double blind random technique, seven patients were given 30 mg/kg body weight or methylprednisolone IV before anesthesia and eight were given a placebo. Half of all the patients had morphine anesthesia and half had halothane.

Cardiopulmonary bypass was run at 2.5 to 3.0 L/min/m² except when on partial bypass when the rate was set in relation to the patient's capabilities. Acid-base balance was maintained by adjusting gas flows and administering sodium bicarbonate as necessary. Bentley or Harvey oxygenators were used with filters in the suction and perfusion lines.

During the course of the study, certain bloods were tested for ventricular depressant activity using a Langendorff preparation: a spontaneously beating isolated rabbit heart was perfused under constant pressure, temperature, and pH. Developed tension was measured by a transducer and coronary flow collected directly. Fifty ml of Feigin's glucose electrolyte solution was altered with randomly selected mixtures of 46 ml of

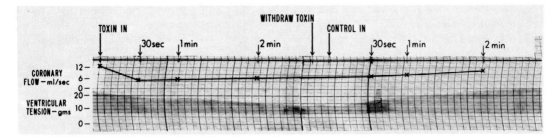

FIG. 2. Effect of CVTF on ventricular contractility in the isolated beating rabbit's heart, perfused under constant pressure. At "Toxin In," infusion is started, prepared with 4 cc of plasma and 46 cc of Feigin's glucose-electrolyte solution. At "Control In," infusion is started of 50 cc of Feigin's glucose-electrolyte solution, while the ventricular depressant effect of the first infusion is still present. The electrolyte concentrations of these two infusions are only slightly different. Note the recovery of ventricular tension despite the infusion of the control solution.

Feigin's solution and 4 ml of treated test plasma, so that each heart was its own control (Fig. 2).

RESULTS

On Induction

PTLF results were as follows: absent in 10; + in 6; ++ in 3; +++ in 4; ++++ in 1. CVTF was essentially absent except in two patients with the same levels (++++ and +++ respectively) they had of PTLF. Both patients had severe ventricular disease (one had aortic stenosis and one had coronary occlusive disease) but did not have cardiac outputs lower than other patients who did not have CVTF in their plasma at this stage.

Prime

To our surprise, in view of our previous experience with freshly drawn donor blood, PTLF and CVTF were found in the priming solution in at least half of the cases:

	PTLF	CVTF
−	9	13
+	4	3
++	4	4
+++	5	3
++++	2	1

Although the blood added was by definition "fresh," it was never straight from a donor and, on several occasions, consisted of packed cells or reconstituted whole blood. In one patient with a +++ level of CVTF in the prime, the high plasma potassium and RBC sodium and low

RBC potassium suggested poor red cell preservation despite the apparent two-day age of the blood. These chance observations led to a study of PTLF and CVTF as well as white-cell lysosomal enzymes, beta glucuronidase, D-cathepsin, and acid phosphatase in stored CPD and ACD human and dog blood (McConn and Nagler, 1973; Kennish et al, 1974). PTLF by the frog bioassay appeared from the second day in human blood and the fourth day in dog blood. CVTF was also found early but reached critical levels by the sixth or seventh day of storage. Beta glucuronidase and acid phosphatase levels were also raised, the former reaching levels seen in man in irreversible shock. The Langendorff preparation showed a decrease in developed tension by the fifth day. All samples were positive on repeated trials by the sixth day.

Beginning and End of Bypass

Five minutes after the beginning of bypass and at the end of bypass, varying from 40 minutes to 240 minutes, including partial bypass, the results for PTLF were as follows:

	Beginning	End
−	9	13
+	4	3
++	4	4
+++	5	3
++++	2	1

Those patients with high titers on induction tended to retain them at the start of bypass. A high level in the prime was usually associated with a high level at the beginning of bypass. In three patients with known poor ventricular function (cardiac outputs in two being 1.56 and 1.84

L/min just prior to bypass) and low systemic pressures after induction, there were striking changes from low to high titers during the period of not more than one hour between anesthetic induction and the institution of bypass. However, there were other patients with similar clinical circumstances (one with a cardiac output of 1.6 L/min) who did not increase their PTLF titers. A +++ titer of CVTF was present at the beginning of bypass in one patient, J.D., the patient with +++ levels, both on induction and in the priming fluid.

By the end of bypass, PTLF assay results were generally lower. High titers were seen in two patients in whom, because of poor ventricular function, prolonged partial bypass was necessary in order to "wean" them from the pump. One of these, J.D., was also the only patient in the series to have a low flow of 2.1 L/min/m² and a low mean arterial pressure of 40 mm Hg during perfusion. The other was a patient, L.R., with a greatly dilated, poorly contractile ventricle, who had developed a ++++ level of PTLF by the beginning of bypass. By the end of the very difficult weaning period after bypass, this had become converted to a +++ level of CVTF. These two patients had +++ levels of CVTF also. High PTLF titers were seen also in one patient who received 8 units of blood during bypass, and in the only cyanotic child in the series, in whom the hematocrit, which had been 70 at the start of bypass, was still 50 at the end, but CVTF was absent in these patients. Duration of bypass had no effect on the level of PTLF or CVTF at the end of bypass.

End of Operation

Five patients who had had PTLF levels of zero to ++ at the end of bypass had developed levels of +++ by the end of the operation. These patients were bleeding more than usual and received 3 to 5 units of blood during this period. One of these had +++ levels of CVTF in addition to PTLF. However, two other patients who received similar amounts of transfusion had no rise in PTLF or CVTF titers. Two patients, including J.D., with +++ levels at the end of bypass were still at those levels, and one with a +++ level fell to + by the end of anesthesia. CVTF was inadvertently not measured in L.R., who almost certainly still had high, if not higher, levels at that time, since he had had +++ levels at the end of bypass, was still in a profound low cardiac output state, and died a few hours later with intractable left ventricular failure. CVTF

was still at +++ levels in J.D. so that there were certainly two patients, and probably three, who had +++ levels of CVTF at the end of anesthesia.

Twenty-four Hours after Surgery

PTLF was present in four of 13 patients who were tested 24 hours postoperatively. Titers were ++ in one, +++ in two, and ++++ in one. Two patients had low cardiac output syndrome, and two had had larger than usual amounts of transfusion. CVTF was present at +++ levels in two of these patients: J.D., who remained in profound cardiogenic shock, and another who had received a large volume of blood. In the sense that cold, poorly perfused extremities with large arteriovenous oxygen differences are features of "shock," the patients with low cardiac output syndromes were in shock, although their blood pressures were maintained above 100 mm of mercury systolic.

Correlations

In general terms, there appeared to be correlations between the presence of PTLF and CVTF in these patients and low cardiac output and/or blood transfusion. The factors were seen to develop between induction and bypass when the cardiac output was low, during a low-flow, low-pressure perfusion (in which only two units of blood were used) and postbypass; and, postoperatively, in the presence of low cardiac output states. These correlations were not absolute: It is not possible as yet to quantify the exact degree, type, and duration of low cardiac output state in these patients that will inevitably cause the development of PTLF or CVTF. Similarly, while the factors have unquestionably been shown to be present in donor blood and to increase progressively with storage under good conditions, the titers present in the prime were quite variable even though the single units used were allegedly more or less equally fresh. Some patients who received as much as 5 units of blood did not develop high titers, but, nevertheless, when larger amounts of blood were transfused, high titers were always seen.

No correlation was found with duration of bypass: On the contrary, cardiopulmonary bypass, *per se*, appeared to result in a lowering of beginning bypass titers of PTLF or CVTF, although, as has already been pointed out, low perfusion pressure and flow and larger than usual blood use may result in high titers at the end of perfusion.

Within the obvious limitation of the small sample sizes, there were no correlations with type of anesthesia (morphine or halothane), type of oxygenator (Harvey with 1:1 or Bentley with 3:1 gas:blood flow ratios), type of pathology, acid-base balance, pulmonary arteriovenous shunting, concentrations of white cell lysosomal enzymes (beta glucuronidase and D-cathepsin), or the administration of 30 mg/kg of methylprednisolone or a placebo.

Correlations with mortality must be made with the levels of CVTF and not with PTLF since the latter is not itself active on the heart and circulation but is only a precursor. In the study on shock patients already mentioned (Nagler and Levenson, 1973), $+++$ levels were associated with death within 24 hours. In this study, $++++$ levels of CVTF were present once in the bypass priming solution: The patient had cleared this by the end of bypass and although a $+++$ level appeared 24 hours after postoperative transfusion of more than five units of stored blood, it had cleared by 48 hours. Three patients had $+++$ levels of CVTF in the priming fluid. Two of these cleared without incident as the cases proceeded. One was the patient J.D., with a subsequent low flow and low pressure perfusion, who can be described completely and suitably at this point.

This patient was the only one in the series to have a $+++$ level of CVTF at the beginning of bypass. At the end of his cardiopulmonary bypass, $+++$ levels of CVTF were still present. It is notable that his peripheral vascular resistance during bypass was the lowest of any patient in this series. It remained low at the end of anesthesia when the cardiac output was also low. At this stage, it was quite clear that despite triple artery bypass grafting with excellent flows in all three veins, the patient had suffered a severe depression of ventricular function. Left atrial filling pressures were extremely high and responded acutely to small alterations in blood volume, and the systolic and mean blood pressures were low. There was no evident ischemia or infarcted tissue visible on exterior inspection of the heart, and subendocardial infarction was diagnosed. The patient continued in this low cardiac output state for three days. CVTF levels reached $++++$ on the second day, and death occurred 24 hours later. At autopsy the grafts were patent but there was a massive left ventricular subendocardial infarction. Thus, in this case, the ultimate postoperative increase in CVTF levels could be fairly well correlated with the prolonged cardiogenic

shock exhibited by the patient. This continued despite the use of intraaortic balloon pumping. However, it should be noted that there were other patients with lower cardiac outputs (some with lower and some with higher peripheral resistances) at the end of operation who had not by that time developed $+++$ titers of CVTF and who went on to complete recovery.

One other patient besides J.D. had a $+++$ level of CVTF at the end of bypass. This was the patient with aortic insufficiency and extremely severe ventricular dysfunction who had developed a $++++$ level of the precursor PTLF by the beginning of bypass. He died six hours after surgery with a progressively rising left atrial pressure, falling cardiac output and systemic pressure, without further examination of CVTF levels.

At the end of operation, excluding the patient just discussed who would presumably have had a continued high level of CVTF, there was only one other patient besides J.D. who had a $+++$ level at the end of anesthesia. This dropped to $++$ after 24 hours, and the patient went on to a complete recovery. Hypovolemia and hypotension were present temporarily in this case, and large-volume transfusions were given.

In summary, one patient had $+++$ levels of CVTF at every phase of his operation and went on to die of a massive subendocardial infarction. One patient had developed a $+++$ level by the end of bypass and died early in left ventricular failure and cardiogenic shock. Four other patients had $++++$ (once) or $+++$ (twice) levels either in the priming fluid or at the end of the operation, and all survived.

DISCUSSION

Several questions are raised by this investigation:

1. What is the relationship of CVTF to the myocardial depressant factor (MDF) of Lefer and Glenn?
2. What is the mechanism of production of PTLF and CVTF in surgical patients?
3. What is the significance of the presence of PTLF and CVTF in cardiopulmonary bypass patients?

The first two questions are subjects of continued investigations in our laboratories. It should be noted here that MDF has a molecular weight of 1,000 and does not produce cardiac arrest in the frog-heart preparation. The question of the mechanism of production in clinical situations has become complicated by the finding of PTLF and CVTF in stored blood. For the low cardiac output status due to hemorrhage, blood transfusion is appropriate therapy so that it is difficult to define whether factors found are endogenous or exogenous. The clinical data from this study show that ordinary cardiopulmonary bypass does not contribute to their production but that a persistent low cardiac output state, even in the absence of hemorrhage and significant transfusion, will result in the appearance of the factors in both precursor and potent forms. Although *in vitro* the importance of white cell enzymes in the conversion of PTLF to CVTF is critical, it is not clear what happens *in vivo*.

From a practical clinical point of view it can be stated that precursor or potent forms of a cardiac toxin may appear and develop in cardiac surgical patients who are in low cardiac output states and are receiving large volumes of stored blood. Since the potent form depresses ventricular function, it is entirely possible that there will be further aggravation of low cardiac output states, possibly to the point of irreversibility. Quantification of this toxin at present is crude, and delineation of the precise circumstances that will result in the appearance of PTLF and its conversion to CVTF is so imperfect as to allow only the broadest kind of prediction of its presence in a given case. The morals are almost trite and have been principles of good cardiac surgical management since its inception: anticipate, prevent, and abort the development of low cardiac output states; prevent hemorrhage and arrest it before massive transfusion is needed.

SUMMARY

A heat-stable nondialysable polypeptide occurs in precursor and active forms in the blood of experimental animals and patients in irreversible shock. The active form is vasoactive and cardiotoxic. The precursor is activated *in vitro* by incubation with white cell lysates or acid phosphatase. Both precursor and toxin develop progressively in stored blood. When maximum toxic activity is found in patients in a variety of kinds of shock, death has ensued within 24 hours.

The precursor was found in at least half of a group of patients undergoing major surgery under cardiopulmonary bypass. Its appearance was related to low systemic blood flow and large transfusions before, during, and after bypass. Significant levels were seen in about a quarter of the patients. In these patients, the potential for conversion to the toxic factor existed and the most potent cause for this would appear to have been prolongation of low flow states. Fortunately, this apparently happens only rarely, but when the cardiovascular toxic factor does appear, it can only serve to aggravate the situation by its ventricular depressant action and contribute to making it irreversible.

References

Greenbaum LM, Freer R, Chang J: PMN-kinin and kinin metabolizing enzymes in normal and maligant leukocytes. Br J Pharmacol 36:623, 1969

Kennish A, Yellin E, Nagler A, McConn R: Myocardial toxic factor in stored blood. Accepted for presentation at SAMA-UTMB Student Research Forum, 1974

Lefer AM, Glenn TH: Congress on shock in low and high flow states. Pub by Excerpta Medica. International Congress 247:88–105, 1971. Lillehei W, Stubbs SS (eds)

McConn R, Nagler A: Unpublished observations, 1973

Nagler AL, Levenson SM: Presence of a passively transferrable lethal factor in the blood of rats in severe hemorrhagic shock. J Trauma 12:608, 1972

Nagler AL, Levenson SM: The nature of the toxic material in the blood of rats subjected to irreversible hemorrhagic shock. Submitted for publication, 1974

Yellin E, Kennish A, Gowda R, Nagler A, Frater RWM: Unpublished observations 1973

59

PROPRANOLOL IN CARDIOVASCULAR SURGERY

Alexander Romagnoli, Phiroze B. Sabawala,
and Arthur S. Keats

In 1948, Ahlquist[1] compared the pharmacological effects of several catecholamines and sympathomimetic compounds and proposed that peripheral adrenergic receptors be divided into two types, alpha and beta, corresponding almost invariably to excitatory and inhibitory responses. Alpha receptors respond by vasoconstriction and beta receptors by a positive chronotropic and inotropic cardiac effect, vasodilation, bronchial relaxation, mobilization of free fatty acids, muscle glycogenolysis, and a rise in circulating lactic acid. Strong evidence supporting the existence of at least two adrenergic receptors did not appear until 1958, when Powell and Slater[2] studied several catecholamine analogues and found that dichloroisoproterenol (DCI) had strong and selective beta receptor blocking activity. DCI blocked the positive inotropic effect of epinephrine, norepinephrine, isoproterenol, and the response to sympathetic ganglion stimulation but did not alter the effect of calcium ions, digitalis, theophylline, or glucagon. Continued studies led to the discovery by Black and Stephenson[3] in 1962 of propranolol, an effective beta blocker with more specific activity than DCI.

PHARMACOLOGY OF PROPRANOLOL

As used clinically, propranolol is a racemic compound with all blocking activity residing in the levo isomer. The block produced is competitive and can be be overcome by large doses of isoproterenol. Studies of a large number of compounds with beta blocking activity (Table 1) indicated that the degree of block of specific actions of epinephrine by these compounds was not uniform. Some compounds primarily block cardiac effects with little effect on bronchial receptors (see practalol in Table 1) whereas others have little effect on the heart and a marked effect on the bronchi and peripheral vascular bed (see butoxanine in Table 1). This led to the suggestion that beta receptors be further subdivided into $beta_1$, stimulation of which was responsible for the cardiac actions of epinephrine, and $beta_2$, responsible for bronchial dilation, vasodilation, and the metabolic effects of epinephrine. These blocking agents possessed varying degrees of local anesthetic activity and block nerve transmission by membrane stabilization, preventing the ion fluxes responsible for nerve propagation. By analogy the same effect applies to the conducting tissue of the heart and accounts for the antiarrhythmic effects of drugs such as procaine and lidocaine. Racemic propranolol therefore acts through its levo isomer to block both B_1 and B_2 receptors. B_1 receptor blockade leads to decreased myocardial function. Blockade of the B_2 receptor leads to bronchoconstriction, vasoconstriction, and prevents the rise in free fatty acids, blood glucose, and lactic acid that follows epinephrine administration. These metabolic changes result from muscle glycogenolysis, since liver glycogenolysis is known to be responsible to alpha stimulation. Both isomers have local anesthetic activity equivalent to lidocaine and are as effective as lidocaine in reversing arrhythmias caused by catecholamines, digitalis, and hydrocarbon anesthetics.[4] The actions of propranolol are summarized in Table 2. An ill-defined central nervous system effect also occurs and is currently being explored.

The intensity of the changes brought about by beta blockade is related to the degree of sympathetic activity present at the time of propranolol administration. Thus, propranolol may induce profound circulatory changes in patients with conges-

TABLE 1. Several Characteristics of Compounds with Beta Blocking Activity

DRUG	POTENCY[a]	MEMBRANE ACTIVITY[b]	RELATIVE BLOCKING POTENCY OF RECEPTORS $B_1:B_2$ [c]	AGONISTIC ACTIVITY[d]	HALF LIFE ORAL ROUTE (hours)
Propranolol	1.0	+	1:1	no	3
L–Propranolol	1.0	+	1:1	no	3
D-Propranolol	0	+	0	no	3
4-Hydroxy- Propranolol	1.0	+	1:1	+	–
Practolol	4	no	8:1	+	7
Pronethalol	0.1	+	1:1	no	–
Butoxanine	–	no	1:20	no	–
Satolol	.8	no	1:1	no	–
Oxprenolol	1.0	+	5:1	+	0.75
Alprenolol	1.0	+	1:1	++	–
DCI	0.1	+	1:1	+++	–

[a] *Relative activity in blocking isoproterenol tachycardia.*
[b] *Measured in terms of local anesthetic activity.*
[c] *Ratio of block of cardiac effects (B_1) to block of other effects (B_2).*
[d] *Stimulation of beta receptors before block.*

tive heart failure known to have high sympathetic tone, whereas only small circulatory changes are produced in animals that have been catecholamine-depleted by reserpine. One consequence of the block of muscle glycogenolysis is the prolongation of the hypoglycemic effect of insulin. Several instances of severe hypoglycemia with blood sugar levels less than 20 mg percent have been reported both in diabetic and normal patients during propranolol therapy. Propranolol also masks the signs of hypoglycemia attributable to epinephrine release, thus confusing its diagnosis.

TABLE 2. Actions of Racemic Propranolol

B_1 receptor block
Decreased heart rate and cardiac output
Decreased myocardial oxygen uptake and work
Decreased coronary blood flow
Antiarrhythmic

B_2 receptor block
Bronchoconstriction
Vasoconstriction
Decreased glycogen activation in sketetal muscle by epinephrine (FFA, glucose, lactic acid)

Membrane stabilizing (local anesthetic) effect
Decreased heart rate
Increased P-R interval
Antiarrhythmic

CNS effects
Tranquilizer
Decreased Parkinsonian tremor

Propranolol given by mouth is readily absorbed and extensively biotransformed in the liver before reaching the systemic circulation. Early and variable biotransformation accounts in part for the vast difference in dose necessary to achieve an adequate blockade among patients.[5] Oral doses necessary to achieve a therapeutic effect vary from 30 to 300 mg per day. After oral administration, significant quantities of a metabolite, 4-hydroxy-propranolol, are found in the circulating blood, and this metabolite is equipotent to propranolol in beta blocking activity (Table 1). No 4-hydroxy-propranolol is found after intravenous administration, suggesting that it is produced by the liver only after some favored pathway of metabolism is saturated with propranolol.[6] Variation in the degree of production of 4-hydroxypropranolol after oral administration may account for the large range of oral doses necessary for a therapeutic effect and the difficulties in correlating propranolol blood levels with degree of beta blockade in many circumstances. The half life of 4-hydroxypropranolol is somewhat shorter than that of propranolol. Propranolol is metabolized only by the liver, and less than 1 percent of administered propranolol is excreted unchanged in urine and feces. It is also excreted in the bile and reabsorbed, a factor contributing to prolongation of its half life, estimated as 3 to 4 hours after a single oral dose, and possibly as long as six hours after chronic oral administration.[7] Since initial hepatic metabolism is bypassed, intravenous propranolol is effective in doses of 0.5 mg or less with an estimated therapeutic effect of only 30 minutes.

Side effects are reported by 25 to 50 percent of patients taking propranolol by mouth. Most are mild, transient, and dose related, usually consisting of diarrhea, dizziness, lightheadedness, bradycardia, impotence, and bronchospasm. Cardiac failure [8] has been reported in less than 0.5 percent and in as much as 7 percent of patients treated with propranolol.[9] This failure, however, responds well to digitalis. Greenblatt and Koch-Weser [10] observed 9.3 percent adverse reactions in 268 hospitalized patients; a few were life threatening such as congestive heart failure or heart block, and none were fatal.

USE IN CARDIOVASCULAR SURGERY

Preoperative Propranolol

Propranolol is used in the therapy of several diseases in patients who may ultimately be candidates for surgical treatment. These include patients with angina pectoris (with or without infarction) with valvular disease, with dissecting aneurysms of the thoracic aorta, and with cyanotic congenital heart disease.

By decreasing cardiac work, propranolol effectively decreases the incidence and severity of anginal attacks. Propranolol achieves a slower heart rate by increasing the degree of atrioventricular block and by preventing the tachycardia associated with endogenous catecholamine release of emotional or physical activity. The rationale for the use of propranolol in patients with dissecting aortic aneurysm is based not only on its ability to decrease blood pressure by lowering cardiac output, but also on its ability to decrease the force of cardiac ejection. Prokop et al [11] proposed that the rate of rise of aortic pressure rather than the hypertension *per se* provides the thrust that dissects away the intima. Decreasing the ejecting force of the heart by propranolol decreases this dissecting force. In both tetralogy of Fallot and idiopathic hypertrophic subaortic stenosis, sympathetic stimulation is postulated as an important mechanism leading to outflow obstruction. Propranolol clearly reduces frequency and severity of cyanotic spells in children with infundibular stenosis.[12]

In view of the well-known direct myocardial depressant effects of most general anesthetic agents, it was thought that administration of general anesthesia to patients chronically treated with propranolol would be exceptionally hazardous. Myocardial depression manifested as congestive heart failure or profound hypotension resistant to conventional treatment, as well as depression of normal homeostatic mechanisms responsive to intraoperative hemorrhage or change in body position or temperature were anticipated. In 1972, Viljoen et al [13] described four patients who could not be resuscitated after aortocoronary bypass operations and ascribed these events to the preoperative use of propranolol. They therefore advocated two weeks of abstinence from propranolol before exposure to a general anesthetic. Recently acquired data tend to support a more moderate view that propranolol be discontinued only 24 to 48 hours before any contemplated general anesthetic since little if any propranolol effects can be observed after that time.

Faulkner et al [14] were unable to find propranolol in the plasma or atrial tissue of eight patients 36 to 48 hours after withdrawal from chronic propranolol therapy, and atrial strips from four of these patients had normal responses to norepinephrine. In two of three patients withdrawn from daily oral doses of 80 to 240 mg of propranolol for 24 hours, the heart rate response to isoproterenol was normal. Our experience has been similar. Twelve of 18 patients withdrawn from oral propranolol for 24 hours had no measurable *plasma levels*. To eliminate the possibility that patients without measurable plasma propranolol levels had persistent block from some as yet unknown metabolite, 15 patients withdrawn from propranolol therapy for 24 hours were given isoproterenol 3 μg intravenously, and the heart rate response was measured. The resulting increase in heart rate was identical to the increase of a group of healthy subjects and to a comparable group of patients with arteriosclerotic heart disease who had not previously received propranolol.

Withdrawal of propranolol for periods longer than 24 hours may have its own hazards. Myocardial infarction has been reported in several patients after acute withdrawal. We observed two patients who developed recurrent ventricular fibrillation when withdrawn from propranolol for more than 24 hours. Administration of intravenous propranolol was effective in converting fibrillation to sinus rhythm when lidocaine, potassium, and countershock repeatedly failed to sustain defibrillation.[15]

Arrhythmias

Serious tachyarrhythmias occur frequently during anesthesia for cardiac operations. Johnstone first reported that propranolol reversed arrhythmias appearing during halothane or cyclopropane anesthesia in patients free of cardiac disease.[16] He recommended propranolol 2 to 5 mg intravenously to control potentially dangerous arrhythmias. McClish claimed similar success in treating cardiac irregularities during anesthesia for open heart operations.

We too have used propranolol intravenously and successfully to treat 239 acute arrhythmias appearing during anesthesia in patients with heart disease (Table 3). We accomplished this, however, by doses much smaller than recommended by the above authors. Our patients included 13 with congenital defects, 86 with acquired valve disease, and 140 with arteriosclerotic heart disease. Only arrhythmias that led to significant hypotension were treated with propranolol. When not associated with hypotension, they were untreated or re-

sponded to a single intravenous dose of lidocaine. In 38 of the 239 treated patients, tachyarrhythmia, either atrial, junctional, or ventricular, occurred before induction of anesthesia (Fig. 1). The remainder appeared during anesthesia and were primarily ventricular arrhythmias precipitated by specific maneuvers, such as anesthetic induction, tracheal intubation, surgical incision, sternotomy, or insertion of caval catheters. Ventricular fibrillation was the commonest arrhythmia and appeared for varying periods during cardiopulmonary bypass, in almost all adults after cross-clamping of the aorta and before anoxic arrest supervened. With restoration of coronary circulation at the end of bypass, almost all adult patients again exhibited ventricular fibrillation. Most commonly, treatment with a single DC shock after a variable period of coronary perfusion was successful. In the occasional patient, however, fibrillation persisted or re-

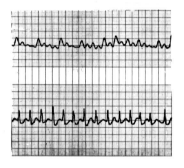

♂ 52 YRS. ASHD SOON AFTER INDUCTION
ACUTE AT. FIB. H.R. >150 B.P. $^{70}/_{50}$ TORR

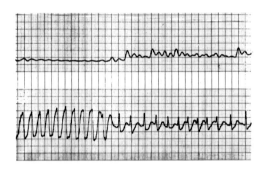

VENT. TACH. REVERTS TO AT. FIB. AS PROPRANOLOL 0.4mg
TAKES EFFECT   B.P. FROM <10 TORR TO $^{70}/_{50}$ TORR

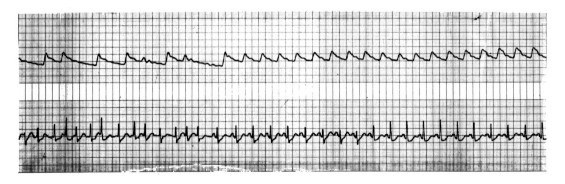

AT. FIB. H.R. >120 PROPRANOLOL 0.4mg AGAIN CONVERTS TO S.R. HR 100 B.P. $^{90}/_{60}$ TORR

FIG. 1. Upper left: Male, 52 years, with severe arteriosclerotic heart disease, developed acute atrial fibrillation immediately after induction of anesthesia; heart rate greater than 150/min, blood pressure less than 70/50 torr, quickly followed by ventricular tachycardia. Upper right: As propranolol 0.4 mg intravenously takes effect, the ventricular tachycardia is converted to atrial fibrillation —blood pressure less than 10 torr to 70/50 torr. Lower: In less than 5 minutes, additional propranolol 0.4 mg was given; this changed the atrial fibrillation to sinus rhythm—Heart rate 100/min, blood pressure 90/60 torr.

TABLE 3. Life-Threatening Arrhythmias in 239 Cardiac Surgical Patients (Propranolol 0.4–1.0 mg IV)

ARRHYTHMIAS	NO. PTS.	SUCCESS RATE (%)
Sinus, atrial, or nodal tachycardia	46	100
Ventricular tachycardia	12	100
Multifocal extrasystoles	2	100
Supraventricular extrasystoles	4	100
Ventricular extrasystoles	29	68
Acute atrial fibrillation	10	100
Chronic atrial fibrillation	58	72
Ventricular fibrillation	78	100

curred after several DC shocks. Successful defibrillation in all of these latter patents was eventually achieved after propranolol administration and further DC shock (Fig. 2).

The fact that most arrhythmias were of acute onset and were precipitated by some anesthetic or surgical maneuver, rather than the result of intrinsic cardiac disease, probably contributed to our high success rate. Our patients, however, also included 87 with chronic arrhythmias of more than three months duration and are listed in Table

3 under ventricular extrasystoles and chronic atrial fibrillation. In these the criterion of successful treatment was a return to preoperative rhythm and not conversion to normal rhythm. The indication for propranolol was a large increase in frequency of premature ventricular contractions or a rapid ventricular rate with atrial fibrillation. Successful treatment reduced ventricular rates with considerable improvement in blood pressure. We considered the contraindications to this method of treating life threatening arrhythmias of acute onset as bradycardia (ventricular rate less than 80/min), heart block, or other conduction defects with slow ventricular rates, asthma, hypokalemia, and hypoglycemia.

We also measured plasma levels of 24 patients following single intravenous doses of propranolol 0.5 mg, our commonest therapeutic dose. Plasma propranolol peaked one minute after intravenous administration and disappeared from the circulation in five minutes. Despite this, the antiarrhythmic effect persisted for approximately 30 minutes in patients in whom the arrhythmia recurred. There seems therefore little hazard of prolonged effect in the event of inadvertent overdosage. In any case, the effect of propranolol can

ECG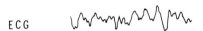

After bypass. Recurrent (5+)
After Lidocaine and
D.C. Shocks

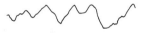

After Propanolol 0.4 mg

ECG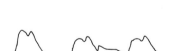

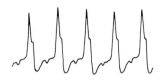

BP

After additional Propanolol 0.2 mg
and DC Shocks

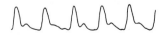

Fifteen minutes later
Epinephrine drip 8 µg/ml

FIG. 2.   Male, 68 years, with arteriorsclerotic heart disease after vein bypass of three coronary arteries. Coming off cardiopulmonary bypass there was recurrent ventricular fibrillation in spite of several doses of lidocaine followed by DC shock each time. Propranolol 0.6 mg in two doses first slowed the ventricular fibrillation, then allowed a countershock to establish a synchronous contraction of the myocardium. Minutes later an epinephrine drip (8 µg/ml) maintained a regular rhythm 84/min, and a blood pressure 100/70 torr. Note the catecholamine administration after partial beta blockade elicits only a positive inotropic effect.

be antagonized by isoproterenol or epinephrine although somewhat larger than usual doses may be required (Figure 2). Fenyvesi and Hadhazy [18] reported that propranolol consistently produced a greater degree of chronotropic than inotropic blockade in animals. Our experience in cardiovascular surgical patients tends to support this observation.

Myocardial Rigor ("Stone Heart")

A rare complication of open-heart operations that utilize anoxic cardiac arrest is the occurrence of myocardial contracture affecting only the left ventricle and variously termed myocardial rigor or "stone heart." We reported encouraging early results [19] in preventing myocardial rigor if propranolol 0.4 to 0.7 mg was given just before bypass and moderate systemic (32 C) and topical cardiac hypothermia were used. Myocardial rigor is most likely to occur in patients with aortic valvular disease associated with pulmonary wedge pressure greater than 45 torr, or left ventricular end diastolic pressure greater than 20 torr, or aortic valve gradients in excess of 75 torr. These conditions predispose to concentric left ventricular hypertrophy with potential for subendocardial ischemia.

Some collateral evidence tends to provide a rationale for propranolol prophylaxis. We have shown that the duration of ventricular fibrillation after crossclamping the aorta is 42 percent shorter in a propranolol pretreated group than in a comparable control group. Hottenrott et al [20] recently demonstrated that ventricular fibrillation not only increased oxygen consumption over the empty beating heart during cardiopulmonary bypass, but fibrillation also diverted blood away from the subendocardial muscle. Although this may not damage normal hearts, he suggested fibrillation may lead to subendocardial injury in markedly hypertrophied ventricles. The anoxic arrested heart is preferable to a fibrillating or an empty beating heart, because oxygen consumption is even lower and the risk of subendocardial damage even less. Additionally, propranolol has been shown to reduce significantly the incidence of myocardial necrosis after episodes of myocardial ischemia. Possibly propranolol exerts a protective effect under circumstances of anoxic cardiac arrest.

During the past year, six instances of myocardial rigor occurred in 2,000 patients undergoing open-heart operations. Four were treated by propranolol after the onset of rigor and the contracture disappeared in all four. None received propranolol prophylactically. One patient survived only two days, but the other three left the hospital improved. Rigor was discovered after bypass in three patients. The other occurred before cardiopulmonary bypass and was treated with propranolol 1.0 mg intravenously while the circulation was supported manually and cardiopulmonary bypass was rapidly instituted.

CONCLUSIONS

Withdrawal of preoperative propranolol for more than 24 hours is not necessary and may be dangerous for some patients. Of 15 patients withdrawn from preoperative propranolol therapy for 24 hours, no propranolol could be found in their plasma and no residual beta blockade could be demonstrated by isoproterenol challenge.

Of 239 consecutive patients with life-threatening tachyarrhythmias during cardiac operations, propranolol invariably resulted in an improvement in cardiac performance and, in most, a return to sinus rhythm.

In four patients with myocardial rigor recognized during open-heart operations, propranolol was effective in relaxing the contracture and three of these survived.

Propranolol is a safe and valuable antiarrhythmic drug in anesthetized patients, provided small intravenous doses are used.

References

1. Ahlquist RP: Study of adrenotropic receptors. Am J Physiol 153:586, 1948
2. Powell CE, Slater IH: Blocking of inhibitory adrenergic receptors by dichloro analog of isoproterenol. J Pharmacol Exp Ther 122:480, 1958
3. Black JW, Stephenson JS: Pharmacology of new adrenergic beta-receptor-blocking compound (nethalide). Lancet 2:311, 1962
4. Harrison DC: Circulatory effects and clinical uses of beta-adrenergic blocking drugs. Monograph, Excerpta Medica, Amsterdam, 1972
5. Evans GH, Shand DC: Disposition of propranolol VI. Independent variation in steady-state circulating drug concentrations and half-life as a result of plasma drug binding in man. Clin Pharmacol Ther 14:494, 1973
6. Fitzgerald JD, O'Donnell SR: Pharmacology of 4-hydroxypropranolol, a metabolite of propranolol. Br J Pharmacol 43:222–35, 1971
7. Colhart DJ, Shand DG: Plasma propranolol levels in the quantitative assessment of B-adrenergic blockade in man. Br Med J iii:731, Sept., 1970
8. Stephen SA: Unwanted effects of propranolol. Am J Card 18:463, 1966
9. Amsterdam EA, Gorlin R, Wolfson W. Evaluation of longterm use of propranolol in angina pectoris. JAMA 210:103, 1969
10. Greenblatt DJ, Koch-Weser J: Adverse reactions to propranolol in hospitalized medical patients: a re-

port from the Boston collaborative drug surveil-lance program. Am Heart J 86:478, 1973

11. Prokop EK, Palmer RF, Wheat MW Jr: Hydrody-namic forces in dissecting aneurysms. Circulation 38 (suppl VI):158, 1968

12. Van Der Horst RL, Winship WS, Gotsman MS: Beta-adrenergic blockade in the relief of paroxysmal cyanotic spells in tricuspid atresia. S Afr Med J 46:494, 1971

13 Viljoen JF, Estafanous F, Kellner GA: Propranolol and cardiac surgery. J Thorac Cardiovasc Surg 64:826–30, 1972

14. Faulkner SL, Hopkins JT, Boerth RC, Young JL, Jellett LB, Nies AS, Bender HW, Shand DG: Time required for complete recovery from chronic pro-pranolol therapy. N Engl J Med 289:607, 1973

15. Romagnoli A, Sabawala PB: The danger of pre-operative withdrawal of propranolol. Cardiovasc Diseases Bulletin of THI 1:15, 1974

16. Johnston M: Propranolol prevents cardiac reaction to acidosis. Br J Anaesth 40:1008, 1968

17. McClish A: Place of I.V. propranolol in the treat-ment of arrhythmias during and after anesthesia for cardiac surgery. Can Med Assoc J 99:388, 1968

18. Fenyvesi T, Hadhazy P: Action of Isoprenaline and B-blocking agents on stroke volume regulation. J Pharmacol 22:105, 1973

19. Cooley DA, Romagnoli A, Reul GJ, Wukasch DC, Kabbani SS, Allmendinger P, Sandiford F, Hallman GL, Norman JC: Stone heart: prevention by in-duced myocardial hypothermia. Presented at the American College of Chest Physicians, Toronto, October 21–25, 1973

20. Hottenrott CE, Towers B, Kurkji HJ, Maloney JS, Buckberg G: The hazard of ventricular fibrillation in hypertrophied ventricles during cardiopulmonary bypass. J Thorac Cardiovasc Surg 5:742, 1973

60

APPLICATION OF THE SUPPLY-DEMAND RATIO FOR THE EARLY POSTPERFUSION DETECTION OF SUBENDOCARDIAL ISCHEMIA

PETER A. PHILIPS and
ALFONSO M. MIYAMOTO

Left ventricular subendocardial necrosis, a direct result of subendocardial ischemia, occurs frequently following cardiopulmonary bypass and may be responsible for more patient deaths than is currently recognized (Taber, 1967; Najafi, 1969). This lesion is caused by a discrepancy between the oxygen needs of subendocardial muscle and the available blood supply. If sole reliance is placed upon systemic arterial pressure and central venous pressure monitoring, factors contributing to decreased subendocardial flow may go unrecognized.

Myocardial oxygen supply, or the flow of blood to the subendocardial layers, occurs predominantly during diastole. Factors occurring in the immediate postoperative period which raise the oxygen demand of the heart and simultaneously lower diastolic pressure, raise left ventricular end diastolic pressure (LVEDP), or decrease diastolic time can lead to subendocardial ischemia and myocardial failure.

Monitoring the supply-demand ratio (EVR), defined as the ratio of the diastolic pressure time index (DPTI) divided by tension time index (TTI) (Buckberg, 1972), in the immediate postperfusion period is an excellent method of determining subendocardial perfusion. Diastolic pressure time index describes the pressure time events during diastole, and, as shown by Buckberg, accurately estimates diastolic and subendocardial blood flow. Myocardial oxygen requirements are directly related to the area under the systolic pressure curve (Sarnoff, 1958), and where TTI is the determinant of factors regulating demand, the ratio of DPTI to TTI should provide an accurate estimate of the oxygen supply-demand relationship.

MATERIALS AND METHODS

Forty-two consecutive open cardiac repairs utilizing cardiopulmonary bypass, hypothermia, and anoxic arrest were performed. A hemodilution prime consisting of Isolyte S, albumin, dextrose, insulin, KCL, heparin, and staphcillin was used. Radial artery (systemic) pressure, supply-demand ratio (EVR), left atrial (LAP) and right atrial (RAP) pressures, blood gases, urinary output, and electrolytes were recorded intraoperatively and for three days postoperatively.

The study group included 20 mitral, six aortic, five combined aortic and mitral, three mitral and tricuspid, five coronary artery bypass, and three ASD procedures. There were 13 valve replacements, four commissurotomies, and three annuloplasties in the mitral series. Of the five combined aortic and mitral procedures, three were double valve replacements and two were mitral commissurotomies with aortic valve replacements. There were two combined mitral and tricuspid replacements, and one tricuspid annuloplasty and mitral valve replacement. The coronary series consisted of one single left anterior descending (LAD) saphenous vein bypass, two combined LAD and right coronary, and two LAD and circumflex bypass combinations. One underwent a left internal mammary artery implant to the LAD, and a saphenous vein bypass graft to the circumflex coronary artery. Ages ranged from 8 to 66, with a mean age of 37.

Changes in subendocardial blood flows were followed by monitoring EVR (Fig. 1). The area

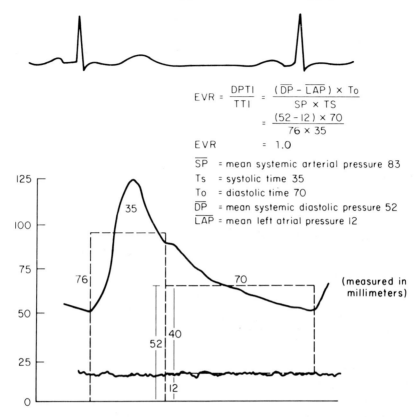

$$EVR = \frac{DPTI}{TTI} = \frac{(\overline{DP} - \overline{LAP}) \times T_o}{SP \times T_S}$$

$$= \frac{(52-12) \times 70}{76 \times 35}$$

$$EVR = 1.0$$

$\overline{SP}$ = mean systemic arterial pressure 83
T_s = systolic time 35
T_o = diastolic time 70
$\overline{DP}$ = mean systemic diastolic pressure 52
$\overline{LAP}$ = mean left atrial pressure 12

(measured in millimeters)

FIG. 1. Components of EVR (supply-demand ratio) derived from indices obtained from systolic and diastolic pressure measurements.

under the radial artery diastolic pressure curve was calculated by an analog computer or measured by planimetry, and the mean left atrial pressure (LAP) subtracted, giving DPTI. Similarly, the analog computer or planimetry of the area under the radial artery systolic pressure curve was used to obtain TTI. The EVR was recorded at 15-minute intervals in the operating room and continuously in the intensive care unit, using an on-line digital computer. All data was analyzed for statistical significance using the paired t-test.

The intraaortic balloon was put in place when left atrial pressures rose above 25 mm Hg, and EVR remained below 0.8 for more than 30 minutes after cessation of cardiopulmonary bypass. Earlier application was initiated when it was apparent that the patient could not be weaned from bypass (Fig. 2), or persistent arrhythmias made maintenance of good cardiac function difficult. In two cases, augmentation was begun six hours and 14 hours following surgery when LA pressures rose above 30 mm Hg, systemic pressures fell below 85 mm Hg systolic and electrocardiographic evidence of ischemia was noted (Fig. 3). In both instances, clinical low cardiac output was mani-

fested by increasing restlessness and mental obtundation, decreasing urinary output, cool mottled extremities, and moist skin. This decline in clinical status was associated with a fall in EVR to below 0.8.

RESULTS

Thirty-two patients with an average postperfusion EVR of 0.9 or greater had uneventful postoperative recoveries. There were 11 patients in whom IABC was used. Each patient had preoperative ECG and vectorcardiographic changes indicative of hypertrophy or myocardial ischemia (Table 1). There were six with enlarged hypertrophic left ventricles, two with severe coronary artery disease, and three had massive right and left atrial and ventricular enlargement. During cardiopulmonary bypass, hypothermia to 26 C, an average anoxic time of 45 minutes, and rewarming to 34 C before weaning from bypass was standard procedure for these patients. Total bypass time ranged from 99 to 150 minutes (average time, 125 minutes).

A

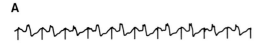

B

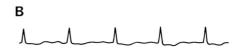

4 hrs. augmented time   EVR = 1.05

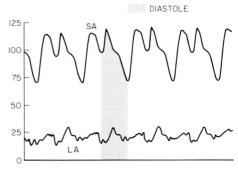

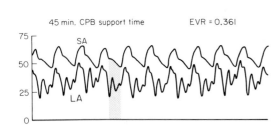

FIG. 2.   A. 45 minutes of cardiopulmonary bypass support time. Factors contributing to poor subendocardial perfusion are markedly elevated LA pressure, low systemic pressure, and rapid cardiac rate. EVR: 0.361.   B. Four hours of balloon augmentation. LA pressures below 25 mm Hg; good diastolic augmentation; cardiac rate slow with narrowed QRS, S-T segments back to the isoelectric line confirm better myocardial perfusion. EVR: 1.05.

Although systemic pressures in this group averaged 90/65 mm Hg, average LA pressures remained above 32 mm Hg, and EVRs were all below 0.7. In seven survivors, the average EVR (Table 2) rose to 1.18 p < 0.0004), average LA pressure fell to 21.0 mm Hg (p < 0.0046), and enhanced coronary perfusion was confirmed by improvement in cardiac rhythm and electrical conductivity. Subendocardial ischemia was considered the cause of the low output syndrome, and intra-aortic balloon counterpulsation was used to wean from cardiopulmonary bypass and improve cardiodynamics. Improved clinical status paralleled the improvement in rhythm and conductivity.

In four others, despite early application of IABC, EVR remained below 0.6 and all died. At

A

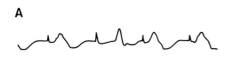

EVR = 0.663

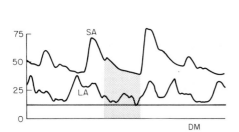

B

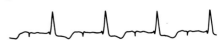

EVR = 1.03   AUGMENTED DIASTOLE

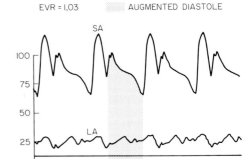

FIG. 3.   A. Four hours postreplacement of aortic valve. LA pressure above 25 mm Hg, decreased diastolic pressure, widened ejection time, and deterioration of rhythm and conductivity on ECG. EVR: 0.66.   B. Two hours of IABC. Improvement in left atrial and systemic pressures and ECG. EVR: 1.03.

TABLE 1. Clinical Findings of Seven IABC Survivors

PT.	AGE	DIAGNOSIS	ECG AND VECTOR-CARDIOGRAM	OPERATION	FINDINGS	IAPB ASSIST
LK	45	Aortic stenosis	LVH	AVR	Bicuspid aortic valve, massive LVH	48 hrs
JK	57	Triple vessel CAD	LVH, anteroseptal inferior wall infarct	SVG-Circu and RCA	Severe triple vessel disease	48 hrs
AP	37	Aortic insufficiency, mitral stenosis	LVH	MVR	Minimal AI, calcific MS	48 hrs
DM	45	Aortic stenosis mitral stenosis	RVH, LVH	AVR, mitral commissurotomy	Calcific MS, massive LVH	72 hrs
PG	36	Aortic stenosis, mitral stenosis	LVH	AVR, MVR	Calcific AS, MS, massive LVH	48 hrs
JH	23	Aortic insufficiency, sinus valsalva aneurysm	LVH, left atrial enlargement	AVR, exclusion of SVA	Bicuspid aortic valve SVA	72 hrs
RT	47	Mitral stenosis	RVH, left atrial enlargement	MVR	Calcific MS	6 hrs

All seven had evidence of left or right ventricular hypertrophy by ECG or vectorcardiogram. Aortic valve disease was present in five. IABC time averaged 56 hours.

necropsy, two had extensive myocardial necrosis, one had evidence of subendocardial ischemia with patchy necrosis and fibrosis, and one succumbed from predominant right heart failure secondary to end-stage mitral valve disease.

DISCUSSION

The low cardiac output syndrome occurring after open intracardiac procedures is a manifestation of impaired cardiac performance and is associated with significant postoperative morbidity and mortality. The syndrome is often associated with elevated mean left atrial pressure and thus, left ventricular end diastolic pressure (LVEDP) and lowered arterial pressures (Kirklin, 1967). With elevations in LVEDP and systemic pressures (afterload), there is an increase in myocardial oxygen demand as oxygen consumption is increased (Sarnoff, 1958; Braunwald, 1973).

Ischemia, more than any other single factor, appears to be the most common cause of the low cardiac output syndrome (Buckberg, 1972a). Good

TABLE 2. Pre- and Postballoon Augmentation Data from Seven Survivors

PT.	PATHOLOGY–SURGERY	PREAUGMENTATION					POSTAUGMENTATION				
		SA	LA	TTI	DPTI	EVR	SA	LA	TTI	DPTI	EVR
LK	AS–AVR	65/48	37	3.7	1.4	0.378	115/117[a]	20	11.0	11.6	1.05
JK	triple-vessel disease– double-vein bypass	100/57	25	7.4	6.2	0.838[c]	135/120[a]	25	8.2	10.5	1.28
AP	AI/MS–MVR	102/55	35	9.0	6.0	0.666	125/120[a]	25	9.5	12.0	1.26[a]
							125/ 87[b]		10.5	11.5	1.09[b]
DM	AS–AVR	70/52	32	7.1	5.6	0.780	135/100[a]	25	8.8	12.0	1.36
PG	MS/AR–MVR/AVR	66/41	25	5.7	6.0	1.05[d]	110/ 87[a]	20	9.0	12.0	1.33
JH	AI–AVR	110/5	28	10.3	7.0	0.678	140/135[a]	12.5	13.0	16.5	1.26[a]
							140/ 98[b]		12.0	11.0	0.92[b]
RT	MS–MVR	60/50	42	6.9	2.7	0.390	70/ 72[a]	20	7.6	6.3	0.83

[a]*Augmented.*
[b]*Unaugmented.*
[c]*Immediate postop.*
[d]*Early augment.*

Greatest changes are seen in LA and diastolic pressures; DPTI, and EVR. The preaugmentation combination of high LA and low mean diastolic pressures are factors contributing to subendocardial ischemia.

TABLE 3. Average Pressures, Indices, and EVR of Seven Survivors Showing Improvement in All Parameters Measured, following Application of IACB

	PREAUGMENTATION	POSTAUGMENTATION	P-VALUE
LA	32.00 mm Hg	21.07 mm Hg	0.0046
Systolic	81.86 mm Hg	117.14 mm Hg	0.0021
Diastolic	53.86 mm Hg	105.86 mm Hg	0.0002
TTI	7.16 cm^2	9.59 cm^2	0.0182
DPTI	4.99 cm^2	11.43 cm^2	0.0003
EVR	0.68	1.18	0.00004

Greatest changes are seen with diastolic pressure, DPTI, and EVR.

subendocardial perfusion is necessary if the heart is to sustain the workload imposed following operation. Early recognition of an ischemic myocardium is imperative if proper therapy is to be initiated in time to prevent necrosis.

Reliance upon systemic arterial pressure and central venous pressure in the postperfusion period may result in delayed diagnosis and treatment of myocardial ischemia. The work of Buckberg and colleagues has confirmed the efficiency of the supply-demand ratio (EVR) as an indicator of subendocardial perfusion. Results obtained from physiologic stress experiments designed to alter DPTI by increasing LA pressure, and thus LVEDP, decreasing diastolic pressure, increasing systolic ejection time, and decreasing diastolic time, verified that subendocardial perfusion and potential ischemia could be predicted from indices derived from systolic and diastolic pressure measurements (Buckberg, 1972b). Correlation of hyperemic response following periods of anoxia, with subendocardial-subepicardial flow ratios, proved DPTI:TTI a highly accurate determinant of subendocardial

ischemia. Below a given ratio for the experimental model, subendocardial blood flow decreased. The flow of coronary blood became predominantly systolic, and although in some instances there was increased coronary flow, the distribution was subepicardial.

The applicability and reliability of EVR as a monitoring modality for subendocardial ischemia and cardiac function was verified by the observance of the supply-demand ratio in the clinical setting. With the use of a simple analog computer, on-line digital EVR's were obtainable on a beat-by-beat basis. The average hemodynamic data and its statistical significance for the seven balloon pump survivors prior to and after balloon augmentation is presented in Table 3. The greatest change was seen in diastole and DPTI, reflected by a significant rise in EVR. Mean DPTI (Fig. 4) rose from preaugmentation levels of 1,010 to 2,357 mm Hg sec after augmentation (Fig. 5). The EVR rose from a mean of 0.608 prior to augmentation to 1.12 following augmentation. Enhanced coronary perfusion was confirmed by improvement in cardiac

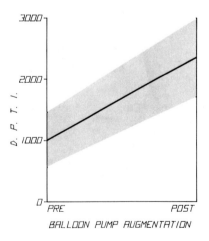

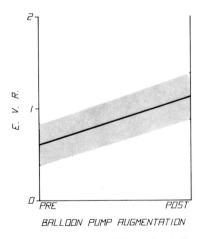

FIG. 4. Significant increase in mean DPTI during balloon augmentation. This figure illustrates in mm Hg sec an increase in diastolic filling time and pressure. Shaded area shows ± one standard deviation.

FIG. 5. Similar increase in EVR during balloon augmentation reflecting improved subendocardial perfusion. Shaded area shows ± one standard deviation.

rhythm and electrical conductivity with loss of ischemic S-T wave depression on ECG noted on all cases in which they had been present prior to IABC. The marked improvement in the clinical status of these patients correlated significantly with the rise in EVR, confirming the reliability of this ratio as a guide to the detection of subendocardial ischemia.

References

Braunwald E, Maroko PR: Protection of the ischemic myocardium. Hospital Practice 8:61–74, 1973

Buckberg GD, Fixler DE, Archie JP, et al: Experimental subendocardial ischemia in dogs with normal coronary arteries. Circ Res 30:67–81, 1972a

Buckberg GD, Towers B, Paglia DE, et al: Subendocardial ischemia after cardiopulmonary bypass. J Thorac Cardiovasc Surg 64:669–84, 1972b

Kirklin JW, Rastelli GC: Low cardiac output after open intracardiac operations. Prog Cardiovasc Dis 10:117–22, 1967

Najafi H, Henson D, Dye WS, et al: Left ventricular hemorrhagic necrosis. Ann Thorac Surg 7:550–61, 1969

Sarnoff SJ, Braunwald E, Welch GH, et al: Hemodynamic determinants of oxygen consumption of the heart with special reference to the tension-time index. Am J Physiol 192:148–56, 1958

Taber RE, Morales AR, Fine G: Myocardial necrosis and the postoperative low-cardiac-output syndrome. Ann Thorac Surg 4:12–28, 1967

61

IMPROVED PATENCY OF CORONARY DOUBLE GRAFTS WITH BILATERAL INTERNAL MAMMARY ARTERIAL ANASTOMOSES

George Schimert, Djavad Arani, Ivan L. Bunnell,
David G. Greene, Ravinder Tandon, Thomas Z. Lajos,
Arthur B. Lee, Jr., and Bernardo Vidne

INTRODUCTION

Bypass grafting is useful to alleviate angina pectoris in patients with significant occlusive lesions in the proximal segments of major coronary arteries. Adequate distal coronary lumina and run-off are essential to the success of this procedure. In the past, saphenous vein grafts have been inserted extensively as conduits of arterial blood.[7,17] However, the observed failure rate of these grafts due to clotting or degenerative changes has suggested the use of arterial structures for this purpose.[1,8,12,14,15] The location, availability, and relative lack of pathologic changes within the wall of the internal mammary artery makes this vessel particularly attractive as a coronary bypass graft.[2,11,18] Elimination of one anastomotic suture line, uniform lumen, comparable size, resistance to kinking, and preservation of pulsatile blood flow are unique to this technique.

Anastomosis of the left internal mammary artery to the left anterior descending coronary artery is the easiest to perform and appears to be the most favored combination. However, the left internal mammary artery also can be used to graft the diagonal and the marginal branches. The right internal mammary can be used to graft the midsection of the right coronary artery and can also be used to graft the left anterior descending coronary artery in patients without excessive cardiac enlargement. Neither the right nor the left internal mammary artery will reach the distal right or the terminal circumflex coronary artery. These vessels must be grafted, if necessary, by saphenous vein grafts or more recently by free radial artery grafts.

This report examines our results in 44 patients with double internal mammary artery grafts and their combination with saphenous vein grafts or free radial artery grafts. Patients requiring additional corrective surgery such as aneurysmectomy, excision of akinetic segments, closure of ventricular septal defects, and valve replacement, have been excluded from this series.

METHODS AND MATERIALS

All patients reported had cardiac work-up including coronary arteriography and ventriculograms at the Buffalo General Hospital by the same diagnostic group. Of the 44 patients who were operated upon, 42 presented themselves with chest pain. One of the two patients who had no chest pain had fainting spells attributed to congenital aortic stenosis, and one patient was referred because of suspicion of a ventricular aneurysm developing three months after a myocardial infarct. There were 40 males and four females with ages ranging from 32 to 68 years. The average age was 52 years. All patients with chest pain were in the New York State Heart Association Classification Stage III or IV. They had severe angina pectoris, often associated with dyspnea, and most had been unable to work for a long period of time prior to operation. Angina at rest and nocturnal angina were commonly present. All patients were on strict medical programs but had failed to achieve significant improvement. Twenty-one patients had one or more myocardial infarcts prior to cardiac catheterization, and one additional patient developed myocardial infarction waiting for surgery. Seven patients were in some degree of congestive heart

TABLE 1. Preoperative Clinical Symptoms in 44 Patients

Angina on exercise	42
Angina at rest	22
Heart failure	7
Arrhythmias	5
Preinfarction angina	11

failure; five of these had recurrent severe tachyarrhythmias. Eleven patients had preinfarction angina with increasing frequency and severity of attacks (Table 1). One patient's left ventricular failure was aggravated by aortic insufficiency, and another patient had heart failure because of an associated large sinus venosus type of atrial septal defect. Eighteen patients suffered from moderate to severe hypertension, and seven patients had been treated for diabetes (Table 2).

TABLE 2. Associated Disease in 44 Patients

Hypertension	18
Diabetes	7
Aortic stenosis[a]	1
Aortic insufficiency[a]	1
ASD sinus venosus type[b]	1

[a] Valve replacement was not indicated.
[b] Concomitantly closed.

Preoperative coronary arteriograms and ventriculograms were essential to establish surgical indications. Coronary arteriograms were done in frontal, lateral, left, and right anterior oblique and a half axial views[4] in order to separate the proximal portions and superimposing branches of the left main coronary artery. All views were taken both by cineangiography as well as by large cut films. Patients with 75 percent or greater decrease in cross-sectional lumen of major coronary arteries were selected for surgery (Table 3). In complete obstruction, retrograde filling and visualization of the distal vessel were considered necessary for a bypass graft. The contractility of the left ventricle as measured by ventriculograms was considered the most important single determination to assess

TABLE 3. Surgical Indications in 44 Patients

Angina with 75 percent or more coronary obstruction	42
No angina with 75 percent or more coronary obstruction in young patients	2[a]

[a] One suspected congenital aortic stenosis; one suspected ventricular aneurysm.

left ventricular function and operative risk. Left ventricular cineangiograms were made in both the right anterior oblique and the left anterior oblique positions in all patients. A thorough appraisal of the state of left ventricular contractility was made by end-diastolic and end-systolic measurements. Estimation of forward flow was expressed by ejection fraction. Left ventricular volumes were determined by the single plane cineangiographic method previously described by Greene and associates,[10] the measurement of left ventricular volume by the single plane cineangiographic method was applied with caution in subjects whose noncontractile segments may have altered critical dimensions. We, therefore, present our figures only as relative indications of cavity volume particularly in patients with grossly enlarged hearts.

Patients with more than 50 percent ejection fractions were considered to have good ventricular function. Patients with ejection fractions between 50 and 35 percent have been judged to have fair ventricular functions. Patients with ejection fractions below 35 percent were judged to have poor ventricular function. In these 44 patients, according to these criteria, 18 had good, 18 had fair, and eight patients had poor ventricular function (Table 4). Patients with fair and poor ventricular functions had variable amounts of diffuse scarring of the left ventricular muscle or had segmental impairment of the contractility localized to the anterolateral and/or the diaphragmatic surfaces of left ventricle. Five patients of the seven treated for cardiac failure were in the poor ventricular function group.

As previously stated, 11 patients were judged to have accelerated or unstable angina and were classified as patients having impending infarction. We believe that this is a distinct group that needs immediate attention. We have included in this group patients with angina pectoris not relieved by usual medical treatment and patients with worsening of an established angina pattern with respect to its tempo or severity. Electrocardiographic findings of myocardial ischemia, such as ST segment depression and T-wave inversions often associated with transient enzyme elevations confirmed this diagnosis in the majority of the

TABLE 4. Diseased Vessels Observed during Coronary Arteriography

Double-vessel disease	10
Triple-vessel disease	27
Quadruple-vessel disease	7

TABLE 5. Assessment of Left Ventricular Function by Ejection Fraction (EF)

	NO. PTS.
EF good (better than 50 percent)	18
EF fair (between 50 and 35 percent)	18
EF poor (less than 35 percent)	8

TABLE 6. Surgical Procedure

	NO. PTS.	DOUBLE INT. MAMM. ARTERY	SAPH-ENOUS VEIN	TOTAL NO. GRAFTS
Double graft	20	20	–	40
Triple graft	20	20	20	60
Quadruple graft	4	4	8	16
Total	44	44 (88 IMA)	28	116

patients. At least four of the patients in this group had main left coronary artery lesions with additional lesions in the left anterior descending or a diagonal branch, the circumflex or the right coronary artery. That coronary arteriography and ventriculography can be performed safely during the phase of impending myocardial infarction is reinforced by the fact that no complications were encountered in any of the 11 patients studied.

By selection, all patients had multivessel disease necessitating the insertion of multiple grafts. Generally, only vessels were grafted that were judged to have suitable size and adequate runoff. Four of seven patients with extensive coronary artery disease received quadruple bypass grafts. Three-vessel disease was present in 27 patients; 20 of these had triple grafts. Two-vessel disease was present in 10 patients, and all of these had double-bypass grafts (Table 5). In order of importance, the first- and second-choice vessels were preferentially grafted by internal mammary arteries. Third- and fourth-choice vessels received saphenous vein bypass grafts. Therefore, 28 vein grafts were inserted in addition to the 44 double internal mammary grafts in 44 patients. The total number of all types of grafts inserted were 116 (Table 6). One additional patient, not yet restudied, had double internal mammary artery grafts to branches of the left coronary artery and a free radial artery graft to the right coronary artery.

OPERATIVE TECHNIQUE

The operative technique utilized in this series of 44 patients was essentially the same. Moderate hypothermia (30 to 32 C), electrical fibrillation, and venting of the left ventricle have been employed. Aortic cross-clamping has been minimized. Perfusion flow rates have been approximately 2.2 L/m². The heart is exposed through a median sternotomy. Dissection of the mammary arteries is greatly facilitated by the Favaloro self-retaining sternal retractor.[6] The internal mammary artery is dissected as a pedicle containing the vein, fascia, and muscle, from the sixth intercostal space

back almost to its subclavian origin. At this point, the right recurrent laryngeal nerve may be seen; this structure must be protected. This careful proximal dissection is necessary if the artery is to reach the circumflex branches behind the heart or if the right internal mammary artery is to cross the midline to the left anterior descending on its branches. The dissection is performed by electrocautery. A needle tip is used with moderate cautery intensity (Bovie® setting 30-35, manufactured by Ritter Company). A long longitudinal incision is made, 1 cm, medial to the artery, starting at a level corresponding to that of the fourth costal cartilage. The mammary artery is then cleared of adventitia and pedicle tissue for 1 cm proximal to its end. A bevel is produced by making a 5 mm longitudinal incision of the cut end with minimal trimming of the corners. Dilatation of the artery with probes may dissect the intima and is therefore avoided.

If the coronary artery is not clearly identified, the epicardial and subepicardial fat are dissected off the anterior surface, but the vessel is never mobilized from its bed. After opening the artery by a hook knife (#12 Bard Parker), the arteriotomy is elongated to 4 mm.

The anastomosis is performed with 7-0 interrupted sutures; each suture is tied before the next is inserted. If the circumflex and anterior descending artery are to be grafted, the left mammary is used for bypass of the circumflex or its branches. When the right coronary artery is involved or more than two bypasses are to be done to branches

TABLE 7. Postoperative Re-catheterization Findings in 43 Patients

GRAFT	TOTAL	PATENT		OCCLUDED	
		No.	%	No.	%
Internal mammary artery	86	83	96.5	3	3.5
Saphenous vein	28	25	89.3	3	10.7
Total	114	108	95	6	5

of the left coronary, a saphenous vein and (recently) a radial artery graft are used.

Intraoperatively and postoperatively, patients are treated with Oxacillin or other appropriate antistaphylococcal agents. All patients have received oral anticoagulants, unless there were some contraindications.

RESULTS

All 43 surviving patients underwent recatheterization between 10 to 15 days postoperatively. For the results of postoperative angiography, see Table 7. In the cineangiographic visualization of the total group of 115 bypass grafts, 108 were patent. From the group of 86 internal mammary artery bypass grafts, only three were closed (3.5 percent). These include one left internal mammary artery graft to the first diagonal branch and two right internal mammary artery grafts to the anterior descending artery. From the group of 28 saphenous vein grafts, three were closed (10.7 percent); these include one to the circumflex and two to the right coronary artery. No patients had more than one graft occluded. Electrocardiographic evidence of new myocardial infarctions was noted in six patients (13.6 percent) three of whom were found to have one occluded graft. All but one apparently had had silent infarction. It is important to emphasize that these patients with electrocardiographic signs of myocardial infarction had postoperative courses and clinical improvement similar to the patients without QRS changes.

It is interesting to note that only three of the six patients with one graft occluded showed electrocardiographic evidence of myocardial infarction; the site of infarction as determined by electrocardiography was in the area of distribution of the grafted coronary artery.

Only one patient had signs and symptoms in addition to electrocardiographic changes suggesting myocardial infarction. This patient died 10 days postoperatively due to irreversible cardiogenic shock.

The postoperative clinical outcome for the 44 patients is summarized in Table 8. Forty-three of these patients gradually improved or were entirely angina free. Of these, 38 have returned to full-time work and/or full physical activity.

DISCUSSION

Direct coronary artery surgery is currently performed with excellent results. The criticism of

TABLE 8. Postoperative Clinical Results in 44 Patients

	NO. PTS.	%
Death	1	2.2
No angina at rest	43	98
Minimal angina on exercise	9	20
Return to work and/or physical activity	30	68
Postoperative myocardial infarction[a]	6	14

[a]Silent: 5; fatal: 1.

surgical results is not so much in reference to the early acute salvage in this critical group of patients but to late patency. In animal experiments, Hirose[16] found great discrepancy in the rate of patency between internal mammary and vein grafts. In addition, the vein bypass grafts showed fibrotic changes at six months postoperatively. In clinical experience, follow-up arteriograms, nine to 12 months after coronary bypass, have shown patency rates of 80 to 85 percent when an autogenous saphenous vein was used as a graft, compared with a 98 percent patency rate when the internal mammary artery was used to bypass obstructions of the coronary artery.[5,12,13]

The results above are considered to be due to the following reasons.

It is our impression that the first important factor is the size of the vein graft. Vein segments more than twice the diameter of coronary artery segments often manifest slow, turbulent flow on early angiograms and stenosis or occlusion on late angiograms. On the contrary, the diameter of the internal mammary artery more closely approximates that of the recipient coronary artery, resulting in a higher velocity of flow than with large saphenous grafts. The slow flow rate produced by this discrepancy unquestionably has been responsible for many early graft closures.[19]

In using the internal mammary artery, only one anastomosis instead of two is required. In addition, arteries constitute better arterial grafts than do veins because the arterial graft does not have to undergo arteriolization changes such as intimal fibrous proliferation that may occur in venous grafts.[1,3,8,9,12,14,15,20] Also, the artery-to-artery anastomosis theoretically has greater longevity than does an artery-vein anastomosis, and this particular systemic artery (internal mammary) is relatively free from atherosclerosis, except in some diabetic patients. No matter what graft is chosen, grafts that are too long show a tendency toward acute angulation and filling defects, and thrombi are frequently seen at points of angulation. Also, grafts that are noted in the operating room to be short or to have torsion of the axis are prone to show stenosis on early angiograms.

In our opinion, 2 to 3× magnification is helpful in performing anastomosis of coronary arteries in the 0.5 to 1.0 mm range, but an end-to-side graft can be constructed to most coronary arteries without magnification with the interrupted suture technique.

We have found that the left internal mammary artery can be used to bypass the left anterior descending, the circumflex, and its branches. The right internal mammary artery must be used to graft the left anterior descending when it is necessary to use the left internal mammary artery to graft the proximal circumflex and its branches or the diagonal branch of the left anterior descending. When more than two bypasses must be done, we have used alternative procedures, such as saphenous vein grafts. In patients with varicose veins or surgically removed saphenous veins, the radial artery was recently used. Our initial experience from these first 44 cases of double mammary-coronary arterial anastomoses has been gratifying. The simplicity of the technique and the favorable clinical and angiographic results warrant its continued practice as either a primary or substitute method of direct myocardial revascularization.

SUMMARY

During the year 1973, double internal mammary artery bypass grafts were placed in 44 patients. In 28 of these patients, an additional one or two saphenous vein grafts were performed. In addition to the double internal mammary grafts, 20 patients had triple- and four patients had quadruple-coronary-bypass grafts. Angina pectoris was the primary indication for surgery.

Comparative evaluation of the postoperative cineangiograms demonstrated a patency rate of 96.5 percent for the internal mammary artery bypass grafts and 89.3 percent for the saphenous vein grafts.

Double internal mammary artery to coronary artery grafting has become our preferred method for bypassing multiple vessel coronary artery occlusion.

References

1. Adam M, Michael BF, Lambert CJ, Geisler GP: Long-term results with aorto-coronary artery bypass vein grafts. Ann Thorac Surg 14:1, 1972
2. Bailey CP, Hirose T: Successful internal mammary coronary artery anastomosis using a mini-vascular suture technique. Int Surg 49:416, 1968
3. Bourassa MG, Lesperance J, Campeau L, Simard P: Factors influencing patency of aortocoronary vein grafts. Circulation 45 (Suppl I):79, 1972
4. Bunnell IL, Greene DG, Tandon RN, Arani D: The half axial projection: a new look at the proximal left coronary artery. Circulation 48:1151, 1973
5. Edwards WS, Lewis CE, Blakeley WR, Napolitano L: Coronary artery bypass with internal mammary and splenic artery grafts. Ann Thorac Surg 15, no 1, 1973
6. Favaloro RC: Unilateral self-retaining retractor for use in internal mammary dissection. J Thorac Cardiovasc Surg 43:864, 1967
7. Favaloro RG: Saphenous vein autograft replacement of severe sequential coronary artery occlusion operative techniques. Ann Thorac Surg 5:334, 1968
8. Flemma RJ, Johnson WD, Lepley D, et al: Late results of saphenous vein bypass grafting for myocardial revascularization. Ann Thorac Surg 14:232, 1972
9. Gleen WWL: Some reflections on the coronary bypass operation. Circulation 55:869, 1972
10. Greene DG, Carlisle R, Grant C, Bunnell IL: Estimation of left ventricular volume by one-phase cineangiography. Circulation 35:61, 1967
11. Green GE, Spencer FC, Tice DA, Stertzer SH: Arterial and venous microsurgical bypass grafts for coronary artery disease. J Thorac Cardiovasc Surg 60:491, 1970
12. Green GE: Internal mammary artery-to-coronary artery anastomosis. Ann Thorac Surg 14:260, 1972
13. Green GE: Rate of blood flow from the internal mammary artery. Surgery 70:809, 1971
14. Grondin CM, Meere C, Castonguay Y, Lepage G, Grondin P: Progressive and late obstruction of an aortocoronary venous bypass graft. Circulation 43: 698, 1971
15. Hamaker WR, Doule WF, O'Connell TJ, Gomez AG: Subintimal obliterative proliferation in saphenous vein grafts. Ann Thorac Surg 13:488, 1972
16. Hirose T: Discussion of 8
17. Johnson WD, Flemma RJ, Lepley D, Ellison E: Extended treatment of severe coronary artery disease: a total surgical approach. Ann Surg 170:460, 1969
18. Kolossev VI: Mammary artery-coronary anastomosis as a method of treatment for angina pectoris. J Thorac Cardiovasc Surg 54:535, 1967
19. Loop FD, Effler DB, Spampinato N, Groves LK, Cheanuechai C: Myocardial revascularization by internal mammary artery grafts. J Thorac Cardiovasc Surg 63:674, 1972
20. Vlosaver Z, Edwards JE: Pathologic changes in aortic-coronary arterial saphenous vein grafts. Circulation 44:719, 1971

62

THE TECHNIQUE OF PREPARATION AND CONSTRUCTION OF INTERNAL MAMMARY-CORONARY ARTERY GRAFT AND ANASTOMOSES

Meredith L. Scott, Noel Mills,
John Ochsner, and Robert D. Bloodwell

INTRODUCTION

The one-year occlusion rate of saphenous veins used as aortocoronary bypass grafts has been reported up to 20 and 35 percent (Bourassa, Lesperance, et al, 1972; Walker, Friedberg, et al, 1972). In contrast, the patency rate of internal mammary artery bypass to coronary arteries has been above 95 percent (Edwards, Lewis, et al, 1973; Green, 1972). Although bypass grafts using either of these autologous vessels have been exceedingly successful in myocardial revascularization, the quest for more assured long-term patency prompts the development of improved techniques in graft preparation and in performing the anastomosis. The development of the internal mammary to coronary artery graft has as its basis the vast experience of peripheral vascular surgery, cardiopulmonary bypass technology, microsurgical techniques, and the evaluation of previous myocardial revascularization procedures.

Historical Aspects

The experiences with the Vineberg procedure (Favaloro, Effler, et al, 1968; Vineberg, 1946; Vineberg and Walker, 1964) of indirect myocardial revascularization using the internal mammary artery have been essential to direct coronary anastomosis using that vessel. Absolon and Lillehei were the first to demonstrate the feasibility of direct internal mammary and carotid to coronary artery anastomoses in dogs (Absolon, Lillehei, et al, 1956). The left subclavian artery was tied to assure flow through the end-to-end suture anastomosis from the internal mammary artery to the left coronary artery. Thrombosis was regularly seen since heparin was not employed. Julian recognized the desirability of a dry, quiet field and used cardiopulmonary bypass and induced asystole in similar experimental direct grafts (Julian, Lopez-Belio, et al, 1957). In 1960, Goetz reported the first successful anastomosis in a patient using a nonsuture technique employing a tantalum ring between the right internal mammary artery and the right coronary artery (Goetz, Rohman, et al, 1961) (Fig. 1).

Several years passed until in 1966 the Russian surgeon Kolessov (Kolessov, 1967) performed internal mammary artery to a right coronary artery bypass in six patients, five of whom obtained excellent clinical results. He used an interrupted suture technique (Fig. 2). His report was not immediately influential in causing other surgeons to employ this procedure since saphenous vein grafts were being introduced and enjoying a good early patency rate. Charles Bailey was the first United States surgeon to perform mammary-to-coronary grafting using suture anastomosis in February of 1968 (Bailey and Hirose, 1968). He recently presented the angiograms of this patient six years postoperatively with a patent functioning graft to the right coronary artery (Bailey, unpublished as of 2/74, from the Meeting of the Society of Thoracic Surgeons, Los Angeles, California, January 1974). This operation was followed 21 days later by Green, who employed optical assistance in making the anastomosis (Green, Stertzer, et al, 1968). His group accumulated the first large series of patients treated by this technique, demonstrating the efficacy of internal mammary artery to coronary bypass grafting. The reported patency rate of these grafts compared to that experienced after saphenous vein grafting by the same group

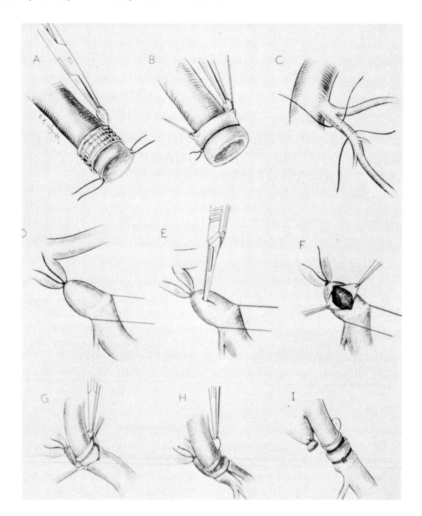

FIG. 1. Diagram of technique of first successful anastomosis of mammary to coronary artery in a patient, showing use of tantalum ring technique (Reproduced by permission of RH Goetz, M Rohman, JD Haller, R Dee, SS Rosenak, J Thorac Cardiovasc Surg 41, 1961).

influenced most surgeons to attempt to duplicate his work (Green, 1972).

Microsurgery as an extension of Halsted's surgical principles of gentle handling and exceedingly accurate approximation of tissues was furthered by Jacobson in the development of microvascular surgery (Jacobson, 1971). The development of microvascular instruments (like those used in ophthalmology) such as needle holders, forceps, holding and retaining probes, etc has proven extremely useful in mammary-coronary surgery (Fig. 3).

General Considerations of Technique

Certain general considerations are very important, if not essential, in performing this pedicled coronary bypass graft. Although many types of suture material have been used for anastomosis of the internal mammary artery to the coronary artery, #6-0 and #7-0 polypropylene monofilament suture on a swaged cardiovascular needle has been a great advance, if not a necessity (Fig. 4). However, many surgeons have had good results with silk and other materials (Loop, Effler, et al, 1971).

We prefer optical assistance with a two- to four-power lens as an essential element of the technique for successful anastomosis (Spencer, 1971). Several surgeons have described performing anastomosis of an internal mammary artery without optical assistance (Loop, 1973b). This seems to be an unnecessary and unrealistic approach to a very difficult anastomosis. The surgeon should be able to inspect and handle with confidence the friable intima of both internal mammary artery and coronary artery. Previous experience in microvascular surgical techniques by

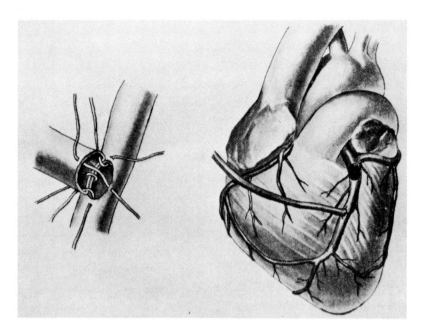

FIG. 2. Technique used in first reported mammary-coronary artery anastomosis in patients (Reproduced by permission of VI Kolessov, J Thorac Cardiovasc Surg 54, 1967).

Jacobson dictates the use of optical assistance in performing anastomoses of this size. He stated, "Anyone who has worked with arteries in the 1-2 mm diameter range realizes that it is simply not possible to perform satisfactory anastomosis with the unaided eye" (Jacobson, 1971). He also feels that technical failure in anastomosis can be virtually eliminated with application of these more precise techniques. The use of an operative microscope is probably unnecessary and too restrictive in the cardiovascular microsurgery where anastomoses are in the 1 to 3 mm range.

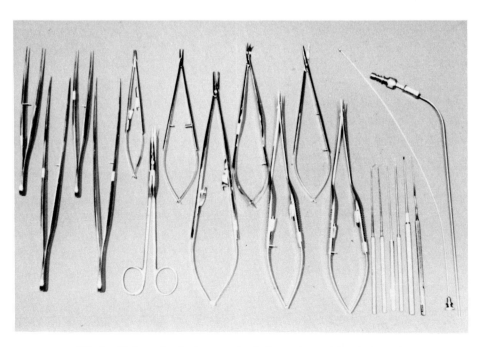

FIG. 3. Photograph of microvascular instruments used in anastomosis.

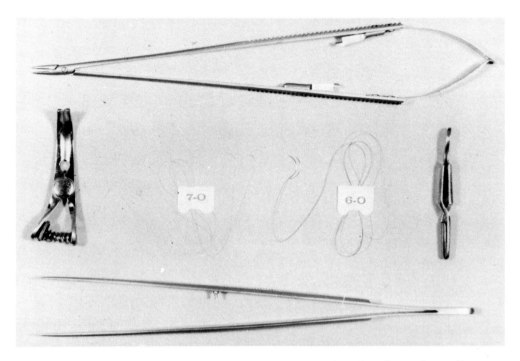

FIG. 4. Small gauge polypropylene monofilament suture and small cardiovascular needle.

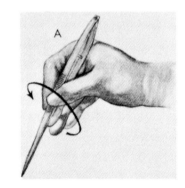

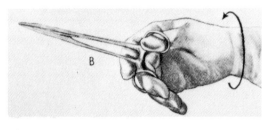

FIG. 5. Diagram illustrating comparison between fingertip (A) and wrist motion (B) while directing a needle holder.

The use of the Castroviejo (Castroviejo, 1952) needle holder is based on the principle that an instrument held by the thumb and forefinger gives much better control of the motion of the needle holder tip (and utilizes the homunculus to its fullest) than a standard needle holder, whose motion depends on gross wrist action. A comparison can be made between writing with a pencil grasped in your hand versus writing with a pencil grasped with the thumb and forefinger (Fig. 5). Employment of the "lathe rest principle" using a fulcrum for the needle holder or other instrument minimizes hand tremor during small vessel anastomosis.

The Favaloro retractor, which was designed to assist in taking down the internal mammary artery pedicle, gained wide usage during the Vineberg procedure (Favaloro, 1967). It was designed to produce a lateral rather than anterior retraction on the sternum. Another retractor fashioned from a lithotomy leg holder and a loop of steel wire attached to two rake retractors provides greater anterior retraction. This gives a better exposure of the internal mammary artery pedicle than the Favaloro retractor, especially of the first intercostal artery, which is extremely important in the preparation of this graft. The development of the cold light fiber optic headlamp in neurosurgery has been extremely useful in the course of the

small branches coming from the internal mammary artery and especially the final anastomosis.*

Specific Considerations of Preparation of the Internal Mammary Artery Pedicle and Anastomosis

Exposure is provided by median sternotomy. The pericardium may or may not be open. However, we have found if one opens the pericardium at the outset, the pericardium and the lung, with its overlying pleura, may drop away from the dissected area to facilitate exposure of the chest wall containing the mammary artery without entry through the pleura. This also permits inspection of the coronary arteries for disease and evaluation of lengths of the internal mammary artery necessary to bypass any lesions present. The internal mammary artery is dissected free from the chest wall from the diaphragm to the subclavian artery.

A combination of hemostatic techniques is employed. The electrocautery is employed to remove the parietal fascia and small intercostal veins. Care is taken not to use the electrocautery too close to the parent vessel, and the intensity is carefully regulated. The concomitant internal mammary veins may or may not be taken with the artery. The large intercostal branches of the internal mammary artery are individually ligated proximally with #0000 silk sutures and distally with silver clips. Cautery is also used in the distal intercostal vessels to assure hemostasis. The artery itself is never handled with the forceps; only the perivascular tissue is touched. If the forceps do grasp the vessel, the chance of dissection of the intima due to an intimal flap is great. Division and ligation of the first intercostal artery is important. Two possibilities may be detrimental to the graft if this is not done: (1) kinking, which can occlude the graft, at this point may occur as it comes away from the anterior thoracic wall and (2) "intercostal steal" can occur if this large intercostal branch is not ligated. After the graft is prepared, either a small #20 Teflon needle or a #20 needle with a finely polished, silver soldered blunt tip is introduced into the distal end of the internal mammary artery under direct vision employing optical assistance and microvascular instruments. A dorsal slit including all layers of the artery, and including the intima, is made to assure that one is introducing the tip of the catheter into the lumen of the artery.

This is essential in avoiding dissection of the intima. After the needle or Teflon cannula is introduced under direct vision, full-strength papaverine is introduced under a small amount of pressure to dilate the vessel all the way to the subclavian artery. Soft clamp or finger pressure is applied at the junction of the internal mammary to the subclavian artery. This procedure assures dilatation of the entire vessel. This is essential in obtaining adequate caliber and also ensures an intact graft. If one encounters a leak, the point of injury is sutured with optical assistance, using #7-0 or #6-0 polypropylene suture. In the past, some surgeons (Loop, Effler, et al, 1971) have dilated the internal mammary artery with a metal probe. We have found this to be disastrous and do not recommend it. Certain other surgeons who previously recommended this no longer utilize the technique. At this point, the internal mammary artery is allowed to bleed freely into a graduated cylinder. Mills and Ochsner found that flows obtained from these grafts are similar to the ones obtained initially by Green with a mean of approximately 100 to 130 cc/min flow (Green, 1971; Mills and Ochsner, 1973). We do not use an internal mammary-artery graft if there is less than 75 cc/min flow. This procedure is accomplished only after the internal mammary artery has been dissected free from the surrounding structures and dilated and the patient has been heparinized to assure no thrombosis within the graft while preparations for the cardiopulmonary bypass are being made. The Teflon needle is either left attached to the vessel or removed at this point. The distal vessel is left intact beyond the site selected for the anastomosis, so one may grasp this area with forceps for retraction. Only adventitia of the artery at the anastomotic site should be touched with the forceps during the anastomotic procedure.

Mammary Anastomosis to Coronary Artery

The mammary artery is opened on its dorsal surface and the anastomosis is performed in the following fashion. The coronary artery is opened for a distance of approximately 3 to 5 mm. With a double-armed #7-0 polypropylene suture on a fine cardiovascular needle, a mattress suture is begun in the internal mammary artery proximally and carried to the proximal end of the arteriotomy in the coronary artery (Fig. 6). A narrow mattress suture is used in order not to compromise the anastomosis. It will allow intimal approximation of the arterial walls. The sutures are tied and con-

---

* Co-axial lamp, Designs for Vision.

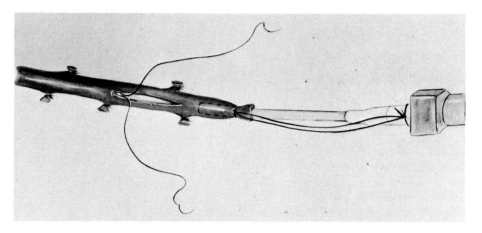

FIG. 6.   Illustration of initial mattress suture of #7-0 polypropylene in opened internal mammary artery.

tinued for one-half of the length of the arteriotomy on the side adjacent to the surgeon (Fig. 7). Slight tension on the suture opens the anastomosis with the other end of the mattress suture, the opposite side is then sewn. Epicardium is included if convenient, but large bites are not taken. As the distal end is approached, the excess internal mammary artery is trimmed off. The suture is continued in a running fashion, or, at times, one or more interrupted sutures are placed at the distal end and tied. The anastomosis is completed by a continuous suture from the distal end back to the middle of the arteriotomy incision. Prior to tying this suture to the first suture, the coronary and internal mammary arteries are checked for patency with small, calibrated probes under direct vision (Fig. 8). Air is evacuated by releasing the soft clamp from the

internal mammary artery and the aortic or soft clamps on the coronary arteries. At times, hemostasis can be obtained by an internal shunt of a small #5 pediatric feeding tube within the coronary artery, these procedures being dictated by individual requirements. The adventitia of the internal mammary artery is tacked to the epicardium of the heart approximately 2 cm from the anastomosis to insure against excessive tension on the anastomosis. This is essential to preservation of the graft (Fig. 9). The graft is inspected as it courses over the edge of the pericardium. If there is tension at this point, a V-shaped opening is made in the pericardium to permit a convenient lie of the internal mammary graft. The coronary arteries that may be bypassed with this technique have been the left anterior descending coronary

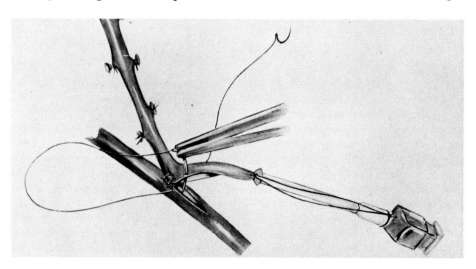

FIG. 7.   Running fine monofilament suture begun along anastomosis of internal mammary to coronary artery.

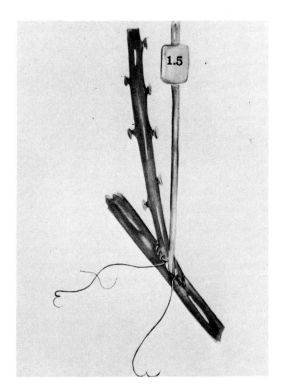

FIG. 8. Near completion of anastomosis of internal mammary to coronary artery with probe-patent coronary lumen.

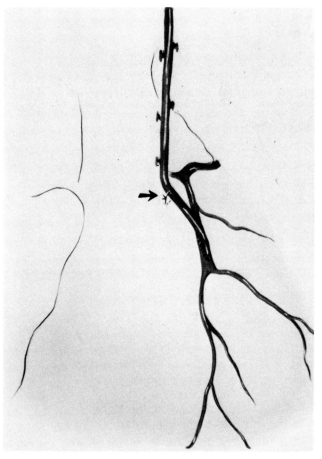

FIG. 9. Completed anastomosis with tacking suture from adventitia of internal mammary artery to epicardium.

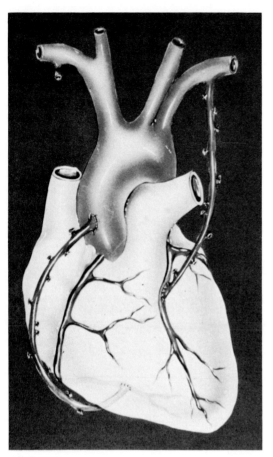

ternal mammary arteries as well as saphenous vein aortocoronary bypass grafts (Fig. 11).

RESULTS

The results of this technique are illustrated in the following series of 184 consecutive cases of internal mammary artery coronary artery bypass grafts performed at the Ochsner Clinic and followed up to 21 months (Mills and Ochsner, 1973). Two hospital deaths occurred among 184 consecutive cases of internal mammary coronary bypass graft, for a hospital mortality of 1.1 percent. One resulted from status asthmaticus and the second from recurrent ventricular arrhythmias. No late deaths occurred during a follow-up period of four to 21 months. No infections were encountered in this series. In five incidences (2.5 percent) the internal mammary artery was found to be too small. Flows measured routinely after cardiopul-

FIG. 10. Illustration of pedicled left internal mammary artery to anterior descending coronary and free graft of right internal mammary to posterior descending coronary artery.

artery, the diagonal branch of the left coronary artery, and the main right coronary artery. The intact internal mammary artery attached to the subclavian artery is restricted by its length to these arteries on the anterior surface of the heart. However, as described by Loop (Loop, 1973a), a free internal mammary artery graft may be fashioned by transecting the parent vessel from the subclavian artery and anastomosing the proximal end to the root of the aorta (Fig. 10). Good length is then obtained with this free graft so that it may be anastomosed to any coronary artery. The proximal anastomosis, however, has been found to be difficult if there is a thick or calcific aorta. This procedure should be considered in patients who do not have adequate veins for grafting or if the internal mammary artery is injured during preparation and sufficient length is not obtained by leaving it attached to the subclavian artery. Several combination grafts are possible using one or both in-

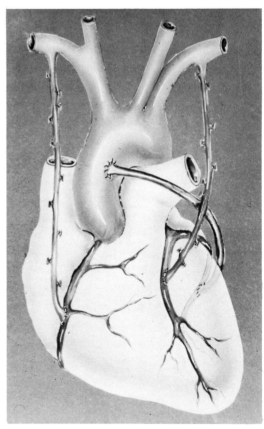

FIG. 11. Diagram of combination mammary and saphenous vein grafting procedure of internal mammary artery to right and left anterior descending and saphenous vein from aorta to circumflex coronary artery.

monary bypass ranged from 45 to 225 ml/min, with a mean of 90 ml/min. Forty-two patients with single or double internal mammary grafts have been submitted to recatheterization at our request from two weeks to one year postoperatively. Only three patients were symptomatic, and we have found some difficulty in acceptance of repeat angiography by asymptomatic patients. No occlusions were demonstrated. Two patients with recurrent angina were found to have distal stenosis of the internal mammary graft. Two were felt to be a narrowing due to technical problems, and a third developed angina, which coincided with resumption of heavy cigarette smoking at three months postoperatively. Repeat catheterization revealed a widely patent functioning graft, and the angina subsided after discontinuation of the use of nicotine. An asymptomatic patient did suffer a catheter-induced dissection of the proximal internal mammary artery graft (Mills and Ochsner, 1973).

DISCUSSION

The advantages of the internal mammary coronary artery graft for myocardial revascularization are as follows:

1. Higher patency rate.
2. Artery-to-artery anastomosis.
3. Comparable size of vessels.
4. Enlargement of the internal mammary artery occurring over months to years with increased demand on it as other arteries in the body have been documented to do when demands on them have been increased.
5. A single anastomosis versus two anastomoses with a vein graft.
6. No leg wound problems.
7. No transfer of graft from one part of the body to another, lessening the chance of infection.

The disadvantages are as follows:

1. Definitely a more tedious dissection to obtain the graft.
2. A more friable vessel.
3. Only two grafts available when multiple grafts are necessary.
4. The length is inadequate for the posterior descending coronary artery anastomoses with the intact internal mammary artery.

The reasons for which we feel the internal mammary artery should sometimes not be used as a coronary artery bypass graft are as follows:

1. Subclavian stenosis or atheromatous disease within the internal mammary artery (we have found atheromatous disease in internal mammary artery very rare, even with severe generalized atherosclerosis in the patient).
2. Inadequate size of the internal mammary artery, less than 2 mm in diameter. We have found that with the above-described method of dilatation of the internal mammary artery, there have been less than 2.5 percent in which the internal mammary artery is not of sufficient size for grafting.
3. The flow into a graduated cylinder is less than 75 cc/min.

With these reservations, the internal mammary artery pedicle graft can supply the heart with as much blood as it will accept. We feel that the internal mammary artery can expand through the years with the demand made upon it by an ischemic myocardium. This conclusion is due to preliminary study on the patent Vineberg procedures eight and nine years postoperatively and with studies on the size of the internal mammary artery used in direct coronary anastomosis, one to two years postoperatively. The flow measurements obtained at the operating table and the flow velocity methods used today have many variables that lead to a wide standard deviation (Furuse, Klopp, et al, 1972). The efficacy of the internal mammary coronary anastomosis will only be borne out through its clinical results. The failures of these grafts are usually due to technical reasons. No intimal hyperplasia has been documented. The preparation of the graft is extremely important in that handling of each branch is almost as essential as the handling of the anastomosis itself. The use of precise microvascular principles will eliminate these problems.

At this phase in the evolution of the coronary bypass operation, the internal mammary artery should be the choice of autogenous graft material utilized in myocardial revascularization whenever possible.

References

Absolon KA, Aust JB, Varco RL, Lillehei CW: Surgical treatment of occlusive coronary artery disease by endarterectomy or anastomotic replacement. Surg Gynecol Obstet 103:180, 1956

Bailey CP, Hirose T: Successful internal mammary-coronary arterial anastomosis using a "minivascular" suturing technique. Int Surg 49:416, 1968

Bailey CP: Discussion of loop. Presented at Meeting of Society of Thoracic Surgeons, Los Angeles, January 1974

Bourassa M, Lesperance J, Campeau L, Simard P: Factors influencing patency of aorto-coronary vein grafts. Circulation 45-46:1–79, 1972

Castroviejo R: Improved needle holders. Trans Am Acad Ophthalmol Otolaryngol 56:929, 1952

Edwards WS, Lewis CE, Blakely WR, Napolitano L: Coronary artery bypass with internal mammary and splenic artery grafts. Ann Thorac Surg vol 15, no 1, January 1973

Favaloro RG, Effler DB, Groves LK, Fergusson DJ, Loazada JS: Double internal mammary artery myocardial implantation: clinical evaluation of results in 150 patients. Circulation 37:549, 1968

Favaloro RG: Unilateral self-retaining retractor for use ics of aorta-to-coronary artery bypass. Ann Thorac Cardiovasc Surg 53:864, 1967

Furuse A, Klopp EH, Browley RK, Gott VL: Hemodynamics of aorta-to-coronary artery bypass. Ann Thorac Surg 14:282, 1972

Goetz RH, Rohman M, Haller JD, Dee R, Rosenak SS: Internal mammary-coronary artery anastomosis: a nonsuture method employing tantalum rings. J Thorac Cardiovasc Surg 41:378, 1961

Green GE, Stertzer SH, Reppert EH: Coronary arterial bypass grafts. Ann Thorac Surg 5:443, 1968

Green GE: Internal mammary artery-to-coronary artery anastomosis. Ann Thorac Surg 14:260, 1972

Green GE: Rate of blood flow from the internal mammary artery. Surgery 70:809, 1971

Jacobson JH II: Microsurgery. Curr Probl Surg, February 1971

Julian OC, Lopez-Belio M, Moorehead D, Lima A: Direct surgical procedures on the coronary arteries: experimental studies. J Thorac Cardiovasc Surg 34:654, 1957

Kolessov VI: Mammary artery-coronary artery anastomosis as method of treatment for angina pectoris. J Thorac Cardiovasc Surg 54:535, 1967

Loop FD, Effler DB, Spampinato N, Groves LK, Cheanvechai C: Myocardial revascularization by internal mammary artery grafts. J. Thorac Cardiovasc Surg 63:674, 1971

Loop FD: The free internal mammary artery bypass graft. Ann Thorac Surg, vol 15, January 1973a

Loop FD: Internal mammary artery grafts without optical assistance. Circulation 48, July 1973b

Mills NL, Ochsner JL: Technique of internal mammary-coronary artery bypass. Presented at the Twentieth Annual Meeting of the Southern Thoracic Surgical Association, Louisville, Ky, Nov 1–3, 1973. Ann Thorac Surg 17:237, 1974

Spencer FC: Binocular loupes (microtelescopes) for coronary artery surgery. J Thorac Cardiovasc Surg 63:163, 1971

Vineberg AM: Development of an anastomosis between the coronary vessels and transplanted internal mammary artery. Can Med J 55:117, 1946

Vineberg AM, Walker J: The surgical treatment of coronary artery heart disease by internal mammary artery implantation. Diseases of the Chest 45:190, 1964

Walker JA, Friedberg HD, Flemma RJ, Johnson WD: Determinants of angiographic patency of aorto-coronary vein bypass grafts. Circulation 45:86, 1972

63

RIGHT INTERNAL MAMMARY ARTERY FOR CORONARY BYPASS

Hendrick B. Barner

INTRODUCTION

Saphenous vein is commonly utilized for coronary reconstruction, but it has a significant closure rate, whereas the internal mammary artery (IMA) has a minimal early and late failure rate (Green, 1972). The left IMA is suitable for reconstruction of the left anterior descending (LAD) and circumflex coronary arteries (CCA). The right coronary artery (RCA) and LAD can be bypassed with the right IMA. Because use of the right IMA has not been emphasized, this experience is reported.

CLINICAL MATERIAL

During the interval from August 1, 1972 to November 30, 1973, 80 patients (Table 1) have had coronary reconstruction with the right IMA. Angina pectoris was the indication for operation in all patients. Angina was considered to be unstable in eight patients. A ventricular aneurysm was resected in one instance, and the aortic valve was replaced in another. One or more myocardial infarctions had occurred in 32 patients.

TABLE 1. Age and Sex Distribution

AGE (years)	MALE	FEMALE	TOTAL
30–40	7	1	8
41–50	31	2	33
51–60	23	10	33
61–70	5	1	6

Supported in Part by U.S. Public Health Service Grant HL-06312.

Single coronary bypass was required in four patients, double in 48, triple in 25, and quadruple in three. The left IMA was used 75 times, and saphenous vein was used 32 times, for a total of 187 grafts or 2.3 grafts per patient.

METHODS

All patients had coronary cineangiography and left ventricular angiography preoperatively. Stenosis of 75 percent or greater was considered to be significant. Arteries with lesser degrees of obstruction were occasionally bypassed when operation was indicated for a significant lesion in another vessel.

The IMA was mobilized as a pedicle graft from the first to the fourth or fifth intercostal space, using hemostatic clips to control branches. Great care was taken to avoid touching the IMA with forceps because intimal fracture had been recognized on three occasions when forceps were inadvertently placed across the IMA. The IMA was sized with probes of 1.5, 2.0, or 2.5 mm prior to making the anastomosis, and free flow was measured for a 20-second interval. The anastomosis entailed a 5 to 8 mm coronary arteriotomy, sizing of the coronary, spatulation of the graft, and two running sutures of 7-0 Dacron. Operating loupes of 2.5x were used. It was necessary to use the right IMA as a free graft in 13 instances in which it would not reach the anastomotic site (Barner, 1973a). Saphenous vein grafts were anastomosed to the ascending aorta, and the coronary anastomosis was made with the same technique as for IMA grafts. Mechanical endarterectomy of the distal RCA was necessary 10 times.

The operating procedure involved a disposable bubble oxygenator, moderate hemodilution,

TABLE 2. Graft Patency at Postoperative Catheterization

	RCA		LAD		DIAGONAL		CCA		TOTAL	
	Patent	No	Patent	No	Patent	No	Patent	No	Patent	No
RIMA	55	57	8	8	5	5	–	–	68	70
LIMA	–	–	53	56	1	2	7	7	61	65
VEIN	–	–	–	–	1	1	15	17	16	18

hypothermia of 29.5 C, electrically induced cardiac fibrillation, and intermittent aortic cross-clamping (not in excess of 40 minutes). Protection of the myocardium during cross-clamping was accomplished by the use of crushed ice made from lactated Ringer's solution.

After discontinuation of cardiopulmonary bypass, and when the patient was hemodynamically stable, the graft flow was measured with an electromagnetic flow probe. Mean arterial pressure was measured electronically with a strain gauge and 16-gauge radial artery cannula. Resistance (mmHg/ml/min) of the IMA to free flow and coronary resistance to anastomotic flow were calculated as the quotient of mean arterial pressure (mmHg) and flow (ml/min).

RESULTS

Six hospital deaths (7.5 percent) occurred in males having two (one patient), three (four patients), or four (one patient) grafts. Two deaths in the operating room were due to ventricular irritability; the others occurred two to five days after operation due to respiratory insufficiency (one), left ventricular failure (two), and arrhythmia (one).

There were two late deaths, one due to renal failure at three months and one at eight months, probably on a cardiac basis. One female patient had recurrence of angina despite patent grafts noted at the one-year postoperative catheterization.

There were three instances of mediastinal infection requiring sternal debridement. All patients healed their wounds, and two had patent grafts, but one died of renal failure (late death).

Postoperative catheterization demonstrated patency of 68/70 (97 percent) right IMA grafts, 61/65 (94 percent) left IMA grafts, and 16/18 (89 percent) vein grafts (Table 2). One-year catheterization revealed patency of 16/16 right IMA grafts, 14/14 left IMA grafts, and 3/3 vein grafts.

Free graft flow and graft resistance were not different for right and left IMA grafts (Fig. 1).

Resistance of the IMA correlated well with internal diameter (Fig. 2).

Anastomotic flow and resistance were not different for the right IMA-RCA and for the left IMA-LAD (Fig. 3). However, when the right IMA-LAD (11 grafts) was compared with the left IMA-LAD (59 grafts), there was a significant difference in flow (34 ± 5 ml/min versus 58 ± 4 ml/min, $p < 0.001$) and resistance (2.65 ± 0.33 mmHg/ml/min versus 1.81 ± 0.16 mmHg/ml/min, $p < 0.05$), as shown in Figure 4.

When internal diameter of the IMA was compared with coronary internal diameter, it was found that 35 percent of the right IMAs and 12 percent of the left IMAs were smaller than the coronary to which they were anastomosed (Table 3).

TABLE 3. Relationship between IMA and Coronary Internal Diameter[a]

	RIMA	LIMA
IMA = coronary	34	44
IMA > coronary[b]	17	20
IMA < coronary[b]	27	9

[a] *As measured with probes in 0.5 mm gradations.*
[b] *Difference in size was never more than 0.5 mm.*

DISCUSSION

Available data indicate a one-year patency of 95 percent when the left IMA is utilized for LAD reconstruction (Barner, 1974; Green, 1972; Kay et al, 1974; Singh et al, 1973). This contrasts with a one-year patency of 70 to 80 percent for saphenous vein (Anderson et al, 1971; Cooley et al, 1973; Flemma et al, 1972; Grondin et al, 1972; Kaiser et al, 1972). The demonstrated usefulness of the left IMA led to use of the right IMA for coronary reconstruction.

It was apparent that right and left IMA size, and therefore resistance to flow, were not different (Fig. 1). Similarly, when coronary flow and resistance for the RCA and LAD were compared,

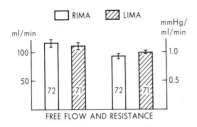

FIG. 1. Mean free flow ($\pm$ 1SEM) (left ordinate) and mean graft resistance ($\pm$ 1SEM) (right ordinate) are shown for right IMA (open bars) and left IMA (shaded bars). The number of grafts is indicated in each bar.

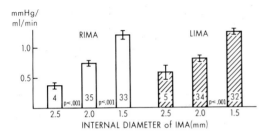

FIG. 2. Mean resistance ($\pm$ 1SEM) of right IMA grafts (open bars) and left IMA grafts (shaded bars) is related to graft diameter shown beneath each bar. The number of grafts is indicated in each bar and significant p values are shown.

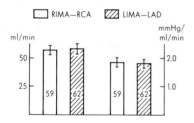

FIG. 3. Mean anastomotic flow ($\pm$ 1SEM) (left ordinate) and mean anastomotic resistance ($\pm$ 1SEM) (right ordinate) are shown for right IMA–RCA grafts (open bars) and left IMA–LAD grafts (shaded bars). The number of grafts is indicated in the bars.

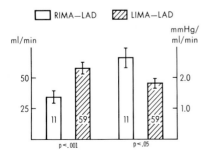

FIG. 4. Mean anastomotic flow ($\pm$ 1SEM) (left ordinate) and mean anastomotic resistance ($\pm$ 1SEM) (right ordinate) are shown for right IMA–LAD grafts (open bars) and left IMA–LAD grafts (shaded bars). The number of grafts is indicated in each bar and significant p values are shown.

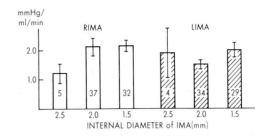

FIG. 5. Mean anastomotic resistance ($\pm$ 1SEM) for right IMA grafts (open bars) and left IMA grafts (shaded bars) is related to graft diameter shown beneath each bar. The number of grafts is indicated in each bar and significant p values are shown.

there was no difference between the right and left IMA (Fig. 3). When the right IMA was utilized for LAD reconstruction, there was greater resistance to anastomotic flow than for the left IMA (Fig. 4). This difference may reflect the small number of right IMA-LAD grafts (11), but probably also reflects the greater length of the right IMA that is necessary to reach the LAD, in contrast to the relatively short length of the left IMA. Comparison of the right and left IMA for diagonal artery reconstruction yielded no statistically significant difference for anastomotic flow and resistance, but the number of grafts was small. Thus, on a hemodynamic basis the right IMA was as adequate for RCA bypass as was the left IMA for LAD bypass.

Although the right IMA was smaller than the coronary to which it was anastomosed 35 percent (Table 3) of the time, this was not reflected in the hemodynamic data and, therefore, may be of no significance. This contention is supported by Figure 5, in which anastomotic resistance is related to graft diameter. There is no statistical difference within the right IMA grafts. This indicates that coronary resistance, *not* IMA resistance, is dominant under basal conditions. This was also true for the left IMA grafts; and although the 2.0 mm grafts appeared to have lower anastomotic resistance, this is not statistically significant (p. > 0.05). Thus, IMA resistance does not appear to be significant under conditions of basal flow, but during coronary vasodilation, the IMA imposes significant resistance to flow (Barner, 1973b).

Perhaps the greatest drawback to use of the right IMA is the anatomic fact that it frequently will not reach beyond the acute margin, although in some individuals it will reach the origin of the posterior descending artery. Therefore, it may not be possible to bypass all disease in the RCA, or, if it is to be bypassed, a free graft will be necessary (Barner, 1973a). At present the experience with free IMA grafts has been satisfactory, with patency of all grafts that have been studied early (10/10) and at one year (3/3). However, the IMA-aortic anastomosis is tedious.

Other considerations in IMA-coronary bypass are longer operating time, longer pump time, and longer aortic cross-clamping time, which are, perhaps, reflected in a greater hospital mortality and a greater incidence (4 percent versus 1 percent) of mediastinal wound infection. If these trends should prove to be real, they should dictate selective use of the IMA. Up till the present, the IMA has been used in all patients without selection. Furthermore, every IMA that was mobilized was utilized, except one that had a diminished flow due to atherosclerosis, and three with recognized iatrogenic intimal fractures (Barner, 1974).

SUMMARY

Coronary bypass with right IMA in 80 patients having 75 left IMA grafts and 32 vein grafts resulted in a 6 percent hospital mortality and two late deaths. Comparison postoperatively and at one year of graft patency, graft internal diameter, graft flow and resistance, and anastomotic flow and resistance revealed no significant difference between the right and left IMA. The right IMA was less suitable for reconstruction of the RCA than was the left IMA for the LAD because of the greater length of graft needed. Use of the right IMA as a free graft may be necessary to bypass all disease.

References

Anderson RP, Hodam R, Wood J, Starr A: Direct revascularization of the heart. J Thorac Cardiovasc Surg 63:353, 1971

Barner HB: The internal mammary artery as a free graft. J Thorac Cardiovasc Surg 66:219, 1973a

Barner HB: Blood flow in the internal mammary artery. Amer Heart J 86:570, 1973b

Barner HB: The value of internal mammary artery bypass. In Vogel JHK (ed): Integrated Medical-Surgical Care in Acute Coronary Artery Disease. Basel, S. Karger, 1975 (in press)

Cooley DA, Dawson JT, Hallman GL, et al: Aortocoronary saphenous vein bypass. Ann Thorac Surg 16: 380, 1973

Flemma RJ, Johnson WD, Lepley D, et al: Late results of saphenous vein bypass grafting for myocardial revascularization. Ann Thorac Surg 14:232, 1972

Green GE: Internal mammary artery–coronary artery anastomosis: Three year experience with 165 patients. Ann Thorac Surg 14:260, 1972

Grondin CM, Castonguay YR, Lesperance J, et al: Attrition rate of aorta to coronary artery saphenous vein grafts after one year. Ann Thorac Surg 14:223, 1972

Kaiser GC, Barner HB, Willman VL, et al: Aortocoronary bypass grafting. Arch Surg 105:319, 1972

Kay EB, Naraghipour H, Beg RA, et al: Internal mammary artery bypass graft—long-term patency rate and follow-up. Ann Thorac Surg 18:269, 1974

Singh H, Flemma RJ, Tector AJ, Lepley D and Walker JA: Direct myocardial revascularization. Arch Surg 107:699, 1973

64

PHYSIOLOGIC LIMITATIONS OF INTERNAL MAMMARY ARTERY AS CORONARY BYPASS

Harjeet Singh, Robert J. Flemma,
Alfred J. Tector, and Derward Lepley

INTRODUCTION

Advocated by Green in 1970,[3] internal mammary artery coronary artery anastomosis has quickly found favor in the revascularization procedures of the myocardium because

1. it requires only one distal anastomosis;
2. it is an arterial channel that frequently matches the coronary artery in size, and it is allegedly better able to withstand hemodynamic stress than a vein graft; and
3. the long-range patency rate is higher compared to vein grafts.[1,3,9]

Notwithstanding such obvious advantages, which led Edwards et al[2] to advocate use of splenic artery grafts, it is pertinent to establish that the internal mammary artery provides for adequate flow and that myocardial function is preserved. Certain physiologic questions arise with the use of the internal mammary as a bypass conduit.

1. Can patency be equated with adequacy of flow?
2. Can a peripheral arterial vessel meet the peculiar requirements of the myocardium and its predominantly diastolic flow?

CLINICAL MATERIAL

Pertinent observations were derived from evaluation of 52 patients who underwent left internal mammary artery-coronary (LIM) bypass. Forty-seven of 252 IMA-coronary bypasses performed were restudied at periods ranging from three weeks to two years postoperatively (mean 5.6 months). Five other patients whose IMA-coronary bypass appeared to yield insufficient flow leading to severe postoperative complications are also included in this study.

Clinical Observations Related to Adequacy of LIM Blood Flow (Table 1)

COMPARISON OF VEIN GRAFT AND LEFT INTERNAL MAMMARY ARTERY FLOW. Post-bypass flow has been measured in thousands of vein grafts and has been found to average 65 ml/min.[8] Flows in 94 LIM-LAD bypasses were significantly lower at 45 ml/min.[4] Of additional significance is the higher range of flow in the vein graft when compared to the LIM. Also of theoretical importance is the fact that a 3 to 4 mm vein graft when attached to the ascending aorta has an average maximal unimpeded flow of 800 to 1,400 ml/min while the usual 2 to 2.5 mm mammary artery has a maximal unimpeded flow of 60 to 150 ml/min.

TABLE 1. Comparison of Bypass Flow

	NO. GRAFTS	MEAN FLOW
Vein	400	64 ml/min (10–220)
Mammary	94	44 ml/min (10–70)

OBSERVATIONS RELATED TO A STUDY OF COMPARATIVE FLOWS IN PATIENTS WITH AN ELEVATED LEFT VENTRICULAR END DIASTOLIC PRESSURE (LVEDP). The left internal mammary to left

557

anterior descending flow (LIM-LAD) in 22 patients with an elevated LVEDP actually dropped from the mean value of 45 to a mean of 35 ml/min, while 32 vein grafts in this group maintained a mean of 66 ml/min despite the increase in elevated EDP (Table 2).

Of less accuracy, but perhaps of more clinical significance is the operating room experience with three patients who had undergone LIM-LAD anastomoses. Following discontinuance of bypass, they developed akinesia of the anterior myocardium, hypotension, and arrhythmias. In these three patients bypass was reinstituted and saphenous vein bypass grafts were placed to the LAD coronary artery. The LIM-LAD anastomoses were all inspected, probed, and found to have no technical aberrations explaining the difficulties. In one patient the LIM bypass flow had been measured at 35 ml/min prior to the hypotension and dyskinesia of the anterior myocardium. When the vein graft was established as the bypass to the LAD, the flow in this vessel was measured after successful bypass at 120 ml/min. The inference that the lower LIM flow was inadequate is difficult to avoid in this and in the other two patients in which the additional saphenous vein grafts led to successful retrieval of deteriorating situations.

In contrast to these successful procedures, there were two patients who expired early in our series and were found to have thrombi in the LAD coronary arteries distal to patent LIM-LAD anastomoses. Autopsy revealed massive anteroseptal infarctions, and in both cases, collateral circulation from the other coronary arteries had been jeopardized seriously. In one, the right coronary artery was so diffusely diseased that it was not bypassed, and in the other there was an 80 percent stenosis of the circumflex coronary vein bypass graft, making the only available circumflex coronary blood supply inadequate to supply the anterior descending in a retrograde manner. Our suspicion that vein bypasses to other vessels acted to compensate for the inadequacy of mammary flows, was verified when we examined postoperative ventricular function in eight patients in this group with combined LIM-LAD anastomoses and additional vein bypass grafts. This study correlated mammary flow as well as postoperative left ventricular angiography. In the eight patients with normal preoperative ventricular contraction, LIM-LAD bypass, and other bypass grafts, the postoperative ventriculogram in two revealed significant anterior wall deterioration dysfunction despite the patent LIM bypass. The interesting point is that the associated vein grafts had closed, and, despite a patent LIM, the myocardial distribution supplied by the LIM had de-

TABLE 2. Bypass Flow in Twenty Patients with Raised LVEDP

PROCEDURE	NO.	MEAN FLOW (ml/min)
LIM-LAD	22	35.5 ± 12
Aorto to cor. VG	32	66.0 ± 13

teriorated. Also of interest in this group of eight patients was the fact that in two patients the LIM had either an 80 percent anastomotic stenosis or closure, but the vein bypass graft had excellent flow and patency. However, there was no deterioration of the area supplied by the occluded LIM anastomosis. The vein grafts had compensated with two collaterals with excellent flow, preventing deterioration of the LAD myocardial distribution.

DISCUSSION

These observations provide data to suggest that LIM coronary bypass has less flow than a vein graft. This low flow in the IMA has been observed by others.[6] The high patency of LIM must be considered and then one must try to balance these drawbacks of both bypass vessels. It is felt that when the "high-flow" situation is anticipated, the vein graft will provide more adequate revascularization. In support of this is the fact that the vein graft patency in bypasses with flows measured over 70 ml/min, there is a late patency of 90 percent. Thus, higher vein graft flow is associated with higher patency as well as adequacy. Also, the presence of an increased LVEDP would mitigate against the use of the mammary as a bypass conduit and suggests use of a vein, since the pressure gradient is decreased and thus there is a decrease in flow. In the anticipated "low-flow" situation, the mammary offers both patency and adequacy of flow and is recommended as the bypass conduit of choice. To optimize our use of bypass alternatives, these views plead the next question as to the preoperative determination of high-flow vs low-flow situations. From our previous experience with flows, we have noted that the site of the LAD obstruction and the distal ventricular contractility provide key determinants of the flow measured at operation. Kaplitt[5] has suggested a more quantitative classification based on the size of the vessel, location of the obstruction, condition of the distal vessel and myocardium, or the SLD classification, which, when used preoperatively and at operation, correlates well with flow. This quantitation may be used effectively in conjunction with our experience to plan more effectively the bypass conduits that offer both adequacy and patency, thus optimizing the results of myocardial revascularization.

The mechanism of low flow in the IMA has been attributed to shorter diastolic filling time.[10] It would also depend on the temporal relationship of the phasic flow in the IMA to the pressure sequences in the ventricles. As most of the perfusion of the myocardium occurs during diastole, lower diastolic flow in the internal mammary artery, particularly during tachycardia with attendant decreases in diastolic filling time, conceivably could leave a large mass of myocardium underperfused. We reported previously a consistent finding that under optimal flow conditions, the LAD coronary had greater flow than the similar right coronary artery when vein grafts were used. The finding was later confirmed by the study of Moran et al.[7] Here we report consistently small flows in the IMA-LAD anastomosis under the most optimal conditions, leading to fatal results in two patients and near catastrophe in three at the time of surgery. There would be nothing wrong in the rationale or application of IMA for direct revascularization if it is realized that flow in it is dependent on its length, cross-sectional area, and the diastolic flow it provides to the myocardium; and that it needs to be tempered to a small mass of myocardium, which can then be effectively revascularized.

SUMMARY

Four sets of clinical data and observations have been presented that suggest that although the LIM as a coronary bypass delivers superb patency rates, these may not be *a priori* equated with adequacy of flow; and in certain situations, it may be grossly inadequate to the point of detriment. A method for detecting the situations in which the LIM may be inadequate is suggested; this may enable the surgeon to select judiciously the most efficacious bypass vessel and optimize the results of myocardial revascularization with the criteria of both patency and adequacy.

References

1. Edwards WS, Blakeley WR, Lewis CE: Technique of coronary bypass with autogenous arteries. J Thorac Cardiovasc Surg 65:2, 272, 1973
2. Edwards WS, Lewis CE, Blakeley WR, Napolitano L: Coronary artery bypass with internal mammary and splenic grafts. Ann Thorac Surg 35:15, 1, 1973
3. Green GE, Stertzer SA, Gordon RB, Tice DA: Anastomosis of internal mammary artery to distal left anterior descending coronary artery. Circulation (Supp II)41:79, 1970
4. Johnson WD, Flemma RJ, Lepley D: Determinants of blood flow in aorto-coronorary saphenous vein bypass grafts. Arch Surg 101:6, 806, 1970
5. Kaplitt MJ, Frantz SL, Beil AR: Analysis of intra-operative coronary angiography in aorto-coronary bypass grafts. Presented at American Heart Association, Atlantic City, NJ, 1973
6. Loop FD, Spampinato N, Cheanvechai C, Effler DB: The free internal mammary artery bypass graft. Use of the IMA in the aorto-to-coronary artery position. Ann Thorac Surg 15:1, 50, 1973
7. Moran JM, Chen PY, Rheinlander HF: Coronary hemodynamics following aorto-coronary bypass graft. Arch Surg 539:103–5, 1971
8. Singh H, Flemma RJ, Tector AJ, Lepley D, Walker JA: Determinants in the choice of vein graft or internal mammary artery in direct myocardial revascularization. Arch Surg 107:5, 1973
9. Spencer FG, Green GE, Tice DA, Glassman EC: Bypass grafting for disease of coronary arteries. Ann Surg 173:6, 1971
10. Wakabayashi A, Beron E, Lov MA, Mino JY, DaCosta IA, Connolly JE: Physiological basis for the systemic to coronary artery bypass graft. Arch Surg 100:1, 17, 1970

65

COMPARISON OF NORMOTHERMIC AND HYPOTHERMIC ANOXIC CARDIAC ARREST IN AORTOCORONARY ARTERY BYPASS

George J. Reul, Jr., Joseph Meyer, Frank M. Sandiford, Don C. Wukasch, John C. Norman, and Denton A. Cooley

INTRODUCTION

Anoxic cardiac arrest is necessary for the adequate performance of certain cardiac operations. In particular, it has been useful in coronary artery surgery because of the dry, immobile operative field it creates, which is necessary for an accurate anastomosis. To avoid anoxic injury in an already ischemic myocardium, alternate techniques have been designed. There are surgeons who prefer the "safety" of the beating heart with or without cardiopulmonary bypass. Unfortunately with this technique not only is the quality of the anastomosis jeopardized but the ischemic heart, with one of its major coronary arteries isolated and occluded, must maintain cardiac output. Others prefer induced ventricular fibrillation by electrical or hypothermic techniques.[2-6] During ventricular fibrillation, the myocardium is perfused and accurate anastomosis may be accomplished. However, oxygen utilization may be increased;[7] myocardial perfusion may be poorly distributed, especially in the hypertrophied myocardium;[8] ultrastructural damage may occur;[9] and the coronary artery must be occluded without injury.

Hypothermia has been used to protect the myocardium during anoxic cardiac arrest.[10-15] Myocardial ultrastructure, short-term and long-term myocardial function, and myocardial metabolism are favorably affected by the use of hypothermia. We have utilized normothermic anoxic arrest for aortocoronary artery bypass.[16-19] This report compares results of aortocoronary artery bypass under normothermic anoxic arrest to results obtained under hypothermic anoxic arrest.

CLINICAL MATERIAL

The study consisted of the retrospective analysis of 659 patients who underwent aortocoronary artery bypass grafts (ACB) over two separate time periods. The first group of patients (Group I) underwent coronary artery bypass grafts through December 1970 under normothermic conditions prior to our use of hypothermia. Results in that study have been reported previously.[1] The operative procedure was similar in 200 patients who comprised the second group (Group II). These patients underwent ACB with aortic occlusion under hypothermic conditions. The 200 patients in Group II were a consecutive series of patients operated upon in 1973. Ancillary procedures such as ventricular aneurysm resection or valve replacement were excluded so that only isolated ACB grafts were analyzed. Most patients in both groups had both the distal and proximal anastomoses placed during one aortic occlusion. For some patients, the aortic occlusion time represented the total anoxic arrest time for individual aortic occlusions.

The preoperative symptoms were similar in both groups (Table 1). In most patients the primary indications for ACB were the presence of either angina alone or angina plus myocardial infarction. Preoperative congestive heart failure was present in 21 percent of the normothermic and 20 percent of the hypothermic group, and previous myocardial infarction was present equally in both groups. Elevated left ventricular end-diastolic pressure was present in more patients in Group II. New York Heart Association Func-

TABLE 1. Preoperative Characteristics

	NORMO-THERMIC (percent)	HYPO-THERMIC (percent)
Angina alone	34	35
Angina + myocardial infarct	38	39
Angina + CHF + MI	15	17
Myocardial infarct	3	6
Angina + CHF	6	3
CHF alone	4	–
Congestive heart failure	21	20
Previous MI	56	62
Elevated LVEDP	40	53
NYHA Functional Class		
I	3	1.5
II	26	12.5
III	49	59.5
IV	22	26.5
Number of patients	454	200

tional Classification (Table 1) was relatively the same in both groups, most patients being in Functional Class III and IV. Both groups of patients were similar in respect to preoperative symptoms, functional classification, presence of previous myocardial infarction, and congestive heart failure.

On the other hand, the groups were not alike when the number of arteries bypassed were analyzed. The patients in Group II had more major arteries involved per patient. They also had more grafts done per diseased artery. Thus, more complete operations were done in Group II (Table 2). Seventy-five percent encroachment upon the lumen of a major coronary artery was considered to be a significant lesion. In Group II, 68 percent of the patients had significant obstruction of three major coronary arteries as compared to 47 percent in Group I. Single-vessel disease was present in 17 percent in Group I and only 3 percent in Group II. Furthermore, 55 percent of Group I received

TABLE 2. Arterial Disease and Grafts

	NORMO-THERMIC (percent)	HYPO-THERMIC (percent)
Arteries obstructed		
One	16.9	3
Two	30.6	21
Three	46.7	67.5
Four	5.8	8.5
Number of grafts		
One	55	6.5
Two	43	35
Three	2	52.5
Four	–	6

only one ACB graft while 6.5 percent of the patients in Group II received only one graft. Three or more bypass grafts were done in 58.5 percent of the patients in Group II and in only 2 percent of the patients in Group I. This reflected a further awareness of the importance of the completeness of the operation with increasing experience.

OPERATIVE TECHNIQUE

The operative technique utilized has been previously reported.[16-19] All patients had aortocoronary artery bypass grafts using a reversed saphenous vein. During simultaneous preparation of the vein, the patient was placed on total cardiopulmonary bypass with aortic cannulation for arterial return. Noncolloid glucose with lactated Ringer's prime was used in all patients. Flow rates from 40 to 55 ml/kg/Hg were maintained. A left atrial or left ventricular vent was used. Anoxic arrest was accomplished by aortic occlusion. In most instances, both the distal and the proximal anastomoses were accomplished during a single aortic occlusion. A separate aortotomy was made for each individual vein graft. The distal anastomosis was accomplished with continuous 6-0 polypropylene.* Standard intraoperative and postoperative care was given, including the use of vasopressors (epinephrine, isoproterenol, norepinephrine) or intraortic balloon counterpulsation to support low cardiac output. In Group II, the heat exchanger varied according to the oxygenator used. For general hypothermia, an esophageal temperature of 30 C was obtained. The rate of cooling ranged from .22 to 1.4 C/min with a mean of approximately 0.55 C/min. As soon as the aorta was cross-clamped, rewarming was begun at a rate of 4.3 to 14.6 minutes per degree centigrade, or a mean of approximately 8 min for each degree centrigrade of rewarming.[20] Topical hypothermia was accomplished by irrigating the heart just prior to aortic occlusion with one liter of normal saline solution cooled to approximately 12 C. This solution was removed after initial instillation, and no more solution was added during the procedure. An average intramyocardial temperature of approximately 26 C resulted.

METHODS

Both patient groups were analyzed with respect to immediate or operating-room death, 30-

* Prolene, Ethicon Laboratories, Sommerville, N.J.

day mortality, and complication rate. Electrocardiograms were obtained immediately after surgery and up to seven days postoperatively. These were analyzed for the appearance of new Q-waves and ischemic changes. If new Q-waves appeared, myocardial infarction was diagnosed. If the blood pressure was supported by vasopressors (epinephrine, isoproterenol, or norepinephrine), a low-output state existed. If electrocardiographic changes of myocardial infarction were present with clinical low output, myocardial infarction with low cardiac output was diagnosed. Subendocardial ischemia was diagnosed on the electrocardiogram when there were nonspecific changes of possible ischemia following surgery. Intramyocardial temperatures were obtained in 20 patients under general and topical hypothermia or normothermia. The anoxic arrest time was recorded for each patient as a total arrest time. In some patients in Group I, anoxic arrest times were occassionally interrupted between anastomoses; however, in Group II the anoxic arrest period was uninterrupted.

In 20 Group II patients, coronary sinus blood samples were obtained before anoxic arrest (control), immediately following anoxic arrest, and for five-minute intervals up to 20 minutes following aortic clamp release. Simultaneous arterial samples were obtained. The blood was analyzed for potassium, calcium, phosphorus, lactate, pyruvate, SGOT, CPK, and LDH concentrations. In addition, SGOT and CPK were analyzed from one through five days following ACB.

RESULTS

The overall operative mortality in both groups was different (Table 3). In Group I (normothermia), there were 29 operative deaths in 454 patients (6.3 percent) as compared to three deaths in the 200 patients in Group II (1.5 percent). In Group I, ten patients died in the operating room following unsuccessful coronary artery bypass. Eight of these patients had myocardial pump failure due to inadequate output on discontinuation of cardiopulmonary bypass. One had preoperative myocardial infarction, and the other had aortic dissection. Thirteen patients died in the postoperative period from myocardial infarction either incurred at operation or shortly after surgery. Six additional patients died from other causes.

In Group II (hypothermia), there were only three operative deaths. One patient died because of low cardiac output in the operating room. The second patient died on the 16th postoperative day

TABLE 3. Myocardial Complications

	NORMO-THERMIC (%)	HYPO-THERMIC (%)
Electrocardiogram	36.7	20.5
Subendocardial ischemia	30	10
Myocardial infarction	6.7	10.5
Arrythmia	21	15
Nonfatal clinical complications	3.2	8.5
Low cardiac output	1.0	3.5
Low cardiac output + MI	2.2	5
Mortality	6.3	1.5
Immediate	2.2	0.5
Operative		
Myocardial	2.9	0.5
Other	1.2	0.5

from myocardial infarction. The patient also suffered a hemorrhagic cerebral infarction shortly after surgery. The third patient died on the 14th postoperative day following a neurological complication because of preexisting cerebrovascular disease but was in good cardiac condition at the time of death. Thus, there were two myocardial deaths in the Group II patients (1 percent).

In Group I, nonfatal clinical myocardial complications were present in 45 patients (9.9 percent) (Table 3). The low-cardiac-output state occurred in four patients (1 percent); myocardial infarction with low cardiac output in 10 (2.2 percent) and myocardial infarction as diagnosed by postoperative electrocardiogram in 31 patients (6 percent). In Group II, there were seven patients with low cardiac output (3.5 percent), 10 with low cardiac output plus the electrocardiographic diagnosis of MI (5 percent), and 21 patients with possible myocardial infarction as diagnosed by electrocardiogram (10.5 percent). Subendocardial ischemia was present in 30 percent of the normothermic group and 10 percent of the hypothermic group. Although the overall mortality rate in the normothermic group was higher than the hypothermic group, the incidence of nonfatal clinical myocardial complications was higher in the hypothermic group. The incidence of electrocardiographic changes of subendocardial ischemia, however, was decreased in the hypothermic group. Ventricular or supraventricular arrhythmias were present in 21 percent of Group I and 15 percent of Group II (Table 3).

The noncardiac complications were not markedly different in either group except for an increased incidence of respiratory problems in the normothermic group (Table 4). Most respiratory

TABLE 4. Noncardiac Complications

	NORMO-THERMIC (percent)	HYPO-THERMIC (percent)
Respiratory	16	5
Hemorrhage	2	2
Infection	2	1
Neurologic	1	3
Psychiatric	1.5	1
Renal	0.5	0.5
Pulmonary embolus	0.2	0.5

complications were atelectasis and hypoxemia requiring prolonged intubation. Tracheostomy was done only in 1 percent of each group. Postoperative hemorrhage requiring re-exploration occurred in only 2 percent of both groups indicating that hypothermia did not result in increased bleeding tendency. Furthermore, the amount of blood required following cardiopulmonary bypass was not different in either group. The serum glutamic oxaloacetic transaminase (SGOT) and creatinine phosphokinase (CPK) were not markedly elevated (Fig. 1). The peak CPK value (300 U) occurred two days after surgery. The highest SGOTs (120 U, 130 U) were on the first and second days after surgery. The SGOT, LDH, and CPK enzyme levels did not correlate with low cardiac output or myocardial damage in these patients.

MYOCARDIAL TEMPERATURE

The intramyocardial temperature following anoxic arrest was variable. In the normothermic group, the myocardial temperature dropped to 32 C within five to ten minutes and returned to 34 C on aortic clamp release (Fig. 2). In some instances of normothermic arrest, the myocardial temperature dropped to 30 C and returned to normal within ten minutes of renewal of normothermic perfusion. With general hypothermia to 30 C (esophageal temperature), the heart temperature generally paralleled the esophageal temperature (Fig. 3). The heart temperature frequently reached 30 C; however, it gradually returned to 35 C, along with the esophageal temperature, and at the renewal of normothermic perfusion on aortic clamp release, the temperature rose significantly to equal the esophageal temperature. In patients who received general hypothermia and topical lavage at the time of aortic occlusion, the myocardial temperature remained about 30 C during most of the period of anoxic arrest (Fig. 4). On reinstitution of normothermic perfusion into the coronary arteries at the time of clamp release, the temperature again returned to 35 C. Thus, it appeared that general hypothermia and topical lavage with iced saline caused the longest interval of myocardial hypothermia, which usually lasted the

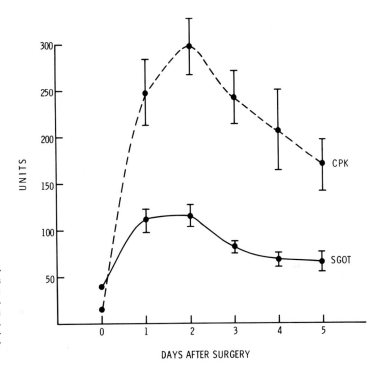

FIG. 1. The serum enzymes following surgery are shown as means and standard deviation in 20 patients who received coronary bypass with anoxic cardiac arrest and hypothermia. The highest mean CPK level was under 300 units, and the highest SGOT was 130 units.

DAYS AFTER SURGERY

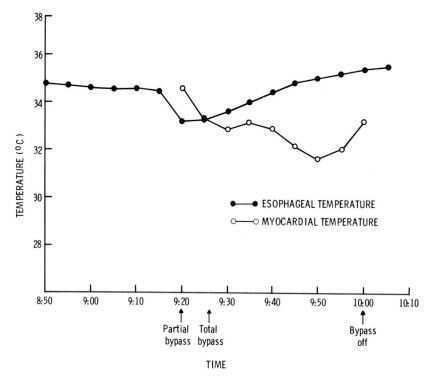

FIG. 2. Myocardial and esophageal temperatures are shown in a patient who had normothermic ischemic arrest for the performance of two aortocoronary artery bypass grafts. In general the myocardial temperature was unpredictable under normothermic conditions.

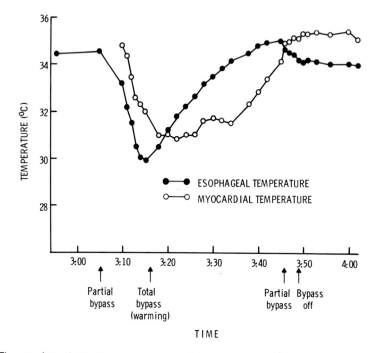

FIG. 3. The esophageal temperature is compared to the myocardial temperature in a patient in general hypothermia at an esophageal temperature of 30 C. Rewarming was done at the time of aortic occlusion. The myocardial temperature did not coincide with the esophageal temperature and in fact was warmer than 30 C. This once again demonstrates unreliability of myocardial temperature prediction in the absence of direct monitoring.

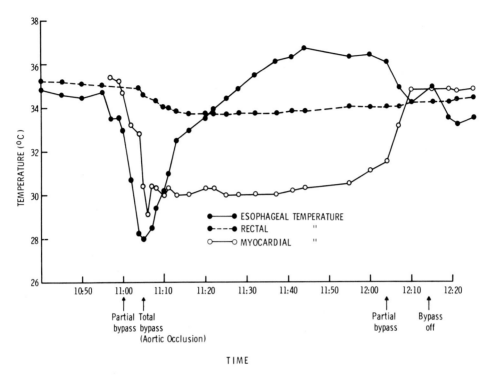

FIG. 4. The combination of general hypothermia and topical hypothermia are shown here. Note the prolonged decreased myocardial temperature after topical application that was applied shortly before aortic occlusion.

entire anoxic period. Nevertheless, it is difficult to predict actual myocardial temperature on the basis of rectal or esophageal temperature.

BLOOD CHEMISTRY

Paired coronary sinus and arterial blood levels were taken in patients who had normothermic arrest up to 30 minutes (Group I), hypothermic arrest from 30 to 60 minutes (Group IIA), and hypothermic arrest for greater than 60 minutes (Group IIB). There was little difference in the coronary sinus potassium, calcium, phosphorous, and serum enzyme levels (Fig. 5). No significant difference in lactate/pyruvate quotients were obtained (Fig. 6). Paired samples of arterial pH, carbon dioxide tension, and oxygen tension were compared to the coronary sinus levels and demonstrated the changes anticipated in the coronary sinus effluent at the time of aortic clamp release. The coronary sinus effluent dropped to a

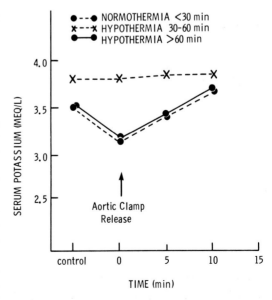

FIG. 5. Coronary sinus serum potassium levels are compared in normothermic and hypothermic patients. There is no significant difference in the three groups.

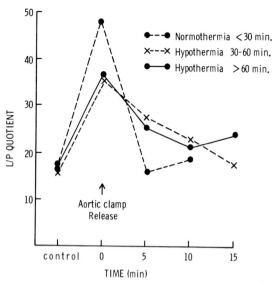

FIG. 6. The lactate/pyruvate quotient is shown in the three groups of patients. There is no significant difference in the normothermic group and the hypothermic group at different intervals. At aortic clamp release there was significant elevation of lactate/pyruvate quotient in the coronary sinus.

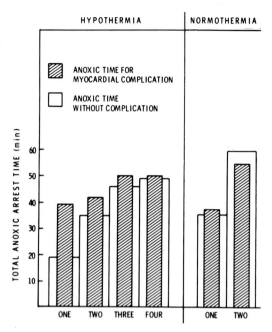

FIG. 8. Anoxic time for myocardial complications and the mean anoxic time without complication are compared in the two groups of patients. Anoxic arrest time for 1, 2, 3, and 4 grafts is shown. Patients without complications had anoxic arrest time similar to those with complications.

mean of pH 7.0 but rapidly returned to normal on reinstitution of coronary perfusion (Fig. 7).

ANOXIC ARREST TIME

It is of importance to correlate complications and death with anoxic arrest time. The anoxic arrest time obviously varies with the severity of the underlying coronary artery occlusive disease,

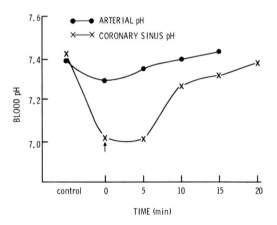

FIG. 7. The arterial pH is compared to the coronary sinus pH in a patient who had hypothermic anoxic arrest. At the time of aortic clamp release, marked zero, the pH approached 7. Within 5 minutes, it began an upward swing and at 10 minutes reached 7.25. Within 20 minutes the pH was normal.

the technical difficulty of the operation, and the number of bypass grafts placed. The mean anoxic arrest times for one, two, three, and four graft procedures varied by approximately five to ten minutes (Fig. 8). In the hypothermic group only one patient with a single bypass graft had a complication, and that ischemic arrest time was 39 minutes.

The mean anoxic arrest times of patients who had no mortality or myocardial complications were 44.3 minutes in Group I and 39 minutes in Group II (Table 5). All patients who expired in

TABLE 5. Total Anoxic Arrest Time Related to Complications

	NORMO-THERMIC (min)	HYPO-THERMIC (min)
No mortality or complications	44.3	39
Nonfatal clinical complications	66.3	45
Myocardial infarct (EKG)	36.8	43.5
Low cardiac output with MI	56.7	50
Mortality	59.2	51
Immediate	56.6	50
Operative (myocardial)	60	52

the immediate or operative period had mean anoxic arrest times over 50 minutes. Patients who had nonfatal low cardiac output with myocardial infarction had mean anoxic arrest times of 56.7 minutes in Group I and 50 minutes in Group II. Patients who had the diagnosis of myocardial infarction on electrocardiographic findings only without low cardiac output did not have prolonged anoxic arrest times when compared to the group without complications. Mean anoxic arrest times were slightly elevated in both groups of patients who had serious complications.

With respect to the nonfatal myocardial complications related to anoxic arrest time, the two groups paralleled the percent of complications that occurred at the various anoxic times (Fig. 9). At 20 minutes of anoxic arrest, 13.3 percent of the patients had complications in Group I whereas 22 percent had complications in Group II. Percent of complications remained the same until the interval of 40 to 49 minutes, at which time 13 percent of Group I had complications, as opposed to 28 percent in Group II. The percent nonfatal myocardial complications remained the same until 70 to 79 minutes, where the complications exceeded safe limits at 67 percent (two out of three patients) in Group II and 30 percent (six out of 20) in Group I. Therefore, a marked rise occurred at 70 to 79 minutes, but only four patients in Group II and 37 patients in Group I had anoxic arrest times over 70 minutes.

DISCUSSION

Both groups of patients were similar with respect to the preoperative symptoms and the presence of congestive heart failure or previous myocardial infarction. Slightly more patients in the hypothermia group had elevated left ventricular end diastolic pressure. The hypothermic group also had more patients who were NYHA Functional Class III and IV. The major differences in both groups, other than the use of hypothermia, were the amount of coronary artery disease present and the number of multiple-graft procedures done. The hypothermic group had more multiple-vessel disease in addition to the higher incidence of elevated LVEDP and previous myocardial infarction. Complete revascularization was accomplished in more patients in the hypothermic group in that over half of the patients had three or more grafts. This alone could account for the decreased mortality in the hypothermic group. On the other hand, there is strong evidence by controlled experimental procedures that hypothermia protects the myocar-

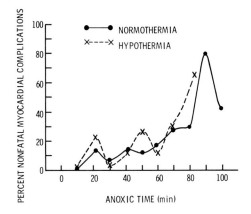

FIG. 9. The percent of nonfatal myocardial complications is compared in the normothermic and hypothermic patients at different anoxic arrest times. There is a relatively equal percent of complications up to approximately 60 minutes, after which the slope rises to a significant percent of complications.

dium during anoxic arrest. It can therefore be assumed that hypothermia reduced immediate mortality previously attributed to left ventricular pump failure occurring during operation and decreased the early operative mortality from acute myocardial infarction.

Failure to achieve reduction in nonfatal clinical complications was related neither to anoxic arrest time nor to the presence of hypothermia *per se*. On careful analysis of the data, it can be seen that there are discrepancies between the patients with myocardial infarctions and subendocardial ischemia in the two groups; ie more patients had subendocardial ischemia in the normothermic group and more patients had the electrocardiographic diagnosis of myocardial infarction in the hypothermic group. The difficulty of diagnosis of myocardial infarction in the postoperative period is well known.[21-23] The interpretation of the electrocardiograms was not done by one person but by a number of cardiologists; therefore, there may have been some variability in the diagnosis. Nevertheless, the immediate and operative mortality was decreased.

The possibility of permanent myocardial damage inflicted upon the heart during anoxic arrest has been expressed.[1] At a later date subendocardial hemorrhagic necrosis may result in subendocardial fibrosis, or localized areas of infarction may result in fibrosis and decreased ventricular function. Our late follow-up did not indicate that there was a decrease in ventricular function following coronary artery bypass in the asymptomatic patient. Our data correlated well with that of others in that ventricular function postoperatively was directly related to the amount of coronary artery involvement, previous state of the myocardium, and the presence of congestive heart failure.[24-26]

Correlation of the length of anoxic arrest time with ventricular function, myocardial ultrastructure, and myocardial metabolism has been experimentally and clinically attempted.[1,10-15] It appears that 30 minutes of normothermic ischemic arrest is safe at least in the experimental animal and that 60 minutes of hypothermic arrest is well tolerated in the experimental animal.[27] Heart transplant preservation chambers have preserved hearts for hours in an isolated state. In our attempt to analyze myocardial metabolism at the time of aortic cross-clamp release, it appeared that hypothermic cardiac arrest up to one hour was safe. There appeared to be no difference between normothermic cardiac arrest at 30 minutes and the hypothermic cardiac arrest at 60 minutes. Any derangements in myocardial metabolism that were apparent were not statistically significant. Return to normal mean levels usually resulted in five to ten minutes following aortic clamp release.

Despite the widespread use of anoxic cardiac arrest, few proposals of safe time limits of aortic occlusion have been reported.[1] Our previous data with normothermic arrest seem to point to a safe anoxic arrest interval of 45 minutes. We could not correlate myocardial complications or death with anoxic arrest time until the interval over 60 minutes. In shorter time intervals, complications were relatively the same for 20 to 60 minutes in both hypothermic and normothermic anoxic arrest. It is true that the immediate mortality and the operative mortality groups both had mean anoxic arrest times over 50 minutes. This probably is a reflection of other factors that have been shown to be determinants in operative mortality. Multiplicity and severity of coronary artery involvement and technical difficulty at time of operation prolonged anoxic arrest time. On the other hand, electrocardiographic evidence of myocardial infarction in the postoperative period was not related to a prolonged anoxic arrest time; however, in patients with low cardiac output with myocardial infarction in both groups, mean anoxic arrest times were again above 50 minutes.

Of further importance was the demonstration that hypothermia did not cause significant postoperative complications. Postoperative hemorrhage was not a problem in either group of patients. Infection was not increased by hypothermia. Hypothermia prolonged cardiopulmonary bypass slightly for cooling and rewarming purposes. Slight hypothermia (34 to 36 C) at the end of the surgical procedure occurred in most patients despite rewarming, and this could be a potential problem in the immediate postoperative period because of the increased tendency for arrhythmias and possible ventricular fibrillation. The incidence of these events was not increased by the use of hypothermia.

An interesting facet of the study was the unpredictability of myocardial temperature by the technique used. General hypothermia failed to maintain the myocardial temperature within the range of the esophageal temperature in most cases. Topical cooling with iced saline did prolong hypothermia throughout the entire anoxic arrest period in most instances. Intramyocardial temperature should be monitored if accurate myocardial temperature is desired.

Our present technique has been altered somewhat from the technique herein reported in that total aortic occlusion time has been further reduced. After each distal anastomosis, the aortic clamp is released to allow coronary perfusion. Proximal anastomoses are accomplished under partial cardiopulmonary bypass or no bypass. Anoxic arrest times have been shortened, and air introduction into the coronary arteries has been avoided.

SUMMARY

In an attempt to establish the efficacy of hypothermia during anoxic cardiac arrest, two similar groups of patients were compared. The first (Group I) had coronary artery bypass procedures under normothermic conditions with anoxic cardiac arrest. The second (Group II) had similar procedures under hypothermic condition. Hypothermia was achieved by general body hypothermia with iced saline lavage. Average intramyocardial temperatures were 26 C, though they were difficult to predict, especially when topical hypothermia was not utilized. Myocardial metabolism was measured at the time of aortic clamp release and on shorter intervals thereafter. Thirty minutes of normothermic arrest appeared to parallel changes that occurred with 60 minutes of hypothermic arrest. Nonfatal cardiac complications were not increased in normothermic, whereas there was a 1.5 percent increase in the hypothermic group. The immediate mortality and operative mortality related to myocardial failure were decreased. Besides hypothermia, another factor in the reduction of mortality was the completeness of the revascularization procedure in that over half the patients had three or more bypass grafts in the hypothermic group. Nonfatal myocardial complications were not decreased by hypothermia, but electrocardiographic changes of subendocardial ischemia were somewhat decreased.

The anoxic arrest interval could not be correlated with increased myocardial complications until approximately 60 minutes in both the normothermic and hypothermic groups. On the other hand, the mean anoxic arrest time was over 50 minutes in surviving patients with postoperative low cardiac output and in the patients who expired from low cardiac output or myocardial infarction. It would appear that anoxic cardiac arrest time should be as short an interval as possible and certainly should be less than 50 minutes. In an attempt further to reduce myocardial complications and operative mortality, intermittent anoxic occlusion has been utilized in a subsequent series of patients, and this has accomplished a reduction in the myocardial complications following surgery.

Anoxic cardiac arrest has been shown to be quite satisfactory within the limits described. General and topical hypothermia have decreased operative mortality. The technical accuracy afforded by hypothermic anoxic cardiac arrest is far superior to any other techniques for aortocoronary artery bypass.

References

1. Reul GJ Jr, Morris GC Jr, Howell FJ, Crawford ES, Sandiford FM, Wukasch DC: The safety of ischemic cardiac arrest in distal coronary artery bypass. J Thorac Cardiovasc Surg 62:511–21, 1971
2. Senning, A: Ventricular fibrillation during extracorporeal circulation. Acta Chir Scand (Suppl) 171:1, 1952
3. Wilson HE, Dalton ML, Kiphart RJ, Allison WM: Increased safety of aorto-coronary artery bypass surgery with induced ventricular fibrillation to avoid anoxia. J Thorac Cardiovasc Surg 64:193–202, 1972
4. Stoney RJ, Zanger LCC, Roe BB: Myocardial metabolism and ventricular function before and after induced ventricular fibrillation. Surgery 52:37–46, 1962
5. Urschel HC, Razzuk MA, Nathan MJ, Miller ER, Nicholson DM, Paulson DL: Combined gas (CO_2) endarterectomy and vein bypass graft for patients with coronary artery disease. Ann Thorac Surg 10:119–31, 1970
6. Favaloro, RG, Effler DB, Groves LK, Sheldon WC, Sones FM Jr: Direct myocardial revascularization by saphenous vein graft: present operative technique and indications. Ann Thorac Surg 10:97–111, 1970
7. Jardetzky O, Greene EA, Lorber V: Oxygen consumption of the completely isolated dog heart in fibrillation. Circ Res 4:144–47, 1956
8. Hottenrott CE, Towers B, Kurkji HJ, Maloney JV, Buckberg G: The hazard of ventricular fibrillation in hypertrophied ventricles during cardiopulmonary bypass. J Thorac Cardiovasc Surg 66:742–53, 1973
9. Hayward RH, Martt JM, Brewer LM, Inmon TM, Best EB: Surgical correction of the vena cava-

bronchovascular complex: developmental pulmonary, arterial and venous anomalies with accessory diaphragm. J Thorac Cardiovasc Surg 64:203–10, 1972
10. Shumway NE, Lower RR, Stofer RC: Selective hypothermia of the heart in anoxic cardiac arrest. Surg Gynecol Obstet 109:750–54, 1959
11. Heimbecker RO, Lajos TZ: Ice-chip cardioplegia. Arch Surg 84:148–58, 1962
12. Griepp RB, Stinson EB, Shumway NE: Profound local hypothermia for myocardial protection during open-heart surgery. J Thorac Cardiovasc Surg 66:731–41, 1973
13. Stemmer EA, Aronow WS, and Connolly JE: Abstracts: Coronary Artery Medicine and Surgery Conference, Houston, February 21–23, 1974
14. Willman VL, Howard HS, Cooper T, Hanlon CR: Ventricular function after hypothermic cardiac arrest. Arch Surg 82:140–47, 1961
15. Ebert PA, Greenfield, LJ, Austen WG, Morrow AG: Experimental comparison of methods for protecting the heart during aortic occlusion. Ann Surg 155:25–32, 1962
16. Reul GJ Jr, Johnson WC, Lepley DW Jr: Aortocoronary vein bypass grafts combined with multiple arterial implants in treatment of coronary artery disease. Rev Surg 27:52–58, 1970
17. Reul GJ Jr, Morris GE Jr, Howell JF, Crawford ES, Sandiford FM, Wukasch DC: Experience with coronary artery grafts in the treatment of coronary artery disease. Surgery 71:586–93, 1972
18. Reul GC Jr, Morris GC Jr, Howell JF, Crawford ES, Stelter WJ: Current concepts in coronary artery surgery: a critical analysis of 1,287 patients. Ann Thorac Surg 14:243–59, 1972
19. Hall RJ, Dawson JT, Cooley DA, Hallman GL, Wukasch DC, Garcia E: Coronary artery bypass. Am Heart Assoc Monograph 41:146–50, 1972
20. Reed CC, Phillips PA, Coleman PA, Clark DK, Migliore JJ, Cooley DA: A disposable heat exchanger for normothermia and hypothermia: evaluation and utilization in avoiding ischemic contracture of the heart (Stone Heart). The Le Journal 1:4–6, 1972
21. Klein HO, Gross H, Rubin IL: Transient electrocardiographic changes simulating myocardial infarction during open-heart surgery. Am Heart J 79:463–70, 1970
22. Dixon SH, Limbird LE, Roe CR, Wagner GS, Oldham N Jr, Sabiston DC Jr: Recognition of postoperative acute myocardial infarction: application of Isoenzyme techniques. Circulation 47 and 48:137–40, 1973
23. Bassan MM, Oatfield R, Hoffman I, Matloff J. Swan HJC: New Q waves after aortocoronary bypass surgery: unmasking of an old infraction. N Engl J Med 290:349–53, 1974
24. Chatterjee K, Swan HJC, Parmley WW, Sustaita H, Marcus H, Matloff J: Depression of left ventricular function due to acute myocardial ischemia and its reversal after aortocoronary saphenous vein bypass. N Engl J Med 286:1118–22, 1972
25. Rees G, Bristow JD, Kremkau EL, Green GS, Herr RH, Griswold HE, Starr A: Influence of aortocoronary bypass surgery on left ventricular performance. N Engl J Med 284:1116–20, 1971
26. Mailhot J, Sandler H, Harrison DC: Left ventricular function following coronary bypass surgery. Circulation 44 Suppl 2:196–210, 1971
27. Cullum PA, Bailey JS, Branfoot AC, Pemberton MJ, Redding VJ, Rees JR: The warm ischaemic time of the canine heart. Cardiovasc Res 4:67–72, 1970
28. Bjork VO, Fors B: Induced cardiac arrest. J Thorac Cardiovasc Surg 41:387–94, 1961

29. Mundth ED, Sokol DM, Levine FH, Austen WG: Evaluation of methods for myocardial protection during extended periods of aortic crossclamping and hypoxic cardiac arrest. Bulletin de la Société Internationale de Chirurgie 4:227–35, 1970

30. Hoelscher B, Just OH, Merker HJ: Studies by electron microscopy on various forms of induced cardiac arrest in dog and rabbit. Surgery 49:492–99, 1961

31. Miller DR, Rasmussen P, Klionsky B, Cossman EP, Allbritten FF Jr: Elective cardiac arrest: its effect on myocardial structure and function. Ann Surg 154:751–68, 1961

66

SELECTIVE DEEP HYPOTHERMIA OF THE HEART DURING AORTOCORONARY SURGERY

Edward A. Stemmer, Wilbert S. Aronow, Peter McCart, Claude Oliver, and John E. Connolly

In 1956 Moulder and Thompson commented that it was surprisingly simple to work directly with the coronary arteries if the aorta was cross-clamped and the heart stopped. Anoxic arrest to provide a dry, quiet operative field (Bloodwell et al, 1958) has been employed successfully in many patients but can produce measurable and sometimes permanent myocardial damage if the period of normothermic ischemia exceeds 30 minutes (Ebert et al, 1962; Reis et al, 1969). Since many patients who are candidates for coronary arterial surgery have already sustained significant myocardial damage and may have borderline adequate myocardial functional reserve, surgeons have sought operative techniques that would avoid or minimize further injury to the myocardium. Understandably, most of the techniques developed to protect the myocardium employ coronary perfusion, hypothermia, or a combination of these two modalities. This report describes our laboratory and clinical experience with continuous cold perfusion of the coronary arteries.

In our animal studies we compared the effectiveness of four methods of myocardial preservation: (1) continuous, normothermic coronary perfusion through the aortic root, (2) direct (selective) coronary perfusion with cold blood, (3) continuous cold coronary perfusion through the aortic root, and (4) topical deep hypothermia of the myocardium without coronary perfusion. The effectiveness of each of these techniques was evaluated in terms of ability to maintain structural and functional integrity of the myocardium. Our clinical experience consists of 81 patients in whom cold aortic root perfusion was employed for valvular and coronary arterial surgery.

METHODS

Animal Studies

All studies were performed on mongrel dogs anesthetized with sodium pentobarbital and ventilated by means of a volume-controlled respirator. Median sternotomy was performed in each animal. A bubble oxygenator with an integral heat exchanger was employed with standard cannulations for cardiopulmonary bypass. When the coronary circulation was separately perfused, an additional heat exchanger was placed in the coronary circuit. The left ventricle was vented in all animals on bypass. All experiments were divided into a two-hour base-line period, a two-hour test period according to the protocol described below, and a two-hour recovery period. All animals were given heparin (5 mg per kilogram) during the test period, after which heparinization was reversed by protamine sulphate. Arterial pressure, central venous pressure, electrocardiogram, urinary output, body temperature, intramyocardial temperature, and arterial and venous PO_2, PCO_2, and pH were monitored in each animal. Cardiac outputs by dye-dilution techniques were determined during the base-line period, at the end of the test period, and at the end of the recovery period. Full-thickness samples of the right and left ventricular myocardium were obtained for electron microscopy from each animal during the base-line period and at the end of the test and recovery periods. Multiple sections of each sample were examined. When the coronary circulation was separately perfused, both pressure and flow in the coronary circuit were monitored. Coronary sinus flow was measured in each animal. Percentage survival was calculated for each group studied. The animals were divided into five groups as follows:

GROUP I: OPEN-CHEST CONTROL DOGS. Fifteen dogs were prepared as described above except that the animals were not placed on bypass. The experimental period was divided into three 2-hour segments for purposes of measuring cardiac output and obtaining myocardial biopsies.

GROUP II: TWO HOURS OF NORMO-THERMIC (37 C) BYPASS WITH NORMO-THERMIC ROOT PERFUSION. After a two-hour base-line period, 15 dogs were placed on cardiopulmonary bypass for two hours. During bypass the ascending aorta was cross-clamped and the coronary arteries were perfused at 37 C through a cannula inserted into the ascending aorta. The root perfusion pressure was maintained at 80 mm Hg, and a separate circuit and pump were used for the coronary line. Body temperature was maintained at 37 C rectally by means of a separate heat exchanger in the systemic circuit. After two hours, the root perfuser was removed, the aorta unclamped, and the animal weaned from bypass. Observations were continued for two hours postbypass.

GROUP III: TWO HOURS OF NOR-MOTHERMIC BYPASS WITH HYPOTHER-MIC ROOT PERFUSION. Same as Group II except that root perfusion temperature was maintained at 15 C for the two-hour test period. Rewarming of the heart was accomplished in five to ten minutes before bypass was discontinued.

GROUP IV: TWO HOURS OF NOR-MOTHERMIC BYPASS WITH SELECTIVE HYPOTHERMIC CORONARY PERFUSION. After a two-hour base-line period, 15 dogs were placed on cardiopulmonary bypass for two hours. During bypass the ascending aorta was cross-

FIG. 1. Facing page: Electron micrograph of a biopsy taken from the left ventricle of a control animal during the baseline period. The nucleus, nuclear chromatin, and myofibrillar arrangement are clearly visible. The section is normal. Original magnification X24,000.

clamped and the aortic root opened. Separate cannulas were inserted into the right and left coronary arteries, and perfusion at 15 C continued for the two-hour bypass (test) period. Coronary perfusion pressure was maintained at 80 mm Hg. Body temperature was maintained at 37 C rectally. After the test period the coronary cannulas were removed, the aortic incision was closed, and the cross-clamp was removed, allowing the heart to rewarm. After weaning from bypass, observations were continued during the two-hour recovery period.

GROUP V: TWO HOURS OF NOR-MOTHERMIC BYPASS WITH TOPICAL MYOCARDIAL HYPOTHERMIA. Cardiopulmonary bypass was instituted in 20 dogs after a two-hour base-line period. The ascending aorta was then cross-clamped for 120 minutes, and the pericardial cavity was filled with saline slush replenished as necessary. The aortic clamp was then removed and the iced saline in the pericardium was evacuated. Rewarming was accomplished in five to ten minutes. Bypass was discontinued, and a two-hour recovery period was begun. Body temperature was maintained at 37 C rectally during bypass.

CLINICAL STUDIES

Normothermic bypass with hypothermic root cooling was employed in 41 patients in whom aortocoronary bypass was performed. After total cardiopulmonary bypass was instituted in these patients, the ascending aorta was cross-clamped, a number 12 arterial cannula was inserted into the

TABLE 1. Laboratory Studies

EXPERIMENT	NO. ANIMALS	% SURVIVAL	CARDIAC OUTPUT (percent change)		
			Baseline	Test	Recovery
Control animals (open chest only)	15	100	100	96	83
Bypass–2 hours, 37 C root perfusion	15	80	100	95	75
Bypass–2 hours, 15 C root perfusion	15	100	100	80	98
Bypass–2 hours, 15 C selective coronary perfusion	15	67	100	70	80
Bypass–15 C, topical hypothermia, no coronary perfusion	20	80	100	75	40

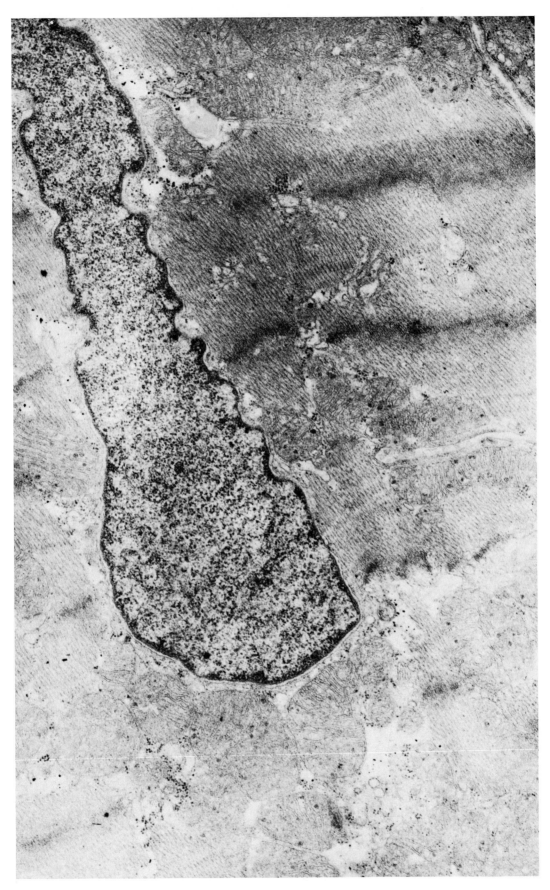

aortic root through a stab wound and cold coronary perfusion was started employing a separate coronary circuit and heat exchanger. The left ventricle was vented routinely. Intramyocardial temperature was monitored continuously. All distal dissections and anastomoses were completed. Root cooling was then discontinued and the proximal anastomoses were accomplished using the root-cooling site for one of the aortic anastomoses. The aortic clamp was then removed, and the heart was rewarmed.

This group was studied for ease of weaning from bypass, death in the operating room, death postoperatively, and the occurrence of nonfatal myocardial infarction.

Cold coronary perfusion was employed during valve replacement in 40 patients. The aortic valve was replaced in 26 patients, the mitral valve in 11, and both the aortic and mitral valves in two patients. Closure of an acquired VSD with resection of a ventricular aneurysm were performed in addition to mitral valve replacement in one patient.

RESULTS

Table 1 compares survival and changes in cardiac output among the five experimental groups. The survival data include all animals. The measurements of cardiac output, however, are averages only of those values obtained from animals surviving the six-hour experimental period. Cardiac outputs are expressed as percentage of base line (100 percent) since absolute values varied with the size of the animal.

Group I

All of the control animals survived the six-hour experiment. All animals demonstrated a slow but steady decline in cardiac output during the six hours. This was almost certainly related to body temperature, which averaged 33 to 35 C at the end of six hours.

As might be expected there was some variation in the ultrastructural detail of the myocardium, depending upon the area sampled, but no significant changes were observed over the six-hour period. Figure 1 demonstrates a low-power view of a control sample. The nucleus is well defined with finely divided, evenly distributed, nuclear chromatin. Figure 2 reveals mitochondria lying between well-ordered myofibrils. The mitochondria are distinct, regular, and sharply demarcated. The cristae arranged in parallel folds within the mitochondria are crisp and detailed. Surrounding

the cristae is the characteristically evenly distributed granular matrix of the mitochondrion. The Z and H bands of the myofibrils are well ordered and clearly visible. Abundant stainable glycogen appears as small, dark, round densities in the spaces about the mitochondria and myofibrils. While these sections were taken from open chest controls, they are typical of controls taken from each of the experimental groups.

Group II

Three of these animals could not be weaned from bypass following two hours of normothermic root perfusion resulting in an 80 percent survival rate. Cardiac output of the surviving animals in this group approximated control values immediately following bypass but were consistently depressed by the end of the two-hour recovery period (Table 1). While the mean value of 75 percent does not differ greatly from the 83 percent observed in the control animals at the end of the recovery period, the difference is probably more important than it seems since the Group II animals were warmed during the test period.

Electron microscopic studies further support our impression that artificial perfusion of the coronary arteries at normothermia resulted in some impairment of myocardial function. Figure 3 is a medium-power view of the nucleus and mitochondria of a section taken at the end of two hours of normothermic root perfusion. The nucleus is well defined, but there is a minor degree of clumping of the nuclear chromatin. Distinct margination of the chromatin is visible along the nuclear boundary. Similarly, distinct although relatively minor abnormalities are apparent in the mitochondria, with smudging of the matrix and distortion, separation, and fragmentation of the cristae. Small vacuoles are visible within the mitochondria. Abundant stainable glycogen is apparent. The myofibrils appear normal. While these ultramicroscopic changes are very probably reversible, they are distinctly abnormal.

Group III

All 15 animals survived normothermic bypass with two hours of continuous hypothermic root perfusion. At the end of the test period the average cardiac output was below control levels, most likely because myocardial temperatures were still below body temperatures at this point. During the recovery period, however, cardiac output rose to control levels. The continued improvement in cardiac output observed in those animals contrasts

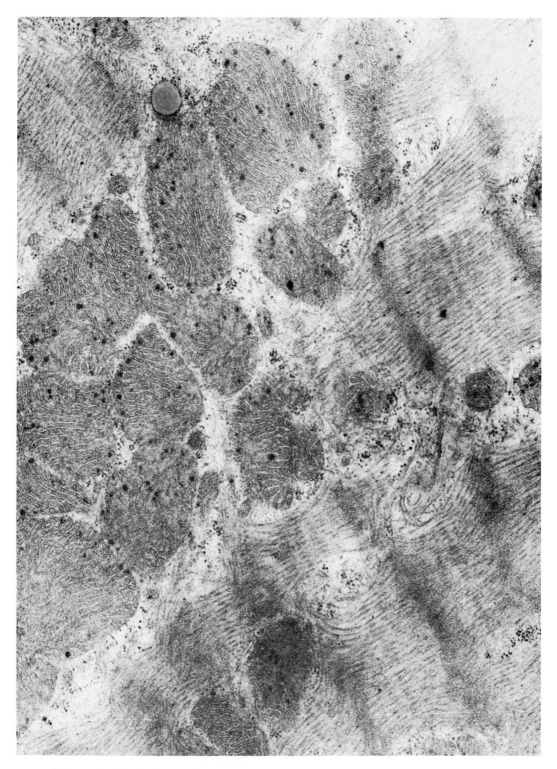

FIG. 2. Details of mitochondrial structure in a control sample. The mitochondria are regular with clearly outlined, folded cristae. There is abundant stainable glycogen (small dark spots about mitochondria and myofibrils). The section is normal. Original magnification ×24,000.

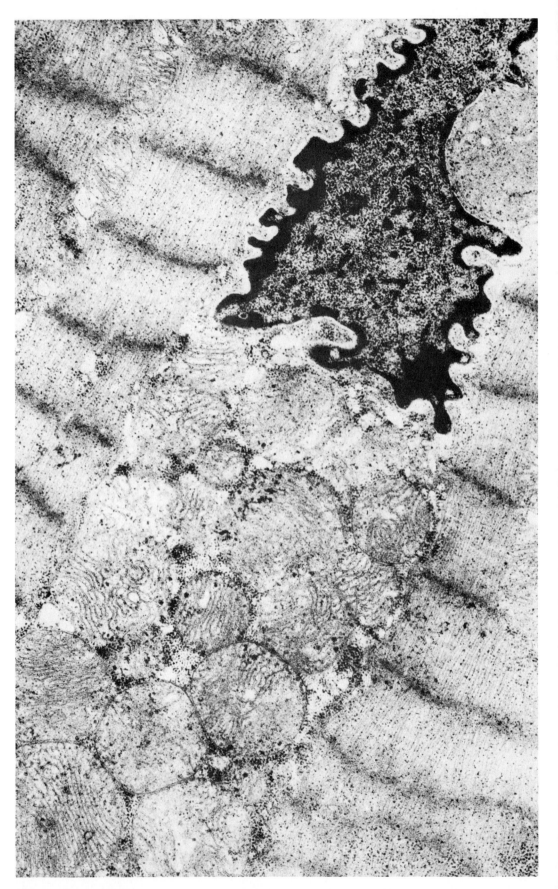

FIG. 3. Facing page: Overview of nucleus and mito-chondria following two hours of normothermic perfu-sion. There is a minor degree of clumping of the nuclear chromatin. There is margination of the nuclear chromatin. Some abnormalities are present within the mitochondria (see text). Abundant stainable glycogen is present. Original magnification X24,000.

with the progressive deterioration of cardiac output observed in animals protected by normothermic root perfusion (Group II) or topical hypothermia without coronary perfusion (Group V).

Figures 4 and 5 are sections of myocardial biopsies taken at the end of two hours of cold root perfusion. The nucleus, nucleolus, mitochondria, stainable glycogen, and myofibrils are strikingly normal.

Group IV

The poor survival in the group (67 percent) was due almost entirely to technical problems in perfusing the circumflex and/or right coronary ar-teries. At the end of the test period those animals surviving two hours of hypothermic perfusion of the individually cannulated arteries had the lowest cardiac outputs of any of the five groups. Surpris-ingly, the cardiac output of these animals im-proved rather than deteriorated during the recovery period.

Electron microscopic studies of the myo-cardium at the end of the test period (Figure 6) demonstrate an essentially normal nucleus but markedly damaged mitochondria with swelling and vacuolization. There is fragmentation, disorganiza-tion, and destruction of the cristae with clearing of the mitochondrial matrix. All of these changes are typically the result of hypoxia and inadequate perfusion. It is apparent that stainable glycogen is decreased. The myofibrillar pattern is not well visualized in this section.

Group V

Immediate survival following two hours of topical hypothermia without coronary perfusion was as good as that following normothermic root perfusion and better than that after attempts at selective cold coronary perfusion. Cardiac output immediately postbypass was also acceptable (75 percent of base-line). However, cardiac output in the topical hypothermia group fell to 40 percent of base-line values during the two-hour recovery period in striking contrast to results after hypo-thermic root perfusion (Group III). In the latter animals cardiac output continued to rise during the recovery period.

Abnormalities of the myocardial ultrastruc-ture in this group reflect the functional changes. Figure 7 is a control section of the mitochondria in this group. Sharp, clear definition of the folded cristae is apparent, as is the abundant stainable glycogen. Following two hours of topical hypo-thermia without coronary perfusion the mitochon-dria are still relatively normal (Figure 8), but some clumping of the nuclear chromatin is ap-parent. Most striking, however, is the nearly com-plete disappearance of stainable glycogen. At the end of the two-hour recovery period (Figure 9), there are readily visible abnormalities of the ultra-structure with swelling of some mitochondria and vacuolization and destruction of others, disruption of the cristae, clearing of the matrix, and general-ized intracellular edema. Little stainable glycogen remains. There are distortion and irregularity of the myofibrils. The ultrastructural changes ob-served after two hours of topical hypothermia in-dicate progressive myocardial deterioration and damage. It is noteworthy that the functional changes (cardiac output) in this group paralleled the structural changes.

Table 2 summarizes our clinical experience with selective hypothermic perfusion of the heart. There have been a total of 81 patients operated upon employing this technique. Aortocoronary by-pass procedures were performed in 41 patients, while replacement of one or more valves was per-formed in 40 patients. Seventy-eight of the 81 pa-tients were easily weaned from bypass. Three pa-tients required pump support for 30 to 60 minutes before they could be weaned. Two of these pa-tients were in frank pulmonary edema at the time of valve replacement, while the third patient developed a brief period of anterior myocardial asynergy as the result of inadequate perfusion of the left anterior descending artery during aortic valve replacement. Nevertheless, all three patients left the hospital alive.

TABLE 2. Clinical Studies

	NO.	%
Valve replacements	40	
Failure to wean from bypass	0	
Deaths in operating room	0	
Postoperative deaths	3	7.5
Aortocoronary bypass	41	
Failure to wean from bypass	0	
Deaths in operating room	0	
Postopeative deaths	1	2.5
Nonfatal myocardial infarction	4	10.0
Total number of patients	81	

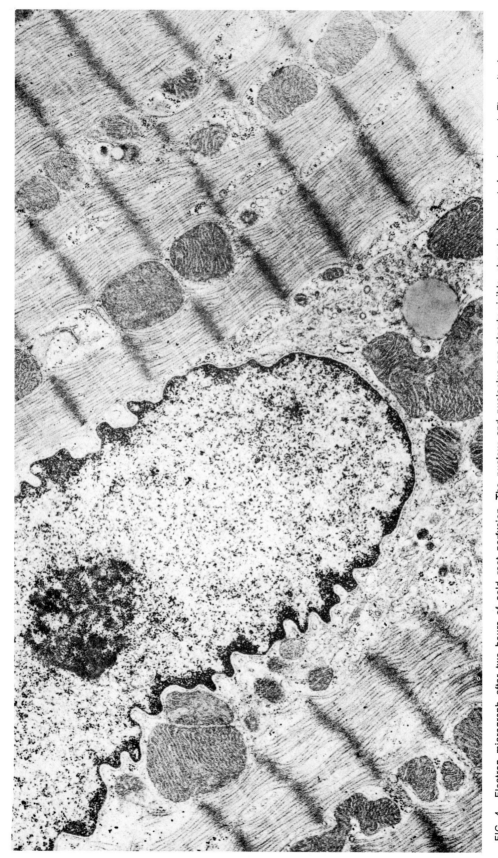

FIG. 4. Electron micrograph after two hours of cold root perfusion. The nucleus and nucleolus are clearly visible, sharply demarcated, and normal. The mitochondria are similarly sharp, regular, and well defined. The cristae within the mitochondria are crisp, regular, and intact. The mitochondria are evenly distributed between the myofibrils. The myofibrils are regular and well demarcated, with clearly apparent Z-bands (heavy transverse bands). Abundant stainable glycogen is visible. The section is normal. Original magnification ×16,800.

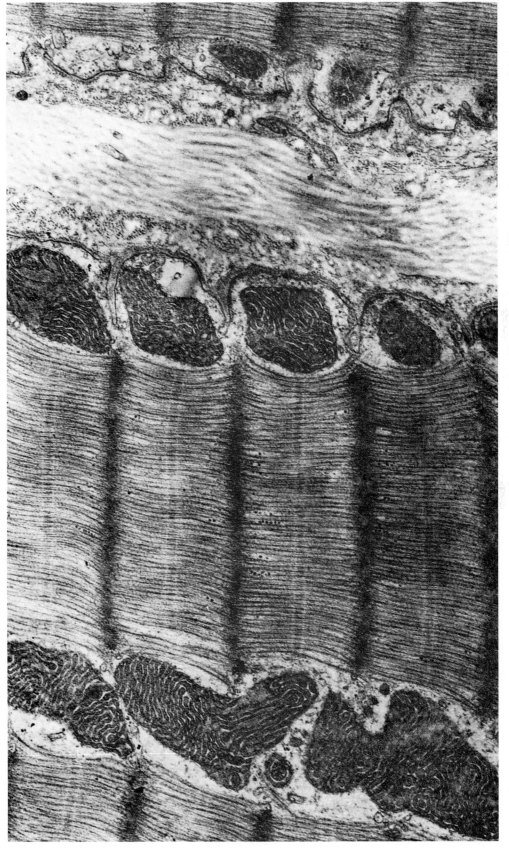

FIG. 5. Closer view of mitochondria from myocardium after two hours of cold root perfusion. The section is normal. The wavy, linear structure to the right is a capillary. Original magnification ×24,000.

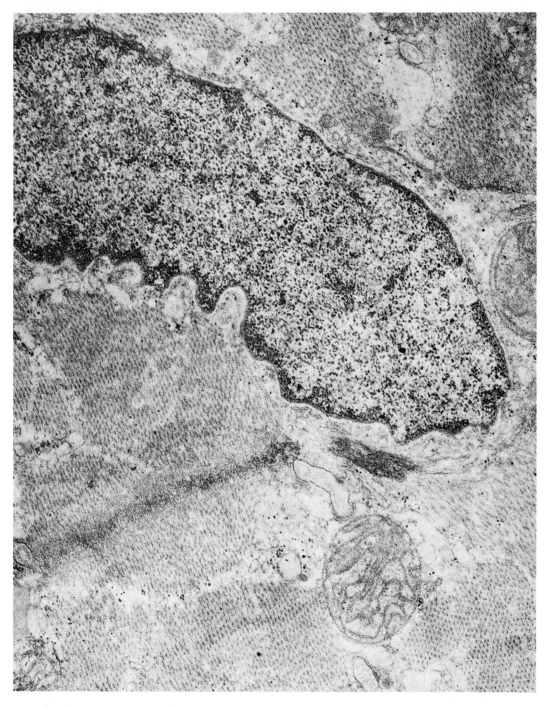

FIG. 6. Appearance of nucleus and mitochondria after two hours of selective cold perfusion of coronary arteries. The nucleus is essentially normal, but there is moderately severe mitochondrial damage (see text). Original magnification ×24,000.

FIG. 7. Facing page: Control section during baseline period prior to topical hypothermic arrest of the heart. The section is essentially normal. Note abundant stainable glycogen (small dark spots). Original magnification ×61,500.

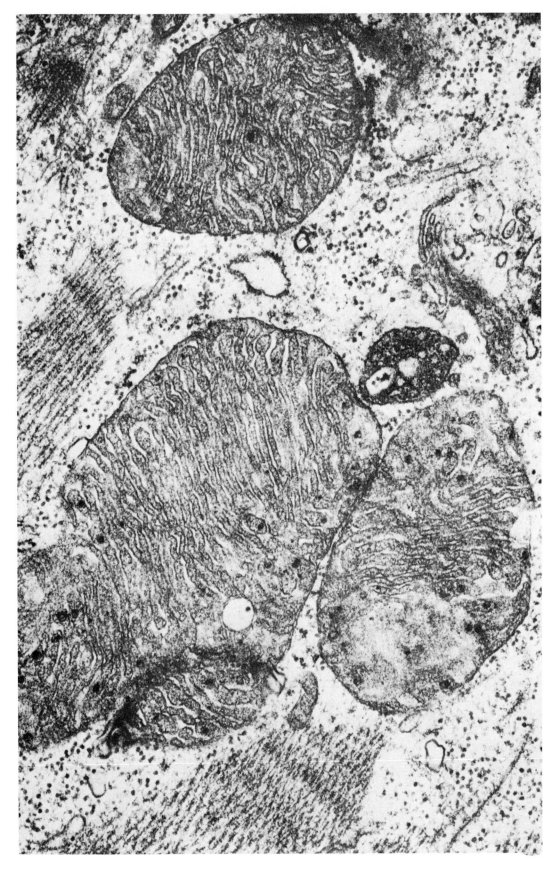

581

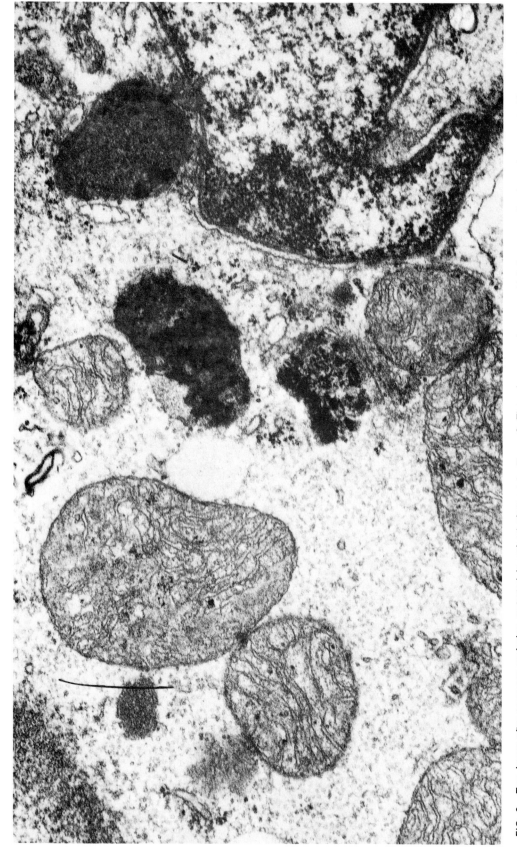

FIG. 9. Two hours after coronary perfusion restarted in animal pictured in Figure 8. There is severe damage, which is progressive from that seen in Figure 8 (see text). Original magnification ×61,500.

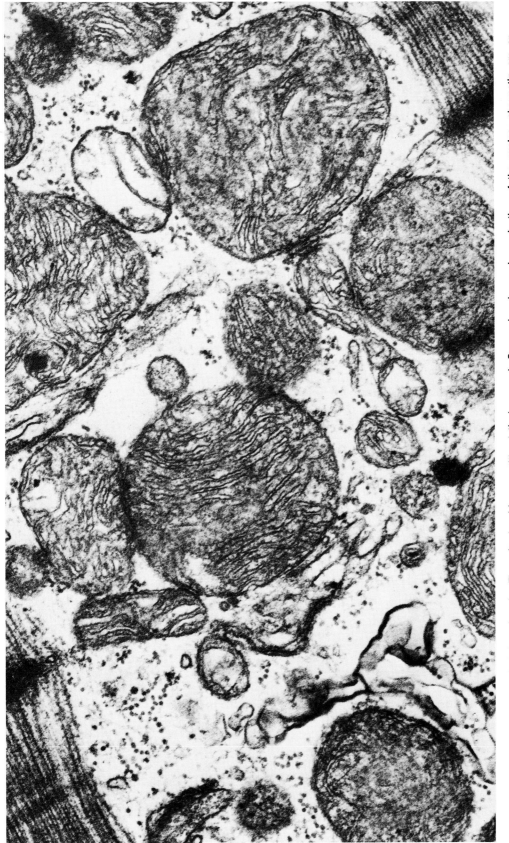

FIG. 8. After two hours of topical hypothermia. The mitochondria are still relatively normal. Some clumping and margination of the nuclear chromatin are apparent. Note almost complete disappearance of stainable glycogen. Original magnification ×61,500.

There were no intraoperative deaths. Two patients died of low cardiac output, three and 23 days following mitral valve replacement. Markedly elevated pulmonary artery pressures were present in both patients preoperatively. One 79-year-old patient died following a myocardial infarction 11 days after aortic valve replacement. A fourth patient suffered a myocardial infarction 11 days after aortic valve replacement. A fourth patient suffered a myocardial infarction during coronary arterial surgery and died three days later. Thus, in this series there was a 7.5 percent operative mortality for valve replacement and a 2.5 percent operative mortality for coronary arterial bypass.

Four of the 40 patients (10 percent) surviving coronary arterial surgery developed nonfatal myocardial infarction sometime during the surgical hospitalization. The criterion for myocardial infarction was development of new, significantly abnormal Q-waves.

DISCUSSION

In 1950 Bigelow et al demonstrated experimentally that general body hypothermia extended the period of time that the brain (and other organs) would tolerate circulatory arrest. Since that time, mild hypothermia (30 C) has become a common modality in cardiac surgery, but deep systemic or regional hypothermia has not gained wide acceptance. Even the advocates of hypothermic myocardial protection do not agree upon the most advantageous level of hypothermia, the duration of protection afforded, or the most effective method of inducing hypothermia. Gollan et al (1955) reported complete recovery of animals cooled to 5 C. Connolly et al (1965) reported that animals undergoing 45 minutes of complete circulatory arrest at 4 to 6 C recovered without cardiac or neurologic damage. Urschel and Greenberg (1960) stated that myocardial temperature must be below 10 C if the heart is to tolerate ischemic arrest longer than 30 minutes. However, Fuquay et al (1962) observed that myocardial ischemia at 10 C resulted in more severe metabolic acidosis than did ischemia at 20 C or 37 C. Braimbridge et al (1973) reported that intermittent coronary perfusion at 10 to 15 C produced histologically significant myocardial damage while intermittent perfusion at 30 C did not. Sanmarco et al (1969) found that myocardial temperatures of 30 C did not increase tolerance of the heart to ischemia. How well deep hypothermia protects against ischemia is similarly unsettled. Griepp et al (1973) believe that the heart will tolerate 90 min-

utes of ischemic arrest with an intramyocardial temperature of 15 to 20 C. Kay et al (1961) reported that protection provided by topical hypothermia was unpredictable but that temperatures of 6 to 12 C provided no more than 60 minutes of myocardial protection against ischemia. Speicher et al (1962) reported that exposure of the heart to saline slush for more than 60 minutes could cause fatal myocardial damage. Urschel and Greenberg (1960) state that cold cardioplegia will protect the heart for at least two hours. Methods for inducing myocardial hypothermia range from topical cold saline (Hurley et al, 1964) to coronary perfusion with cold Ringer's lactate (Urschel and Greenberg, 1960), coronary perfusion with cold blood (Kay et al, 1961), or total body hypothermia (Willman et al, 1961).

In an earlier study we demonstrated that hypothermia did extend the length of time that the heart could tolerate ischemia and still recover sufficient function to maintain an acceptable cardiac output (Stemmer et al, 1973). Nevertheless, a heart arrested by cold suffers from ischemia unless it is perfused. In the current study, sections of myocardium taken from animals after two hours of hypothermic ischemia revealed a substantial decrease in stainable glycogen as well as mitochondrial abnormalities clearly indicating that at 15 C the metabolic processes in the myocardium continue at a rate sufficient to deplete the myocardial energy sources. Progression of the ultrastructural changes after two hours of reperfusion certainly suggests that the two-hour period of anaerobic metabolism was not just a physiological response but had resulted in significant myocardial injury.

While coronary perfusion would seem to be the obvious solution to problems of myocardial ischemia, our study indicates that artificial coronary perfusion at body temperatures is not the equivalent of normal (anatomic) coronary perfusion. Both survival and cardiac output were clearly impaired after two hours of normothermic root perfusion (Group II, Table 1). Distinctly abnormal ultrastructural changes were found in these animals, but widespread mitochondrial defects were not observed, nor was stainable glycogen depleted. Imbalance of blood flow/oxygen demand or maldistribution of blood flow as reported by Hottenrott et al (1973) seems the most likely explanation for failure of normothermic coronary perfusion to meet the metabolic demands of the myocardium. Failure of mechanical coronary perfusion to provide safe, effective myocardial protection has also been reported clinically (Ramsey et al, 1967; Fishman et al, 1968; Kay et al, 1968).

When it is necessary to interrupt normal

coronary circulation it would seem logical to employ a combination of hypothermia to reduce the oxygen demand of the myocardium and coronary perfusion to supply the reduced oxygen requirement of the myocardium. Theoretically, such a technique would avoid the potential myocardial damage of ischemic cold arrest and at the same time reduce the possibility of myocardial injury due to maldistribution of coronary blood flow. Furthermore, the possibility of mechanical injury of the coronary arteries could be avoided if aortic root perfusion were employed instead of individual coronary arterial cannulation. Finally, selective cooling of the coronary circuit with rewarming of the systemic circulation would avoid the potential problems of systemic hypothermia (bleeding, metabolic acidosis, acute circulatory failure, prolonged pump time).

In our animal studies, continuous cold perfusion of the coronary arteries via the aortic root (Group III) consistently produced better results than either topical hypothermia (without coronary perfusion) or continuous normothermic root perfusion. All animals undergoing cold root perfusion survived the six-hour experiment. The cardiac output of these animals remained normal, as did the myocardial ultrastructure.

The advantages of cold perfusion of the aortic root during clinical coronary arterial bypass surgery have been impressive. The heart is flaccid, motionless, and collapsed. Moreover, the heart can be displaced out of the dry pericardium without concern that rewarming of the heart will occur or that coronary blood flow will be further compromised by distortion of diseased coronary vessels. The latter point is important since we have noted in patients that the root pressure necessary to maintain stable blood flow must be substantially increased when the heart is displaced out of the pericardium. Multiple proximal anastomoses can be easily and precisely accomplished while the ascending aorta is cross-clamped and the myocardium is protected by deep hypothermia. We believe it is better to continue to perfuse the myocardium while the coronary arterial dissections and distal anastomoses are completed, but in five patients we interrupted the root perfusion for as long as 45 minutes to accomplish difficult anastomoses or perform coronary endarterectomy. At a myocardial temperature of 8 to 12 C (the usual temperature reached during cold root perfusion), these interruptions of coronary flow have been without sequelae. Our 10 percent incidence of postoperative myocardial infarction is the same as that reported by Hultgren et al (1971) and well below that reported in most series (Williams et al, 1973).

Cold coronary perfusion seems to be an effective method for preserving existing myocardial function during cardiac surgery. It should be particularly useful in poor-risk patients or those in whom maximal preservation of myocardial function is essential for survival. Patients with low ejection fractions, borderline or frank congestive failure, or impending infarction or those in whom multiple cardiac procedures are planned are candidates for the use of this technique.

SUMMARY

Techniques ranging from normothermic arrest of the heart to total body hypothermia have been advocated when the coronary circulation is interrupted during cardiac operations. This study evaluated and compared the effects of three techniques of deep hypothermia of the heart on survival, function, and structural integrity of the canine myocardium.

Topical cooling with saline slush, cold selective coronary perfusion, and cold aortic root perfusion were the techniques studied. All three methods of myocardial preservation yielded good survival. Recovery of myocardial function was 40 percent of normal after two hours of topical hypothermia, 80 percent of normal after two hours of cold selective coronary perfusion, and 98 percent of normal following two hours of cold aortic root perfusion. Ultrastructural damage was greatest in hearts with the poorest recovery and least when there was good myocardial recovery.

Cold root perfusion seems to be an effective method for preserving existing myocardial function. The technique is particularly applicable in patients with poor myocardial function, impending infarction, or multiple cardiac lesions.

ACKNOWLEDGMENT

This study was supported in part by the Long Beach Heart Association and the Children's Heart Foundation of Southern California.

References

Bigelow WG, Callaghan JC, Hopps JA: General hypothermia for experimental intracardiac surgery. Ann Surg 132:531, 1950

Bloodwell RD, Goldberg LI, Braunwald E, et al: Myocardial contractility in man: the acute effects of digitalis, sympathomimetic amines and anoxic arrest. Surg Forum 9:532, 1958

Braimbridge MV, Darracott S, Clement AJ, Bitensky L, Chayen J: Myocardial deterioration during aortic valve replacement assessed by cellular biological tests. J Thorac Cardiovasc Surg 66:241, 1973

Connolly JE, Roy A, Guernsey JM, Stemmer EA: Bloodless surgery by means of profound hypothermia and circulatory arrest. Ann Surg 162:724, 1965

Ebert PA, Greenfield LJ, Austen WG, Morrow AG: Experimental comparison of methods for protecting the heart during aortic occlusion. Ann Surg 155:25, 1962

Fishman NH, Youker JE, Roe BB: Mechanical injury to the coronary arteries during operative cannulation. Am Heart J 75:26, 1968

Fuquay MC, Bucknam CN, Frajola WJ, Sirak HD: Myocardial metabolism in the hypothermic bypassed heart. J Thorac Cardiovasc Surg 44:649, 1962

Gollan F, Grace JT, Schell MW, Tysinger DS, Feaster LB: Left heart surgery in dogs during respiratory and cardiac arrest at body temperatures below 10°C. Surgery 38:363, 1955

Griepp RB, Stinson EB, Shumway NE: Profound local hypothermia for myocardial protection during open-heart surgery. J Thorac Cardiovasc Surg 66:731, 1973

Hottenrott CE, Towers B, Kurkji HJ, Maloney JV, Buckberg G: The hazard of ventricular fibrillation in hypertrophied ventricles during cardiopulmonary bypass. J Thorac Cardiovasc Surg 66:742, 1973

Hultgren HN, Miyagawa M, Buck W, Angell WW: Ischemic myocardial injury during coronary artery surgery. Am Heart J 82:624, 1971

Hurley EJ, Lower RR, Dong E Jr, Pillsbury RC, Shumway NE: Clinical experience with local hypothermia in elective cardiac arrest. J Thorac Cardiovasc Surg 47:51, 1964

Kay EB, Head LR, Nogueira C: Direct coronary artery perfusion for aortic valve surgery. JAMA 168:1767, 1968

Kay EB, Nogueira C, Suzuki A, Postico J, Mendelsohn D: Myocardial protection during aortic valvular surgery. Ann Surg (Suppl) 154:159, 1961

Moulder PV, Thompson RG: Protection of heart under hypothermia with acetylcholine arrest. Proc Soc Exper Biol Med 92:49, 1956

Ramsey HW, de la Torre A, Linhart JW, Wheat MW Jr: Complications of coronary artery perfusion. J Thorac Cardiovasc Surg 54:714, 1967

Reis RR, Staroscik RN, Rodgers BM, Enright LP, Morrow AG: Left ventricular function after ischemic cardioplegia. Arch Surg 99:815, 1969

Sanmarco MF, Marquez LA, Hall C, et al: Myocardial contractility following cardiopulmonary bypass with and without myocardial ischemia. Ann Thorac Surg 8:237, 1969

Speicher CE, Ferrigan L, Wolfson RK, Yalav EH, Rawson AJ: Cold injury of myocardium and pericardium in cardiac hypothermia. Surg Gynecol Obstet 114:659, 1962

Stemmer EA, McCart P, Stanton WW, Thibault W, Connolly JE: Functional and structural alterations in the myocardium during aortic crossclamping. J Thorac Cardiovasc Surg 66:754, 1973

Urschel HC, Greenberg JJ: Differential cardiac hypothermia for elective cardioplegia. Ann Surg 152:845, 1960

Williams D, Iben A, Hurley E, et al: Myocardial infarction during coronary artery bypass surgery. (Abstr) Am J Cardiol 31:164, 1973

Willman VL, Howard HS, Cooper T, Hanlon CR: Ventricular function after hypothermic cardiac arrest. Arch Surg 82:120, 1961

67

MANAGEMENT OF THE STENOTIC LEFT MAIN CORONARY ARTERY AND IMPAIRED LEFT VENTRICLE WITHOUT ISCHEMIC ARREST

Maruf A. Razzuk, Harold C. Urschel, Richard E. Wood, Robert Sloan, and Raymond Belanger

Direct myocardial revascularization in patients with major stenoses of the left main coronary artery or impaired left ventricles (classes III and IV) secondary to coronary artery disease is associated with high operative mortality, 12 percent [5,8] and 15 to 35 percent, respectively, significantly higher than that for any other coronary lesion. This high mortality, as well as postoperative myocardial failure, reflects ischemic injury sustained by the heart whose function should have improved from the operation. Ischemia may result from hypotension during anesthetic induction or aortic cross-clamping during cardiopulmonary bypass.

To combat anesthetic induction hypotension, the extracorporeal system is primed and put on standby with the femoral vessels exposed concomitantly with the median sternotomy. Should hypotension ensue, circulatory assist by femoral-to-femoral bypass is instituted.

To circumvent intraoperative ischemia that results from anoxic arrest often required during left coronary anastomoses, the technique of initial insertion of an aortocoronary vein graft into a diseased right coronary artery has been employed. The proximal anastomosis is placed high on the ascending aorta to provide space for proximal aortic cross-clamping.

This technique has been employed successfully in 24 patients undergoing myocardial revascularization with no operative mortality; 10 had left main artery stenosis and 14 had class III and IV ventricles.

CLINICAL MATERIAL

Twenty-four patients were treated with this technique. Ten had greater than 75 percent obstruction of the left main coronary artery and greater than 75 percent narrowing in one, two, or all three of the coronary vessels. Fourteen had triple-vessel disease with impairment of the left ventricle (class III and IV), as evidenced by LVED > 20, ejection fraction < 0.45, elevation of pulmonary artery pressure, reduced cardiac output, and three or more areas of dyssynergy on the ventriculogram. Of the 14 cases of impaired ventricle, one was an acute myocardial infarction and was operated six hours after onset; two had aneurysms that were concomitantly resected; and three had distal CO_2 (gas) endarterectomy with proximal vein graft of diffusely diseased anterior descending coronary artery.

The right coronary artery was diseased in all patients. It was grafted first and both coronary and aortic anastomoses completed. The left coronary grafts were inserted next. Average flow values in the graft were obtained with the heart fibrillating (120 cc/min), the heart fibrillating and aorta cross-clamped proximal to graft (120 cc/min), and the heart beating (60 cc/min).

TECHNIQUE

Because of the higher risk in these patients during anesthetic induction, the extracorporeal system is primed first and the femoral vessels are exposed simultaneously with the median sternotomy. Should hypotension or progressive cardiac ischemia occur, extracorporeal circulation is instituted rapidly through the femoral vessels; otherwise, routine cannulation of the ascending aorta and both vena cavae through the atrium is performed. A left ventricular sump is routinely inserted via the right superior pulmonary vein to assure constant ven-

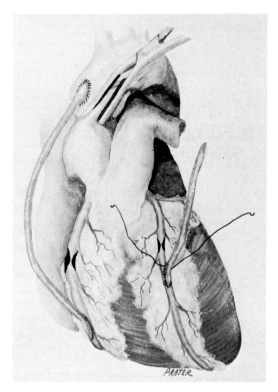

FIG. 1. Diagram illustrating right aortocoronary vein graft with proximal anastomosis placed high on the aorta to allow proximal cross-clamping.

DISCUSSION

Major stenosis of the left main coronary artery and impaired left ventricle (classes III and IV) secondary to coronary artery disease are associated with significantly high operative mortality.

Hearts afflicted with these lesions seem to have increased vulnerability to anesthetic induction and hypotension is not uncommonly encountered. Readiness to institute circulatory assist through femoral-to-femoral cardiopulmonary bypass helps prevent evolving catastrophes.

Intraoperative ischemia incurred by the myocardium as a result of ischemic arrest needed to provide quiet heart to facilitate performing the coronary anastomoses, particularly in the circumflex system, contributes to the high mortality and postoperative morbidity in this type of lesion. Local hypothermic cardioplegia or moderate hypothermia and hemodilution offer some protection to the myocardium during ischemic arrest. However, as an alternative approach, the new technique of flow augmentation by the initial placement of a right aortocoronary graft has been employed in this series of 24 patients. Ten had major left main artery stenosis, and 14 had class III and class IV ventricles. There was no operative mortality or postoperative morbidity except for postoperative low cardiac output syndrome in one patient who had an evolving myocardial infarction prior to surgery.

This technique of coronary flow augmentation, when a well-developed collateral circulation is present, immediately improves the reduced perfusion pressure in the coronary bed beyond the obstruction, avoids acute total ischemia of the myocardium, and prevents vascular stasis, which otherwise would result from ischemic arrest. These factors—namely, reduced perfusion pressure, acute ischemia, and vascular stasis—are known to produce relative ischemia of the endocardium and have been identified as factors leading to left ventricular subendocardial hemorrhagic necrosis and low output syndrome after open-heart operations.[1,2,6]

The coronary perfusion pressure, which is reduced in the distal coronary bed because of the obliterative process, sustains a further decrement during cardiopulmonary bypass. The endocardium suffers a greater degree of ischemia when ventricular fibrillation is instituted because the gradient of flow seems to favor the epicardium. However, flow measurement obtained intraoperatively on the right graft, which is employed to provide coronary flow augmentation, showed a greater degree of flow

tricular decompression. While on total cardiopulmonary bypass, the heart is electrically fibrillated and immediately the right aortocoronary vein graft inserted. The proximal anastomosis is placed high on the aorta to allow ample space for proximal aortic cross-clamping (Fig. 1). The coronary anastomoses of the left coronary arteries are completed with the heart fibrillated and, if necessary, the aorta is cross-clamped proximal to the right graft take-off. The aortic anastomoses are inserted after cessation of the cardiopulmonary bypass.

RESULTS

Six patients, two with left main artery stenosis and four with impaired left ventricle, required femoral-to-femoral circulatory assist because of complicating hypotension early during the operation. There was no operative mortality or postoperative morbidity, except for postoperative low cardiac output syndrome in one patient who had an evolving myocardial infarction prior to operation, which required supportive medical therapy for 12 hours with subsequent complete recovery.

during fibrillation than when the heart was beating.

The effect of increases in transmyocardial tension caused by fibrillation may play a greater role in impeding coronary flow in the normal or hypertrophic ventricle [2,7] than in the thin ventricle with coronary artery disease. In the latter type, ventricular transmural tension resulting from fibrillation may interfere less with coronary flow; hence more blood might reach the subendocardial plexus, which attains a large capacity in severe obliterative coronary disease.[3,4]

Experience with this series indicates the value of preparedness for institution of circulatory assist by means of femoral-to-femoral cardiopulmonary bypass in instances of anesthetic induction hypotension, and the advantage of coronary flow augmentation by initial placement of right aorto-coronary graft, which affords protection during ischemic arrest.

SUMMARY

The high mortality associated with revascularization of left main coronary stenoses and impaired left ventricles (classes III and IV) has been significantly reduced by combating hypotension during anesthetic induction and preventing ischemia resulting from anoxic arrest, often needed to facilitate the insertion of the left coronary anastomoses. This has been achieved by (1) readiness to institute circulatory assist by means of femoral-to-femoral cardiopulmonary bypass and (2) augmentation of coronary flow through immediate insertion of aorto-to-right coronary artery vein graft where anatomy permits.

References

1. Becker LC, Fortruih NJ, Pitt B: Effect of ischemia and antianginal drugs on the distribution of radioactive microspheres in the canine left ventricle. Circ Res 28:263, 1971
2. Becker RM, Shizgal HM, Dobell ARC: Distribution of coronary blood flow during cardiopulmonary bypass in pigs. Ann Thorac Surg 16:228, 1973
3. Estes EH, Entman ML, Dixon HB, Hackel DB: Vascular supply of the left ventricular wall: anatomic observations plus a hypothesis regarding acute events in coronary artery disease. Am Heart J 71: 58, 1966
4. Fulton WFM: The dynamic factors in enlargement of coronary arterial anastomoses and paradoxical changes in the subendocardial plexus. Br Heart J 26:39, 1964
5. Johnson WD, Kayser KL: An expanded indication for coronary surgery. Ann Thorac Surg 16:1, 1973
6. Moir TW, de Bra DW: Effect of left ventricular hypertension, ischemia and vasoactive drugs on the myocardial distribution of coronary flow. Circ Res 21: 65, 1967
7. Najafi H, Lal R, Khalili M, Serry C, Rogers A, Haklin M: Left ventricular hemorrhagic necrosis. Ann Thorac Surg 12:400, 1971
8. Zeft HJ, Manley JC, Huston JH, Tector AC, Johnson WD: Direct coronary surgery in patients with left main coronary artery stenosis. Circulation 46 (Suppl II):II-50, 1972

68

THE USE OF DISTAL RIGHT CORONARY ENDARTERECTOMY AND SAPHENOUS CORONARY BYPASS TO DECREASE TOTAL GRAFTS AND EXTEND OPERABILITY IN PATIENTS WITH CORONARY ARTERY DISEASE

Eugene Wallsh, Gerald Weinstein, Andrew J. Franzone, and Simon H. Stertzer

The surgical treatment of severe coronary artery disease is frequently impeded by diffuse disease in one or more vessels, making them unsuitable for bypass grafting. The distal half of the main right coronary artery is especially prone to narrowing at the crux of the heart, where it begins its course into the posterior and posterolateral left ventricle.[1] The atrioventricular continuation of the dominant right coronary artery beyond the posterior descending coronary artery is frequently obstructed at its origin. Distal right coronary artery endarterectomy combined with saphenous vein aortocoronary bypass to that vessel is used to extend operability in a diffusely involved right coronary artery. The diseased circumflex system is then revascularized via the right coronary artery through its atrioventricular groove branch, thereby avoiding a separate circumflex bypass. This report presents 29 patients treated with this technique.

MATERIAL AND METHODS

A series of 29 male patients is presented. Each patient clinically had severe angina or angina at rest. They were treated medically preoperatively with propranolol and combinations of long- and short-acting nitrates. Treatment was considered unsuccessful either because of intolerance to medication or intensification of symptoms. Each patient had coronary angiograms and left ventriculography. The common feature in this series is complete or near complete obstruction of a dominant right coronary artery extending to the crux of the heart.

Visualization of the atrioventricular groove branch beyond the crucial obstruction was variable. A portion of the posterior descending coronary artery was frequently visualized via collaterals from the left coronary artery and rarely by antegrade filling from the right coronary artery. Twenty-four patients, in addition, had greater than 70 percent stenosis in both the left anterior descending and left circumflex coronary arteries (Table 1). Three patients of this group had left mainstem lesions. Two patients required segmental left anterior descending endarterectomies. Four patients of the reported group had significant lesions only in the left anterior descending coronary artery in addition to right coronary artery obstruction. One patient had only left circumflex obstruction in addition to right coronary artery obstruction. In patients with left circumflex disease, the vessel was usually diffusely involved.

The patients' ages ranged from 42 to 74 (mean 55) years. Seventeen (59 percent) had previously documented myocardial infarctions. Ten patients (35 percent) demonstrated abnormal glucose tolerance tests or elevated fasting blood sugars. Six (21 percent) were hypertensive clini-

TABLE 1. Distribution of Obstructed Vessels

No. PTS.	RCA 100%	LAD >70%	LCAA >70%
24	+	+	+
4	+	+	
1	+		

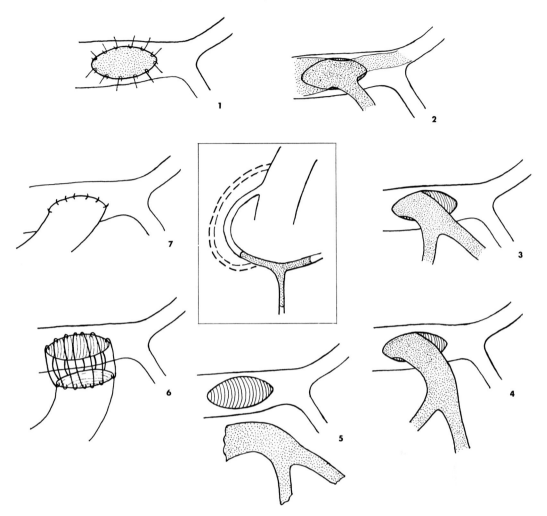

FIG. 1. Technique of distal right coronary artery endarterectomy and vein bypass. (1) Preplacement of interrupted sutures at endarterectomy site. (2)–(5) Delivery of endarterectomy specimen. (6) and (7) Completion of distal vein bypass.

cally. Nine (31 percent) had ventriculographic evidence of dyskinesia associated with elevated left ventricular end diastolic pressures. One patient required surgical resection of a portion of the posterior ventricular wall. Pre- and postoperative ECG's were followed in all patients.

The surgical technique was uniform in all patients (Fig. 1). Complete or partial cardiopulmonary bypass was employed following systemic heparinization. The ascending aorta was always the site of arterial cannulation. Venous return was separately brought out of both cavae via the right atrium. The left ventricle was vented at its apex. Left atrial pressure was continuously monitored by display on a video console.

A Bentley® bubble oxygenator was used primed with a nonblood protein-electrolyte solu-

tion. The patient was maintained normothermic during the procedure.

Aortic cross-clamping was assiduously avoided. When technically possible, continuous fibrillation was never allowed to persist throughout the bypass. Currently, the briefest periods of electrical fibrillation are used.

The obstructed right coronary artery is always the first level approached. A distal endarterectomy with saphenous coronary bypass is constructed. A longitudinal incision is made one centimeter proximal to the crux in the main right coronary artery. The incision is deepened through the outer coats of the vessel until the atheromatous core is clearly demonstrated. A brushing motion with a small curved scalpel helps with this maneuver. Before any further core mobilization is at-

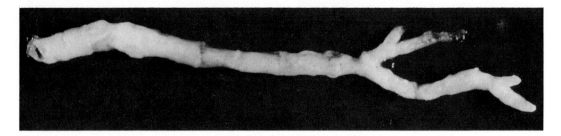

FIG. 2.   Endarterectomy specimen. Actual size.

tempted, interrupted 5-0 Tevdek® sutures are placed through the developed circumferential lip at the endarterectomy site. Care is taken to include the adjacent edge of the incised epicardium in the suture to aid in obtaining a hemostatic anastomosis. Because the lumen of the right coronary artery is not entered nor is the diseased core extensively mobilized, suture placement is done in a bloodless field. Following this, the core is mobilized. The distal portion is removed first. Mild traction is placed on the core. The most important maneuver for successful extraction is the progressive separation of the superficial layers from the core rather than traction removal. Excessive traction can cause fracture of the specimen, leaving thickened intima distally. When the bifurcation of the right coronary artery is encountered, each limb is removed separately. The proximal specimen is formed by amputation of the core 1 to 2 cm proximal to the arteriotomy incision. Extensive proximal removal of the core is unnecessary but was performed early in the series.

Confirmation of complete core removal distally is essential and is suggested by the production of backbleeding from the distal segment. The extracted specimen should have thin, translucent tapering ends (Fig. 2). Following endarterectomy, the outer layers are soft and pliable. The insertion of a narrow suction into the distal lumen produces intussusception of the distensible vessel toward the suction. Fragments of ragged wall can be visualized and removed. Palpation along the posterior descending artery and the atrioventricular groove branch may detect retained plaques. The use of a Fogarty balloon catheter has thus far been unnecessary.

Following confirmation of complete core removal, the previously placed sutures are used to construct an end-to-side anastomosis with the spatulated end of a segment of reversed saphenous vein. Probing the outlet of the anastomosis is unnecessary and unwise. The sutures on the coronary side are placed in a bloodless field; therefore misplacement is unlikely. Probing the thin-walled

coronary can result in perforation and a dissecting hematoma.

The proximal aortic anastomosis is constructed within a partially occluding vascular clamp using interrupted 5-0 Tevdek® sutures. Air is carefully vented from the bypass graft prior to establishment of blood flow.

The bypass to the left anterior descending coronary artery is constructed using interrupted 6-0 Tevdek® sutures distally and interrupted 5-0 Tevdek® sutures for the aortic anastomosis. A portion of the aortic wall is excised at the site of proximal anastomosis.

A Statham electromagnetic flow probe and console is used to determine blood flows in the grafts at the end of the procedure.

RESULTS

In this group of 29 patients, there was one operative death (3.4 percent) (Table 2). This occurred in a severely hypertensive patient with massive left ventricular hypertrophy. The surgical technique prior to and including this patient's operation used continuous induced electrical fibrillation. The patient developed a so-called stone heart and could not be weaned from bypass even

TABLE 2. Procedures and Results

PROCEDURE	NO. PTS.
DRCAE and DSCAB	28 (+ 2 LADE, 1 VR)
DRCAE and SSCAB	1
Hospital deaths	1 (3.4%)
Postop ECG infarcts	9 (32.2%)
RCA graft flows	25–200 (74) ml/min

DRCAE: distal right coronary artery endarterectomy; DSCAB: double saphenous coronary artery bypass; LADE: left anterior descending coronary artery endarterectomy; VR: ventricular resection; SSCAB: single saphenous coronary artery bypass; RCA: right coronary artery.

after balloon counterpulsation. The use of electrical fibrillation has subsequently been limited.

Graft flow rates varied from 25 to 200 ml/min (mean flow 74 ml/min). Only three flows were less than 40 ml/min. The single early closure occurred in a patient having an operative flow of 25 ml/min. The graft was probe patent at surgery without evidence of retained plaque within the vessel. This patient had ventricular arrhythmias prior to surgery. He remained without angina for three months following surgery, suddenly developing severe angina with ST segment elevations. Repeat catheterization failed to demonstrate either left anterior descending or right coronary artery grafts. At reoperation, the right coronary artery graft was closed and contained organized thrombus, indicating early closure. The endarterectomized site was patent and had scent backbleeding. Because of the original poor flow, suggesting poor runoff, no attempt was made to reconstruct the right coronary artery bypass. The LAD graft was patent with low flow. The proximal graft was severely narrowed where it was entrapped in dense scar beneath the sternum. This graft was revised producing a flow of 120 ml/min. The patient remained without angina for four months when he suddenly expired, presumably from an arrhythmia. A postmortem examination was not obtained. This was the only late death.

Six patients have been followed for more than 18 months, 10 patients for more than one year, and 12 patients for more than three months. Four patients (14 percent) have persistent mild angina easily controlled with long-acting nitrates whereas the remainder are asymptomatic.

There have been no late myocardial infarctions in this series. Postoperatively nine (32 percent) patients developed ECG changes consistent with intraoperative myocardial infarction, which usually were localized to the inferior wall. One patient developed transient ventricular arrhythmias postoperatively, whereas the others remained asymptomatic.

The only operative complication directly attributable to the endarterectomy was the development of large hematomas at the operative site in two (6.9 percent) patients. It is significant that preoperatively both of these patients clinically had sudden accelerations in their angina. At surgery, the epicardial fat over the endarterectomy site contained many small blood vessels. The fat clung tenaciously to the coronary vessel, which also had distended small blood vessels on its outer wall. It was difficult to demarcate accurately the endarterectomy plane in these vessels; once located, the remainder of the core extraction distally was routine (Fig. 3). The site of the arteriotomy was ragged and awkward to close hemostatically. Attempts to secure the bleeding with sutures while on bypass were unsuccessful. The bleeding stopped spontaneously with the administration of protamine. Within one hour, the large hematoma was smaller. Flows in the right coronary artery grafts while on bypass were below 40 ml/min. With the subsiding hematoma, flows in both grafts were found to be 60 ml/min. Both these patients developed ECG changes of a posterior wall infarction and are currently asymptomatic. The findings of adherent, neovascularized epicardium and poorly defined layers in the arterial wall were also seen in several other patients with clinical evidence of accelerated angina. The significance is unknown. The relationship to abnormal glucose tolerance or hypertension is variable.

At this time, five patients have had postoperative (mean eight months) angiograms. Four showed patency of both grafts including widely patent endarterectomized segments. One patient,

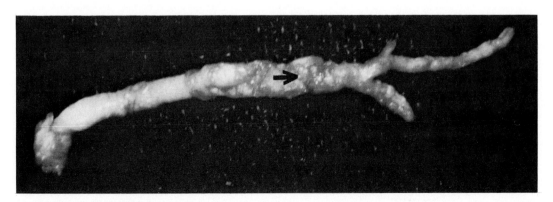

FIG. 3. Endarterectomy specimen. Arrow indicates poorly demarcated endarterectomy plane. Actual size.

who has been without angina, failed to demonstrate either left anterior descending or right coronary artery grafts.

DISCUSSION

The extensive use of selective coronary arteriography revealed patterns of obstructive coronary disease not previously appreciated, ie, a high incidence of distal lesions and diffuse sclerosis of the right coronary artery.[1] The right coronary artery is involved in 80 to 90 percent of all cases of coronary artery disease and is frequently the most extensively involved vessel.[2,3,4] In order to increase operability of this type of right coronary artery, several groups combined the technique of endarterectomy and saphenous coronary bypass to the right coronary artery with impressive results and satisfactory long-term patency.[1,2,5,6,7]

This report supports the view that operability in patients with severe disease of the right coronary artery is enhanced using distal right coronary artery endarterectomy and saphenous coronary bypass. With careful attention to the technical details of endarterectomy, and strict avoidance

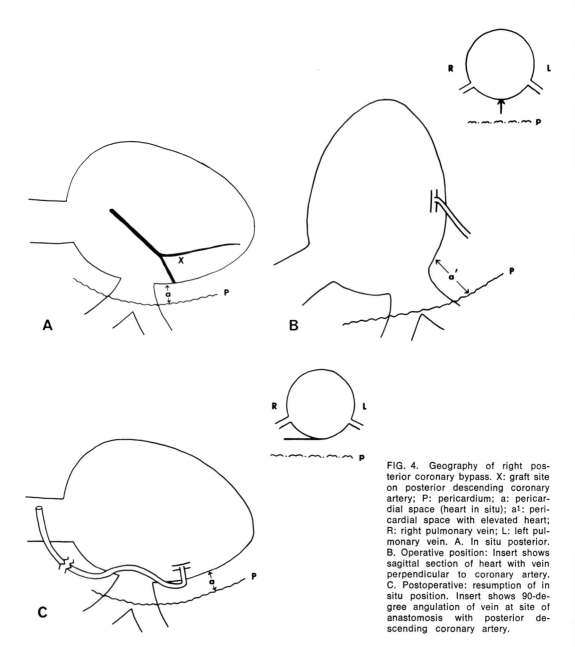

FIG. 4. Geography of right posterior coronary bypass. X: graft site on posterior descending coronary artery; P: pericardium; a: pericardial space (heart in situ); a1: pericardial space with elevated heart; R: right pulmonary vein; L: left pulmonary vein. A. In situ posterior. B. Operative position: Insert shows sagittal section of heart with vein perpendicular to coronary artery. C. Postoperative: resumption of in situ position. Insert shows 90-degree angulation of vein at site of anastomosis with posterior descending coronary artery.

FIG. 5. Photograph of angulated vein graft to left marginal coronary artery. SC: saphenous coronary bypass; a: angulated site; A: anastomosis; M: distal marginal coronary artery; RV: right ventricle; LV: left ventricle.

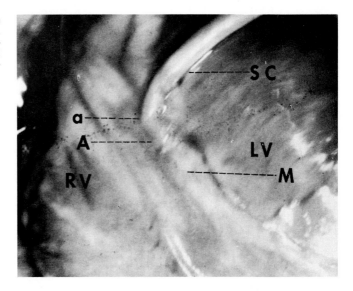

of intraoperative anoxia and fibrillation, a low mortality can be expected. The single operative death in the reported 29 patients was a massive subendocardial infarction in a patient with hypertensive myocardial hypertrophy resulting clinically in a "stone heart" and power failure after cardiopulmonary bypass. This heart was electively fibrillated during the construction of the coronary bypasses and endarterectomy. Recent reports emphasize the hazard of using this technique.[8]

The use of distal right coronary artery endarterectomy and saphenous coronary bypass can decrease the number of grafts necessary in patients with a dominant right coronary system and obstructive disease of the left circumflex coronary artery. This possibility was first suggested by Robinson.[9]

Historically, at the inception of coronary bypass surgery, patients were chosen with localized high-grade proximal obstruction restricted to one or two vessels. As good clinical results, low mortality, and long-term graft patency were established, patients with more extensive and diffuse disease were operated upon. It was generally accepted that each obstruction should be bypassed.[10] The necessity for this approach is questioned by the angiographic finding of nonfunctioning grafts in asymptomatic patients suggesting collateral perfusion from the remaining patent grafts. In addition, it has been our impression that there is an increased tendency for graft closure in bypasses directly into the descending posterior circulation, both left and right. We believe the geography of this circulation predisposes bypasses to a high closure rate (Figs. 4 and 5). A bypass graft placed near the origin of right posterior descending coronary artery or the marginal branches of the circumflex makes an almost 90-degree angle at the anastomosis with the coronary artery passing around the pulmonary veins and superior vena cava on the right and around the pulmonary artery with its pericardial reflection on the left. The predisposition to thrombosis would depend on several factors including flow rate. However, the posterior graft angulation is a constant source of turbulence and is technically difficult to avoid.

The application of the distal right coronary artery endarterectomy and saphenous coronary bypass can avoid the need for posterior grafts by perfusing the left circulation via the atrioventricular groove branch of the right coronary artery. The saphenous coronary bypass graft is aligned parallel to the main right coronary artery at the crux and, therefore, avoids angulation at the anastomosis (Fig. 6). In addition, the increased graft flow produced by opening the atrioventricular groove branch following endarterectomy may inhibit graft closure from low flow into a single, small, right posterior descending coronary artery with limited runoff.

The 29 patients in this report had severe intractable angina including rest angina. Diffuse coronary disease and complete obstruction of the right coronary artery were characteristic of this series. Twenty-four patients (83 percent) had involvement of the three major coronary artery branches. Three patients had left coronary mainstem lesions.

There was one operative death and one late death. Of the nine patients who developed ECG changes consistent with intraoperative infarction, only one developed transient ventricular irrita-

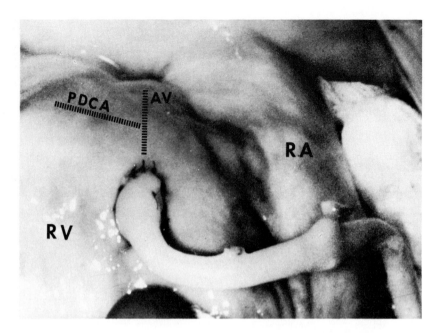

FIG. 6. Photograph of distal portion of saphenous coronary bypass endarterectomy site on right coronary artery demonstrating alignment of graft to coronary vessel. RA: right atrium; RV: right ventricle; AV: atrioventricular continuation of right coronary artery; PDCA: posterior descending coronary artery. Hatched lines: representation of distal right coronary artery and terminal division.

bility. There were no other early or late sequelae. We believe the high rate of intraoperative infarction (32.2 percent) is related to the critical coronary circulation as well as to the operative technique. Two patients in this series developed ST segment elevations shortly after traction sutures were used to steady the right coronary artery during the endarterectomy. When traction was discontinued, the changes subsided. Following rapid construction of the distal saphenous coronary bypass, the graft was temporarily perfused through the proximal vein orifice. This technique was used in order to minimize anoxia in the distribution of the vessel. Neither patient developed significant ECG changes. Among the nine patients developing ECG changes, two developed hematomas that interfered with graft flow. A third patient was hypotensive following surgery because cortisone was inadvertently withheld. This patient had been receiving steroids for ulcerative colitis. It would appear that interruption of coronary blood flow in these patients with severely diminished coronary circulation was responsible for the ECG changes. This suggests that intraoperative infarctions can be avoided by alteration in the surgical technique, ie, minimal local anoxia during graft construction.

Of the survivors, 86 percent are asymptomatic and 14 percent have mild persistent angina.

All surviving patients have experienced significant improvement over their preoperative state.

SUMMARY AND CONCLUSION

Distal right coronary endarterectomy and saphenous coronary bypass were used to extend operability and decrease the number of grafts in 29 patients with a dominant right coronary artery. Indications for surgery were intractable angina and rest angina. Features of this group include involvement of the anterior descending coronary artery, left circumflex coronary artery, and near or complete occlusion of a dominant right coronary artery including the atrioventricular branch. The proximal posterior descending coronary artery was usually involved. A coronary bypass to the anterior descending coronary artery, as well as a distal right coronary endarterectomy and saphenous coronary bypass performed at the crux of the dominant right coronary artery, were the only procedures performed. The endarterectomy opens the atrioventricular branch supplying the left circulation, as well as providing flow into the posterior descending coronary artery. Twenty-eight patients survived (mortality: 3.4 percent), four of whom developed mild angina. The use of distal right coronary endarterectomy appears to increase the operability and decrease the use of triple grafts in patients with advanced disease, without increasing the surgical risk.

References

1. Cohen L: Surgical Treatment of Acute Myocardial Ischemia. Mt Kisco, Futura, 1973, pp. 44–63
2. Groves LK, Loop FD, Silver GM: Endarterectomy as a supplement to coronary artery-saphenous vein bypass surgery. J Thorac Cardiovasc Surg 64:514–22, 1972
3. Robinson G, Kaplitt MJ, Philips P, Patel B: Complete surgical correction of the totally occluded and diffusely diseased right coronary artery. J Thorac Cardiovasc Surg 60:504–9, 1970
4. Effler DB, Sones FM Jr, Favaloro R, Groves LK: Coronary endarterectomy with patch-graft reconstruction. Ann Surg 162:590–601, 1965
5. Danielson GK, Gan GT, David GD: Early results of vein bypass grafts for coronary artery disease. Mayo Clin Proc 48:487–91, 1973
6. Urschel HC, Razzuk MA: Reconstruction of the left anterior descending coronary artery. JAMA 216:141–43, 1971
7. Urschel HC, Razzuk MA, Wood RE, Paulson DL: Distal CO_2 coronary artery endarterectomy and proximal vein bypass graft. Ann Thorac Surg 14: 10–15, 1972
8. Hottenrott CE, Towers B, Kurkji HJ, et al: The hazard of ventricular fibrillation in hypertrophied ventricles during cardiopulmonary bypass. J Thorac Cardiovasc Surg 66:742–53, 1973
9. Urschel HC, Razzuk MA, Nathan MJ, et al: Combined gas (CO_2) endarterectomy and vein bypass graft for patients with coronary artery disease. Ann Thorac Surg 10:119–30, 1970
10. Johnson WD, Flemma RJ, Lepley D Jr, Ellison EH: Extended treatment of severe coronary artery disease. Ann Surg 170:460–70, 1969

69

THE ROLE OF ENDARTERECTOMY IN CURRENT MYOCARDIAL REVASCULARIZATION

Edward B. Diethrich, Bicher Barmada, David Goldfarb, and Martin J. Kaplitt

Aortocoronary artery bypass is employed in many centers for the relief of symptoms related to coronary arterial obstruction. Postoperative follow-up studies have documented its success, showing a five-year patency rate (75 percent) with low incidences of mortality and morbidity (Reul et al, 1972; Griffith et al, 1973; Rees et al, 1971).

The combined application of bypass with coronary endarterectomy has increased still further the number of patients to be benefited by operation. Even in the presence of total occlusion of the proximal arterial segment, a distal obstructing core can be removed, and revascularization can be provided through a reversed autogenous saphenous vein grafted to the endarterectomized segment.

In our experience, carbon dioxide gas has been a useful tool in the endarterectomy procedure. Its application to coronary endarterectomy was begun in 1967 (Sawyer et al, 1967a and b) after it was proven successful in opening peripheral vessels over long distances (Kaplitt et al, 1971a and b). Reopening of the full length of a totally occluded or diffusely diseased coronary artery, especially the right, was shown to be possible with this technique, with the added benefit of preservation of the arterial side branches. While this capability led to the greater success of coronary endarterectomy and to more favorable results than obtained with mechanical procedures, there were still some drawbacks to its application, including incomplete distal endarterectomy, residual proximal core, stenosis of the arteriotomy, and extra-adventitial dissection (Absolon et al, 1971). These problems caused early investigators to abandon total endarterectomy of the coronary arteries in favor of distal endarterectomy with bypass (Urschel et al, 1969, 1971). Our application of this procedure and follow-up evaluations of its efficacy have given certain indications for its most appropriate uses.

MATERIAL AND METHODS

Between August 1971 and June 28, 1973, four hundred patients at the Arizona Heart Institute received aortocoronary bypass grafts with reversed segments of autogenous saphenous vein. Fifty-eight of those patients (14 percent) underwent combined carbon dioxide gas endarterectomy with bypass, sometimes of more than one coronary artery. The percentages of distribution of the disease among the three major coronary arteries and the number of endarterectomies performed are summarized in Table 1. The age range of patients treated was from 32 to 75 years, with 18.1 percent in their fourth decade of life and 56.3 percent in their fifth. A summary of the bypass grafts performed in conjunction with carbon dioxide gas endarterectomy and their distribution in the coronary arterial circulation is presented in Tables 2 and 3. In one patient, the endarterectomy of the right coronary artery was closed by vein patch-graft angioplasty, and a saphenous vein was grafted

TABLE 1. Summary Distribution of Carbon Dioxide Gas Endarterectomy to Coronary Arteries in 58 Patients Requiring Bypass Grafts of One or More Coronary Arteries

LOCATION	NO. ENDARTERECTOMIES	% OF TOTAL
RCA	56	91.8
LAD	3	4.9
CFX	2	3.3
Total	61	100.0

RCA: right coronary artery; LAD: left anterior descending coronary artery; CFX: circumflex coronary artery.

TABLE 2. Distribution of Saphenous Vein Bypass Grafts Used in Conjunction with Carbon Dioxide Gas Endarterectomy in 58 Patients

BYPASS TYPE AND LOCATION	NO. BYPASSES	ENDARTERECTOMY LOCATION	NO. ENDARTERECTOMIES	NO. PTS.
Single				
RCA	14	RCA	15	14
LAD	3	LAD	2	3
Double				
RCA and LAD	64	RCA and LAD	32 and 1	32
RCA and CFX	2	RCA	1	1
Triple				
RCA and LAD and CFX	21	RCA and CFX	7 and 2	7
Quadruple				
RCA and LAD and CFX and CFX(Bi)	4	RCA	1	1
Total	108		61	58

RCA: right coronary artery; LAD: left anterior descending coronary artery; CFX: circumflex coronary artery; CFX(Bi): bifurcation of the circumflex coronary artery.

TABLE 3. Summary Distribution of Saphenous Vein Bypass Grafts in 58 Patients Requiring Carbon Dioxide Gas Endarterectomy of One or More Coronary Arteries

LOCATION	NO. BYPASSES	% OF TOTAL
RCA	55	50.9
LAD	43	39.8
CFX	10	9.3
Total	108	100

RCA: right coronary artery; LAD: left anterior descending coronary artery; CFX: circumflex coronary artery.

from the ascending aorta to the left anterior descending coronary artery. In all other cases, the distal segment of one or more coronary arteries was endarterectomized, with subsequent vein graft to the endarterectomized segment. Immediately after suspension of cardiopulmonary bypass, 89.6 percent of the patients were evaluated arteriographically to determine the radiographic patency of the graft(s) and the quality of the distal runoff. In addition, flow rates and pressure gradients across the bypassed and endarterectomized arteries were measured.

In association with distal carbon dioxide gas endarterectomy, segmental endarterectomy to the left anterior descending coronary artery was performed in four cases using conventional methods. In another four cases, associated cardiac lesions were also treated during operation for myocardial revascularization. In one of these patients a dyskinetic left ventricular apex was plicated; in two others, left ventricular aneurysms were resected; and a fourth underwent aortic valve replacement.

RESULTS

Fifty patients had an excellent postoperative course and were discharged in good condition. Four patients died (6.9 percent), two of them of severe cardiac lesions that had been associated with preoperative ventricular failure. From six months to one year following operation, three others died at home. Four patients experienced postoperative complications, including secondary wound closure requiring reoperation in two cases, and two cases of myocardial infarction, one of which was uncomplicated. The other patient with a myocardial infarction had the further complication of associated arrhythmia, which necessitated the insertion of a permanent transvenous pacemaker (Table 4).

TABLE 4. Postoperative Complications in Patients with CO_2 Gas Endarterectomy

COMPLICATIONS	NO. PTS.
Disruption of sternal wound	2[a]
Myocardial infarction	1
Myocardial infarction with arrhythmia leading to insertion of pacemaker	1

[a]*One patient also had V + P for bleeding stress ulcer.*

TECHNICAL CONSIDERATIONS

Experience from other series of patients has proved that coronary endarterectomy with carbon dioxide gas is feasible, even in the presence of extensive and diffuse arterial disease. Attention to technical details, however, is mandatory if satisfactory results are to be obtained. The occasional observer may look upon the procedure as one of technical simplicity because in many instances it is accomplished quickly and without difficulty.

Although the coronary artery to be treated is occluded or severely involved with diffuse atherosclerosis, cardiopulmonary bypass should be established because the injected carbon dioxide gas rapidly passes into the coronary arterial circulation through the side branches and the distal collateral channels that it opens. A high carbon dioxide concentration in the coronary circulation causes bradycardia with a resultant decrease in cardiac output.

While there are several tested methods of performing coronary carbon dioxide gas endarterectomy, there is one that we have found to be superior. The procedure is begun with palpation of the distal portion of the artery to be treated. If the extension of the disease core is found to require the application of carbon dioxide gas, the gas is introduced subadventitially using a 25-gauge needle at a flow rate of 15 liters per minute along a short length of the distal segment (Fig. 1). When either the left anterior descending or the circumflex coronary artery is being treated, the artery should be cross-clamped just beyond its bifurcation. A longitudinal arteriotomy is then made at the point at which the gas has been introduced,

FIG. 2. Facing page: Intraoperative angiogram showing patent vein graft and good distal anastomosis.

and the adventitial layer is retracted with fine stay sutures. A specially designed gas spatula of appropriate size is then inserted distally between the obstructing core and the adventitia. The carbon dioxide gas can thus be delivered to the most distal ramification of the artery. Once this has been accomplished, gentle traction on the core will deliver the entire diseased specimen with its tapered end and its intact side branches. When the intimal core is removed through the arteriotomy, good back flow of blood can be observed within the artery. When a particularly long core is present (the length varies from 2 cm to 10 cm), some resistance may be encountered. This problem is best solved by introducing additional gas more distally with either a 25-gauge or a 26-gauge needle. Forcing the gas spatula may result in extraadventitial dissection, which will cause technical failure of the operation.

After the endarterectomy is complete and good back flow has been demonstrated, the bypass is begun. A reversed segment of autogenous saphenous vein is sutured end-to-side to the arteriotomy with No. 5-0 monofilament material. The proximal end of the vein graft is then sutured to the ascending aorta in the routine end-to-side manner. This technique is equally applicable to the left anterior descending and the circumflex coronary arteries.

EVALUATION

In all 58 cases of endarterectomy with bypass, intraoperative studies were conducted immediately after discontinuation of cardiopulmonary bypass. The testing included cineangiography, blood flow measurement through both the vein graft and the endarterectomized segment, and pressure-gradient recordings in the vein graft.

The methods and materials applied in the conduct of the intraoperative cineangiography have been described elsewhere (Diethrich et al, 1972). Of the 49 grafts tested in this manner, all were immediately patent with good distal anastomosis (Fig. 2). Four cases in which the right coronary artery was treated showed poor distal runoff (Fig. 3).

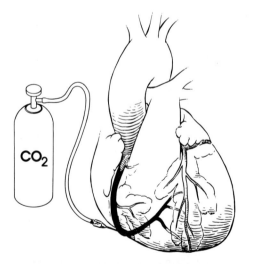

FIG. 1. After the extent of the disease core has been determined, carbon dioxide gas is introduced subadventitially through a 25-gauge needle at a flow of 15 liters per minute along a short length of the distal arterial segment.

FIG. 3. Facing page: Intraoperative angiogram showing patent vein graft with poor distal runoff.

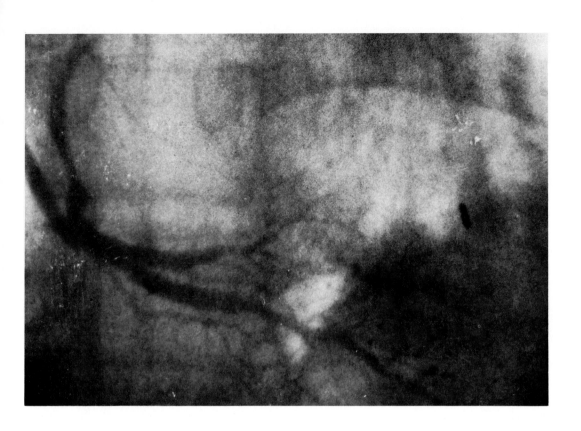

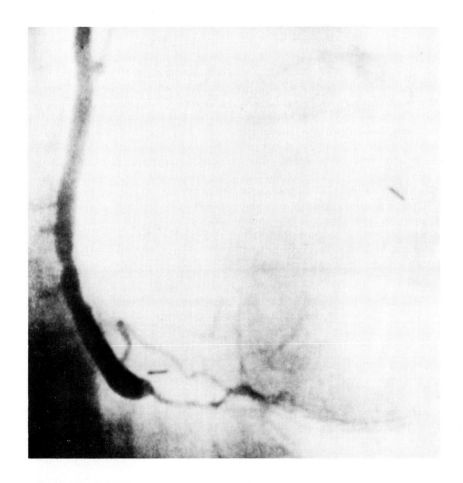

TABLE 5. Postoperative Follow-up of Patients with CO_2 Gas Endarterectomy

	CLINICALLY		TREADMILL		RECATHETERIZATION 1 YEAR LATER
	3 mos	1 yr	3 mos	1 yr	
Improved	28	22	16	8	4 patients with all grafts patent
Nonimproved	1	4	4	1	1 patient with occluded graft but patent
Equivocal	2	–	1	2	endarterectomized segment; 1 patient
					with grafts open (at autopsy)
Total	31	26	21	11	6 patients

Flow studies were carried out in 45 of the 58 cases. A Statham electromagnetic flow probe and meter were used to demonstrate immediate restoration of flow (average of 57 cc/min) through all endarterectomized arteries. This figure compares favorably with flow measurements obtained from venous bypass grafts sutured to non-endarterectomized arteries. Flows as high as 115 to 140 cc/min were observed in over 15 cases of right coronary artery endarterectomy with bypass.

The pressure gradient for the bypass graft was measured intraoperatively in 44 of the 58 patients. Comparative studies were performed with the graft occluded and with it open and showed a range of 0 to 124 mm Hg and an average gradient of 47 mm Hg.

FOLLOW-UP

Fifty-four patients were discharged in good condition 10 days after surgery. Of these, 31 were evaluated three months postoperatively. Maximum-stress exercise testing was negative or showed improved exercise tolerance in 16 of the 21 patients who underwent that type of evaluative study (Table 5).

One year after operation 26 patients were reevaluated; 23 were clinically asymptomatic and had negative stress electrocardiograms. Five underwent repeat arteriography, which revealed patent grafts with good distal runoff in four cases (Fig. 4,

Table 6). The fifth had an occluded right coronary artery graft, but excellent retrograde distal filling of the endarterectomized segment was observed to come from the left anterior descending coronary artery. Three patients died six, seven, and 11 months postoperatively of unrelated causes.

DISCUSSION

With the rapid increase in the number of candidates for direct myocardial revascularization, there is a need to investigate all possible methods of increasing blood flow through the coronary circulation. The most effective treatment of coronary arterial disease is the immediate reestablishment of pulsatile blood flow. The restoration of vascular continuity between the aorta and the distal coronary vascular bed has been achieved with autogenous saphenous vein grafts and with endarterectomy. The combined approach to revascularization has further increased the number of patients who can be treated by the direct approach.

From its inception in 1968, carbon dioxide gas endarterectomy has not gained wide acceptance, primarily because many failures have been associated with high mortality rates. The condition of the arterial lining after endarterectomy caused concern and pessimism regarding long-term patency of the vessel, but our series indicates that careful attention to the technical application of the procedure will usually assure complete re-

TABLE 6. Follow-up on all CO_2 Gas Endarterectomy Patients One Year after Operation (August 1971 to January 1974)

	AUG 71 TO JULY 73	AUG 73 TO JAN 74	TOTAL	%
Aortocoronary bypass	400	114	514	100
CO_2 Gas endarterectomy	58	12	70	13.6
Mortality	4	1	5	7.1
Morbidity	4	0	4	5.7
Recatheterization	5(+1)[a]	5	10	1.3
Open grafts	4(+1)[a]	4	8	80

[a]*One patient was found to have patent graft at autopsy seven months after surgery. He died of unrelated causes.*

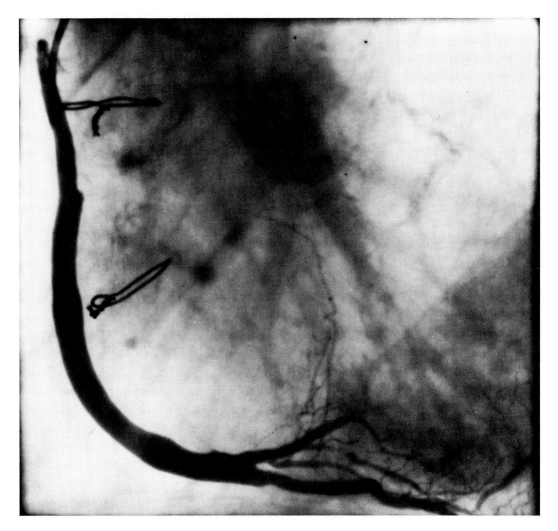

FIG. 4. Arteriogram 2 years after operation, showing patent vein graft and good distal runoff.

moval of the obstructing core with resultant good back flow.

Because long-term patency is the primary concern, intraoperative arteriography with pressure and flow studies are necessary indicators of the potential for long-range success. Studies demonstrating good distal runoff with high flow rates through the graft (above 40 cc/min) correlate with adequate distal cleanout and are predictive of long-term patency. On the other hand, poor distal runoff and flow rates below 30 cc/min are associated with inadequate removal and late occlusion of the graft.

Several groups of investigators reported their experience with the carbon dioxide gas endarterectomy technique in a combined report on 177 patients presented at the 37th Annual Meeting of the American College of Chest Physicians.

The patency rate for these combined series was as high as 90 percent for right coronary artery endarterectomy after the first postoperative month. Follow-up arteriography between one and two years after operation showed a reduction in patency from 50 to 60 percent.

Our experience has given several examples of multiple narrowing of the proximal and middle segments of arteries that appeared at follow-up one year after surgery to be normal and patent (Fig. 5). Two years after the operation, these segmental narrowings were observed to have progressed to total obstruction of the vessel (Fig. 6). In those cases in which this was seen to occur, however, the distal right and posterior descending coronary arteries were not affected. Although this is usually not apparent with right coronary arteriography, it can be observed when the left coronary

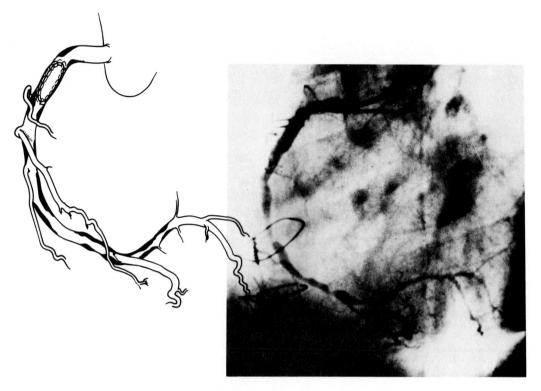

FIG. 5. Follow-up arteriogram taken one year after surgery, showing slight segmental occlusion of the vein graft.

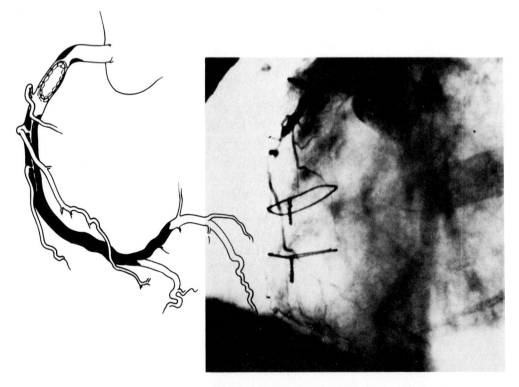

FIG. 6. Follow-up arteriogram taken 2 years after operation showing total occlusion of the vein graft that was only partially occluded one year earlier (see Fig. 5.)

artery is injected and fills the other vessels in retrograde fashion.

Because this phenomenon has been consistently observed when an artery is totally occluded or distally involved, we have adopted as routine the modified approach of carbon dioxide gas endarterectomy of the distal artery, with venous bypass from the aorta to the endarterectomized segment (Absolon et al, 1971). This technique obviates the need for removing the proximal obstructing core and assures a satisfactory inflow through the venous graft to the cleared distal artery. By avoiding blind endarterectomy through a proximal arteriotomy, the possibility of leaving atherosclerotic material at the bifurcation of the right coronary artery is reduced.

A recognized theoretical disadvantage of the bypass technique is that it eliminates all proximal side branches of the right coronary artery. Provision of adequate inflow to the left coronary circulation may, however, maintain collaterals that serve to keep the side branches open.

Once carbon dioxide gas endarterectomy with bypass had been demonstrated to be an effective means of restoring the function of the right coronary artery, its application was extended to the left coronary artery as well. In one case, both the left anterior descending coronary artery and the distal right coronary artery were endarterectomized and double vein grafts were applied. Two other cases involved simple left anterior descending endarterectomy with bypass.

Later the treatment was applied to the circumflex coronary artery, in spite of its difficult anatomical position. We have had two cases of combined circumflex-right coronary endarterectomy. In both cases, vein grafts to the endarterectomized segments of both vessels showed good angiographic runoff, and an excellent flow rate was observed in one case.

The use of the combined procedure of endarterectomy and saphenous vein bypass grafting has increased the number of candidates for direct coronary arterial surgery. It is apparent, as indications for the application of coronary arteriography are becoming liberalized, that the number of patients presented for operation is increasing. Originally the operation was limited to those patients with discrete proximal lesions in one of the main coronary arteries. Now, obstructing lesions in all areas of the coronary arterial tree are being bypassed. The preoperative coronary arteriogram frequently fails to reveal the presence of atherosclerotic disease at the proposed site of distal anastomosis. Under these circumstances, local endarterectomy will provide a suitable graft site. We had four such cases in our series, and segmental endarterectomy permitted satisfactory anastomosis to the distal left anterior descending coronary artery.

Because carbon dioxide gas endarterectomy is not always the appropriate treatment for coronary atherosclerosis, patients should be evaluated carefully before selection. The candidate for this type of surgery should have certain disease characteristics. First, he should have dominant right coronary circulation in which the right coronary artery is the primary source of blood supply to the posterior left ventricle and is directly connected with the posterior descending coronary artery. Second, the right coronary artery should be either totally occluded or severely affected by diffuse atherosclerosis. Proximal, middle, and even distal isolated lesions can be satisfactorily bypassed, using a reversed autogenous saphenous vein graft, so endarterectomy is not necessary in such cases. When the disease is extensive, however, even to the point that the posterior descending coronary artery is involved, application of the carbon dioxide gas endarterectomy technique will restore blood flow through the vessel by permitting extraction of the central obstructing core and opening of multiple arterial side branches.

SUMMARY

The combined technique of carbon dioxide gas endarterectomy with reversed autogenous saphenous vein bypass to the endarterectomized segment has been generally effective in our series of 58 patients. Proper evaluation for candidate selection is critical, and careful attention to the technical aspects of the endarterectomy procedure is essential to its long-term success. Intraoperative angiography and flow and pressure gradient tests performed in 49 of the 58 cases proved to be indicative of the actual long-term results observed at follow-up three months, one year, and two years postoperatively. The mortality rate in the series was 6.9 percent, with four immediate postoperative deaths and three late deaths, six, seven, and 11 months after surgery. Of the 26 patients reevaluated one year after operation, 23 were asymptomatic under maximum-stress exercise conditions. Five patients were recatheterized, and one right coronary artery bypass graft was seen to be occluded. In spite of this loss of patency, blood flow through the endarterectomized segment was supplied in distal retrograde fashion from the left.

The addition of carbon dioxide gas endarterectomy to the bypass technique provides a means of surgical treatment of coronary atherosclerosis that has greatly increased the number of patients who can be helped by direct coronary revascularization.

References

Absolon KB, Lewis EH, Bashour F: Simultaneous peripheral coronary endarterctomy and bypass graft in coronary artery obstruction. Surg Gynecol Obstet 132:1083–85, 1971

Diethrich EB, Kinard SA, Scappatura E, et al: Intraoperative coronary arteriography. Am J Surg 124:815–18, 1972

Griffith LSC, Achuff SC, et al: Changes in intrinsic coronary circulation and segmenta; ventricular motion after coronary bypass graft surgery. N Engl J Med 288:589–95, 1973

Kaplitt MJ, Philips P, Patel B, Robinson G: Coronary gas endarterectomy. Procedure of choice for diffuse coronary artery disease. JAMA 215:913–15, 1971a

Kaplitt MJ, Robinson G: Coronary gas endarterectomy. Am Heart J 81:136–40, 1971b

Reis G, Bristow JD, Kremkau EL, et al: Influence of aortocoronary bypass surgery on left ventricular performance. N Engl J Med 284:1116–20, 1971

Reul GJ, Morris GC, Jr, Howell JF, et al: Current concepts in coronary surgery: a critical analysis of 1,287 patients. Ann Thorac Surg 14:243–59, 1972

Sawyer PN, Kaplitt MJ, Sobel S, Dimaio D: Application of gas endarterectomy to atherosclerotic peripheral vessels and coronary arteries. Circulation (Suppl I):163–68, 1967a

Sawyer PN, Kaplitt MJ, Sobel S, et al: Experimental and clinical experience with coronary gas endarterectomy. Arch Surg 95:736–42, 1967b

Urschel HC, Razzuk MA, Miller ER, et al: Vein bypass graft and carbon dioxide gas endarterectomy for coronary artery occlusive disease. JAMA 210:1725, 1969

Urschel HC, Razzuk MA: Reconstruction of the left anterior descending coronary artery. Proximal vein bypass and distal gas endarterectomy. JAMA 16:141–43, 1971

70

A PROGNOSTIC INDEX FOR PREDICTION OF AORTOCORONARY BYPASS GRAFT CLOSURE WITH SPECIAL REFERENCE TO ENDARTERECTOMY

VICTOR PARSONNET, LAWRENCE GILBERT,
and ISAAC GIELCHINSKY

The reputation of the saphenous vein aortocoronary bypass hinges, in large part, on the long-term patency of the graft. At one year the sum of the immediate and late closures varies between 5 and 35 percent.[1,4,9,10] At least some of these failures have been caused by a degenerative process of subintimal proliferation.[7]

It appears that the results of direct anastomosis of the internal mammary artery are statistically better than the vein bypass.[6] There is a possibility that case selection invalidates direct comparison of one method with the other. One difference that is immediately obvious is seen in a report of a series of internal mammary artery bypass procedures where endarterectomy was *never* performed, while in our experience endarterectomy is necessary in 20 percent of cases (or about 10 percent of vessels). Thus in comparing one type of procedure to another one must evaluate features of prognostic importance, such as collateral and competitive circulation, graft flow rates, the diameters of the vein and artery, and the severity and distribution of the arteriosclerotic lesion.

An intuitive reaction is to regard the problem of early graft closure as more or less predictable. Surely all of us have inserted a bypass into a severely diseased artery, knowing that the probability of short-term, let alone long-term patency, was extremely poor.

To test this hypothesis, we use a prognostic index that assigns point values, or demerits, for difficulties encountered at surgery. The intent of this report is to describe this index, to indicate some of the early results of the study, and to evaluate in more detail one of the factors that has been said to increase the chance of graft closure, namely endarterectomy.

METHOD

The scoring of the index was designed to give a value of 10 as a "perfect" bypass, and zero to one with no chance of remaining patent. Although the total number of possible demerits exceeds 10, initial experience with the index has shown that it is hard to accumulate a total of 10 points, except in disastrous situations. The values for the deductions are estimates based upon information found in the literature, and upon surgical judgment. In approximate order of importance, determinants of patency were the following:

1. Competitive flow. This judgment was difficult to quantify, but estimates of the amount of competitive flow were based upon the volume of flow from the open arteriotomy, the presence or absence of reactive hyperemia, and the increase of flow that followed compression of the proximal artery (one to three demerits).
2. Endarterectomy. Establishment of demerit values were based upon the technical difficulty encountered, the ease of extraction of the atheromatous plug, and the presence of distal intimal flaps (one to two demerits).
3. Uncorrected proximal or distal stenosis (one to two demerits).
4. Miscellaneous factors. Various less common technical factors may come into play, such as difficulty in performance of the anastomosis, extra suture lines in the vein (for reinforcement of an anastomosis, Y-grafts, shortening or lengthening the bypass), atheromatous

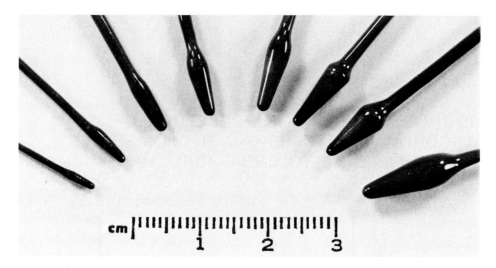

FIG. 1. Calibrated, flexible probes used in aortocoronary bypass (manufactured by United States Catheter and Instrument Corporation, Billerica, Massachusetts).

debris in the anastomotic lumen (one to two demerits).

5. Small artery or vein. The external diameter of the vein was measured or estimated from the size of the flow probe that fit comfortably on the vessel. The arterial lumen was measured with intraluminal calibrated probes shown in Figure 1 (one to two demerits).

6. Blood flow. When the index was first used, blood flow in the graft of less than 30 cc was counted as a demerit, but in the present index it was excluded for reasons explained below (Table 1).

The sum of the demerits for each bypass was subtracted from the perfect score of 10. Following aortocoronary bypass and just before closure of the sternum, flow in the bypass graft was measured with a Statham electromagnetic square wave flow meter * with flow probes of 2 to 4 mm ID, most commonly 3 mm. Blood flow and mean systemic arterial blood pressure were measured simultaneously. Reactive hyperemia was measured after 10 to 30 seconds of occlusion of the bypass graft.

* Statham Flowmeter Model No. SP 2201.

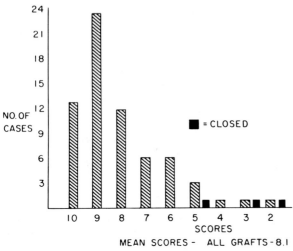

MEAN SCORES -   ALL GRAFTS - 8.1

LAD - 8.0

R - 8.0

C - 8.3

PERFECT SCORE IN ONLY 1/5

FIG. 2. Index scores in 66 cases. Note that there were 6 with scores of 5 or less, and closures occurred only in that group.

TABLE 1. Scoring for Coronary Artery Reconstruction

| | RECIPIENT ARTERY | | |
	LAD	R	C
Diameter of artery (mm)	2.0	2.5	2.5
Diameter of vein (mm)	3.0	3.0	3.0
Mean blood flow (and R.H.)	50 + 20	25 + 10	15 + 0
Prognostic index (0-10)	7	6	4
Technical defect (demerits)			
Competition (1–3)	–	–	3
Artery diameter			
<2.0 (1)	1	–	–
<1.5 (2)	–	–	–
Vein diameter >3.5 (1)	–	–	–
Endarterectomy (1–3)	–	2	–
Technical difficulty (1–3)	1	–	1
Extra suture lines (1–2)	–	–	–
Debris in lumen (1)	–	1	–
Vein length, too long/too short (1–2)	–	–	1
Kink or twist in vein (1)	–	–	1
Absent proximal runoff (1)	–	1	–
Stenosis of distal runoff (1–2)	–	–	–
Vein pathology (1–2)	1	–	–
Total demerits	3	4	6

Before discharge from the hospital, usually within 10 to 14 days, a postoperative graft angiogram was performed.

The quality of the bypass graft at angiography is also evaluated, using another index system similar to one described by Prian and Diethrich, but discussion of this index is not pertinent to this report.[3]

RESULTS

Sixty-six grafts have been studied in 34 patients (Table 2). The arteries most commonly bypassed were the LAD and right (44 percent and 35 percent respectively), and the most frequent combinations were the LAD and right, or

TABLE 2. Graft Patency in Patients with Prognostic Index (2/1/1974)

	NO.	%
Patients in Series	240	
Patients with prognostic index	34	
Grafts	66 (1.9/pt.)	
Closures	3	4.2

TABLE 3. Location of Grafts (2/1/1974)

AREA	NO.	%
LAD	29	44
R	23	35
C	12	18
D	2	3

LAD-circumflex-right (Table 3). There was an average of 1.9 grafts per patient.

Mean arterial flow in a slightly larger series of grafts (including the 66 in this study) was 54 cc per minute, with no significant difference between the arteries bypassed (Table 4).

TABLE 4. Graft Flows (2/1/1974)

ARTERY	NO. CASES	RANGE	MEAN
LAD	35	0–140	53.3
R	31	12–130	51.4
C	15	10–140	56.5
D	2	16–155	–
Total	83	0–155	54.0

The mean prognostic index was 8.1 for all vessels, with no difference between the vessels (Figure 2). Perfect scores were slightly more common in the left anterior descending artery but were recorded in only 20 percent of the bypasses. Deductions were most commonly taken for competitive flow and small artery size (Table 5).

TABLE 5. Reasons for Demerits (2/1/1974)

REASON	NO. CASES
Competitive flow	20
Small artery (<2.5 mm)	20
One-way runoff	10
Debris in distal lumen	8
Endarterectomy	6
Technical features[a]	16

[a]*Extra suture lines; difficult anastomosis, kinks in vein, distal stenosis, vein pathology or size.*

There were six cases that had index value of 5 or less, and all three of the graft closures occurred in that group. With respect to flow, all three failures occurred when the flow was less than 30 cc per minute, actual values being 8, 10, and 22 cc per minute (Fig. 3). Other features in common in the three occluded vessels were small caliber of the recipient artery in three, and absence of retrograde flow in two (Table 6). Two of the grafts that occluded were one in a double bypass, and one in a triple bypass.

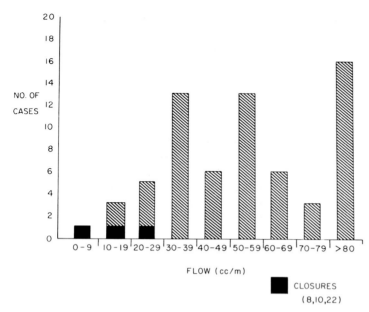

FIG. 3. Mean graft flow. Closures occurred only in grafts with flows of less than 30 cc/min.

DISCUSSION

All the technical flaws shown in Table 5 will produce impairment of flow by various mechanisms, such as impedance of run-off, turbulence, thrombosis on roughened surfaces or suture lines, or peripheral embolization. Therefore, although measurement of flow alone is essential in predicting graft patency, it does not reveal the *reasons* for low flow.[11] For example, demerits were frequently taken because the recipient artery was too small. An artery of less than 1.5 mm in diameter may contribute to graft occlusion because of both inadequate runoff and difficulty in performing a technically perfect anastomosis. This one observation has already led to modification of our operative technique, where the left anterior descending anastomosis is now performed as proximal on the artery as possible where the artery is likely to be large.

Competitive flow through the host vessel is detrimental to prolonged patency of the graft, and

this suggests that careful judgment must be used in selecting the arteries to be bypassed. Intraoperative identification of competitive flow can be assessed by comparing the mean intraluminal pressure distal to the temporarily occluded graft, to the mean pressure in the opened and functioning graft (which pressure will be the same as the coronary artery pressure proximal to the stenosis). Competition can also be assessed by the less quantitative method of observing the volume of flow through the arteriotomy, measuring the increase in mean graft flow while compressing the proximal side of the recipient artery, and by demonstrating absence of reactive hyperemia. Elimination of the problem of competing flows is probably not possible, because the selection of the artery to be bypassed is based on preoperative evaluation of the arteriogram and because there is no convenient way to assess the degree of stenosis at the operating table without actually opening the artery. Once this is done, bypass, rather than repair of the arteriotomy, is preferable. Thus if only one vessel is chosen for bypass and there proves to be significant competitive flow, the wisdom of the choice must be ques-

TABLE 6. Analysis of Closures (2/1/1974)

PT.	AGE/SEX	ARTERY	FLOW CC/M	PROBLEMS ENCOUNTERED	SCORE
GD	61/M	Lat. br. of circ (1 of 3)	10	Small artery (1.0–1.5mm), 2 extra suture lines to lengthen graft	2
NU	53/M	LAD (1 of 2)	8	Small artery (<1.5 mm), no retrograde arterial flow	3
JO	54/F	LAD (1 of 2)	22	Endarterectomy, small artery (<1.5 mm), no retrograde arterial flow	5

FIG. 4. Mean flows in 6 endarterectomized right coronary arteries were the same as flow in right coronary arteries without endarterectomy.

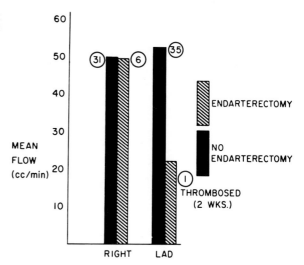

tioned, and the coronary arteriogram must be restudied for other reasons to account for the symptomatology.

The relative importance of endarterectomy remains an unresolved problem. Demerits were assigned to it based on reports in the literature that indicate a higher incidence of closure in these vessels.[2,5,8] In our experience, however, both in long-term patency and in seven early cases reported in this study, endarterectomy did not appear to be a serious threat to graft patency. In 42 endarterectomized vessels in 41 patients, closure occurred in 5.5 percent of cases before discharge from the hospital (Table 7). Blood flow was measured in seven of the endarterectomized vessels (Fig. 4). In the six to the right coronary artery, mean flow was 50.3 cc per minute, which was the same as the mean flow in all bypasses without endarterectomy (54 cc per minute). The one closure of the seven in which flow was studied occurred in the left coronary artery where there was poor runoff, with a flow of only 22 cc per minute.

The distal coronary artery is particularly suitable for endarterectomy, because the atheromatous plug is easily dissected free from the adventitia (Fig. 5), and the distal plugs found at the bifurcation of the right coronary and posterior descending branch can be extracted without leaving loose intimal flaps. This type of plaque formation is less often found in the left anterior descending coronary artery. Thus, we do not hesitate to perform endarterectomy, and we find that it is necessary in approximately 10 percent of vessels, resulting in excellent flows, and postoperative arteriograms reveal adequate runoff.

FIG. 5. A, B. Drawing of technique for removal of atheromatous plug from distal right coronary artery. When the plug is extracted from each branch with care, formation of distal flaps of intima can be avoided. C. Removed distal cores.

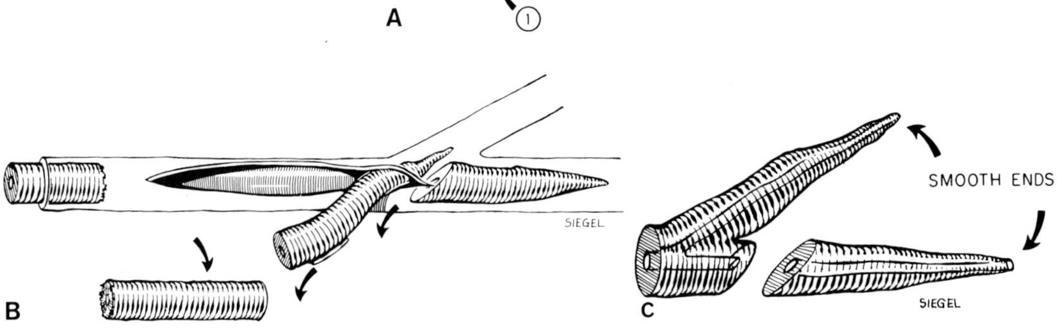

TABLE 7. Endarterectomy Results (12/31/1973)

BYPASSED ARTERIES	NO. GRAFTS	NO. ENDARTERECTOMIZED	OCCLUSION
LRC	27	9	(1: LAD occlusion not endarterectomized)
LR	34	17	0
LR	8	4	1
LR	2	2	0
RC	8	4	0
L	1	1	0
R	5	5	2
Total	85	42	3 (7.1%)
Right coronary			2/36 (5.5%)
LAD			1/6

Whether to perform an endarterectomy on the distal right coronary artery is a matter of judgment, particularly when the opened artery reveals a thick atheromatous core in which there remains a patent lumen. In such an instance, endarterectomy will be performed if manipulation of the artery begins to loosen the core, in which case there is danger of subsequent dissection and graft occlusion, and if 2 mm probes (Fig. 1) cannot be passed into all major runoff branches, of which there are usually two.

Demerits for low graft flow are no longer added to the demerits for other technical problems, because it is apparent that a detriment in flow *already* represents the sum of the other problems. Thus patency can be predicted on the basis of demerits for technical flaws, from volume of flow in the graft, and from both. (The present index that reflects all this information is seen in Table 1.) It is anticipated that the use of the index will in future studies show the reasons for eventual graft closures, especially when combined with a prospective, graded assessment of the postoperative graft angiogram. It will be especially important to define the incidence and significance of subintimal fibrosis of the vein bypass that may eventually come into play to account for late graft closures.

SUMMARY

The results of this study tend to support the belief that technical factors clearly identifiable at surgery are predictive of early graft closure. Furthermore, our experience indicates that endarterectomy performed in a distal right coronary artery does not contribute to an increased closure rate. How all the factors listed in the index relate to graft closure at six months and one year and how many closures are caused by subintimal fibrosis remains to be seen.

ACKNOWLEDGMENT

The authors gratefully acknowledge the assistance of Mrs. Toni Hartmann and Miss Anne Brenner for collection and compilation of the data.

References

1. Bourassa P, Lespérance J, Campeau L, Simard P: Factors influencing patency of aortocoronary vein grafts. Circulation (suppl 1) 45–46:78, 1972
2. Diethrich E, Kinard S, Friedewald V, Prian G. CO_2 gas endarterectomy: an appraisal of its current role in coronary artery surgery. Chest 62:362, 1972
3. Prian GW, Diethrich EB: True measurement of blood flow in long-term aortocoronary bypass graft. Am J Surg 125:331, 1973
4. Favalaro RG, Cheavnechai D: Myocardial revascularization by the saphenous vein graft technique. Geriatrics 27:80, 1972
5. Groves LK, Loop FD, Silver GM: Endarterectomy as supplement to coronary artery-saphenous vein bypass surgery. J Thorac Cardiovasc Surg 64:514, 1972
6. Hutchinson JE III, Green GE, Mekhjian HA, Kemp HG: Coronary bypass grafting in 376 consecutive patients, with three operative deaths. J Thorac Cardiovasc Surg 67:7, 1974
7. Johnson D, Hoffman JF Jr, Flemma RJ, Tector AJ: Secondary surgical procedure for myocardial revascularization. J Thorac Cardiovasc Surg 64:523, 1972
8. Kaplitt MJ, Robinson G: Evaluation of gas endarterectomy in the surgical treatment of diffuse coronary artery disease. Circulation (suppl 2) 43–44:694, 1971
9. Lespérance J, Bourassa MG, Biron P, Campeau L, Saltiel J: Aorto to coronary artery saphenous vein grafts: preoperative angiographic criteria for successful surgery. Am J Cardiol 30:459, 1972
10. Morris GE Jr, Reul GJ, Howell JR, Crawford ES, Chapman DW, Beagley HL, Winters WL, Peterson PK, Lewis JM: Follow-up results of distal coronary artery bypass for ischemic heart disease. Am J Cardiol 29:180, 1972
11. Walker JA, Friedberg D, Flemma RJ, Johnson WD: Determinants of angiographic patency of aortocoronary vein bypass grafts. Circulation (suppl 1) 45–46:72, 1972

71

USE OF METHYLPREDNISOLONE IN IMPROVING LONG-TERM PATENCY OF VEIN GRAFTS

Stephen L. Frantz, M. Oka, Raj K. Gandhi,
Stanley Gross, Arthur R. Beil, Jr.,
and Martin J. Kaplitt

INTRODUCTION

The saphenous vein has been used for by-passing diseased portions of the arterial system since Linton first popularized this operation in 1955.[1] From the advent of coronary artery bypass surgery in 1964, some of the intriguing phenomena affecting these grafts have become more apparent.[2] With the elimination of technical errors and the use of severely diseased veins, most problems are dependent on the distal runoff. Despite this vascular surgical axiom, we have been puzzled by the unexpected closure of vein grafts in some vessels and the unexpected patency in others. Also, there has been much discussion over the progression of disease in vein grafts and with the type of conduit to be used for the bypass. It has been our feeling that if the distal runoff is excellent, vein graft patency and flow will also be excellent. However, in those vessels where the distal runoff is only adequate and the flows are marginal, further exploration of methods of insuring patency are required. We have attempted to evaluate the effect of methylprednisolone sodium succinate * on vein grafts in dogs.

MATERIAL AND METHODS

Twelve mongrel dogs were studied to evaluate the effects of methylprednisolone on the healing and patency rate of vein interposition grafts.

* Solu-Medrol®.

Under sterile conditions, the cephalic vein was removed from the front leg of all animals and used as an interposition graft in the femoral arteries. The animals were treated with 600,000 units of procaine penicillin prior to surgery and for the following three days. The dogs were divided into four groups:

Group I (4 dogs): Represented the controls.
Group II (4 dogs): The veins were soaked in a solution of 125 mg methylprednisolone in 2 cc of heparinized Ringer's Lactate. 500 mg of methylprednisolone was given intravenously during surgery and 8 mg per day was given orally during the postoperative period. This dosage was continued until exploration at 8 to 10 weeks.
Group III (2 dogs): Treated as in Group II, but the methylprednisolone was discontinued after one month. The dogs were sacrificed three months after surgery.
Group IV (2 dogs): Treated as Group II with methylprednisolone continued for three months, at which time the femoral areas were explored. After exploration, the femoral areas were closed with the dogs given procaine penicillin 600,000 units, for three days. No methylprednisolone was administered following this exploration, and the femoral areas were explored again at six weeks.

RESULTS

Group I

A. *Patency of graft*: 50 percent: two dogs patent; two dogs occluded.

B. *Quality of pulsation:* Barely pulsatile in the patent grafts; graded 1+ (out of four).
C. *Appearance of vein graft and relation to surrounding tissue:* All grafts were densely adherent to surrounding tissues and shriveled in appearance. Histologically, the vein walls were thicker—primarily in the adventitial layer. No appreciable intimal or medial hypertrophy (Figs. 1–4).

Group II

A. *Patency of graft:* 100 percent: four dogs patent
B. *Quality of pulsation:* Bounding pulse; graded 4+ (out of four)
C. *Appearance of vein graft and relation to surrounding vessels:* All grafts were easily distinguishable from surrounding tissues. There were no dense adhesions, and the grafts had a normal soft venous appearance and consistency. Histologically, the medial layer appeared to be somewhat hypertrophied (Figs. 5–7).

Group III

A. *Patency:* 100 percent closed
B. *Quality:* No pulsation
C. *Appearance:* Similar to Group I

Group IV

A. *Patency:* All patent (two dogs), and grafts remained patent after six weeks without methylprednisolone.
B. *Quality:* 4+
C. *Appearance:* Same as Group II

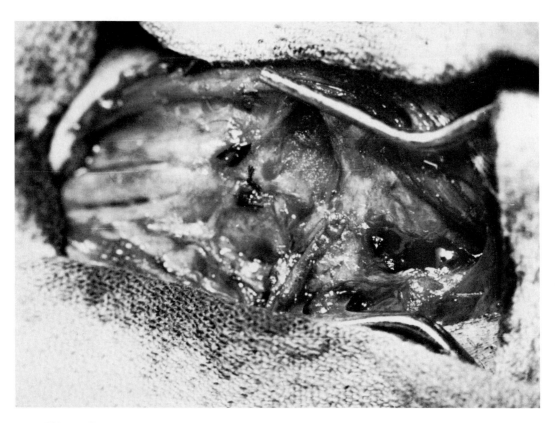

FIG. 1. The vein *in situ* in the nontreated dog. The scar tissue is noted to obscure completely the femoral artery and interposition vein graft. The femoral vein is visualized.

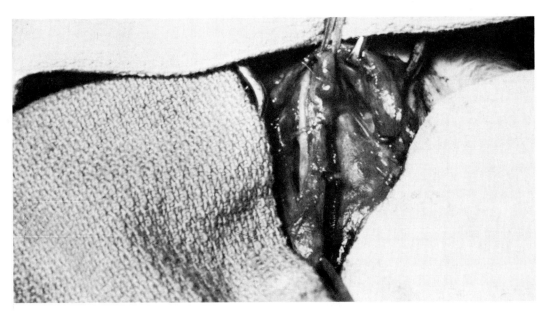

FIG. 2. This shows the vein graft after tedious dissection. It was palpated to be firm, thick-walled, and completely occluded.

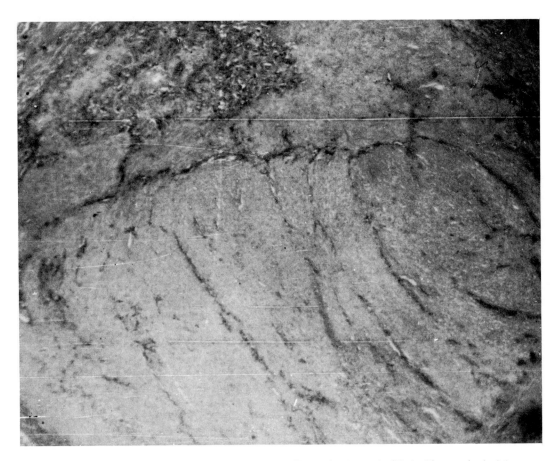

FIG. 3. A section through a nontreated vein graft. The entire lumen is filled with organized clot. There is no evidence of thickened intima or media.

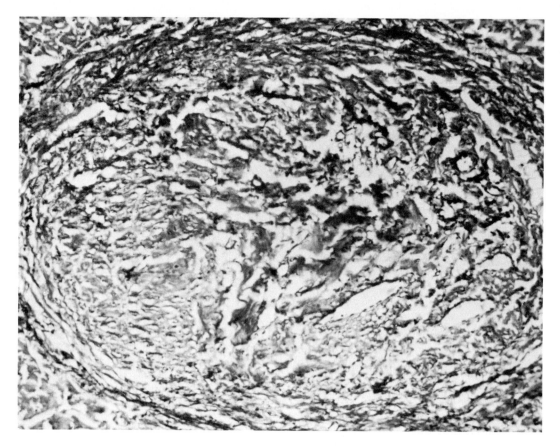

FIG. 4. A section through a nontreated vein graft (trichrome stain). There is some recanalization of the organized clot.

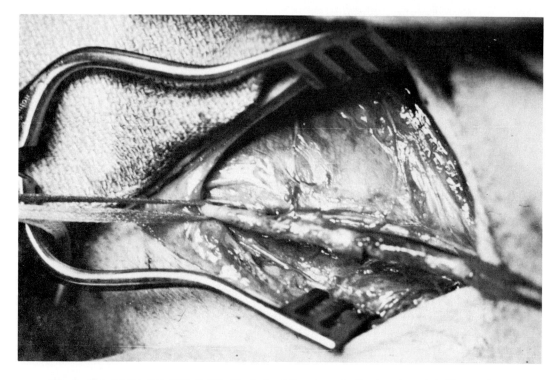

FIG. 5. The treated vein graft *in situ*. The lack of fibrosis and adhesions is noted. The specimen was easily dissected from its surrounding tissue.

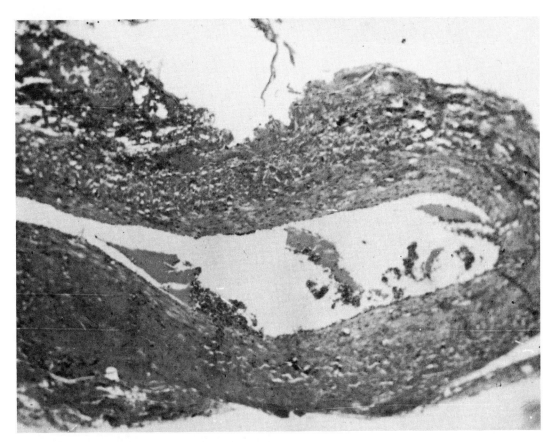

FIG. 6. A section through a widely patent vein graft in a dog treated with methylprednisolone. There is no evidence of intimal hypertrophy, but some slight thickening of the media.

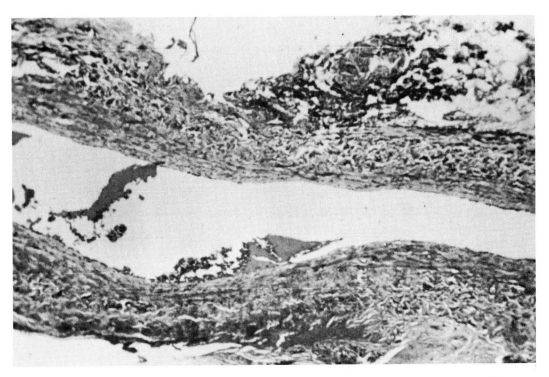

FIG. 7. A section of a treated vein graft with a trichrome stain—again showing wide patency. The media is slightly thickened.

DISCUSSION

The effect of methylprednisolone on the patency and quality of vein interposition grafts in dogs was quite dramatic. The magnitude of pulsation in those controls whose grafts remained patent was severely impaired. The gross specimens of the nontreated animals showed vessels that had lost their normal contours in the midst of dense scar tissue and were greatly adherent to the surrounding structures. The treated grafts, however, were not adherent and had the appearance of patent pulsatile vein grafts. Histologically, there was no appreciable difference in the layers of the veins; in fact, the media of the treated veins were thicker than the controls. This suggests that the normal progression of the vein arterialization continues and that the effect of methylprednisolone is not on the structure of the vein layers but on other factors. Recent electron microscopic studies have shown that stress can cause the intravascular aggregation of platelets, and this has been proposed as a possible etiology of some myocardial infarctions.[3] It has also been shown by Ashford et al that there is significant platelet aggregation at sites of minimal endothelial injury.[4] Several investigators have shown that methylprednisolone prevents the aggregation of platelets by decreasing peripheral resistance, lowering platelet adhesiveness, and inhibiting the release of 1- serotonin by ADP.[5,6] Also the antiinflammatory effect of the glucocorticoids is well known, and Llao and Associates have shown this in the prevention of intestinal adhesions.[7]

Since these mechanisms may be only part of the answer, other areas of consideration in determining the cause of the phenomenon noted in the present study are streaming potentials, intimal electronegative charges, vein enzyme changes, and tagged steroid experiments.

It is our feeling that the patency and flow of vein grafts are primarily dependent upon the distal runoff. It is propitious for the surgeon to choose carefully the vessels for bypass surgery so that he is not confronted by those situations in which the runoff is poor. However, in coronary artery surgery in particular there are circumstances in which the surgeon is faced with less than ideal conditions. The flows may be poor, the vessels may be smaller than anticipated, or (if angiography is available in the operating room) the runoff may not be as extensive as predicted. In these marginal situations it may be advantageous to use methylprednisolone to help ensure the patency of vein grafts. It is probable that Class IV vessels (those vessels that are very small, whose runoff is very poor, or that contain diffuse disease) should not be bypassed; and if grafts are attempted, no adjunct will help keep them open.[8] However, particularly in Class III vessels and in some Class II vessels, methylprednisolone may make the difference between patency and closure. Furthermore, it is widely accepted that flow rates are critical in predicting vein graft patency. It is our feeling that those grafts that have flows of less then 60 cc/min are likely to close. The effect of methylprednisolone may again improve the patency rate in these cases.

References

1. Linton RR: Some practical considerations in surgery of blood vessel grafts. Surgery 38:817, 1955
2. Garret HE, Dennis EW, Debakey ME: Aortocoronary bypass with saphenous vein graft: seven-year followup. JAMA 223, 7:792, 1973
3. Haft JI, Fami K: Stress and the induction of intravascular platelet aggregation in the heart. Circulation 48:164, July 1973
4. Ashford RP, Friedman DG: Platelet aggregation at sites of minimal endothelial injury. Am J Pathol 53:599, 1968
5. Pierce CH, Gutelius JR: Effects of glucocorticoids on platelet junction in experimental shock. Pharmacologist 13:318, 1971
6. Tamari Y: Personal communication, New York 1974
7. Llao SK, Suchiro GT, McNamara JJ: Prevention of postoperative intestinal adhesions in primates. Surg Gynec Obstet 137:816–18, Nov 1973
8. Kaplitt MJ, Frantz SL, Beil AR: Analysis of intraoperative coronary angiography in aortocoronary bypass grafts. Circulation (suppl 2) 50:141, 1974

72

LONG-TERM FOLLOW-UP OF CORONARY VEIN BYPASS GRAFTS: APPRAISAL OF FACTORS INFLUENCING PATENCY

Harold C. Urschel, Maruf A. Razzuk, and Richard E. Wood

The major objective of direct myocardial revascularization is to reestablish adequate blood flow to the viable myocardium, which is jeopardized by significant atherosclerotic obstructive coronary artery disease. Direct coronary artery surgery aims to improve the quality of life and postpone or prevent death, myocardial infarction, and its complications. The success of this surgical endeavor can only be assured by prolonged patency of the reconstructed conduits. These techniques [19,20] allow the least margin of error of any current surgical procedure because of the size of the vessels involved and the ominous result of failure.

To assess the critical factors that influence graft patency, the physiologic, pathologic, and technical aspects (Table 1) of 1,150 saphenous vein bypass grafts and 65 carbon dioxide gas endarterectomies in 561 patients were evaluated over a five-year period. The important physiologic factors include pressure-resistance-flow relationship (Poiseuille's law), tension-radius effect (law of Laplace), tension-length effect (Hooke's law), the velocity-cross-sectional area effect on flow, defined in the equation of continuity, and the effect of cardiac cycle. Important pathophysiologic factors influencing patency are competitive flow either between the artery and graft or between different grafts, extent of outflow tract disease, status of collateral circulation, postoperative bleeding and infection, and the postcardiotomy syndrome. Critical technical considerations involve the selection and preparation of the vein bypass graft, construction of the aortic and coronary anastomoses, and the performance of technically complete and safe endarterectomy when indicated.

For significant proximal coronary artery stenoses with adequate distal vessels, saphenous vein bypass grafts provide optimal myocardial revascularization.[21] For diffusely diseased or occluded vessels not amenable to saphenous vein bypass grafting, distal carbon dioxide gas endarterectomy has been employed with proximal vein bypass grafts for inflow.[19,24] Constant reassessment of the hemodynamic and technical factors involved with these procedures is mandatory for the achievement of the optimal objectives of direct myocardial revascularization.

Although coronary bypass grafts differ from those placed in the femoropopliteal area in that the coronary grafts are shorter, are placed in an anatomically different area, and are exposed to a negative intrathoracic pressure, by extrapolation of the

Table 1. Factors Influencing Patency of Aortocoronary Saphenous Vein-Bypass Grafts

I.   Physiologic
  1. Poiseuille's Law: $F = P/R$
  2. Cardiac cycle
  3. Equation of continuity: $F = v \times A \text{ cm}^2$
  4. Hooke's Law: tension – length
  5. Laplace's Law: tension – length
II. Pathologic
  1. Competitive flow
    a. Coronary lesion
    b. Outflow tract
    c. Collateral vessels
  2. Postcardiotomy syndrome
  3. Infection
III. Technical
  1. Aortic anastomosis
  2. Vein graft
  3. Coronary anastomosis

long-term results of Darling and associates[5] (65 percent), 10- to 20-year patency rates for femoral grafts can be expected in coronary vein grafts if proper attention is given to the important factors influencing patency.

CLINICAL MATERIALS AND OBSERVATIONS

From 1968 to 1974 there were 1,150 vein grafts and 65 carbon dioxide gas endarterectomies performed on 561 patients. Since 1968 twenty total carbon dioxide gas endarterectomies were performed in the right coronary artery from the aorta to the distal radical arteries. Subsequently, 45 carbon dioxide gas endarterectomies were performed on distal coronary vessels, with proximal vein bypass grafts for inflow. In this latter group, there were 33 left anterior descending (LAD), 10 distal right and posterior descending, and two circumflex carbon dioxide gas endarterectomies. The advantages of such a procedure include the safe revascularization of a left coronary artery branch without jeopardizing an uninvolved vessel or requiring difficult technical proximal endarterectomy behind the pulmonary artery, elimination of proximal blind endarterectomy to the aorta, and substitution with high-flow vein graft inflow for simple arteriotomy closure, all of which previously contributed to failure of total vessel endarterectomy and its application to the crucial left system.[19]

In our experience, mechanical endarterectomy is not as safe as gas endarterectomy because it is not as complete, opens fewer collateral channels, and risks creating a distal plaque that will occlude the vessel on reinstitution of blood flow. Local endarterectomy in the area of the vein graft should be avoided, since it is difficult to provide a satisfactory ending in such a small vessel (compared to the good results in the larger vessels such as the carotid artery).

Intraoperative blood flows were measured in over 700 grafts with the Micron electromagnetic flowmeter. The mean flow in the right coronary artery grafts averaged 70 cc per minute (range, 10 to 135 cc per minute); in left anterior descending grafts, it averaged 95 cc per minute (range, 20 to 250 cc per minute); and, in circumflex grafts, it averaged 80 cc per minute (range, 10 to 180 cc per minute). Mean flows of less than 20 cc per minute were associated with a high rate of occlusion. Pressures were measured in the graft and coronary artery beyond the stenosis to determine the pressure gradients across the lesion. It was diffi-

cult to record a significant number of flows in the coronary arteries because the necessary dissection might jeopardize some branches. In the multiple-vein graft procedures, flows were measured concomitantly in the grafts, and in each graft alone while the other grafts were temporarily occluded to ascertain the collateral circulation between one system and another, and whether competitive flow existed. Flows were also measured after injection of 15 mg of Papaverine into the graft. This usually increased flow from 50 to 100 percent in the graft for a period of five to 20 minutes.

Angiographic reevaluation of the grafts was carried out, when possible, prior to the patient's leaving the hospital or within the first few months after discharge and subsequently at yearly intervals. Of the 532 vein grafts restudied in the early period, 474 were patent (80 percent); 25 distal gas endarterectomies with proximal vein grafts were all patent (100 percent); and of the 18 total right gas endarterectomies restudied, 12 were patent (75 percent). Over one year, 170 were restudied, 153 being patent (90 percent); 65 were studied over two years, with 60 patent (93 percent); and 42 were studied over three years, and 38 were patent (91 percent). Seven grafts have been found to be patent over five years.

PHYSIOLOGIC FACTORS

The overall determinant of flow through the surgically reconstructed arterial system is based on the sum of all factors influencing Poiseuille's law (flow = pressure/resistance) (Fig. 1). All physiologic, pathologic, and technical factors relate to various components of this law, and the summation of their effects on pressure and resistance determines flow. While it can be argued that Poiseuille's law applies to steady-state laminar flow of a Newtonian fluid[14] not strictly present in direct coronary artery surgery, this and the other theoretical laws of physics explain the hemodynamic data, and there is close correlation between experimental data and these theoretical laws.[3]

The normal cardiac cycle influences flow through the coronary arteries and thus through the vein bypass grafts, as can be observed in Fig. 2. The predominant flow occurs during the diastolic phase of the cycle, with slightly different flows for the right and left coronary arteries. However, during systole, there is an increase in tissue pressure surrounding the small vessels, which reduces their transmural pressure even to below zero for the left coronary vessels. They are also temporarily occluded. This intermittent increase in re-

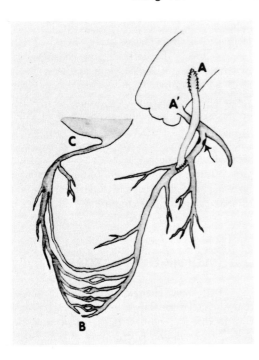

FIG. 1. Poiseuille's law expressing flow as the ratio between pressure and resistance. The stenosis (arrow) in the artery makes the total resistance (A'RC) in the A'–B–C system greater than ARC in the A–B–C system. Extrapolating flow from the formula F = Δ P/R gives higher value of flow through the vein graft. Poiseuille's law:

$$F_{VG} = \frac{PA - PC}{ARC = ARB + BRC} > F_{CA} = $$

$$\frac{PA' - PC}{A'RC = A'RB + BRC}$$

FIG. 2. Cardiac cycle and vein graft flow, illustrating the effect of cardiac cycle on coronary blood flow. Flow in the left coronary artery falls during isometric contraction period and is even retrograde for a short time. During ejection, flow rises (a), then falls again, probably because ventricular pressure and therefore tissue pressure are still rising, producing more impingement on small vessels. Only after ventricular pressure has fallen (b) (isometric relaxation period) does flow rise again (c). As a result of lower right ventricular pressure, these effects are less marked on right coronary flow.

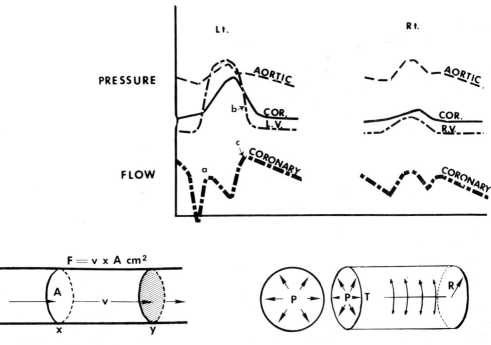

FIG. 3. Equation of continuity expressing flow as the product of velocity and the cross-sectional area. A reduction in the lumen reduces the total sum of V × A cm². This is operational in the coronary artery when the proximal stenosis reduces the lumen by 70 percent of its cross-sectional area. F: flow; V: velocity; and A: area.

FIG. 4. Laplace's Law expressing tension as being proportional to the product of the pressure and radius. Increase in the graft intraluminal pressure increases tension and stretch of the smooth muscles of the vein, which may increase the contractility, leading to medial hypertrophy and consequently possible narrowing of the vein lumen. P: pressure; T: tension (dynes per centimeter of length); and R: radius.

sistance to flow of the coronary vascular bed may contribute to thrombosis in a traumatized vein graft or a technically poor anastomosis, particularly during episodes of hypotension in the period following the operation.

A second important consideration with regard to flow involves the equation of continuity ($F =$ velocity $\times$ the area cm ^{2}) (Fig. 3). This operates in the coronary artery in relation to the proximal stenosis, which must reduce the lumen by 70 percent of its cross-sectional area in order to decrease the flow, and to the diameter of the bypass conduit as well as the coronary artery distal to the stenosis. This inverse relationship of velocity to cross-sectional area was reviewed by Furuse and associates,[9] who showed experimentally that a bypass conduit to the proximally diseased coronary artery of a 2 mm internal mammary artery had a velocity of 37 cm per second, a distal vein with a 3 mm diameter had a velocity of 16 cm per second, and a 6 mm proximal vein had a velocity of 4 cm per second, while the distal coronary artery with a 1.5 mm diameter had a velocity of 62 m per second. The flow through this graft system was 65 cc per minute. An advantage of a higher velocity is that the sheer stress is greater at the vessel wall and anastomosis, which decreases the tendency for platelet and fibrin deposition and thus thrombosis.

The pressure and tension effect as expressed by Laplace's Law (Fig. 4) may cause long-run changes in the vein. It is possible that the sudden exposure of the vein graft to the high aortic pressure causes increased tension and stretch of the smooth muscle in the vessel wall, which in turn may cause changes in the contractile elements, permitting stronger contractions, which may lead, in due time, to anatomic hypertrophy of the media and, consequently, possible narrowing of the lumen. This type of mechanism has been put forward by Simeone[18] to explain the medial hypertrophy observed in arteries after sympathetic denervation.

The tension-length effect (Hooke's law) occurs when elastic tissue is stretched; tension is developed proportionally to elongation. A change in the elasticity as a result of an increase in collagenous fibers in the wall of the vein graft, as occurs in traumatically prepared veins, causes increased tension at a lesser degree of stretch. This results in an increased velocity as well as resistance to flow. The increased resistance may chronically compromise the flow and consequently lead to thrombosis.

These physiologic factors are important in the selection of conduit and in determining the

optimum size for a vein bypass graft. The general feeling is that vein bypass grafts should be 4 to 6 mm to provide the optimal cross-sectional area so that inflow is not limited and, at the same time, to avoid too large a cross-sectional area with a lower velocity that might encourage relative degree of stasis and subsequent occlusion. The internal mammary artery, which is used when an adequate vein is not available, has a small cross-sectional area with an inherent higher velocity, which improves patency; however, in certain situations, it may not provide adequate inflow for the distal coronary system. The conduit should be slightly larger (1 to 2 mm) than the artery grafted.

PATHOLOGIC FACTORS

Pathologic changes, whether secondary to the atherosclerotic disease or complicating the reconstructive procedure such as postoperative bleeding or infection and postcardiotomy syndrome, influence both the early and the late graft patency. The assessment of the outflow tract (Table 2) and the collateral circulation plays an important role in deciding which reconstructive procedure to use and, subsequently, its future patency. Poor outflow tracts have been associated with both low flow and low patency rates.

The competition between proximal conduits, ie, grafts and arteries, for the distal arterial bed may create a state of competitive flow that may jeopardize the patency of one of the inflow conduits. The prevalence and outcome of such a condition is determined by the inflow, the magnitude of the proximal arterial occlusion, and the extent of collateral circulation. Competitive flow may

TABLE 2. Classification of Outflow Tract on Basis of Angiographic and Operative Assessment

GRADE	DESCRIPTION
1. Excellent	Isolated segment lesion; soft pliable distal vessel
2. Very good	Isolated segmental lesion; some thickening of distal vessel
3. Good	Isolated segmental lesion; occasional distal plaques
4. Poor	Diffusely scalloped but patent lumen
5. Very poor	Totally and diffusely occluded vessel

Vein bypass grafts are used for 1, 2, and 3 outflow tracts, whereas distal CO_2 endarterectomy and proximal vein graft are used for 4 and 5.

occur between (1) graft and artery, (2) grafts to different branches of the same vascular bed with good intercoronary collateral vessels, and (3) grafts to different vascular beds with good intercoronary collateral vessels.[26,27]

Competitive Flow

Although flows could not be measured directly in the coronary arteries in most cases, a measurement of the pressure gradients across the coronary artery obstruction was recorded. The pressure in the vein graft distal to the last valve was measured with the vein open (reflecting aortic pressure) and with the vein graft clamped (reflecting coronary artery pressure). Pressure gradients ranged from 0 to 110 mm Hg. In one patient's right coronary artery distal to the obstruction, the pressure was 90/60 mm Hg with the graft open and 40/0 mm Hg while the vein graft was temporarily occluded (Table 3). This suggested a tight proximal lesion with minimal degree of competitive flow. In the same patient, pressure was measured in the LAD coronary artery distal to the obstruction. A pressure value of 90/60 mm Hg was recorded with the graft both open and occluded. This suggested that the pressure in the distal vessel was not decreased and that some degree of competitive flow between the LAD and its vein graft was present. Although the patency of vein grafts could not be correlated directly to these pressure measurements as it would with reduced flows below 20 cc per minute, the pressure measurement can give some indication of the status of competition between the coronary artery and its vein graft. Selmonosky and Ellison [16] have shown that collateral circulation does not influence coronary artery pressure distal to a stenosis in acute experimental situations; however, in chronic states, this may be a factor. Experimenal studies by

Furuse and associates [9] have shown that most of the blood flows through a vein graft used as a bypass for a normal coronary artery; whereas Kakos and associates [11] demonstrated a more equal distribution between the two in a similar situation. The principle of competitive flow between vein graft and coronary artery suggests that it is not advisable to bypass stenoses less than 50 percent, because flow will be decreased in both conduits, potentially leading to adverse conditions that could produce thromboses in either graft or artery and jeopardizing a stable situation with adequate flow.

Dilatation of a proximal stenosis increases competitive flow between the coronary artery and vein graft and is contraindicated except to increase flow to another distal vessel where there remains an even more proximal obstruction that is not dilated. This is demonstrated in the totally occluded or diffusely diseased distal vessel, which is treated by proximal vein bypass graft and distal carbon dioxide endarterectomy, leaving the proximal coronary artery obstruction intact. Early restudy demonstrates 100 percent patency in 25 such vessels.

Tight coronary artery lesions have been observed to occlude in early postoperative studies following placement of a high-inflow vein bypass graft, presumably on the basis of competitive flow from the vein graft.[11] This occurs less frequently in the coronary system than in the femoral arteries, probably because of constant to-and-fro blood movement during systole and diastole.

Competitive flow may exist between grafts to different vascular beds or different grafts to the same vascular beds, which have good intercoronary collateral channels. Although collateral circulation may be suspected by the preoperative coronary angiogram, the actual variation in flow can be measured at the operating table when more than one vein bypass graft is placed. Flow is determined in each graft, while the other is open and temporarily occluded. Table 4 demonstrates that the LAD graft increased both its mean and systolic flow when the right graft was occluded. The right graft increased its mean and systolic flow as well

TABLE 3. Competitive Flow between Graft and Artery

GRAFT	FLOW		PRESSURE	
	Both Open	One Clamped	Graft	Coronary Artery
Rt	100/25	100/25	90/60	40/0
LAD	75/0	75/0	90/60	90/60

The pressure gradient between right artery and its graft suggests a tight proximal lesion with minimum degree of competitive flow, whereas the equal pressures in both the LAD and its graft indicate the presence of competition. Rt: right coronary artery; LAD: left anterior descending artery.

TABLE 4. Competitive Flow between Grafts

GRAFT	BOTH OPEN	ONE CLAMPED
LAD	110/37	150/45
Rt	75/10	100/23

As one graft is temporarily occluded, flow increases in the other, indicating competition between grafts for the vascular beds.

when the LAD graft was occluded. However, the sum total of both grafts was greater with regard to systolic and mean flow than was present in either graft alone, suggesting either that the intercoronary collateral vessel was not adequate to carry the whole flow or that the single conduit was not of adequate size to provide the volume of flow for the two vascular beds.

Competitive flow between vein grafts is important to consider in deciding the number of grafts to be placed into an individual patient with more than one vessel involved with severe coronary artery disease. One point of view suggests that all arteries with significant obstruction should be bypassed by placing as many as six grafts into a diseased heart. This philosophy suggests that each vessel is independent, and it disregards the presence of intercoronary collateral or competitive flow between the vein grafts. It encompasses the position that because of some "unknown factor" that is causing failure of vein grafts, the more grafts placed, the greater the chance for more of them to remain patent. On the other end of the spectrum is the philosophy that too many vein grafts jeopardize each other if good intercoronary collateral circulation is present and that an adequate number to provide the maximum flow needed for the left ventricle should be placed, but not more than would jeopardize any of the other grafts. With this approach, revascularization is done in only the three major systems, taking advantage of intercoronary collateral circulation and not jeopardizing further veins by competitive flow. This would also assume that the grafts in combination would provide an adequate amount of flow for the left ventricle. The decision in each case depends on careful evaluation of the preoperative coronary angiogram, selection of the appropriate dominant vessels to be treated, and the estimation of flow during the operation. By employing distal gas endarterectomy and proximal vein graft, all the major systems can be revascularized directly, and many intercoronary collateral vessels can be opened at the time of surgery in the diffusely diseased vessels, eliminating the necessity of revascularizing smaller diseased vessels, which leads to an increased incidence of occluson.[19,24]

The number and placement of grafts with specific anatomic lesions is determined by the number of obstructive lesions and the significance of the vessels involved. For a left main coronary artery stenosis, with a large LAD artery and a small circumflex artery, a single graft to the LAD artery should be adequate to revascularize the diseased system because of retrograde flow from the LAD into the small circumflex (Fig. 5A). Should the circumflex be "balanced" or "dominant," certainly two vein grafts would be placed to assure adequate inflow to the system. If an additional lesion in either the left anterior descending or circumflex should be present in combination with the left main lesion, a graft to the circumflex and distally in the LAD would be indicated (Fig. 5B). If two lesions are present in a vessel, the distal lesion, if it is short, may be "bridged" with a vein graft (Fig. 5C and D) or can be dilated if it is long (Fig. 5E and F) in order to provide retrograde as well as distal flow from the single vein graft. Another technique employed occasionally in multiple stenoses is a distal end-to-side anastomosis with a side-to-side anastomosis to the most distal obstruction (Fig. 5G). This is yet to be evaluated by long-term patency, and one anastomosis could jeopardize the other with regard to patency. If the disease is diffuse, it is our policy to endarterectomize the major portion of the distal vessel and to place a proximal vein graft.

Postoperative Hemorrhage, Infection, and "Cardiotomy" Syndrome

If the chest and mediastinum are not well evacuated, significant postoperative hemorrhage not only jeopardizes the early course of coronary vein bypass grafts as a result of hypotension tamponade and potential thrombosis of the vein graft but it also reduces the chance for long-term patency. The remaining hematoma may organize and produce severe fibrosis that could entrap the grafts and encroach on their lumina. In six patients with significant postoperative hemorrhage, the patency rate was 60 percent.

To reduce the chance for postoperative hemorrhage, the use of fresh autogenous blood transfusions at the conclusion of the procedure has been employed in the last 100 cases. At the beginning of the procedure, 1,000 cc of the patient's blood are removed through the monitoring arterial catheter prior to heparinization and collected in acid citrate dextrose (ACD) plastic bags. This volume is replaced by cross-matched homologous blood. The fresh, autogenous blood is kept at room temperature and transfused into the patient following heparin reversal at the end of the procedure. This provides fresh blood with preserved cellular elements, particularly platelets, not subjected to the pump-oxygenator.[25] Compared to the previous 100 instances, in which the average blood loss postoperatively was 950 cc per patient with three severe bleeding episodes requiring reoperation, the last 100 patients given fresh autogenous blood had an average blood loss of 450 cc per patient with only one severe bleeding episode requiring reoperation.

The presence of mediastinal and sternal infection occurred in four patients with one death, but it uniformly led to occlusion of all vein grafts. This is a disappointing catastrophe that should be avoided at all costs. Two of the four had previous double internal mammary artery implantation procedures with decreased blood supply to the area of previous sternotomy. Ideally, in this situation, the sternal edges should be cleaned back to normal tissue prior to closure.

The "postcardiotomy" syndrome is another postoperative pathological entity that influences graft patency. This has been clinically documented in six patients; four subsequently had occluded vein grafts after having demonstrated early patency. This syndrome has been recognized from four days to nine months following surgery. It should be treated vigorously with steroid therapy to prevent thrombosis of the grafts. The symptoms and signs include increased incisional pain, fever of unknown origin, and, occasionally, increased pleural fluid. Pericardial "rub" is not of diagnostic value in these cases.

Two patients had undergone operation three months following myocardial infarctions, and at operation, a severe postmyocardial infarction syndrome (Dressler's) was found in both patients. In one case, the severity was such that no vein grafts were placed, and the operation was performed electively at a later date following steroid therapy. In the second case, revascularization and ventricular aneurysmectomy were performed because of the severe disability of the patient. Steroid therapy was started immediately after surgery and continued for five months with satisfactory results.

TECHNICAL FACTORS

Technical factors that influence vein graft patency can be divided into those that influence the (1) aortic anastomosis, (2) selection and preparation of the vein graft, and (3) coronary anastomosis and extent of disease in the outflow tract.

Aortic Anastomosis

A variety of techniques have been employed since 1968 for the aortic anastomosis. Grafts to the right coronary artery are sutured through a longitudinal slit to the ascending aorta, brought directly around the right coronary artery groove to the distal vessel or posterior descending branch.

This has continued to provide satisfactory patency. Originally, left coronary artery grafts were sutured to the aorta through a longitudinal slit, then looped cephalad, and brought in a gentle U-shaped curve to the LAD or circumflex coronary arteries. Several occlusions were thought to be related to the position of these loops during the sternal closure. Since 1971 grafts to the left coronary artery branches have been sutured at right angles to the ascending aorta, after a small button of aortic wall (Fig. 6A and B) has been removed. The graft is directed in a gentle curve to the appropriate distal vessel.

Originally, separate anastomoses were used for each graft. Subsequently, J and Y configuration grafts, as well as a single side-to-side aortic anastomosis with two distal limbs were tried.[22] All of these demonstrated an increased occlusion rate, so since 1972 a separate aortic anastomosis for each graft has been used when possible. In 25 J-, Y-, or U-shaped grafts with a single aortic takeoff, the early patency rate was 75 percent, which is significantly lower than for a single takeoff for each distal graft. A decreased patency rate has also been observed with multiple distal branches from a single aortic anastomosis in other series.[28] Good early patency for "snake" grafts with multiple distal anastomoses has been reported by Sewell.[17]

Originally, the aortic anastomoses were placed prior to cardiopulmonary bypass, and the distal anastomoses to the coronary artery were placed during cardiopulmonary bypass. Although this procedure was usually satisfactory, an inappropriate vein length occasionally resulted. For the last three years, the patient has been placed on cardiopulmonary bypass, the distal graft has been sutured first to the coronary artery, and the patient then has been taken off cardiopulmonary bypass (possible in over 90 percent of the patients); the length of the graft is measured with the heart beating, and the proximal aortic anastomosis is performed with the use of a side-occlusive aortic clamp without the necessity of cardiopulmonary bypass. In cases in which the ventricular function is extremely poor, both distal and proximal anastomoses are performed on cardiopulmonary bypass.

In two cases, one because of an aneurysm and the second because of a dissection following placement of the vein grafts, the ascending aorta was resected and replaced with an interposed Teflon graft, and the saphenous veins were anastomosed to the prosthetic material without jeopardizing subsequent patency. In a third patient, the proximal aorta was extremely diseased, calcific, and of "eggshell" consistency. The internal mam-

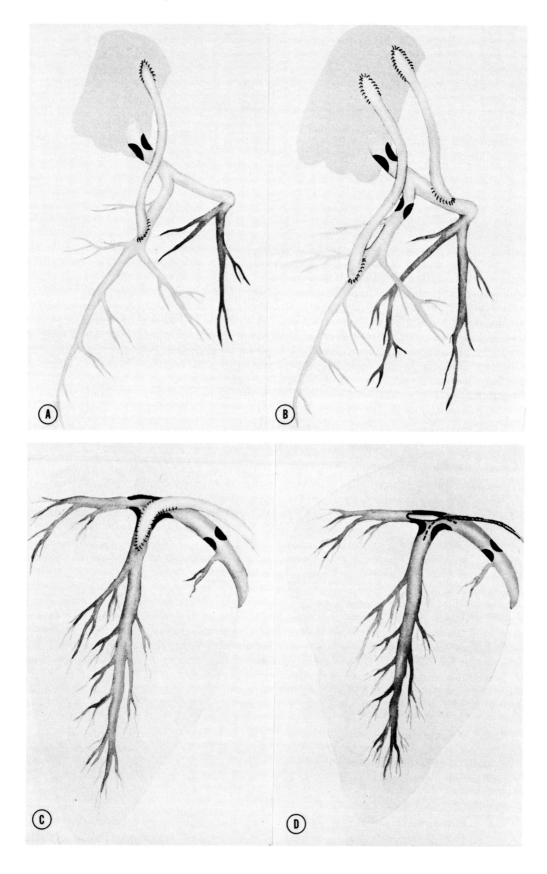

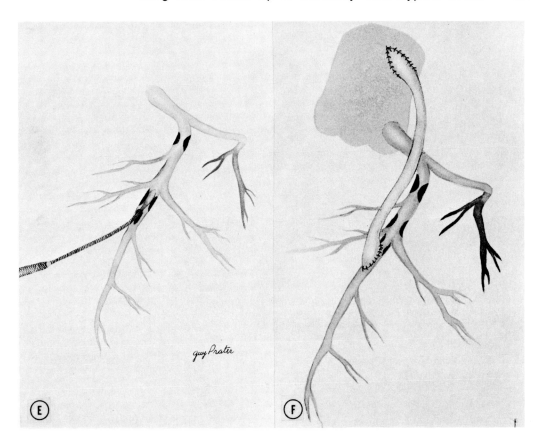

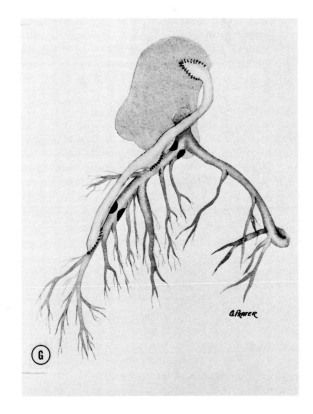

FIG. 5. A through D. A single-vein bypass graft is sufficient in revascularizing
the left coronary system in case of left
main coronary artery lesion, a large
LAD, and a small circumflex artery. The
latter vessel is perfused by retrograde
flow. If the circumflex artery is "balanced" or dominant, two grafts to both
the LAD and the circumflex arteries
should be placed. B. A lesion in either
the LAD or circumflex artery in combination with a left main lesion requires two
vein bypass grafts to both the LAD and
the circumflex arteries. C and D. If two
lesions are present, the distal short
lesion is bridged with a vein graft (C).
If this distal lesion is at a bifurcation as
in distal right coronary artery, the anastomosis is extended beyond the stenosis
over the posterior descending artery
(C) and the other branch is dilated (D).
If two lesions are present, the distal
lesion can be dilated if long (E), and
then a vein graft is placed distal to the
distal lesion (F).   G. Side-to-side and
end-to-side anastomoses with a single
graft, a technique occasionally used for
multiple stenoses.

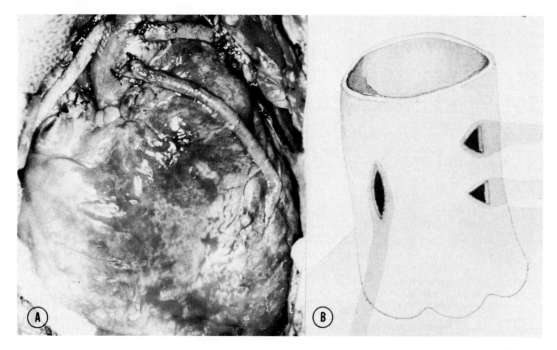

FIG. 6. Grafts to the left coronary artery are sutured at a right angle to the ascending aorta (A) after the excision of a small button of the aortic wall (B). Grafts to the right coronary artery are sutured to the aorta through a linear aortotomy (B).

mary arteries were used as direct grafts to the coronary arteries, obviating proximal aorta suture.

Vein Graft Selection and Preparation

Although this is one of the most important steps in direct revascularization, the selection and preparation of the autogenous saphenous vein is often inappropriately relegated to the least experienced member of the team. Ideal size of the vein graft is 4 to 6 mm in diameter. The average vein employed ranged between 4 and 8 mm in diameter. "Arterialization" of the vein occurs in time, due to exposure to high intraluminal pressures, which in the thigh position has involved thickening of all layers of the graft wall.[6] If the vein is smaller than 4 mm, the normal "arterialization" process can potentially narrow the inflow beyond the needs of the coronary artery outflow tract. It is planned that the inflow will be slightly greater than the outflow at all times and will not be a limiting factor in the supply of blood to the ischemic myocardium. On the other hand, the ultimate lumen should approach as nearly as possible the smallest diameter that will provide this adequate flow, so as to allow maximum velocity and provide the optimum flow characteristics for patency.

The saphenous vein is an ideal autogenous conduit, since the upright posture produces some thickening of the wall, which will tolerate the intraluminal arterial pressure without dilatation in its new position. On the other hand, the wall thickening should not be so great that it decreases normal elastic components or significantly encroaches upon the internal diameter. If the vein is diseased or it appears that the wall is markedly thickened, the vein should not be used. In borderline or normal cases, a small segment is taken from each end of the vein and sent to pathology for a frozen section in order to evaluate any significant disease process or thickening of the wall. The part of the leg selected for the donor site is also an important factor when considering the wall thickness of the vein. The thigh is usually the ideal site, as described by Linton and Darling[13] because the vein is of adequate size with the minimum thickness of the wall to internal diameter ratio. The lower leg veins are of adequate size on the outside; however, the wall generally tends to be thicker in proportion to the lumen. These are used only as second choices for autogenous grafts.

The ideal incision is one that will allow easy harvesting, without undue trauma, pulling, or manipulation of the vein. This involves longer incisions than would ordinarily be necessary for a stripping procedure. Veins examined under the microscope, which were taken through small incisions with long bridges, have more intimal cracks and damage than those taken through longer incisions with short skin bridges (Fig. 7A and B). Handling of the veins is extremely important; dissection should be minimal and the branches should be ligated and divided atraumatically. Forceps and encircling silk sutures and other traumatic techniques should be avoided, because wall damage, particularly to the intima, will lead to progressive narrowing and ultimate occlusion (Fig. 7C and D). The vein should be gently removed with its periadventitial tissues preserved. The vein is left in continuity until time to prepare and insert it; the distal end is divided first, followed by the proximal end. The vein is cannulated with a Marks needle through its distal lumen and gently perfused with room-temperature heparinized Hank's Solution, which is corrected to body pH and osmolality. Overdistention is to be avoided. Although the vein is cleaned adequately to allow normal distention, the periadventitial tissue is not completely removed circumferentially because this will destroy the vasa vasora, expose the external elastic membrane (Fig. 7E and F), and produce a higher subsequent incidence of fibrosis.[2] Blood supply to the vein in the transplanted position is by diffusion through the intima and surrounding tissues prior to its taking on a new blood supply through the periadventitial tissues and revascularization of the vasa vasora. Therefore, it is important not to strip it clean. The ideal situation is to have constant perfusion of the vein in its extracorporeal position until its insertion, so that metabolites can be eliminated and normal milieu provided for minimal enzyme destruction, loss of fibrinolysin, and cell degeneration. No long-term studies have been evaluated to determine the actual length of time and under what circumstances a vein can be left out of the body without affecting its normal healing response in a transplanted autogenous position. Unfortunately, thick-walled veins comparable to those of the saphenous system are not available in experimental animals. The data for homograft veins are meager and not well controlled, and at this time, it is not considered a satisfactory primary graft. Experimentation currently with regard to banking of veins, prolonged preservation, and other procedures is in progress.

Initially, the distal end of the vein is split longitudinally and the length of the anastomosis is decided and tailored as a "cobra head," as described by Linton and Menendez[12] for coronary artery anastomosis. The proximal anastomosis is constructed by splitting the vein equidistant, but not tailoring it, and suturing it to the aorta. Care should be taken not to invert the vein edge into the aorta, not to flatten or twist it, and to achieve the intima-to-intima approximation during the anastomosis and without much infolding of tissue. Occasionally, a valve will be present at the distal anastomosis, which should be excised. If any rough surfaces are present, the vein should be shortened and a new area chosen, particularly for the distal coronary anastomosis.

No one has yet demonstrated whether competent valves in the vein transplanted to the coronary system are good or bad. The internal mammary artery, either in the Vineberg position or as a direct anastomosis to a coronary artery, has no valves, and "to-and-fro" flow occurs through the cardiac cycle. This has been alleged to be the reason for higher patency. In a vein graft, the valve, if present between the aorta and coronary artery, prevents the flow of blood retrograde during systole. This possibly increases the pressure in the coronary system at the end of systole and early diastole, which may be an advantage, or it may contribute to occlusion if all the other technical aspects of the system are not ideal. It is possible that in the future valves should be removed. In the group of 25 patients treated with single-vein "U"-grafts, in which the double-limb distal veins were placed with a side-to-side aortic anastomosis in the middle of the vein graft, the valves were destroyed under direct vision by inversion in some cases or by blind destruction in others. The fact that one or more limbs of these occluded in a higher percentage of cases than in grafts with a single aortic anastomosis suggests that they do contribute to graft failure to some degree or that removal of them is traumatic enough to increase the occlusion rate.

If a satisfactory vein is not available, the internal mammary artery may be employed with direct coronary artery anastomosis,[10] the vessel may be endarterectomized, a homograft vein employed, or a bovine heterograft inserted.

Coronary Anastomosis

Another critical aspect of conduit patency and adequate flow is careful evaluation of the outflow tract distal to the coronary artery obstruction and selection of the proper sites for vein graft anastomosis. From the angiogram, the outflow tract is graded from I to V, I being an isolated proximal lesion with an adequate distal vessel, and V being very poor outflow, with totally occluded, diffusely diseased, and, therefore, inappropriate for vein graft (Table 2). Vein bypass

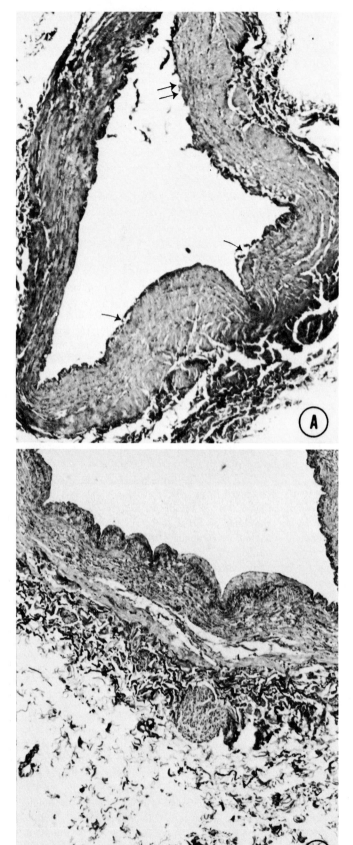

FIG. 7. A. Microscopic section of a vein removed through multiple incisions and umbilical tape used for traction during excision. Notice fragmentation of intima (single arrows) and denudation in some areas (double arrows). B. Section of another vein removed atraumatically through long incisions. Notice an intact intima and preservation of vasa vasora and periadventitial tissue.

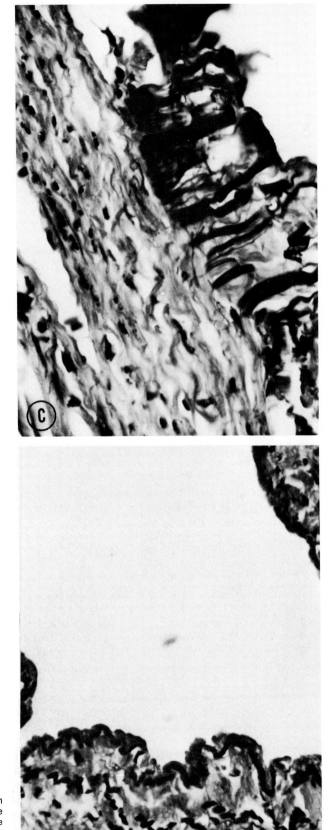

FIG. 7. C. Microscopic section of a vein manipulated with DeBakey forceps. Notice distortion of the internal elastic membrane giving a "brush" effect. Similar pattern was noticed upon using a hard-toothed bull-dog clamp. D. Elastic tissue stain of a vein for comparison. Notice the preserved pattern of the internal elastic membrane.

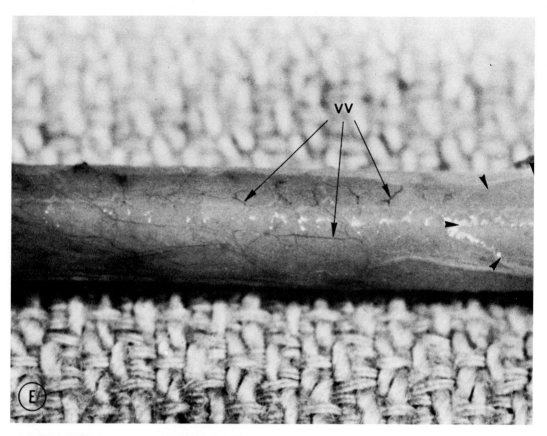

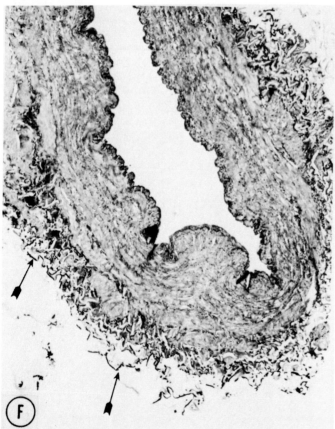

FIG. 7. E. Saphenous vein showing preserved vasa vasora (VV). Arrow tips point to an area deeply stripped of adventitial tissue. F. Microscopic section of a saphenous vein atraumatically removed (note preserved intima), but deeply stripped. Notice absence of periadventitial tissue and vasa vasora. Stripping was carried down to the external elastic membrane (arrows). Compare with Fig. 7B.

grafts alone are only used in excellent or very good outflow tracts (I to III). If the coronary vessel is severely diseased and small, carbon dioxide gas endarterectomy is performed distally and a proximal vein graft placed into the distal endarterectomized segment. An anastomosis to a small vessel (less than 1.5 mm), such as a diagonal branch of the LAD or distal posterior descending coronary artery, or a severely diseased vessel has a decreased flow and patency.[1] From the angiogram, the sites of anastomoses are selected and enlarged pictures are available in the operating room for constant referral. At the time of surgery, selection of a soft, pliable segment of the distal vessel, as far proximal as possible, distal to the coronary artery anastomosis, is made. If possible, the vein is inserted in a subepicardial area rather than an intermuscular segment. An acute angle of the vein to the artery is better than a perpendicular anastomotic angle with regard to flow characteristics. Construction of a "cobra head," as described by Linton and Menendez,[12] is ideal. Redundancy is avoided to prevent kinking and to minimize eddy currents. Interrupted sutures have been used in the past; however, continuous running sutures with small "bites" are felt to provide the highest patency. The advantage of the interrupted sutures is that they are often more expeditious to perform in difficult positions; however, to take advantage of a reduced time, a shorter anastomosis with a less acute angle to the coronary artery is necessary. This does not have as ideal flow characteristics as a flatter, less beveled anastomosis, which would require more interrupted sutures and decrease its advantage over the continuous running technique.

If the outflow tract is diffusely diseased or occluded, or if the vein graft flow is less than 20 cc per minute, a distal endarterectomy is performed by occluding the proximal vessel to avoid gas dissection and utilizing the technique previously described for gas endarterectomy distally.[19] The vein graft is then placed in the proximal arteriotomy, leaving the obstruction intact proximal to the anastomosis in order to avoid any competitive flow from the coronary artery that may jeopardize patency. Early restudy has substantiated the validity of this approach.

During distal coronary anastomosis under normothermic perfusion, the aorta is cross-clamped to provide a smaller, still heart and a bloodless field, particularly for the circumflex and left anterior descending arteries. A vent is placed through the apex of the left ventricle or into the left atrium via the right superior pulmonary vein. Electric fibrillation is instituted to stop the heart following aortic cross-clamping. Following suture of all distal anastomoses, the patient is removed from bypass.

Appropriate vein length is determined, and the proximal anastomosis is performed off cardiopulmonary bypass (in approximately 90 percent of the patients).

In certain specific situations where aortic cross-clamping with normothermic anoxic arrest might increase the risk, such as (1) a left main coronary artery stenosis, (2) functional left main coronary stenosis with tight lesions of the proximal LAD and circumflex, (3) patients with acute myocardial infarction in the early stage, requiring surgery, (4) ventricular aneurysms requiring cross-clamping, and (5) impaired left ventricles, we have determined the collateral circulation from the right to the left coronary arterial system by angiography. If good collaterals are present, the distal graft to the right coronary artery is placed first and attached to the aorta without aortic cross-clamping. The aorta is then cross-clamped proximal to the aortic takeoff of the right coronary graft, allowing perfusion of the left ventricle through the collateral circulation from the right during the distal left coronary anastomoses or opening of ventricular aneurysms. This technique has been employed in over 20 patients without mortality in these higher-risk groups and without evidence of significant infarction, except for those who were being operated on for an already evolving myocardial infarction.

Hemodilution of 50 to 75 percent is used for cardiopulmonary bypass with 3 mg of heparin per kilogram of body weight every two hours plus added potassium.

Anticoagulant agents are not used postoperatively, and aspirin and Persantine are being evaluated for their effect on the antiplatelet adhesive factor as it may relate to patency.

Use of coronary bypass grafts in patients with preinfarctional angina has been substantiated.[8] Its use in the occasional patient with myocardial infarction that is evolving in the hospital—either after coronary angiogram or in a situation where its onset can be determined, such as in the catheterization lab or coronary care unit—has been rewarding in our experience and in certain other centers.[4] When cardiogenic shock is present, the intraaortic balloon is used to stabilize the patient, either for coronary arteriography and surgery or for surgery alone in a certain specific ideal anatomic situation where bypass grafting can appear to benefit and prevent the extension of the infarct or limit the area of ischemia surrounding an infarct. Where large infarctions are present with mediocre to poor vessels and cardiogenic shock exists, results have not been as good with direct, immediate revascularization.[15]

The importance of subendocardial infarction

as a warning and indication for angiography has been established.[7] The rich collateral circulation to the subendocardial layer can be jeopardized by such an infarction. Depending on the anatomy and the coronary occlusions or stenoses (many of these have not had occlusions), transmural infarctions can evolve subsequently and can be prevented by revascularization surgery.

References

1. Bourassa MG, Lesperance J, Campeau L, Simard P: Factors influencing patency of aortocoronary vein grafts. Circulation (Suppl I) 45-46:1–79, 1972
2. Brody WR, Angell WW, Kosek JC: Changes in vein grafts following aortocoronary bypass induced by pressure and ischemia. Am J Pathol 66:111, 1972
3. Burton AC: Physiology and Biophysics of the Circulation. Chicago, Year Book Medical Publishers, 1968
4. Cheanvechai C, Effler DB, Loop FD, et al: Emergency myocardial revascularization. Am J Cardiol 32:901, 1973
5. Darling RC, Linton RR, Razzuk MA: Saphenous vein bypass grafts for femoropopliteal occlusive disease: a reappraisal. Surgery 61:31, 1967
6. DeWeese JA, Terry R, Barnes HB, Rob CG: Autogenous venous femoropopliteal bypass grafts. Surgery 59:28, 1966
7. Eliot RS, Holsinger JW: A unified concept of the pathophysiology of myocardial infarction and sudden death. Chest 62:4, Oct 1972
8. Favaloro RG, Effler DB, Cheanvechai C, et al: Acute coronary insufficiency (impending myocardial infarction and myocardial infarction): surgical treatment by the saphenous vein graft technique. Am J Cardiol 28:598–607, 1971
9. Furuse A, Klopp EH, Browley RK, Gott VL: Hemodynamics of aorto-coronary bypass: experimental and analytic studies. Ann Thorac Surg 14:282, 1972
10. Green GE, Spencer FC, Tice DA, Stertzer SH: Arterial and venous microsurgical bypass grafts for coronary artery disease. J Thorac Cardiovasc Surg 60:491, 1970
11. Kakos GS, Oldham NH Jr, Dixon SH, et al: Coronary artery hemodynamics after aortocoronary artery vein bypass. J Thorac Cardiovasc Surg 63:839, 1972
12. Linton RR, Menendez CV: Arterial homografts: a comparison of the results with end-to-end and

end-to-side vascular anastomosis. Ann Surg 142:568, 1955
13. Linton RR, Darling RC: Autogenous saphenous vein bypass grafts in femoropopliteal obliterative arterial disease. Surgery 51:62, 1962
14. McDonald DA: Blood flow in arteries. London, Edward Arnold, 1960
15. Mundth ED, Buckley MJ, Leinbach RC, et al: Myocardial revascularization for the treatment of cardiogenic shock complicating acute myocardial infarction. Surgery 70:78–87, 1971
16. Selmonosky CA, Ellison RG: The role of the coronary collateral circulation in the pressure changes distal to an acute coronary occlusion. Surgery 71:283, 1972
17. Sewell WH: Improved coronary vein graft patency rates with side-to-side anastomoses. Ann Thorac Surg 17:538, 1974
18. Simeone FA: Intravascular pressure, vascular tone, and sympathectomy. Surgery 53:1, 1963
19. Urschel HC Jr, Razzuk MA: Reconstruction of the left anterior descending coronary artery: repair with proximal vein bypass graft and distal gas endarterectomy. JAMA 216:1, 1971
20. Urschel HC Jr, Miller ER, Razzuk MA, Alvares JF: Vein bypass graft and carbon dioxide gas endarterectomy for coronary artery occlusive disease. JAMA 210:1725, 1969
21. Urschel HC Jr, Miller ER, Razzuk MA, et al: Aorta to coronary artery vein bypass graft for occlusive disease. Ann Thorac Surg 8:114, 1969
22. Urschel HC Jr, Razzuk MA, Nathan MJ, Ginsberg RJ, Paulson DL: Direct and indirect myocardial revascularization: follow-up and appraisal. Surgery 68:1087, 1970
23. Urschel HC Jr, Razzuk MA, Nathan MJ, et al: Combined gas (CO_2) endarterectomy and vein bypass graft for patients with coronary artery disease. Ann Thorac Surg 10:119, 1970
24. Urschel HC Jr, Razzuk MA, Wood RE, Paulson DL: Distal CO_2 coronary artery endarterectomy and proximal vein bypass graft. Ann Thorac Surg 14:1, 1972
25. Urschel HC Jr: Autogenous blood transfusions to reduce postpump hemorrhage. Unpublished data
26. Urschel HC Jr, Razzuk MA, Wood RE, Paulson DL: Factors influencing patency of aortocoronary artery saphenous vein grafts. Surgery 72:6, 1972
27. Urschel HC Jr: Factors influencing flow of aortocoronary artery saphenous vein grafts. Dallas Med J 59:316, 1973
28. Walker JA, Friedberg HD, Flemma RJ, Johnson WD: Determinants of angiographic patency of aorto-coronary vein bypass grafts. Circulation (Suppl I) 45-46:1–86, 1972

73

SIMULTANEOUS MYOCARDIAL REVASCULARIZATION AND VALVE REPLACEMENTS

Derward Lepley, Harjeet Singh,
Robert J. Flemma, and Alfred J. Tector

INTRODUCTION

Various studies have documented the high incidence of coronary artery disease and rheumatic heart disease occurring together.[2,6,7] That coronary artery disease itself leads to mitral insufficiency needing valve replacements on occasions is also apparent.[1,4,14] The difficulty of perfusing the myocardium through atherosclerotic coronary arteries during valve replacement in the past led to significant myocardial damage[8,13] resulting in high operative mortality and failure to improve in the long-term hemodynamic status of these patients.[11] A previous study described the method of simultaneous myocardial revascularization and valve replacement.[3] The initial mortality in our hands was high. The continuing improvement in our results prompted us to review our patients again. The aim of the study presented here was to determine whether the reduction in mortality in our patients was due to improvement in myocardial protection during cardiopulmonary bypass.

CLINICAL MATERIAL

Thirty-eight patients underwent cardiopulmonary bypass for valve replacement and vein graft procedures from January 1, 1971 through December 31, 1973. Their ages ranged from 43 to 70 years with a mean age of 56 years. Four patients were female. Twenty-seven patients presented with Grade IV, NYHA classification, cardiac failure; and 21 patients gave a history of myocardial infarction. Severe generalized reduction in myocardial contractility at angiography was seen in five patients. The left ventricular end-diastolic pressure was raised above 15 mm Hg in 17 patients. Table 1 shows the procedures performed in 38 patients. Thirty-two patients had single-valve replacement with single- or double-vein graft procedures. Five had double-valve replacement with single- or triple-graft insertions.

High-flow cardiopulmonary bypass with a Temptrol * oxygenator was used in all cases. Group I was comprised of the first 31 patients. Except for two patients in whom the severity of coronary artery disease had been underestimated at angiography, the sequence of events at cardiopulmonary bypass was similar. Vein graft procedures were performed first with the heart being perfused through the newly constructed vein grafts, and then valve replacements were carried out.[3] However, in the two patients in whom coronary artery disease was thought to be minimal, valve replacements were executed first. Failure to come off bypass and palpation of disease in coronary vessels led to subsequent vein graft procedures. Autopsy revealed severe diffuse coronary vessel disease in these two patients. Seven patients operated on in 1973 comprised Group II. After the myocardium had been cooled to 30 C via a heat exchanger, topical cooling with 4 C of Ringer's lactate was carried out in these patients. Emphasis was placed on cooling the inside of the left ventricle in an attempt to lower the temperature in the septum to below 10 C. There were nine patient deaths; two in whom coronary artery disease was thought to be minimal at angiography proved to be severe at autopsy. Valve replacement in these two patients was accomplished without particular attention to coronary artery disease. The

* Product of Travenol.

TABLE 1. Procedures and Operative Mortality

| | N | SINGLE | | | DOUBLE | | | | TRIPLE | % MORT. |
		LAD	CX	RC	CX RC	LAD RC	LAD Diag.	LAD CX	RC + LAD + Circ.	
MVR	14[2]	6[2]	2	1	2	3	–	–	–	14
AVR	19[6]	10[3]	1[1]	4[4]	–	1[1]	2	1	–	30
MVR + AVR	3[1]	1	–	1	–	–	–	–	1[1]	20
MVR + TA	2	1	–	–	–	–	–	–	1	
Totals	38[9]	18[5]	3[1]	6[1]	2	4[1]	2	1	2[1]	
Percent Mortality			26			11			50	

Bracketed number indicates operative mortality, described as death within one month of operation.

TABLE 2. Causes of Death

	NO. DEATHS	CAUSE
At operation	5	Myocardial damage during cardiopulmonary Bypass (two patients CAD not fully recognized at angiography; one patient perioperative MI)
1–3 weeks postop.	3	Two MI; one arrhythmia
3–6 weeks postop.	1	Further MI

TABLE 3. Yearly Mortality

	1970	1971	1972	1973
No. cases done	13	15	11	12
No. deaths	7	6	3	0
Percent mortality	54	40	27	0

TABLE 4. Group I: Valvular Pathology and Mortality

	NO. PTS. STUDIED	NO. PTS. EXPIRED	% MORT.
Mitral valves	15	3	
Rheumatic	11	1	9 (DVR)[a]
Papillary muscle infarction	2	2	100
Ruptured chordae	2	0	0
Aortic valves	16	6	
Calcified aortic stenosis	11	5	45
Mainly incompetence	5	1	17
Total	31	9	

[a]*DVR: includes one double valve replacement.*

causes of death and yearly mortality are listed in Tables 2 and 3, respectively.

RESULTS

There was no mortality in patients comprising Group II. Our mortality in Group I correlated with the following features:

Clinical Profile: Table 4 shows that age over 60 years correlated with higher mortality ($p = < 0.005$). A history of congestive cardiac failure and myocardial infarction, with or without angina, and cardiac output below 2.0 $L/m/m^2$ had similar correlation with high mortality (Table 5). The prognosis was severely compromised if the left ventricular end-diastolic pressure was raised at rest and if left ventricular angiography revealed a poorly contracting muscle (Table 5).

Procedures Carried out: Significantly higher mortality was present in the aortic valve replacement group undergoing graft procedures. Mitral valve replacement and simultaneous revascularization carried a much lower mortality. The two patients in whom coronary artery disease was underestimated at angiography and in whom valve replacements were carried out before vein grafts were inserted died. These were desperate efforts to improve circulation after a great deal of bypass time.

Valvular Pathology: Table 4 shows that posterior myocardial infarction with papillary muscle infarction and severe mitral regurgitation carried high mortality when valve replacement and vein graft procedures were performed. Similarly, calcific aortic stenosis with left ventricular hypertrophy and fibrosis, and small aortic annulus had a high mortality in our hands.

TABLE 5. Clinical and Catheterization Data and Operative Mortality in Group I Patients

CLINICAL DATA	NO. PTS. STUDIED	NO. PTS. EXPIRED	STATISTICAL SIGNIFICANCE
Age			$p < 0.005$ ($y^2 = 11.33$)
Below 60 yrs	22	2	
Above 60 yrs	9	7	
History (CCF + MI + angina)	3	3	$p < 0.025$ ($y^2 = 6.45$)
PAP			not significant
Below 60 mm Hg	24	5	
Above 60 mm Hg	7	4	
CI			$p < 0.025$ ($y^2 = 6.45$)
Below 2.0 L/M/M^2	3	3	
Above 2.0 L/M/M^2	28	6	
LVEDP[a]			$p < 0.005$ ($y^2 = 9.41$)
Below 15 mm Hg (at rest)	16	1	
Above 15 mm Hg (at rest)	14	8	
LV angiography			$p < 0.05$
Good LV	21	4	
Poor LV (generalized)	5	4	

[a]*LV not entered in one patient.*

Mode of Myocardial Protection: In Group II, all patients, despite considerably worse preoperative function as compared to patients in Group I, survived. The cardiac index in these patients ranged from 1.38 to 1.9, and left ventricular end-diastolic pressure varied between 8 and 35 mm Hg (mean values 23). However, cardiopulmonary bypass time and aortic cross-clamp time were shorter. Improvement seen in our latest figures (Table 3) can only be attributed to better myocardial protection during cardiopulmonary bypass. In experimental anoxic arrest in the canine myocardium in our laboratory, better preservation of functions was uniformly obtained by this method of cooling even at 90 minutes of aortic occlusion time. Causes of death in nine patients as shown in Table 2 indicate that myocardial damage during perfusion and myocardial infarction in the postoperative period were the major causes of death (55 percent).

DISCUSSION

Our overall mortality of 22 percent closely reflects the experience of Merin[10] and associates who described a mortality of 24 percent in 50 patients studied. It compares unfavorably to that reported by Loop et al.[9] Our study, however, did not include patients undergoing mitral commissurotomy and vein graft procedures in whom results are significantly better.

There was no mortality in those patients whose myocardium had been topically cooled as described. In those with coronary perfusion through newly constructed vein grafts, our mortality was related to older age, lower cardiac output, raised left ventricular end-diastolic pressure, and generalized impairment of left ventricular contractility at angiography (Table 5). Significantly higher mortality was encountered in patients with severe calcific aortic stenosis, diffuse myocardial fibrosis, and smaller aortic annulus. Mortality was also appreciably higher in those with severe mitral incompetence due to papillary muscle infarction as part of posterior myocardial infarction. Improvement in mortality noted recently in our patients is believed to be due to better myocardial protection during cardiopulmonary bypass procedures. The mode utilizing myocardial cooling to 30 C from the heat exchanger and, thereafter, topical cooling with 4 C lactated Ringer's solution has been detailed by others.[12,15] We emphasize that in order to prevent subendocardial necrosis in the hypertrophied left ventricle, both the inside and outside of the left ventricle needs to be rapidly cooled to septal temperatures of below 10 C.[5] Outside cooling of the myocardium failed to lower septal temperatures below 18 C, and, hence, the subendocardium was still vulnerable if the ischemic period was prolonged. Although our initial method of simultaneous myocardial revascularization and valve replacement proved successful in those with relatively better function, it clearly had its limitations in those with poor function, atherosclerotic coronary arteries, and a grossly hypertrophied left ventricle.

With topical cooling, the myocardium seems to be protected irrespective of whether there are lesions that cannot be bypassed or diffuse lesions, even when these have been underestimated by angiography. Hence, myocardial revascularization and valve replacement can be carried out under optimal surgical conditions. Furthermore, complications and limitations of coronary perfusion in a hypertrophied nonbeating heart with atherosclerotic coronary arteries are obviated.

The cause of death in nine patients was attributed to myocardial damage incurred during cardiopulmonary bypass and myocardial infarction at or soon after surgery. The importance of coronary angiography in patients undergoing valve surgery is highlighted because 12 of 38 patients (32 percent) had no angina despite severe coronary artery disease. Again the two patients in whom coronary artery disease was underestimated at angiography but proved to be actually severe at surgery died. The symptom complex of congestive cardiac failure with previous myocardial infarction, with or without angina, and the presence of severe coronary artery disease was associated with appreciable mortality. Hence, coronary angiography becomes mandatory in all patients undergoing valve replacement. It is our belief that in order to produce satisfactory long-term results in patients undergoing valve replacement and vein graft procedures, care of the myocardium during cardiopulmonary bypass becomes the single most important factor.

CONCLUSIONS

Continuing reduction in our mortality led us to review our patients. Factors such as age and poor left ventricular function were significantly related to mortality. Aortic stenosis with massive left ventricular hypertrophy and small aortic annulus had high mortality. In 55 percent of those who died, mortality could be attributed to myocardial damage during cardiopulmonary bypass.

The improvement in mortality is thought to be due to attention given to myocardial protection during simultaneous valve replacement and myocardial revascularization.

References

1. Burch GE, De Pasquale NP, Phillips JH: Clinical manifestation of papillary muscle dysfunction. Arch Intern Med 112:112, 1963
2. Coleman EH, Soloff LA: Incidence of significant coronary artery disease in rheumatic valvular heart disease. Am J Cardiol 25:401, 1970
3. Flemma RJ, Johnson WD, Lepley D, Auer JE, Tector AJ, Blitz J: Simultaneous valve replacement and aorto-coronary saphenous vein bypass. Ann Thorac Surg 12, no 2:163, 1971
4. Fluck DC: Acute mitral incompetence after acute myocardial infarction with successful early treatment by mitral valve prosthesis. Lancet 2:1052, 1966
5. Greenberg JJ, Edmunds LH: Effect of ischemic temperature on left ventricular function and tissue O² tension. J Thorac Cardiovasc Surg 42:84, 1961
6. Lewis RC, Creus HB, Shirey EK: Angina pectoris and aortic valve disease. Presented before the 120th Annual Convention of Am Med Assoc, Atlantic City, NJ, 1971
7. Linhart JW, Torre A, Ramsey HW, Wheat MW: Significance of coronary artery disease in aortic disease in valve replacement. J Thorac Cardiovasc Surg 55:811, 1968
8. Linhart JW, Wheat MW: Myocardial dysfunction following aortic valve replacement. J Thorac Cardiovasc Surg 54:259, 1967
9. Loop FD, Favaloro RG, Shirey EK, Groves LK, Effler DB: Surgery for combined valve and coronary artery disease. JAMA 220:372, 1972
10. Merin G, Danielson GK, Wallace RB, Rutherford BD, Pluth JR: Evaluation of combined one stage coronary artery and valve surgery. Circulation Supp II-110, 46:4, 1972
11. Peterson CR, Herr R, Crisera RV, Starr A, Bristow JD, Griswold HE: Failure of hemodynamic improvement after valve replacement surgery. Ann Intern Med 66:1, 1967
12. Shumway NE, Lower RR, Stoffer RC: Selective hypothermia of the heart in anoxic cardiac arrest. Surg Gynecol Obstet 109:715–54, 1959
13. Singh HM, Horton EH: Myocardial damage and valve replacements. Thorax 89:26, 1971
14. Spencer FC, Rappert EH, Stertzer SH: Surgical treatment of mitral insufficiency secondary to coronary artery disease. Arch Surg 95:853, 1967
15. Urschel HC, Greenberg JJ: Differential hypothermic cardioplegia. Surg Forum 10:506, 1959

74

SURGERY FOR 26 PATIENTS WITH SIGNIFICANT MITRAL INSUFFICIENCY DUE TO CORONARY ARTERY DISEASE

Tohru Mori, Pablo Zubiate,
A. Michael Mendez, and Jerome Harold Kay

INTRODUCTION

With the introduction of coronary artery bypass surgery, the simultaneous surgical treatment of valvular heart disease and coronary artery disease is possible.[1] Following the initial high mortality of this type of surgery,[2] a lower mortality has been presented in recent papers.[3,4] These papers,[1-4] however, have been concerned primarily with rheumatic valvular disease incidentally combined with coronary artery disease. The purpose of this report is to describe the operative and follow-up results of patients having combined coronary artery disease and associated significant mitral insufficiency due to coronary artery disease with or without prior myocardial infarction.

MATERIAL AND METHODS

Since 1969, twenty-six patients have been operated upon with mitral insufficiency due to coronary artery disease—seventeen men and nine women, ranging in age from 51 to 76 years, with an average age of 60. Preoperative chest X-rays, electrocardiography, coronary cineangiography, right and left heart catheterization, and left ventriculography were performed on all patients.

From 1969 to 1970, six patients had mitral valve surgery alone (Group I). From 1970 to 1973, twenty patients had mitral valve surgery as well as revascularization (Group II). All operative

procedures were performed employing anoxic arrest at normothermia. Mitral repair was performed for mitral insufficiency with or without torn chordae tendineae using the technique previously described by Kay et al, in 1965.[5] For mitral valve replacement, a Kay-Shiley disc valve with muscle guard[6] was used. Coronary revascularization was performed using saphenous vein bypass, except in one patient, in whom the left internal mammary artery was anastomosed to the left anterior descending coronary artery. All patients were followed to the present time.

Group I

The six men were between 51 and 76 years of age, and all had typical angina (Table 1). Three had histories of myocardial infarctions. In five patients, angina or myocardial infarction pre-

TABLE 1. Preoperative Evaluation of 26 Patients

	GROUP I[a]	GROUP II[b]
Age	51–76	51–73
Preoperative angina		
Present	6	19
Absent	0	1
Preoperative myocardial infarction	3	15
PA pressure, systolic/ mean (mm Hg)	43–97 (63)	24–119 (45)
LVEDP (mm Hg)	11–20 (16)	10–35 (24)
Ejection fraction	0.63–0.70 (0.68)	0.15–0.67 (0.40)

[a]Mitral valve surgery only. Men: 6; women: 0.
[b]Mitral valve surgery with coronary revascularization. Men: 11; women: 9.

Aided by a grant from the Children's Heart Foundation of Southern California and the Los Angeles Thoracic and Cardiovascular Foundation.

639

ceded the occurrence of a murmur. In one patient, the relation of the murmur to the occurrence of angina was unknown. Two patients were NYHA function class III, and four patients were in class IV. The systolic pulmonary artery pressure ranged from 43 to 97 mm Hg (average 63 mm Hg), and the mean pulmonary artery pressure ranged from 22 to 53 mm Hg (average 36 mm Hg). The left ventricular end-diastolic pressure varied from 11 to 20 mm Hg (16 mm Hg average). The ejection fraction of this group was essentially normal, between 0.63 and 0.7. Cineangiography revealed the following obstructions: right coronary artery, six patients; left anterior descending, three patients; circumflex, five patients.

Group II

The 11 men and nine women in this group were between 51 and 73 years of age. Nineteen had typical anginal pain, and 15 gave a history of myocardial infarction confirmed by electrocardiography. In 18 patients, an apical systolic murmur was heard after occurrence of anginal pain or myocardial infarction. In two of the 20 patients, the onset of mitral insufficiency in relation to angina could not be determined.

Preoperatively, one patient was in NYHA class II, 10 patients in class III, and nine patients in class IV. The systolic pulmonary artery pressure ranged from 24 to 119 mm Hg (average 45 mm Hg), and the mean pulmonary artery pressure ranged from 16 to 80 mm Hg (average 37 mm Hg). The left ventricular end-diastolic pressure ranged from 10 to 35 mm Hg (average 24 mm Hg). The ejection fraction varied from 0.15 to 0.67. Three patients had an ejection fraction of 0.10 to 0.20, seven an ejection fraction of 0.25 to 0.40, and eight an ejection fraction of 0.45 to 0.70 (normal). In two patients, the ejection fraction was not measured.

Cineangiography revealed obstruction of the right coronary artery in 16 patients, of the left anterior descending coronary artery in 10 patients, and of the circumflex coronary artery in nine patients.

Operative Results (Table 2)

GROUP I.   Coronary revascularization was not performed in this group of six patients. Four patients had mitral valve repair, with no deaths. Torn chordae tendineae or ruptured head of the papillary muscle associated with a dilated annulus were present in these four cases. The mitral valve was replaced in two of the six patients, with one

TABLE 2. Operative Results and Findings

	GROUP I (6 patients)		GROUP II (20 patients)	
	No.	Deaths	No.	Deaths
Mitral valve surgery				
Replaced	2	1	3	1
Repaired	4	0	17	2
Hospital deaths	1	17%	3	15%
Pathologic finding				
Dilated annulus	2	–	13	
Torn chordae tendineae with dilated annulus	4	–	7	–

hospital death. Both of the patients with mitral valve replacement had a dilated annulus, without torn chordae tendineae. Repair could not be accomplished in these two patients.

GROUP II.   In this group of 20 patients, a total of 40 bypass grafts were performed. Nine patients had a single graft, four had double grafts, and the remaining seven had three or more grafts. There were three hospital deaths (15 percent) in this group of patients. Low cardiac output complicated with bacteremia caused death in one patient. In another, death was thought to be due to insufficient coronary blood flow following anastomosis of the left internal mammary artery to left anterior descending coronary artery.

Seventeen of these 20 patients (85 percent) had mitral valve repair with two hospital deaths (12 percent). Torn chordae tendineae with a dilated annulus was noted in five of these patients (29 percent) and a dilated annulus without torn chordae tendineae in 12 patients (71 percent). In three patients (15 percent), repair of the mitral valve did not seem feasible, and the mitral valve was, therefore, replaced with a Kay-Shiley disc valve with a muscle guard. There was one death in these three patients. Two had torn chordae tendineae with a dilated annulus, and the other had dilated annulus with stretched chordae tendineae.

Follow-Up Results

GROUP I.   Follow-up in this group was from 14 to 51 months postoperatively (average, 40 months). Five of the six patients survived the immediate postoperative period. Follow-up was complete. There were two late deaths, one of which was due to myocardial infarction three months after surgery. The second death was in a patient who died suddenly eight months post-operatively. The remaining three patients are surviving: Two are in NYHA class I and are free of angina; one remains in class III and continues to have angina.

GROUP II. Follow-up for this group was from six to 23 months (average 12 months) postoperatively. Seventeen of 20 patients in this group were discharged from the hospital and have survived six months or more after surgery. There was one late death due to sudden arrhythmia. Of the surviving 16 patients, nine are in NYHA functional class I, and seven are in class II (Table 3). Postoperative recurrence of anginal pain was seen in three patients.

DISCUSSION

With the possibility of coronary arteriography and saphenous vein bypass operations, it is possible to replace or repair the mitral or aortic valve as well as perform coronary revascularization with no added risk. Several papers [7,8] have been published that discuss the possibility of coronary revascularization in patients with aortic valve disease and coronary artery disease. Recently, Oury et al (1973) [3] reported good results of combined surgery for rheumatic mitral valvular and coronary artery disease. However, in their patients with mitral valve dysfunction due to late sequelae of coronary artery disease, the late follow-up results were poor.[3] Loop et al in 1972 [4] also reported on

TABLE 3. Follow-up Results: NYHA Functional Classification

GROUP I
(3 patients)

| | | From | | |
	I	II	III	IV
To I	–	–	1	1
To II	–	–	–	–
To III	–	–	1	–
To IV	–	–	–	–

GROUP III
(16 patients)

| | | From | | |
	I	II	III	IV
To I	–	–	4	5
To II	–	1	4	2
To III	–	–	–	–
To IV	–	–	–	–

patients undergoing mitral surgery and revascularization and reported only two late deaths in 19 patients followed.

In this paper, we reported 26 cases with significant mitral valve insufficiency due to coronary artery disease. In Group I, only mitral valve surgery was performed; but in Group II, coronary artery revascularization was performed in conjunction with mitral valve surgery. The overall hospital mortality in these two groups was similar (Group I, 17 percent; Group II, 15 percent). In this small series, the mortality of mitral valve replacement was higher than the mortality of mitral valve repair (mitral valve repair, 10 percent; mitral valve replacement, 40 percent).

The chance of emboli with repair is negligible compared to that with replacement. We feel strongly that for patients with pure mitral insufficiency, with or without torn chordae tendineae, mitral valve repair (rather than replacement) is the procedure of choice.

Although a history of previous myocardial infarction was not an important factor in determining the hospital mortality,[9] ejection fraction was. Of the four hospital deaths in the 26 patients operated upon, two were in-patients with an ejection fraction of 0.10 to 0.20. Revascularization is important for long-term survival. In those patients in whom only mitral valve surgery was performed, there were two deaths out of five patients discharged from the hospital. In addition, one of the surviving three patients has angina and is still in NYHA class III. In those patients undergoing revascularization as well as mitral valve surgery, there was only one death in 17 patients discharged from the hospital. In addition, there was significantly more clinical improvement in the function of those patients with revascularization compared to those without.

SUMMARY

Twenty-six patients with combined mitral and coronary artery disease were divided into two groups, and the follow-up results of both groups were reported. In Group I, only mitral valve surgery was performed. In Group II, mitral valve surgery was performed along with coronary artery revascularization. The hospital mortality was the same (15 percent). In both groups, the hospital mortality was higher in mitral valve replacement than in mitral valve repair.

Follow-up data revealed a higher incidence of late mortality in patients without revascularization. The main cause of death was myocardial infarction.

It would appear that for the patient with significant mitral insufficiency due to coronary artery disease, combined mitral and coronary artery surgery is mandatory.

References

1. Coleman EH, Soloff LA: Incidence of significant coronary artery disease in rheumatic valvular heart disease. Am J Cardiol 25:401, 1970
2. Flemma RJ, Johnson WD, Lepley D Jr, et al: Simultaneous valve replacement and aorta-to-coronary saphenous vein bypass. Ann Thorac Surg 12:163, 1971
3. Oury JH, Quint RA, Angell WW, et al: Coronary artery vein bypass grafts in patients requiring valve replacement. Surgery 72:1037, 1972
4. Loop FD, Favaloro RG, Shirey EK, et al: Surgery for combined valvular and coronary heart disease. JAMA 220:372, 1972
5. Kay JH, Tsuji HK, Redington JV: The surgical treatment of mitral insufficiency associated with torn chordae tendineae. Ann Thorac Surg 1:269, 1965
6. Kay JH: The muscle guard for mitral valve prostheses. Arch Surg 98:626, 1969
7. Linhart JW, de la Torre A, Ramsey HW, et al: The significance of coronary artery disease in aortic valve replacement. J Thorac Cardiovasc Surg 55:811, 1968
8. Nakib A, Lillehei CW, Edwards JE: The degree of coronary atherosclerosis in aortic valvular disease. Arch Pathol, 80:517, 1965
9. Merin G: Giuliani ER, Pluth JR, et al: Surgery for mitral valve incompetence after myocardial infarction. Am J Cardiol, 32:322, 1973

75

SURGICAL THERAPY OF ACUTE VENTRICULAR ANEURYSMS

Frederick B. Parker, Jr., John F. Neville, Jr.,
E. Lawrence Hanson, and Watts R. Webb

The therapy of ventricular aneurysms has been well accepted for many years. Since the initial work by Bailey (Bailey and Gilman, 1957), thousands of patients have been aided by surgical excision. Chronic congestive failure and peripheral emboli remain the primary indications for surgery. Most aneurysms can be described as chronic. They form slowly and become symptomatic many weeks to months following an acute myocardial infarction. The acute ventricular aneurysm, we feel, is an entity unto itself and should be treated in an active, more aggressive manner (Parker and Webb, in press). In the acute ventricular aneurysm, there appears to be a more rapid dilatation of the involved myocardium. This causes a markedly reduced stroke volume and an acutely elevated end diastolic pressure with early, severe pulmonary edema. They may also present with hypotension and oliguria much like the patient in cardiogenic shock. Unlike chronic aneurysms, temporary medical measures, including digitalis and diuretics, are to no avail in relieving pulmonary edema. Unless aggressive therapy intervenes, these patients will succumb to irreversible left ventricular failure.

Acute occlusion of a major coronary vessel without the presence of previously formed collateral channels sets the stage for formation of an acute ventricular aneurysm. The vessel usually involved is the left anterior descending coronary artery, and the occlusion most frequently occurs just distal to its takeoff from the main left coronary artery. Septal and diagonal branches of the left anterior descending vessel are frequently involved, resulting in damage to a large area of anterolateral ventricle and septum. This transmural infarct initially demonstrates akinesis, but as the ischemia progresses to necrosis, the ventricular wall loses support. Dilatation follows and the dilated, non-contractile area of ventricle develops paradoxical motion. With systole, the aneurysmal area expands or paradoxes and, thus, receives blood to the detriment of the systemic circulation. Cardiac output necessarily falls. In diastole, the remaining sequestered blood from the aneurysm as well as the left atrial discharge results in an increased resting ventricular volume. There then occurs overall left ventricular dilatation and a further rise in left ventricular end diastolic pressure. A vicious cycle ensues, and the resting ventricular pressure soon enters pulmonary edema range. Klein, Herman, and Gorlin (1967) have shown that a left ventricular aneurysm must involve more than 20 percent of the left ventricular surface to cause increased left ventricular end diastolic pressure and volume. They postulate that the reason for left ventricular dilatation is inability of myocardial fibers to shorten enough to maintain a normal stroke volume following a large infarct. Therefore, in an attempt to increase cardiac output, left ventricular dilatation generally occurs by the Starling mechanism.

Any patient who has sustained a significant myocardial infarction and develops severe left ventricular failure a few days to weeks following the occlusion must be suspected of having an acute ventricular aneurysm. In this situation, correct diagnosis becomes imperative. Cardiac catheterization including coronary arteriography and left ventriculography must be immediately performed. There is little doubt that the risk of angiography in these acutely ill patients is greatly increased. We have found intraaortic balloon counterpulsation (IABP) to be extremely effective in preparing these acutely ill patients for emergency catheterization and possible surgery (Parker, Neville, et al, 1974). When it becomes apparent that medical therapy is ineffective, IABP is immediately instituted. Clinical signs of an improved cardiac output almost immediately occur. The major reason for this appears to be the reduction in left ventricular afterload provided by the balloon assist. Blood pressure and urine output increase, and left ventricular end diastolic pressure falls (pulmonary artery wedge pressure). With clinical improvement, cardiac catheterization can be performed with a reduced risk. In spite of the sometimes remarkable clinical improvement following commencement of IABP, we have made it a policy to perform cardiac catheterization with the intraaortic balloon in place and functioning. This gives further protection during catheterization.

Widespread coronary artery disease in these patients is a common finding. Coronary angiography allows proper assessment of the coronary arteries. Careful evaluation of the ventricle is essential. An acute aneurysm usually is found on the anterolateral ventricular wall. A large, akinetic paradoxing area is the hallmark of this entity. If other major areas besides the acute aneurysm are nonfunctional due to previous infarcts, surgical intervention may be fruitless. We have followed the suggestions of Sanders and associates (Sanders, Buckley, Leinbach, et al, 1972) in evaluating the feasibility of surgery in patients with severely compromised left ventricular function. They have arbitrarily divided the ventricle into six major areas and feel that at least four of these areas must have adequate contractility for the patient to survive operative intervention. If the patient meets these stringent criteria, surgery is elected. Many may also require coronary bypass procedures if high-grade lesions are present in the coronary vessels. Most will require IABP in the postoperative period as left ventricular function recovers.

SURGICAL TECHNIQUE

Surgery is performed through a midline sternotomy. Cardiopulmonary bypass is instituted by obtaining venous return from two cannulae in the right atrium. Arterial return is through a cannula in the ascending thoracic aorta. As bypass commences, the intraaortic balloon is removed. By the temporary clamping of the graft through which the balloon is placed at its connection to the femoral artery, postoperative counterpulsation is readily available. After bypass begins, the heart is fibrillated and the aneurysm excised. Close attention should be paid to the interventricular septum. If there are areas of fresh necrosis, particularly near the apex, cognizance of the possibility of for-

mation of an acute ventricular septal defect is important. Sutures can be placed that exclude this area during the aneurysm repair. Following excision of the infarcted aneurysmal area, careful suture placement is essential. The friability of the base of a recent infarct cannot be overemphasized. Our technique in ventricular closure involves placement of horizontal mattress sutures carefully tied over Teflon pledgets. The surrounding myocardium of an acute aneurysm lacks the firm fibrous ring so often found at the base of a chronic aneurysm. If the sutures are tied too tightly, the soft myocardium may be torn and overwhelming hemorrhage ensue. Following completion of the initial row of sutures, a more superficial running suture further ensures hemostasis. A left ventricular vent is utilized at the apex of the suture line until the heart is defibrillated and the patient is removed from bypass. If coronary artery bypass grafting is indicated, it is performed following completion of the aneurysm excision. Careful attention is paid to the left atrial pressure as bypass is discontinued. Usually it is in the elevated range (20 mm Hg or greater), and, if so, we elect commencement of IABP as bypass is discontinued. Left atrial pressure has proven most useful as a guide to patient management in the postoperative period. As the patient's left ventricular performance improves, this is reflected in a reduced left atrial pressure. The patient is slowly weaned from IABP when left atrial pressure can be maintained at 20 mm Hg or less and there is clinical evidence of adequate cardiac output (blood pressure, urine flow, etc). During convalescence, ventricular arrhythmias are common. The serum potassium level must be maintained at high levels and ventricular suppressive therapy utilized to prevent fatal arrhythmias. Continuous respiratory support has also been necessary. With meticulous attention to detail, a significant percentage of these patients will survive.

CLINICAL EXPERIENCE

In the last 18 months, we have seen five patients with acute ventricular aneurysms (Table 1). There were four males and one female, ages ranged from 51 through 68. All were transferred to our hospital following onset of acute pulmonary edema following a myocardial infarction. The onset of left ventricular failure varied from 11 to 63 days following the infarction. Chest X-ray revealed severe pulmonary edema in each case (Fig. 1). The electrocardiogram revealed an acute anterolateral infarct in all patients. Initial management consisted

TABLE 1. Clinical Material

PT./AGE	FAILURE OCCURRENCE FOLLOWING INFARCTION	EKG	BLOOD PRESSURE	PAWP[a]	X-RAY
AS/52	37 days	Anterolateral infarct	90/60	30	Severe pulmonary edema
DS/67	40 days	Anterolateral infarct	80/60	21	Severe pulmonary edema
CH/55	63 days	Anterolateral infarct	90/60	27	Massive pulmonary edema
DQ/57	11 days	Anterolateral infarct	90/70	25	Severe pulmonary edema
TM/68	14 days	Anterolateral infarct	100/70	25	Severe pulmonary edema

[a]Pulmonary artery wedge pressure.

TABLE 2. Clinical Course

PT.	IABP[a] (preop/postop)	SURGICAL PROCEDURE	RESULT
AS	1 day/1 day	Aneurysm resection	Home–return to work
DS	1 day	Aneurysm and CVG[b] to LCCA[c]	Died at surgery–irreversible ventricular fibrillation
CH	2 days/2 days	Aneurysm resection	Home–doing well
DQ	11 days/5 days	Aneurysm resection	Home–doing well
TM	Balloon not used	Aneurysm resection	Home–doing well

[a]Intraaortic balloon counterpulsation.
[b]Coronary vein graft.
[c]Left coronary circumflex artery.

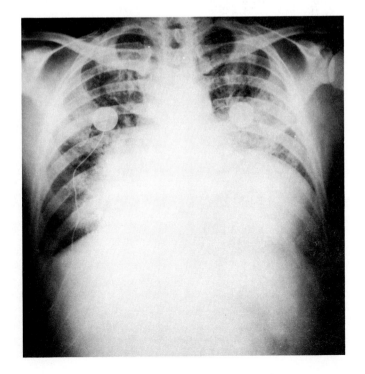

FIG. 1. Typical chest X-ray of patient admitted with rapid onset of left ventricular failure secondary to an acute ventricular aneurysm following anterior myocardial infarction (Patient A.S.).

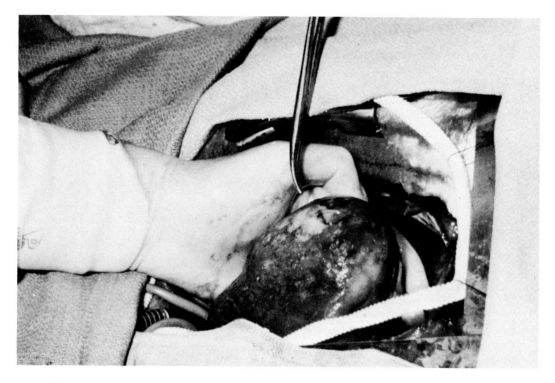

FIG. 2. Demonstration of acute aneurysm at surgery (patient DQ) 13 days following acute anterior myocardial infarction. Following excision, he has made a successful recovery.

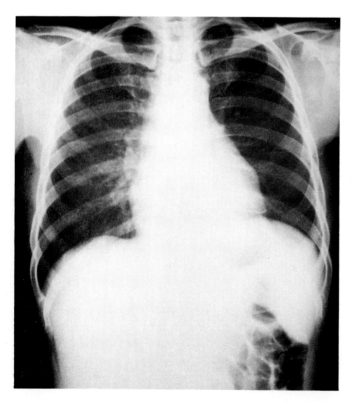

FIG. 3. Chest X-ray of patient (A.S.) one month following discharge from hospital after successful excision of an acute ventricular aneurysm.

of rapid digitalization and diuretics (Furosemide and/or Ethacrynic Acid). In each case, medical therapy was unsuccessful, and the severe left ventricular failure persisted. Following this, intraaortic balloon counterpulsation was begun on four of the five patients. Four of the patients underwent cardiac catheterization within four days of hospital admission, while one patient was catheterized 12 days after hospitalization. All patients had anterior ventricular aneurysms in the distribution of the left anterior descending coronary artery. The left anterior descending coronary artery was completely occluded in each case. Three patients also had high-grade occlusive lesions in branches of the circumflex coronary artery. The right coronary artery was without significant lesions in all patients. Left ventricular end diastolic pressure ranged between 20 and 30 mm Hg. In all patients, the remaining left ventricle appeared to function adequately.

At operation, all patients had acute ventricular aneurysms (Fig. 2). Surgery consisted of aneurysm resection in all five patients. One patient also had a saphenous vein graft performed to the left coronary circumflex artery but died at surgery of irreversible ventricular fibrillation. Three of the remaining four patients had continuation of IABP for three to five days following operation. The four surviving patients were discharged from the hospital and are doing well (Fig. 3). Follow-up is from 6 to 18 months (Table 2).

SUMMARY

We are convinced that the acute ventricular aneurysm is a definite entity. Treating this problem to a successful conclusion requires alert and aggressive management. Importance of cardiac catheterization to assess correctly the operability of the clinical situation cannot be overemphasized. The advent of intraaortic balloon counterpulsation has provided significant support to the patient in severe left ventricular failure unrelieved by medical means. By utilization of the proper facilities, a significant percentage of these acutely ill patients may be properly salvaged.

References

Bailey CP, Gilman RA: Experimental and clinical resection for ventricular aneurysm. Surg Gynecol Obstet 104:539–42, 1957

Klein MD, Herman MV, Gorlin R: A hemodynamic study of left ventricular aneurysm. Circulation 35:614–30, 1967

Parker FB Jr, Neville JF Jr, Hanson EL, Webb WR: Intra-aortic balloon counterpulsation and cardiac surgery. Ann Thorac Surg vol 17 2:144, Feb 1974

Parker FB Jr, Webb WR: Surgery in acute coronary problems. Webb, WR (ed): Acute Ventricular Aneurysms. New York, Medcom Press, 1974

Sanders CA, Buckley MJ, Leinbach RC, et al: Mechanical circulatory assistance: Current status and experience with combining circulatory assistance, emergency coronary angiography and acute myocardial revascularization. Circulation 45:1292, 1972

76

ANEURYSMECTOMY AND BYPASS GRAFTS FOR POSTINFARCTION VENTRICULAR ANEURYSMS

Alfred J. Tector, David G. DeCock, Roger Gabriel,
Robert J. Flemma, and Derward Lepley

INTRODUCTION

Ventricular aneurysm is one of the most frequent complications of myocardial infarction. Congestive heart failure, embolization, and arrhythmias are indications for surgery. Since the first aneurysm resection by Cooley[1] using cardiopulmonary bypass, operative mortality has progressively decreased as reported by Loop (6.8 percent)[2] and Merin (17 percent).[3] This report summarizes our experience over the past two years of treating left ventricular aneurysms by resection of the aneurysm and bypassing all significant obstructions in the coronary arteries.

METHODS

Clinical Findings

Forty-six patients underwent left ventricular aneurysm resection during the past two years. Twenty-seven patients had one documented myocardial infarct and 18 had multiple heart attacks. Fifteen patients had congestive heart failure, nine had recurrent dysrhythmias, and 39 had severe angina. One patient had mitral insufficiency secondary to papillary muscle infarction, and another had rheumatic heart disease with aortic stenosis.

Cardiac Catheterization

Cardiac catheterization and coronary arteriograms were performed on all patients. All aneurysms in the series involved the apex and anterior wall of the left ventricle. Left anterior oblique and right anterior oblique ventriculograms were obtained in order better to assess the extent of the myocardial damage. An obstructed left anterior descending coronary artery was the most frequent cause of the aneurysm; however, most of the patients had lesions in multiple vessels (Table 1).

TABLE 1. Extent of Atherosclerosis

VESSEL	OCCLUSION	SEVERE STENOSIS >70 (percent)	MOD. STENOSIS <70 (percent)
LAD	31	10	1
Circ.	2	19	16
RCA	5	23	9

Average resting left ventricular end diastolic pressure (LVEDP) was 14.3 mm Hg (4 to 44), and the average cardiac index (C.I.) was 2.9 (1.9 to 4.1) (Table 2).

TABLE 2. Hemodynamic Data

LVEDP	NO. PTS.	CI[a]	NO. PTS.
0–10	16	<1.5	1
11–20	20	1.6–2.5	13
21–30	9	2.5–3.5	20
>50	1		

[a]*Data unavailable in 20 patients.*

Technique

Antibiotics and digitalis were administered one day preoperatively and 48 hours postoperatively. Morphine anesthesia was usually administered. The heart was exposed through a median sternotomy incision, and reversed saphenous vein bypasses were sutured into the ascending aorta. Cardiopulmonary bypass was instituted utilizing total hemodilution and normothermia. The ascending aorta was cross-clamped before incising the aneurysm in order to prevent the possibility of embolization, as 18 of our patients had mural thrombus.

We resected as much of the aneurysm as possible, leaving a rim of scar for suturing. The ventricle was closed with interrupted and, more recently, running Teflon-bolstered sutures. Care was taken not to injure the anterior papillary muscle. If the ventricular septum was infarcted the sutures were placed to exclude its lower portion from the left ventricular chamber. Thirty-seven patients had one (16 patients), two (18 patients), or three (3 patients) saphenous vein grafts anastomosed to all the significantly obstructed coronary arteries. In 14 patients the left anterior descending coronary artery was bypassed even though its distal portion was involved in the aneurysm if its proximal segment was a good vessel. One of the patients had an aneurysm involving most of the anterior wall of his left ventricle associated with mitral insufficiency. He would not come off cardiopulmonary bypass until after his mitral valve was replaced with a no. 27 Bjork-Shiley prosthesis in the subannular position. Another patient had resection of a stenotic aortic valve and replacement with a no. 25 Bjork-Shiley prosthesis as well as resection of his aneurysm.

RESULTS

There was one operative death, for an operative mortality of 2.2 percent, and one late death, for a total mortality of 4.5 percent. The early death occurred in a patient who had an extensive aneurysm resected and a vein graft to his circumflex coronary artery. The patient could not maintain an adequate output after coming off cardiopulmonary bypass, and at postmortem the remaining left ventricle was diffusely fibrotic. The late death occurred two months postoperatively in a patient who had had severe diffuse coronary atherosclerosis of all vessels necessitating a right coronary endarterectomy at operation. One vein graft had been placed end-to-side to a circumflex marginal branch and side-to-side to the diagonal branch. This graft closed proximally, resulting in

closure of both grafts and a fatal myocardial infarction.

Ten patients have undergone postoperative catheterization studies from 4 to 24 months. Little change in hemodynamics was found; however, none of the patients were in congestive heart failure. Eight patients were relieved completely of their angina, and two reported a significant decrease in their angina. Eighty percent of the vein grafts studied were patent.

DISCUSSION

Survival following aneurysm resection is related to the degree of viability of the remaining left ventricle. The bypassing of all significant coronary artery lesions and the adherence to certain technical points are also responsible for lower mortality following aneurysm resection. It is sometimes difficult to estimate on the left ventriculograms the degree of contractility in the heart muscle not involved in the aneurysm. Frequently, a left anterior oblique ventriculogram as well as a right anterior oblique view give a better estimate of septal contractility. Repeating the ventriculogram after giving the patient nitroglycerine and observing him for increase in contractility has been helpful in some instances.

Patients with (1) aneurysms, (2) large, dilated poorly contracting hearts, and (3) either left main stenosis or severe diffuse coronary atherosclerosis are poor candidates for surgery. The patient in our study who died early had left main disease and a large dilated akinetic left ventricle. The patient who died late had severe diffuse coronary atherosclerosis. He also had a proximal closure of an end-to-side, side-to-side graft resulting in closure of two bypass grafts. This is one objection to this technique.

Bypassing all significant coronary artery lesions improves contractility of ischemic areas. We recommend bypassing the left anterior descending coronary artery if it supplies diagonal or septal branches. Mitral valve replacement was essential in the patient who had mitral insufficiency and a large left ventricular aneurysm. This can easily be accomplished through a left ventricular approach. Cross-clamping the ascending aorta helps to prevent embolization of mural thrombi. Resection of as much of the aneurysm as possible should give a better hemodynamic result. A continuous suture closure is preferable to interrupted sutures because it is more hemostatic and rapid.

CONCLUSIONS

1. Forty-six patients underwent left ventricular aneurysm resection and bypass grafts to all significant coronary artery lesions with a 2.2 percent early and 4.5 percent late mortality.
2. Angina was relieved or reduced in many of the patients; hemodynamics were not altered; and 80 percent of the vein bypass grafts were patent from four to 24 months postoperatively.
3. Patients with large, dilated, poorly contracting left ventricles or severe diffuse coronary atherosclerosis are poor surgical candidates.
4. Bypassing all significant coronary artery lesions and observance of a few technical features increases survival.

References

1. Cooley DA, Collins HA, Morris, GC, Chapman DW: Ventricular aneurysm after myocardial infarction: surgical excision with the use of temporary cardiopulmonary bypass. JAMA 167:557, 1958
2. Loop FD, Effler DB, Navia JA, Sheldon WC, Groves LK: Aneurysm of the left ventricle: survival and results of a ten-year experience. Ann Surg 178:399, 1973
3. Merin G, Schattenberg TT, Pluth, JR, Wallace RB, Danielson GK: Surgery for postinfarction ventricular aneurysm. Ann Thorac Surg 15:588, 1973

77

RESECTION OF LEFT VENTRICULAR ANEURYSM: REPORT OF 277 PATIENTS

Frank M. Sandiford, George J. Reul, Jr., John T. Dawson,
Don C. Wukasch, Luigi Chiariello, Grady L. Hallman,
and Denton A. Cooley

INTRODUCTION

Ventricular aneurysm has been defined by Edwards[1] as a protrusion of a localized portion of the external aspect of the ventricle with corresponding projection of the ventricular cavity. If the dilatation increases during systole, a paradoxical movement of the ventricle is said to be present and the aneurysm is referred to as dyskinetic. As more experience is gained in the diagnosis and treatment of ischemic heart disease and its complications, less difficulty is encountered, both in the cardiac catheterization laboratory and in the operating room, in differentiating between hypokinetic or akinetic areas of the ventricular myocardium and a true ventricular aneurysm.

Nearly all ventricular aneurysms are located in the left ventricle and result from stenotic or occlusive arteriosclerotic coronary artery disease (CAD), most frequently of the anterior descending branch of the left coronary artery.[2,3] Estimated to occur in three to 38 percent of patients who survive a major myocardial infarction,[4-6] ventricular aneurysms may appear as early as two days or as late as 10 years after the ischemic episode.[4,7]

Indicative of the poor prognosis for patients with postinfarction ventricular aneurysm who are treated medically is a mortality two to three times higher than that observed in patients who do not develop ventricular aneurysm after myocardial infarction.[5]

Intracavity mural thrombi, although almost always present at surgery, are reported to occur generally in up to 50 percent of the patients studied and become clinically significant as thromboembolism occurs in more than five percent of patients with ventricular aneurysm.[2,8]

Symptoms of congestive heart failure with or without angina are present in most patients with left ventricular aneurysm. Angina is a predominant manifestation in about 20 percent of the patients, and ventricular tachyarrhythmias occur in a smaller percentage.[9-12]

In recent years, extensive analysis of the hemodynamic effects of ventricular aneurysm has been pursued by a number of investigators.[13-16] A better understanding of the impairment of cardiac function caused by development of ventricular aneurysm has led to an aggressive surgical approach in the treatment of left ventricular aneurysm (LVA), as pioneered by us[17-22] and others[23-28] in the last 15 years.

Since the advent of coronary arteriography[29] and aortocoronary bypass (ACB) surgery, a more comprehensive evaluation of patients with ventricular aneurysm has become necessary, and the need for extended surgical treatment combining aneurysmectomy with coronary revascularization has become apparent. Our experience with 277 patients who underwent surgical treatment of LVA from January 1958 to July 1973 was reviewed to evaluate the efficacy of ACB and concomitant resection of an LVA.

MATERIAL AND METHODS

In this series of 277 patients, 101 underwent resection of an LVA without myocardial revascularization during the period from January 1958 to December 1969 (group I). From 1969

TABLE 1. Left Ventricular Aneurysm

	GROUP I	GROUP II	GROUP III
Procedure	LVA resection alone	LVA resection with ACB	LVA resection alone
Time period	1/58 to 12/69	12/69 to 7/73	12/69 to 7/73
No. of patients	101	125	51
Total: 277			

to July 1974, 125 patients underwent LVA resection combined with ABC (group II). During the same period, 51 patients had LVA resection alone because associated coronary lesions were not amenable to bypass (group III) (Table 1).

Age and sex distribution was similar in all three groups. Included were 246 men and 31 women, a ratio of eight to one, who ranged in age from 38 to 65 years with a mean age of 56 years. All patients had experienced at least one clinically documented myocardial infarction.

Among groups I and II, in accordance with the New York Heart Association functional classification,[30] 28 percent of the patients were in class IV, 65 percent in class III, and seven percent in class II. In contrast, 86 percent of patients in group III were in class III, 12 percent were in class IV, and two percent were in class II.

Symptoms of congestive heart failure were present in 95 percent of the patients in groups I and III, and in 66 percent of the patients in group II. Angina was significant in 35 percent of group I, 90 percent of group II, and 26 percent of group III (Fig. 1).

Diagnostic evaluation of patients with LVA included left heart catheterization, left ventriculography, and selective coronary arteriography. Over 75 percent of all patients with LVA were found to have multiple-vessel CAD. The coronary arteriograms were scored according to the method of Friesinger and associates.[31] The mean score for group II was 9.5 and group III was 6.5.

Symptomatic patients who had a reasonable residual area of functional left ventricle were selected for surgical treatment. In all patients in group II, at least one distal coronary vessel was suitable for bypass in addition to the LVA resection.

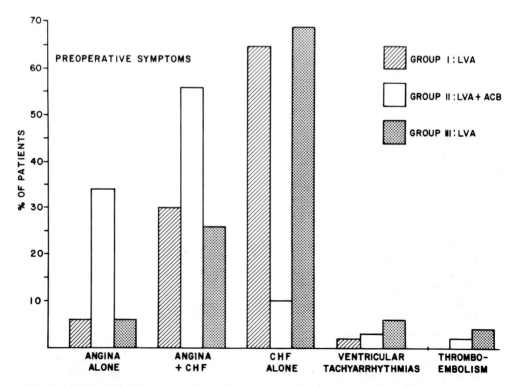

FIG. 1. Presenting symptoms in patients with left ventricular aneurysm (LVA). ACB: Aortocoronary bypass.

Group I

This group consisted of 101 patients who underwent LVA resection without myocardial revascularization during the "pre-ACB" period from 1958 to December 1969. Of these patients, 65 percent had symptoms of congestive heart failure, 30 percent had congestive heart failure and angina, and only five percent experienced angina as the only major presenting symptom. In two patients, intractable ventricular tachyarrhythmias were prevalent.

Of the 60 patients who underwent selective coronary arteriography, multiple-vessel coronary artery disease was present in 77 percent, and total occlusion of a major vessel to the area of the ventricular aneurysm was found in 23 percent. The average left ventricular end-diastolic pressure (LVEDP) was above 20 mm Hg.

These 101 patients represent a heterogeneous group in the "pre-ACB" era, not uniformly investigated, and include patients with and without concomitant severe CAD.

Group II

Resection of an LVA and ACB were performed concomitantly in 125 patients from December 1969 to July 1973. Angina was the major presenting symptom in 90 percent and was associated with congestive heart failure in 56 percent of these patients. Congestive heart failure alone was present in 10 percent. Four patients had ventricular tachyarrhythmias, and three had symptoms of systemic embolism.

Single-plane ventriculography and selective coronary arteriography were performed in all patients. Most of the patients in group II (96 percent) had significant occlusive disease in at least one vessel, in addition to occlusion in the one tributary to the area of the LVA. Severe triple-vessel involvement occurred in 24 patients, and significant stenosis of the left main coronary artery was noted in 20 percent (Table 2). The mean coronary artery score was 9.5, and the mean LVEDP was 24 ± 9 mm Hg.

In 86 patients ejection fractions were calculated, and a mean value of 37 percent was found. The average area of the aneurysm was estimated to be 40 percent of the area of the functional ventricle. In 25 percent of the patients, the aneurysm was as large as, or larger than, the

TABLE 2. Group II. Left Ventricular Aneurysm, Arteriographic Findings

	NO. PTS	%
Single vessel	5	4
Double vessel	96	77
Triple vessel	24	19
Total	**125**	**100**
Significant left main stenosis	25	20
Complete proximal occlusion	81	65
Without distal filling	39	
With some distal filling	42	
Stenosis > 90%	34	27
Stenosis < 90%	10	8
Total	**125**	**100**

functional ventricle. Arteriographic analysis of the main vessel to the area of the LVA demonstrated that complete occlusion was present in 81 patients (65 percent). In about half of these (42/81), some distal filling was seen. A stenosis of more than 90 percent was present in 34 patients (27 percent) and less than 90 percent in 10 patients (eight percent) (Table 2). The degree of vascular stenosis was not found to be related to the size of the LVA.

In over 90 percent of this group, the aneurysm was located in the anteroapical area (74 patients) or apical area alone (39 patients) of the left ventricle. The aneurysm was inferoposterior in seven cases and lateral in five (Fig. 2). Seven patients with anteroapical aneurysms also had evidence of inferoposterior akinesia.

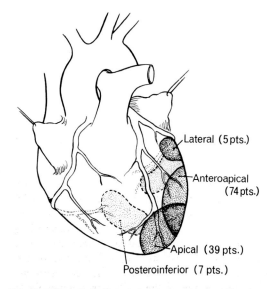

FIG. 2. View of the heart showing anatomical location of left ventricular aneurysm in 125 patients of group II.

TABLE 3. Group II: Left Ventricular Aneurysm, Arteries Involved versus Arteries Grafted

ARTERIES INVOLVED	CONCOMITANT PROCEDURE			
	Single ACB	Double ACB	Triple ACB	Total
Single	5[a]			5
Double	59	37[a]		96
Triple		16	8[a]	24
Total	64	53	8	125

[a]*All diseased arteries grafted in 40 percent of patients.*

Among the 125 patients in this group in whom LVA resection was performed, 64 underwent single ACB, 53 had double ACB, and eight underwent triple ACB. Double ACB was performed in 37 patients for double-vessel CAD and in 16 for triple CAD. Single ACB was performed in 59 patients with double CAD and in only five with single-vessel disease (Table 3). In 27 patients, a vein graft was placed to the left anterior descending coronary artery, which was a tributary to the area of the aneurysm. One patient with posterioinferior LVA underwent resection of the aneurysm, ACB to the left anterior descending coronary artery, and mitral valve replacement. A second patient required a mitral valve replacement and associated ACB to the right coronary artery.

Group III

The 51 patients in this group underwent LVA resection without concomitant myocardial revascularization from December 1969 to July 1973. Congestive heart failure was predominant in 95 percent, and associated angina was present in 26 percent of the group. Three patients had severe tachyarrhythmias, and two had evidence of peripheral thromboembolism.

Associated multiple-vessel CAD was either absent or hemodynamically insignificant. The mean coronary artery score was 6.5, and the average LVEDP was 22 ± 8 mm Hg. The major vessel supplying the area of the ventricular aneurysm was occluded in about half of the patients. In 94 percent, the aneurysm was located in the anterior or apical area, and the left anterior descending coronary artery was involved. There were two aneurysms of the lateral wall, and one was located in the posteroinferior area of the left ventricle. The average size of the LVA was comparable to that observed in group II.

SURGICAL TECHNIQUE

Operation was performed through a median sternotomy. After the pericardial cavity was entered, the dense adhesions over the aneurysm were left undisturbed until cardiopulmonary bypass was begun and the ascending aorta cross-clamped to prevent embolization from mural thrombi frequently found within the aneurysm. Cardiopulmonary bypass was instituted by venous cannulation of the superior and inferior vena cava through the right atrium, and the ascending aorta was cannulated for arterial return. As has been the custom at our institution since 1962, hemodilution perfusion techniques were employed in all patients. Disposable plastic bubble oxygenators were used, primed with five percent dextrose in Ringer's lactate solution. In the past, normothermia has been used at our hospital, but more recently, in an effort to avoid or minimize possible damage to already ischemic hearts from even a brief period of ischemic cardiac arrest, general body hypothermia to approximately 28 to 30 C is induced, and local cardiac cooling with iced saline solution is now routinely employed. The aorta was then cross-clamped and the left side of the heart decompressed with a sump placed through the right superior pulmonary vein into the left atrium. Dissection of the aneurysm from the pericardium was then performed, and the aneurysm was opened. The laminated clots and mural thrombi were carefully evacuated, fully exposing the extent of the aneurysm. The aneurysmal wall was then excised, preserving a sufficient rim, usually of dense fibrotic scar tissue, for reapproximation.

The amount of resection varied with the size, extent, and location of the aneurysm. Unless a mitral valve replacement was to be performed, the area of insertion of the papillary muscles was carefully avoided. In the resection of anteroapical and lateral aneurysms, an adequate residual left ventricular cavity was usually preserved when insertion of the papillary muscles was taken into consideration. This was not necessarily applicable in aneurysms of the posterior or inferior wall. When mitral regurgitation was present due to mechanical distortion of the papillary muscle attachment, it was possible—on two occasions—to restore, by ventriculoplasty, partial competence of the mitral valve. In two patients with posterior LVA, replacement of the mitral valve was necessary. The Cooley-Cutter mitral prosthesis [32] was inserted and easily secured to the mitral annulus through the left ventriculotomy.

When ACB was indicated as a concomitant procedure, the saphenous vein was prepared by distending the vein with autologous, heparinized blood instead of saline solution, to prevent damage to the wall by overdistention and saline extravasation.[22] The vein bypass graft was attached to the distal vessel and the ascending aorta with continuous suture technique. Each graft was attached to the ascending aorta separately.

Endarterectomy of the distal right coronary artery in association with ACB was necessary in 22 patients. Plication of the aneurysm was done in 25 patients who had small aneurysms when there was no discernible evidence of intercavitary clots. In half of these patients, the size of the aneurysm was less than 15 percent of the functional ventricle.

Cross-clamping the aorta and inducing ischemic cardiac arrest provided an optimal, dry, and motionless operating field for best recognition of the structures involved. Intermittent release of the aortic clamp was desirable, especially in patients with a high coronary artery score and multiple ACB, as long as one was careful to avoid or minimize repetitive coronary air embolism. For this purpose, we developed a special aspirating slit needle that was connected to low-pressure suction and inserted into the ascending aorta. Ventricular closure was usually accomplished with continuous and interrupted 1-0 and 2-0 black silk sutures. On several occasions, a saphenous vein bypass graft was placed to the distal right coronary artery with the patient in total cardiopulmonary bypass, but without cross-clamping the aorta.

RESULTS

In all three groups, early deaths were due primarily to acute or progressive myocardial failure or were secondary to recurrent myocardial infarction. Electocardiographic evidence of myocardial infarction in the early postoperative period was seen in 10 percent of the patients in group II and in 25 percent of group I. Other significant post-operative complications included arrhythmias, congestive heart failure, and postpericardiotomy syndrome. Clinical improvement was apparent in most survivors of all groups. Follow-up data were obtained from six months to 12 years postoperatively in over 75 percent of the patients surviving the operation. The average follow-up period of time was eight years in group I, three years in group II, and two years in group III.

Group I

An early mortality (30 days or less) of 19.8 percent (20 patients) occurred among those 101 patients who underwent LVA resection from 1958 to 1969. Most of the patients who died (18/20) had preoperative clinical or angiographic evidence of severe CAD. Neither of two patients who had predominant intractable preoperative ventricular tachyarrhythmias survived the operation.

Of the survivors 25 percent developed electrocardiographic evidence of myocardial infarction in the early postoperative period. Symptoms of congestive heart failure decreased in 60 percent, and angina was relieved or significantly decreased in 25 percent of the survivors. The late mortality was 38.8 percent (31/81), and most of the 31 deaths occurred within eight years after operation.

Group II

The early mortality in 125 patients following LVA resection and ACB was 12.8 percent (16/125). Of the two patients who had a concomitant mitral valve replacement, one died in the early postoperative period because of intractable congestive heart failure. All three patients who underwent operation within 30 days after acute myocardial infarction died in the early postoperative period.

In this group, the highest mortality was observed among patients who had double ACB (18.8 percent), and the lowest mortality was among those who had single ACB (7.8 percent) (Table 4). Furthermore, of the patients who underwent double ACB and died, 50 percent had triple-vessel disease. All five patients who died after single ACB had double-vessel disease. Only one of eight patients who underwent triple ACB for triple-vessel CAD died (12.5 percent).

A definite relationship between mortality and coronary artery score was found among the patients in group II. The average coronary artery

TABLE 4. Group II: Left Ventricular Aneurysm, Operative Mortality

CONCOMITANT PROCEDURE	NO. PTS.	DEATHS	%
Single ACB	64	5	7.8
Dougle ACB	53	10	18.8
Triple ACB	8	1	12.5
Mitral valve replacement	2	1	50.0
Total	125	16	12.8

score was 11.8 among patients who died and 8.9 among the survivors. A notably high incidence of left main coronary artery lesion (28.6 percent) occurred in those patients who did not survive the operation.

In four of the 16 patients who died, the aneurysm was located in the inferoposterior wall of the left ventricle. Also, in four of the 16 patients who died (25 percent), endarterectomy of the right coronary artery, in association with ACB, was necessary. One patient in group II survived mitral valve replacement, resection of anterolateral LVA, and ACB to the left anterior descending coronary artery.

Eleven patients (10 percent) showed electrocardiographic evidence of postoperative myocardial infarction in the early period after surgery. The infarctions occurred in areas supplied by stenotic vessels that had been bypassed at the time of the operation. All of these patients recovered from this complication.

Symptoms of congestive heart failure were decreased in 82 percent, and angina was relieved or significantly decreased in 85 percent of the survivors.

Twelve patients underwent postoperative angiographic studies on an average of 8.2 months after surgery. The LVEDP was observed to be significantly reduced in eight patients, remained unchanged in three, and became worse in one. An impressive threefold increase in the ejection fraction was seen in two patients, and significant improvement was noted in six. Late mortality was 10.1 percent, with most deaths occurring in the first two years after the operation.

Group III

Three of 51 patients undergoing LVA resection without ACB died following the operation (5.9 percent). One of these patients had severe

preoperative ventricular tachyarrhythmias that were not relieved by LVA resection. One patient with marked mitral regurgitation and LVA of the lateral wall died of myocardial failure. Another patient had a postoperative cerebral infarct.

In most patients surviving the operation, symptoms of congestive heart failure were decreased (85 percent) and angina was relieved or significantly reduced (92 percent). Only three patients (6.3 percent) died of myocardial infarction within two years of the operation.

COMMENT

Improved surgical techniques and a more comprehensive evaluation of all patients with ventricular aneurysms appear to be responsible for the reduction in mortality from 19.8 percent to 10.7 percent following LVA resection since 1969 (Table 5). The presence of significant concomitant CAD in vessels other than those supplying the area of the aneurysm enables better selection of those patients in whom a combined ACB procedure is indicated.

Following resection of a ventricular aneurysm, rapid hemodynamic improvement will occur, provided the residual myocardium is not ischemic. The association of ACB with resection of LVA is aimed at improving the blood supply to the residual left ventricle when concomitant CAD is present. In our series of 277 patients with LVA, the lowest early and late mortalities, and the best long-term results were seen in patients with occlusion of a single vessel and otherwise normal coronary arteries. Severe concomitant CAD with a high coronary artery score would be expected to

TABLE 5. Left Ventricular Aneurysm Mortality

	GROUP I	GROUP II	GROUP III
No. of patients	101	125	51
Operative mortality (30 days)	20 (19.8%)	16 (12.8%)	3 (5.9%)
Late mortality	31 (38.8%)	11 (10.1%)	3 (6.3%)
Overall operative mortality		39/277 (14%)	
Operative mortality since 1969		19/176 (10.7%)	

TABLE 6. Left Ventricular Aneurysm

	GROUP I	GROUP II	GROUP III
No. of patients	101	125	51
Mean coronary artery score	–	9.5	6.5
Mean LVEDP	>20	24 ± 9	22 ± 8
Left main lesion	–	20%	–
Multiple-vessel disease	77%[a]	96%	–
Early mortality	19.8%	12.8%	5.9%
Late mortality	38.8%	10.1%	6.3%
CHF improved	60%	82%	85%
Angina relieved or significantly improved	25%	85%	92%[b]

[a]*In those 60 patients who underwent coronary arteriography.*
[b]*Angina was present with CHF in 26 percent of patients.*

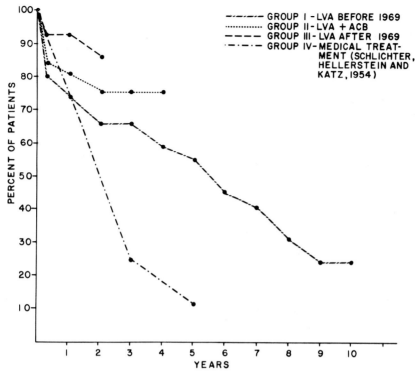

FIG. 3. Known late mortality in patients with left ventricular aneurysm resection (three groups) and with medical treatment alone (group IV).

increase the surgical mortality in patients with left ventricular aneurysm. In fact, the association of ACB in patients in group II led to an early mortality about twice (12.8 percent) that of group III (5.9 percent) but was still significantly different from the higher mortality (19.8 percent) in patients in group I (Table 6). In group II patients, the highest mortality (18.8 percent) was observed among those who underwent double ACB, and in half of these, associated triple CAD was present. Also, all five patients who died following single ACB had double CAD.

A corresponding lower mortality in those patients of group II who underwent revascularization of all diseased arteries would seem to justify the rationale for a "complete" operation. Factors other than a high coronary score—that is, left main lesion, posterior or inferior location of LVA, necessity for endarterectomy (25 percent), and mitral valve replacement—have significantly affected operative mortality. The length of the follow-up was not comparable because of the time lapse difference after the operation among the survivors of groups I and those of groups II and III. However, data thus far accumulated on late mortality in patients operated on before and after 1969 appear to demonstrate the validity of combined ACB and aneu-

rysmectomy in improving late results in patients with LVA (Fig. 3).

References

1. Edwards JE: An Atlas of Acquired Disease of the Heart and Great Vessels, vol 2: Coronary Arterial Diseases, Systemic Hypertension, Myocardiopathies, the Heart in Systemic Disease, and Cor Pulmonale Acute and Chronic. Philadelphia, WB Saunders 1961, p. 615
2. Dubnow MH, Burchell HB, Titus JL: Postinfarction ventricular aneurysm: a clinicomorphologic and electrocardiographic study of 80 cases. Am Heart J 70:753–60, 1965
3. Abrams DL, Edelist A, Luria MH, Miller AJ: Ventricular aneurysm: a reappraisal based on a study of sixty-five consecutive autopsied cases. Circulation 27:164–69, 1963
4. Applebaum E, Nicolson GHB: Occlusive disease of the coronary arteries: an analysis of the pathological anatomy in 168 cases with electrocardiographic correlation in 36 of these. Am Heart J 10:662–80, 1935
5. Schlicter J, Hellerstein HK, Katz LN: Aneurysm of the heart: a correlative study of one hundred and two proved cases. Medicine (Baltimore) 33:43–86, 1954
6. Cheng TO: Incidence of ventricular aneurysm in coronary artery disease: an angiographic appraisal. Am J Med 50:340–55, Mar 1971
7. Crawford DW, Barndt R Jr, Harrison EC, Lay FYK: A model for estimating some of the effects of aneurysm resection following myocardial infarc-

tion: preliminary clinical confirmation. Chest 59: 517–23, 1971

8. Bjork VO: Ventricular aneurysm. Thorax 19:162–65, 1964

9. Wasserman E, Yules J: Cardiac aneurysm with ventricular tachycardia. Ann Intern Med 39: 948–56, 1953

10. Couch OA: Cardiac aneurysm with ventricular tachycardia and subsequent excision of aneurysm. Circ 20:251–53, Aug 1959

11. Ritter ER: Intractable ventricular tachycardia due to ventricular aneurysm with surgical cure. Ann Intern Med 71:1155–57, Dec 1969

12. Magidson O: Resection of post myocardial infarction ventricular aneurysms for cardiac arrhythmias. Chest 56:211–18, 1969

13. Greenwood WJ, Aldridge HE, Wigle ED: The nature of the disorder of function in chronic postinfarction aneurysm of the left ventricle. Can Med Assoc J 92:611–14, 1965

14. Gorlin R, Klein MD, Sullivan JH: Prospective correlative study of ventricular aneurysm: mechanistic concept and clinical recognition. Am J Med 42: 512–31, 1967

15. Klein MD, Herman MV, Gorlin R: A hemodynamic study of left ventricular aneurysm. Circulation 35: 614–30, 1967

16. Berman DA, Grismer JT: Postmyocardial infarction syndrome followed by left ventricular aneurysm with papillary muscle dysfunction. Am J Cardiol 25:349–52, Mar 1970

17. Cooley DA, Collins HA, Morris GC Jr, Chapman DW: Ventricular aneurysm after myocardial infarction: surgical excision with use of temporary cardiopulmonary bypass. JAMA 167:557–60, May 1958

18. Cooley DA, Henly WS, Amad KH, Chapman DH: Ventricular aneurysm following myocardial infarction: results of surgical treatment. Ann Surg 150:595–612, 1959

19. Chapman DW, Amad K, Cooley DA: Ventricular aneurysm: fourteen cases subjected to cardiac bypass repair using the pump oxygenator. Am J Cardiol 8:633–48, Nov 1961

20. Cooley DA, Hallman GL, Henly WS: Left ventricular aneurysm due to myocardial infarction. Arch Surg 88:114–21, 1964

21. Cooley DA, Hallman GL: Surgical treatment of left ventricular aneurysm: experience with excision of post-infarction lesions in 80 patients. Prog Cardiovasc Dis 11:222–28, 1968

22. Cooley DA, Dawson JT, Hallman GL, Sandiford FM, Wukasch DC, Garcia E, Hall RJ: Aortocoronary saphenous vein bypass. Ann Thorac Surg 16:380–90, Oct 1973

23. Cathcart RT, Fraimow W, Templeton JY III: Postinfarction ventricular aneurysm: four year followup of surgically treated cases. Dis Chest 44:449–56, 1963

24. Favaloro RG, Effler DB, Groves LK, Westcott RN, Suarez E, Lozada J: Ventricular aneurysm—clinical experience. Ann Thorac Surg 6:227–45, 1968

25. Johnson WD, Flemma RJ, Lepley D Jr, Ellison EH: Extended treatment of severe coronary disease: a total surgical approach. Ann Surg 170:460–70, Sept 1969

26. Iben AB, Pupello DF, Stinson EB, Shumway NE: Surgical treatment of postinfarction ventricular septal defect. Ann Thorac Surg 8:252–62, 1969

27. Rossi NP, Flege JB Jr, Ehrenhaft JL: Surgically treatable complications of myocardial infarction. Surgery 65:118–26, Jan 1969

28. Machleder HI, Mulder DG: Surgical treatment of ventricular aneurysms. Am J Surg 121:720–23, June 1971

29. Sones FM Jr, Shirley ER: Cine coronary arteriography. Mod Concepts Cardiovasc Dis 31:735–38, 1962

30. Nomenclature and criteria for diagnosis of diseases of the heart and blood vessels, 6th ed. New York, New York Heart Association, 1964

31. Friesinger GC, Page EE, Ross RS: Prognostic significance of coronary arteriography. Trans Am Assoc Physicians 83:78–92, 1970

32. Cooley DA, Okies JE, Wukasch DC, Sandiford FM, Hallman GL: Ten-year experience with cardiac valve replacement: results with a new mitral prosthesis. Ann Surg 177: no 6 818–26, June 1973

78

RESECTION OF POSTINFARCTION ANEURYSMS OF THE LEFT VENTRICLE

WILLIAM A. GAY, JR., and PAUL A. EBERT

Acute myocardial infarction results in formation of an aneurysm of the left ventricle in 12 to 15 percent of cases.[1,12] The usual clinical course is for the patient to exhibit moderate to severe left ventricular failure during the recovery phase of infarction, then to progress to chronic heart failure for months or years afterward. Until the recent advances in acute coronary care, many of these patients did not survive the early postinfarction period. The majority of these individuals can benefit from excision of their aneurysm at some time during the course of their disease. The purpose of this chapter is to report operative experience with 53 patients undergoing resection of left ventricular aneurysms and the factors influencing timing of operation and selection of concomitant procedures.

The ages of the 53 patients ranged from 51 to 68 years, with a mean age of 58. There were 48 males and five females. All 53 patients were symptomatic, 31 (58 percent) were class III (NYHA), and 22 (42 percent) were class IV. Congestive heart failure was present in 46 (83 percent) patients; 26 (49 percent) had experienced arrhythmias (life-threatening in 10) and 20 (38 percent) had angina.

All patients except one had left ventriculography and coronary arteriography preoperatively. In that patient a Swan-Ganz catheter was advanced through the right heart chambers, where the presence of a ventricular septal defect was documented by blood oxygen content and pressure tracings. The aneurysm was located in the apical-anterior area in all 53 patients, and the left anterior descending coronary artery was found occluded in all. In 20 patients (38 percent) the right and circumflex coronaries were free of significant occlusive disease. The right coronary, along with the LAD, was significantly involved

in 14 patients (26 percent), and both the right and circumflex were affected in five (10 percent). There was "diffuse" occlusive disease involving the right and circumflex in 14 patients (twenty-six percent). Significant aortic stenosis (gradient > 50 mm Hg) was present in two patients and gross mitral regurgitation in an additional two.

The interval between myocardial infarction and operation ranged from eight days to seven years, but no patient was subjected to elective operation earlier than four weeks following infarction. There were five patients whose clinical condition made it necessary to undertake operation urgently prior to that time. Four of the five were suffering incapacitating and progressive heart failure, and the other was experiencing a series of uncontrollable life-threatening arrhythmias. The infarct-to-operation interval was two months to seven years in the remaining 48 patients, and surgery was undertaken on a more elective basis in this group, even though many were in severe chronic heart failure.

Of the 53 patients undergoing operation, 50 are surviving two months to five years following their procedure. There were two early deaths (one intraoperative and one two days postoperative) and one late death (seven months postoperative). Of the 50 survivors 24 (48 percent) had only an aneurysmectomy, while 14 (28 percent) had an additional right coronary bypass, and five (10 percent) had both right and circumflex coronary bypasses accompanying resection of the aneurysm. Three patients had closure of VSD, two had aortic valve replacement, and two had mitral valve replacements.

Both of the early deaths occurred in patients undergoing operation on an urgent basis within four weeks of their infarctions. One died intraoperatively during an attempt at resection of a large anteroseptal aneurysm and closure of a VSD. The patient had been in refractory cardiogenic shock for 24 hours preoperatively and could not sustain himself without cardiopulmonary bypass. With the use of intraaortic balloon counterpulsation, it is quite possible that this patient might have survived. The other early death occurred in a 60-year-old patient operated upon three weeks following a massive myocardial infarction. His initial postinfarction course had been uncomplicated, but he soon began to manifest severe heart failure, which could not be managed with drugs. He improved within 24 hours of the institution of intraaortic balloon support and underwent ventriculography and coronary arteriography. Although most of his left ventricle was moving paradoxically, an attempt at ventricular resection and revascularization of a near totally blocked right coronary was deemed advisable. In spite of continuous balloon support, he survived for only 48 hours after surgery. Retrospectively, the extent of left ventricular damage was probably beyond surgical relief. The single late death was due to heart failure in a 57-year-old patient who had extensive myocardial fibrosis in addition to a discrete aneurysm that had been resected seven months previously. This patient also had diffuse occlusive disease of both his circumflex and right coronary arteries rendering them unfit for bypass. He improved in the early postoperative period but then reverted to chronic progressive heart failure. All 50 of the survivors were improved by at least one functional class, and many were able to return to gainful employment following operation.

Although some patients with left ventricular aneurysms may not become symptomatic for several years following their myocardial infarctions,[5] this course of events seems now to represent the exception rather than the rule. Due, in large measure, to improvements in care of patients with acute myocardial infarctions, many individuals with large infarcts are now surviving the rhythm and failure problems that would have caused their death a few years ago. These patients, with a significant (usually 20 percent or more)[8] portion of their left ventricle infarcted, are the ones who develop congestive heart failure during the recuperative period. A large percentage of patients in this category (75 percent) will have a localized area of left ventricular dysfunction.[3] Although there are some proponents of early resection of these dyskinetic areas,[9] most surgeons prefer to delay surgery for two to three months after acute infarction.[4,6,10,11,13] This period allows the development of firm scar tissue about the edges of the aneurysm, thus facilitating

suturing of the ventricular wall. The absence of operative mortality in those patients undergoing surgery longer than four weeks after their infarction in the present series substantiates this approach.

With all 53 aneurysms located in the distribution area of the left anterior descending coronary artery, it was not surprising to find this vessel occluded in each instance. The incidence of diffuse multiple vessel involvement of 26 percent in this series is somewhat higher than that reported in other clinical series,[3,7] but strikingly lower than a previously reported autopsy series.[5] The 38 percent incidence of relatively normal right and circumflex coronaries was surprisingly high when compared with the report of Kitamure et al[7] but was lower than the occurrence of single-vessel occlusive disease reported by Baxley and Reeves.[3] Certainly, ventriculography and coronary arteriography are necessary in order to plan intelligently any form of surgical therapy in these patients.[2] Significant occlusive lesions outside the area of aneurysm should be bypassed[4,6,9,10,11,13] because it seems that this favorably alters the long-term outlook for patients in whom a leading cause of death is a subsequent myocardial infarction.

Although the risk of clinically significant arterial embolization is small[5,12] the occurrence of mural thrombi of considerable size within ventricular aneurysms is quite high.[5] With the shaggy, loosely attached clot present within the ventricular cavity, opening of the ventricle and manual removal of this material not only avoids intraoperative embolization but also significantly reduces the risk of postoperative emboli. No embolic episodes have occurred in the series reported herein, either intra- or postoperatively.

SUMMARY

Fifty-three patients have had excision of left ventricular aneurysms with two early deaths and one late death. Both early deaths occurred in patients operated on less than one month after acute myocardial infarction. The late death occurred seven months postoperatively in a patient with severe diffuse ventricular fibrosis, in addition to a discrete aneurysm. Whenever possible, resection of ventricular aneurysms should be undertaken no sooner than four weeks (and preferably 12 weeks) from the time of acute infarction. At the time of aneurysmectomy, bypass grafts should be placed to vessels outside the area of the aneurysm that have significant occluding lesions. To reduce the risk of intra- and postoperative embolization of mural thrombotic material, the aneurysm should be opened, and the thrombus evacuated.

References

1. Abrams DL, Edelist A, Luria MH, Miller AJ: Ventricular aneurysm: a reappraisal based on a study of sixty-five consecutive autopsied cases. Circulation 27:164, 1963
2. Baron MG: Post infarction aneurysm of the left ventricle. Circulation 43:762, 1971
3. Baxley WA, Reeves TJ: Abnormal regional myocardial performance in coronary artery disease. Prog Cardiovasc Dis 13:405, 1971
4. Cokkinos DV, Hallman GL, Cooley DA, Zamalloa O, Leachman RD: Left ventricular aneurysm: analysis of electrocardiographic features and postresection changes. Am Heart J 82:149, 1971
5. Davis RW, Ebert PA: Ventricular aneurysm: a clinical-pathological correlation. Am J Cardiol 29:1, 1972
6. Hazan E, Bloch G, Rioux C, et al: Surgical treatment of aneurysm and segmental dyskinesia of the left ventricular wall after myocardial infarction. Am J Cardiol 31:708, 1973
7. Kitamura S, Kay JH, Krohn BG, Magidson O, Dunne EF: Geometric and functional abnormalities of the left ventricle with a chronic localized noncontractile area. Am J Cardiol 31:701, 1973
8. Klein MD, Herman MV, Gorlin R: A hemodynamic study of left ventricular aneurysms. Circulation 35:614, 1967
9. Kluge TH, Ullal SR, Hill JD, Kerth WJ, Gerbode F: Dyskinesia and aneurysm of the left ventricle: surgical experience in 36 patients. J Cardiovasc Surg (Torino) 12:273, 1971
10. Merrin G, Schattenberg TT, Pluth JR, Wallace RB, Danielson GK: Surgery for postinfarction ventricular aneurysm. Ann Thorac Surg 15:588, 1973
11. Mundth ED, Buckley MJ, Daggett WM, Sanders CA, Austen WG: Surgery for complications of acute myocardial infarction. Circulation 45:1279, 1972
12. Schlicter J, Hellerstein HK, Katz LN: Aneurysm of the heart. Medicine 33:43, 1954
13. Stoney WS, Alford WC Jr, Burrus GR, Thomas CS Jr: Repair of anteroseptal ventricular aneurysm. Ann Thorac Surg 15:304, 1973

79

COMBINED REVASCULARIZATION AND ANEURYSMECTOMY: RATIONALE AND RESULTS

U. F. Tesler, J. Fernandez,
D. P. Morse, and G. M. Lemole

The effectiveness of simultaneous coronary revascularization by saphenous vein bypass graft and resection of postinfarction ventricular aneurysm was evaluated in 45 patients.

The late mortality following aneurysmectomy alone is high and attributable to the diffuse obstructive lesions usually present in the remaining coronary circulation.

Each patient in this series had severe obstructive disease of the left anterior descending coronary artery and of one or both of the other major coronary arteries.

In addition to resection of the ventricular aneurysm, the left anterior descending coronary artery was bypassed in 32 cases, the right in 21, the circumflex in four, and a diagonal in one; 31 patients had a single graft, 12 had two, and one had three grafts inserted. Six patients required concomitant valve surgery, four of them for papillary muscle dysfunction. Preoperatively, 36 of the 45 patients had congestive heart failure, 15 had repeated episodes of pulmonary edema, and 35 had severe angina.

Perioperative mortality was four out of 45 cases. There were no late deaths.

Twenty-one patients became completely asymptomatic and 20 more were considerably improved. Angina was relieved in all cases. Further use of the combined procedure is recommended.

Resection of left ventricular aneurysm usually produces significant clinical and hemodynamic improvement; however, the long-term prognosis of patients who have resection of ventricular aneurysm is largely dependent upon the extent and progression of occlusive disease present in the portions of the coronary arterial tree other than the branch whose occlusion caused the aneurysm formation.

The ideal surgical situation of a discrete ventricular aneurysm, secondary to the occlusion of a single coronary artery branch, is rarely present.

Since the development of myocardial revascularization surgery, simultaneous performance of coronary artery bypass has represented, in selected cases, the logical extension of aneurysmectomy, in an attempt to improve both the performance of the residual myocardium and the long term prognosis.

In this report, we describe our experience with 45 patients in whom simultaneous resection of ventricular aneurysm and coronary artery bypass was performed.

CLINICAL MATERIAL

There were 39 men and six women. The average age was 50.3 years. Of the 45 patients, 36 had congestive heart failure, either alone (10 cases) or combined with angina pectoris (26 cases). Angina pectoris was the main symptom of another nine patients. Among the group of patients with congestive heart failure, 15 had had repeated episodes of acute pulmonary edema.

Severe arrhythmias were observed in five patients who also had failure: two had an episode of ventricular fibrillation prior to surgery and were resuscitated; one had runs of ventricular tachycardia resistant to medical therapy and persistent over a three-day period. This represented an imperative indication for emergency surgical treatment. Two patients had previous insertions of permanent pacemakers for complete heart block. In addition, four patients had severe mitral regurgitation secondary to papillary muscle dysfunction, and two had aortic stenosis. All of these patients required surgical correction.

Physical findings in most cases were consistent with the presence of ventricular aneurysm and congestive heart failure. In every case the electrocardiogram showed evidence of an old myocardial infarction and often suggested the presence of a ventricular aneurysm in the precordial leads. Radiographic examination of the chest was generally abnormal and suggested ventricular aneurysm; in one case, however, the heart silhouette appeared normal, and in two additional cases the chest roentgenograms indicated nonspecific cardiomegaly.

All patients who were not disabled by chest pains or congestive heart failure at rest, had a 7 percent grade treadmill exercise test preoperatively. Their limitations were documented by their inability to walk at rapid rates. Eight could walk only at 1 mph, 12 were able to attain 2 mph, and only five could reach the 3 mph level. Ten developed angina pectoris with exercise, eight became short of breath, and seven had both angina and shortness of breath. Premature ventricular beats appeared in three patients, and another had a brief run of atrial tachycardia. Exercise-induced ST segment elevations, though often present, were not uniformly seen, perhaps reflecting the inability of these patients to attain higher levels of exercise.

All patients had cardiac catheterization, left ventriculograms, and selective coronary arteriography. A moderate-to-marked elevation of the left ventricular end-diastolic pressure and obvious impairment of the efficiency of contraction of the left ventricle due to the presence of the aneurysm was demonstrated in all. The status of the individual coronary arteries as visualized by selective coronary arteriograms is tabulated in Table 1.

It can be noted that the anterior descending coronary artery was totally occluded in 33 cases and significantly in 12 others (Fig. 1). Although in 11 of the 33 cases the vessel was totally obliterated, retrograde filling was observed in the other 22 through collateral circulation (Figs. 2, 3). This collateral filling occurred via the diagonal, the right conus or right marginal branches, and the septal perforators. The circumflex or marginal system was totally or significantly obstructed in 29 cases. The right coronary artery was significantly involved in 19 cases. In 15 patients, subtotal occlusion of all three major coronary arteries was demonstrated. In addition to visualization of the aneurysm in all cases, most patients showed evidence of mural thrombi in the left ventriculogram.

OPERATIVE FINDINGS

In all cases the aneurysmal wall was fibrotic. In 41 patients, the anterolateral wall of the left ventricle was the major site of involvement. In 11 patients there was also significant involvement of the apex, and in six the septum was massively involved. Four patients had major involvement of the posterior-inferior ventricular wall. In two of these there was severe mitral regurgitation secondary to papillary muscle dysfunction. (In the other two cases of posterior ventricular aneurysm, the posterior papillary muscle was not involved.)

The size of the aneurysm varied from 4×5 cm to a huge thin-walled sac. The number of clots was variable. In four cases there were no discernible mural thrombi. Besides the two cases with posterior-inferior ventricular aneurysms, there were two other patients with severe mitral insufficiency due to fibrosis and dysfunction of the papillary muscles. In yet another two cases, concomitant calcific aortic stenosis was present.

SURGICAL TREATMENT

Simultaneous aneurysmectomy and aortocoronary artery bypass with reversed saphenous vein graft was performed in all cases using extracorporeal circulation, intermittent ischemia, and topical cardiac cooling with iced saline. The left anterior descending artery was bypassed in 32 cases, the right in 21, the circumflex marginal system in four, and a diagonal artery in one (Fig. 4). Thirty-one patients had a single graft, 12 had two, and one had three grafts inserted. Six patients had concomitant prosthetic valve replacements, two in the aortic and four in the mitral area employing the Bjork-Shiley and the Beall prosthesis respectively.

RESULTS

Two of the patients died on the first postoperative day of arrhythmias and hypotension refractory to any medical treatment. One of these was a patient who had had ventricular fibrillation on admission to the hospital. Autopsy showed that the two vein grafts were patent (to the anterior descending and marginal arteries) but that there was severe occlusive disease beyond each site of anastomosis.

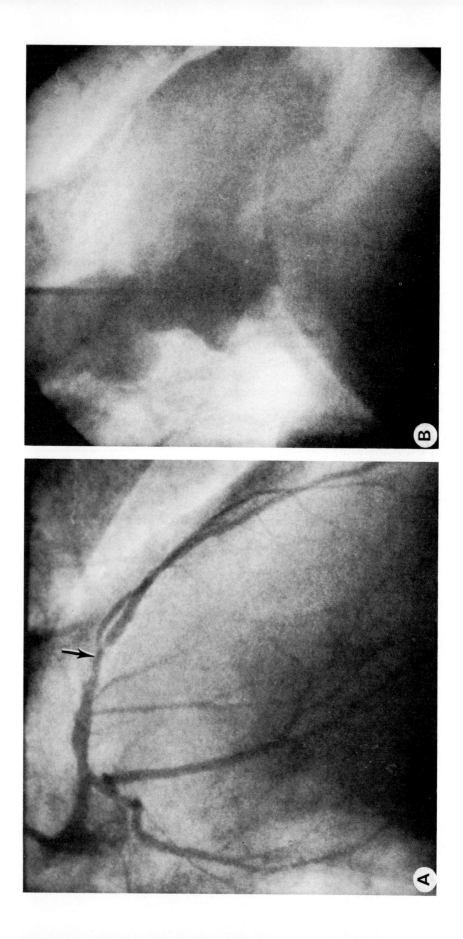

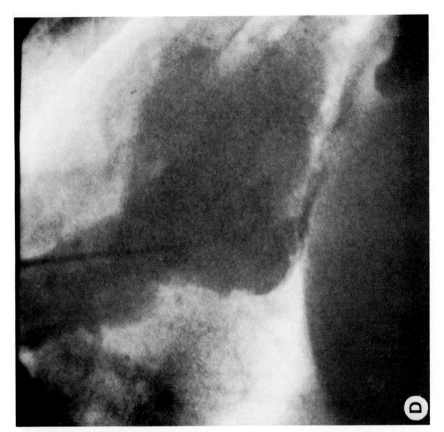

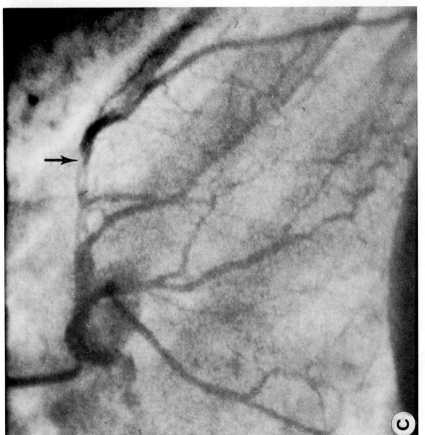

FIG. 1. A, C, E. Selective left coronary arteriograms in the RAO projection demonstrate localized subtotal occlusion of the anterior descending coronary artery in each of three patients with distal patency. B, D, F. Corresponding left ventriculograms in the RAO projection in the same patients demonstrate the presence of aneurysm with the suggestion of thrombi in B and D. Resection of the aneurysm combined with the saphenous vein bypass graft to the distal left anterior descending coronary artery was performed in each case. Continued on next page.

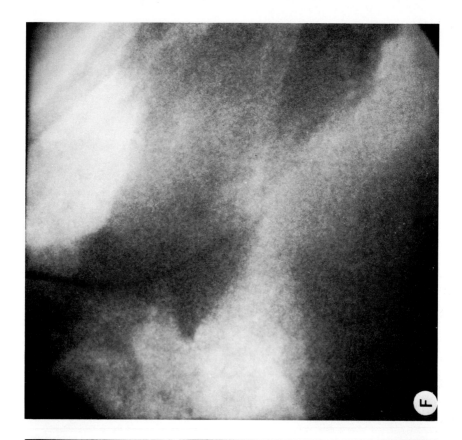

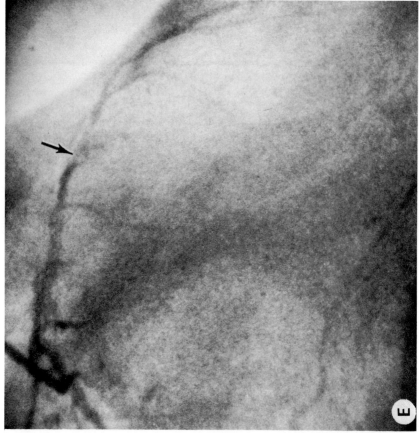

Another patient died suddenly 10 days postoperatively of massive pulmonary embolism as demonstrated at autopsy.

A fourth patient died of congestive heart failure 45 days after operation, following a stormy postoperative course, complicated by infection and recurrent sternal dehiscence.

In half of the patients, the immediate postoperative course was essentially uneventful, and their excellent condition allowed early discharge from the hospital. Three patients required reoperation for bleeding. One patient had a delayed recovery of consciousness 24 hours after the operation and has subsequently done well. Congestive heart failure was the major postoperative problem in eight patients, requiring prolonged medical therapy in the hospital. Arrhythmias in the immediate postoperative period were observed in 11 patients but were controlled with medications.

All patients have been closely followed in the out-patient clinic for an average time of two years. There have been no late deaths. Twenty-one patients are completely asymptomatic. Fourteen more are markedly improved and are quite active. Of the remaining six patients, all are improved over their preoperative status, but three of them continue to have mild failure with shortness of breath on exertion and moderate dependent edema.

Graded postoperative exercise tests were performed six to 12 months after surgery on 20 patients who had undergone combined aneurysmectomy and aortocoronary bypass. These tests measured their ability to perform exercise and showed their maximum heart rate as well as other electrocardiographic changes. The results were compared to the same patients' preoperative performance, and related both to the change in symptomatology and the angiographic demonstration of graft patency.

In seven of these patients, preoperative tests could not be performed because of the severity of congestive heart failure and/or of angina at rest.

The improvement over the preoperative status of these 20 patients was documented by their increased ability to walk in some and at more rapid rates in others. Of the seven patients who could not be exercised preoperatively, four could walk at 3 mph, two were able to attain 2 mph, and one attained 1 mph. Similar improvement was noted in the patients who had been tested preoperatively, and who, in general, could attain a higher level of exercise with freedom from angina. It is apparent that such improvement may be related to the effect of resection of the aneurysm alone and does not represent evidence of effective

revascularization of the residual ischemic myocardium.

Postoperative cardiac catheterization was performed in 10 patients after an average interval of 18 months. Six of these patients were asymptomatic, and four had residual or recurrent symptoms.

In five of the six asymptomatic patients, patency of the grafts was demonstrated (right in two cases, LAD in three cases). In the sixth asymptomatic patient, the graft (to the LAD) was occluded. Thus, the remission of the angina and failure is attributed to the improved efficiency of contraction that follows aneurysm resection.

Occlusion of the grafts (both to the right coronary and the LAD) was demonstrated in two of the other four cases in whom repeat catheterization was performed because of a recurrence of symptoms.

In another two patients restudied postoperatively with recurrent congestive heart failure, the grafts were patent. One of these had a mitral prosthesis and a right coronary bypass. The other had two coronary arteries bypassed. We feel that the failure in these two patients was due to inadequate residual myocardial reserve.

DISCUSSION

The presence of a ventricular aneurysm is responsible for an increased workload of the left ventricle and a decrease of its efficiency. When aneurysmal involvement is 20 percent or more of the surface of the left ventricular wall, hemodynamic abnormalities will necessarily be produced (Klein et al, 1967).

The factors responsible for such derangement are numerous: first, the presence of a paradoxically pulsing chamber that sequesters the blood in systole, decreasing forward flow, and returns it to the ventricle during diastole, thus increasing the end-diastolic volume; second, the increased diameter of the ventricle. In fact, it has been demonstrated mathematically by applying Laplace's Law (Burch et al, 1965; Burton, 1957) that a ventricle that has a diameter twice normal must generate four times as much force to maintain the same systolic pressure. Third, the diminished rate of fiber shortening decreases efficiency. This can be demonstrated by the increased tension-time index, and reflects, with fair approximation, the increased oxygen consumption that appears to be directly related to the size of the dyskinetic area (Pairolero et al, 1970; Heimbecker et al, 1967).

The operation eliminates the inelastic sac

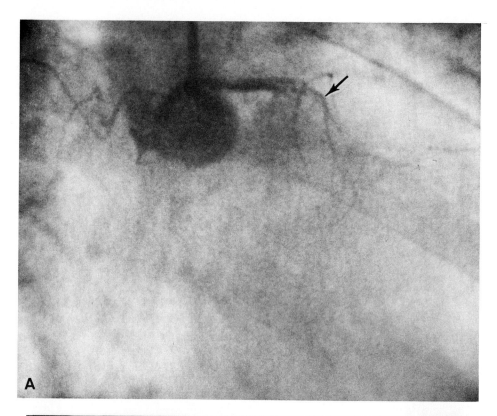

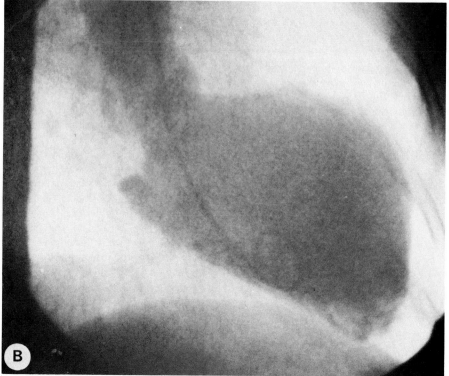

FIG. 2. A. Injection of left main coronary artery shows complete occlusion of the anterior descending and circumflex branches. B. Ventriculography demonstrates a large smooth-walled aneurysm of the left ventricle in this patient (RAO projection).

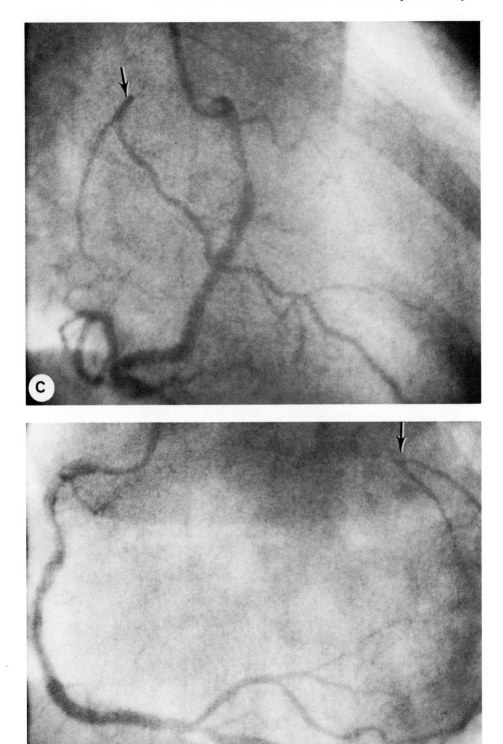

FIG. 2. C, D. RAO and LAO projection of right coronary arteriogram in the same patient showing retrograde filling of the left anterior descending artery.

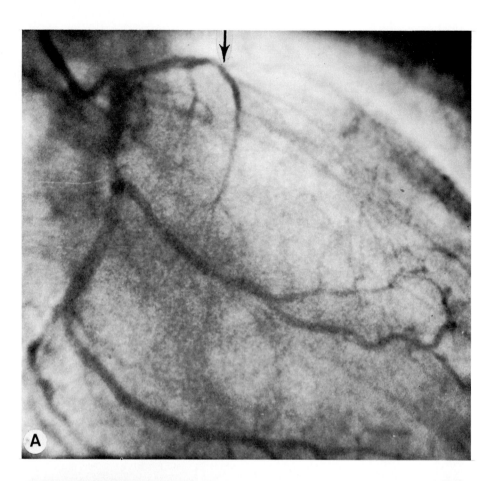

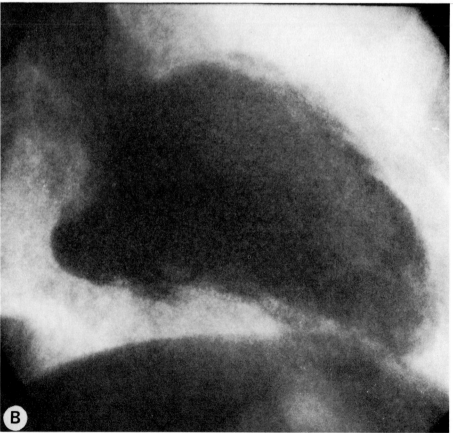

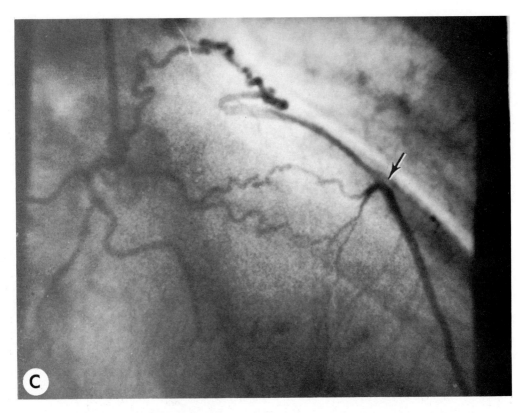

FIG. 3. A and B on facing page. A. Left coronary injection in RAO projection demonstrates complete occlusion of left anterior descending coronary artery with a distal lesion in the circumflex. B. Left ventriculography: There is an aneurysm of the anterolateral wall of the left ventricle (RAO projection). C. Right coronary injection results in retrograde filling of the distal left anterior descending coronary artery.

and reduces the size of the ventricular cavity, thus decreasing the dissipation of energy. As less wall tension is needed to generate the same amount of intracavity pressure, oxygen consumption is reduced, and myocardial metabolism is improved.

In general, in the numerous series of ventricular aneurysmectomies that have been published, the hemodynamic and the clinical results have been favorable. This has occurred both with closed (Likoff and Bailey, 1955; DeCamp, 1956; Petrovsky, 1962) and with open techniques (Cooley et al, 1958; Effler et al, 1963; Favaloro et al, 1968; Cooley and Hallman, 1968; Key et al, 1968; Kay et al, 1970; Schattenberg et al, 1970; Tich et al, 1970; Graber et al, 1972; Najafi et al, 1973). The immediate hemodynamic improvement (Greenwood et al, 1965; Harmans et al, 1969; Kay et al, 1970; Tesler et al, 1971; Hazan et al, 1973) has, however, been accompanied by long-term results that have not been as encouraging. The early postoperative mortality, ranging between 8 and 25 percent, has been followed by a late mortality as high as 50 percent in three years (Schattenberg et al, 1970). The poor rate of late

mortality has generally been attributed to recurrent myocardial infarction (Gorlin et al, 1967; Cooley and Hallman, 1968; Favaloro et al, 1968; Schattenberg et al, 1970; Graber et al, 1972; Najafi et al, 1973).

In the presence of left ventricular aneurysm, the importance and extent of coronary artery disease is shown by the significant incidence of severe involvement of multiple coronary vessels (Graber et al, 1972; Cooley 1973; Loop et al, 1973). This finding has been confirmed in our series (Table 1). Besides important obstructive disease of the left

TABLE 1. Angiographic Findings in 45 Patients with Postinfarction Ventricular Aneurysm

DEGREE OF OBSTRUCTION	ARTERY INVOLVED		
	LAD	RCA	Circ.
Complete obliteration	11	2	6
Complete occlusion with retrograde filling	22	5	7
Severe narrowing (over 80%)	12	12	16
Moderate narrowing (60-80%)	0	15	6

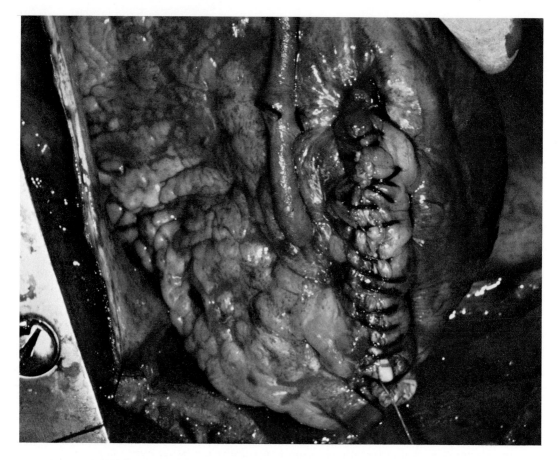

FIG. 4.   Operative photograph of heart showing reserved saphenous vein bypass graft to left anterior descending coronary artery and suture line following resection of left ventricular aneurysm.

anterior descending coronary artery, all patients had severe obstruction of one or both of the other major coronary arteries.

The risk of surgery seems to be dependent not so much on the characteristics of the aneurysm itself but rather on the severity of the concomitant occlusive disease in the coronary arteries not directly involved in the aneurysm formation (Favaloro et al, 1968; Johnson and Lepley, 1970; Milstein 1970; Graber et al, 1972). Further, the long-term prognosis of patients who have resection of ventricular aneurysm appears to be largely dependent upon the extent, distribution, and progression of occlusive disease present in the portions of the coronary arterial tree other than that branch whose occlusion caused the aneurysm formation. Since the availability of myocardial revascularization procedures, their simultaneous employment in association with ventricular aneurysm resection represents a logical attempt to improve those results. The validity of this assumption is confirmed by the fact that the late results of aneurysmectomy

combined with saphenous vein bypass grafting have been found to compare favorably with the late results of aneurysmectomy alone (Loop et al, 1973; Spencer, 1973).

In a series of 35 patients who had aneurysmectomy alone at this institution, prior to the advent of coronary bypass surgery, hospital mortality was 15 percent and late mortality (within two years from surgery) was 12 percent. In contrast, there was no late mortality in the present series, during the same time period (Figure 5).

The high incidence of obstruction in remote coronaries (Table 1) coupled with the consistent dyskinetic areas seen in the left ventriculogram adjacent to the aneurysm, supports the impression that around the area of totally infarcted muscle that becomes fibrotic, there is usually a zone of chronically ischemic but viable myocardium.

The difficulty in distinguishing areas of complete loss of muscle from ischemic zones and the problem in defining exactly the size and limits of the aneurysm further point to the frequent pres-

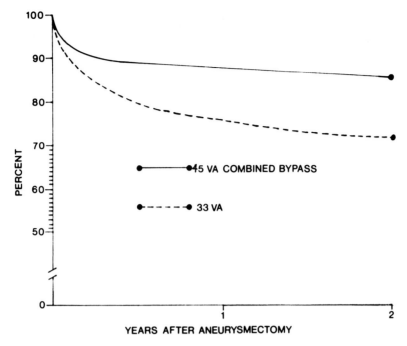

FIG. 5. Survival after aneurysmectomy alone compared to survival after combined aneurysmectomy and revascularization.

ence of both types of abnormal ventricular wall in these patients.

The significant disparity in the incidence of ventricular aneurysm in the reported series (3.5 to 38 percent) (Applebaum and Nicholson, 1935; Schlichter et al, 1954) is in great part due to the differences in anatomical or functional diagnostic criteria. Edwards defined ventricular aneurysm as the protrusion of a localized portion of the external surface of the ventricle accompanied by a corresponding protrusion of the ventricular cavity. If this strict definition is adopted, the incidence of ventricular aneurysm (Dubnow et al, 1965) is far less than the incidence of ventricular aneurysm diagnosed by means of cineangiographic studies (Gorlin et al, 1967). Confirmation of this statistical ratio was obtained by the study of Mourdjinis et al, who, out of 112 patients admitted to a coronary care unit with acute myocardial infarction, found a 14 percent incidence of postinfarction ventricular aneurysm by functional criteria (based on clinical electrocardiographic and radiological evidence), but only three cases of true ventricular aneurysm in accordance with Edwards's anatomic criteria.

Further, the lack of reliable correlation between the angiographic picture of dyskinesia and the operative findings of full thickness scar, has been a confusing and not exceptional observation

in our own, and in others', experience (Gorlin et al, 1967; Favaloro et al, 1968; Graber et al, 1972). Angiographic findings suggestive of ventricular aneurysm may, in fact, correspond to an area of ischemic but viable myocardium, indistinguishable from the surrounding tissue, either by gross or microscopic examination (Gorlin et al, 1967; Favaloro et al). This question will probably be better clarified by measurement of myocardial capillary perfusion by means of isotope techniques that have been recently described and that are presently being evaluated clinically in our center and others.

The problem has practical importance. It may be plausible that chronic ischemia may cause localized disturbances of contraction of viable myocardial tissue, with the consequent functional and hemodynamic behavior of a true ventricular aneurysm (Gorlin et al, 1967). In view of the available evidence of improvement of myocardial contractility with revascularization procedures (Johnson and Lepley, 1970; Hairston et al, 1973; Moran et al, 1973), the question has to be raised whether or not in such cases the appropriate surgical management should not be a revascularization procedure associated with, or even in lieu of, the excision of the dyskinetic area.

In the presence of true ventricular aneurysm, associated stenotic lesions of remote coronary artery branches, by causing chronic myocardial ischemia, may induce dyskinesia of portions of viable myocardium and thus aggravate the hemodynamic derangement. It follows that surgical treatment in these cases should not be limited to the excision of the fibrous area but should also include revascularization of the ischemic myocardium. Earlier attempts using internal mammary implants in such cases (Favaloro et al, 1968; Loop, 1971) have given way to saphenous vein bypass grafting (Johnson and Lepley, 1970; Tich et al, 1970; Tesler et al, 1971; Hazan et al, 1973; Najafi et al, 1973; Stoney et al, 1973).

Considering the high incidence of severe involvement of portions of the coronary arterial tree remote from the aneurysm area, the comparatively small number of combined aneurysmectomy and vein grafting recently reported in other large series (Reul et al, 1972) is surprising. Although some authors (Stoney et al, 1973) have abandoned attempts to preserve the anterior descending coronary artery in patients with an anterior ventricular aneurysm, our experience has shown, to the contrary, that in at least 32 out of 45 cases of left ventricular aneurysm, the anterior descending coronary artery, although proximally obstructed, was patent distally, was filled through collaterals, and could be revascularized (Table 2). Patency of the graft and satisfactory myocardial perfusion were demonstrated in those cases that were studied postoperatively by angiocardiography. The functional significance of this is obvious, as it is well known that this artery, besides supplying the anterior surface of the left ventricle by means of its diagonal branches, also supplies the anterior two-thirds of the ventricular septum by means of its numerous septal branches (James, 1961). The importance of revascularization of such branches has recently been emphasized by Johnson, who has measured flows up to 80 ml/min in grafts electively anastomosed to the first septal branch. Further, it has been noted (Spencer, 1973) that surgical obliteration of the left anterior descending coronary artery during aneurysmectomy is associated with severe arrhythmias postoperatively.

The question has been raised (Graber et al, 1972) as to whether the increase in the magnitude of the operation adversely affects operative mortality. This has not been so in our experience, nor in that of others (Merin et al, 1973). On the contrary, with the increased number of combined revascularization procedures, there has been a corresponding decline in operative mortality (Loop, 1971; Spencer, 1973).

It has been observed (Kluge et al, 1971) that in some instances resection of the aneurysm

TABLE 2. Combined Aneurysmectomy and Aortocoronary Bypass in 45 Patients

	NO.
Artery involved	
LAD	32
RCA	21
Circ	4
Diagonal	1
Associated Procedures	
Mitral valve replacement	4
Aortic valve replacement	2

alone was not sufficient to restore enough myocardial efficiency for an effective circulation until establishment of coronary artery bypass produced striking improvement of myocardial contractility. It has also been stated, in retrospect (Johnson and Lepley, 1970), that several deaths following ventricular aneurysmectomy would have been prevented if direct coronary surgery had been performed simultaneously. Thus, the tendency is emerging to revascularize every coronary vessel that shows significant obstruction, whether near or remote from the aneurysm itself (Merin et al, 1973; Cooley, 1973; Spencer, 1973).

With the limitations due to the relatively short follow-up in our series (average two years), we feel that our experience has been successful in relieving both angina and failure in a group of severely disabled patients with advanced coronary artery disease and, therefore, supports further use of combined simultaneous aneurysmectomy and revascularization procedures in selected cases.

References

Appelbaum E, Nicholson GHB: Occlusive disease of the coronary arteries: an analysis of the pathological anatomy in 168 cases with electrocardiographic correlation in 36 of these. Am Heart J 10:662, 1935

Burch GE, DePasquale NP, Cronvich JA: Influence of ventricular size on the relationship between contractile and manifest tension. Am Heart J 69:624, 1965

Burton A: The importance of shape and size of the heart. Am Heart J 54:801, 1957

Cooley DA: Discussion paper by Loop FD et al. Ann Surg 178:404, 1973

Cooley DA, Collins HA, Morris GC, Chapman DW: Ventricular aneurysm after myocardial infarction: surgical excision with the use of temporary cardiopulmonary bypass. JAMA 167:557, 1958

Cooley DA, Hallman GL: Surgical treatment of left ventricular aneurysm: experience with excision of post-infarction lesions in 80 patients. Prog Cardiovasc Dis 11:222, 1968

DeCamp PT: Excision of an aneurysm of the left ventricle. Ochsner Clinic Reports 2:38, 1956

Dubnow MH, Burchell HB, Titus JL: Post-infarction ventricular aneurysm. Am Heart J 70:753, 1965

Edwards JE: An atlas of acquired diseases of the heart and great vessels. Philadelphia, Saunders, 1961, vol II, p 615

Effler DB, Westcott RN, Groves LK, Scully NM: Surgical treatment of ventricular aneurysm. Arch Surg 87:249, 1963

Favaloro RG, Effler DB, Groves LK, Westcott RN, Suarez E, Lozada J: Ventricular aneurysm. Clinical experience. Ann Thorac Surg 6:227, 1968

Gorlin R, Klein MD, Sullivan JM: Prospective correlative study of ventricular aneurysm: mechanistic concept and clinical recognition. Am J Med 42:512, 1967

Graber JD, Oakley CM, Pickering BN, Goodwin JF, Raphael MJ, Steiner AE: Ventricular aneurysm: an appraisal of diagnosis and surgical treatment. Br Heart J 34:830, 1972

Greenwood WF, Aldridge HE, Wigle ED: Nature of the disorder of function in chronic post-infarction aneurysm of the left ventricle Can Med Assoc J 92:611, 1965

Hairston P, Newman WH, Daniell HB: Myocardial contractile force as influenced by direct coronary surgery. Ann Thorac Surg 15:364, 1973

Harmans MA, Baxley WA, Jones WB, Dodge HT, Edwards S: Surgical intervention in chronic post-infarction cardiac failure. Circulation 39, Suppl 1:91, 1969

Hazan E, Block G, Rioux C, Louville Y, Cirotteau Y, Mathey J: Surgical treatment of aneurysm and segmental dyskinesia of the left ventricular wall after myocardial infarction. Am J Cardiol 31:708, 1973

Heimbecker RD, Chen C, Hamilton N, Murray DWG: Surgery for massive myocardial infarction: an experimental study of emergency infarctectomy. Surgery 61:51, 1967

James TN: Anatomy of the coronaries. New York, Hoeber, 1961

Johnson WD, Lepley D: An aggressive surgical approach to coronary disease. J Thorac Cardiovasc Surg 59:128, 1970

Kay JH, Dunne E, Krohn BG, Tsugi HK, Redington JV, Mendez A, Dykstra P, Magidson D: Left Ventricular excision, exclusion or plication for akinetic areas of the heart. J Thorac Cardiovasc Surg 59:139, 1970

Key JA, Aldridge HE, MacGregor DC: The selection of patients for resection of left ventricular aneurysm. J Thorac Cardiovasc Surg 56:477, 1968

Klein MD, Herman MV, Gorlin R: A hemodynamic study of left ventricular aneurysm. Circulation 35:614, 1967

Kluge TH, Ullal SR, Hill JD, Kerth WJ, Gerbode F: Dyskinesia and aneurysm of the left ventricle: surgical experience in 36 patients. J Cardiovasc Surg 12:273, 1971

Likoff W, Bailey CP: Ventriculoplasty: excision of myocardial aneurysm: report of a successful case. JAMA 158:915, 1955

Loop FD, Effler DB, Navia JA, Sheldon WC, Groves LK: Aneurysms of the left ventricle: survival and results of a ten year surgical experience. Ann Surg 178: 399, 1973

Loop FD: Ventricular aneurysmectomy. Surg Clin North Am 51:1071, 1971

Merin G, Schattenberg TT, Pluth JR, Wallace RB, Danielson GK: Surgery for post-infarction ventricular aneurysm. Ann Thorac Surg 15:588, 1973

Milstein BB: Exploring surgical treatment for myocardial infarction. Br Heart J 32:421, 1970

Moran SV, Tarazi RC, Urzua JU, Favaloro RG, Effler DB: Effects of aorto-coronary bypass on myocardial contractility. J Thorac Cardiovasc Surg 65:335, 1973

Mourdjinis A, Olsen E, Raphael MJ, Mounsey JPD: Clinical diagnosis and prognosis of ventricular aneurysm. Br Heart J 30:497, 1968

Najafi H, Serry C, Dye WS, Javid H, Hunter JA, Goldin MD, Julian OC: Surgical management of complications of myocardial infarction. Med Clin North Am 53:205, 1973

Pairolero PC, McCallister BD, Hallermann FJ, Ellis FHJ Jr: Experimental production and hemodynamic effects of left ventricular akinesis. Am J Cardiol 25: 120, 1970

Petrovsky BV: Surgery for aneurysm of the heart after myocardial infarction. Arch Surg 84:35, 1962

Reul GJ, Morris GC, Howell JF, Crawford ES, Stelter WJ: Current concepts in coronary artery surgery: a critical analysis of 1287 patients. Ann Thorac Surg 14:243, 1972

Schattenberg TT, Giuliani ER, Campion BC, Danielson GK: Post-infarction ventricular aneurysm. Mayo Clin Proc 45:13, 1970

Schlichter J, Hellerstein HU, Katz LN: Aneurysm of the heart: a correlative study of one hundred and two proved cases. Medicine 33:43, 1954

Spencer, FC: Discussion paper by Loop DF et al. Ann Surg 178:404, 1973

Stoney WS, Alford WC Jr, Burrus GR, Thomas CS Jr: Repair of anteroseptal ventricular aneurysm. Ann Thorac Surg 15:394, 1973

Tesler UF, Hallman GL, Cooley DA: L'aneurisma post-infartuale del ventricolo sinistro. Esperienza in 134 casi operati. Minerva Chir 26:1001, 1971

Tich DA, Cheng TO, Dolgin M: Surgical treatment of post-myocardial infarction scars (ventricular aneurysms). Am Heart J 80:282, 1970

80

CORONARY ARTERY SURGERY AND CONGESTIVE HEART FAILURE

GEORGE C. MORRIS, JR.

INTRODUCTION

Since 1968, worldwide experience has been obtained in the surgical treatment of coronary artery disease. Bypass grafts from the aorta to coronary artery utilizing reversed saphenous vein have become standard procedures with low mortality and excellent postoperative results. Despite a vast and ubiquitous surgical exposure to this approach in treatment, many unresolved problems remain. If lack of cohesiveness or clinical uniformity is an indicator of such problems, then case selection should figure high among the unresolved questions in this area.

Differences in case selection of patients with coronary artery disease for coronary surgery span every parameter of the problem. Perhaps the widest divergence concerns poor left ventricular function or congestive heart failure.[1,3,4,7-9,11,13,15-18] At one end of the clinical spectrum, some surgeons limit the scope of surgery to patients with good ventricular function while, at the opposite end, others maintain a very aggressive approach with little patient selection. Obviously, if the surgical approach could demonstrate its effectiveness and reasonable risk, the terminal heart cases would be the most rewarding from an operative point of view. If experience would indicate a promise of improvement for the patient with poor left ventricular function with current bypass techniques, opinion might drift in an operative direction. The purpose of this report is to provide an analytic comparison of patients with preoperative congestive heart failure and patients with normal or nearly normal left ventricular function.

CLINICAL MATERIAL

Through January 1974, we had operated on 1,196 patients with coronary artery bypass procedures for coronary artery disease. In this group, 21 percent of the patients had preoperative symptoms of congestive heart failure (treated by digitalis and diuretics) with left ventricular end-diastolic pressures over 20 mm Hg, poorly contracting ventricles, and decreased ventricular function. It is significant to note that less than 2 percent of the patients had failure without angina and all others had congestive heart failure with moderate or severe angina categorized as Class III or IV. Hence, evaluation of the failing heart without angina is not a consideration in this study. In considering end-stage coronary artery disease, congestive heart failure was the most common element (21 percent of 1,196 patients), and functional Class IV angina without failure was the other major factor (17 percent).[11]

OPERATIVE TECHNIQUE

All aortocoronary artery bypass grafts were performed utilizing total cardiopulmonary bypass with hemodilution and disposable bubble oxygenator, as previously described.[5,10,12] Ischemic arrest by aortic occlusion was utilized for distal anastomosis.[14] Separate aortic origins were made with all grafts necessary for total correction of the occlusive lesions. No form of left ventricular assistance was employed after completion of the operative procedure.

RESULTS

Thirty-day hospital mortality for the entire group of 1,196 patients was 3.5 percent. For patients with preoperative congestive heart failure, mortality was 8.4 percent (Table 1).

TABLE 1. Percent Mortality Related to Disease

	%
All Patients	3.5
Ventricular Aneurysm	8.3
Congestive Heart Failure	8.4
Mitral Valve Replacement	26.6
Emergency	34.0

Late mortality in the congestive heart failure patients was essentially similar to the overall group of 1,196 patients. Patients in both groups have been followed for periods up to six years and show little difference, both showing an approximate yearly attrition of about 2.5 percent (Fig. 1).

COMPARATIVE ASSESSMENT AFTER OPERATION

Postoperative cinearteriography, left ventriculography, and cardiodynamic studies have been limited, for the most part, to selected patients, or to those returning with problems or change in status and, therefore, have not been considered statistically. Despite the fact that most patients studied had problems after operation, graft assessment has shown a satisfactory patency (Table 2).

TABLE 2. Coronary Artery Bypass Assessment of Graft Patency

	NO.	%
Total Number Patients	1,196	
Postoperative Arteriography	130	11.0
Patients with an open graft	121	94.0
Grafts studied	226	–
Grafts occluded	22	9.7
Patients with an occluded graft	24	18.0

Among the 130 patients having cinearteriography, 94 percent had at least one open graft with an overall graft occlusion rate of 9.7 percent. There appeared to be little difference in the occlusion incidence in patients with congestive heart failure and other patients.

Comparative studies of left ventriculography and end-diastolic pressure showed only minimal-to-moderate improvement despite generally significant to striking clinical improvement. Several case illustrations are helpful in elaboration of this apparent dichotomy between measurable hemodynamic improvement and clinical improvement.

CASE 1: *A 28-year-old male, presented with a history of disabling angina and dyspnea, had been unresponsive to medical treatment for one year. Catheterization showed total occlusion of the proximal left anterior descending coronary artery. Left ventricular function was very poor, with a large adynamic apex. A single left coronary bypass was performed in March 1971 and was followed by complete relief of symptoms. Follow-up catheterization in February 1972 showed an open graft and improved left ventricular function with a reduction in LVEDP from 18 to 5 mm Hg (Fig. 2).*

CASE 2: *A 47-year-old male presented with a history of two previous myocardial infarctions, severe angina, and congestive heart failure. Despite digitalis and diuretics, he had been unable to work for one year. The patient was refused surgical treatment in two other centers. Catheterization showed total occlusion of the proximal left anterior descending coronary artery and 95 percent proximal stenosis of the dominant left circumflex coronary artery. Left ventricular function was very poor, with an end-diastolic pressure of 30 mm Hg. Double left coronary artery bypass was performed in August 1971. Since operation, the patient has been free of angina and working full time without*

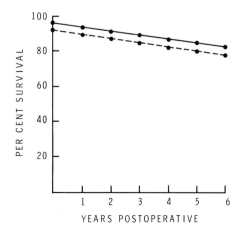

FIG. 1. Postoperative Survival. Comparison of yearly attrition rates from deaths of all causes between all patients (solid line) and patients with preoperative congestive heart failure (broken line) following coronary artery bypass.

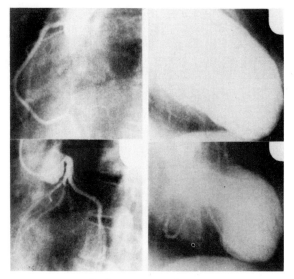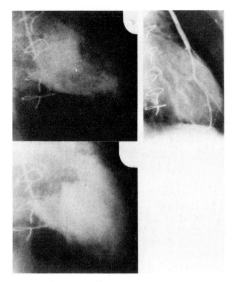

Before operation   1 year after operation

FIG. 2. Cinearteriograms and ventriculograms in 28-year-old male totally disabled one year by angina and dyspnea. Note improvement in ventriculogram and LVEDP after single bypass to totally occluded left anterior descending coronary artery. LVEDP dropped from 18 to 5mm Hg.

significant symptoms. The patient continues with digitalis and the occasional use of diuretics. Follow-up catheterization three years after operation showed both grafts open, little change in left ventricular function, and end-diastolic pressure still elevated to 30 mm Hg. (Fig. 3).

CASE 3: *The history of this 58-year-old male re-*

vealed four myocardial infarctions. Despite digitalis and diuretics, he was unable to work because of dyspnea. Intractable angina led to catheterization, showing total proximal occlusion of the dominant right coronary artery and total occlusion of the left anterior descending proximal to the first diagonal branch. Left ventricular function was very poor with end-diastolic pressure of 35 mm

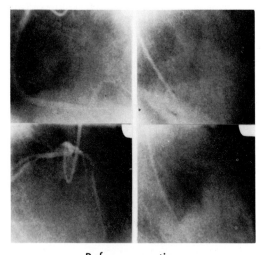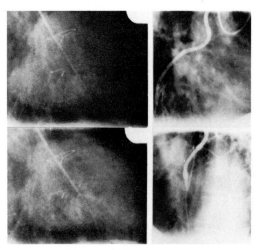

Before operation   3 years after operation

FIG. 3. Cinearteriograms and ventriculograms in 47-year-old male before operation and three years after operation. Note functioning grafts to totally obstructed left anterior descending and stenotic dominant left circumflex coronary arteries. Despite patient's remarkable symptomatic improvement, ventricular function appears only slightly improved.

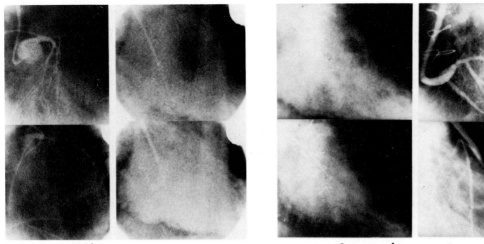

Before operation   3 years after operation

FIG. 4. Cinearteriograms and ventriculograms in 58-year-old male with intractable angina and congestive heart failure. Note total occlusion of dominant right coronary and left anterior descending coronary artery. Note moderately improved left ventricular function nearly three years after operation. Patient has been relieved of all cardiac symptoms.

Hg. *Bypass grafts in April 1971 to the posterior descending division of the right coronary artery and first diagonal branch of the left anterior descending coronary artery were inserted, followed by an uneventful recovery, with relief of angina. He returned to full-time work. One episode of supraventricular tachycardia led to follow-up catheterization in November 1973, in another center revealing open grafts and continued impaired left ventricular function but reduction of the end-diastolic pressure to 18 mm Hg (Fig. 4).*

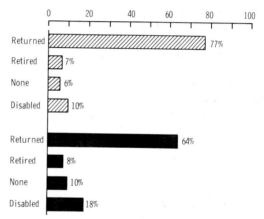

Returned 77%
Retired 7%
None 6%
Disabled 10%

Returned 64%
Retired 8%
None 10%
Disabled 18%

FIG. 6. Postoperative work assessment. Graphs compare work assessment after coronary artery bypass between all patients (shaded bars) and those with congestive heart failure (black bars).

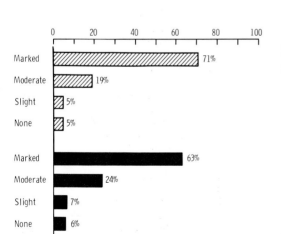

Marked 71%
Moderate 19%
Slight 5%
None 5%

Marked 63%
Moderate 24%
Slight 7%
None 6%

FIG. 5. Postoperative improvement. Graphs compare degree of improvement after coronary artery bypass as assessed by cardiologists between all patients (shaded bars) and those with congestive heart failure (black bars).

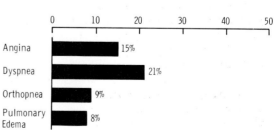

Angina 15%
Dyspnea 21%
Orthopnea 9%
Pulmonary Edema 8%

FIG. 7. Postoperative symptoms: congestive heart failure. Graphs showing major residual cardiac symptoms in patients with preoperative congestive failure following coronary artery bypass.

Improvement after operation as assessed by the attending cardiologists showed very little difference between the average of all patients and those with preoperative congestive heart failure (Fig. 5). The latter group showed an 8 percent lower incidence of marked improvement but a 5 percent higher incidence of moderate improvement than the overall group. Those showing slight or no improvement were nearly the same for both groups.

After operation, return-to-work status is more meaningful than a general clinical assessment and has been analyzed for two groups (Fig. 6). It must also be remembered that the congestive heart failure group was severely, if not totally, disabled prior to operation. In this connection, therefore, it is remarkable that 64 percent of the congestive failure group returned to work, compared to 77 percent of the overall series, and only 18 percent remained disabled, compared to 10 percent for all patients. In truth, something should be said for the 18 percent still disabled but alive, since many might have been expected to die without surgical intervention.[2,6]

Residual symptoms in patients with preoperative congestive heart failure were minimal (Fig. 7). Essentially, all patients suffered from angina prior to operation, while only 15 percent experienced angina after operation. Some degree of exertional dyspnea remained in 21 percent of patients and orthopnea in 9 percent. At least one episode of pulmonary edema was observed in 8 percent.

DISCUSSION

After six years (1968–74) of experience with coronary bypass procedures during which a consistently aggressive approach has been directed at left ventricular dysfunction, a knowledgeable perspective has been gained. Overall hospital mortality has been reduced to 8.4 percent for patients with congestive heart failure and in the past two years has been even less. Late mortality appears to parallel the overall group, with an attrition rate of about 2.5 percent per year, certainly less than might be anticipated without operation.

Statistical analysis of left ventricular functional changes following revascularization in patients with congestive failure has not been possible. However, in the minority of patients in whom comparative ventricular function studies are possible, improvement has not been great, ranging from very modest to moderate. Relief of angina

in patients with congestive failure was observed in 85 percent. Undoubtedly, the most impressive change in patients with poor ventricular function and least subject to skepticism has been the return-to-work status of 64 percent following operation.

The question as to which patients with congestive failure present an unacceptable operative risk has been most important in this clinical study. Left ventricular ejection fraction and end-diastolic pressure are relative guides and have not been reliable in answering the central question, Which patient will fail to come off the pump? Experience has shown that more consistent probability in determining this question can be gleaned from cinearteriography. The cardinal factor in answering this central question is whether or not significant improvement in coronary blood flow to the left ventricle can be achieved by operation. The patient with total proximal occlusion in the left coronary circulation with open distal vessels can be expected to do well after bypass despite very poor ventricular function. In contrast, the patients without proximal total occlusion with multiple areas of stenosis and very poor ventricular function may represent an unacceptable threat as an operative mortality.

SUMMARY

An attempt to evaluate the results of coronary artery bypass in patients with congestive heart failure has been made in terms of operative mortality, late mortality, symptomatology, and work status.

1. Among 1,196 surgical patients, 21 percent presented with congestive heart failure before operation. Results of operation in these patients with poor left ventricular function compared favorably with those having good ventricular function with respect to relief of angina and return-to-work status.
2. Operative mortality was 8.4 percent for the failure group compared to 3.5 percent for the overall group.
3. Late mortality was similar for both groups, with an average attrition rate of 2.5 percent per year.
4. Improvement in left ventricular dynamics ranged from very modest to only moderate in patients with congestive heart failure.

Operative mortality can be reduced to less than 8 percent in patients with congestive heart failure if bypass to open left coronary vessels can be achieved beyond areas of proximal total occlusion.

References

1. Cooley DA, Dawson JT, Hallman GL, et al: Aorto-coronary saphenous vein bypass. Ann Thorac Surg 16:380, 1973
2. Diethrich EB, Liddicoat JE, Kinard SA, DeBakey ME: An analysis of operated and non-operated patients and documented coronary artery disease. J Thorac Cardiovasc Surg 57:115, 1969
3. Favaloro RG, Effler DB, Groves LK, Sheldon WC, Sones FM: Direct myocardial revascularization by saphenous vein graft. Ann Thorac Surg 10:97, 1970
4. Flemma RJ, Johnson WD, Lepley D, et al: Simultaneous valve replacement and aorta-to-coronary saphenous vein bypass. Ann Thorac Surg 12:163, 1971
5. Howell JF, Reul GJ, Morris GC, Crawford ES: Surgical treatment of coronary artery disease. Tex Med 67:48, 1971
6. Johnson WD, Hughes RK: An expanded indication for coronary surgery. Ann Thorac Surg 16:1, 1973
7. Lefemine AA, Moon HS, Flessas A, Ryan TJ, Ramaswamy K: Myocardial resection and coronary artery bypass for left ventricular failure following myocardial infarction. Ann Thorac Surg 17:1, 1974
8. Manley JC, Johnson WD, Flemma RJ, Lepley DW: Objective evaluation of the effects of direct myocardial revascularization on ventricular function utilizing ergometer exercise testing (Presented at 20th Annual Scientific Session of American College of Cardiology, 1971)
9. May AM: Results of national survey, coronary artery surgery, 1970 (presented to Symposium on Direct Coronary Artery Surgery sponsored by American College of Chest Physicians, October 25, 1971)
10. Morris GC, Howell JF, Crawford ES, et al: The distal coronary bypass. Ann Surg 172:652, 1970
11. Morris GC, Howell JF, Crawford ES, Reul GJ, Stelter W: Operability of end stage coronary artery disease. Ann Surg 175:1024, 1972
12. Morris GC, Reul GJ, Howell JF, et al: Follow-up results of distal coronary artery bypass for ischemic heart disease. Am J Cardiol 29:180, 1972
13. Mundth E, Harthorne JW, Buckley MJ, Dinsmore R, Austen WG: Direct coronary artery revascularization in the treatment of cardiac failure. Arch Surg 103:529, 1971
14. Reul GJ, Morris GC, Howell JF, et al: The safety of ischemic cardiac arrest in distal coronary artery bypass. J Thorac Cardiovasc Surg 62:511, 1971
15. Reul GJ, Morris GC, Howell JF, et al: Coronary artery bypass in totally obstructed major coronary arteries. Arch Surg 102:373, 1971
16. Reul GJ, Morris GC, Howell JF, Crawford ES, Stelter WJ: Emergency coronary artery bypass grafts in the treatment of myocardial infarction. Circulation (Suppl III) 67-68:117, 1973
17. Saltiel J, Lesperance J, Bourassa MG, et al: Reversibility of left ventricular dysfunction following aortocoronary bypass grafts. Am J Roentgenol Radium Ther Nucl Med 110:739, 1970
18. Spencer FC, Green GE, Tice DA, et al: Coronary artery bypass grafts for congestive heart failure. J Thorac Cardiovasc Surg 62:529, 1971

81

CORONARY ARTERY SURGERY FOR THE PATIENT WITH DRASTIC IMPAIRMENT OF LEFT VENTRICULAR FUNCTION

PABLO ZUBIATE, JEROME HAROLD KAY, YOUNG TSO LIN, A. MICHAEL MENDEZ, and EDWARD F. DUNNE

Revascularization of the ischemic heart with reversed saphenous vein autografts and internal mammary anastomosis has proven an acceptable procedure, with low mortality and improvement for the majority of patients with angina pectoris. However, there are few reports of coronary artery surgery for patients with marked impairment of left ventricular function. Spencer (1971), Siderys (1972), and Johnson (1970) [1,2,3] reported their experiences with coronary artery bypass grafting in patients with congestive heart failure or impaired function of the left ventricle.

This report is on our experience with myocardial revascularization of 144 patients with marked impairment of left ventricular function, as revealed by an ejection fraction of 0.05 to 0.20 (normal: 0.70).

From August 1969 to January 1974, there were 144 patients operated upon for occlusive coronary artery disease with marked impairment of left ventricular function and an ejection fraction of 0.05 to 0.20. This group represented 9 percent of the 1,573 patients operated upon for coronary artery disease during this period. The ages ranged from 37 to 76 years (average 56 years). Of the patients, 123 were men and 21 were women. Fifty-two patients were 60 years or older, and 92 were 59 years or younger. Review of past history revealed that 95 percent of the patients had angina pectoris and 95 percent had a documented myocardial infarct. The 5 percent without a history of myocardial infarct were operated upon for preinfarction angina. All 144 patients were in congestive heart failure, which was either controlled by a strict medical regimen or was unresponsive to medical treatment. All patients had forward angi-

ography to determine the function of the left ventricle, followed by coronary arteriography. Left ventricular end-diastolic pressure ranged from 13 mm Hg to 68 mm Hg, with a mean of 26 mm Hg.

The number of grafts inserted depended upon the vessels potentially suitable for grafting. This was determined by the preoperative arteriograms as well as feasibility at the time of surgery. Thirty-nine patients had one graft, 63 had two grafts, 35 had three grafts, and seven had four grafts. In the 144 patients, there were a total of 296 reversed saphenous vein grafts and two internal mammary artery grafts. In addition to the bypass grafts, 45 patients had additional procedures performed. Sixteen patients had excision of an aneurysm, and 14 had exclusion or plication of an akinetic or dyskinetic area of the left ventricle.[4,5] Seven patients had mitral annuloplasty, and two had mitral valve replacement. One with mitral annuloplasty and one with mitral valve replacement had excision of a left ventricular aneurysm as well. Four patients had aortic valve replacement, one of whom also had replacement of the ascending aorta along with the aortic valve replacement. One had a pericardiectomy, and another patient had closure of an atrial septal defect.

RESULTS

There were 41 hospital deaths in these 144 patients (28 percent) and 16 late deaths after discharge from the hospital (11 percent), with a total mortality of 39 percent, while 87 (61 percent) survived.

Fifty-two patients were over 60 years of age,

and 19 (36 percent) of these died in the hospital. There were three deaths (6 percent) following discharge from the hospital, and 30 patients were living (58 percent). Twenty-two of the 92 patients (24 percent) 59 years of age or less died during surgery or postoperatively. There were 13 (14 percent) additional deaths after discharge from the hospital, and 57 (62 percent) survived. Of the 45 patients of all ages with vein grafts plus additional procedures, the hospital death rate was approximately 1.5 times greater than that of patients with vein grafts only (38 percent as compared to 24 percent). The late death rate was about the same (13 percent as compared to 10 percent) (Table 1).

TABLE 1. Mortality Comparison in Patients with Vein Grafts and Associated Procedures

	REVASCULARIZATION ONLY		REVASCULARIZATION PLUS ASSOCIATED PROCEDURES	
	No.	%	No.	%
Hospital deaths	24	24	17	38
Late deaths	10	10	6	13
Living	65	66	22	49
Total	99	100	45	100

All of the hospital deaths appeared to be related to a low cardiac output secondary to poor contractility of the left ventricle and progression of the preoperative cardiac failure. Of particular importance is the fact that in the last year—January 1, 1973 to January 1, 1974—33 consecutive patients of all ages were operated upon, with only three hospital deaths, a mortality of 9 percent. Of these 33 patients, 19 were between the ages of 39 and 59 with two deaths and 14 patients were between 60 and 69 with one death. We think the reason for this marked improvement in mortality in this last group of 33 critically ill patients is due to the increased experience of the surgeons.

FOLLOW-UP

Thirty-seven patients, 12 over 60 years of age and 25 less than 59 years of age, underwent repeat forward cineangiography and coronary arteriography 13 to 590 days postoperatively. The average interval was 178 days. Eighty-three vein grafts had been inserted into these 37 patients, and 71 were patent (86 percent). The ejection fraction increased from a preoperative 0.16 ± 0.03 to postoperative 0.27 ± 0.07. This value was statistically significant ($p < 0.001$). Left ventricular end-diastolic pressure was 6 mm Hg to 28 mm Hg, with a mean of 15 mm Hg. In 26 patients (70 percent), the ejection fraction increased; in 10 patients (27 percent) it remained unchanged; and in one patient (3 percent) it decreased. Of the 37 patients restudied, 29 (78 percent) were subjectively improved. The procedures performed on the group of patients restudied are shown in Figure 1. Forty-seven of the 50 patients not restudied stated that they were significantly improved in the relief of angina and experienced increased ability to participate in physical activity (Table 2). Interestingly, when a patient did not obtain a good result,

TABLE 2. Follow-up of Relief of Angina in 87 Patients

	NO.	%
No angina postoperatively	69	79
Mild to moderate improvement	11	13
Unchanged from preoperation	7	8

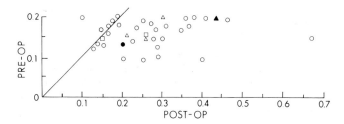

EJECTION FRACTION 0.2 OR LESS

INCREASED	26/37 - 70%	VEIN GRAFTS ONLY	30 PT. ○
UNCHANGED	10/37 - 27%	ANEURYSMECTOMY	1 PT. ▲
DECREASED	1/37 - 3%	RESECTION OR PLICATION	3 PT. △
GRAFT PATENCY	71/83 - 86%	ASD	1 PT. ●
		MITRAL REPAIR	2 PT. □

FIG. 1. Revascularization: Postoperative studies in 37 patients aged 44 to 68 years.

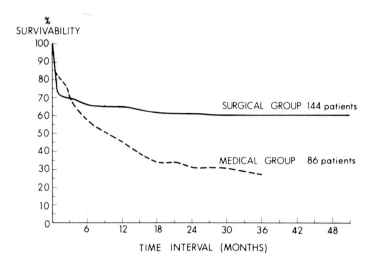

FIG. 2. Medical and surgical survival of patients with ejection fraction of 0.10 to 0.20 (actuarial curve).

he and his physician wanted postoperative studies performed. In contrast to this, if a patient did well after discharge from the hospital it was difficult to have him return for study. Both the physician and the patient were so pleased with the patient's improved postoperative status that they felt restudy was not indicated.

Eighty-six patients with an ejection fraction of 0.10 to 0.20 were treated medically from August 1969 to January 1974. These patients were not operated upon for one of three reasons: (1) the patient refused surgery; (2) the patient did not have graftable vessels; or (3) the patient died prior to admission. Sixty-one patients (71 percent) died during the period of this study (Fig. 2).[8]

DISCUSSION

The value of bypass grafting for patients with occlusive coronary artery disease and marked impairment of left ventricular function has been considered uncertain. It has been thought that marked impairment of left ventricular function prohibited surgery because of a very high surgical mortality, with little, if any, chance for improvement in heart function, in the patient's clinical status, or in his chance for longevity.

In 1971, Spencer, Green, Tice, et al[1] reported on 40 patients operated upon for congestive heart failure. This was considered severe or intractable in 23 patients, moderate in 11, and mild in six. Twenty-five of the 40 patients were living at the time this article was written. It was felt that little objective improvement could be expected in severe congestive failure following bypass grafting.

Mundth, Harthorne, et al (1971)[6] reported on 40 patients with ischemic cardiomyopathy and

cardiac failure due to coronary artery disease who had undergone direct coronary arterial revascularization. The left ventricular end-diastolic pressure was elevated (greater than 12 mm Hg) in all patients and was associated with left ventricular dilatation. Left ventricular contractility was assessed to be markedly reduced in 23 patients (58 percent). Five of these patients underwent postoperative angiography. They concluded that because of the virtually hopeless prognosis of this group of patients and the encouraging early results of direct coronary artery surgery, as reported in their series, continued application of this mode of treatment in selected cases was indicated.

Siderys, Pittman, and Herod (1972)[2] reported on 32 patients with severe left ventricular impairment. These patients had left ventricular end-diastolic pressures of 25 mm Hg and/or ventriculograms that revealed severe diffuse evidence of poor function. The operative mortality was 31 percent. Two-thirds of the patients had evidence of decreased left ventricular end-diastolic pressures postoperatively, while one-half showed definite improvement of their ventriculograms. The surprising factor postoperatively was the apparent clinical improvement in these patients.

The ejection fraction of the left ventricle is a good indicator of left ventricular function. The determination of left ventricular function must be done before coronary arteriography, since injection of dye into the coronary arteries may produce a temporary but significant depression in the left ventricular function and ejection fraction. The ejection fraction not only must be determined before coronary arteriography, but it should be done by injecting dye into the superior or inferior vena cava to prevent the frequent ventricular premature contractions that occur with a left ventricular ejection and result in a false determination of the ejection fraction.

All of these patients had marked impairment of left ventricular function. They had pronounced congestive failure and were markedly symptomatic. We have noticed that if the ejection fraction is 0.20 or less, the patient is severely symptomatic and difficult to control with medical treatment. On the other hand, once the ejection fraction is 0.25 or greater, the patient is easier to manage medically and is able to participate in a more normal existence and even return to a sedentary job; this has been true in 51 of these patients following surgery. Although the ejection fraction following surgery may still be far below normal for these patients, it may represent a 1.5 to 2-fold, or even greater, improvement in the function of the heart. It was not unusual to see the ejection fraction in these patients increase from 0.10 to 0.25 or from 0.15 to 0.25 or 0.40. One cannot expect an ejection fraction of 0.10 or 0.15 to return to normal, since there is a great deal of scar tissue replacement in the myocardium of these patients. However, in one patient, the ejection fraction did increase from 0.15 preoperatively to 0.67 postoperatively.

In our series, surgery was offered to all patients no matter how low the ejection fraction or how old or debilitated the patient. The only patients not operated upon were those refusing surgery or those without a graftable vessel. Of the patients with an ejection fraction 0.10 to 0.20 treated medically, there were 61 deaths in 86 patients (a mortality of 71 percent). Bruschke, Proudfit, and Sones (1973)[7] reported a mortality of 84 percent over a five-year period of patients with coronary artery disease and congestive failure. They did not specify the ejection fraction for these patients.

As we operated upon these patients during the past four years, it became apparent that each year our surgical mortality was decreasing significantly. We felt that with the increasing experience, our group could operate on terminal patients with an acceptable mortality rate. This was borne out by a hospital mortality of three patients in 33 (nine percent) operated upon from January 1, 1973 to January 1, 1974, as compared to six deaths in 15 operations (40 percent) during the first year. It is our strong conviction that if the patient with an ejection fraction of 0.10 to 0.20 can be operated upon with less than a 25 percent surgical risk, then surgery is indicated, since the quality of life is considerably enhanced. It would also appear that the life span may be significantly improved.

SUMMARY

The surgical mortality for 144 patients with drastic impairment of the left ventricular function undergoing coronary artery surgery during the past four years was 28 percent (41 patients). The late mortality during this five-year period was 11 percent (16 patients). The majority of the surviving patients restudied showed improvement in the left ventricular ejection fraction. There were only three hospital deaths in the 33 (9 percent) patients operated upon with an ejection fraction of 0.10 to 0.20 from January 1, 1973 to January 1, 1974. In contrast to this, 86 patients were treated medically, with 61 deaths during the same four-year period, for a medical mortality of 71 percent. It is felt that these patients with marked depression in ejection fraction should be operated upon if the revascularization can be done with a low mortality.

References

1. Spencer FC, Green GE, Tice DA, et al: Coronary bypass grafts for congestive heart failure: a report of experiences with 40 patients. J Thorac Cardiovasc Surg 62:529, 1971
2. Siderys H, Pittman JN, Herod G: Coronary artery surgery in patients with impaired left ventricular function. Chest 61:483, 1972
3. Johnson D, Flemma RJ, Manley JC, Lepley D: The physiologic parameters of ventricular function as affected by direct coronary surgery. J Thorac Cardiovasc Surg 60:483, 1970
4. Kay JH, Dunne E, Krohn BG, et al: Left ventricular excision, exclusion, or plication for akinetic areas of the heart. J. Thorac Cardiovasc Surg 59:139, 1970
5. Kitamura S, Echevarria M, Kay JH, et al: Left ventricular performance before and after removal of the noncontractile area of the left ventricle and revascularization of the myocardium. Circulation 45:1005, 1972
6. Mundth ED, Harthorne JW, Buckley MJ, Kinsmore R, Austen WG: Direct coronary arterial revascularization: treatment of cardiac failure associated with coronary artery disease. Arch Surg 103:529, 1971
7. Bruschke AVG, Proudfit WL, Sones FM Jr: Progress study of 590 nonsurgical cases of coronary disease followed 5–9 years: II: ventriculographic and other correlations. Circulation 47:1154, 1973
8. Armitage P: Survivorship tables. Chapter 14 in P Armitage, Statistical Methods in Medical Research. New York, John Wiley and Sons, a Halsted Press Book, 1971, pp. 408–14

82

VENTRICULAR SEPTAL RUPTURE, SECONDARY TO MYOCARDIAL INFARCTION

Roberto Lufschanowski, Paolo Angelini, Robert D. Leachman, Grady L. Hallman, and Denton A. Cooley

Rupture of the ventricular septum, one of the most dramatic complications of ischemic heart disease, has been recognized in autopsy material since the last century.[1] Only in recent years has the clinician been sharing with the pathologist a direct interest in this condition. The first clinical analysis was published in 1934[2] and the first reported surgical repair in 1954.[3] At the present time, sufficient cases have been collected to demonstrate the ominous natural prognosis of ventricular septal rupture. The diagnosis can be suspected with reasonable accuracy on clinical grounds and confirmed by simple hemodynamic procedures. A problem still unsolved is the optimal time for surgical repair. Previous studies[4,5] favored a tendency to delay any surgical procedure until two months after the rupture. An earlier report from this institution[3] described our first experience with this problem. Our experience has now increased with 14 more cases.

MATERIAL AND METHODS

This series consists of 15 cases. Each was operated on for repair of the ventricular septal rupture, confirming the original diagnosis by the operative findings. Most of the patients were referred for surgical evaluation from other institutions. Our experience, therefore, cannot be used to establish the actual incidence of ventricular septal rupture after myocardial infarction, since it is preselected in the sense that the majority of patients (10 cases) were admitted not less than 25 days after infarction.

Hemodynamic studies were performed in 12 instances. Due to the critical condition of many of these patients and because the great majority of them were studied before coronary surgery was performed at this institution, selective coronary angiography was done in only eight. Retrograde arterial catheterization with left ventricular angiography was performed in nine patients. Only three patients died in the immediate postoperative period. At the time of discharge, every patient was reevaluated clinically for evidence of residual ventricular septal defect.

FINDINGS

In these 15 patients, there were three females and 12 males, ranging in age from 47 to 71 years. Mean age was 59 years. Every patient had a single episode of myocardial infarction. None had a previous history of angina or cardiac murmurs. One had diabetes mellitus, one had gout, and none had systemic hypertension.

Clinical evidence of rupture of the ventricular septum appeared in 10 cases before the fourth day following the acute myocardial infarction (Table 1). In patient 9, the clinical pattern changed two weeks after the infarction. Case 7 was referred to us because of the onset of severe and progressive congestive heart failure, 10 years after his only myocardial infarction. At operation, organized fibrous tissue was found surrounding large, multiple perforations of the lower septum, giving the microscopic impression of old infarctions.

The clinical course of these patients after ventricular septal rupture, was dramatic, essentially because of rapid and progressive congestive heart failure (10 cases), or low output syndrome,

TABLE 1. Ventricular Septum Defect (VSD) Postacute Myocardial Infarction

PT.	SEX	AGE	MURMUR (days)	OPERATION
1	M	49	4	2 mos
2	M	47	3	5 days
3	M	52	5	2 mos
4	F	68	1	6 mos
5	M	63	2	1 mos
6	M	49	3	1 mos
7	M	60	?	?
8	F	65	8	25 days
9	M	71	12	2 mos
10	F	60	3	2 mos
11	M	69	8	3 mos
12	M	59	1	3 days
13	M	65	3	21 days
14	M	51	3	6 mos
15	M	53	3	4 days
Mean		59	4.2	83 days

which in four patients evolved into severe shock (cases 2, 6, 12). Since these two clinical patterns are common in cases with severe myocardial infarction, an important clinical diagnostic finding is the presence of a hyperdynamic heart, which is rather atypical in severe ischemic heart disease. A harsh systolic murmur, frequently accompanied by a thrill, was found in all patients.

The plain X-ray of the chest showed nonspecific signs such as cardiomegaly and pulmonary congestion. Increased pulmonary flow was usually difficult to recognize in the usual roentgenograms because the signs of passive venous congestion predominated.

The electrocardiogram did not offer specific patterns in ventricular septal rupture and only showed the localization of the infarcted area, frequently suggesting the presence of a ventricular aneurysm. In 11 cases, there were electrocardiographic signs of inferior infarction and, in 11 cases, signs of anterior infarction. In seven cases, they were coexistent, so that in only five cases was a single infarcted area present.

Cardiac catheterization was performed in all but two patients (Table 2). In 13 cases, dye dilution curves consistent with a left-to-right shunt at the ventricular level were obtained. The pulmonary blood flow was calculated to vary between two and six times systemic flow (mean 3:1).

The pulmonary arterial wedge pressure was elevated in every patient, with a range of 17 to 45 mm Hg and a mean for the group of 24 mm Hg. The main pulmonary artery systolic pressure ranged between 44 and 100 mm Hg with a mean for the group of 61 mm Hg.

In only five cases, retrograde arterial catheterization was performed, and left ventricular angiograms were obtained. Selective coronary arteriography was performed in two cases. In one of them there was evidence of triple-vessel disease of severe degree, and in the other the right coronary artery was completely occluded with the left coronary essentially normal. Left ventriculography confirmed the presence of a ventricular septal defect, usually near the apex, and always in the muscular septum. Aneurysm of the left ventricle coexisted in three cases in this group.

The left ventricular phase of pulmonary angiograms was equally sensitive in detecting the presence of a ventricular septal defect. Operative findings in these patients are described in Table 1.

TABLE 2. VSD Postacute Myocardial Infarction Hemodynamics

PT NO.	CLASS	QP:QS	PCW (mm Hg)	PA SYST	OUTCOME
1	IV	2.4:1	−	−	Died, 45 days
2	Shock	−	−	−	Died same day
3	IV	2.5:1	25	59	64 mos
4	III	3.4:1	17	29	50 mos
5	III, VF	5:1	18	60	Died same day
6	Shock	2:1	17	44	25 mos
7	III	2.5:1	20	70	Died, 18 mos
8	III	2:1	20	48	10 days
9	III	2:3:1	25	75	8 mos
10	III	2.6:1	28	55	12 mos
11	III	2:1	45	100	20 mos
12	Shock	−	−	−	Died, 11 days
13	IV, VF	5:1	22	70	1 mo
14	IV	2:1	27	67	1 mo
15	Shock, VF	6:1	28	58	Died same day
Mean		3:1	24	61	5 hosp deaths

SURGICAL TECHNIQUE

Because of progressive cardiogenic shock, unresponsive to medical treatment, three cases were operated upon as an emergency (Table 3). One of them had to be put on partial bypass before the cardiac procedure could be started (#8). Another patient (#5) had ventricular fi-

brillation during the induction of anesthesia, and extracorporeal circulation was started immediately.

The approach to the ventricular septum was through a right ventriculotomy in six cases, left ventriculotomy in seven, and combined in two. An Ivalon sponge was used as patching material in the first case, in 1956. In seven other cases, the patch was made of Dacron. In the remaining four cases only sutures were used.

TABLE 3. Postoperative Results after Surgery for Ventricular Septal Rupture

YR. OF OP.	SURGICAL FINDING	VENTRI-CULOTOMY	USE OF PATCH	ANEURS-MECTOMY	RESULTS	POSTOP. FOLLOW-UP
1956	2 cm VSD–posterior; small posterior aneurysm of LV	RV	Yes	No	Persistent murmur; CHF and pulmonary infection	Died, 45 days
1958	3 cm VSD–anterior; massive anterior infarct	RV	Yes	Yes	Persisting shock	Died same day
1967	1 cm VSD–inferior; small inferior aneurysm	RV	No	No	Hemodynamically and clinically very favorable (class I-II)	64 mos
1967	Multiple small VSD's (high–lat.); small aneurysm	LV RV	No	Yes	Alive and well (class I–II)	50 mos
1968	1.5 cm VSD–apical; anterolateral infarct	RV	No	No	Persisting Shock and ven. fib.	Died same day
1968	1.5 cm VSD–apical	RV	Yes	No	Satisfactory (class II); VSD murmur	25 mos
1969	Single VSD from LV; anterior aneurysm	RV	No	No	Normal dynamics by cath. no VSD-working without limitation	Died suddenly after 18 mos
1969	2 cm VSD–anterior; anterior aneurysm	LV	Yes	Yes	No murmur at discharge (no late follow-up)	10 days
1970	1 cm VSD–apical; apical aneurysm	LV	Yes	Yes	No murmurs (class II)	8 mos
1970	Small VSD–posterior; small posterior aneurysm	LV	Yes	No	2/6 murmur (class II)	12 mos
1970	1 cm VSC–apical; apical aneurysm	LV	Yes	Yes	No murmur (class I-II)	20 mos
1971	3 cm VSD–mid; diffuse hypokinesia	LV	Yes	No	Murmur–renal failure; low output–ven. fib.	Died, 11 days
1973	10 mm muscular VSD; ant-lat. aneurysm with clots	LV	Yes	Yes	Doing well	
1973	Cribiform VSD; 5 X 8 cm ant-lat aneurysm	LV	Yes	Yes	Doing well	
1973	Necrotic post. wall; post. wall VSD	RV LV	Yes	Yes	Infarctectomy	Died at surgery

In the three cases (2, 12, 15) operated upon within the first five days after the infarction, the defects were large, the infarcted areas were extensive, and it was difficult to find healthy tissue for satisfactory suture of the patch.

Ventricular aneurysms of the free wall of the left ventricle were excised in five cases that had a left ventricular approach. In the remaining cases with this type of ventriculotomy and in all of those in which a combined approach was used, the ventricle was entered through the infarcted area. In a single case, direct suture repair of the rupture was performed from both the right and the left sides of the septum (#7). In case 10, a fresh infarction involved a major part of the septum, and the anterior wall of the right and left ventricles. In this case, infarctectomy was performed on both sides of the septum, and the free walls of the ventricles were resutured to the septum.

RESULTS

The overall operative mortality in this series is 20 percent (3/15). Two other patients died in the hospital before discharge 11 and 45 days postoperatively. One of the two operative deaths was that of an extremely ill patient who entered the surgical suite having an episode of ventricular fibrillation unresponsive to medical treatment. The second operative death occurred in a patient who required emergency partial bypass with femoro-femoral perfusion for treatment of progressive cardiogenic shock. In both, the left ventricular myocardium was diffusely and severely compromised, and no effective contractions could be obtained after extracorporeal circulation was discontinued.

The late hospital deaths were due to a moderately severe low output syndrome with secondary renal failure in one patient (#8) and progressive respiratory and cardiac failure in another (#11). An autopsy was obtained in three of these five cases and showed a satisfactory repair of the ventricular septal defect in one case (#5), and a partial reopening of the ventricular septal defect in the other two. In case 8 an abscess at the patch site was found.

Of the 10 patients who left the hospital (average postoperative hospital stay of nine days), only one had a II out of VI systolic murmur, without thrill. At one year of follow-up, which did not include hemodynamic studies, X-rays showed a great improvement in signs of congestive heart failure and cardiomegaly, and correlated with the absence of significant functional limitations. In six of the remaining seven cases who had follow-up clinical evaluation, there were no signs of congestive heart failure on physical examination and x-ray. Three of these patients are still partially limited by dyspnea on exertion (functional Class II) and have been maintained on digitalis and diuretic treatment. None had experienced new episodes of myocardial infarction after an average 31-month period of observation (ranging from 10 to 50 months). Patient 7 had a smooth and favorable course for 18 months after surgery when he suddenly died. No autopsy was obtained.

DISCUSSION

The natural history of ventricular septal rupture secondary to myocardial infarction has already been well-described in the literature.[6,7,8] Two extreme variants can be outlined for practical purposes. The first corresponds to a case of acute myocardial infarction, which is eventually complicated by severe and rapidly progressive congestive heart failure with low-output syndrome. The short-term prognosis with this clinical pattern is poor. The second variety is that of a stable acute myocardial infarction, with the clinical findings of a ventricular septal defect developing during the first few days after infarction, and complicated by moderate congestive heart failure. Although there are evidently many intermediate forms between these two extremes, this simplification should be borne in mind when treating an individual case of ventricular septal rupture. The diagnostic and therapeutic procedures will eventually vary according to these two different patterns. It is our opinion that in cases with severe acute compromise of the hemodynamic status, the diagnostic studies should be restricted to a few essential and rapid tests. Besides the electrocardiogram and X-ray examination of the chest, a simple right heart catheterization is usually sufficient to confirm the diagnosis of left-to-right shunt. The two patients in this series who presented with cardiogenic shock were not catheterized and were transferred to the operating room as emergencies a few hours after admission. On the other hand, in cases with a relatively smooth postinfarction course and with signs of congestive heart failure responsive to medical treatment, it is advisable to wait for the optimal time for surgical repair, which is usually considered to be two to three months following the infarction. In our own experience, one month after the infarction the fibrous scar is already well developed and permits a safe suturing of the defect (cases 2, 3, 5, and 13). In these circumstances, hemodynamic studies should be performed and must include left and right heart catheterization with selective coronary and left ventricular angiography.

The surgical approach to the ventricular septal defect has to be selected for the individual case. In general, it is safe to close this type of ventricular septal defect through a left ventricular approach since it is easier to localize the rupture and to insert the sutures of the patch. This approach is also advised because of the general principle that a communication between two cavities at different pressures should be closed from the high-pressure side. In fact, the left surface of the septum is essentially smooth, while the right has trabeculations and recesses. A left ventriculotomy, on the other hand, can decrease the contractility of an already diseased left ventricle. Since a left ventriculotomy through healthy tissue should be avoided, this approach is best justified in those cases in which an infarcted area is present in the anterior or apical regions of the left ventricle. In cases with posterior or exclusively septal infarctions, the right ventriculotomy is probably more convenient. Recently, Shumaker [9] suggested an incision in the posterior wall of the right ventricle in posterior defects.

The relationship between the ventricular septal rupture and the conduction system is not usually a problem, as the great majority of the perforations are found in the lower two-thirds of the septum. The right ventriculotomy leads to a right bundle branch block pattern of no real significance, as these are not true bundle lesions but only peripheral blocks, and atrioventricular conduction is essentially unaltered. [10]

The choice of using a patch versus direct suture of the defect is decided by the individual findings. When the ventricular septal defect is small and well-circumscribed by strong fibromuscular tissue, simple closure is consistently successful. Otherwise a patch, eventually combined with reinforcement of the tissue by sutures, should be used. In cases of very extensive perforations, the insertion of two patches, one on each side of the septum, may be necessary.

Since the indication of ventricular septal rupture repair is heart failure, the elimination of the diastolic overload of the left ventricle is always beneficial. Other surgical procedures, such as aneurysmectomy, infarctectomy, plastic repair of the mitral valve, and aortocoronary bypass, can also be performed according to the individual situation. This multiplicity of approaches not only will improve the late prognosis but also the operative risk, especially in cases operated on during cardiogenic shock, where the restoration of cardiac reserve is very important following the operative trauma.

We believe that the diagnosis of postinfarction rupture of the interventricular septum is an almost unequivocal indication for surgical repair. The natural history of this complication of myocardial infarction has proved to be extremely ominous with a survival rate of only 10 to 20 percent two months after the perforation. Our experience, however, is not truly representative of the unselected population of ventricular septal ruptures because only a few cases were followed in our institution from the time of the acute infarction. The majority were referred for surgical treatment at a later time. Several other patients not included in this series were referred as emergency cases in cardiogenic shock and died on admission or a few hours after admission before surgical repair. Even with these limitations, it is interesting to notice the absence of predisposing factors in our series. None of our cases had a history of hypertension, nor of multiple infarctions, two major risk factors for complications of myocardial necrosis. No specific review of these factors is available at the present time with regard to VSR, but they are expected to be similar to those of cardiac rupture. [11]

Compared with the reported natural history, our surgical mortality is low in the cases operated upon in the post acute phase (one month after the infarction). Of the 12 cases in this group, we had two deaths, one being that of a patient operated on in 1956, the first open-heart operation in our series. The three cases treated as emergencies in the first few days after the infarction, because of cardiogenic shock unresponsive to medical treatment, died in the immediate postoperative hours with persistent low output syndrome and arrhythmias. This group is too small for significant conclusions but shows that the surgical risk is very high under these circumstances, especially if the shunt is not the main determinant of the poor performance of the heart. The review of the literature presented by Kitamura et al [12] in 1971 showed that of 65 patients reported to have had a ventricular septum repair, 21 were operated on within the first month after infarction. Of these, only five (30 percent) were alive at the time of the report.

References

1. Latham PM: Lectures on Subjects Connected with Medicine, Comprising Diseases of the Heart (vol. 2). London, Longman, Brown, Green and Longmans, 1946, p 108
2. Sager RV: Coronary thrombosis: perforation of infarcted inverventricular septum. Arch Intern Med 53:140, 1934
3. Cooley DA, Belmonte BA, Zeis LB, et al: Surgical repair of ruptured interventricular septum following acute myocardial infarction. Surgery 41:930, 1957
4. Friedberg CK: Diseases of the heart. Philadelphia, Saunders Co., 1966, p 856
5. Davison T, Degenshein GA, Yuceoglu YZ, et al: Repair of ventricular septal defect following myocardial infarction. Ann Surg 160:33, 1964
6. Sanders RJ, Kern WH, Blount SG Jr: Perforation of the interventricular septum complicating myocardial infarction: a report of eight cases, one with cardiac catheterization. Am Heart J 51:736, 1956
7. Oyomada A, Queen FB: Spontaneous rupture of the interventricular septum following acute myocardial infarction with some clinicopathological observations on survival in five cases. Presented at Pan Pacific Pathology Congress, Tripler US Army Hospital, 1961
8. Lee WY, Cardon L, Slodki SJ: Perforation of infarcted interventricular septum. Arch Intern Med 109:731, 1962
9. Shumaker HB: Suggestions concerning operative management of postinfarction septal defects. J Thorac Cardiovasc Surg 64:452, 1972
10. Massig GK, James TN: Conduction and block in the right bundle branch: real and imagined. Circulation 45:1, 1972
11. Lewis A, Burchell HB, Titus JL: Clinical and pathologic features of postinfarction cardiac rupture. Am J Cardiol 23:43, 1969
12. Kitamura S, Mendez A, Kay JH: Ventricular septal defect following myocardial infarction: experience with surgical repair through a left ventriculotomy and review of literature. J Thorac Cardiovasc Surg 61:186, 1971

83

MANAGEMENT OF THE RUPTURED VENTRICULAR SEPTUM
Early and Late Results

GEORGE E. REED, LUIS E. CORTES,
ARTHUR C. FOX, and EPHRAIM GLASSMAN

INTRODUCTION

Rupture of the interventricular septum following myocardial infarction is generally a rapidly lethal event. The majority of untreated patients survive for a few days, and fewer than 15 percent survive more than two months.[12] If surgery is to produce significant salvage, it must be focused on the 24 percent of patients who will die within the first 24 hours or the additional 40 percent who succumb in the ensuing two weeks.[11]

We analyzed the experience at the New York University Medical Center along with other published cases in an attempt to identify which group should be operated upon without delay and in which group operation could be safely postponed until the time when technical conditions would be optimal.

CLINICAL EXPERIENCE

Between January 1969 and December 1972, eleven patients with rupture of the interventricular septum were admitted to New York University Hospital. In 1969 and 1970, five patients were treated after transfer here because of rapid hemodynamic deterioration. Three patients had repair of the perforation within hours of admission to the hospital from two to 10 days after rupture of the septum; none survived (Table 1). A fourth patient (IG) had equal pressures in pulmonary and systemic circuits and had pulmonary artery banding in an effort to gain time until definitive repair was possible; he did not survive. Because of the lack of success in the operative management

of these four very ill patients, we developed a technique for temporary closure of ventricular septal defects by inflation of a balloon inserted transvenously.[10] The fifth patient (TMc) was treated medically in preparation for an attempt at balloon closure of the septal defect. She died before this could be attempted.

In 1971 and 1972, seven operations were performed in six patients with rupture of the interventricular septum and all survived. In one patient (TT), the rupture probably resulted from a crushing chest injury that had occurred 17 years before.

ANALYSIS OF RESULTS

Age and Sex

There was little age difference between the survivors, who ranged from 51 to 72 years, and the nonsurvivors, who were from 52 to 70 years of age. There were two women among those who survived, and a third woman died without operation.

Interval between Infarction and Rupture

The time of perforation was generally well documented, although the dating of the infarct was less exact. The diagnosis of septal rupture was made from 24 hours to 35 days following infarction. At operation in patient SF, one day after rupture of the septum and two days after infarction, there was extensive necrosis of the left ventricle and the odor of gangrene permeated the operating room when the pericardium was opened.

**TABLE 1. Comparison of Survivors and Nonsurvivors after Surgical Treatment
of Ruptured Ventricular Septum**

PT.	AGE/SEX	DATE OF OR	MI→VSD	MI→OR	SHUNT	PA PRESSURE	BP	LA OR LVED
Nonsurvivors								
JB	52/M	2/27/69	10 days	12 days	–	–	70/–[a]	–
IK	68/M	6/13/69	3 days	19 days	3.5:1	80/–	90/–[a]	–
SF	56/M	10/10/69	1 day	2 days	–	–	60/–[a]	–
IG	67/M	11/7/69	2 days	3 days	4.0:1	60/40	60/–[a]	–
TMc	70/F	No op	6 days	d. 11 days	4.0:1	45/13	80/55[a]	17[b]
Survivors								
LM	68/M	10/8/71	35 days	37 days	2.7:1	52/23	95/60	23[c]
RH	60/F	1/27/72	Not known	3 mos	3.0:1	56/20	80/54	26[c]
VI	72/M	2/25/72	44 days	11 days	3.3:1	60/14	95/75	–
TT[d]	54/M	5/24/72	17 yrs	17 yrs	–	140/40	130/90	15[c]
MW	51/M	8/8/72	7 days	5 wks	2.5:1	79/25	105/72	24[c]
MW	51/M	9/20/72	3 days	5 wks	–	90/–	90/–	–
AM	58/F	10/31/72	5 days	5 wks	–	64/12	93/61	22[c]

[a]On pressors.
[b]Wedge.
[c]LVED.
[d]Crushing chest injury.

**TABLE 2. Coronary, Clinical, and Hemodynamic Status of Patients with
Ruptured Ventricular Septum**

PT.	BUN	CREAT.	CORONARY LESIONS	LV CONTRACTILITY	MENTAL STATUS	URINE OUTPUT	ADDITIONAL PROCEDURES
Nonsurvivors							
JB	46	–	Not studied	Poor at op	Moribund	Anuric	Excision of necrotic infarct
IK	210	–	Autopsy: LAD–90% stenosis; RCA–moderate stenosis	Poor at op	Moribund	Oliguric	Excision of necrotic infarct
SK	38	2.6	Autopsy: LAD–occluded; RCA–severe stenosis	Poor at op	Moribund	Anuric	Excision of necrotic infarct
IG	–	–	Not studied	–	Stuporous	Anuric	PA banding only
TMc	198	6.4	Autopsy: LAD–occluded	–	Stuporous	Anuric	No operation
Survivors							
LM	130	2.4	LAD-occluded	Fairly good	Clear	Oliguric	LV Aneurysmectomy
RH	20	0.8	RCA–occluded; LAD–90% stenosis	Fairly good	Clear	Adequate	Mitral annuloplasty Saphenous bypass to LAD
VI	102	1.9	Not studied	Good at op	Stuporous	Anuric	LV Aneurysmectomy
MW	43	1.6	PD[a]–occluded; LAD–severe stenosis	Good	Clear	Adequate	Saphenous bypass to LAD
MW	27	1.5	Not restudied	Good	Clear	Adequate	LV Aneurysmectomy
AM	32	1.0	LAD–occluded	Good	Stuporous	Adequate	LV Aneurysmectomy

[a]PD: posterior descending branch of right coronary artery.

At the other extreme was patient LM, in whom perforation is thought to have occurred 35 days following infarction. In one patient (RH) who developed mitral regurgitation following infarction, the septal defect was recognized only at cardiac catheterization, and its duration was not known.

Interval between Infarction and Operation

There was a substantial difference in the time from infarction to operation, which ranged from 11 to 37 days for the survivors, as compared with the nonsurvivors for whom this interval was from 2 to 19 days (Table 1). Operation was performed on the day of transfer to this hospital on all patients who died and immediately following cardiac catheterization in three of the five who survived. The need for immediate operation was dictated in each instance by the rapid hemodynamic deterioration of the patient and could not be postponed until a more advantageous time. Each of these patients was hypotensive despite infusions of pressors; all but one were oliguric or anuric, and six were comatose or stuporous (Table 2). The oldest patient was the earliest survivor. (Operation was done 11 days after infarction.) In only two patients was a scheduled operation performed. One patient (MW) was treated on a day-to-day basis for a predetermined period of five weeks, after which time operation was performed. When the shunt recurred, he was again managed in the same way for an additional five weeks. At the second operation, a posterior aneurysm was found at the site of previous repair. This could have resulted from extension of his infarction in the period surrounding operation or could have been produced by ischemia from the mattress sutures placed through the ventricular wall during the repair of the defect. A second patient (LM), also operated upon five weeks after infarction, has a recurrent murmur.

A review of the cases reported for whom this information is available,[13,5,6,4,7,2] including the present series, shows that of 21 patients operated upon less than three months after infarction, 10 patients had residual or recurrent shunts. Contrary to the reported rates at which infarcts heal,[9,8] RH, who had operation three months after infarction, still had necrosis near the site of perforation.

It was not possible in our own experience to delay operation electively until three months after infarction although it may be that such a delay permits more complete and permanent repair of the defect.

Size of Pulmonic-to-Systemic Shunt

The average ratio for pulmonic-to-systemic flow in the nonsurvivors was 3.8; for the survivors it was 2.9 (Table 1). The effect of a large shunt on survival, however, cannot be deduced from the experience to date. Campion's series[2] had an average shunt ratio of 3.7; two patients with ratios of 4.6 and 6.6 survived to be operated upon five months and three months, respectively, after infarction.

In our series, one patient had hemoptysis and another had a septic pulmonary infarct that progressed to empyema and a broncho-pleural fistula. The latter patient later required pulmonary resection and decortication. Both of these events may have resulted from embolization of necrotic tissue from the septum via the large left-to-right shunt.

Pulmonary Artery Pressure

Pulmonary artery systolic pressure equaled 78 percent of systemic pressure in the nonsurvivors and 73 percent in survivors. The range of pressures within each group was the same (Table 1).

Coronary Artery Lesions

The location and severity of coronary stenoses were identified in three patients at autopsy and in four of the survivors by preoperative coronary angiography. There was no obvious correlation between the distribution of the lesions and survival (Table 2).

Left Ventricular Function

Left ventricular function was assessed preoperatively by left ventricular end diastolic pressure (LVEDP) and ventriculography. In four patients, LVEDP ranged from 22 to 26 mm Hg (Table 1). Although LVEDP was elevated in each, contractility of the left ventricle appeared fairly good despite the presence of aneurysms in three patients and moderate mitral regurgitation in a fourth. This was a striking contrast to the inadequate contractility of the left ventricle observed at operation in patients who died.

Associated Procedures

In addition to repair of the ventricular septal defect, necrotic tissue was excised in three of the nonsurvivors. A fourth patient had only pulmonary artery banding. His preoperative pulmonary artery pressure was equal to systemic pressure and pulmonary artery banding was performed to decrease pulmonary flow. The immediate result was dramatic, with a fall in the pulmonary artery pressure to 30/18. The systemic pressure rose to 80/60 and the right ventricular pressure was 80/5. The low end diastolic pressure in the right ventricle probably reflected good right ventricular function. The immediate effect was a decrease in pressor requirements and an increase in urine flow. However, these salutory effects were transient and the patient succumbed.

Among those who survived repair of the septal defect, four patients had left ventricular aneurysmectomies. In one, a saphenous vein bypass graft was inserted into the left anterior descending coronary artery. In a fifth patient, mitral annuloplasty was performed and a saphenous vein graft was inserted into the left anterior descending coronary artery. Two patients had significant disease only of the left anterior descending. Both had aneurysms as well as septal perforations, indicating that the entire distribution of the anterior descending had been infarcted. There seemed little point in revascularizing this area.

Surgical Technique

The technique used for repair of the septal defects in this series is based on a few concepts and some simple principles:

1. All sutures were buttressed (with Teflon felt) on all sides of the myocardium.
2. Patch material was cut generously so that sutures (#0 and #1 nonabsorbable material) were placed well back from the defect. Occasionally, the muscle was of questionable viability even at a distance from the perforation.
3. Mattress sutures were used with 8 mm separating the two limbs of each suture and with 4 mm distance between adjacent sutures.
4. The cut edges of the ventricular wall were often everted to form the two sides of a sandwich with the Teflon felt septum as the filler. After placement of interrupted horizontal mattress sutures, the cut edge was oversewn with continuous sutures.

We avoided incision in the left ventricle through viable muscle when coronary angiography demonstrated that a significant source of blood would be interrupted. In patient MW, who was operated on twice, the septal defect was initially approached through the right atrium by detaching the tricuspid valve in order to reach the posterior-inferior aspect of the septum, where a linear tear was present. Coronary angiography in this patient had demonstrated occlusion of the posterior descending coronary artery and a 90 percent stenosis of the left anterior descending coronary artery. The anterior and posterior walls of the left ventricle were being supplied almost entirely from the circumflex coronary artery, and an incision through the left ventricle might have seriously compromised blood flow.

DISCUSSION

Although the consensus of the literature is to delay operation until fibrosis of the infarct has occurred, there have been other proponents of early operation.[1,3] The timing of surgery is usually dictated by the clinical situation. When the patient develops signs of left ventricular failure such as hypotension with continued need for pressors or oliguria and a rising BUN, operation should be performed without delay. Such patients are unlikely to survive to the optimum two-to-three-month stage. Since technical benefits from a better infarct scar probably do not accrue before this time has elapsed, there appears to be no gain in delaying operation by a shorter interval.

Effective forward flow remained adequate for long periods in those patients who lived to have elective operation two or more months after infarction. The clinical event that ultimately brought most of them to operation was right ventricular failure. Initially, the increased flow and pressure work was well tolerated by the right ventricle and the pulmonary vasculature. Failure of the right ventricle seems to occur relatively late. This was true in a series reported by Campion,[2] in which operation was performed between 2.5 months and 32 months after infarction. In the present series, left ventricular failure was prominent in all patients who died and in those survivors who required early operation.

All patients should be studied by coronary angiography and left ventriculography. In our experience, the prognosis is not made worse by the presence of ventricular aneurysm or mitral regurgitation. Indeed, each of the survivors had one of these additional complications of myocardial infarction. Complete assessment of the coronary circulation is necessary to plan properly the operative approach to the defect and to determine the need for coronary revascularization. Incision should be made through aneurysmal or infarcted tissue, sparing contracting myocardium to which the blood supply from one side may have been compromised. Where high-grade stenosis or occlusion is demonstrated in vessels with adequate distal lumens, revascularization should be considered. Survival is possible with operation early after infarction if left ventricular contractility is reasonably spared by the infarction and preserved during operation.

References

1. Allen P: Discussion of paper by Iben AB, Pupello DF, Stinson EB, Shumway NE: Surgical treatment of postinfarction ventricular septal defects. Ann Thorac Surg 8:252, 1969
2. Campion BC, Harrison CE, Giuliani ER, Schattenberg TT, Ellis FH: Ventricular septal defect after myocardial infarction. Ann Intern Med 70:251, 1969
3. Cooley DA, Belmonte BA, Zeis LB, Schnur S: Surgical repair of ruptured interventricular septum following acute myocardial infarction. Surgery 41:930, 1957
4. Daggett WM, Burwell LR, Lawson DW, Austen WG: Resection of acute ventricular aneurysm and ruptured interventricular septum after myocardial infarction. N Engl J Med 283:1507, 1970
5. Daugherty HK, Robicsek F, Mullen DC: Post-infarction ventricular septal defect: a major surgical emergency. N C Med J 30:433, 1969
6. Gerard FP: Ventricular septal rupture secondary to coronary occlusion. Angiology 21:116, 1970
7. Iben AB, Pupello DF, Stinson EB, Shumway NE: Surgical treatment of postinfarction ventricular defects. Ann Thorac Surg 8:252, 1969
8. Levene SA, Brown CL: Coronary thrombosis; its various clinical features. Medicine 8:245, 1929
9. Mallory GK, White PD, Salcedo-Salgar J: The speed of healing of myocardial infarction. Am Heart J: 18:647, 1939
10. Mills NL, Vargish T, Kleinman LH, Bloomfield DA, Reed GE: Balloon closure of ventricular septal defect. Circulation (Suppl I) 13, 14:111, 1971
11. Oyamada A, Queen FB: Spontaneous rupture of the interventricular septum following acute myocardial infarction with some clinicopathological observations on survival in five cases. Presented at Pan Pacific Pathology Congress, Tripler US Army Hospital, October 12, 1961
12. Sanders RJ, Kern WH, Blount SG: Perforation of the interventricular septum complicating myocardial infarction. Am Heart J 51:736, 1956
13. Shumacker HB: Suggestions concerning operative management of postinfarction septal defects. J Thorac Cardiovasc Surg 64:452, 1972

84

SUCCESSFUL IMMEDIATE REPAIR OF ACQUIRED VENTRICULAR SEPTAL DEFECT AND SURVIVAL IN PATIENTS WITH ACUTE MYOCARDIAL INFARCTION SHOCK USING A NEW DOUBLE-PATCH TECHNIQUE

A. B. Iben, R. R. Miller, E. A. Amsterdam,
E. J. Hurley, J. A. Bonanno, G. K. Hilliard,
C. Caudill, D. Williams, R. Zelis,
and D. T. Mason

Emergency operative restoration of normal cardiac hemodynamics is necessary for improved survival following postinfarction ventricular septal perforation.[1] Previously, operations to close septal lesions were attempted only after medical therapy failed or at the end of a three-to-six-week delay when the patient's condition was thought to be more stable and the zone of infarction was less friable. These methods resulted in a high mortality. Use of assist devices for substantial periods followed by surgical treatment does not improve survival chances.[2] Such support during short periods for the purpose of safe conduct of catheterization and surgical scheduling may be useful.[3]

Our experience with 13 patients having secondary septal perforations formed the basis for the development of operative techniques applicable at any stage of the disease. They are most successful, however, when used as soon as the septal defect is recognized.

PATHOPHYSIOLOGY

The defect usually involves the apical portion of the muscular septum, but the surrounding infarction is often extensive, involving large portions of the septum and the left ventricular free wall.[4] Occasional perforations are found at any point along the posterior wall.

The magnitude of the left-to-right shunt is often large, usually in excess of a pulmonary-to-systemic flow ratio of 2:1.[5] The presence of an akinetic or aneurysmal ventricular wall together with the transeptal shunt results in biventricular failure, pulmonary edema, and cardiogenic shock.

OCCURRENCE

Rupture of the ventricular septum is not common, but it is a dramatic complication of acute myocardial infarction and occurs within 4 to 12 days of infarction. Its incidence is 1.2 percent.[6] It produces 1 to 2 percent of all deaths from myocardial infarction.[7,8,9] Mortality is reported to be 24 percent within 24 hours, with the majority of patients dying within one week.[10] Fewer than 7 percent live for one year.

CLINICAL MATERIAL

Among the first nine cases operated upon from two days to six weeks following defect formulation, five survived. Failures within this group resulted from early surgical technical problems, postoperative cardiac pump failure, and pulmonary and renal complications resulting from ill-advised delays of operative intervention. The 10th patient deserves presentation because of complications resulting from a delay in surgical intervention.

The subsequent three consecutive patients in this series were operated upon 18 hours, six days, and 12 hours after appearance of their lesions. Following extensive infarct resection of the free wall and septum and cardiac reconstruction they are alive and well 14 months, 12 months, and 18 months since operation.

CASE REPORTS

CASE 10 SW: *This 58-year-old white female was admitted from another hospital following eight days of serious illness resulting from ventricular septal perforation. At admission she barely had perceptible pulses and blood pressure. Chest examination revealed a holosystolic murmur and thrill. Her renal performance was decreased, and a peritoneal dialysis catheter was inserted. Pulmonary edema and pneumonia were established. Operation was performed without difficulty.*

The postoperative course was complicated by continued renal failure and increasing ventilation problems. Cardiotonic drugs were successful in re-establishing cardiac output, but the patient died on the 13th postoperative day of failure of multiple organ systems.

CASE 11 AF: *This 67-year-old male entered the emergency room of the Sacramento Medical Center with a five-day history of midback pain and nausea that culminated on the admission day with excruciating substernal pain. Examination revealed a pale, diaphoretic man in severe pain. Blood pressure by palpation was 85 mm Hg. Electrocardiogram revealed an anteroseptal infarction. Following the ECG the patient developed ventricular fibrillation from which he was immediately resuscitated using one 400-watt second dc countershock.*

Cardiac examination revealed the thrill and murmur typical of septal rupture. Right and left

heart catheterization confirmed the diagnosis (Table 1).

Surgical repair followed the catheterization. The procedure began, with norepinephrine infusion needed to provide barely discernible pulses. Isoproterenol was used for 12 hours postoperatively. The postoperative course was otherwise uneventful.

CASE 12 GC: *This 51-year-old woman had no previous cardiac complaints but was diabetic and hypertensive for four years prior to admission. An anteroseptal myocardial infarction was diagnosed electrocardiographically soon after her admission for anterior crushing chest pain and dyspnea. Seventeen hours after admission she became hypotensive concomitant with the onset of a loud pansystolic murmur. The diagnosis of VSD or possible mitral regurgitation necessitated her transfer. Upon admission to our hospital, examination revealed a disoriented, cold, and diaphoretic woman with a cuff blood pressure of 70 mm Hg obtainable by palpation and a heart rate of 110. Jugular venous distension was present at 30 degrees with visible "A" and "V" waves. Cardiac findings were consistent with those of septal perforation. These included a left lower parasternal systolic lift, a systolic thrill, and a grade 4/6 harsh pansystolic murmur.*

Norepinephrine was started, and the patient underwent cardiac catheterization. A 2.6:1 pulmonic-to-systemic flow ratio was measured. Left ventricular cineangiography displayed immediate biventricular opacification and a large akinetic area in the left ventricular anterior-apical wall. She was taken immediately to the operating room with the norepinephrine infusion running.

The infarcted septum including a 1.5 cm defect and the akinetic free wall were resected. Repair was easily achieved. Inotropic medications

TABLE 1. Most Recent Patients Operated on for Acquired Ventricular Septal Defect

	CASE NO. 11 AF		CASE NO. 12 GC		CASE NO. 13 RB	
	Preop	**Postop**	**Preop**	**Postop**	**Preop**	**Postop**
HR	135	104	122	106	94	82
BP (mm Hg)	68/54	124/67	72/54	115/68	112/62	152/69
RA						
mm Hg	8	4	9	3	16	3
O_2 sat percent	51	73	72	76	47	69
RV (mm Hg)	46/16	24/7	31/17	26/5	62/16	21/6
PA						
mm Hg	42/24	24/9	31/12	62/12	62/19	21/10
O_2 sat percent	84	72	89	76	87	68
PAW	22	6	13	9	26	6
CI (L/min/M²)	—	2.1	—	4.1	—	2.7
P:S flow (L/min)	5.1/1	1/1	2.8/1	1/1	6.0/1	1/1

were utilized for 36 hours following surgery. Thereafter, her course was uneventful, with discharge from the hospital on the 14th postoperative day.

CASE 13 RB: *This 68-year-old woman was transferred to the University of California, Davis, Sacramento Medical Center six days after admission to another hospital for acute anterior wall infarction. During that hospitalization, early signs of congestive heart failure were complicated by atrial tachyarrhythmias and the onset of a harsh-grade 4/6 pansystolic precordial murmur. Following a course of digitalis and diuretics to which there was no response, she was transferred with a diagnosis of mitral regurgitation.*

Examination revealed a blood pressure of 100/60 mm Hg, distended jugular veins to the mandibular angle at 80 degrees, and moist inspiratory rales throughout both lung fields. Moderate dependent edema was present. The typical lower left sternal border thrill was present, and pansystolic precordial murmur was heard. Because of hypotension, oliguria, and a further clouded sensorium, immediate right heart catheterization was performed. A pulmonic-to-systemic flow ratio of 6:1 was measured. Complete cardiac catheterization studies (Table 1) showed biventricular failure.

Resection and repair were carried out immediately, with an uncomplicated postoperative course. Discharge was on the 15th postoperative day.

PROCEDURE

With the patient heparinized and placed on cardiopulmonary bypass using standard caval and aortic cannulation, caval tourniquets are applied and the heart is fibrillated electrically. Coronary perfusion proceeds normally through the aortic root.

A longitudinal incision is placed in the left ventricle in the area observed previously to be akinetic and near the point of maximum thrill intensity. Most of the akinetic left ventricular free wall is resected. The septal defect is measured, and all infarcted septal muscle is debrided.

Two pieces of one-eighth-of-an-inch-thick Teflon felt are cut so that they are 2.5 cm larger overall than the defect in the septum. The patch edges are curved to approximate the contour of the posterior cardiac wall. Using a series of horizontal mattress sutures, the residual septum is sandwiched between the two felt bolster patches. Thereafter, two rectangular felt bolsters are cut for use on the epicardial surface of the left and right ventricles. A structural row of interrupted mattress sutures align,

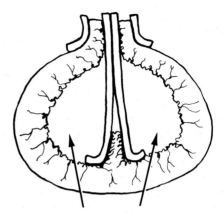

FIG. 1.   Reconstructed ventricles (arrows).

in everting fashion, the ventricular walls against the septal prosthesis (Fig. 1). A running hemostatic suture line may be placed over the entire ventricular closure.

RESULTS

Three patients, two in the seventh decade and one in the sixth decade of life, underwent emergency repair of postinfarction septal perforation. All survived with little difficulty. Postoperative catheterizations revealed no residual shunt as measured by all available methods. Normal cardiac output was noted along with vigorously contracting left ventricles.

DISCUSSION

This aggressive approach to resection of infarcted myocardium was adopted when four of five consecutive patients were treated successfully in this manner for cardiogenic shock and electrical instability that resulted following free-wall infarction. Infarctectomy was performed within four hours of infarct on one patient, in one week with two others, and within three weeks with two. The only nonsurvivor required mitral valve replacement and repair of a walled-off perforation of the posterior cardiac wall just below the atrioventricular groove.

Acute septal rupture is characterized by abrupt clinical deterioration associated with sudden onset of a left precordial thrill and a holosystolic murmur. Cardiac dysfunction becomes manifest when ventricular asynergy involves 20 percent of the left ventricle. Added to this is the sudden occurrence of a left-to-right intracardiac shunt that further decreases left ventricular output. Such markedly decreased cardiac output produces severely reduced perfusion of the heart and all organ systems. It is for this reason that the use of prolonged temporizing measures following recognition of these lesions increase morbidity and mortality.

Operation with the techniques described results in permanent closure. Resection of asynergic free wall is known to improve ventricular function.[11,12]

Debridement of necrotic and poorly perfused septal tissue makes it possible to apply sutures in viable muscle. The double patch described above is used more easily than a left-sided patch placed with individually bolstered sutures. The rebuilt septum does not result in a greater decrease in left ventricular chamber size than would occur from the free wall resection alone. There is no tension at the suture lines.

A posterior perforation, especially when located high on the septum, is best approached through a right ventriculotomy as we described earlier.[13] Resection of the posterior ventricular wall, most notably in the area near the atrioventricular groove, is avoided unless perforation appears imminent.

Heart block was not present in this entire series in spite of the wide resection of septal tissue. Postoperative ventricular irritability was not seen.

If cardiac catheterization and coronary arteriography does not endanger the patient, it may be performed. Coronary arterial lesions may be found that require bypass procedures. At times, the suddenness of decompensation following septal rupture requires operative intervention without complete catheterization assessment of cardiac dynamics. The obvious clinical diagnosis and the possible fatal consequences preclude any efforts short of emergency operative correction. The alternative diagnosis, mitral insufficiency from papillary muscle dysfunction, can be diagnosed and treated intraoperatively.

CONCLUSION

Three patients, two of them in cardiogenic shock and one in cardiac failure with severe pulmonary edema, underwent successful emergency repair of postinfarction septal perforation. This proven technique allows for a sound repair at any time and includes patients in a moribund condition following septal disruption. Operation at the earliest possible time significantly increases survival from a serious and, obviously, surgical disease.

References

1. Iben AB, Lurie AJ, Chung G, Holmes S, Hurley EJ: Emergency infarctectomy and repair of postinfarction ventricular septal defects. (Presented at Society of Thoracic Surgeons meeting in Los Angeles, January 1974)
2. Buckley MJ, Mundth ED, Daggett WM, et al: Surgical management of ventricular septal defects and mitral regurgitation complicating acute myocardial infarction. Ann Thorac Surg 16:598, 1973
3. Buckley MJ et al: Discussion of emergency infarctectomy and repair of post-infarction ventricular septal defects, at Society of Thoracic Surgeons meeting in Los Angeles, January 1974
4. Swithinbank JM: Perforation of the interventricular septum in myocardial infarction. Br Heart J 21: 562, 1959
5. Selzer A, Gerbode F, et al: Clinical hemodynamic and surgical considerations of rupture of the ventricular septum after myocardial infarction. Am Heart J 78:598, 1969
6. Johnson WD, Flemma RJ, et al: Extended treatment of severe coronary artery disease: a total surgical approach. Ann Surg 170:460, 1969
7. London RE, London SB: Rupture of the heart. A critical analysis of 47 consecutive autopsy cases. Circulation 31:202, 1965
8. Ross RM, Young JA: Clinical and necropsy findings in rupture of the myocardium: a review of 43 cases. Scott Med J 8:222, 1963
9. Lee WY, Cardon L, et al: Perforation of infarcted septum. Arch Intern Med 109:731, 1962
10. Sanders RJ, Kern WH, et al: Perforation of the interventricular septum complicating myocardial infarction. Am Heart J 51:736, 1956
11. Schimert G, Falsetti HL, Bunnell IL, et al: Excision of akinetic left ventricular wall for intractable heart failure. Ann Intern Med 70:437, 1969
12. Lichtlen P: The hemodynamics of clinical ischemic heart disease. Ann Clin Res 3:333, 1971
13. Iben AB, Pupello DF, et al: Surgical treatment of postinfarction ventricular septal defects. Ann Thorac Surg 8:252, 1969

85

SURGICAL MANAGEMENT OF CORONARY ARTERY ANEURYSMS

SETH BEKOE, G. J. MAGOVERN, G. A. LIEBLER,
F. R. BEGG, and S. B. PARK

The marked increase in coronary artery surgery during the past few years can be attributed to the development and popularization of cinecoronary arteriography (Sones, Shirey, 1962). This procedure has been responsible for the premortem recognition and understanding of the many pathological conditions of the coronary arteries. One such condition is coronary artery aneurysm, an entity first described by Bougon in 1812. The report was a postmortem finding, as were nearly all the approximately 100 cases subsequently described up to 1967, when Sherkat et al diagnosed, by aortography, aneurysms of both coronary arteries in a nine-month-old boy. Recent reports have indicated premortem diagnosis and attempts at surgical correction when indicated (Konecke et al, 1971; Sayegh et al, 1968; Cafferky et al, 1969; Ghahramani et al, 1972; Ebert et al, 1971; Dawson and Ellison, 1972; Mattern et al, 1972).

The present report is based on studies of five patients recently evaluated for surgical correction of coronary artery disease in our institution and include a review of the literature.

CASE REPORTS

CASE 1: This patient was a 57-year-old male who sustained a myocardial infarction in 1963. He recovered successfully and was placed on anticoagulant therapy for two years. He did well until May 1972, when he began to have recurrent angina pectoris on exertion. Coronary arteriography was performed in August 1972 and revealed a saccular aneurysm as well as a proximal occlusion of the left anterior descending coronary artery (LAD), diffuse disease of the circumflex coronary artery (CCA), and total occlusion of the right coronary artery (RCA) (Figs. 1 and 2). Physical

examination was essentially negative. He had a regular rhythm and no murmur. Laboratory tests showed hyperthyroidism, and the electrocardiogram (EKG) revealed left ventricular hypertrophy. He was treated with I¹³¹ and was considered euthyroid in December 1972, but he still complained of angina pectoris on exertion. On January 26, 1973, he was operated upon and had left internal mammary artery (LIMA) bypass to the LAD. The saccular aneurysm of the LAD was dissected out and excised at the neck; the base was sutured. The wall of the aneurysm was thin and soft, and the lumen did not contain thrombi. Postoperatively he did well without complications except for recurrence of the hyperthyroidism, which necessitated another dose of I¹³¹. He was discharged after 20 days, free of angina. Reexamination one year after surgery showed a patent anastomosis between the LIMA and LAD and a satisfactory repair of the aneurysm (Fig. 3).

CASE 2: A 52-year-old man sustained a myocardial infarction in February 1973, requiring 17 days of hospitalization. A month later, after successful recovery under medical management, he underwent selective cinecoronary arteriography. This showed subtotal occlusion of the LAD, a fusiform aneurysm 1 cm from the ostium of a small nondominant RCA, and diffuse disease of the CCA without any localized stenotic lesion. On examination prior to surgery, he was found to be normotensive. Laboratory investigations showed normal cardiac enzymes and a normal EKG tracing; the lipid profile was within normal limits. At operation on April 30, 1973, he had LIMA bypass to the LAD beyond the obstructive lesion; the entire aneurysmal portion of the RCA was dissected and the roof of the aneurysm excised. A previously prepared, reversed autogenous saphenous vein was fashioned to the size of the defect in the RCA and anastomosed end-to-side. The proximal aortic anastomosis was made in routine

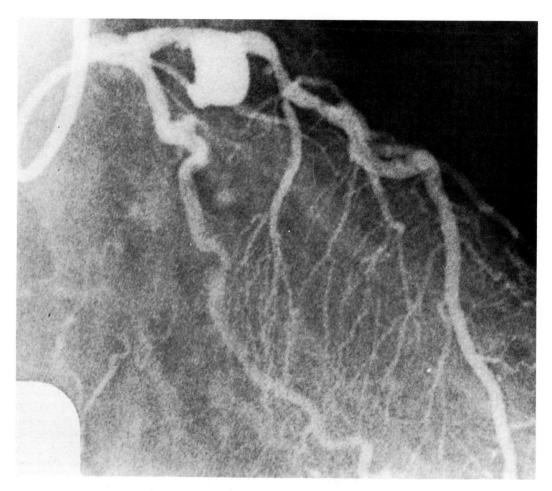

FIG. 1. Left coronary arteriogram in the right anterior oblique projection showing aneurysm of the LAD (Case 1).

fashion. The aneurysm measured 1.8 cm in length and had calcified plaques in the wall. There was no thrombus in the lumen. The patient was discharged after 11 days following an uncomplicated recovery. Six months after operation, an angiographic study showed a patent LIMA graft to the LAD. The aneurysm had been well repaired, and the saphenous graft to the RCA was occluded 1 cm beyond the anastomosis.

CASE 3: *A 57-year-old man was admitted to the hospital on April 21, 1973, with a history of myocardial infarction six months previously. He denied angina but complained of progressively worsening pain in the left arm radiating to the hand during the preceding four months. The pain was not related to use of the extremity or position of the hand but was initiated by exertion. He was normotensive, and no abnormal findings were elicited on examination. Glucose tolerance was abnormal, but the lipid profile was normal. His EKG showed nonspecific T-wave changes. Coronary arteriography showed aneurysms of the RCA and*

CCA (Fig. 4). There was no localized obstructive lesion of the coronary arteries, and the left ventriculogram was normal. He was not considered a surgical candidate and was placed on anticoagulant medication.

CASE 4: *A 52-year-old male had myocardial infarction in February 1968. He recovered without major complications and was well until February 1970, when he had recurrent angina pectoris. Coronary arteriography performed in March 1970 was reported as showing minimal diffuse disease. The patient was managed medically with initial improvement but in January 1973, his symptoms became worse. Repeat coronary arteriography showed surgically correctable stenotic lesions involving the RCA and LAD. There was a stenotic lesion of the CCA with an aneurysm distal to the stenosis (Fig. 5). On examination he was found to be moderately obese and normotensive. The electrocardiogram showed nonspecific T-wave changes, and his lipid profile was abnormal. At operation, March 22, 1973, autogenous vein grafts were uti-*

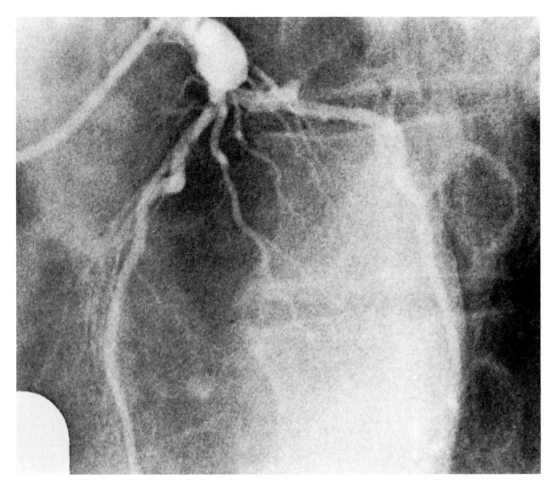

FIG. 2. Left coronary arteriogram in the left anterior oblique projection demonstrating aneurysm and stenotic lesion of LAD (Case 1).

lized to bypass the lesions on the RCA and LAD. The proximal CCA was dissected to identify the aneurysm. It was incised and the wall was found to be smooth without plaques of calcification. There were no thrombi. The redundant anterior wall was excised, and a portion of autogenous vein was fashioned and sutured end-to-side to the defect in the artery, thus bypassing the stenosis as well. The postoperative period was complicated first by pulmonary insufficiency necessitating extra efforts to maintain adequate blood gases. The patient also developed a psychosis that responded to medication. He subsequently developed thrombophlebitis of the left leg, which was successfully treated with parenteral anticoagulation. Coronary angiograms 10 months postoperatively showed patent grafts to the LAD and CCA and an adequate repair of the aneurysm (Fig. 6).

CASE 5: A 59-year-old male was admitted with an 18-month history of exertional angina pectoris, occasional nocturnal chest pains, and a well-documented hiatal hernia. Physical examination was within normal limits. Chest roentgenography was normal, and the electrocardiogram, including a Master's test, was negative. He was found to have hyperlipidemia and type II hyperlipoproteinemia. Cardiac enzymes were not elevated. Coronary arteriography showed a dominant RCA and aneurysms of the proximal LAD and CCA (Figs. 7 and 8). Both the left ventricular end-diastolic pressure and the left ventriculogram were normal. There was no discrete stenotic lesion. He was not considered a surgical candidate, and anticoagulation was recommended.

DISCUSSION

The basis for aneurysm formation is a structural weakening of the wall of the coronary artery. This weakening can result from destruction of the musculo-elastic elements secondary to the atherosclerotic process, or from inflammatory diseases such as necrotizing arteritis, syphilis, or mycotic

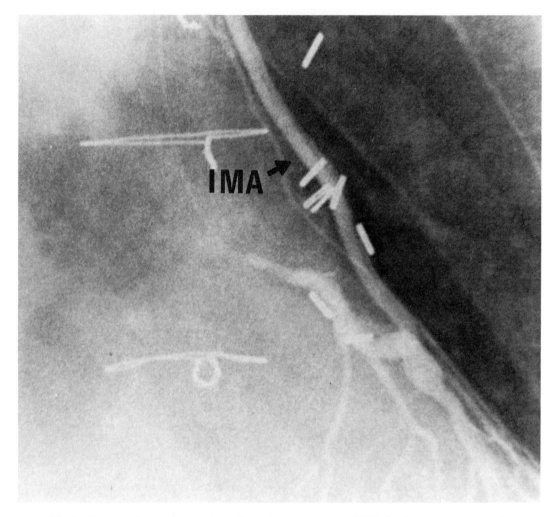

FIG. 3.   Postoperative arteriogram via the internal mammary artery (IMA) showing patent anastomosis between LIMA and LAD and satisfactory repair of aneurysm (Case 1).

embolic phenomena. It may also be present as a congenital defect or may result from trauma. Thus coronary artery aneurysms have been classified as atherosclerotic, syphilitic, mycotic, embolic, congenital, traumatic, and so forth (Konecke et al, 1971; Daoud et al, 1963; Plachta and Speer, 1958).

The majority of reported cases have been of atherosclerotic origin. Fifty-two percent of 89 cases reviewed by Daoud et al (1963) were in this category. The five cases in our series were all atherosclerotic aneurysms. This type of aneurysm tends to occur in older patients who usually have other manifestations of atherosclerosis including obstructive lesions of the coronary arteries or of other arteries. Of particular interest were eight out of 10 patients described in detail by Daoud et al (1963) who had associated aneurysms of the abdominal aorta. Most of the reported cases have

been single aneurysms, but multiple aneurysms do occur as have been noted in two of our patients and by others (Scott, 1948; Sayegh, 1968; Crocker et al, 1957; Plachta and Speer, 1958).

Congenital aneurysms have variously been reported to represent between 15 and 20 percent of all aneurysms of the coronary arteries (Daoud et al, 1963). They have been reported both in children and adults, and some have been associated with venous communications. The latter are not considered true aneurysms since the observed aneurysmal dilatations are secondary to the high flow-through fistula (Crocker et al, 1957; Ebert et al, 1971).

The occurrence rate of mycotic aneurysms of the coronary arteries is reported as 11 percent by Daoud et al (1963). As pointed out recently by Crook et al (1973), subacute bacterial endocarditis may give rise to mycotic aneurysms of

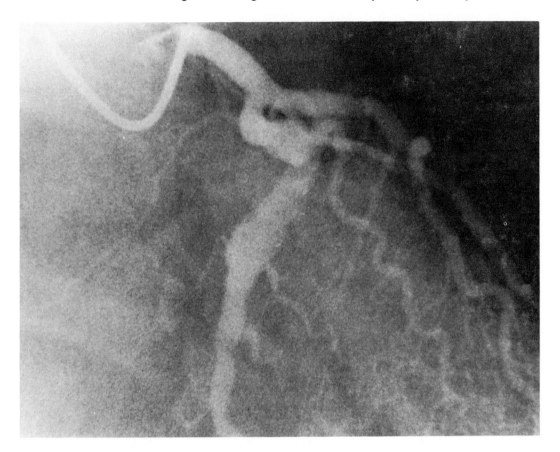

FIG. 4. Left coronary arteriography in the right anterior oblique projection showing aneurysm of the CCA (Case 3).

the coronary arteries. The pathogenesis of these aneurysms is the same as in other parts of the body; viz, a source of infection and previous damage to the vascular wall by either atherosclerosis, trauma, or congenital defects (Weintraub and Abrams, 1968).

The exact incidence of coronary artery aneurysms is not known. It has been estimated to be one in every 500 coronary artery examinations at the Cleveland Clinic (Eisinger and King, 1966). Daoud et al (1963), in a study of 694 hearts at autopsy, found 10 cases. The five cases reported in this series were encountered during the course of 1,500 arteriographic studies from August 1972 to July 1973.

Statistical distribution between the right coronary artery and the left coronary artery and its branches has been reported to be equal (Daoud et al, 1963). In the present series, however, there were two in the right coronary artery, one in the left main coronary artery, one in the anterior descending, and three in the circumflex branch (Table 1).

Most aneurysms are found within the first

2 cm from the origin or from a major branch of the coronary artery (Packard and Weschler, 1929). They give rise to nonlaminar flow with turbulence and eddy currents (Ebert et al, 1971) resulting in the deposition of laminated clot in the sac (Scott, 1948; Forbes and Bradley, 1960; Sayegh et al, 1968; Eisinger and King, 1966). Distal embolization from clots has been demonstrated by clinical, electrocardiographic, and arteriographic studies (van den Broek and Segal, 1973). Cases of total occlusion of the artery distal to the aneurysm have also been documented (Ghahramani et al, 1972, Mattern et al, 1972).

TABLE 1. Distribution of Coronary Artery Aneurysms in This Series

PT.	RCA	LCA	LAD	CCA
WC		X		
JB	X			
JK	X			X
ES				X
CW			X	X

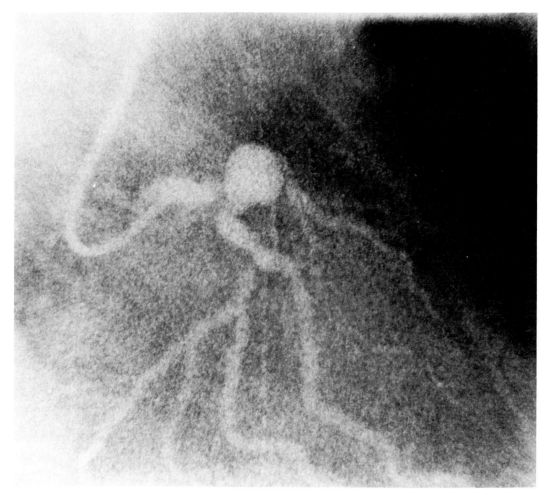

FIG. 5. Left coronary arteriogram in the right anterior oblique projection showing aneurysm of the CCA (Case 4).

Rupture resulting in acute cardiac tamponade and death was reported by Packard and Weschler. An intramural aneurysm of the left anterior descending coronary artery without connection either to a vein or to any cardiac chamber, but causing reverse flow, was reported by Bjork and Bjork (1967).

In general, however, the clinical manifestations of coronary artery aneurysms are the same as those resulting from ischemic heart disease. Most patients have presented with recurrent angina pectoris and past histories of myocardial infarction as demonstrated in the present series. But some patients have died from other causes without any apparent symptoms from their aneurysms (Daoud et al, 1963).

Specific clinical findings have not been associated with coronary artery aneurysms except in cases of congenital aneurysms with fistulous communications with which a precordial murmur has been reported (Grob and Kolb, 1959).

As noted above, premortem diagnosis of aneurysm of the coronary arteries was first made in 1967 by Sherkat et al, using aortography. Calcifications in the wall of the aneurysmal sac can be recognized on plain chest roentgenography (Anderson and Wennerold, 1971; Barclay et al, 1964) but differentiation between aneurysmal dilatation and calcification in the wall of a stenotic atherosclerotic coronary artery would be difficult without coronary arteriography. This diagnostic tool (Sones and Shirey, 1962) remains the investigative mainstay of coronary artery disease.

The complications enumerated above indicate the need for treatment in order to prevent their occurrence. Anticoagulation therapy has

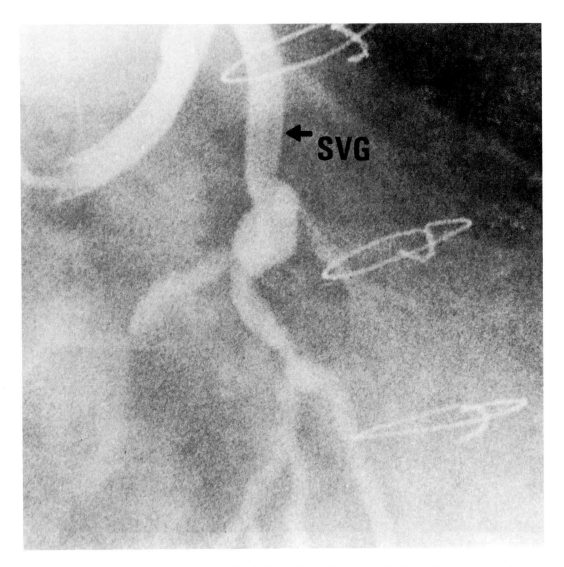

FIG. 6. Postoperative arteriogram in the right anterior oblique view via the saphenous vein graft (SVG) showing patent anastomosis and adequate repair of aneurysm (Case 4).

been recommended when surgical intervention is contraindicated as in two of the cases presented in this series.

Surgical procedures for the management of coronary artery aneurysms, as reported previously and in this presentation, include resection of the aneurysm and interposition of autogenous vein graft (Ebert et al, 1971; Dawson and Ellison, 1972), bypass of the aneurysm with saphenous vein graft (Ghahramani et al, 1972), excision of the roof of the aneurysm with the vein graft anastomosed to that area, and repair of a saccular aneurysm by lateral aneurysmorrhaphy. Bjork and Bjork (1967) reported the closure of the neck of

a saccular aneurysm with suture obliteration of the aneurysm for an intramural aneurysm that caused coronary artery steal syndrome.

Certainly no single procedure can be utilized in all cases. The surgical procedure should be individualized, taking into consideration the coronary artery involved, the location of the aneurysm, the probable etiological factors and associated lesions as demonstrated by arteriography. Total excision of an aneurysm of the anterior descending coronary artery with interposition of a saphenous vein graft might result in occlusion of septal perforators and subsequent infarctions as noted by Dawson and Ellison (1972). However,

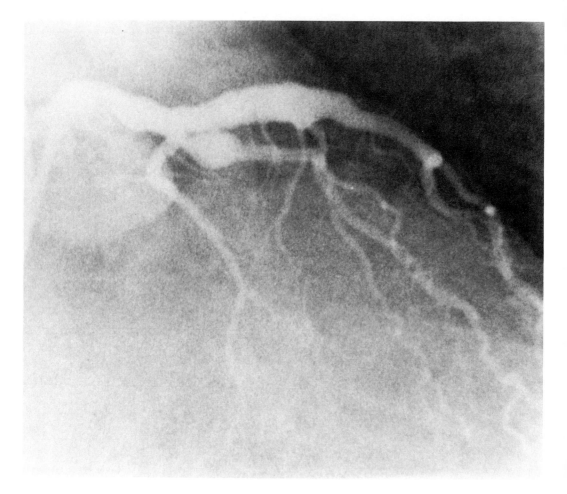

FIG. 7. Left coronary arteriogram in the right anterior oblique view demonstrating aneurysms of the LAD and LCA (Case 5).

such a method may be quite acceptable in the proximal circumflex branch of the left coronary artery as successfully reported by Ebert et al (1971), and possibly this may be used for aneurysms of the right coronary artery. Excision of the roof and inspection of the lumen of the aneurysm with implantation of autogenous vein grafts, as described in case 4, seems preferable to mere bypass of the aneurysm. However, bypassing a completely thrombosed and occluded aneurysm with good runoff is a logical approach (Ghahramani et al, 1972). Lateral aneurysmorrhaphy may be indicated in a large saccular aneurysm, but one must be careful and not compromise the lumen of the artery. Roof patching and ligation of the coronary artery proximal to the aneurysmal dilatation (Grob and Kolb, 1959) have a doubtful place in the treatment of coronary artery aneurysms.

References

Anderson M, Wennevold A: Aneurysm of the hepatic artery and of the left coronary with myocardial infarction. Scand J Thorac Cardiovasc Surg 5:172, 1971

Barclay CC, Glenney WR, Hobbs RE, et al: Aneurysm of the coronary artery, a case report. Am J Roentgen 91:1315, 1964

Bjork VO, Bjork L: Intramural coronary artery aneurysm: a coronary artery steal syndrome. J Thorac Cardiovasc Surg 54:50, 1967

Bougon A: Arterial aneurysm of the heart. Bibliotti Med 37:183, 1812 (cited by Packard and Weschler)

Cafferky EA, Crawford DW, Turner AF, Lau FYK, Blankenhorn DH: Congenital aneurysm of the coronary artery with myocardial infarction. Am J Med Sci 257:320, 1969

Crocker DW, Sobin S, Thomas WC: Aneurysms of the coronary arteries. Report of three cases in infants and review of the literature. Am J Pathol 33:819, 1957

Crook BRM, Raftery EB, Oram S: Mycotic aneurysms of coronary arteries. Br Heart Journal 35:107, 1973

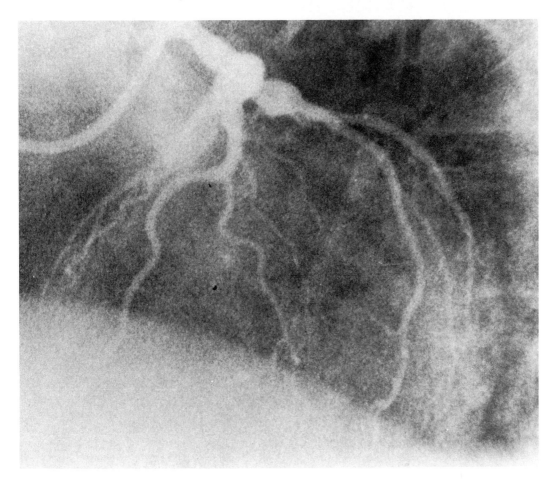

FIG. 8.   Left coronary arteriogram in the left anterior oblique projection showing aneurysms of LAD and LCA (Case 5).

Daoud AS, Pankin D, Tulgan H, Florentin RA: Aneurysms of the coronary artery: report of ten cases and review of literature. Am J Cardiol 11:228, 1963

Dawson JE, Ellison RG: Isolated aneurysm of the anterior descending coronary artery surgical treatment. Am J Cardiol 29:868, 1972

Ebert PA, Peter RH, Gunnells JC, Sabiston DC: Resecting and grafting of coronary artery aneurysm. Circulation 45:593, 1971

Eisinger G, King AB: Precipitous death in a police officer due to coronary artery aneurysm (report of a case). Bull Johns Hopkins Hosp 119:161, 1966

Forbes G, Bradley A: Coronary artery aneurysm. Br Med J 2:1344, 1960

Ghahramani A, Iyengar R, Cunha D, Jude J, Sommer L: Myocardial infarction due to congenital coronary arterial aneurysm (with successful saphenous vein bypass graft). Am J Cardiol 29:863, 1972

Grob M, Kolb E: Congenital aneurysm of the coronary artery. Arch Dis Child 34:8, 1959

Konecke LL, Spitzer S, Mason D, Kasparian H, James PM: Traumatic aneurysm of the left coronary artery. Am J Cardiol 27:221, 1971

Mattern AL, Baker WP, McHale JJ, Lee DE: Congenital coronary aneurysm with angina pectoris and myocardial infarction treated with saphenous vein bypass graft. Am J Cardiol 30:906, 1972

Packard M, Weschler HF: Aneurysm of the coronary arteries. Arch Intern Med (Chicago) 43:1, 1929

Plachta A, Speer FD: Aneurysm of the left coronary artery—review of literature and report of three cases. Arch Pathol (Chicago) 66:210, 1958

Sayegh S, Adad W, Macleod CA: Multiple aneurysms of the coronary arteries. Am Heart J 76:252, 1968

Scott DH: Aneurysm of the coronary arteries. Am Heart J 36:403, 1948

Sherkat A, Kavanagh-Gray D, Edworthy J: Localized aneurysms of the coronary arteries. Radiology 89:24, 1967

Sones FM, Shirey DK: Cine coronary arteriography. Mod Concepts Cardiovasc Dis 31:735, 1962

van den Broek H, Segal BL: Coronary aneurysms in a young woman: angiographic documentation of the natural course. Chest 64:136, 1973

Weintraub RA, Abrams HL: Mycotic aneurysms. Am J Roentgen 102:354, 1968

86

COMPLICATIONS OF CORONARY BYPASS SURGERY

Hooshang Bolooki, Abelardo Vargas, Ali Ghahramani
with technical assistance of Adrianne Fried

INTRODUCTION

Coronary bypass operations are being employed with increasing frequency for coronary artery disease at all stages. The procedure, technically, is relatively straightforward, and the results in thousands of patients have shown a high success rate in alleviating angina pectoris.[9,11,12] However, in spite of its wide acceptance as an established coronary surgery procedure, only brief reports of its complications have been published.[1,2] The purpose of this study was to evaluate the type and incidence of cardiac complications in a group of patients undergoing this operation.

METHODS AND MATERIALS

The patients were selected from 170 patients who were operated upon at Jackson Memorial Hospital-University of Miami School of Medicine during May 1970 through May 1972. All patients initially received complete hemodynamic studies and cardiac catheterization with selective coronary angiograms while they were mildly sedated. The hemodynamic studies included measurement of intracardiac pressures with a catheter transducer (Millar, Houston, Texas). An index of left ventricular (LV) contractility (Vmax) was obtained by using the three component muscle model and the formula dP/dt/kp.[3,13] Where dP/dt is the rate of LV pressure rise and P is the developed left ventricular pressure in the course of

the isometric contraction. The left ventricular stiffness was calculated as the ratio $\Delta P/\Delta t$,[8] where ΔP is the average change in the left ventricular diastolic pressure and Δv is the instantaneous left ventricular diastolic volume change. Cardiac output studies were done by using the Fick principle; blood samples were drawn from the pulmonary artery and from the ascending aorta for measurement of oxygen content, and the oxygen consumption was measured by direct respirometry methods.

Rigid criteria were used in selection of patients for surgery. Only those who were unresponsive to vigorous medical treatment, including isosorbide trinitrate and propranolol when indicated, and those who anatomically exhibited coronary artery lesions greater than 80 percent of the diameter, with acceptable distal vessels and run-off, were selected for aortocoronary bypass operation.

Briefly, the procedure was done by removing a segment of the saphenous vein, and after the side branches were ligated, the segment was interposed between the ascending aorta and the obstructed coronary artery. The procedure was done under total cardiopulmonary bypass with the pump primed with Ringer's lactate. The pump flow rate was maintained at 2.4 L/min/m^2 at normothermia. Usually the proximal anastomosis was done first, and coronary ischemia was not induced. Depending upon the number of grafts, duration of cardiopulmonary bypass varied from 45 to 120 minutes.

Intraoperative monitoring of the LV pressure was done in most patients by a pressure catheter transducer (Millar) left in situ for six days. Postoperatively, all patients had 12 lead EKG routinely. With observation of any significant EKG changes, serum enzyme studies were carried out for three consecutive days.[5] Serum enzyme studies included creatine phosphokinase (CPK), glutamic oxaloacetic transaminase (GOT), hydroxybutric de-

Supported in part by a grant from NHLI 13978-03 and Eli-Lilly Research Laboratories, Indianapolis. Dr. Bolooki is a Research Career Development Awardee, NHLI Grant HL 70670-02.

hydrogenase (HBD), and lactic dehydrogenase (LDH).

The patients discharged from the hospital were followed up in an outpatient clinic. Upon development of any complications, they were re-admitted to the hospital for the purpose of diagnostic studies. Follow-up cardiac catheterization studies were done within four weeks to four months after the operation, and methods similar to preoperative procedure were employed. All patients received prophylactic antibiotic treatment with sodium cephalothin * 2 gm into the heart-lung machine, followed by 1 gm intravenously every four hours for two days. This was followed by two days of treatment with cephalexin † 500 mgm oral every four hours.

RESULTS

Our overall operative mortality for patients undergoing coronary bypass grafts for various stages of coronary artery disease has been 5 percent (8 of 170 patients). Two patients developed suture abscesses in the lower area of skin incision and required wound drainage and debridement. There were no other infectious complications.

In Table 1, the clinical course of the 11 patients (6 percent) who developed perioperative cardiac complications *early* (up to 24 hours) after aortocoronary bypass procedure is shown. In Table 2, the hospital course of four other patients (2 percent) developing similar complications *late* postoperatively is given. Most complications were in the form of cardiac dysrhythmia because of transmural acute infarcts (nine patients) or in the form of electrocardiographic changes compatible with subendocardial ischemia (six patients). In patients who were awake after surgery, these complications usually were associated with recurrence of chest pain followed by rhythm disturbances and moderate hypotension.

Changes in Cardiac Rhythm

As shown in Table 1, all 11 patients developing cardiac complications *early* after aortocoronary bypass procedure had evidence of atrial or ventricular rhythm disturbances. Six patients had significant premature ventricular contractions requiring repeated administration of antiarrhythmic

* Keflin, Eli-Lilly Research Laboratories.
† Keflex, Eli-Lilly Research Laboratories.

drugs. The remaining five patients developed atrial tachycardia in the form of fibrillation or flutter, which responded to digitalis therapy or electric countershock. Two of the four patients who developed *late* cardiac complications (Table 2) also showed evidence of atrial and ventricular premature contractions, and both developed cardiac arrest requiring external cardiac massage for 30 to 45 minutes. In two patients in the *late* group cardiac dysrhythmias were not recorded. At times cardiac dysrhythmias were accentuated with associated hypokalemia, but improved after correction.[4]

Changes in Blood Pressure

Eight of 11 patients in the *early* complication group had sudden hypotension and two others were hypotensive immediately after discontinuation of cardiopulmonary bypass and required vasopressor therapy. In these patients, cardiogenic shock and pump failure eventually caused their demise (Table 1). The decrease in blood pressure in the other patients usually occurred suddenly in the first few hours after surgery. This lasted only for one to two hours and responded to volume loading. Cardiac dysrhythmia caused hypotension in three patients.

Electrocardiogram

Nine of the 11 patients with *early* cardiac complications showed electrocardiographic evidence of transmural acute myocardial infarction, which usually involved the anterior wall of the left ventricle at the region of the left anterior descending coronary (LAD), (Fig. 1). In one patient (AG) the infarct involved the anterior wall while the right coronary artery was grafted. The LAD in this case, angiographically had minimal disease. Another patient (TS) developed subendocardial infarction over the anterior wall of the left ventricle three months postoperatively. In this man, the coronary graft to the acute marginal branch of circumflex artery was patent at restudy. In this case, the anterior descending coronary artery (less than 1 mm) was not found suitable for bypass grafting.

Coronary Arteriograms

Eight of the nine surviving patients in the *early* complication group had postoperative cardiac catheterization. Of the 16 grafts, eight were closed or could not be selectively catheterized. All four patients in the *late* complication group had postoperative cardiac catheterization, and three had

TABLE 1. Clinical Course in Patients Developing Cardiac Complications Early after AC Bypass Procedure

PT.	AGE/SEX	LOCATION GRAFT	ARRHYTHMIA	BP	LOCATION MI ON EKG	CORONARY ANGIOGRAM	OUTCOME
EM	42/M	LAD and RC	PVC	90/60	Ant-lat. post wall transmural	Both grafts patent LV dyskinesis	Symptomatic follow-up 2 yrs progressive CAD
FM	41/M	LAD, AM	PVC	Normal	Lat wall subendocardial	Both grafts closed	Follow-up 2 years working, no angina, progressive CAD
MD	52/F	LAD, Diag	Atrial tachy	Normal	Ant wall subendocardial	Diag. graft closed	4-mo followup, no angina
RP	62/M	LAD, Diag	Atrial tachy	80/50	Ant wall transmural	LAD graft closed, open diag. graft, LV aneurysm	Asymptomatic 15-mo follow-up
GL	56/M	LAD	PVC	80/50 (shock)	Ant wall transmural	Patent graft LV aneurysm	Asymptomatic 1-yr follow-up
LP	54/F	LAD, RC	Atrial tachy.	Normal	Ant wall subendocardial	LAD graft closed	Asymptomatic 28-mo follow-up
DM	56/F	LAD, AM	Atrial tachy.	90/60	Ant wall transmural	LAD graft closed, dyskinesis	Symptomatic mildly, 2-yr follow-up
FL	54/F	LAD, Diag	PVC	90/60	Ant wall transmural	LV aneurysm narrowed LAD graft closed diag	Symptomatic
AG	52/M	RC	Atrial tachy	90/60	Ant wall transmural	Graft patent	Died 1 mo later of GI hemorrhage
LB	61/F	LAD	PVC	80/50 (shock)	Ant wall transmural	—	Died, LAD graft closed
OK	58/F	LAD, AM, RC	PVC	80/60 (shock)	Ant-lat. wall transmural	—	Died, LAD graft closed

LAD: left anterior descending coronary artery; RC: right coronary artery; AM: acute marginal branch of circumflex coronary; Diag: diagonal branch of the anterior descending coronary; CAD: coronary artery disease; GI: gastrointestinal; LV: left ventricular; PVC: premature ventricular contractions; MI: myocardial infarction.

TABLE 2. Clinical Course in Patients Developing Complications Late after AC Bypass Procedure

PT.	AGE/SEX	GRAFTS TO:	ARRHYTHMIA	BP	LOCATION MI ON EKG	CORONARY ANGIOGRAM	OUTCOME
PL	38/F	LAD	–	Normal	Ant wall transmural 3 mos postop	Graft closed	Asymptomatic 2.5-yr follow-up, progressive CAD
TS	58/M	AM	None	Normal	Ant wall subendocardial 3 mos postop	Patent graft, LV dyskinesis	Asymptomatic 10-mo follow-up, progressive CAD
WU	35/F	LAD	PVC, cardiac arrest	–	Ant wall subendocardial 3 mos postop	Graft closed	Died 6 mos postop suddenly, progressive CAD
DA	62/F	LAD	PAC and PVC, cardiac arrest	–	Ant wall subendocardial 1 wk postop	Graft closed, LV dyskinesis	Asymptomatic 16-mo follow-up

LAD: left anterior descending coronary artery; AM: acute marginal branch of circumflex coronary; PVC: premature ventricular contractions; LV: left ventricular; CAD: coronary artery disease; MI: myocardial infarction.

TABLE 3. Hemodynamic Findings in Patients Developing Myocardial Infarction after A-C Bypass Procedure

PT.	CI L/min/M² #1	#2	PA-mm Hg #1	#2	PR Dyne/cm⁻⁵ #1	#2	EdP (mm Hg) #1	#2	Vmax (circ/sec) #1	#2	dp/dt mm Hg/sec #1	#2	Δp/Δv mm Hg/cc #1	#2	HR/min #1	#2
EM	3.0	2.5	13	15	1,315	1,561	8	13	4.2	3.0	2,717	1,973	0.14	0.14	70	73
FM	3.9	3.1	13	19	791	929	8	21	4.1	2.1	1,909	1,470	0.10	0.28	72	66
MD	3.1	3.1	14	18	1,247	1,500	13	17	2.0	1.3	3,127	2,482	0.12	0.59	100	100
RP	2.2	2.4	16	20	1,681	1,400	13	17	3.4	2.0	1,984	1,183	0.26	0.18	72	80
GL	2.3	2.5	11	18	1,730	1,867	3	27	1.6	1.38	2,159	1,802	0.15	0.46	90	90
LP	4.0	2.0	17	17	1,380	3,180	13	11	4.2	2.4	3,385	1,751	0.07	0.11	66	58
DM	3.5	2.8	17	14	2,520	2,910	6	12	3.8	2.3	3,055	2,027	0.08	0.53	100	102
FL	4.2	2.7	13	15	1,516	2,114	2	10	1.82	1.70	1,705	1,773	0.24	0.43	120	120
TS	2.6	1.85	11	12	1,565	2,260	14	22	3.0	2.85	1,837	1,290	0.12	0.25	72	92
WU	3.8	2.4	14	20	877	1,493	14	13	2.68	2.88	893	1,192	0.14	0.20	80	95
DA	–		–		–		6	16	1.83	1.82	925	1,030	–		90	100
Mean	3.26	2.54	13.9	16.8	1,462	1,921	9.0	16.3	2.96	2.16	2,235	1,697	0.14	0.32	84	88
± SE	0.23	0.13	0.69	0.85	153	222	1.3	1.5	0.31	0.18	224	127	0.02	0.05	5	5
P Value	<0.01		<0.01		<0.2		<0.005		<0.05		<0.05		<0.001		n.s.	

The data obtained from preoperative cardiac catheterization studies (#1) and follow-up studies (#2) within four weeks to three months after the operation. CI: cardiac index; PA: pulmonary artery pressure; PR: peripheral resistance in dyne/sec/Cm⁻⁵; Edp: left ventricular end-diastolic pressure; Vmax: maximal velocity of contractile element during isometric contraction (13); dp/dt: maximal rate of rise of left ventricular pressure; Δp/Δv: and index of left ventricular stiffness (8); HR: heart rate. The statistical analysis for these values was done by comparison of paired data sampling method.

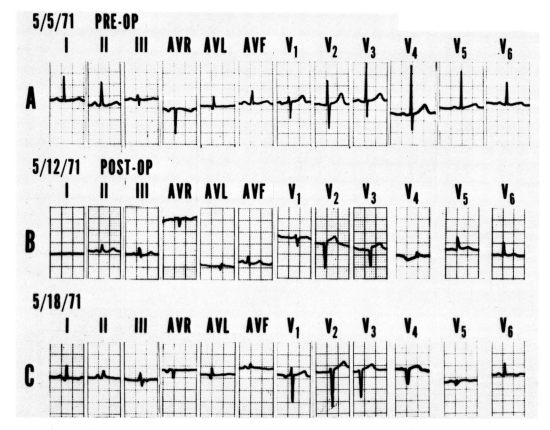

FIG. 1. Serial 12 lead electrocardiograms in a patient who developed anterior-wall myocardial infarction (Q-wave in I, AVL, V2, V3, V4, and V5) after double aortocoronary (A-C) graft. Vein graft to anterior descending was closed but the one to its diagonal branch was patent. Patient had a large anterior-wall aneurysm at postoperative studies.

closed grafts. Overall, of 20 grafts at restudy, 11 were closed, but five patients (of 12 studied) had at least one patent graft.[4] Progression of coronary artery disease was seen in five patients. The two patients who died in the early postoperative period were found to have closed LAD grafts at autopsy. The patient (AG) who died one month postoperatively due to upper gastrointestinal hemorrhage had a patent graft at autopsy.

Left Ventricular Angiograms

Five of the eight patients in the *early* complication group had left ventricular dyskinesia and aneurysm formation. In two of these patients, one-year follow-up studies were also done, and in one (EM) an improvement in the ventricular contraction was noted in spite of progression of coronary artery disease.[4] In patients in the *late* group, two had dyskinetic areas of the anterior wall of the left ventricle.

Hemodynamic Studies

The hemodynamic data for the 11 patients who had postoperative complete cardiac catheterization are shown in Table 3. One patient (PL) of the *late* group had angiograms only. In all patients, there was a significant decrease in cardiac index with a marked increase in left ventricular end-diastolic pressure (Fig. 2). The pulmonary artery pressure, the peripheral resistance and left ventricular stiffness ($\Delta P/\Delta v$) also increased significantly. Myocardial contractility Vmax and dP/dt were decreased markedly ($p < 0.01$) (Fig. 2).

Serum Enzyme Studies

There was a significant increase in the serum enzymes, especially serum CPK and HBD, to levels four to 10 times normal in patients de-

FIG. 2. Hemodynamic findings in patients developing complications after aortocoronary (AC) bypass operations are shown. In the upper panel, myocardial contractility index (Vmax), left ventricular diastolic stiffness ($\Delta p / \Delta v$), and rate of left ventricular pressure rise (dp/dt) are shown. Below, changes in cardiac index (CI), left ventricular end-diastolic pressure (EDP), and peripheral resistance (PR) are depicted. The points and vertical bars indicate mean and one standard deviation for each parameter. Statistical analysis of the data for preoperative (before) and postoperative (after) values showed significant changes for all parameters.

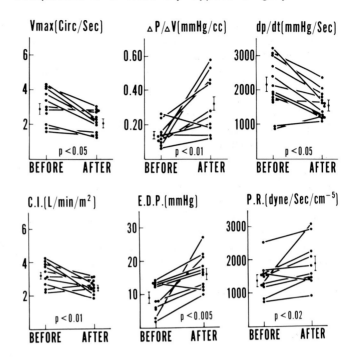

veloping myocardial infarction early after aortocoronary bypass graft. A detailed account of the significance of serum enzymes on diagnosis of myocardial infarction after direct coronary surgery has been reported.[5]

DISCUSSION

The procedure of aortocoronary bypass grafting has become an accepted method of treatment of advanced coronary artery disease. This procedure in a selected group of patients with the so-called acute cardiac ischemia or preinfarction angina may alter the prognosis of the disease process and improve the depressed left ventricular function.[6,7,10] However, development of acute myocardial infarction due to either a technical mishap or closure of the saphenous vein graft due to accommodation or arterialization of the vein graft in patients undergoing direct coronary surgery is a disturbing complication. The results of our study indicate that the overall incidence of acute myocardial infarction in patients undergoing this procedure is 6 percent and may produce only transient clinical signs. For this reason, development of this complication may go unrecognized. Since this is a significant morbidity, it should be detected in all patients who undergo this type of operation. Our study indicates that a routine postoperative EKG is mandatory to the care of all these patients and would establish the

diagnosis in most cases. Aside from technical mistakes, one possible reason for development of ischemia and infarction in patients undergoing myocardial revascularization is poor coronary microperfusion. This assumption was based on our experience with two patients (EM and GL, Table 1) who developed left ventricular infarction and dyskinesia in spite of patent grafts. Another reason is the unreliability of coronary arteriography in recognizing the extent of coronary lesions. The intraoperative decrease in coronary blood flow within areas of the myocardium supplied by diseased coronary vessels may induce myocardial infarction. This factor could have played a role in two patients who developed myocardial infarction at areas where coronary branches were not bypassed (AG and TS).

In patients undergoing the procedure of direct myocardial revascularization, development of early or late myocardial infarction due to, or independent of, graft closure requires early diagnosis. In these patients, complications inherent to the use of cardiopulmonary bypass such as bleeding diatheses, respiratory failure, and dysrhythmia are also seen. The present study shows that the clinical course of the majority of patients developing myocardial infarcts sustained dysrythmias or hypotension or both. Furthermore, in these patients, more than half of the vein grafts were found to be occluded. Thus, development of hypotension and dysrhythmia when not associated with hypovolemia or hypokolemia should raise the suspicion of a more serious complication and should lead to serial EKG and serum enzyme tests in order to confirm the diagnosis.

Although the present studies indicate a marked decrease in all parameters of left ventricular function after myocardial infarction, most surviving patients have remained asymptomatic. We have reasoned that the disappearance of symptoms in our patients was possibly related to an improvement in myocardial blood supply due to the patency of at least one vein graft in some of these patients as well as possibly being due to infarction of the ischemic segments. While aortocoronary bypass grafting remains a useful procedure in selected patients, the incidence of 5 percent operative mortality and 6 percent myocardial infarction development as seen in our series, indicates the need for careful selection of the patients for this operation.

SUMMARY

Among 170 patients undergoing aortocoronary bypass surgery, 11 (5 percent) developed acute myocardial infarction within 24 hours after surgery. An additional four patients (2 percent) developed myocardial infarction within three months after discharge. Clinically, acute myocardial infarction was suspected because of sudden transient hypotension associated with dysrhythmia, angina, or cardiac arrest that responded to conventional therapy. Elevation of serum enzymes with acute EKG changes were also observed. Three patients died (20 percent mortality). In 12 patients, cardiac catheterization studies were performed within two to 10 weeks after the incident. Eleven of the 20 grafts were found occluded, and progression of coronary occlusive disease was seen in five. There was a marked decrease in left ventricular function, contractility, and compliance in all patients with left ventricular aneurysm formation or dyskinesia. Eight of these patients were asymptomatic. The results indicate that after coronary surgery, a combination of sudden arrhythmia and transient hypotension may indicate perioperative development of acute myocardial infarction. Also, in spite of a depressed cardiac function, most surviving patients remain angina free.

References

1. Achuff S, Griffith L, Humphries JON, et al: Myocardial damage after aorto-coronary vein bypass surgery. (Abstr) J Clin Invest, 51:1a, 1972
2. Alderman EL, Enright LP, Cohn LH, et al: Detection of myocardial infarction following coronary-saphenous graft surgery by ECG and serum enzyme changes. (Abstr) Circulation 44, Suppl II:134, 1971
3. Bolooki H, Sommer LS, Faraldo A, et al: The significance of serum enzyme studies in patients undergoing direct coronary artery surgery. J Thorac Cardiovasc Surg 65:836, 1973
4. Bolooki H, Rubinson RM, Michie DD, et al: Assessment of myocardial contractility after coronary bypass grafts. J Thorac Cardiovasc Surg 62:543, 1971
5. Bolooki H, Sommer LS, Ghahramani A, et al: Complications of coronary bypass surgery. Circulation Suppl III, 47–48:120, 1973
6. Bolooki H, Vargas A, Ghahramani A, et al: Aorto-coronary bypass graft for preinfarction angina. Chest 61:247, 1972
7. Chatterjee K, Swan HJC, Parmley WW, et al: Depression of left ventricular function due to acute myocardial ischemia and its reversal after aorto-coronary saphenous vein bypass. N Engl J Med. 286:1118, 1972
8. Diamond G and Forrester JS: Effects of coronary artery disease and acute myocardial infarction on the left ventricular compliance in man. Circulation 45:11, 1972
9. Favaloro RG, Effler DB, Groves LK, et al: Severe segmental obstruction of the left main coronary artery and its divisions: Surgical treatment by the saphenous vein graft technique. J Thorac Cardiovasc Surg 60:469, 1970
10. Favaloro RG, Effler DB, Cheanvechai C, et al: Acute coronary insufficiency (impending myocardial infarction and myocardial infarction): surgical treatment by saphenous vein graft technique. Am J Cardiol, 28:589, 1971
11. Johnson WD, Flemma RJ, Lepley D Jr: Direct coronary surgery utilizing multiple-vein bypass graft. Ann Thorac Surg 9:436, 1970
12. Reul GJ, Morris GC, Jr, Howell JF, et al: Current concepts in coronary artery surgery: a critical analysis of 1,287 patients. Ann Thorac Surg 14:243, 1972
13. Sonnenblick EH, Parmley WW, Urschel CW, et al: Ventricular function: evaluation of myocardial contractility in health and disease. Prog Cardiovasc Dis 12:449, 1970

87

PERIOPERATIVE INFARCTION IN DIRECT CORONARY SURGERY

Its Pathoetiology

Robert J. Flemma, Harjeet M. Singh, Alfred J. Tector, and Derward Lepley

INTRODUCTION

The significant incidence of myocardial infarction (MI) following coronary graft surgery is beginning to be recognized. Thus, Sheldon,[8] Hultgren,[5] and Morris[6] reported an incidence of 9 percent, 10 percent, and 11 percent, respectively, associated with this type of surgery. However, the mechanism of infarction associated with direct revascularization of the myocardium remains unknown.[3] The fact that MI occurs in 0.66 percent of patients undergoing any type of surgery without previous history of MI, and a tenfold increase in this incidence occurs in those with previous history of MI may be particularly relevant. The very high incidence of MI following Vineberg's procedure involving the tunneling of the myocardium is more readily understandable.[4,5,9] We have been prompted to look into the genesis of MI in the group of patients undergoing direct revascularization of the myocardium on two accounts:

1. The common finding that infarction does not occur more frequently in grafts that are occluded at autopsy than in those that are patent suggests other reasons for MI in this group of patients.
2. Although MI associated with coronary bypass graft surgery is usually well tolerated with low fatality rate, it may contribute to absence of angina in the postoperative period and may be claimed to be the result of successful surgery rather than being further damaging to myocardial function.

The purpose of the present study was to recognize factors in the genesis of MI in this group of patients with particular reference to pre- and intraoperative features.

METHODS AND MATERIALS

Three groups of patients undergoing direct myocardial revascularization with the aid of cardiopulmonary bypass were studied.[1]

Group A: This group consisted of 90 consecutive patients undergoing coronary bypass graft procedures for coronary artery disease in whom MI had been excluded by all criteria.

Group B: This group was comprised of 25 patients with proven diagnosis of MI on the basis of electrocardiogram (EKG), vectorcardiography, and enzyme changes. These 25 patients were reported by Silberman[10] from a study of 300 patients at our center.

Group C: These were 34 patients with triple-vessel disease who showed no evidence of MI on the basis of the above changes. This group is particularly susceptible to MI as shown in the study of Brewer et al.[3] The group was compared to Group B patients with regard to the number of vein graft procedures and graft flows (Table 5).

Clinical

History was elucidated regarding duration and severity of angina, presence of preinfarction angina, and number of episodes of proven infarctions. The preinfarction state in this study was defined as increasing frequency and/or severity of angina.[7] Selective coronary angiograms, LV angiograms, and left ventricular end diastolic pressures (LVEDP) were available in all patients. At operation, the presence of diffuse disease was noted. It was recorded if all disease was bypassed. Graft flows were monitored at the end of the operation using electromagnetic flow probes. The procedure for cardiopulmonary bypass was standard in all patients. The aorta was cross-clamped for the distal anastomoses only. The duration of cardiopulmonary bypass, total, and each period of aortic cross-clamp time were noted.

Criteria for Diagnosis of Myocardial Infarction

The diagnosis of MI was arrived at with the aid of pre- and postoperative vectorcardiographic changes, serial electrocardiography, and serum enzymic changes as shown in Table 1.

TABLE 1. Basis of Diagnosis of Myocardial Infarction in 25 Patients

DIAGNOSIS	NO. PTS.
EKG changes with enzymic changes	5
EKG and vector changes with enzymic changes	12
Vector changes with enzymic changes	5
At operation	1
At necropsy	2

EKG's were only taken as positive when new pathological Q-waves appeared. No value was attached to ST- and T-wave changes in arriving at the diagnosis. In five cases where the vectors were positive for the diagnosis of MI and EKG changes were nonspecific, serum enzymes were

in the diagnostic range. Values of SGOT greater than 90 units, LDH greater than 900 units, and CPK greater than 200 units in conformance with other studies [2,4,5,7,9] were deemed diagnostic particularly when these remained persistently elevated after 24 hours of surgery or showed a secondary rise in the postoperative period. Vectorcardiographic changes confirming the diagnosis of MI were arrived at by two cardiologists independently of each other. In one patient it was apparent that MI had occurred at the time of surgery before going on cardiopulmonary bypass from the cyanotic discoloration in the distribution of the left anterior descending artery. This area was plicated and the patient made an uneventful recovery. In two patients, the diagnosis was confirmed at necropsy.

Statistical Analysis

Groups A and B were compared on the basis of (1) distribution of coronary artery disease, diffuseness of disease, and whether the lesions were amenable to bypass at operation; (2) preoperative left ventricular angiograms and LVEDP; and (3) cardiopulmonary bypass and aortic cross-clamp time. Comparison between Groups B and C was made on the basis of graft flows and number of bypass grafts performed. X^2 values were obtained for independent variables in Groups A and B, and in Group B and C from observed and expected values. Yates correction was applied and P-values were then arrived at. Only values below 0.05 were significant.

RESULTS

The age and sex ratio did not vary significantly in the three groups. There were 11 females in the control Group A. The age ranged from

TABLE 2. Distribution of Coronary Artery Disease, Diffuseness of Disease and Inability to Bypass at Operation in A and B Groups

	GROUP A (90 pts.)	GROUP B (25 pts.)	STATIS. SIGNIF.
Distribution of disease			
Single-vessel disease	14	2 (8%)	—
Double-vessel disease	42	4 (16%)	—
Triple-vessel disease	34	19 (76%)	<0.01 $X^2 = 11.67$
Diffuse disease	26	18 (72%)	<0.001 $X^2 = 15.25$
Disease not bypassable at operation	8	12 (48%)	<0.001 $X^2 = 21.33$

TABLE 3. Left Ventricular Angiograms and LVEDP in Groups A and B Patients

	GROUP A	GROUP B	STATIS. SIGNIF.
LV Angiograms			
Good left ventricle	51	2	
Abnormal ventricle			
Apical lesion	0	2	
Ant. wall lesion	12	9	P <0.001
Post. wall lesion	15	10	X² = 16.61
Generalized	3	2	
LVEDP			
Normal with stress	56	4	
Abnormal with stress	24	16	P <0.001
			X² = 14.65
Abnormal at rest	10	5	

TABLE 4. Length of Pump Runs and Aortic Cross-Clamp Time in Groups A and B Patients

	GROUP A	GROUP B	STATIS. SIGNIF.
Pump Runs			
Less than 90 mins	62 pts.	8 pts.	p < 0.01
More than 90 mins	28 pts.	17 pts.	X² = 9.68
Total Aortic Cross-Clamp Time			
Less than 60 mins	78 pts.	10 pts.	p < 0.001
More than 60 mins	12 pts.	15 pts.	X² = 15.37
Average duration of each period of aortic cross-clamp time	17.6 ± 4.5	21.5 ± 6.5	— —

31 to 69 years with half the patients in the 51-to-60-year group and a third in the 41-to-50-year bracket. The duration of angina and the number of previous episodes of proven MI were similar in the three groups. However, there was significant variation in the incidence of preinfarction angina in the three groups. Group A had an incidence of preinfarction angina of 21 percent; Group B, 60 percent; and Group C, 28 percent.

Table 2 shows that a significantly higher number of patients in Group B had triple vessel and diffuse disease than in Group A. More patients in Group B did not have all disease bypassed as compared to Group A and C patients. Both the left ventricular angiogram and LVEDP reveal that significantly more patients in Group B had poorer left ventricular function as compared to Group A patients (Table 3). Group B patients also had longer pump runs and longer periods of aortic cross-clamp time (Table 4).

Table 5 indicates that patients in Group B had more procedures performed than patients in Group A, but fewer than patients in Group C. Blood flows in Group C, particularly in the in-

TABLE 5. Procedures Performed and Vein Graft Flows in Groups A, B, and C

	GROUP A (90 pts.)	GROUP B (25 pts.)	GROUP C (34 pts.)
Procedures			
Vein grafts	159	48	88
IMA direct	47	16	24
No. procedures per pt.	2.28	2.6	3.28
Flows			
Mean vein graft flow	63 mls	59 mls	66 mls
Mean IMA flows	45 mls	41.5 mls	56 mls

ternal mammary arteries, were considerably higher than in Group B as well as the control Group A.

In the genesis of inferior or posterior infarction as shown in Table 6, severe triple-vessel disease with hypokinesia of posterior and inferior segments seemed to be the main prerequisites. Triple-vessel disease was not universally present in those suffering anterior infarctions, although

**TABLE 6. Comparison between Patients
Sustaining Anterior and Posterior
or Inferior Infarcts**

	ANT.	POST. OR INF.
No. Pts.	15	10
History of Preinfarction	10	4
Distribution of CAD		
Single	2	
Double	4	
Triple	9	10
Left ventricular angiogram		
Hypokinesia	10	7

most patients had hypokinesia of anterior segments
preoperatively.

DISCUSSION

Our incidence of MI of 8 percent is comparable to other studies. We confirm that vectorcardiography adds to the accuracy of the diagnosis.[10]
The combination of vectorcardiography with serial
EKG and enzyme changes in this study most
likely reflects a near true incidence of MI. EKG
alone would have underestimated the incidence.
Myocardial infarction in our patients was reasonably well tolerated. There were, however, two
deaths, and four patients complained of angina
postoperatively. The absence of angina in others
may be due to infarction of muscle that was previously ischemic and the cause of the anginal pain.
More objective testing should reveal whether there
is improvement in myocardial function in this
group of patients.

Our study in general supports the work of
Brewer et al.[3] At particular risk are those patients
with relatively poor left ventricular function, with
diffuse triple-vessel disease, who did not have all
disease bypassed, and were subjected to longer
cardiopulmonary bypass and aortic cross-clamp
times. These patients ultimately had lower graft
flows. We believe that that significantly higher
graft flows and attempts to bypass all obstructive
disease guarded against MI in those patients who
had triple-vessel disease. The lower graft flows in
those who sustained MI may indicate a causal relationship or the presence of diffuse disease. It is
reasonable to argue that the lower graft flows were
the result of MI itself.

The location of the area of infarction is very
likely dependent on the distribution of coronary
artery disease and the area of hypokinesia preoperatively. Perhaps the site is made particularly vul-

nerable by periods of perfusion and aortic cross-
clamping. Although this hypothesis accounts for
the genesis of MI in most of this group of patients, the risk of MI is particularly acute at the
time of induction of anesthesia and the period
immediately following.[11] Thus, at least one patient in our group developed MI before cardiopulmonary bypass could be instituted. The successful outcome after plication of the infarction
and direct revascularization of the myocardium
suggests that an early and more aggressive approach to the surgical treatment of acute MI may
be beneficial. The number of patients who develop infarction at or just prior to the induction
of anesthesia is conjectural. Our system of excluding from surgical lists those who have enzyme
changes in the period before surgery does not
entirely exclude that group of patients who either
have infarctions immediately before surgery or at
the time of induction of anesthesia. Although MI
is better tolerated by these patients, it is nevertheless a hazard of this type of surgery.

CONCLUSIONS

1. Significantly more patients sustaining
   acute MI postoperatively presented with
   preinfarction angina and had severe
   triple-vessel disease. A greater number
   had poor left ventricular function on
   angiography and elevated LVEDP.
   More patients had diffuse disease that
   was not amenable to bypass.
2. Patients sustaining MI had more graft
   procedures than the control group, but
   fewer than those who had triple-vessel
   disease but no MI. They had longer
   cardiopulmonary bypass and aortic
   cross-clamp times. Mean flows in vein
   grafts and the internal mammary artery
   bypasses were lower than in the control
   groups.
3. Those sustaining inferior or posterior
   infarctions invariably had severe three-
   vessel disease. Preoperatively, contractile
   lag in the affected segments was frequently observed during ventriculography.

References

1. Alderman GL, Matloff HJ, Wexler L, Shumway NE,
   Harrison DC: Results of direct coronary artery
   surgery for the treatment of angina pectoris. N
   Engl J Med 288:535, 1973
2. Baer H, Blount S: The response of SGOT to open
   heart operation. Am Heart J 60:867, 1960

3. Brewer D, Bilbro R, Bartel A: Myocardial infarction as a complication of coronary bypass surgery. Circulation 47:58, 1973
4. Diethrich EB, Liddicoat JE, Alessi FJ, Kinard SA, DeBakey MD: Serum enzyme and electrocardiographic changes immediately following myocardial revascularization. Ann Thorac Surg 5:195, 1968
5. Hultgren NH, Miyagawa M, Buck W, Angell WW: Addendum to ischemic myocardial injury during coronary artery surgery. Am Heart J 82:624, 1971
6. Morris CC, Reul GJ, Howell JF: Follow-up results of distal coronary artery bypass for ischemic heart disease. Am J Cardiol 29:180, 1972
7. Scanlon PJ, Nemickas R, Moran JF, Talano JV, Pifarre R: Accelerated angina pectoris: clinical, hemodynamic, arteriographic and therapeutic experience in 85 patients. Circulation, January 1973
8. Sheldon W, Favaloro R, Sones FM, Effler D: Reconstructive coronary artery surgery—venous autograft technique. JAMA 213:78, 1970
9. Shirey EK, Proudfit WL, Sones FM: Serum enzyme and electrocardiographic changes after coronary artery surgery. Diseases of the Chest 57:122, 1970
10. Silberman J, Friedberg D: Pre- and postoperative vectorcardiograms in diagnosis of myocardial infarction. Personal communications
11. Topkins MJ, Artusio JF: Myocardial infarction and surgery—five year study. Anesth Analg 43:716, 1964

88

ACUTE MYOCARDIAL INFARCTION DURING SURGERY FOR CORONARY ARTERY DISEASE

Herbert N. Hultgren, R. Shettigar, James F. Pfeifer,
William W. Angell, and Martin M. Lipton

It is now well recognized that acute intra-operative myocardial infarction is a significant complication of coronary artery surgery. Supporting evidence consists of the appearance of typical ECG signs of acute infarction in the immediate postoperative period accompanied by abnormal elevation of serum enzymes.[1-3] In fatal cases autopsy studies have confirmed the diagnosis of acute infarction. In addition, many patients exhibit abnormalities in T-waves and ST segments associated with abnormal enzyme elevations that probably represent lesser degrees of acute infarction with an intramural or subendocardial location. The term "acute ischemic injury" has been applied to such occurrences.[1]

The purpose of this study was to determine the incidence of acute infarction and acute ischemic injury in the following four operative interventions for coronary artery disease:

1. Internal mammary implants for stable angina.
2. Saphenous vein bypass grafts for stable angina.
3. Saphenous vein bypass grafts for unstable angina or the impending myocardial infarction syndrome.
4. Saphenous vein bypass grafts performed in conjunction with valve replacement surgery or commissurotomy.

The present study has the following features, which permit a valid comparison between the four procedures:

1. All operations were performed by the same operating team using similar techniques of cardiopulmonary bypass and vein bypass grafting.

2. The group of patients studied did not have other surgical procedures performed, such as resection of ventricular aneurysms or endarterectomy.
3. Selection of patients for internal mammary implants and vein bypass grafts was performed using a standard protocol that excluded patients with persisting evidence of left ventricular failure, left ventricular aneurysm, or other features associated with a high operative mortality.
4. Pre- and postoperative evaluation of the electrocardiograms and serum enzymes was carried out by a single group of observers using similar methods and criteria.

For these reasons the present study should present a reasonably accurate comparative evaluation of the incidence of myocardial infarction and ischemic injury occurring in the four groups of patients evaluated.

MATERIALS AND METHODS

Electrocardiograms were recorded on all patients prior to surgery and daily thereafter for seven days. All tracings were reviewed independently by two observers using the following criteria for the diagnosis of acute myocardial infarction or acute ischemic injury:

Infarction. Appearance of significant, persistent Q-waves or of QS deflections associated with characteristic changes in the ST segment and with T-waves.

Ischemic Injury. (1) Flat ST segment depression of greater than 2 mm in left ventricular leads, lasting more than 48 hours; (2) deep T-wave inversions persisting for more than 48 hours; (3) ventricular arrhythmias, such as ventricular tachycardia or ventricular fibrillation; and (4) absence of recent significant Q-waves or QS deflections.

The following serum enzyme determinations were performed preoperatively and postoperatively on days 1, 2, 3, 6, and 10: serum glutamic oxalacetic transaminase (SGOT), lactic dehydrogenase (LDH), and creatine phosphokinase (CPK). Upper limits prior to operation were considered to be 40, 350, and 60 units, respectively. Standard analytical methods were employed.[4-6]

It is well known that cardiac and coronary surgery will result in an increase in serum enzymes during the immediate postoperative period in the absence of evidence of myocardial infarction or acute ischemic injury. Previous studies from our hospital suggest that acceptable criteria for abnormal rises in serum enzymes in the immediate postoperative period consist of CPK values exceeding 200 units, SGOT values exceeding 90 units, and LDH values exceeding 900 units.[1]

These values may differ in other hospitals since they are dependent, in part, upon the surgical technique employed including the duration of cardiopulmonary bypass, aortic cross-clamp time, and the clinical status of the patients.

RESULTS

Internal Mammary Implants

A total of 40 consecutive patients were studied: 38 were males and two were females. The mean age was 50 years (range, 35 to 69). All had stable angina of at least six months duration. None had persistent symptoms of LV failure.

Thirty-five had treadmill tests, and 30 (75 percent) were positive. Twelve had right heart catheterization studies and none had a PA wedge pressure exceeding 16 mm at rest. Twenty-six (65 percent) had ECG evidence of prior myocardial infarction. All had coronary arteriography that revealed severe coronary artery disease involving at least two major vessels in all patients. Surgery was performed from October 1965 to August 1971. The surgical technique employed has been previously described.[7] Twenty-seven had single and 13 had double implants.

ECG evidence of acute myocardial infarction was observed in the immediate postoperative period in 11 patients (27.5 percent), and evidence of acute ischemic injury was observed in 12 patients (30 percent).

Data on SGOT levels are available in 31 patients, LDH in 29, and CPK in eight patients.

SGOT levels exceeded 90 units in 11/31 patients (35 percent), LDH levels exceeded 900 units in 10/29 patients (35 percent), and CPK levels exceeded 200 units in three/eight patients (38 percent).

Acute infarction patterns plus abnormal levels of either SGOT or LDH occurred in eight patients. Normal enzyme levels were seen in two, and no enzyme data were available in one patient.

Acute ischemic injury patterns plus abnormal levels of either SGOT or LDH were seen in six patients. Four had normal enzymes, and two had no enzyme data available.

If one examines the abnormal elevations of either SGOT or LDH observed in 15 patients, one sees that there were associated ECG signs of either acute infarction or ischemic injury in 11 patients (27 percent). Enzyme data are summarized in Table 1.

The 30-day operative mortality in 40 patients was 10 percent (four deaths). All four deaths were clearly due to intraoperative infarction with characteristic ECG changes in four patients and abnormal rises in SGOT and LDH

TABLE 1. Serum Enzyme Abnormalities in Internal Mammary Implant Surgery (40 Patients)

	ECG ABNORMALITIES		ABNORMAL ENZYMES			
	No.	%	SGOT > 90	N.D.	LDH > 900	N.D.
Acute infarction	11	27.5	5	3	7	3
Ischemic injury	12	30.0	4	3	4	2
Neither of above	17	42.0	0	3	0	5

N.D.: not determined.

TABLE 2. Enzymes in Saphenous Vein Bypass Grafts (112 patients)

	ECG ABNORMALITIES		ABNORMAL ENZYMES			
	No.	%	SGOT > 90	N.D.	LDH > 900	N.D.
Acute infarction	16	14.4	14	1	9	4
Ischemic injury	25	22.4	8	1	5	9
Neither of above	71	63.2	10	7	3	34

N.D.: not determined.

in three patients. One patient died 36 hours after surgery, and no enzymes were obtained.

Saphenous Vein Bypass Grafts for Stable Angina

A total of 112 consecutive patients was studied. All were males. The mean age was 51 years (range 33 to 63). All had stable angina of at least six months duration. None had persistent symptoms of LV failure. Forty-six (41 percent) had ECG evidence of prior myocardial infarction. The clinical characteristics of these patients were similar to those in the internal mammary implant series since the criteria of selection for surgery were similar. Forty-one patients had multistage treadmill tests prior to surgery, and 27 (68 percent) had positive tests. Seventy-three patients had right heart catheterization studies performed prior to surgery. Only two (three percent) had a PA wedge pressure exceeding 20 mm at rest. In 69 patients the mean ejection fraction was 62 percent (range 89 to 22). The operative technique employed has been previously described.[8] None of the patients had procedures other than vein bypass grafts performed. Single grafts were used in 32 patients, double grafts in 58, and triple grafts in 20. The mean cardiopulmonary bypass time was 103 minutes (range 190 to 31), and the mean aortic cross-clamp time was 17 minutes (range 5 to 46).

RESULTS. ECG evidence of acute myocardial infarction was found in 16 patients (14.4 percent), and evidence of acute ischemic injury was found in 25 patients (22.4 percent).

Data on SGOT levels are available in 103 patients, LDH in 62, and CPK in 30 patients.

SGOT levels exceeded 90 units in 35/103 patients (34 percent); LDH levels exceeded 900 units in 16/62 patients (26 percent); and CPK levels exceeded 200 units in eight of 30 patients (27 percent).

Acute infarction patterns plus abnormal levels of SGOT or LDH occurred in 14 patients.

Normal enzyme levels were seen in one, and no enzyme data are available in another patient.

Acute ischemic injury patterns plus abnormal levels of either SGOT or LDH were seen in nine patients. In 12 patients enzymes were within normal limits, and no enzyme data are available in one patient.

In 38 patients who had an abnormal elevation of either SGOT or LDH there were 27 (71 percent) who had ECG signs of acute infarction or ischemic injury. Enzyme data are summarized in Table 2.

The 30-day operative mortality in 112 patients was 2.7 percent (three deaths). In two patients death was clearly due to extensive myocardial infarction manifested by typical ECG changes and abnormal elevations of serum enzymes. One patient died of deteriorating left ventricular function in the operating room.

Unstable Angina

A total of 40 patients were studied—38 males and two females. The mean age was 54 years (range 35 to 72). All had unstable angina with a duration of acute symptoms of one to 180 days prior to hospital entry. Four general clinical presentations were observed:

1. Stable angina of more than six months duration with a recent increase in severity—28 patients (70 percent).
2. Acute coronary insufficiency or rest angina—nine patients (23 percent).
3. Recent onset of angina within 90 days of hospital entry—three patients (8 percent).
4. Angina with episodes of ventricular tachycardia or ventricular fibrillation—two patients (5 percent).

All patients had acute, transient electrocardiographic changes during chest pain compatible with myocardial ischemia. These changes consisted of:

TABLE 3. Serum Enzyme Abnormalities in Surgery for Unstable Angina (40 patients)

	ECG ABNORMALITIES		ABNORMAL ENZYMES			
	No.	%	SGOT > 90	N.D.	LDH > 900	N.D.
Acute infarction	8	20	5	0	4	0
Ischemic injury	6	16	2	0	3	0
Neither of above	26	70	4	1	3	2

N.D.: not determined.

1. Deep T-wave inversion—17 patients (43 percent).
2. ST segment depression—14 patients (35 percent).
3. ST segment elevation—nine patients (23 percent).
4. Lesser T-wave inversion—five patients (12 percent).
5. Ventricular arrhythmias—two patients (5 percent).

None of the patients had clinical evidence of an acute myocardial infarction as evidenced by the appearance of diagnostic Q waves and evolutionary ST-T-wave changes or diagnostic serum enzyme elevations. None of the patients had symptoms of persistent left ventricular failure. Nineteen (48 percent) had ECG evidence of healed myocardial infarction. All patients had coronary arteriography. Severe coronary disease involving at least two major coronary vessels was present in all patients. Twenty-six patients (65 percent) had moderate abnormalities in left ventricular contraction and the mean ejection fraction determined in 20 patients was 69 percent (range 33 percent to 88 percent).

Surgery was performed between February 1971 and January 1974. All patients except two had saphenous vein bypass grafts without endarterectomy or other procedures. The mean pump bypass time in 33 patients was 107 minutes (range 29 to 235), and the mean aortic cross-clamp time in 17 patients was 17 (range 5 to 71). Eight had single grafts, 20 had double grafts, and 10 had triple grafts.

RESULTS. ECG evidence of acute myocardial infarction was observed in the immediate postoperative period in eight patients (20 percent), and evidence of acute ischemic injury was observed in six patients (16 percent).

Data on SGOT levels are available in 38 patients and LDH in 36 patients. Data on CPK changes were incomplete and will not be evaluated.

SGOT levels exceeded 90 units in 9/38 patients (24 percent), and LDH levels exceeded 900 units in 10/36 patients (28 percent).

ECG evidence of acute infarction plus abnormal levels of either SGOT or LDH were observed in six patients (15 percent). Both enzymes were within normal limits in two patients.

ECG evidence of acute ischemic injury plus abnormal levels of either SGOT or LDH were observed in four patients (10 percent). In two patients both enzyme levels remained within normal limits.

If one examines the abnormal elevations of either SGOT or LDH observed in 14 patients, one sees that there were ECG signs of acute infarction or acute ischemic injury in 10 patients. Additional data are summarized in Table 3.

The 30-day operative mortality in 40 patients was 2.5 percent (one death). This death occurred in the operating room because the patient was unable to maintain a suitable blood pressure. No autopsy was obtained.

Combined Bypass Graft and Valve Replacement Surgery

A total of 44 consecutive patients were studied. The mean age was 58.5 years (range 43 to 81). Forty patients were males and four were females. The primary indication for surgery was valvular heart disease. Vein bypass graft surgery was performed because of the presence of significant obstructive lesions of major coronary arteries demonstrated by selective coronary arteriography. In most patients symptoms were primarily related to valvular heart disease, but in

TABLE 4. Valve Replacement Operations

	NO.
Aortic valve replacement	32
Mitral valve replacement	5
Mitral and aortic valve replacement	2
Other valve operations	5

TABLE 5. Saphenous Vein Bypass Grafts and Valve Replacement Surgery (44 patients)

| | ECG ABNORMALITIES | | ENZYME ABNORMALITIES | | | |
	No.	%	SGOT > 90	N.D.	LDH > 900	N.D.
Acute infarction	10	23	7	1	7	1
Ischemic injury	17	39	13	0	12	2
Neither of above	17	48	7	1	5	2

N.D.: not determined.

many patients angina was probably due to the associated coronary disease.

The operations performed are summarized in Table 4. Twenty-nine patients had single-vein bypass grafts, 14 had double grafts, and one had a triple graft. Mean bypass time was 135 minutes (range, 52 to 247 minutes). Mean aortic cross-clamp time in 35 patients was 42 minutes (range, 10 to 87 minutes).

The operative technique employed in the valve replacement operation has been previously described.[8]

RESULTS. ECG evidence of acute intra-operative myocardial infarction was found in 10 of 44 patients (23 percent), and evidence of acute ischemic injury was noted in 17 patients (39 percent).

Data on SGOT levels are available in 41 patients, and LDH in 38. Data on CPK levels are incomplete.

SGOT levels exceeded 90 units in 27 patients (66 percent) and LDH exceeded 100 units in 23 patients (60 percent).

Acute infarction patterns plus abnormal levels of either SGOT or LDH occurred in eight patients (18 percent). Two patients had enzyme levels within normal limits. Acute ischemic injury patterns plus abnormal levels of either SGOT or LDH occurred in 14 patients (32 percent). Three patients had enzyme levels within normal limits.

If one examines the abnormal elevations of either LDH or SGOT that were observed in 30 patients one sees that in 23 (77 percent) there were ECG signs of either acute infarction or ischemic injury. Additional enzyme data are summarized in Table 5.

Five operative deaths (30-day) occurred for a mortality of 11.2 percent. Three deaths occurred in association with ECG and serum enzyme evidence of acute intraoperative myocardial infarction.

DISCUSSION

Most previous reports of intraoperative myocardial infarction during coronary surgery have only identified patients who had the appearance of ECG abnormalities compatible with acute transmural myocardial infarction. In this study and in previous studies from this hospital an additional group of patients have been identified who have had ECG evidence of acute ischemic myocardial injury.[1] Electrocardiographic abnormalities in this group have consisted of changes in the T-waves and ST segments compatible with severe ischemia or injury and, in some patients, recurring episodes of ventricular tachycardia or AV block. Such changes occurring in the presence of abnormal elevations of serum enzymes strongly suggest that subendocardial, intramural, or diffuse, focal infarction is probably present. Table 6 illustrates the incidence of abnormal serum enzymes in patients with ECG changes of acute transmural infarction, ischemic injury patterns, and neither of these ECG changes in the immediate postoperative period. In patients without such ECG changes, abnormal rises of either SGOT or LDH were observed in only 16 percent and 11 percent respectively. In patients with ischemic injury patterns abnormal rises of SGOT or LDH occurred in 48 percent and 51 percent respectively. These data should be compared with that from patients with typical ECG signs of transmural infarction

TABLE 6. Total Group: Abnormal Enzymes in Patients with Acute Infarction, Acute Ischemic Injury, and Neither

ECG CHANGES	SGOT ↑ %	LDH ↑ %
Acute infarction	78	73
Ischemic injury	48	51
Neither of above	16	11

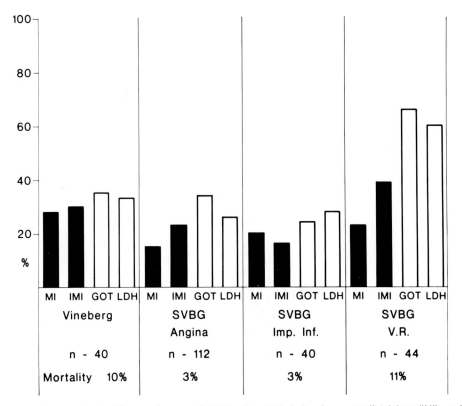

FIG. 1. Comparative incidence of myocardial infarction (MI), ischemic myocardial injury (IMI), and abnormal elevations of SGOT (GOT) and LDH in four operations for coronary artery disease. Imp. inf.: impending infarction.

where the incidence of abnormal SGOT and LDH levels were 78 percent and 73 percent respectively. These data support the validity of identifying acute ischemic injury as a complication of coronary surgery and indicate that in approximately 50 percent of such episodes acute myocardial infarction is probably present, based on the presence of associated elevations in serum enzymes. It would appear, therefore, that the true incidence of acute myocardial infarction associated with coronary surgery is probably higher than generally reported. In the present study, for example, if one considers only patients with acute infarct patterns and ischemic injury patterns who have SGOT levels as elevated as patients with acute infarction, the incidence becomes 58/167 (35 percent) instead of 31/167 (19 percent).

Additional support for this view can be obtained by inspection of Table 7 and Figure 1. In each operation the incidence of abnormal enzyme elevations is greater than the incidence of acute myocardial infarction, and in two operations (vein bypass grafts for stable angina and vein bypass grafts and value replacement surgery)

TABLE 7. Comparative Incidence of Myocardial Infarction and Ischemic Injury in All Four Groups

	NO.	AMI %	AII %	SGOT ↑ %	LDH ↑ %
IMI	40	27.5	30.0	35	35
Stable AP	112	14.4	22.4	34	26
Unstable AP	40	20.0	16.0	24	28
VR + SVBG	44	23.0	39.0	66	60
VR only[a]	126	7.0	30.0	32	37

[a]Ref. 9.

the incidence of abnormal enzyme elevations is approximately equal to the sum of the acute infarcts and acute ischemic injury episodes.

Serum enzyme data in the present study have several limitations. Isoenzymes (myocardial components) for CPK and LDH were not determined. Total CPK values are unreliable and do not correlate well with ECG changes, probably due to the effect of skeletal muscle CPK. LDH values may be high due to hemolysis in addition to myocardial infarction. SGOT values are probably most reliable since very few patients with right ventricular failure and hepatic congestion or necrosis were subjected to surgery. Such patients were confined to the group of patients having combined valve replacement surgery and vein bypass grafts. Only 4/44 (9 percent) of these patients had right ventricular failure prior to surgery and preoperative serum enzymes were normal in these patients.

It is evident fom Figure 1 that the highest incidence of acute infarction and acute ischemic injury was observed in patients who had internal mammary implants or vein bypass grafts associated with valve replacement surgery. Several reasons may be given for the high incidence of these complications observed with internal mammary implants. The patients represent the early, initial experience with the operation; hence, the surgical technique may not have been optimal. Internal mammary implantation does not provide the immediate revascularization that vein bypass graft surgery does. The internal mammary implant operation causes considerably more epicardial and myocardial damage in the creation of the myocardial tunnel than does the vein bypass graft technique.

The high incidence of infarction, ischemic injury, and enzyme elevations in the group of patients having combined valve replacement surgery and vein bypass grafts is probably due, in part, to the longer period of cardiopulmonary bypass required for the combined procedure. It has

been previously shown that valve replacement surgery alone, even in the absence of significant coronary artery disease, may be accompanied by acute infarction, ischemic injury, or abnormal rises in serum enzymes.[9] These complications tended to occur more frequently in patients with double valve replacement operations and with prolonged periods of cardiopulmonary bypass. These data are summarized in Table 8.

In the group of patients having valve replacement surgery and bypass grafts, the mean cardiopulmonary bypass time in 16 patients who had acute infarction or ischemic injury with abnormal enzymes was 156 minutes compared to 104 minutes in seven patients who had none of these complications.

Most of the data presented in this study relate to the *incidence* of intraoperative infarction and acute ischemic injury in the four types of operations. The amount of myocardial necrosis occurring with such episodes can be roughly related to the magnitude of the enzyme elevation associated with the ECG changes. These data are indicated in Table 9. The mean elevation of serum enzymes for patients with ECG signs of acute infarction or ischemic injury patterns are indicated for each operation. It is evident that the highest mean levels of SGOT and LDH were observed

TABLE 9. Magnitude of Serum Enzyme Rises

OPERATION	SGOT		LDH	
	Acute Infarcts	Ischemic Injury	Acute Infarcts	Ischemic Injury
Implants	167	153	1,305	1,219
Impending infarction	215	95	804	843
SVBG–angina	194	94	1,434	810
SVBG + VR	353	210	1,710	1,420

in patients who had combined vein bypass grafts and valvular surgery. This difference is at a significant level (P = < 0.012). Thus, the combined operation is not only associated with the highest *incidence* of intraoperative infarction and ischemic injury but also with the highest levels of SGOT and LDH, which indicate a greater amount of myocardial necrosis.

Acute intraoperative myocardial infarction is not only an important nonfatal complication of coronary surgery but is also an important cause of death, since nine of the 13 deaths occurring in the combined series of 236 patients were associated with clear evidence of recent myocardial infarction.

TABLE 8. Cardiopulmonary Bypass Time and Aortic Cross-Clamp Time in Patients with Valve Replacement and Bypass Grafts, Bypass Grafts Alone (Stable Angina) and Valve Replacement Surgery Alone

	BYPASS TIME (min.)	CROSS-CLAMP TIME (min.)
VR + SVBG	135	42
VR alone	88	43
SVBG alone	103	17

References

1. Hultgren H, Miyagawa M, Buck W, Angell WW: Ischemic myocardial injury during coronary artery surgery. Am Heart J 82:624, 1971
2. Dixon S Jr, Limbird L, Roe C, Wagner G, Oldham H Jr, Sabiston D Jr: Recognition of postoperative acute myocardial infarction. Circulation 48:Supp III:137, 1972
3. Brewer D, Bilbro R, Bartel A: Myocardial infarction as a complication of coronary bypass surgery. Circulation 57:58, 1973
4. Reitman S, Frankel S: A colorimetric method for the determination of serum glutamic pyruvic transaminases. Am J Clin Pathol 28:56, 1957
5. Cobaud P, Wroblewski F: Colorimetric measurement of lactic dehydrogenase activity of body fluids. Am J Clin Pathol 30:234, 1958
6. Rosalki S: An improved procedure for serum creatine phosphokinase determination. J Lab Clin Med 69:696, 1967
7. Hultgren H, Hurley E: Surgery in obstructive coronary artery disease. Advances in Internal Medicine, vol. 9, Chicago 1968 Year Book, Medical Publishers, Inc., pp 107–50
8. Oury J, Quint R, Angell WW, Wuerflein R: Coronary artery vein bypass grafts in patients requiring valve replacement. Surgery 72:1037, 1972
9. Hultgren H, Miyagawa M, Buck W, Angell WW: Ischemic myocardial injury during cardiopulmonary bypass surgery. Am Heart J 85:167, 1973

89

TERMINATION OF POST-OPEN-HEART ATRIAL FLUTTER AND ATRIAL TACHYCARDIA WITH RAPID ATRIAL STIMULATION

David E. Pittman, Jasbir S. Makar,
and Claude R. Joyner

Atrial tachycardia, atrial flutter, and reciprocating tachycardias occur frequently in the early postoperative period after cardiac surgery. These ryhthm disturbances may precipitate or exaggerate critical hemodynamic abnormalities for the patient with preexisting ischemic or valvular heart disease. Aggressive and prompt effective therapy is particularly important in this type of patient.

The etiology of the supraventricular tachycardias have been reviewed by several authors. They have suggested that atrial tachycardia, which was once thought to be due to rapid depolarization from a single atrial focus, frequently results from a "circus" movement of electrical impulses with a reentrant component around the AV node causing reactivation of the atria.[8,14,15,28] Recent evidence also supports the "circus" movement theory to explain the origin of atrial flutter.[24] Junctional tachycardia represents either a perinodal or subnodal focus of pacemaker activity with increased automaticity or a reentrant type activation of the ventricles.[17,29] Since it is now recognized that the AV node has no intrinsic property of spontaneous depolarization, the junctional tissue is apparently the site of depolarization from the rhythm previously designated as "nodal rhythm."

These tachyarrhythmias may be precipitated by many factors that are likely to be present in the patient who has undergone cardiac surgery with cardiopulmonary bypass. The arrhythmias may result from inflammatory changes, pH and electrolyte abnormalities, myocardial ischemia, or systemic hypoxia.

The established methods of treating atrial and junctional tachyarrhythmias includes the use of various antiarrhythmic drugs and/or external countershock. Drug therapy may take a long period to be effective, and proper dosage can be difficult to determine in the patient with decreased cardiac output and compromised hepatic and renal function. Even the proper therapeutic dose of some antiarrhythmic agents may act as a significant cardiac depressant.

Transthoracic external cardioversion has become a well-established method of terminating various supraventricular tachyarrhythmias.[7,10,16, 21,22,25,26,30] When effective, this has the advantage of speed when there is urgent need to terminate a tachycardia. However, the procedure is not without hazard. Complications are especially likely to occur in those patients who have received digitalis prior to electrical countershock.[10,21,25] These patients are subject to having a ventricular arrhythmia precipitated by precordial shock or developing a bradycardia when the rapid rhythm is terminated.

RAPID ATRIAL STIMULATION

Recently, rapid atrial stimulation has been introduced as an alternative method for terminating atrial flutter, atrial tachycardia, and reciprocating tachycardias.[2,3,6,9,12,13,19,27,31] We have reported a series of 32 patients in whom rapid atrial stimulation was used as the method of cardioversion.[20] Fifteen of these patients developed atrial tachycardia or flutter following coronary artery bypass surgery and five following valvular heart surgery. Of the remaining patients, 10 had documented coronary artery disease but had not undergone a revascularization procedure.

TABLE 1. Pertinent Clinical Data after Coronary Artery Surgery

PT. NO.	AGE/ SEX	CARDIAC ARRHYTHMIA	MEDICATION	RATE-PACEMAKER STIMULATION	RESULTS
1	47/M	A. flutter	Digoxin, quinidine	220/min	A. fib. → NSR
2	55/M	A. flutter (recurrent)	Digoxin, propranolol	500/min	A. fib.
3	60/F	A. flutter (recurrent)	Digoxin	150/min	NSR
4	56/M	A. tachy.	Digoxin	150/min	NSR
5	60/M	A. flutter	None	600/min	Unchanged
6	50/M	A. flutter	Digoxin	540/min	A. fib. → NSR
7	54/M	A. flutter	Digoxin	400/min	A. fib. → junctional (atrial pacing → NSR)
8	59/M	A. flutter	Digoxin	800/min	NSR
9	58/M	A. flutter	Digoxin	Mechn. stim	NSR
10	56/M	A. flutter	Digoxin	800/min	Unchanged
11	47/M	A. flutter	Digoxin	500/min	A. fib.
12	60/M	A. flutter	Digoxin	800/min	A. fib.
13	59/M	A. flutter	Digoxin, quinidine	700/min	NSR
14	59/M	A. flutter	Digoxin, inderal	400/min	NSR
15	49/F	A. flutter	Digoxin	400/min	NSR

M: male; F: female; A. fib.: atrial fibrillation; NSR: normal sinus rhythm; A. flutter: atrial flutter; A. tachy.: atrial tachycardia; arrow (→) indicates "spontaneously converted to."
Reprinted with permission from Am J Cardiol 32: 700–6, 1973

The arrhythmia, prestimulation drugs, rate of atrial pacing, and the post-pacing rhythm are summarized in Tables 1 and 2. In 17 of the 32 patients, atrial stimulation caused direct conversion to normal sinus rhythm. In six patients, atrial flutter or tachycardia was converted to atrial fibrillation, which spontaneously converted to normal sinus rhythm. A summary of the results in this series is outlined in Table 3. In only three patients in the study was the tachyarrhythmia un-

TABLE 2. Pertinent Clinical Data in Patients Who Had Not Had Coronary Revascularization

PT NO.	AGE/ SEX	ETIOLOGY	CARDIAC ARRHYTHMIA	MEDICATION	RATE-PACEMAKER STIMULATION	RESULTS
16	59/M	Cardiomyopathy	A. flutter	Digoxin, quinidine	300/min	NSR
17	45/M	Postaortic valve replacement	A. flutter	None	300/min	A. fib.
18	57/M	Postmitral valve replacement	A. flutter	Digoxin	300/min	A. fib. → NSR
19	65/M	Postmitral valve replacement	A. flutter	Digoxin	300/min	A. fib. → NSR
20	51/M	Postaortic valve replacement	A. flutter	Digoxin	150/min	NSR
21	59/M	ASHD	A. tachy. (recurrent)	Digoxin	300/min	NSR
22	59/F	ASHD	A. flutter (recurrent)	Digoxin	300/min	NSR
23	57/M	Idiopathic ? ASHD	A. flutter	Digoxin	150/min	A. fib. → NSR
24	75/M	ASHD	A. flutter	Digoxin	300/min	A. fib.
25	59/M	ASHD	A. flutter	None	540/min	NSR
26	69/F	ASHD	A. tachy.	None	160/min	NSR
27	77/M	ASHD	A. tachy.	Digoxin	300/min	NSR
28	58/M	ASHD	A. tachy.	Digoxin	300/min	NSR
29	42/F	2 yr postop mitral commissurotomy	A. flutter	Digoxin	300/min	A. fib.
30	75/M	ASHD	A. flutter	Digoxin, quinidine	350/min	NSR
31	55/F	Postop bivalve rep.	A. tachy.	Digoxin	800/min	Unchanged
32	60/F	ASHD, chronic lung disease	A. flutter	Digoxin, quinidine	800/min	NSR

M: male; F: female; A. fib.:atrial fibrillation; NSR: normal sinus rhythm; A. flutter: atrial flutter; A. tachy.: atrial tachycardia; ASHD: arteriosclerotic heart disease; arrow (→) indicates "spontaneously converted to."
Reprinted with permission from AM J Cardiol 32:700–6, 1973

TABLE 3. Summary of Results (32 Patients)

RESULTS OF ATRIAL STIMULATION	PATIENTS (No./Total)	% TOTAL
Patients converted directly to normal sinus rhythm	17/32	53.0
Patients converted from atrial flutter to atrial fibrillation	12/32	37.5
Patients subsequently spontaneously reverting from atrial fibrillation to normal sinus rhythm	6/12/32	18.8
Patients remaining in atrial fibrillation (with controlled ventricular rate)	5/12/32	15.6
Patients subsequently converted by precordial shock before discharge	2/12/32	6.3
Patients in whom rhythm unaffected	3/32	9.1
Patients in whom atrial stimulation successful in *terminating* atrial flutter or tachycardia	29/32	90.9

Reprinted with permission from Am J Cardiol 32:700–6, 1973.

affected by rapid atrial stimulation. Since this study, we have incorporated this method into routine use in treatment of post-open-heart supraventricular tachycardias and have continued to find it an extremely valuable and successful method.

METHOD OF RAPID ATRIAL STIMULATION

In our department, cardioversion of the postoperative patient is initially attempted with the transthoracic atrial pacing wires that are implanted during thoracotomy. However, we have found that the success rate is much less with the transthoracic pacing wires than with intraatrial pacing catheters. The possible reasons for this are now being investigated. Either the transthoracic pacing wires are not always in the optimum position or the milliampere (ma) requirement for effective epicardial atrial stimulation is considerably greater than the threshold for intraatrial stimulation. Certainly there is little doubt that proper placement of the transthoracic wire is an important factor.

One can obtain some idea as to the adequate placement of the transthoracic atrial wire by recording a precordial ECG from this wire. Improperly placed wires or dislodgement of the wires from the surface of the atrium will usually yield atrial complexes that are smaller than those obtained from properly placed epicardial or intraatrial wires (Fig. 1)

In the majority of our patients a Cordis 4F bipolar pacemaker wire is inserted percutaneously into the subclavian vein. Passage of the wire into the right atrium is usually performed under fluoroscopic control. However, the wire may be passed "blindly" with electrocardiographic monitoring from the electrode. When fluoroscopy is used, proper apposition of the tip of the electrode to the upper or mid-portion of the right atrial wall is easily assured. In cases performed with electrocardiographic monitoring, proper position is assumed by recording the large P-waves characteristic of the intracavitary right atrial electrocardiogram.

Stimulation of the atrium is accomplished by using a battery powered external pacemaker designed to pace up to 800 beats per minute with a

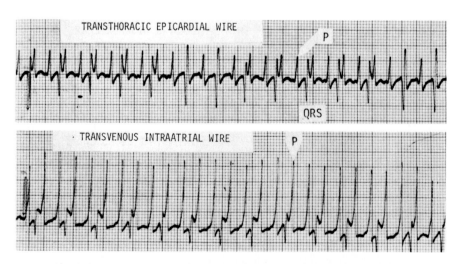

FIG. 1. Tracing illustrating the distinct difference in voltage of P-waves recorded from transthoracic wire (upper tracing) and transvenous wire (lower tracing). Standardization was identical.

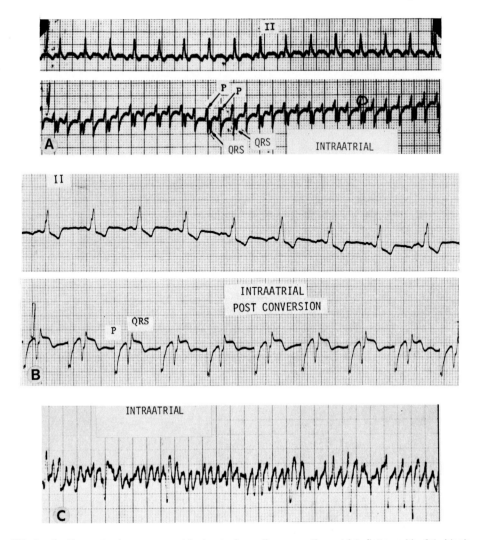

FIG. 2. A. Upper tracing: supraventricular tachycardia suggesting atrial flutter with 2:1 block. Lower tracing: intraatrial electrocardiogram in the same patient defining P-waves very clearly, confirming rhythm to be atrial flutter with an atrial rate of 320/min and a ventricular rate of 160/min (Reprinted with permission from Am J Cardiol 32:700–6, 1973.) B. Intraatrial ECG and Lead II after conversion from atrial flutter showing return of normal sinus rhythm. Note large biphasic P-waves in lower tracing indicating intraatrial position of electrode. C. Intraatrial electrocardiogram taken after rapid atrial stimulation showing characteristic appearance of atrial fibrillation. The patient had atrial flutter before atrial stimulation. (Reprinted with permission from Am J Cardiol 32:700–6, 1973.)

maximum of 25 ma (Medtronic Unit 5800). The stimulation rate is progressively increased from 5 ma until capture of the atrium is accomplished, termination of the tachycardia occurs, or maximum rate and ma is reached without change in the cardiac rhythm. Ten minutes of stimulation at maximal rate and milliamperes is usually performed before failure is accepted. Although a few patients have a sensation of the electrical impulse with higher ma and rate settings, the discomfort has never been severe enough to necessitate abandoning the procedure.

Prestimulation intraatrial leads are routinely taken in all patients. After termination of the atrial stimulation, another intraatrial electrocardiogram is taken to document the rhythm (Fig. 2). Tracings shown in Figure 3 were taken from a 37-year-old female who developed rapid, regular tachycardia several days after open mitral commissurotomy. Intraatrial lead confirmed the rhythm to be atrial flutter. Attempts at conversion using the transthoracic wire were unsuccessful in spite of the use of maximal rate and ma. With a bipolar wire placed under fluoroscopic guidance into the

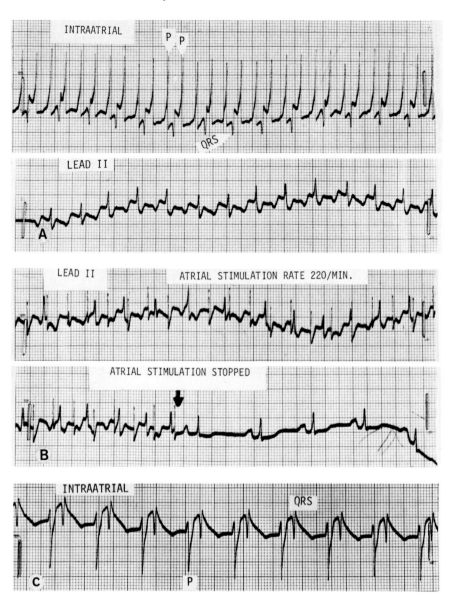

FIG. 3. A. Tracings taken from a patient several days after mitral commissurotomy. Upper tracing: Intraatrial ECG showing tachycardia to be atrial flutter with 2:1 AV conduction. Lower tracing: Lead II in same patient suggesting the diagnosis of atrial flutter. B. Upper tracing: Lead II rhythm strip taken during rapid atrial stimulation with transvenous right atrial electrode. Lower tracing: Continuation of above showing the termination of atrial flutter and return of normal sinus rhythm upon discontinuation of atrial pacing. C. Post-conversion intraatrial ECG confirming change of rhythm to normal sinus.

right atrium, stimulation at a rate of 220 per minute and 12 ma terminated the flutter within 20 seconds, resulting in normal sinus rhythm. Figure 4 illustrates the successful use of rapid atrial stimulation in terminating atrial tachycardia in a patient after coronary bypass graft surgery. In one patient the arrhythmia was converted to atrial fibrillation, which within several minutes sponta-

neously terminated (Fig. 5). This event was followed by sinus arrest and a resultant slow junctional escape rhythm. The patient underwent atrial pacing for 48 hours until sinoatrial nodal function returned and stable normal sinus rhythm was established. This sequence of events illustrates the potential hazard of a bradyarrhythmia developing after cardioversion and is much more likely to occur

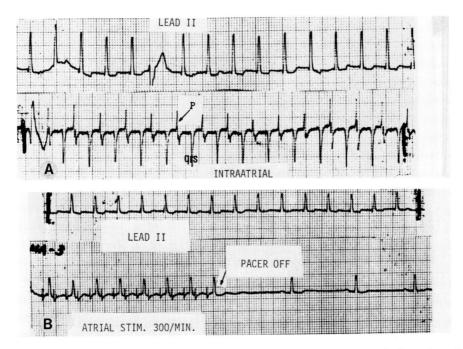

FIG. 4. A. Case 28. Upper tracing: Lead II electrocardiogram showing supraventricular tachycardia at rate of 160/min with no consistent definable P-waves. Lower tracing: intraatrial electrocardiogram showing P-waves with a 1:1 conduction ratio (carotid massage resulted in a transient increase in atrioventricular block, thus confirming the atrial tachycardia and ruling out the possibility of sinus rhythm with a P-R interval). B. Upper tracing: lead II electrocardiogram after attempted conversion at rate of 150/min showing continuation of atrial tachycardia. Lower tracing: Lead II electrocardiogram taken during rapid atrial stimulation at rate of 300/min showing atrial capture with 2:1 atrioventricular conduction and return of normal sinus rhythm on termination of atrial pacing. (Reprinted with permission from Am J Cardiol 32:700–6, 1973.)

in patients who have been treated with multiple cardiac suppressant drugs. This case also exemplifies the benefit of having a pacemaker wire in place for immediate cardiac pacing if necessary.

DIAGNOSTIC VALUE OF INTRAATRIAL ELECTROCARDIOGRAM

In addition to its use in terminating atrial or junctional tachyarrhythmias, the transthoracic epicardial or transvenous intraatrial electrode wire is of value in determining the nature of the arrhythmia. Atrial flutter, especially with persistent 2:1 block may be extremely difficult to diagnose with an external electrocardiogram. The flutter may be confused with a sinus, atrial, or junctional tachycardia (Fig. 1A, 3A, 4A). If aberrant conduction is present, a supraventricular tachycardia may be difficult to differentiate from a ventricular tachycardia. The proper identification of P-waves is almost always possible with the intraatrial ECG. The source and type of tachycardia can then be

defined and the proper therapy undertaken.

Figure 6 shows the ECG monitor strip from a patient who developed a rapid regular tachycardia 10 days after aortic valve replacement. The rhythm was interpreted to be supraventricular tachycardia with aberrant conduction. The intraatrial lead, however, demonstrated that the mechanism was a ventricular tachycardia. Control of the arrhythmia was achieved with intravenous lidocaine and oral procainamide.

MECHANISMS OF ATRIAL STIMULATION

There are probably several mechanisms by which atrial stimulation can effectively terminate various types of supraventricular tachyarrhythmias. These are as follows:

1. Single ectopic pacemaker sites in the atrium or junctional tissue may be overdriven or suppressed by capture with atrial pacing at a faster rate than the

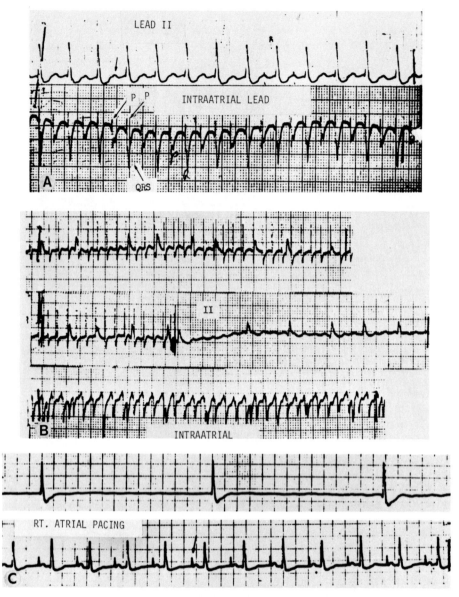

FIG. 5. A. Case 7. Upper tracing: Lead II electrocardiogram showing regular rhythm (rate of 140/min), which would be almost impossible to define as atrial flutter. With position of the P-waves (arrow) and the relatively slow ventricular rate, it is difficult to differentiate the rhythm from sinus tachycardia. Lower tracing: Intraatrial electrocardiogram showing the P-wave not only on the T-wave but also embedded in the initial portion of the QRS complex. This is diagnostic of atrial flutter with rate of 280/min and 2:1 atrioventricular block.   B. Upper tracing: Taken during rapid atrial stimulation of 400/min. Middle tracing: Continuation of strip with resulting rhythm suggesting atrial fibrillation at termination of atrial stimulation. Lower tracing: Intraatrial lead taken immediately after previous strip, showing rapid atrial depolarization at a rate of 400/min representing a definite change from the lower tracing of A. Upper tracing: taken several minutes after B following spontaneous termination of atrial fibrillation with complete silencing of sinoatrial nodal function, and resultant slow junctional or Purkinje rhythm. Lower tracing: atrial pacing accomplished with intraatrial pacing wire previously used for atrial stimulation and left in place in upper right atrium. Note the pacemaker spike (arrow) followed by atrial depolarization and QRS complex. (Reprinted with permission from Am J Cardiol 32:700–6, 1973.)

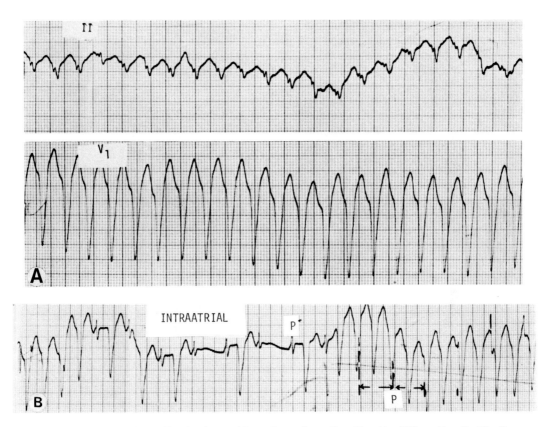

FIG. 6. A. Leads II and V_1 showing rapid regular tachycardia with wide QRS making it difficult to differentiate between supraventricular tachycardia with aberrant conduction or ventricular tachycardia. B. Intraatrial electrocardiogram (taken with transthoracic epicardial wire) showing the tachycardia spontaneously converting to normal sinus rhythm in the midportion of the tracing. There are several nonconducted sinus beats indicating presence of a component of AV block. In the latter portion of the tracing, with recurrence of the tachycardia, P-waves are identified, bearing no relationship to the QRS complexes. The P-waves are indicated by black markers and, when measured, have the same P-P interval as that measured during the return of sinus rhythm. These features are compatible with the diagnosis of ventricular tachycardia.

ectopic focus. Return of sinus rhythm follows termination of the pacing.

2. Termination of fixed (circus or reciprocating) pathway rhythms in the atrium or AV nodal-junctional area may be accomplished by rapid atrial stimulation. If these rhythms are indeed secondary to the "circus" movement phenomenon, electrical atrial stimulation must be capable of depolarizing a part of the pathway that is then refractory to the depolarizing circus wave. This theory would appear to be substantiated by the observations that a single, properly timed stimulus can terminate atrial flutter, and conversion of atrial flutter often occurs with atrial stimulation rates slower than the atrial flutter rate.

Interruption of the ectopic pacemaking activity by either of the above mechanisms will permit a return of normal sinus rhythm or a change to atrial fibrillation. If the resultant rhythm is atrial fibrillation, this may spontaneously convert to normal sinus rhythm, may be later converted precordially, or may be acceptable as a chronic rhythm that can be controlled satisfactorily with digitalis.

ATRIAL STIMULATION VERSUS EXTERNAL COUNTERSHOCK

Cardioversion using transthoracic direct current countershock has been very successful for the treatment of postoperative arrhythmias. However, there is some potential danger in external countershock. The hazard is increased in patients receiving digitalis.[10,21,25] External countershock may uncover latent digitalis toxicity and precipitate disruptive ventricular arrhythmias. The absence of ventricular arrhythmias in our patients having rapid atrial stimulation should be emphasized. We have had no postconversion ventricular or junctional arrhythmias. We feel the safer approach to cardioversion of the postoperative patient is to use rapid atrial stimulation. Precordial shock is employed only if it appears absolutely necessary.

Atrial stimulation avoids direct application of electricity to the ventricular muscle and the relatively small amounts of electrical energy minimizes the chances of precipitating serious dysrhythmias. Another advantage of this method is that it avoids the need for general anesthesia, which is usually administered for external precordial cardioversion.

We routinely leave the atrial wires in place after cardioversion by atrial pacing. Repeated cardioversion may be done in cases of recurrent tachycardia, and the atrial electrode may be used to overdrive subsidiary ectopic beats or for pacing the heart if a bradyarrhythmia develops.

PREVENTING RECURRENCE OF TACHYCARDIA

Atrial tachyarrythmias, especially atrial flutter, are notorious for their tendency to recur after conversion. The tendency of recurrence depends upon many factors influencing the integrity of the cardiac conductive and pacing system. This tendency appears to be enhanced in patients after open-heart surgery. This fact illustrates the usefulness of either having a transthoracic wire left in place at time of surgery or in having a transthoracic wire in the right atrium following successful rapid atrial stimulation cardioversion. With the pacing wire in the right atrium, repeated cardioversion using this method can be accomplished without discomfort, inconvenience, or danger to the patient.

Most patients are also either receiving antiarrhythmic drugs at the time of cardioversion or are placed on appropriate drugs (ie digitalis, procainamide, quinidine, propranolol, dilantin, etc) after cardioversion. This is done in hope of suppressing the tendency of recurrence of the tachycardia. If, however, the rhythm recurs and cannot be adequately suppressed with drug therapy then atrial or ventricular pacing can be used following

termination of tachycardia to "overdrive"-suppress the tachyarrhythmia.[2,4,5,11,32] Pacing should routinely be used in cases of postconversion bradycardia and tachycardia (the so-called bradycardia-tachycardia syndrome).[1,18,23]

SUMMARY

Supraventricular tachyarrhythmias, especially atrial flutter and atrial tachycardia, frequently complicate the postoperative course following open-heart surgery. Serious hemodynamic and circulatory aberrations can result from such uncontrolled tachycardias. Therefore, they deserve an aggressive approach in diagnosis and therapy in an attempt to terminate the tachycardia, reestablish sinus rhythm, and prevent recurrence of the rhythm disturbance.

Previous established modes of therapy have involved use of various antiarrhythmic drugs and precordial countershock. We feel that rapid atrial stimulation should now be considered as a *primary* method of attempting to terminate supraventricular tachycardias in the postoperative patient. Its use has recently been advocated by numerous reports and its efficacy confirmed by our recent experience outlined in this chapter.

We suggest its use because this method represents a successful, convenient, and safe technique for converting supraventricular tachycardias, especially atrial tachycardia and flutter. The numerous advantages of this method, the rationale for its use and its benefits over precordial shock cardioversion have been discussed. Particular consideration should be given to conversion by rapid atrial stimulation in patients with possible digitalis toxicity and in all patients who have atrial flutter, atrial tachycardia, or junctional tachycardia after open-heart surgery.

ACKNOWLEDGMENTS

Appreciation to Mrs. Jacqueline Soltis for her excellent technical and secretarial assistance; Dr. Kian S. Kooros who participated in several of the cases; Dr. George Magovern whose postoperative patients represented a large component of the study; and Ms. Peg Lischner for photographs.

References

1. Adelman AG, Wigle ED: The bradycardia, tachycardia, asystole syndrome: treatment by a pacemaker. Can Med Assoc J 100:75–77, 1969

2. Barold SS, Linhart JW: Recent advances in the treatment of ectopic tachycardias by electrical pacing. Am J Cardiol 25:698–706, 1970

3. Barold SS, Linhart JW, Samet P, et al: Supraventricular tachycardias initiated and terminated by a single electrical stimulus. Am J Cardiol 24: 37–41, 1969

4. Cohen HE, Kahn M, Donoso E: Treatment of supraventricular tachycardias with catheter and permanent pacemakers. Am J Cardiol 20:735–38, 1967

5. DeFrancis NA, Giordano RP: Permanent epicardial atrial pacing in the treatment of refractory ventricular tachycardia. Am J Cardiol 22:742–45, 1968

6. Haft JI, Kosowsky BD, Lau SH, Stein E, Damato AN: Termination of atrial flutter by rapid electrical pacing of the atrium. Am J Cardiol 20:239–344, 1967

7. Halmos PB: Direct conversion of atrial fibrillation. Br Heart J 302–8, 1966

8. Han J: The mechanism of paroxysmal atrial tachycardia: sustained reciprocation. Am J Cardiol 26: 329–30, 1970

9. Hunt NC, Cobb FR, Waxman MD, Zeft HJ, Peter RN: Conversion of supraventricular tachycardias with atrial stimulation. Evidence of re-entry mechanisms. Circulation 38:1060–64, 1968

10. Kleiger R, Lown B: Cardioversion and digitalis. II. Clinical studies. Circulation 33:878–87, 1966

11. Lefemine AA, Low HB, Drux W, et al: Alternating current pacing of the heart to control tachycardias. Vasc Dis 5:48–60, 1968

12. Lister JW, Cohen LS, Berstein EH, Samet P: Treatment of supraventricular tachycardias by rapid atrial stimulation. Circulation 38:1044–59, 1968

13. Massumi RA, Kistin AD, Towakkol AA: Termination of reciprocating tachycardia by atrial stimulation. Circulation 36:637–43, 1967

14. Mendez C, Moe GK: Demonstration of dual AV nodal conduction system in the isolated rabbit heart. Circ Res 19:378–93, 1966

15. Moe GK, Mendez C, Han J: Some features of dual AV conduction system. In Mechanisms and Therapy of Cardiac Arrhythmias (18th Annual Hahneman Lecture: Dreifus LS, Likoff W, eds). NY, Grune-Stratton, 1973, pp 361–72

16. Morris JJ, Peter RH, McIntosh HD: Electrical conversion of atrial fibrillation and immediate and long-term results and selection of patients. Ann Intern Med 65:216–31, 1966

17. Pick A: Recent advances in the differential diagnosis of AV junctional arrhythmias. Am Heart J 76:553–75, 1968

18. Pittman DE: Use of pervenous ventricular demand pacing in the treatment of the bradycardia tachycardia syndrome. Allegheny General Hospital Bulletin 3, January 1973

19. Pittman DE, Makar JS: Atrial tachyarrhythmias: conversion by means of rapid atrial stimulation. Report of two cases. Allegheny General Hospital Bulletin 2:30–37, 1972

20. Pittman DE, Makar JS: Rapid atrial stimulation: successful method of conversion of atrial flutter and atrial tachycardia. Am J Cardiol 32:700–6, 1973

21. Rabbino MD, Likoff W, Dreifus LS: Complications and limitations of direct current countershock. JAMA 190:792–96, 1964

22. Resnekov L, McDonald L: Appraisal of electroconversion in treatment of cardiac dysrrhythmias: Br Heart J 30:786–810, 1968

23. Rokseth R, Hatle L, Gedde-Dahl D, Foss PO: Pacemaker therapy in sino-atrial block complicated by paroxysmal tachycardia. Br Heart J 32:93–98, 1970

24. Rytand DA: The circus movement (entrapped circuit wave) hypothesis and atrial flutter. Ann Intern Med 65:125–59, 1966

25. Szelkely P, Wynne NA, Pearson DT, Batson GA, Sidris DA: Direct current shock and digitalis. A clinical and experimental study. Br Heart J 31: 91–96, 1969

26. Thind GS, Blakemore WS, Zinseer HF: Direct current cardioversion in digitalized patients with mitral valve disease. Arch Intern Med (Chicago) 123: 156–59, 1969

27. Vergara GS, Hildner FJ, Schoenfeld CB: Failure of rapid atrial pacing in the conversion of atrial flutter. Circulation 45:788–93, 1972

28. Wallace AG, Daggett WM: Re-excitation of the atrium. The echo phenomenum. Am Heart J 68: 661–66, 1964

29. Watanke Y, Dreifus LS: Arrhythmias: mechanisms and pathogenesis. In Cardiac Arrhythmias (25th Annual Hahneman Lecture: Driefus LS, Likoff W, eds). NY, Grune-Stratton, 1973, pp 35–54

30. Yang SS, Moranhao V, Manheit R: Cardioversion following open heart valvular surgery. Br Heart J 28:309, 1966

31. Zeft JH, Cobb FR, Waxman MD, Hunt MC, Morris JJ: Right atrial stimulation in the treatment of atrial flutter. Ann Intern Med 70:447–56, 1969

32. Zipes DP, Wallace AG, Sealy WC, Floyd WL: Artificial atrial and ventricular pacing in the treatment of arrhythmias. Ann Intern Med 70:885–96, 1969

90

SURVIVAL FOLLOWING SURGERY FOR END-STAGE CORONARY ARTERY DISEASE

David A. Clark, Robert A. Quint, Robert D. Wuerflein, and William W. Angell

As the indications for coronary artery bypass graft surgery continue to be debated in the literature [1,2,3] and at meetings and seminars throughout the world, several indisputable facts have become apparent. Six hundred thousand persons in the United States die each year of coronary artery disease, a disease of epidemic proportions whose etiology is currently unknown. The medical and surgical approach to coronary artery disease is mainly secondary treatment directed at the alleviation of symptoms caused by the inability of diseased coronary arteries to respond to the oxygen demands of the myocardium and toward the prevention of myocardial infarction with resultant compromised cardiac function. Certain investigators [4,5] have expressed concern that bypass graft surgery may prove to be a procedure popularized and exploited without proper control studies, only to be considered later as of questionable benefit and destined for abandonment. The apparent success of surgery for the relief of angina, and short-term follow-up studies suggesting that revascularization surgery is probably effective in preventing infarction of compromised myocardium have led to a marked increase in the number of cases performed (20,000) in the United States last year. As the number of procedures increase the close follow-up of operated patients becomes vital.

To consider coronary artery disease as a single entity would be a serious error. Coronary artery disease represents a spectrum of diseases, and patients may present at any point along that spectrum. It is important, therefore, to identify various subgroups and subsets of patients with coronary disease and both prospectively and retrospectively consider the benefits of bypass graft surgery in each instance. The purpose of this presentation is to examine a particular subgroup of patients with coronary artery disease. These patients present with "end-stage" coronary artery disease. This group is characterized by preoperative data and by the type of operative procedures that necessarily must be performed. For purposes of definition, included in this group will be patients who not only are demonstrated to have indications for bypass graft surgery but who also have evidence of previously severely compromised coronary circulation as demonstrated by the presence of nonrheumatic mitral regurgitation and/or localized or diffuse severe myocardial fibrosis demonstrated angiographically.

CLINICAL DATA

Surgery was performed on all patients in our series by the same group of surgeons with comparable pre- and postoperative care provided in two separate institutions. In this particular analysis of patients, no attempt was made to separate them by the number of grafts received. Likewise, the "pre-infarction" or "unstable angina" patients were not elected for separate appraisal in the study; this particular subgroup has been discussed at length elsewhere.[6] Following history and physical examinations, all patients underwent cardiac catheterization and selective coronary angiography as well as left ventriculography. Approximately half of the patients were studied by the transfemoral technique and the other half by the Sones brachial approach.[7] Left ventriculography was performed using the biplane technique on approximately half the patients. Statistical data presented was prepared using the life table (actuarial) method of Cutler and Ederer.[8]

Total Patient Experience

During the past four years our group has performed coronary artery bypass graft surgery on 611 patients. Table 1 divides these patients chronologically but does not further define subgroups. Each year the number of procedures has increased. This reflects the acceptance of the procedure by both referring physicians and patients.

Each year the actuarial mortality has decreased. Of the 611 patients, 52 were lost to follow-up or died for noncardiac related reasons and therefore do not appear in subsequent subgroup sets.

TABLE 1. Coronary Artery Bypass Graft Surgery—All Patients

YEAR	TOTAL PTS.	EARLY DEATHS	%	TOTAL DEATHS	%
1970	37	2	5.4	8	21.6
1971	125	5	4.0	10	8.0
1972	175	8	4.5	11	6.2
1973	274	5	1.8	8	2.9
1970–73	611	20	3.2	37	6.0

Coronary Artery Bypass Graft Surgery as an Isolated Procedure

Table 2 lists our experience in a "pure" group of 464 patients whose only surgical procedure was revascularization surgery. This group includes patients with single (112), double (229), and multiple (123) vessels grafted. Even though patients presenting with "unstable angina" and cardiogenic shock are included in this group, it is obvious that both the early (30 days) and one-year mortality rates are significantly lower than the entire group of patients undergoing revascularization surgery. Patients in this group presented primarily with angina, and very few had either symptomatic or hemodynamically demonstrable evidence of congestive heart failure. Left ventricular end-diastolic pressures were nearly always normal (less than 12 mm Hg) and no significant degree of mitral regurgitation was demonstrated in this group of patients.

Patients with End-Stage Coronary Heart Disease, Combination Coronary Heart Disease, and Rheumatic Heart Disease

Table 3 demonstrates our experience with patients who have undergone combined procedures. Patients in both "end-stage" and rheumatic subgroups did not differ with respect to age or sex from the patients who underwent coronary bypass surgery as an isolated procedure.

Patients in the "end-stage" subgrouping uniformly had some component of congestive heart failure and in 70 percent of cases had evidence for mitral regurgitation, both on physical examination and by hemodynamic and angiographic parameters. The average left ventricular end-diastolic pressure at rest was above normal in this subgroup (17 mm Hg) and often rose dramatically (above 25 mm Hg) following left ventriculography. In the normal noncompromised heart, the left ventricular end-diastolic pressure does rise following left ventricular contrast injection but usually no higher than 18 mm Hg. Surgery in this subgroup consisted not only of bypass graft surgery but also additional surgical procedures to repair the effects of advanced coronary disease. Specifically, these patients underwent either mitral valve replacement or repair secondary to ischemic, and not rheumatic, dysfunction and/or the resection of a localized left ventricular aneurysm caused by extensive myo-

TABLE 2. Coronary Artery Bypass Graft Surgery as an Isolated Procedure

YEAR	TOTAL PTS.	EARLY DEATHS	%	DEATHS AT 1 YR.	%
1970	28	2	7.1	4	14.2
1971	99	1	1.0	3	3.0
1972	123	3	2.4	4	3.2
1973	214	2	0.9	5	2.3
1970–73	464	8	1.7	16	3.9

TABLE 3. Coronary Artery Bypass Graft Surgery in Patients with End-Stage Coronary Disease Requiring Valve Repair/Replacement and/or Aneurysmectomy Compared with Bypass Plus Valve Surgery Secondary to Rheumatic Disease

	END-STAGE	RHD
No. pts.	42	53
No. early deaths	6	5
% early mortality	14.2	9.4
Total deaths	15	8
% mortality at 1 yr.	35.7	15.0

cardial fibrosis. Actuarial rates (14.2 percent and 35.7 percent, respectively) are significantly higher than the respective 1.7 percent and 3.9 percent mortality rates in patients undergoing bypass graft surgery as an isolated procedure.

Obviously, the patients in the "end-stage" subgrouping have more cardiac dysfunction and represent a group at high risk if treated medically. While they appear to be risking more with the higher mortality rate with surgery, they also are the group that has more to gain from revascularization of compromised vessels and the repair of valvular or myocardial damage secondary to the previous effect of coronary disease.

Patients with Coronary Artery Bypass Graft Surgery and Rheumatic Heart Disease

Another subgroup of patients undergoing combined procedures is that group of patients with rheumatic, aortic, or mitral valvular disease who also have coronary artery disease requiring revascularization surgery. Table 3 demonstrates that patients in this group, while having a higher 30-day and one-year mortality rate than those undergoing revascularization surgery alone, do not approach the significantly higher mortality figures demonstrated by the patients whose combined procedure was necessitated by the effects of coronary damage to the valve or myocardium. Comparison of the rheumatic group of patients with the "end-stage" group would indicate that the additional surgical manipulation required for valve replacement does not, per se, account for the increased mortality in the "end-stage" subgroup. The "end-stage" patients also require significantly longer periods of pharmacologic and mechanical support for blood pressure and cardiac function in the immediate postoperative period, as well as longer periods of hospitalization, than patients in either the combined coronary and rheumatic heart disease group or the patients undergoing coronary artery bypass grafts alone.

CONCLUSIONS

Table 4 again contrasts the subgroups examined. No significant age or sex difference between the subgroups was demonstrated and no attempt was made to divide the patients into a number of grafts received, "preinfarction" angina, etc.

Within the total group of patients under-

going coronary artery bypass graft surgery, there are definable subgroups with varying morbidity and mortality. The importance of recognizing the inclusion of each individual patient in the appropriate subgroup rather than applying whole group statistics to every patient is obvious. It is also important that each physician group explore its own statistics and apply them rather than utilizing national averages when discussing the procedure of bypass graft surgery with the patient and his referring physician.

TABLE 4. Actuarial Comparison of Patient Subgroups

GROUP	NO.	30-DAY MORTALITY (%)	1-YR. MORTALITY (%)
All patients	611	3.2	6.0
CABG only	464	1.7	3.9
"End-stage"	42	14.2	35.7
RHD + CABG	53	9.4	15.0

Those patients representing "end-stage" cardiac disease as defined by nonrheumatic valvular dysfunction and/or extensive myocardial fibrosis should be made aware of the increased risk of surgery but also appraised that they are at high risk with medical management as well.

The patients with "end-stage" coronary artery disease are preoperatively demonstrable by symptomatic, hemodynamic, and angiographic studies of left ventricular dysfunction and require, in addition to revascularization surgery, the repair or replacement of the mitral valve apparatus and/or the resection of extensively damaged myocardium. These patients represent a high-risk group, and, while not an absolute contraindication to coronary artery bypass graft surgery, the presence of parameters depicting "end-stage" coronary disease should alert the physician to inform the patient of the potential benefits as well as the potentially high mortality of the operation.

Additional and longer-term follow-up is needed to assess both the subjective-functional and objective-hemodynamic benefits of surgery as well as the effect on longevity following revascularization surgery for end-stage coronary artery disease.

References

1. Swan HJC, Chatterjee K, et al: Myocardial revascularization for Acute and Chronic Coronary Heart Disease. Ann Intern Med 79:851, 1973

2. Subcommittee on Coronary Bypass Surgery of the Advisory Committee of the National Heart and Lung Institute, July 1972
3. Cannom DS, Miller DC, Shumway NE, et al: The long-term follow-up of patients undergoing saphenous vein bypass surgery. Circulation 49:27, 1973
4. Selzer A, Keith WJ: Surgical treatment of coronary artery disease: too fast, too soon? Am J Cardiol 28:490, 1971
5. Corday E: Myocardial revascularization: need for hard facts (editorial). JAMA 219:507, 1972
6. Miller DC, Cannom DS, Fogarty TJ, et al: Saphenous vein coronary artery bypass in patients with "pre-infarction angina." Circulation 47:234, 1972
7. Sones FM Jr, Shirey EK: Cine coronary arteriography. Mod Concepts Cardiovasc Dis 31:735, 1962
8. Cutter SJ, Ederer F: Maximum utilization of the life table method in analyzing survival. J Chronic Dis 8:600, 1958

91

LEFT MAIN CORONARY ARTERY DISEASE, I
A Perspective

Henry DeMots, Lawrence I. Bonchek, Joseph Rösch,
Richard P. Anderson, Albert Starr,
and Shahbudin H. Rahimtoola

The incidence of left main coronary artery (LMCA) disease in patients undergoing coronary arteriography varies from 2.5 percent [1] to 5.9 percent.[2] Its frequency in people with coronary artery disease is unknown. Early reports stressed several features that appeared to distinguish the patient with disease of the LMCA from the remainder of patients with coronary artery disease. An increased mortality rate during coronary arteriography and coronary artery surgery and poor survival rates without surgical intervention were reported in these patients. In this chapter we will review the current knowledge about this important subset of patients with coronary artery disease.

CORONARY ARTERIOGRAPHY

Cohen et al, first drew attention to the lethal potential of coronary arteriography in patients with left main coronary artery disease.[1] Similar findings were reported by other investigators.[3,4] Subsequently, however, several groups of patients were examined with a low mortality rate using the Sones technique [5] or a combination of the Sones and Judkins [6] techniques.[8-11] It was suggested that the Sones technique may be preferable when LMCA disease is present because of the higher mortality rate occurring with the use of the Judkins technique.

The 2,100 coronary arteriograms performed between September 1967 and May 1973 at the

University of Oregon Medical School Hospital were examined, and 50 patients with 50 percent or greater narrowing of luminal diameter were found. This degree of luminal narrowing corresponds to 75 percent or greater narrowing of cross-sectional area. The degree of narrowing is associated with a significant reduction in flow.[12,13] A total of 65 coronary arteriograms were performed in these 50 patients. The Judkins technique was used in all patients. In our series, 36 of the 50 lesions were within 12 mm of the coronary ostia and, therefore, within reach of the catheter tip. There were no complications in any study. One patient with ventricular arrhythmias and a large heart had a 50 percent diffuse stenosis of the LMCA, occlusions of all three major coronary arteries, and a left ventricular end-diastolic pressure of 35 mm Hg. He developed ventricular fibrillation six hours after the study, was resuscitated, but died three days later of multiple ventricular tachyarrhythmias. At autopsy, LMCA disease was confirmed, but an acute myocardial infarction was not found.

It is important to use meticulous technique while performing coronary arteriography in patients with LMCA disease.[14] Several technical points need reemphasis. Manipulation of the catheter in the LMCA must be minimized to avoid dislodgement of atheromatous material. All torque should be removed from the catheter when it is in the aortic arch so that it can be advanced to the LMCA without further rotation. Pressure at the catheter tip should be monitored continuously and the catheter removed from the LMCA immediately if damping of pressure occurs. Damping of catheter tip pressure indicates either impingement of the catheter tip against the vessel wall or

Supported in part by Program Project Grant HL 06336 and Graduate Training Grant HL 05791 from the National Heart and Lung Institute.

obstruction of the lumen at the site of stenosis. Subintimal injection may occur with the former catheter position and a rapid, marked fall in coronary blood flow and perfusion pressure with the latter.[15] These precautions are very important because in 72 percent of our patients the lesion in the LMCA was in reach of the catheter tip. Prophylaxis and treatment with atropine of the bradycardia (and subsequent hypotension) is especially important in these patients.

PREDICTION OF LMCA DISEASE

It has been suggested that the presence of severe angina, calcification of the LMCA, and marked exercise-induced ST segment depression allow preangiographic prediction of LMCA disease.[20] We evaluated these parameters in our patients and found severe or unstable angina in 20 (40 percent), calcification of the LMCA in 11 (22 percent), and greater than 2 mm ST segment depression in only one of 13 (6 percent) patients. The predictive value of exercise testing in our patients might have been greater except that we continually monitored the 12-lead electrocardiogram during exercise and stopped the test as soon as diagnostic abnormalities occurred rather than continuing the exercise until a predetermined work load was completed.[16] Continuation of effort after diagnostic abnormalities are present may be dangerous and, in addition, does not discriminate between LMCA disease and widespread disease in other major coronary arteries.[17]

One of the above three features considered suggestive of LMCA disease was present in less than half of our patients. Conversely, in a group of 55 patients with unstable angina reviewed at our hospital, only two had LMCA disease.[18] Therefore, the usefulness of these parameters is limited, and each patient undergoing coronary arteriography must be approached as a patient with possible LMCA disease.

ASSOCIATED CORONARY ARTERY DISEASE

Coexisting coronary artery disease was found in three major vessels in 22 patients, in two vessels in 17, and in one vessel in nine. Isolated LMCA disease was present in only two patients (4 percent). Twenty-nine patients had associated disease of the left anterior descending coronary artery; 34 had associated disease of the left circumflex coro-

TABLE 1. Angiographic Findings

	NO. PTS.
Severity of LMCA stenosis	
50–70%	22
71–95%	28
Involvement of other coronary arteries	
None	2
1 vessel	9
2 vessels	17
3 vessels	22
LAD or LCX	45
LAD	29
LCX	34
RCA	40

nary artery and 40 had associated disease of the right coronary artery (Table 1). Forty-five of 50 patients had associated disease of either the left anterior descending or circumflex coronary arteries. The extensive coexisting disease found in our patients is not unique, as others have reported similar findings.[1,3,19]

An evaluation of the factors affecting survival must consider the effects of coexisting disease. The poor prognosis observed in patients with LMCA disease cannot be attributed solely to the LMCA lesions because multiple-vessel disease without LMCA disease carries a significant mortality. Bruschke et al [19] have shown that the long-term survival of patients with LMCA disease is no worse than patients with three-vessel disease even though most of the patients with LMCA disease also had disease of two or three major coronary arteries. Further, isolated LMCA disease is uncommon and occurred in 4 percent of our patients with LMCA disease.

The extent of coexisting disease may preclude surgery if vessels distal to stenoses are unsuitable for grafting. Each of our 50 patients were evaluated retrospectively by two investigators to determine operability by current criteria [16] *without knowledge of the therapy actually given or its outcome.* Ten of the 50 patients were judged inoperable, eight because distal vessels were unsuitable for grafting and two because of severe left ventricular dysfunction. The number of patients judged inoperable serves as another index of the severity of coexisting coronary artery disease and also identifies a group of patients who are unsuitable for inclusion in a nonsurgical group that is used to compare survival in surgical and nonsurgical patients.

Coexisting disease of the left coronary system, present in 45 to 50 patients, would amplify the effect of the LMCA stenosis because the

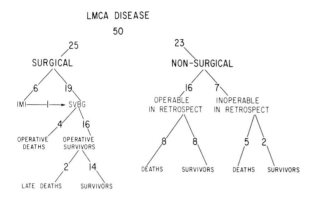

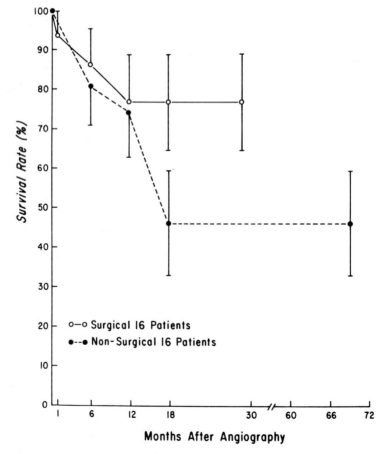

FIG. 1. The number of patients receiving each type of therapy and the number of survivors and deaths in each group are shown in this figure.

hemodynamic effects of stenosis in series are additive as shown by Gould et al, elsewhere in this volume.[21]

The reason for the frequent association of widespread disease of the coronary arteries in patients with LMCA disease is not apparent. Because most available information of survival with LMCA disease is derived from patients with severe coexisting coronary artery disease, these data may not be applicable to patients with isolated LMCA disease or those with minimal coexisting disease.

MEDICAL THERAPY

The largest number of patients with LMCA disease in whom survival has been reported without surgical therapy is a group reported by

FIG. 2. Survival curves determined by the actuarial method are shown for the nonsurgical patients who were suitable for surgery by current criteria and the surgical patients operated after 1970.

Bruschke et al.[19] An actuarially determined survival rate of 37 percent at the end of seven years was found in this group of 76 patients. This was a similar survival rate to that found in patients with three-vessel disease. No attempt was made to exclude inoperable patients, so the value of this group for comparison with surgical patients is limited. Cohen et al[1] and Lavine et al[3] reported a poor prognosis in smaller numbers of patients who were not treated with surgery. However, several of these patients were not operated on because suitable vessels for grafting were not present.

Of our 50 patients, two were lost to follow-up. Twenty-three patients in whom follow-up is available to the present time were treated without surgery for a variety of reasons including patient refusal (Fig. 1). Retrospective analysis of operability as described above shows that seven of these 23 patients were inoperable by current criteria and therefore must be excluded from the comparison of survival in surgical and nonsurgical patients. Four of the seven inoperable patients died within six months and a fifth at 18 months. The remaining 16 patients were considered operable by current criteria. Survival in this group of patients determined by the actuarial method[22] is shown in Figure 2. Eight patients died an average of 10 months following angiography. Eight are still alive after an average survival of nearly four years. The estimated survival at 18 months is 46 percent. If inoperable patients are included in the nonsurgical group, the estimated survival at 18 months is 35 percent.

SURGICAL THERAPY

Operative mortality rates for saphenous vein bypass grafting in patients with LMCA disease have varied widely. Early reports have stressed the high operative mortality rate, which, in a group of patients with both left main coronary artery

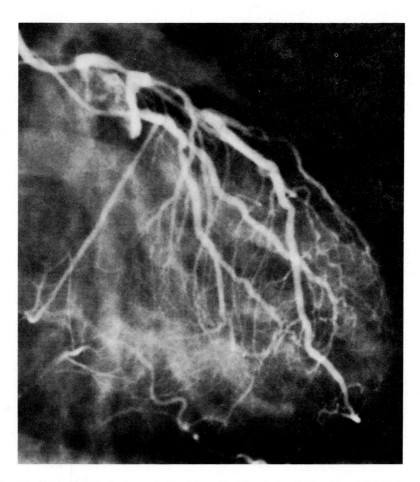

FIG. 3.   Significant disease is shown in the left main, left anterior descending, and left circumflex coronary arteries. A 60 percent stenosis was found in the right coronary artery.

disease and coexisting three-vessel disease, was 37 percent.[19] Pritchard et al[7] have reported an 8 percent mortality rate among 72 patients, and more recently Zeft et al[11] reported a 10 percent mortality rate among 56 patients. Since 1969, 26 patients have received saphenous vein bypass grafts at the University of Oregon Medical School Hospital. Four (15 percent) patients died in the perioperative period. However, three of the four deaths occurred among the first four patients encountered. Twenty-one of the last 22 patients (that is, all patients operated after 1970) have survived surgery, suggesting that the operation can be performed with low mortality (4.5 percent) at the present time.

We have analyzed the long-term effect of surgical therapy on survival by comparing the actuarially determined rate of survival in the surgical patients operated on between January 1971 and May 1973 and our nonsurgical patients, after exclusion of inoperable patients. This comparison is shown in Figure 2. Survival at 18 months in the surgical group is 77 percent and in the nonsurgical group 45 percent. Though the difference appears great, it is still not statistically significant.

FUNCTIONAL CAPACITY OF MEDICAL AND SURGICAL SURVIVORS

Functional improvement occurred in all surgical survivors; 7 of 13 patients (54 percent) are currently asymptomatic (Figs. 3 to 5). Some improvement of angina occurred in several of the

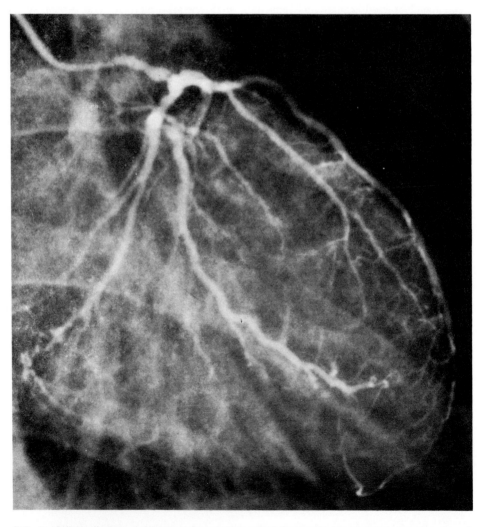

FIG. 4. Diffuse disease of the left main coronary artery frequently accompanies a severe stenosis as seen near the bifurcation in this patient.

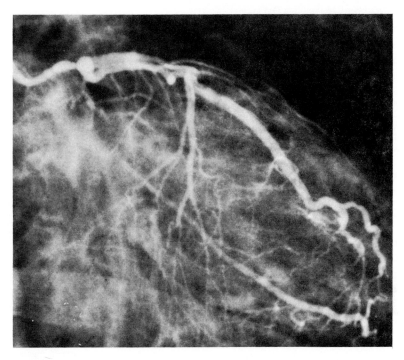

FIG. 5. This patient with a severe LMCA stenosis and significant disease of other coronary arteries is asymptomatic three years after surgery.

nonsurgical survivors, while deterioration occurred in others. None of the nonsurgical patients are free of angina.

CONCLUSIONS

We conclude that coronary arteriography can be performed with low risk even though the preangiographic prediction of the lesion is not reliable. The need for meticulous technique in performing coronary arteriography is important in all patients. Isolated LMCA disease is uncommon or commonly asymptomatic. In symptomatic patients with LMCA disease, the degree and extent of coexisting disease accounts for a significant percentage of patients (20 percent) who are inoperable and also must have an important influence on the natural history of such patients. The survival rate of patients with operable LMCA disease without surgical intervention is poor (46 percent at 18 months) and resembles that of other patients with extensive coronary artery disease. The operative mortality rate at this time is similar to other patients with extensive coronary artery disease and may be as low as 5 percent. Survival of operated patients is 77 percent at 18 months. Although the difference in survival appears large,

it is not yet statistically significant, and more follow-up is required. With medical therapy alone, some patients improve and others deteriorate; none are asymptomatic. Following surgery all patients were functionally improved and more than half were asymptomatic.

References

1. Cohen MV, Cohn PF, Herman MV, Gorlin R: Diagnosis of left main coronary obstruction. Circulation 45:II–57, 1972
2. Proudfit WL, Shirey EK, Sones FM Jr: Distribution of arterial lesions demonstrated by selective cine coronary arteriography. Circulation 36:54, 1967
3. Lavine P, Kimbiris D, Segal BL, Linhart JW: Left main coronary artery disease, clinical arteriographic and hemodynamic appraisal. Am J Cardiol 30:791, 1972
4. Wolfson S, Grant D, Ross Allan M, Colton LS: Risk of death related to coronary arteriography: role of left coronary lesions. (Abstract) Circulation 48:4–88, 1973
5. Sones FM Jr, Shirey EK: Cine coronary arteriography. Mod Concepts Cardiovasc Dis 31:735, 1962
6. Judkins MP: Selective coronary arteriography: I, a percutaneous transfemoral technic. Radiology 89:815, 1967
7. Pichard AD, Sheldon WC, Shinji K, Effler DB, Sones FM Jr: Severe atherosclerotic obstruction of the left main coronary artery: followup results in 176 patients. (Abstract) Circulation 48:4–53, 1973
8. Scanlon PJ, Talano JV, Moran JF, et al: Left main coronary artery disease, II. In Coronary Artery

Medicine and Surgery (Norman JC ed), NY, Apple-ton-Century-Crofts, 1975, pp 751–55

9. Sharma S, Khaja F, Heinle R, Goldstein S, Easley R: Left main coronary artery lesions: risk of catheterization, exercise test and surgery (Abstract) Circulation 48:4–53, 1973

10. Kisslo J, Peter R, Behar V, Barter A, Kong Y: Left main coronary artery stenosis. (Abstract) Circulation 48:4–57, 1973

11. Zeft HJ, Manley JC, Huston JH, Tector AJ, Auen JE, Johnson WD: Left main coronary artery stenosis: results of coronary bypass surgery. Circulation 49:68, 1974

12. May AG, DeWeese TA, Rob CG: Hemodynamic effects of arterial stenosis. Surgery 53:513, 1963

13. Brice JG, Dowsett DJ, Lowe RD: Hemodynamic effects of carotid artery stenosis. Br Med J 2:1363, 1964

14. Rosch J, DeMots H, Antonovic R, Rahimtoola SH, Judkins MP, Dotter CT: Coronary arteriography in left main coronary artery disease. Am J Roentgenol Radium Ther Nucl Med 121:583, 1974

15. Bassan MM, Ganz W, Marcus HS: Effect of left coronary artery catheterization on coronary blood flow. (Abstract) Circulation 48:4–142, 1973

16. Kassebaum DG, Sutherland KI, Judkins MP: A comparison of hypoxemia and exercise electrocardiography in coronary artery disease. Am Heart J 75:759, 1968

17. Cohn PR, Vokonas PS, Most AS, Herman MV, Gorlin R: The diagnostic accuracy of the two-step postexercise electrocardiogram: results in 305 subsets studied by coronary arteriography. JAMA 220:501, 1972

18. Rahimtoola SH, Bonchek LI, Anderson RP, Starr A, Bristow JD: Unstable angina: extended follow-up (1–4 years) after urgent bypass operation. (Abstract) Am J Cardiol 33:174, 1974

19. Bruschke AVG, Proudfit WL, Sones FM: Progress study of 590 consecutive non-surgical cases of coronary disease followed 5–9 years: I arteriographic correlations. Circulation 47:1147, 1973

20. Rosch J, Dotter CT, Antonovic R, Bonchek LI, Starr A: Angiographic appraisal of distal vessel suitability for aortocoronary bypass graft surgery. Circulation 48:202, 1973

21. Gould L, Lipscomb K: Hemodynamics of coronary stenosis, part I: coronary flow reserve as a scriptor of the effects of stenoses on coronary pressure-flow relationships. Symposium on Coronary Artery Medicine and Surgery of the Texas Heart Institute, Houston, Feb 21–23, 1974

22. Cutler SJ, Ederer F: Maximum utilization of life table method in analyzing survival. J Chronic Dis 8:699, 1958

92

LEFT MAIN CORONARY ARTERY DISEASE, II

PATRICK J. SCANLON, JAMES V. TALANO, JOHN F. MORAN,
RIMGAUDAS NEMICKAS, ROLF M. GUNNAR, and ROQUE PIFARRE

The left main coronary artery (LMC) supplies branches to the free wall and apex of the left ventricle and to the interventricular septum. Significant obstruction of this vessel is associated with severe angina, massive myocardial infarction, and sudden death.

Although there are numerous potential causes of obstruction of the LMC, atherosclerosis is by far the most common (Friedberg, 1966). In an analysis of coronary angiograms in 627 patients with 30 percent obstruction of at least one coronary artery, Proudfit et al, 1967, found that 72 patients (11.5 percent) had LMC obstruction of variable degree. In most cases disease in this artery is associated with severe disease of the other major coronary vessels, although occasionally the LMC alone is obstructed by atherosclerosis. Coronary ostial obstruction can occur from other causes. Scharfman et al, 1950, found that 17 percent of patients with syphilitic aortitis, now a rare entity, have ostial narrowing. Enos et al, 1963, reported that arteriosclerosis of the aortic sinuses of Valsalva can result in partial or complete obstruction of the coronary ostia, especially the right coronary.

Angina is the predominant symptom in 90 percent of patients with obstruction of the LMC. Lavine et al, 1972, noted that 47 percent of their 30 patients with LMC disease had a history of acceleration of anginal symptoms during the six months preceding coronary arteriography. Cohen et al, 1972, reported that 38 percent of their 29 patients with angina had dyspnea as a significant symptom. A history of previous myocardial infarction is reported in about 50 percent of patients. Physical findings are nonspecific, with an audible fourth heart sound the most common auscultatory abnormality. Evidence of congestive heart failure is not uncommon.

Resting electrocardiograms often show ischemic ST–T-wave changes and/or old myocardial infarction, although not uncommonly they are normal. Exercise electrocardiograms almost always are normal. Cohen et al found that 14 of 17 patients had greater than 2 mm of ST segmental depression with the double Master's test and suggested that with this finding either LMC disease or proximal disease of all three major coronary arteries is suspect.

Cardiac catheterization frequently demonstrates hemodynamic abnormalities suggestive of left ventricular dysfunction. Cohen et al, 1972, found no correlation between severity of the LMC disease and abnormal hemodynamics.

Coronary arteriography generally reveals significant disease of several coronary vessels. The right coronary artery has 75 percent or more obstruction in the majority of patients. Total obstruction of the LMC artery is rare; such patients appear to survive on the basis of right-to-left collateral circulation. Evidence of intercoronary collaterals is present in about two-thirds of all patients with LMC disease. Calcification of the LMC artery is seen fluoroscopically in about 75 percent of patients. Left ventricular angiography reveals abnormality of left ventricular contraction in approximately 75 percent of patients.

Early studies showed that coronary arteriography was performed at a 10 to 16 percent mortality risk in patients with LMC disease. However Pichard et al, 1973, reported only one death associated with catheterization of 176 patients; several other more recent reports have substantiated a risk of approximately 1 to 2 percent. Though the risk of study appears to be increased in these patients, careful attention to proper coronary angiographic technique should result in an acceptably low mortality for the procedure in relation to the serious nature of the entity itself.

There have been no studies regarding the natural history of LMC disease. Most reports relating to medical versus surgical therapy have been uncontrolled. Pichard et al, 1973, reported one-, two-, and three-year survivals of 88 percent, 83 percent, and 76 percent in 48 patients treated medically. Most other reports suggest that two-year survival is approximately 50 percent for medically treated patients. DeMots et al, 1974, found that, of 16 patients judged operable but treated without surgery, eight died within 18 months, whereas six of 10 patients judged inoperable were dead within 16 months.

Early surgical reports related experience with various techniques for LMC disease. Beck et al, 1965, and Sabiston et al, 1965, reported cases of ostial obstruction of the LMC successfully treated by transaortic proximal coronary endarterectomy. Effler et al, 1965, reported 10 cases of LCA disease treated by endarterectomy and patch graft reconstruction; five died at surgery. Three other patients had transluminal dilation of the proximal left coronary artery, and all survived. Favaloro et al, 1970, stated that the in-hospital mortality rate at the Cleveland Clinic for double internal mammary artery implantation for LCA disease was 23.5 percent.

Since 1967, saphenous vein bypass has been the primary surgical technique for coronary disease. Recent reports suggest a lower follow-up mortality rate for patients treated with coronary bypass than for medically treated patients. Pichard et al reported an in-hospital mortality of 8.2 percent and a three-year survival of 90 percent for 73 patients who had bypass surgery at the Cleveland Clinic. Lavine et al, 1972, had two deaths among 18 patients who had bypass surgery. DeMots et al, 1974, had one operative death and two late deaths among 16 bypassed patients. Other reports have been less optimistic, with surgical mortalities of 30 percent (Sharma et al, 1973), 25 percent (Kisslo et al, 1973), and 22 percent (Cohen et al, 1972).

In general, most authors now recommend bypass surgery, if possible, for symptomatic patients with significant LMC disease. Follow-up data shows significant symptomatic improvement in surgical survivors compared to patients treated medically. Pichard et al, 1973, noted that angina persisted in 89 percent of medical survivors (25 of 28), but in only 28 percent of bypass survivors (16 of 64). It has not been determined whether surgery decreases the probability of late myocardial infarction.

PRESENTATION OF AUTHORS' DATA

From January 1, 1970 to September 1, 1973, a total of 1,178 patients with coronary artery disease were studied by coronary arteriography at the Loyola University Medical Center. Of these, 76 patients were found to have > 50 percent narrowing of the left main coronary artery. Sixty-three were male and 13 were female. The mean age was 54 years (range 35 to 72 years). Eleven patients were 45 years or under.

Precatheterization, a chest x-ray, resting electrocardiogram, SMA–12, cholesterol determination, CPK, SGOT, and LDH were obtained in all patients. Triglyceride levels and lipoprotein typings were obtained in 50 patients. Patients presenting with a syndrome of preinfarction angina prior to catheterization and angiography were usually admitted to the coronary care unit and treated with coronary vasodilators, sedation, anticoagulants, and beta adrenergic blocking agents. Once the presence of a recent myocardial infarction was excluded, these patients were referred for catheterization and coronary arteriography. Two patients developed a myocardial infarction prior to catheterization; however, their clinical picture was so unstable that catheterization and cardiovascular surgery were felt to be necessary for survival. One of these patients had a postmyocardial infarction ventricular septal defect with refractory congestive failure. The other had refractory left ventricular failure following a myocardial infarction, in addition to moderate aortic insufficiency secondary to an earlier dissection of the aorta.

CATHETERIZATION STUDIES

Right heart catheterizations were performed on 75 patients. Left heart catheterization, left ventriculography, and coronary arteriography were done in all 76 patients. Coronary arteriography was performed by the Sones technique in 68 patients, the Judkins technique in seven patients, and both techniques in one. Cardiac outputs were determined by either Fick or dye dilution technique. Ventriculograms were performed in the 30-degree right anterior oblique projection using 40 to 50 cc of contrast material (Renografin 76). When a ventricular aneurysm was present, a second ventriculogram in the left anterior oblique projection was often performed. The coronary vessels that were evaluated were the left main coronary artery, the left anterior descending, the circumflex, the first diagonal, the obtuse marginal, and the right coronary artery. Narrowing of the left main vessel of > 50 percent and 75 percent or greater of the other coronary vessels was considered significant. Each vessel was evaluated for location of obstructing lesions, size of the distal vessel, and whether the obstructed vessels were, by angiographic criteria, bypassable. Based on coronary arteriography the patient was considered operable or nonoperable.

Sixty-seven patients were considered operable by angiography, of whom 53 patients went to surgery. A single bypass was performed in 14 patients, double bypass in 26 patients, triple bypass in 10 patients, and single bypass and endarterectomy in three patients. Aneurysm resection was performed in two patients, infarctectomy in two patients, and a postinfarction ventricular septal defect was repaired in one. During the first year of the study period, four patients had internal mammary artery implants in addition to bypass procedures. In these 53 patients, with 106 significantly obstructed vessels considered bypassable, 99 (93 percent) were actually bypassed.

Follow-up data were obtained through January 1974 from hospital records, contact with referring physicians, and personal patient contact. The mean follow-up period was 18 months with a range of four to 45 months.

RESULTS

The presenting clinical systems were typical angina pectoris in 71 patients (93 percent) and dyspnea on exertion without typical angina in five patients (7 percent). A history of previous myocardial infarction was present in 41 patients (54 percent), of congestive heart failure in 16 patients (20 percent) and of valvular heart disease in three patients (4 percent).

Of the 71 patients presenting with angina, the mean duration of angina was 46 months, ranging from one day to 15 years. Three patients presented with their first symptom of angina one day prior to admission. The anginal pattern was of a stable nature in 38 patients. In 33 patients (43 percent) a clinical picture of preinfarction angina was present. Preinfarction angina was defined as a progressive increase in the severity, duration, and frequency of anginal attacks, frequently associated with rest pain, without electrocardiographic or enzymatic changes of myocardial infarction. The mean duration of preinfarction angina was 3.9 weeks (range, 1 day to 12 weeks).

The risk factors associated with coronary atherosclerosis were found in a high percentage of patients. A history of cigarette smoking of at least one package per day up to 30 days prior to hospitalization was present in 51 patients (67 percent) and a cholesterol greater than 250 mg percent was present in 43 patients (57 percent). Twenty-nine (58 percent) of 50 patients tested had a triglyceride level greater than 200 mg percent. Family history of coronary artery disease was present in 39 patients (51 percent). A history of hypertension was present in 23 patients (30 percent) and diabetes mellitus in six patients (8 percent).

Physical findings in general were nonspecific. There was clinical evidence of congestive heart failure in 17 patients. The heart was normal by chest x-ray in 52 patients (69 percent). Cardiomegaly was present in 23 patients (31 percent). Only two patients had evidence of pulmonary venous congestion on x-ray.

The resting electrocardiogram on the day prior to catheterization was normal in eight patients. In 44 patients (56 percent) old myocardial infarction was present, and two patients had a recent infarction. Location of infarction was inferior in 20 patients, anteroseptal in 14, anterior in six, and true posterior in six. Left ventricular hypertrophy was diagnosed in 23 patients (32 percent), and left atrial enlargement in 14 (18 percent). Conduction abnormalities were present in 24 electrocardiograms. The most common abnormality was left axis deviation, which was present in 10 cases; 1 degree AV block occurred in seven, left bundle branch block in three, right bundle branch block in one, left posterior hemiblock in one, and interventricular conduction delay in two.

RESULTS OF CATHETERIZATION

Table 1 shows the frequency of involvement of the various major coronary vessels. Five patients had isolated left main coronary obstruction. In two-thirds of all the patients three or more other

TABLE 1. Frequency of Coronary Artery Involvement

VESSEL	NO. PTS.
Left main	76
RCA	61
LAD	57
Circ.	38
First diagonal	29
Obtuse marginal	23

coronary vessels were also significantly narrowed. Total obstruction of the left main coronary was seen in two patients. Calcification of the left main coronary artery was visible fluoroscopically in 18 patients (24 percent). Intercoronary collaterals were present in 51 patients. Of 178 major vessels with greater than 75 percent narrowing, 154 (81 percent) were judged bypassable by angiography.

Abnormalities of left ventricular contraction were noted in 63 patients and were considered major in 50. Diffuse hypokinesis was present in 26 patients, segmental hypokinesis in six, and ventricular asynergy in 16. Fourteen patients had a ventricular aneurysm, and one patient had a post-myocardial infarction ventricular septal defect. The mean ejection fraction was found to be 0.44 ± 0.03.

Left ventricular function as assessed hemodynamically was abnormal for the group as a whole. Mean left ventricular end-diastolic pressure (LVEDP) was 14.9 ± 1.0 mm Hg. Mean cardiac index was 2.56 ± 0.08 L/min/m². Estimated cardiac work, determined from the product of cardiac index and mean aortic pressure, was 250 ± 10 units, and mean stroke index was 32 ± 1 cc/beat/m².

One patient died at catheterization; two developed ventricular fibrillation and were successfully resuscitated. One patient developed a cerebral vascular accident. No major complications occurred at catheterization in 72 patients, or 95 percent. Within 24 hours after catheterization two patients sustained a myocardial infarction after uneventful catheterization. One subsequently died. Another patient died suddenly 18 hours after uneventful catheterization, presumably due to a ventricular aneurysm.

RESULTS OF SURGERY

Six of 53 patients (11 percent) died in the hospital following surgery. Eight postoperative myocardial infarctions developed. There were three late deaths in the surgical patients during the follow-up period, for a total mortality of 17 percent. One patient developed a myocardial infarction 14 months postoperatively. Of 44 surgical survivors, 32 (73 percent) are angina free. Nine patients have occasional angina, two continue to have severe angina, and one remains in congestive failure. Ninety-three percent of the survivors, or 78 percent of all patients going to have surgery, have subjective improvement of their symptoms.

MEDICAL PATIENTS

Of 23 patients followed medically, 14 were considered operable but for various reasons did not have surgery. Six deaths were recorded in this group (for a mortality of 43 percent). Two late myocardial infarctions occurred. Nine patients were considered inoperable by angiography; of these five died (56 percent) and one had a late infarction. In all, 48 percent of patients medically treated have died. Of the 12 patients surviving, moderate to severe angina exists in eight. The symptoms were unchanged or worsened in 83 percent. Of all 23 patients treated medically only two are improved.

Thirty-three patients presented with preinfarction angina. Twenty-four patients were bypassed with three postoperative deaths, a 12.5 percent mortality. There were two late deaths for a total surgical mortality of 21 percent. Of nine patients treated medically five have died during the follow-up period for a mortality of 56 percent.

ANALYSIS

Our patients with LMC disease presented with symptoms and findings similar to those reported by others. We could derive no specific clinical factor that might be predictive for LMC obstruction. We did find that clinical evidence of congestive heart failure carried definite prognostic risk. Of six patients with failure who went to surgery, four died, compared to only five deaths among 47 surgical patients without failure (p < 0.01). Nine of 11 medically treated patients with failure have succumbed, compared to only two of 12 without failure (p < 0.01). Patients with preinfarction angina had somewhat higher mortality rates surgically and medically than did the more stable patients, but the differences were not significant.

The surgical patients could be divided into three groups based on the number of coronary vessels involved. All five patients with isolated LMC disease, and all but one of 24 patients with LMC plus three vessel disease, survived surgery. Interestingly, the intermediate group, those with LMC plus one- or two-vessel disease, did significantly worse than those with three-vessel disease, in that eight of 24 died (p < 0.01).

**TABLE 2. Hemodynamic Risk Factors
(Scanlon et al, 1973)**

1. LVEDP > 12 mm Hg
2. Cardiac index < 2.7L/minute/m^2
3. Stroke index < 35 ml/beat/m^2
4. Cardiac work < 240 units
5. Ejection fraction < 50%

Perhaps of importance was that 83 percent of patients with three-vessel disease had collaterals, whereas only 50 percent of these with one- or two-vessel disease had collaterals. However, there was no significant difference, either surgically or medically, between patients with and without collateral circulation, when evaluated without reference to the number of vessels involved. It is difficult to understand why patients with fewer lesions should do worse surgically than those with more diffuse disease.

In another study we found there were five hemodynamic risk factors (Table 2) for patients with preinfarction angina (Scanlon, 1973). Analysis of these factors in the present group of patients revealed that deaths were more common in patients with any specific hemodynamic abnormality, both surgically and medically, but significant risks were found only for surgical patients with an estimated cardiac work (mean aortic pressure x cardiac index) of less than 240 units ($p < 0.05$), and for total groups of patients with low cardiac work ($p < 0.05$), or cardiac index < 2.7 liters/min/m^2 ($p < 0.05$). When patients with four or more hemodynamic risks were compared to those with fewer than four, mortality for the former group was significantly higher surgically, medically, and all together (Table 3).

**TABLE 3. Mortality versus
Multiple Hemodynamic Risks**

	<4 RISKS			4 OR MORE RISKS			
	Pts.	Died	%	Pts.	Died	%	P
Surg.	38	3	8	13	5	38	<0.01
No Surg.	10	2	20	12	8	67	<0.05
Total	48	5	10	25	13	52	<0.001

There was a relationship between the degree of revascularization and the surgical mortality. Of 19 patients with bypass of all obstructed vessels, only one died (5.3 percent), while 8 of 34 patients with incomplete revascularization succumbed (24 percent).

It is concluded that LMC disease is associated with a high risk of myocardial infarction and/or early death. Properly selected patients, based on clinical, arteriographic, and hemodynamic factors, appear to do well surgically, with relatively low mortality and with substantial subjective improvement. To insure maximum benefit from surgery, all obstructed vessels should be bypassed if possible.

References

Beck W, Barnard CN, Schrire V: Syphilitic obstruction of coronary ostia successfully treated by endarterectomy. Br Heart J 27:911, 1965

Cohen MV, Cohn PF, Herman MV, Gorlin R: Diagnosis and prognosis of main left coronary artery obstruction. Circulation 45 (Suppl I):57, 1972

DeMots H, Rösch J, Bonchek LI, et al: Survival in left main coronary artery disease: the role of coronary angiography, coexisting coronary artery disease, and revascularization. Am J Cardiol 33:134, 1974

Effler DB, Sones FM Jr, Favaloro RG, Groves LK: Coronary endarterectomy with patch graft reconstruction: clinical experience with 34 cases. Ann Surg 162:590, 1965

Enos WF, Beyer JC, Holmes RH: Arteriosclerosis of the aortic sinuses. Am J Clin Path 39:506, 1963

Favaloro RG, Effler DB, Groves LK, et al: Severe segmental obstruction of the left main coronary artery and its divisions. J Thorac Cardiovasc Surg 60:469, 1970

Friedberg CK: Diseases of the Heart. Philadelphia, Saunders, 1966

Kisslo J, Peter R, Behar V, Bartel A, Kong Y: Left main coronary artery stenosis. Circulation 48 (Suppl 4): 223, 1973

Lavine P, Kimbiris D, Segal BL, Linhart JW: Left main coronary artery disease. Am J Cardiol 30:791, 1972

Pichard AD, Sheldon WC, Shinji J, Effler DB, Sones FM Jr: Severe arteriosclerotic obstruction of the left main coronary artery: follow-up results in 176 patients. Circulation 48 (Suppl 4):53, 1973

Proudfit WL, Shirey EK, Sones FM Jr: Distribution of arterial lesions demonstrated by selective cine-coronary arteriography. Circulation 36:54, 1967

Sabiston DC, Ebert PA, Friesinger GC, Ross RS, Sinclair-Smith B: Proximal endarterectomy, arterial reconstruction for coronary occlusion at aortic origin. Arch Surg 91:758, 1965

Scanlon PJ, Nemickas R, Moran JF, et al: Accelerated angina pectoris: clinical, hemodynamic, arteriographic, and therapeutic experience in 85 patients. Circulation 47:19, 1973

Scharfman WB, Wallach JB, Angrist A: Myocardial infarction due to syphilitic coronary ostial stenosis. Am Heart J 40:603, 1950

Sharma S, Khaja F, Heinle R, Goldstein S, Easley R: Left main coronary artery lesions: risk of catheterization, exercise test, and surgery, Circulation 48 (Suppl 4):53, 1973

93

REDUCED MORTALITY FOLLOWING REVASCULARIZATION SURGERY FOR LEFT MAIN CORONARY ARTERY STENOSIS

Lawrence H. Cohn and John J. Collins, Jr.

INTRODUCTION

Documented lesions of the main left coronary artery (LCA) have been generally associated with a poor prognosis if treated by medical measures alone. [4,10-12] Since the LCA supplies the major portion of blood to the ventricular septum, left ventricular free wall, apex, and a portion of the inferior aspect of the left ventricle, occlusion of this vessel is often catastrophic. Clinical experience with the surgical treatment of LCA lesions since 1970 has indicated that an aggressive and organized therapeutic approach may reduce the mortality of patients with this lesion.

CLINICAL MATERIAL

From July 1970 to July 1973, there were 290 patients who underwent operations for ischemic heart disease in the Cardiac Surgical Service at the Peter Bent Brigham Hospital. Thirty-eight patients (13 percent) were operated upon with the diagnosis of significant obstructive lesion of the LCA greater than 70 percent. There were five females and 33 males ranging in age from 27 to 67, averaging 53 years. All but one of the patients had a history of disabling angina pectoris. This patient, a 51-year-old asymptomatic executive, was found to have > 4 mm depression of precordial ST segments on electrocardiogram after repeated treadmill exercise testing. Four patients had signs and symptoms of moderately severe left ventricular failure in addition to severe angina pectoris. Previous myocardial infarction

was noted in 20 patients. One patient had associated valvular disease that necessitated simultaneous double-valve replacement. One patient had received an aortic valve three months prior to a second operation. Twelve patients presented with the syndrome of "preinfarction" angina with electrocardiographic changes of precordial ischemia (inverted T-waves) without enzyme or electrocardiographic evidence of a myocardial infarction.

Stress electrocardiography was carried out in 32 patients. In 23 patients (72 percent), a positive exercise test (> 2 mm depression in ST segment) was noted, comparable to the incidence of positive tests in other series [16] (Fig. 1).

Cardiac catheterization, selective coronary angiography, and left ventriculography were carried out in every patient. In 23 patients the LCA obstruction was subtotal (> 90 percent) (Fig. 2), and in 15 patients the obstruction was > 70 percent. Positive exercise tests were noted in every patient with > 90 percent obstruction. Multiple coronary lesions were found in 35 of 40 patients; five patients had only isolated LCA stenosis. Left ventricular hemodynamics and an estimation of left ventricular wall motion indicated that two patients had distinctly abnormal ventricular function with biplane systolic ejection fractions of 25 percent. Two other patients had reasonable ventricular function at catheterization but developed severe depression of ventricular function with the onset of acute coronary occlusion and left ventricular power failure.

Patients with preinfarction angina (12) or acute myocardial infarction and left ventricular power failure (2) were taken directly from the catheterization laboratory, or the area where the acute myocardial infarction developed, to the operating room for emergency operation.

FIG. 1. Electrocardiographic response to a double Master's test in a patient with an isolated 80 percent stenosis of the main LCA. The resting control ECG demonstrates slightly abnormal ST segments. Immediately after (p) exercise, there is obvious 3 to 4 mm R-ST-segmental depression. Ten minutes after administration of TNG (nitroglycerin), 0.3 mg sublingually, the ECG has returned to baseline. (Reproduced with the permission of Cohen et al from Circulation 45:(Suppl 1) 57, 1972.)

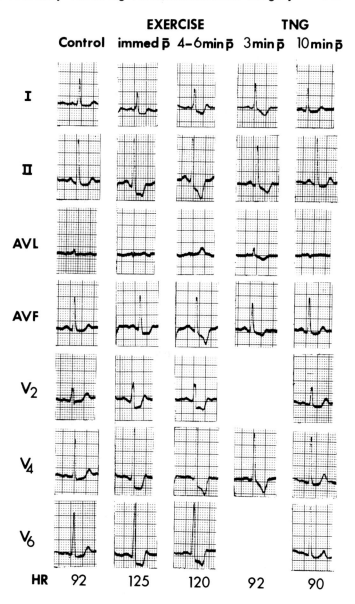

OPERATIVE TECHNIQUE

Operations were carried out with cardiopulmonary bypass, complete hemodilution in a disposable oxygenator, and moderate hypothermia. The prime was composed of 1800 ml lactated Ringer's solution, 200 ml albumin, and 50 ml dextrose to simulate the oncotic pressure of plasma. Phlebotomy and autologous transfusion, ordinarily used in our elective operations, were not used in this precarious patient group. This simple perfusion setup without blood allows for institution of urgent operations without waiting for

blood to be cross-matched.[7] The pump oxygenator is primed and standing by prior to induction of anesthesia.

After total intrathoracic cannulations, the heart is fibrillated electrically, the left ventricle vented, and the left anterior descending coronary artery (LAD) encircled using Silastic® elastomer tapes (Fig. 3), or the aorta is cross-clamped if collateral circulation is excessive and venoarterial anastomosis is carried out as shown. The left internal mammary artery is our vessel of choice for elective LAD bypass and has been used in more than 125 patients undergoing elective coronary revascularization. In this series, four patients had LAD bypass by the left internal mam-

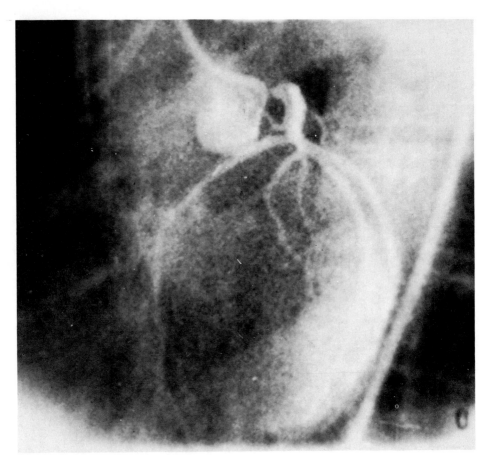

FIG. 2. Left anterior oblique projection after dye injection into the left coronary system demonstrating an 80 to 85 percent ostial narrowing. (Reproduced with the permission of Cohen et al from Circulation 45:(Suppl 1) 57, 1972.)

mary artery. The saphenous vein graft is preferred as a bypass vessel in the emergency cases because the patient's condition is often precarious and may not tolerate the slightly increased operative time associated with the takedown of the left internal mammary artery. Following completion of the anastomosis, the heart is defibrillated, the left ventricular vent is removed, and the patient is weaned off cardiopulmonary bypass utilizing left atrial pressure monitoring if indicated.

The operative procedures are listed in Table 1. Five patients had single bypass grafts to the LAD, 10 patients had grafts to the LAD and left circumflex coronary artery (LCF), 16 patients had LAD and right coronary artery (RCA) grafts, and seven patients had grafts to the LAD, LCF, and RCA. Distal endarterectomy was performed in 13 patients (12 RCA and one LAD). In all, there were 78 grafts in the 38 patients. Currently,

our treatment of choice would be a graft to the LAD and LCF because of the possibility of the progression of the proximal LCA lesion extending to one or the other branch of the LCA after bypass grafting.[2] Concomitant ventricular resection for left ventricular aneurysms was performed in two patients.

TABLE 1. Operative Procedures

Single graft	5
Double graft	26
Triple graft	7
Internal mammary to LAD bypass	4
Endarterectomy	
LAD	1
RCA	12
Ventricular resection	2
Valve replacement	2

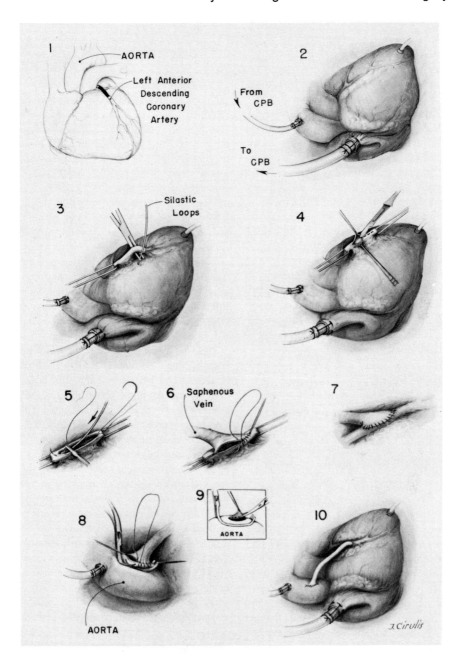

FIG. 3. Cardiopulmonary bypass is established through intrathoracic cannulations and the left ventricle is decompressed via a left ventricular sump catheter (1, 2). The left anterior descending coronary is encircled with Silastic® elastomers without dissecting up the coronary (3). A 0.5–1.0 centimeter incision is made (4). A 6.0 Prolene® suture 36″ long is placed at either apex (5) and the saphenous vein anastomosed by running the sutures down both sides of the arteriotomy (6, 7). The side of the aorta is partially occluded with a Dale® peripheral vascular clamp (8) after a button of aorta is removed (insert, 9). The graft is tailored to loop over the right ventricular outflow tract (1), by occluding the venous return line and distending the right heart momentarily. Note the right-angle takeoff of the aortovenous anastomosis in (10). (Reproduced with the permission of Cohn, from The Surgical Treatment of Acute Myocardial Ischemia, Mount Kisco, NY, Futura Publishing Company, 1974.)

RESULTS

The operative and postoperative results on the 38 patients are summarized in Table 2. There were three operative deaths, for a mortality of 8.0 percent. Two of the three deaths were in patients operated on for LCA disease following acute myocardial infarction with left ventricular power failure. One patient sustained a catheter embolus during coronary angiography and died despite revascularization within two hours of the incident. A second death occurred early in our experience when a patient with LCA stenosis and preinfarction angina was allowed to wait in the hospital four days after catheterization for surgery. The day prior to surgery he collapsed, suffering an acute myocardial infarction, and surgical revascularization was to no avail. The third death occurred because of a massive intraoperative infarction, probably on the basis of poor intercoronary collateralization.

TABLE 2. Postoperative Mortality

INDICATIONS	OP. DEATH	LATE DEATH
PIA	12	0	0
LVPF	2	2	–
Angina	24	1	2
Total	38	3 (8%)	2 (8%)

There have been two late deaths (8.0 percent) in the follow-up period of seven to 42 months (average 18) (Table 3). One patient died of a cerebrovascular accident, and the other had an acute myocardial infarction associated with saphenous vein graft occlusion. Angina has been relieved in 28 patients and is recurrent to a moderate degree in four patients. There was no improvement in one patient, whose LAD graft closed and whose LCF graft remained open. Six patients have been restudied by angiography; three patients had multiple grafts that were patent, one had both grafts open, but progression in the RCA requiring reoperation, and two patients had one of two grafts occluded, one of whom was reoperated upon.

TABLE 3. Clinical Results (7 – 42 Mo. $\overline{18}$)

	NO.	%
Excellent	28	85
Good	4	12
Poor	1	3

DISCUSSION

The incidence of lesions of the LCA is about 10 percent of all significant coronary arterial obstructions by angiography.[12,13] The report by Cohen and coworkers[4] initially stimulated an awareness of the seriousness of LCA lesions during diagnostic and therapeutic maneuvers. In their report, five of 32 patients died during selective injection of the LCA. Lavine et al[11] also documented a 10 percent mortality after catheter studies of the LCA. Since then, modifications in catheter technique have evolved, and this procedure can now be performed with little increased risk over injection of other coronary arteries. With intentional subselective injections using the Judkins technique, the catheterization mortality has fallen to 2.4 percent (1/41).[5] Other groups have also reported improved results and a decreased risk of LCA catheterization.[9,10,12,15]

The medical treatment of LCA stenosis has been documented in only a relatively small number of series. The long-term follow-up, however, indicates from our hospital's experience and that of others[4,5,9,12,14] that medically treated patients with this lesion have a high yearly attrition rate. For example, medical treatment of 10 of 32 patients reported originally by Cohen et al,[4] was associated with a mortality of 50 percent during the first two years of follow-up. In an updated follow-up from this group, actuarial analysis indicates a mortality of 18.8 percent per year over the first four years of follow-up.[5] Medical treatment in 48 patients followed one and one-half years to nine years at the Cleveland Clinic[12] was associated with a mortality of 24 percent at the end of three years. De Mots et al[9] reported a mortality of 54 percent within 1.5 years in their medically treated series of documented LCA stenosis. Medical follow-up of LCA disease with preinfarction angina has substantiated the lethality of this combination. Scanlon and coworkers[14] reported a hospital mortality of 57 percent in these patients similar to the results of Battock et al.[1]

Although the surgical treatment of LCA stenosis carries a slightly higher risk than elective coronary revascularization, the follow-up results in our series and others would appear to be improved over those results obtained by medical treatment alone.[6] While elective coronary revascularization carries a 2 to 3 percent risk in our institution[8] and others,[3] the mortality in this group of 38 patients was 7.9 percent. This compares to the Cleveland Clinic mortality rate of 8.2 percent[12] and that of Johnson and associates of 10.7 percent.[16] Two of the deaths in our series occurred in patients who had evolving acute myocardial infarction with left ventricular power failure. Mortality in the emergency group was 2/14 or 14 percent, but only 1/26 (4 percent) in the group who did not have preinfarction angina or left ventricular power failure.

The precarious state of many of these patients with this lesion, particularly after cardiac catheterization, has prompted us to advise operation within 48 hours or less to patients with this diagnosis because it is often not possible to predict which patient may have surgery delayed. If the patient presents with preinfarction angina or left ventricular power failure, the operating room is set up ahead of the scheduled cardiac catheterization and the patient is taken from the catheterization laboratory to the operating room for the revascularization procedure following angiography.

Operative techniques such as hemodilution and intrathoracic cannulation that speed up operations and allow for initiation of operations without delay have also aided immeasurably in reducing mortality from this serious arteriosclerotic obstruction.

SUMMARY

Left main coronary lesions were diagnosed by angiography and treated by coronary revascularization in 38 patients. The operative mortality was 8.0 percent, and late mortality was 8.0 percent followed from 7 to 42 months, averaging 18 months. The data suggest that early revascularization of LCA lesions will result in a lower mortality and morbidity than medical treatment alone.

References

1. Battock DJ, Steele PP, Davies H: Left main coronary artery disease—is surgery always indicated? Am J Cardiol 33:125, 1974

2. Bousvaros G, Piracha AP, Chaudhry MA, et al: Increase in severity of proximal coronary disease after successful distal aortocoronary grafts. Circulation 46:870, 1972

3. Cheanvechai C, Effler DB, Groves LK, et al: Triple bypass graft for treatment of severe triple coronary vessel disease. Ann Thorac Surg 17:545, 1974

4. Cohen MV, Cohn PF, Herman MV, Gorlin R: Diagnosis and prognosis of main left coronary artery obstruction. Circulation 45, Suppl 1:57 1972

5. Cohen MV, Gorlin R: Main left coronary artery disease: clinical experience, 1964–1973. Chest, 1975 (in press)

6. Cohn LH: The Surgical Treatment of Acute Myocardial Ischemia. Mount Kisco, NY, Futura Publishing Co, 1974

7. Cohn LH, Fosberg AM, Anderson W, Collins JJ: Decreased blood utilization in open-heart surgery. In preparation

8. Collins JJ Jr, Cohn, LH Sonnenblick EH, et al: Determinants of survival following coronary revascularization. Circulation 47–48, Suppl 3:132, 1973

9. De Mots H, Rosch J, Bonchek L, Anderson R, Starr A: Survival in left main coronary artery disease; the role of coronary angiography, coexisting coronary artery disease, and revascularization. Am J Cardiol 33:134, 1974

10. Kislo J, Peter R, Behar V, Bartel A, Kong Y: Left main coronary artery stenosis. Circulation 48, Suppl 4:53, 1973

11. Lavine P, Kimbus D, Segal BL, Linhart JW: Left main coronary artery disease: clinical, arteriographic and hemodynamic appraisal. Am J Cardiol 30:791, 1972

12. Pichard AD, Sheldon WC, Shinji K, Effler DB, Sones FM: Severe arteriosclerotic obstruction of the left main coronary artery: followup results in 176 patients. Circulation 48, Suppl 4:53, 1973

13. Proudfit WL, Shirey EK, Sones FM Jr: Distribution of arterial lesions demonstrated by selective cine coronary arteriography. Circulation 36:54, 1967

14. Scanlon P, Talano J, Moran JF, Gunnar RM: Main left coronary artery disease. Am J Cardiol 33:169, 1974

15. Sharma S, Khaja F, Heinle R, Goldstein S, Easley R: Left main coronary lesions: risk of catheterization, exercise test and surgery. Circulation 48, Suppl 4:53, 1973

16. Zeft HJ, Manley JC, Huston JH, et al: Left main coronary artery surgery: results of coronary bypass surgery. Circulation 44:68, 1974

94

THE PROGNOSIS OF ANGINA PECTORIS: SURGICAL VERSUS MEDICAL RESULTS

Richard P. Anderson, Lawrence I. Bonchek, Shahbudin H. Rahimtoola, and Albert Starr

Does surgical treatment by means of coronary bypass grafting improve the survival of patients with angina pectoris? An answer to this vital and intriguing question must be based on knowledge of the natural history of such patients, but their history is in fact poorly understood. For example, only recently has it been shown that the distribution of obstructing lesions in the major coronary arteries is a far more important determinant of prognosis than is the presence of angina.[1,2] Similarly, the rate of progression of coronary atherosclerosis and the extent of deterioration in ventricular function may be important determinants of long-term survival; yet, at present, these parameters cannot be measured in an entirely satisfactory manner.

Obviously, an accurate comparison of survival following medical or surgical treatment requires that treatment be applied to comparable patient groups in whom favorable and unfavorable prognostic factors are equally distributed or, at least, are readily apparent. The prospective, double-blind clinical trial is the technique most likely to produce parity in treatment groups and to yield a convincing comparison of results. Such studies are now being conducted in several institutions in this country, but until the final results are available, a comparison of medical with surgical treatment must be based on results obtained when either treatment is applied separately.

There are many difficulties inherent in comparing results from retrospective studies. Some are obvious, such as the difficulties in comparing patients from different hospitals treated at different times by different techniques. Other difficulties are more subtle, such as the suspicion that a particular study may contain disproportionate numbers of good- or poor-risk patients, which could bias results. Finally, some difficulties render a study valueless for purposes of survival comparison. An example is the common practice of reporting survival at an average time of follow-up, when all patients have not completed the entire duration of the study, and the distribution of survivors and nonsurvivors in time is not specified.[3]

Nevertheless, when these limitations are kept in mind, a review of the time-related progress of patients with angina pectoris treated with and without surgery promotes an understanding of prognosis and supports some tentative conclusions about the impact of therapy on prognosis.

The survival pattern of angina patients observed in large medical centers prior to 1950 and determined retrospectively provides background information about prognosis unmodified by present-day therapy. The early studies of Richards, Bland, and White[4] from the Massachusetts General Hospital and Block et al[5] from the Mayo Clinic described annual mortality rates of approximately 6 percent (70 percent five-year survival rate) and 9 percent (58 percent five-year survival rate), respectively. Each of these studies described hypertension, cardiac enlargement, and previous myocardial infarction as adverse prognostic factors and reported particularly that the presence of congestive heart failure on entry into the study drastically reduced long-term survival.

In contrast, recent prospective survival studies of persons from large general populations followed from the first appearance of angina suggest a somewhat more favorable prognosis. Frank, Weinblatt, and Shapiro[6] reporting 275 persons

Supported in part by Program Project Grant HL 06336 from the National Heart and Lung Institute.

from the Health Insurance Plan of Greater New York found an approximate 4 percent annual mortality (82 percent 4.5-year survival rate). Nevertheless, this represented a threefold increase in the risk of dying in comparison with an age-comparable subset of men without clinical evidence of coronary artery disease drawn from the same general population. Kannel and Feinleib [7] reporting from the Framingham study also found approximately a 4 percent per year mortality (four-year survival rate: 85 percent for men with uncomplicated angina and 81 percent for men with angina and previous myocardial infarction).

The better survival rates noted above may have resulted, in part, from inclusion of patients with normal coronary arteries since coronary arteriography with documentation of coronary artery disease was not obtained. It has been shown that patients with typical angina pectoris may have normal coronary arteries [8,9,10] and that these patients have a benign course [10,11] with a life expectancy similar to the normal population. [12] The incidence of angiographically normal coronary arteries in angina patients may be as high as 19 percent. [13]

Since survival appears to be little affected by angina without coronary artery disease, it seems most reasonable to compare survival studies only of nonsurgical and surgical patients who have documented obstruction of coronary arteries. At this writing only a few such studies are available for comparison, primarily because both coronary arteriography and direct myocardial revascularization are relatively new techniques and because the unprecedented application of coronary bypass grafting has tended to preempt the nonoperative management of angina. Furthermore, some authors fail to provide time-related data in their reports, so that it is impossible to recalculate survival rates of their patients

in a uniform manner for comparison with other studies.

Reports of angina patients treated with and without operation were selected for comparison of survival rates by the following criteria: documentation of 50 percent or greater obstruction in one or more major coronary arteries in all patients, number of patients greater than 100, follow-up period greater than three years, and availability of complete survival data in relation to time permitting life table analysis. Based on these criteria, three recent survival studies, two concerning patients treated nonsurgically and one concerning patients treated surgically, are available for comparison (Table 1).

The nonsurgical series are those of Friesinger, Page, and Ross [1] from the Johns Hopkins Hospital, and Bruschke, Proudfit, and Sones [14] from the University of Oregon Medical School. [15] These three series differ somewhat in numbers and mean age of patients. Also, the methods of angiographic scoring, while comparable, are not identical. The nonsurgical series are remarkably similar in the proportion of patients having two or more coronary arteries obstructed (69 and 66 percent, respectively), while this proportion is higher (79 percent) in the surgical patients.

The yearly survival rates and standard errors listed in Table 1 were recalculated using actuarial methods [3,16] from data provided in the three reports. The survival rate of surgical patients is better than the survival rate of nonsurgical patients for each yearly interval except the first in the study of Friesinger et al. [1] Differences in four-year survival rates were tested by determining a deviate of the standardized normal distribution (z score) and requiring a value of 1.96 for significance at the 0.05 level. These calculations indicate that the difference in four-year survival rates be-

TABLE 1. Clinical Data and Progress of Patients with Coronary Artery Disease from Three Series

SERIES MANAGEMENT	FRIESINGER ET AL[1] NONSURGICAL	BRUSCHKE ET AL[14] NONSURGICAL	ANDERSON ET AL[15] SURGICAL
No. patients	103	590	532
Percent follow-up	93	97	93
Mean age	41.8	49.7	51.9
Percent vessel involvement			
Single	31	34	21
Double	} 69	46	41
Triple		20	38
Yearly survival rate (±SE)			
1	95.1 ± 2.1%	88.5 ± 1.3%	94.5 ± 1.0%
2	87.3 ± 3.3%	80.8 ± 1.6%	93.2 ± 1.2%
3	81.0 ± 3.9%	74.2 ± 1.8%	92.6 ± 1.3%
4	74.6 ± 4.5%	69.3 ± 1.9%	89.0 ± 2.8%

tween the two series of nonsurgical patients (74.6 percent and 69.3 percent) was not statistically significant (p > 0.05) while the four-year survival rate for the surgical patients (89.0 percent) was significantly higher (p < 0.01) than in either non-surgical series.

Three additional studies of large patient groups with coronary artery disease treated by means of coronary bypass grafting have recently appeared. The results, while not strictly comparable to the studies cited above because of differences in the reporting of data and the analysis of survival, as well as in probable differences in the severity of disease in the study groups, nevertheless, indicated a more favorable prognosis for surgical patients. Thus Sheldon et al [17] reporting on 1,000 patients from the Cleveland Clinic, estimated a four-year survival rate of 82 percent. Cannom et al [18] reporting from Stanford University School of Medicine estimated the three-year survival rate for 400 patients at 94 percent. Cooley et al [19] from the Texas Heart Institute projected survival in 1,105 patients at three years at approximately 85 percent.

The above citations and observations constitute an overview of the reported effects of surgical versus nonsurgical management on the prognosis of patients with angina and coronary artery disease, based on the current state of our knowledge. Although present evidence tends to favor surgical management, it should not yet be construed as definitive. Pending the outcome of randomized clinical trials of surgical and medical treatment, the superiority of one form of therapy over another will continue to be a matter of clinical judgment for the individual clinician.

References

1. Friesinger GC, Page EE, Ross RS: Prognostic significance of coronary arteriography. Trans Assoc Am Physicians 83:78, 1970
2. Oberman A, Jones WB, Riley CP, Reeves TJ, Sheffield LT, Turner, ME: Natural history of coronary artery disease. Bull NY Acad Med 48:1109, 1972
3. Anderson RP, Bonchek LI, Grunkemeier GL, Lambert LE, Starr A: The analysis and presentation of surgical results by actuarial methods. J Surg Res 16:224, 1974
4. Richards DW, Bland EF, White PD: A completed twenty-five year follow-up study of 456 patients with angina pectoris. J Chronic Dis 4:423, 1956
5. Block WJ, Crumpacker EL, Dry TJ, Gage RP: Prognosis of angina pectoris: observations in 6,882 cases. JAMA 150:259, 1952
6. Frank CW, Weinblatt E, Shapiro S: Angina pectoris in men: prognostic significance of selected medical factors. Circulation 47:509, 1973
7. Kannel WB, Feinlieb M: Natural history of angina pectoris in the Framingham study: prognosis and survival. Am J Cardiol 29:154, 1972
8. Likoff W, Segal BL, Kaspar H: Paradox of normal selective coronary arteriograms in patients considered to have unmistakable coronary heart disease. N Engl J Med 276:1063, 1967
9. Kemp HG, Elliot WG, Gorlin R: The anginal syndrome with normal coronary arteriography. Trans Assoc Am Physicians 80:59, 1967
10. Neill WA, Judkins MP, Dhindsa DS, Metcalfe J, Kassenbaum DG, Kloster FE: Clinically suspect ischemic heart disease not corroborated by demonstrable coronary artery disease: physiologic investigations and clinical course. Am J Cardiol 29:171, 1972
11. Bemiller CR, Pepine CJ, Rogers AK: Long-term observations in patients with angina and normal coronary arteriograms. Circulation 47:36, 1973
12. Kemp HJ Jr, Vokonas PS, Cohn PF, Gorlin R: The anginal syndrome associated with normal coronary arteriograms: report of a six year experience. Am J Med 54:735, 1973
13. Scanlon PJ, Nemickas R, Moran JF, Taland JV, Amirparviz F, Pifarre R: Accelerated angina pectoris: clinical, hemodynamic, arteriographic, and therapeutic experience in 85 patients. Circulation 47:19, 1973
14. Bruschke AVG, Proudfit WL, Sones FM: Progress study of 590 consecutive nonsurgical cases of coronary disease followed 5–9 years: I, arteriographic correlations. Circulation 47:1147, 1973
15. Anderson RP, Rahimtoola SH, Bonchek LI, Starr A: The prognosis of patients with coronary artery disease after coronary bypass operations: time-related progress of 532 patients with disabling angina pectoris. Circulation 50:274, 1974
16. Cutler SJ, Ederer F: Maximum utilization of the life table method in analyzing survival. J Chronic Dis 8:699, 1958
17. Sheldon WC, Rincon G, Effler DB, Proudfit WL, Sones Jr FM: Vein graft surgery for coronary artery disease: survival and angiographic results in 1,000 patients. Circulation 47–48:3–184, 1973
18. Cannon DS, Miller DC, Shumway NE, Fogarty TJ, Daily PO, Brown Jr B, Harrison DC: The long-term follow-up of patients undergoing saphenous vein bypass surgery. Circulation 49:77, 1974
19. Cooley DA, Dawson JT, Hallman GL, Sandiford FM, Wukasch DC, Garcia E, Hall RJ: Aortocoronary saphenous vein bypass: results in 1,492 patients, with particular reference to patients with complicating features. Ann Thorac Surg 16:380, 1973

95

UNSTABLE ANGINA: EXTENDED FOLLOW-UP (ONE TO FOUR YEARS) AFTER URGENT BYPASS OPERATION

Lawrence I. Bonchek, Richard P. Anderson, Shahbudin H. Rahimtoola, John H. McAnulty, J. David Bristow, and Albert Starr

Although gratifying early results have been reported following saphenous vein aortocoronary bypass grafting (SVBG) for unstable angina (Lambert et al, 1971; Cheanvechai et al, 1973), long-term follow-up of large numbers of postoperative patients has not yet been reported. In addition, certain reports have suggested that patients with unstable angina should be treated conservatively in the acute phase, since the prognosis after hospitalization is good (Krauss et al, 1972; Fischl et al, 1973). A possible cause of differences in the management regimens that have been suggested is the wide variation in descriptions of the clinical picture that constitutes unstable angina.

We reviewed our experience with patients undergoing emergency SVBG for unstable angina with emphasis upon long-term follow-up. Patients operated upon less than one year before were excluded.

DEFINITION

The term unstable angina is used in this study to denote a clinical syndrome in which anginal episodes begin to occur with *increasing* frequency and/or severity (crescendo), and culminate in *recurrent* attacks of chest pain *at rest* that continue to occur more than 24 hours after hospitalization despite supportive measures. Transient electrocardiographic evidence of myocardial ischemia such as ST depression or elevation, or T-wave

inversion, is almost invariably present during at least one episode of pain. Myocardial infarction (MI) cannot be documented by serum enzyme studies or by electrocardiography. Narrowing of the lumen of one or more coronary arteries by at least 50 percent can be demonstrated angiographically. Patients may or may not have a history of prior chronic angina and/or myocardial infarction.

CLINICAL MATERIAL

Fifty-five consecutive patients with unstable angina as defined above had coronary arteriography and emergency SVBG at the University of Oregon Medical School Affiliated Hospitals from September 1969 to February 1973. All patients had recurrent chest pain at rest for at least 24 hours after admission. There were 38 men and 17 women who ranged in age from 35 to 68 years (mean 53 years). Thirty-four patients had a history of chronic angina with recent acceleration; 21 had their first episode of angina less than three months before admission. Thirteen had ECG evidence of a previous MI, and 11 were chronically hypertensive.

Seventeen patients had a single coronary artery involved, 16 had two, 20 had three, and two had four (including a diagonal branch of the left anterior descending). Single grafts were performed in 28 patients, double grafts in 23, triple grafts in three, and quadruple grafts in one patient. Thus, 87 of 117 arteries with 50 percent or greater narrowing received bypass grafts, and 24 patients had residual disease that could not be or was not bypassed for reasons discussed below.

Supported by Program Project Grant 06336 and NHLI Training Grants HL05791 and HL05693.

METHODS

Preoperative catheterization was performed in all patients and included cinearteriograms, cut-film selective right and left coronary arteriograms in several projections, and left ventricular (LV) cineangiograms by the percutaneous transfemoral approach. Ejection fraction (EF) was calculated by a previously described method (Bristow et al, 1970). ECG's and serum enzyme determinations were obtained upon admission to the hospital and at least daily thereafter until operation. Postoperatively, each patient had serial electrocardiograms and serum enzyme determinations for three or four consecutive days, and weekly thereafter, until discharge. Subsequent ECG's were obtained at periodic follow-up examinations. The diagnosis and electrocardiographic localization of perioperative and postoperative infarction were based on the development of 0.04-sec Q-waves in the appropriate leads according to the criteria of myocardial infarction developed by Gunnar and McConahay and their coworkers (1967; 1970).

Our previously described operative tech-nique, which includes cardiopulmonary bypass with moderate hemodilution and mild hypothermia (30–32 C), was utilized. During the first two years of this experience, few vessels with less than 70 percent obstruction were grafted, and diseased circumflex arteries were not grafted unless they appeared to provide the sole vascular supply to the posterior wall of the heart. Subsequently, all major vessels with 50 percent or greater obstruction were grafted whenever feasible if they supplied areas of viable myocardium (Anderson et al, 1974).

RESULTS

Early Mortality

There were no deaths or major complications (persistent ventricular arrhythmias, emboli, vascular complications, infections) due to emergency coronary arteriography.

There were three operative deaths (5.4 percent). Two patients could not be removed from bypass; one had sustained a cardiac arrest upon entering the operating room. The third death re-

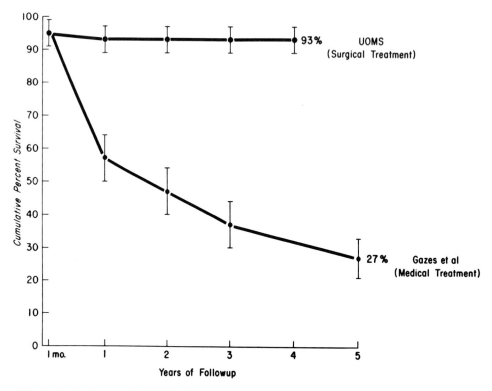

FIG. 1. Survival curves in 55 high-risk patients treated with urgent operations by the authors, and in 54 patients (a high-risk subgroup) treated medically by Gazes and coworkers. The actuarial method was used, and all values are ±1 SE. Calculations include deaths from all causes.

sulted from an aortic dissection caused by the arterial cannula in the ascending aorta.

Late Mortality and Functional Results

Follow-up extends from 12 to 52 months (mean 24 mos). There was only one late death 12 months postoperatively in a 61-year-old woman. She had frequent ventricular extrasystoles and is presumed to have died of an arrhythmia. The survival experience of the entire group is displayed in an actuarial manner in Figure 1. The probability of survival at the end of four years is 93 percent.

Functional classification (FC) was determined by NYHA criteria. Patients were assigned a postoperative FC no higher than that permitted by their general exercise tolerance, even if angina was absent; symptoms of fatigue or dyspnea were also considered. Of 51 survivors, 23 are in FC I, 19 are in FC II, and eight are in FC III. None are in FC IV. One has been lost to follow-up.

Postoperative Angiography

Thirty patients with 51 grafts were studied an average of nine months postoperatively (range, one week to 32 months). Thirty-five grafts (69 percent) were patent and 16 (31 percent) were occluded. Twenty-seven of 30 patients (90 percent) had at least one patent graft.

These results do not reflect a random selection of patients for postoperative studies and were biased against patients with good functional results. Postoperative studies were carried out in 10 of 22 patients (45 percent) in postoperative FC I and in 12 of 18 (67 percent) in FC II. However, eight of eight patients (100 percent) in FC III had postoperative angiography. The overall results of postoperative studies in all patients having SVBG in our institution have been recently presented. An 81 percent graft patency rate was found, with 89 percent of patients having at least one patent graft an average of seven months postoperatively (Bonchek et al, 1974).

Left Ventricular Function

Preoperative and postoperative left ventricular end-diastolic pressure (LVEDP) determinations were available in 20 patients (all values are ± 1 SE). The mean LVEDP preoperatively was 12.2 ± 1.8 (range 2 to 35), and postoperatively it was 12.8 ± 1.1 (range 5 to 25). LV ejection fraction (EF) could be determined pre- and post-

operatively in 10 patients. Mean EF preoperatively was 0.57 ± 0.04 (range 0.37 to 0.72), and postoperatively it was 0.61 ± 0.04 (range 0.46 to 0.79). These differences are not statistically significant (paired T-test, $p > 0.05$).

DISCUSSION

The variation in mortality rates reported with unstable angina patients may be due to the wide range of clinical syndromes encompassed by recent studies. Our definition of unstable angina excludes patients without episodes of pain that persist more than 24 hours after hospitalization and requires that coronary obstruction be demonstrated angiographically.

Gazes and coworkers (1973) have recently provided a long-term study of unstable angina patients treated medically with identification of clinical subgroups and actuarial analysis of late mortality rates. Fifty-four patients were identified as a high-risk subgroup because of continued pain after 48 hours of bed rest. Nineteen of 54 (35 percent) developed an acute MI within three months, and 12 of these 19 (63 percent) died. The probability of surviving three years in this subgroup of 54 patients was 37 percent, and five years 27 percent. These high-risk patients resemble our own very closely, since all but six of our patients had operations more than 48 hours after admission. The actuarial curve depicting survival in Gazes' high-risk subgroup is compared with that of our patients in Figure 1.

It is noteworthy that coronary arteriography was not performed in the patients studied by Gazes and his coworkers. It is widely recognized that patients with presumed angina (even unstable angina) may have normal coronary arteries (Likoff et al, 1967; Neill et al, 1972), and such patients have a benign course and normal life expectancy (Bemiller et al, 1973; Kemp et al, 1973). It seems likley, therefore, that some of the patients in the aforementioned report did not have obstructive coronary artery disease, and their inclusion favorably biased the results of medical therapy.

Comparison of our surgically treated patients with the medically treated patients of Gazes and his coworkers appears to indicate that survival and symptomatic relief are greatly enhanced by SVBG for high-risk patients with unstable angina. It is then pertinent to consider whether coronary arteriography and SVBG should be performed as emergency procedures or following a period of medical management. In this regard Fischl et al

(1973) have analyzed a group of 23 patients with unstable angina ("intermediate coronary syndrome") defined by criteria that closely resemble our own. Twenty received propranolol acutely, 21 subsequently had angiographic demonstration of coronary obstruction, three had urgent operations because they were refractory to medical therapy, and 11 had elective operations one to four weeks after "stabilization" with propranolol. There was one operative death in 14 patients, and three deaths in the nine patients not operated upon. One of the six unoperated survivors and 10 of 13 operated survivors were asymptomatic. They concluded that beta-adrenergic blockade effectively stabilizes most acutely ill patients so that operation can be considered on an elective basis.

Since our experience indicates that in our institution emergency coronary arteriography is not accompanied by increased risk and that—considering the predominance in our series of patients with multiple-vessel disease—the operative and late mortality rates in patients with unstable angina compare favorably with the overall mortality rates for SVBG in our own and other institutions, we prefer to carry out angiography and SVBG urgently. While the graft patency rate in this group is slightly lower than we have observed in our overall experience, the disproportionate number of patients with poor results studied postoperatively probably accounts for this discrepancy (see above). We are particularly concerned that the risk of MI or death in the interval during which patients await elective operation is always present. Of the three deaths in the medically treated patients of Fischl and coworkers, one occurred only one month following the acute episode of unstable angina, and the overall mortality of 33 percent in unoperated patients is unacceptable.

We conclude that for high-risk patients with unstable angina, direct myocardial revascularization on an urgent basis is an effective therapy in terms of early and late survival, prevention of myocardial infarction, and relief of anginal pain.

ACKNOWLEDGMENT

We gratefully acknowledge the invaluable assistance of Mr. Lou Lambert with data collation and analysis.

References

Anderson RP, Rahimtoola SH, Bonchek LI, Starr A: The prognosis of patients with coronary artery disease after coronary bypass operation: time-related progress of 532 patients with disabling angina pectoris. Circulation 50:274, 1974

Bemiller CR, Petine CJ, Rogers AK: Long-term observations in patients with angina and normal coronary arteriograms. Circulation 47:36, 1973

Bonchek LI, Rahimtoola SH, Chaitman BR, et al: Vein graft occlusion: immediate and late consequences and therapeutic implications. Circulation (Suppl 2): 84, 1974

Bristow JD, Vanzee BE, Judkins MP: Systolic and diastolic abnormalities of the left ventricle in coronary artery disease: studies in patients with little or no enlargement of ventricular volume. Circulation 42:219, 1970

Cheanvechai C, Effler DB, Loop FD, et al: Emergency myocardial revascularization. Am J Cardiol 32:901, 1973

Fischl SJ, Herman MZ, Gorlin R: The intermediate coronary syndrome: clinical, angiographic and therapeutic aspects. N Engl J Med 288:1193, 1973

Gazes PC, Mobley EM, Faris HM, et al: Pre-infarctional (unstable) angina—a prospective study—ten year follow-up. Circulation 48:331, 1973

Gunnar RM, Pietras RJ, Blackaller J, et al: Correlation of vector cardiographic criteria for myocardial infarction with autopsy findings. Circulation 35:158, 1967

Kemp HG Jr, Vokonas PS, Cohn PS, et al: The anginal syndrome associated with normal coronary arteriograms: report of a six year experience. Am J Med 54:735, 1973

Krauss KR, Hutter AM, DeSanctis RW: Acute coronary insufficiency: course and follow-up. Arch Intern Med 129:808, 1972

Lambert CJ, Adam M, Geisler GS, et al: Emergency myocardial revascularization for impending infarctions and arrhythmias. J Thorac Cardiovasc Surg 62:522, 1971

Likoff W, Segal BL, Kaspar H: Paradox of normal selective coronary arteriograms in patients considered to have unmistakable coronary heart disease. N Engl J Med 276:1063, 1967

McConahay DR, McCallister BED, Hallermann FJ, et al: Comparative quantitative analysis of the electrocardiogram and the vector cardiogram correlations with the coronary arteriogram. Circulation 42:245, 1970

Neill WA, Judkins MP, Dhindsa DS, et al: Clinically suspect ischemic heart disease not corroborated by demonstrable coronary artery disease: physiologic investigations and clinical course. Am J Cardiol 29:171, 1972

96

PROGNOSIS AFTER SURGERY FOR PREINFARCTION ANGINA

John J. Collins, Jr., Hillel Laks,
and Lawrence H. Cohn

The syndromes of unstable angina pectoris must be carefully classified and defined if semantic confusion is to be avoided in discussing results of various forms of treatment. The surgical experience presented in this chapter includes operations performed upon patients with either crescendo angina or the intermediate coronary syndrome.

Crescendo angina was defined as angina of increasing severity, either acceleration of chronic angina or progression of recent onset of angina with severe pain on minimal exertion or at rest. The intermediate coronary syndrome includes criteria specified by Fischl, Herman, and Gorlin [5] as follows:

1. Recurring episodes of anginal discomfort at rest lasting longer than 20 minutes.
2. Incomplete or no relief by nitrates.
3. Electrocardiographic changes of ischemia in ST and T-wave segments.
4. Absence of elevated enzymes or electrocardiographic changes indicating infarction.

Direct coronary revascularization surgery in patients with crescendo angina and the intermediate coronary syndrome has been proven safe and effective in our experience.

CLINICAL MATERIAL

From July 1970 through December 1973, there were 40 patients who underwent revascularization surgery at the Peter Bent Brigham Hospital for relief of crescendo angina or the intermediate coronary syndrome. This represents 11 percent of the total of 378 patients who underwent direct

coronary revascularization for all indications during this interval. There were 24 patients with the intermediate coronary syndrome and 16 with crescendo angina.

There were 28 males (70 percent) and 12 females (30 percent), ranging in age from 27 to 66 years (mean 51). A history of chronic angina was obtained in 21, with 19 having had recent onset of angina. Documented myocardial infarction had occurred in 16 patients (40 percent) and six had experienced two or more infarctions. Congestive heart failure as evidenced by exertional dyspnea and fluid retention was present in three patients.

All patients underwent cardiac catheterization with left ventriculography and coronary cineangiography. Lesions estimated to obstruct more than 70 percent of the vascular lumen were considered significant. Angiographic findings are outlined in Table 1. There were 13 patients with obstruction in the left main coronary artery. A single significant lesion was found in eight patients, two obstructed vessels in 11, three in 18 patients, and four (including a large diagonal or circumflex marginal) in three patients.

Left ventricular systolic ejection fraction, obtained by techniques previously described,[4] was over 50 percent in 34 patients, between 40 and 49 percent in four patients, and under 40 percent

TABLE 1. Angiographic Findings

	LEFT MAIN	1-VESSEL	2-VESSEL	3-VESSEL	4-VESSEL
ICS	4	5	5	12	2
PA	9	3	6	6	1
Total	13	8	11	18	3

in only two patients. Localized areas of abnormal contractility by ventriculography were noted in 19 patients and diffuse hypokinesis was present in six patients.

All operations were performed using cardiopulmonary bypass with complete hemodilution. Autotransfusion with removal of blood after anesthetic induction for return after cessation of bypass was generally not utilized in patients with the preinfarction syndromes. The technical aspects of surgery and postoperative care remain as previously reported.[2] Intraaortic balloon counterpulsation was not utilized in any of these patients. The number and types of vascular procedures are summarized in Table 2. Single grafts were used in 14 patients, two grafts in 22, and three grafts in four patients. Mechanical endarterectomy was utilized for the distal right coronary artery in 11 patients and for the left anterior descending coronary in two patients. Reversed saphenous vein grafts were used for all bypasses except for nine patients in whom the left internal mammary was directly anastomosed to the left anterior descending coronary artery.

TABLE 2. Coronary Artery Bypass Grafts

	NO.
Single vessel	14
Double vessel	22
Triple vessel	4
Coronary artery endarterectomy	
Right	11
Left	2
Internal mammary artery bypass to LAD	9

There were no in-hospital deaths, and only one death (due to pulmonary embolism) has occurred in the entire series following surgery. Electrocardiographic and enzyme changes characteristic of myocardial infarction developed in three patients (7.5 percent).

Follow-up data were complete for all patients, of whom 28 were more than six months after operation. Mean duration of evaluation after surgery for these 28 patients was 14.3 months with a range of six to 30 months (Table 3).

TABLE 3. Relief of Angina 6 to 30 Months after Operation

	NO.	%
Excellent	18	64
Good	4	14
Fair	3	11
Poor	3	11

Repeat catheterization with angiography of grafts and the native coronary arterial circulation was obtained in only nine patients, including the six patients with persistent or recurrent angina (fair and poor results) (Table 4). Results of the postoperative angiograms are shown in Table 5. In patients with fair or poor results, seven of nine grafts were either stenotic or occluded. In three asymptomatic patients, only one graft of five was occluded or stenotic, and this occurred in a patient having two other perfectly patent grafts.

TABLE 4. Rehabilitation 6 to 30 Months after Operation

Returned to previous occupation	80%
Myocardial infarction	1
Stroke	1
Late death (pulmonary embolism)	1
Required reoperation for angina	2

DISCUSSION

Many differences of opinion among cardiologists and surgeons relative to the merits of medical versus surgical management of myocardial ischemic syndromes stem from nonuniform definition of patient categories. At least some of the confusion seems now to be abating as care is taken to define the anginal syndromes that previously had been collectively termed preinfarction angina. Some cardiologists have observed that the diagnosis of preinfarction angina can be made only in retrospect. Using this technique, questioning 100 patients with infarctions available from 144 consecutive coronary care unit admissions, Solomon, Edwards, and Killip reported 65 patients with prodromal symptoms occurring from 14 hours to two months before the onset of myocardial infarction.[10] Duration of prodromal symptoms was one to six days in 10 patients (65 percent), one to three weeks in 36 (55 percent), and more than three weeks in 18 (28 percent). The incidence of prodromal symptoms was highest (80 percent) in patients who developed anterior infarctions. The most common, and often the only, prodromal symptom was pain—characteristically progressive or crescendo in nature. Other observers have found a lesser incidence of prodromata of myocardial infarction.[9,12] In each study, however, there was no doubt that a substantial proportion of patients had sufficient warning that intervention would have been possible had help been available and had the patients been sufficiently educated to the sig-

TABLE 5. Results of Repeat Catheterization

SUBJECT	POSTOP. PERIOD (mos.)	VESSELS BYPASSED	GRAFTS		RESULTS	REOPERATION
			Occluded	Stenosed		
MM	23	1	1	–	F	IMA implant
PM	23	1	–	1	F	–
CB	1	1	1	–	P	–
WC	5	2	–	1	P	2 grafts
AB	8	2	1	–	F	–
RL	5	2	–	2	F	–
Total (6)	M:13	9	3	4	F-P	2
MC	12	1	–	–	E	–
NY	3	1	–	–	E	–
RB	26	3	1	–	E	–
Total (3)	M:13	5	1	0	E	0

nificance of a change in the pattern of symptoms to seek medical assistance.

The next question, of course, is what proportion of patients reporting definable increases in angina may be expected to experience myocardial infarction soon thereafter. The answer is uncertain because of differences in definition of accelerated angina, crescendo angina, acute coronary insufficiency, and the intermediate coronary syndrome. From a number of reported series, however, a few important points may be ascertained. Krauss, Hutter, and DeSanctis[7] reviewed the courses of 100 patients with acute coronary insufficiency defined as pain lasting at least 30 minutes within 24 hours of admission without electrocardiographic evidence of myocardial infarction. Only 66 of these showed electrocardiographic changes consistent with new ischemia, corresponding with our definition of acute intermediate syndrome. There was only one death during initial hospitalization for medical therapy, and six others developed myocardial infarction. Angiograms were not obtained. At follow-up, an average of 20 months after the episode, 26 patients had died, 21 of cardiac causes. The survival at one year was 85 percent. Patients whose acute episode was superimposed on previous chronic angina fared worse than those with recent onset of symptoms. Gazes and associates[6] reported 10-year survival figures for 140 consecutive patients from a private practice including patients with recent onset angina of progressive severity, crescendo angina superimposed on chronic angina, and prolonged angina occurring at rest. Within 12 months, 25 (18 percent) were dead and about 50 percent had resumed normal activities. Angiograms were not obtained.

Fischl, Herman, and Gorlin[5] reported three deaths in nine patients with the intermediate coronary syndrome during the first 12 months of medical management. From these data, one must conclude that a group of patients with angina pectoris at high risk for early myocardial infarction and death may be identified by clinical criteria that include the previously mentioned outline for the intermediate coronary syndrome. Continuing or recurring pain at rest while hospitalized on maximum medical management (including beta adrenergic blockade) seems to identify a subgroup with an even more grim outlook, but few, if any, studies are available without surgical intervention in these patients. That such patients can be medically treated during the initial episode seems well established from the above studies.[5,7] Despite initial success in relieving pain with medical measures, a high proportion of patients go on to die of myocardial infarction within a few months to a few years.

During the past several years direct coronary revascularization surgery has been increasingly utilized for the preinfarction anginal syndromes in an effort to prolong life as much as to obviate an immediately threatened infarction. Despite a few reports of surgical mortality greater than 10 percent,[3,8] it has become clear that these patients can be operated upon with little more than the two to four percent risk attendant upon operations for relief of chronic stable angina. In the group of 40 patients reported here, there were no in-hospital deaths and only one late death. Similar encouraging results have been reported by others.[1,11]

Successful surgical management in these patients requiring urgent or emergency surgery depends upon several factors. If possible, patients should be brought to a stable condition by bed rest, narcotics, sedatives, vasodilators, and beta adrenergic blockade before catheterization and coronary angiography. Emergency angiograms should be obtained if pain continues or recurs on maximal medical therapy. If angiograms show significant obstruction of the main left coronary artery, or if catheterization was precipitated by failure of medical management, patients should be removed directly from the catheterization laboratory to the operating room. We have had no experience with preoperative use of intraaortic balloon counterpulsation in these patients. Operations have been carried out expeditiously with simple intrathoracic cannulation, total hemodilution using a disposable bubble oxygenator, left ventricular decompression, minimal coronary artery dissection, endarteractomy where necessary to achieve adequate coronary flow, and up to 15 minute periods of ischemic arrest at moderate hypothermia (28 to 30 C). We have not found any great detrimental effect when propranolol is given up to 6 to 12 hours before surgery. Direct anastomosis of the left internal mammary artery to the left anterior descending coronary artery has been utilized with increasing frequency. The time necessary for mobilization of the mammary artery is not excessive, and flows up to 70 ml per minute have been observed. If patients are hypotensive or otherwise unstable, saphenous vein grafts are utilized for all bypasses.

Multiple grafts were used in 26 of these 40 patients including four where circumflex coronary branches were grafted. We feel, however, that restraint is wiser than a compulsive commitment to graft small diagonal and circumflex vessels. Probably nowhere in surgery is the axiom "perfect is the enemy of good" more applicable than in emergency coronary revascularization. If the left anterior descending and the dominant posterior artery are adequately perfused, there is a high likelihood of immediate success, which is, of course, a prerequisite for satisfactory long-term results.

The data reported above, as well as the reports cited, support the conclusion that direct coronary revascularization surgery is more effective than medical management alone in preventing myocardial infarction, prolonging life, and promoting return to a normal life-style during at least the first year after onset of crescendo angina or the intermediate coronary syndrome.

SUMMARY

A group of 40 patients, 24 with the intermediate coronary syndrome and 16 with crescendo angina, have undergone urgent or emergency coronary artery bypass from July 1970 through December 1973, at the Peter Bent Brigham Hospital. There have been no in-hospital deaths and only three myocardial infarctions (7.5 percent). There has been one late death due to pulmonary embolism. In 28 patients followed six to 30 months after operation, one myocardial infarction and one stroke have occurred. Severe persistent or recurrent angina continued in three patients. There were 26 patients with good to excellent relief of angina at an average of 14 months after operation. Return to previous occupation was achieved by 80 percent of patients six months or more after surgery.

References

1. Bertolasi CA, Tronge JE, Carreno CA, Jalon J, Vega MR: Unstable angina—prospective and randomized study of its evolution, with and without surgery. Am J Cardiol 33:201, 1974
2. Collins JJ Jr, Cohn LH, Sonnenblick EH, et al: Determinants of survival after coronary artery bypass surgery. Circulation 47–48, Suppl 3;132, 1973
3. Conti CR, Brawley RK, Griffith LSC, et al: Unstable angina pectoris: morbidity and mortality in 57 consecutive patients evaluated angiographically. Am J Cardiol 32:745, 1973
4. Dodge HT, Sandler H, Ballew DW, et al: The use of biplane angiocardiography for measurement of left ventricular volume in man. Am Heart J 60:762, 1960
5. Fischl SJ, Herman MV, Gorlin R: The intermediate coronary syndrome. Clinical, angiographic, and therapeutic aspects. N Engl J Med 288:1193, 1973
6. Gazes PC, Mobley EM Jr, Faris HM Jr, Duncan RC, Humphries GB: Preinfarctional (unstable) angina—a prospective study—ten year follow-up. Circulation 48:331, 1973
7. Krauss KR, Hutter AM, DeSanctis RW: Acute coronary insufficiency: course and follow-up. Circulation 45–46, Suppl 1:66, 1972
8. Miller DC, Cannom DS, Fogarty TJ, et al: Saphenous vein coronary artery bypass in patients with "preinfarction angina." Circulation 47:234, 1973
9. Mouncey P: Prodromal symptoms in myocardial infarction. Br Heart J 13:215, 1951
10. Solomon HA, Edwards AL, Killip T: Prodromata in acute myocardial infarction. Circulation 40:463, 1969
11. Traad EA, Larsen PB, Gentsch TO, Gosselin AJ, Swaye PS: Surgical management of the preinfarction syndrome. Ann Thorac Surg 16:261, 1973
12. Wood P: Acute and subacute coronary insufficiency. Br Med J 1:1779, 1961

97

PATIENT PROGNOSIS WITH VENTRICULAR ANEURYSM: MEDICAL VERSUS SURGICAL TREATMENT

Mark E. Thompson, Pesara S. Reddy, Eugene P. Haddock,
C. Gerald Sundhal, Donald F. Leon, James A. Shaver,
and Henry T. Bahnson

The occurrence of a ventricular aneurysm as a complication of an acute myocardial infarction has been recognized for a number of years. Hunter first described the pathologic features characteristic of a ventricular aneurysm in the 18th century.[1] It was not until the end of the 19th century that an association between the occurrence of an acute myocardial infarction and the subsequent development of a ventricular aneurysm was noted.[2] From that time until the first surgical procedures designed to alter the natural history of ventricular aneurysm, this complication of acute myocardial infarction remained amenable only to medical treatment.[3,4] In the past decade, however, there has been increasing enthusiasm for surgical intervention in patients with ventricular aneurysms.[5] This view is supported in part by the studies of Schlichter et al, which emphasize the relatively unfavorable prognosis of patients developing this complication of acute myocardial infarction.[6] Likewise, as greater surgical experience is gained and advancements in surgical techniques are available, the feasibility of aneurysmectomy is enhanced. Recent reports by Favaloro et al,[7] Cooley et al,[8] and Johnson et al[9] attest to the role of surgery in the treatment of ventricular aneurysms. By contrast, little information is available concerning the prognosis of patients with ventricular aneurysms who are treated medically.

It is the purpose of this report to summarize the experience gained at the University of Pittsburgh with both medical and surgical treatment of 26 patients found to have ventricular aneurysms.

On the basis of this experience and that reported in the literature, the results of both medical and surgical therapy will be discussed.

MATERIALS AND METHODS

Patients were entered into this study as a result of diagnostic evaluation that was prompted by the onset of increasing angina pectoris or progressive cardiac failure. During the period from April 1969 to May 1972, a series of 26 patients were shown to have left ventricular aneurysms at the time of cardiac catheterization. In all but one of these patients, the asynergic myocardial segment was felt to be secondary to acute myocardial infarction related to arteriosclerotic coronary vascular disease. Of these patients, 12 underwent surgical excision of the asynergic myocardial segment and the remainder of the patients were treated medically. The decision regarding the modality of the treatment was based upon the patients' symptoms and laboratory findings, as well as the anticipated benefit of the treatment regimen. Surgery was recommended for those patients with symptoms of congestive heart failure unresponsive to medical treatment and in whom there was reasonable contractility of the remaining myocardium. Likewise, patients were treated medically if they showed an initially good response or were felt to be otherwise unsuitable for surgical intervention.

The hospital records of all patients were reviewed in order to characterize the clinical and laboratory presentation of each patient. The results of the history and physical examination, electrocardiogram, routine chest X-ray, and cardiac catheterization data were tabulated. The type of ven-

Supported by University of Pittsburgh Grant 2T 12 HE 05678-07.

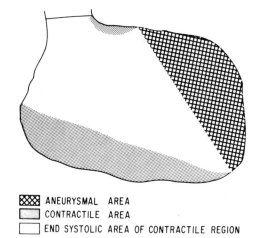

ANEURYSMAL AREA
CONTRACTILE AREA
END SYSTOLIC AREA OF CONTRACTILE REGION

FIG. 1. Analysis of left ventricle geometry was carried out as indicated in this figure. An estimate of the size of the left ventricular aneurysm was made by comparing the diastolic area of the asynergic myocardial segment (cross-hatched area) to the total diastolic left ventricular area determined in the right anterior oblique view by planimetry. The residual area of the contractile portion of the left ventricle (plain area) was assessed by comparing the end systolic area with the end diastolic area of the ventricle after exclusion of the area included in the aneurysmal segment.

tricular aneurysm was classified according to the method proposed by Key, et al.[10] *

An estimate of the size of the left ventricular aneurysm was made by comparing the diastolic area of the asynergic myocardial segment to the total diastolic left ventricular area determined in the right anterior oblique projection by planimetry. Likewise, the residual area of the contractile portion of the left ventricle was assessed by comparing the end-systolic area with the end-diastolic area of the ventricle after exclusion of the area contained in the noncontractile segment (Fig. 1). The angiographic definition of a dyskinetic ventricular segment or an akinetic ventricular segment was used to establish the presence of a ventricular aneurysm.[11] Edward's definition of ventricular aneurysm was applicable to all patients in this study from whom anatomic material was obtained, either at the time of surgery or postmortem examination.[12]

* Type I aneurysms are defined as those located inferior to the insertion of the papillary muscles. Type II aneurysms are defined as those located superior to the insertion of the papillary muscles. Type III aneurysms are defined as those in which a diffuse ischemic myocardiopathy involves a major portion of the left ventricle. The designation *A* refers to the presence of good basilar constrictor activity of the left ventricle. The designation *B* refers to the absence of good basilar constrictor for activity of the left ventricle.

In those patients who underwent surgery, a median sternotomy was performed and cardiopulmonary bypass was used during resection of the ventricular aneurysm. In one patient, concurrent mitral valve replacement was carried out, and in another patient, a Vineberg procedure was also performed. Otherwise, the surgical procedure involved only surgical resection of the aneurysmal area of the left ventricle.

The duration of the observation period for this group of patients was calculated from the time of the most recent myocardial infarction to the cardiac catheterization study and then through the termination of the follow-up period. The follow-up period was terminated with either the death of the patient or known survival until November 1973. Complete follow-up information was available for each patient. The patient's functional class was determined using the guidelines of the New York Heart Association.[13]

RESULTS

Details of the clinical profile for each patient are presented in Tables 1 and 2. The patients ranged in age from 26 to 71 years, at the time of entry into the study. Anginal pain was present in 19 of 26 patients, and shortness of breath on exertion was present in 19 of 26 patients. One patient had recurrent episodes of ventricular tachycardia, and two experienced partial hemiparesis as a result of a systemic embolus. All patients had a history of previous myocardial infarction occurring from one month to 12 years prior to entry into this study. One patient had angiographically normal coronary arteries and was felt to have a ventricular aneurysm, presumably as a result of a coronary embolus that resulted in myocardial infarction. The remainder of the patients were found to have significant occlusive coronary disease.*

In this group, risk factors associated with an increased incidence of coronary artery disease included smoking (more than one pack of cigarettes per day—16/26), a family history of coronary artery disease (16/26), hypertension (blood pressure greater than 140/90—9/26), and an abnormal glucose tolerance (8/26).

At the time of physical examination, 10 of 26 patients had evidence of uncompensated congestive heart failure; 22 of 26 patients had an atrial diastolic gallop; 14 of 26 patients had a

* Defined as at least a 75 percent obstruction of a major coronary artery.

TABLE 1. Clinical Profile: Medical Therapy

PATIENT		FUNCTIONAL CLASS[a]		FOLLOW-UP PERIOD[c]		HEMODYNAMIC DATA			ANEURYSM TYPE[f]	CORONARY ANGIOGRAPHY[g]
Age	Sex	Initial	Current	Total[d]	Cath.[e]	$\overline{PA}$ mm Hg	LVEDP mm Hg	CI L/min/m^2		
41	F	I	I	78	37	–	4	–	Ap. I A	0
43	M	III	III	33	24	50	26	2.0	Ap. I A	1
41	M	III	III	89	29	12	8	2.7	Ap. I A	1
47	M	II	II	36	30	–	11	1.9	Ap. I A	1
26	M	I	III	99	26	12	8	3.0	Ap. I A	1
58	M	II	II	39	34	16	6	3.5	Ap. I A	2
57	M	III	b	17	15	20	12	2.7	Ap. I B	2
48	M	II	II	35	33	18	24	3.1	Post. I A	2
59	M	III	b	28	22	20	14	2.5	Ap. I B	2
54	M	III	III	35	33	20	10	2.2	Ap. I B	2
36	M	III	III	44	36	16	14	4.7	Ap. I A	3
63	M	IV	b	153	9	14	12	1.7	Ap. I B	3
47	M	II	III	36	29	–	14	1.8	Ap. I B	3
46	M	IV	II	60	55	28	18	2.3	Ap. I A	–

[a] New York Heart Association.
[b] Patient deceased.
[c] In months.
[d] Since the most recent myocardial infarction until termination of the follow-up period.
[e] From the time of cardiac catheterization until termination of the follow-up period.
[f] Aneurysm location and type according to Key et al.[10]
[g] Number of major coronary arteries with at least a 75 percent obstruction.

TABLE 2. Clinical Profile: Surgical Therapy

PATIENT		FUNCTIONAL CLASS[a]		FOLLOW-UP PERIOD[d]		HEMODYNAMIC DATA			ANEURYSM TYPE[g]	CORONARY ANGIOGRAPHY[h]
Age	Sex	Initial	Current	Total[e]	Cath.[f]	$\overline{PA}$ mm Hg	LVEDP mm Hg	CI L/min/m^2		
50	M	IV	IV[b]	55	22	50	32	1.9	Ap. I B	1
58	M	III	II	35	33	25	28	2.9	Ap. I A	1
63	M	IV	III	42	38	45	23	3.1	Ap. I B	2
49	M	II	II[b]	57	28	20	18	2.7	Ap. I A	2
49	M	III	III	66	27	20	13	2.8	Ap. I A	2
41	M	IV	II	47	34	40	30	2.0	Ap. I B	–
51	M	IV	IV[b]	36	10	25	19	2.9	Ap. I A	3
59	M	III	II[b]	48	42	14	20	1.3	Ap. I B	–
51	M	IV	c	4	0	35	25	2.3	Ap. I B	2
70	M	IV	c	90	0	20	16	1.9	Post. II B	2
62	M	IV	c	3	2	45	20	1.9	Lat. II B	2
71	M	IV	c	1	0	45	18	1.7	Post. II B	3[i]

[a] New York Heart Association.
[b] Patient deceased, functional class following surgery.
[c] Patient died at surgery or in the immediate postoperative period.
[d] In months.
[e] Since the most recent myocardial infarction until termination of the follow-up period.
[f] From the time of cardiac catheterization until termination of the follow-up period.
[g] Aneurysm location and type according to Key et al.[10]
[h] Number of major coronary arteries with at least a 75 percent obstruction.
[i] Extent of coronary disease determined at postmortem examination.

ventricular diastolic gallop; and 14 of 26 patients had both an atrial and ventricular diastolic gallop.

All patients had electrocardiographic evidence of previous myocardial infarction. The distribution of the abnormal Q-waves in the electrocardiogram corresponded to the site of ventricular aneurysm in all instances. Likewise, there was persistent ST segment elevation in 14 of 15 patients at least six months following the most recent myocardial infarction. There was definite cardiac enlargement in only 10 of the 26 patients assessed roentgenographically. Of the three patients with posterior ventricular aneurysm, two had normal chest X-rays and in the third patient, the posterior aneurysm was obscured by concurrent pericardial effusion.

CARDIAC CATHETERIZATION DATA

All patients underwent cardiac catheterization. In most instances, information regarding pulmonary artery pressure (23/26), cardiac output (25/26), and coronary circulation (22/26) was obtained (Tables 1 and 2). The hemodynamic information obtained at the time of cardiac catheterization for the medically and surgically treated group of patients was as follows: mean pulmonary artery pressure 21 mm Hg vs 32 mm Hg (P < 0.005); mean left ventricular end diastolic pressure 13 mm Hg vs 22 mm Hg (P < 0.005); and mean cardiac index 2.6 1/min/m^2 vs 2.3 1/min/m^2 (P = > 0.2), respectively. These differences in hemodynamic measurements serve to emphasize that the patients ultimately selected for surgery were more severely affected by the presence of the left ventricular aneurysm than the patients treated medically.

An attempt to quantitate the extent of left ventricular asynergy was made by arbitrarily dividing the ventricle into a contractile and noncontractile portion (Fig. 1). The planar area of the asynergic portion of the left ventricle was compared to the total diastolic area of the left ventricle in the right anterior oblique position by planimetry. The result of this calculation was expressed as the percentage of total left ventricular area included in the aneurysmal segment. Similarly, the residual area of the remaining contractile portion of the ventricle was calculated from the ratio of the end systolic area to the end diastolic area of the contractile portion of the left ventricle as determined by planimetry (Fig. 1).

For the group treated medically, the dyskinetic or akinetic area of the left ventricle composed an average of 26 percent of the end diastolic area of the left ventricle. The residual area of the remaining contractile portion of the left ventricle was 79 percent.

For the group treated surgically, the dyskinetic or akinetic area of the left ventricle composed an average of 41 percent of the end diastolic area of the left ventricle. The residual area of the remaining contractile portion of the left ventricle was 79 percent.

In all cases, a left ventriculogram was obtained in the right anterior oblique position, and in two of three patients with a posterior ventricular aneurysm, in the left anterior oblique position as well (Fig. 2 and 3, Tables 1 and 2). The ventricular aneurysm involved the anterior and/or apical portion of the left ventricle in 22 of 26 patients. In one instance a high lateral wall aneurysm was associated with mitral insufficiency. In three patients the diaphragmatic surface was involved with a resulting posterior aneurysm. In the group treated medically, there were 10 patients with Type IA aneurysms. Of this group, one patient had no demonstrable coronary artery disease; four patients had single-vessel disease; two patients had two-vessel disease; and two patients had three-vessel disease. One patient had no assessment of the coronary arteries. There were four patients with Type IB aneurysms. Three of these patients had two-vessel disease and one patient had three-vessel disease.

In the group treated surgically, there were four patients with Type IA aneurysms. In this subgroup, one patient had single-vessel disease; two patients had two-vessel disease; and in one patient, no assessment of the coronary vessels was obtained prior to surgery. Of the five patients with Type IB aneurysms, one patient had single-vessel disease; two patients had two-vessel disease; one patient had three-vessel disease; and one patient had no assessment of the coronary vessels prior to surgery. Of the three patients with Type 2B aneurysms, one had two-vessel disease with mitral insufficiency and two had three-vessel disease. The Type 2B aneurysms included two patients with posterior aneurysms and one patient with a high lateral wall aneurysm.

There was follow-up information available on all patients in this study (Tables 1 and 2). In the group of patients treated medically, two patients were in Class I, four in Class II, six in Class III, and two in Class IV, at the time of entry into the study. At the present time, one patient remains

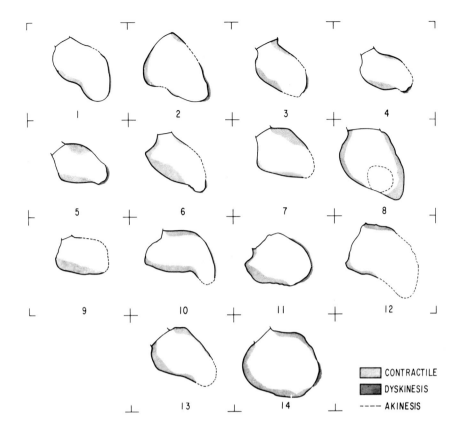

FIG. 2. A graphic representation of each ventriculogram for the medically treated group. An estimate of the degree of ventricular dysfunction may be obtained by comparing the end systolic and end diastolic areas and the degree of ventricular asynergy. Each ventriculogram is designated by a number that corresponds to the numbering in the patient profile chart.

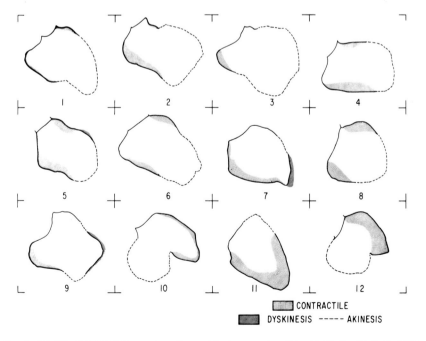

FIG. 3. A graphic representation of each ventriculogram for the surgically treated group. An estimate of the degree of ventricular dysfunction may be obtained by comparing the end systolic areas and the degree of ventricular asynergy. Each ventriculogram is designated by a number that corresponds to the numbering in the patient profile chart.

TABLE 3. Duration of Follow-up

	MEDICAL GROUP		SURGICAL Group	
	No.	Av. Time, Mos. (Range)	No.	Av. Time, Mos. (Range)
Total follow-up period[a]	14	56 (17–153)	12	40 (1–90)
Alive	11	53 (33–99)	4	48 (35–66)
Dead	3	66 (17–153)	8	37 (1–90)
Follow-up since catheterization[b]	14	29 (9–55)	12	20 (0–42)
Alive	11	33 (24–55)	4	33 (27–38)
Dead	3	15 (9–22)	8	13 (0–42)

[a] *Since the most recent myocardial infarction until the termination of the follow-up period.*
[b] *From the time of cardiac catheterization until termination of the follow-up period. The follow-up period after surgery can be accurately calculated from the time of cardiac catheterization since surgery followed cardiac catheterization by less than three months.*

in Class I, four patients are in Class II, six patients are in Class III, and three patients have subsequently died. All deaths in this group were related to the primary underlying cardiovascular disease.

As a group, the patients treated surgically had a great deal more symptomatic limitation than the medically treated group. No patient was in Class I. There was only one patient in Class II. Two patients were in Class III, and the remaining eight patients were in Class IV. Of these eight patients, four were judged to be critically ill at the time of surgery. At the present time, four patients are alive in the surgically treated group. Two of these patients are in Class II, and two are in Class III. Of the patients who survived the immediate postoperative period, two were unimproved and remained in Class IV and two others showing improvement were in Class II, prior to death. Of the deaths in the immediate postoperative period, two were related to myocardial failure, one to a presumed arrhythmia and another to surgical complications. All late deaths in this group were related to the primary underlying cardiovascular disease.

As a group, the 14 medically treated patients had an average follow-up period of 56 months from the time of the most recent myocardial infarction (range 17 to 153 months); and 29 months (range 9 to 55 months) from the time of cardiac catheterization (Table 3). There are presently 11 survivors in this group who have an average follow-up period of 53 months (range 33 to 99 months) from the time of the most recent myocardial infarction and 33 months (range 24 to 55 months) from the time

of cardiac catheterization. Of the three deceased patients in this group, the average survival time was 66 months (range 17 to 153 months) from the most recent myocardial infarction and 15 months (range 9 to 22 months) from the time of cardiac catheterization.

As a group, the 12 surgically treated patients had an average follow-up period of 40 months (range 1 to 90 months) from the time of the most recent myocardial infarction and 20 months (range 0 to 42 months) from the time of cardiac catheterization. Of the four patients currently alive following surgery, the average follow-up period from the time of the most recent myocardial infarction was 48 months (range 35 to 66 months) and was 33 months (range 27 to 38 months) from the time of cardiac catheterization.*

DISCUSSION

Introduction of the cardiopulmonary bypass technique has permitted an increasing number of surgical procedures to be performed for the correction of complications resulting from acute myocardial infarction. Yet the long-term benefit of medical and surgical treatment of ischemic heart disease and its sequelae remains controversial. In an effort to provide more information regarding the prognosis of patients with ventricular aneu-

* In all instances, surgery followed cardiac catheterization by less than three months. Thus, the follow-up period after surgery can be accurately calculated from the time of the cardiac catheterization.

rysms, a detailed account of the clinical course of a small group of patients selected for either medical or surgical treatment is presented.

The clinical profile of patients included in this series is similar to that described in other series.[5,14,15] As was our experience, the patients with ventricular aneurysms generally fall within the fourth to the sixth decade, with males predominating.[16] Our patients, as have others, had persistent symptoms of angina pectoris or congestive heart failure. Although one might expect that peripheral emboli would be a common clinical finding, this has been reported in only a relatively small number of patients.[7] Likewise, serious recurrent rhythm disturbances are infrequently associated with ventrical aneurysms, although dramatic examples of this complication have been reported.[17,18,19]

Increasing emphasis has been placed on the ability to detect the presence of ventricular dysfunction by physical examination. In a prospective study by Gorlin and associates, clues to the presence of ventricular aneurysm were present on physical examination in 75 percent of the patients.[11] Many of the most frequently documented abnormalities in physical examination such as the presence of an abnormal precordial impulse, atrial or ventricular gallops, cardiac murmurs, and signs of congestive heart failure were present in our patients.[15] Noninvasive graphic techniques including apex cardiography and echocardiography have also been useful adjuncts for the detection of ventricular aneurysms.[20,21]

The electrocardiogram was helpful in suggesting the diagnosis of ventricular aneurysm in this group of patients. All patients had electrocardiographic evidence of transmural myocardial infarction that corresponded to the area of the left ventricle in which the aneurysm was demonstrated angiographically.[22] In addition, persistent ST segment elevation for at least six months following the acute myocardial infarction was found in 15 of 16 patients in our group with ventricular aneurysm. In several patients, Gorlin et al have demonstrated elevation of previously normal ST segments during exercise in patients with ventricular aneurysms.[11] On the other hand, Groden and James have indicated that only approximately one-half of the patients with persistent ST segment elevation were subsequently felt to have ventricular aneurysms assessed fluoroscopically.[23] Thus the importance of ST segment elevation may be less useful as a diagnostic aid than previously thought.

The presence of a normal chest X-ray does not exclude the diagnosis of ventricular aneurysm.[24] Often the cardiac silhouette is normal or only minimally enlarged, as it was in 10 of 26 patients in this group. Nevertheless, alterations in the cardiac contour have been emphasized as indicating the presence of ventricular aneurysms. Posterior ventricular aneurysms frequently evade detection by the routine roentgenographic procedures, as was the case in this study. Increased accuracy in the detection of ventricular aneurysm may be attained by using kymographic or fluoroscopic techniques.[25,26] Limitations of noninvasive roentgenographic techniques in the detection of ventricular aneurysm must be appreciated, however, so that left ventriculography will be performed when indicated.[24]

The extent and consequences of left ventricular myocardial asynergy were documented by the hemodynamic studies done in this group of patients. Comparison of the cardiac catheterization results for the medically and surgically treated groups of patients indicate that there was significantly greater elevation of the mean pulmonary artery pressure (21 vs 32 mm Hg $P < 0.005$) and mean left ventricular end diastolic pressure (13 mm Hg vs 22 mm Hg $P < 0.005$) in the group that ultimately underwent aneurysmectomy. These laboratory findings served to emphasize that the group of patients treated surgically was more extensively compromised by the presence of the ventricular aneurysm than in the medically treated group. These findings are consistent with previous observations that indicate that patients with demonstrable left ventricular dyskinesia or akinesia following myocardial infarction tend to have elevated pulmonary artery pressures, elevated left ventricular end diastolic pressure, and decreased cardiac output.[27,28]

Ventriculography is the definitive diagnostic study for the demonstration of left ventricular aneurysms. Gorlin has found that an area of akinesis or dyskinesis most closely correlates with the presence of an anatomically demonstrated left ventricular aneurysm.[11] However, it should be pointed out that the mechanistic definition of ventricular aneurysm and the anatomic definition do not always correlate.[11] When it was possible to correlate the pathologic and angiographic features of the altered left ventricular anatomy in this study, the ventricular aneurysm was found to be composed of a dilated, thin-walled sac composed of fibrous tissue.

The extent of left ventricular involvement by the aneurysmal segment was estimated by planimetry as previously described. The aneurysm occupied approximately 25 percent of the left ventricular planar area in the medically treated group of patients. In a similar study by Klein et al, it was estimated that up to 25 percent of the left ventricular surface area could be involved in aneurysm formation before dilatation and hypertrophy of the remaining myocardium was required in order to compensate for the loss of noncontractile aneurysmal tissue.[29] Such an observation is in keeping with the findings in the medically treated group of patients in this study in whom only modest elevation of intracardiac pressures and modest reductions of cardiac output were present.

By contrast, 41 percent of the left ventricular planar area was included in the left ventricular aneurysm in the group of patients treated surgically. There was a more significant degree of left ventricular functional impairment with greater elevations of intracardiac pressure and greater depressions of cardiac output in this group. Such alterations in cardiac function would be expected in individuals with more extensive left ventricular dysfunction secondary to aneurysm formation.

A great deal of experimental effort has been directed toward correlating the hemodynamic and angiographic features exhibited by patients with left ventricular aneurysms. Recently Parmley et al have indicated that akinesis is the most frequent angiographic abnormality associated with left ventricular aneurysm.[30] In the majority of instances, there is sufficient scar tissue in the wall of the ventricular aneurysm to convert it to an akinetic segment. This relatively noncompliant portion of the left ventricular wall does not alter the left ventricular function as greatly as does a truly paradoxically late-moving portion of the left ventricle. Dyskinesis, on the other hand, is more frequently observed shortly following acute myocardial infarction, prior to extensive fibrosis of the infarcted myocardium. Under these circumstances, there is more severe dissipation of left ventricular contractile energy.

In an effort to quantitate the significance of left ventricular aneurysms, artificial models have been constructed to estimate the anticipated benefits of surgical intervention. Recently, Watson et al [31] and Arthur et al [32] studied the relative volume of a left ventricular aneurysm in relationship to the total left ventricular volume. These studies indicated that the ejection fraction of the residual contractile segment exceeded 45 percent in a majority of the patients who survived surgery and showed improvement. Sander et al have also emphasized that good contractility of the remaining

myocardium is essential for survival of patients operated upon with cardiogenic shock.[33] Estimates of aneurysmal size and segmental shortening of the uninvolved portion of the left ventricle were made in this study. However, in this small series, it was not possible to discern any relationship between these factors and the subsequent outcome of surgical intervention.

Longevity and quality of life are two generally accepted parameters used to judge the overall contribution of any treatment regimen to a patient's well being. In this study, the patients treated medically were less symptomatic than the patients treated surgically. Most patients stabilized with medical management and remained in the same functional class during the period of observation. The extent of disease in the Class III patients made them unsuitable candidates for surgical intervention, and those who were less symptomatic did not warrant surgery.

The longevity of the medically treated patients compared favorably with that of similar patients reported by others. In this study, the average duration of follow-up in all 14 patients from the time of the most recent myocardial infarction until the preparation of this manuscript was 56 months with a range of 17 to 153 months and a median of 39 months. For the three patients who died in the medically treated group, the average duration of survival was 66 months from the time of the most recent myocardial infarction. The deaths in this group were all related to the underlying cardiovascular disease. In the group of 25 medically treated patients with ventricular aneurysms reported by Shattenburg et al, 19 were dead an average of 39 months after the most recent myocardial infarction.[34] At the time of that report, there were only five survivors in that group. The survivors were in Class I or Class II. Deaths in 16 of 19 patients in the medically treated group were directly attributed to recurrent myocardial infarction or congestive heart failure. The overall five-year survival rate for patients with ventricular aneurysm following acute myocardial infarction is in the range of 12 to 27 percent, with an average survival ranging from 2.8 to 4.8 years.[5,6,16,35]

The overall follow-up for the medically treated group following cardiac catheterization was 29 months with a range of nine to 55 months. During this time there were three deaths occurring on the average of 15 months following cardiac catheterization (range nine to 22 months). This information may be compared with the more extensive study recently published by Burschke et al from the Cleveland Clinic. [36] In this report, there was a subgroup of 75 patients who were demonstrated to have an aneurysmal left ventricular segment. This group was further subdivided into 25 patients with a dilated, poorly contractile left ventricle, and 50 patients with segmental asynergy only. The patients with a diffuse ischemic myocardiopathy had a 36 percent five-year survival rate. The remaining 50 patients with localized dyskinesia had a 54 percent five-year survival rate. When one correlates the yearly survival in this group with the number of coronary arteries severely involved in the atherosclerotic process as well as the presence of left ventricular dyskinesia, there was no appreciable difference in the mortality rate between patients with single-, double-, or triple-vessel disease (range 50 to 62 percent five-year survival).

In comparing the five-year survival figure of patients with demonstrated left ventricular aneurysm to those reported in older studies of patients suffering myocardial infarction alone (without specific mention of the presence of a ventricular aneurysm), one appreciates that there is a great deal of overlap in these statistics.[37,38] For example, in patients reported to have infarction alone, the five-year survival rate was 49 to 74 percent, which is similar to that reported by Bruschke et al[36] but considerably better than that reported in the autopsy series.[5,6,16,35]

The group of patients treated surgically were more symptomatic than the medically treated group. A majority of the patients were in Class III or IV at the time of initial evaluation. Postoperatively, there was symptomatic improvement in four of the eight patients. The average period of observation for the surgically treated patients from the time of the most recent myocardial infarction until the termination of the follow-up period was 40 months (range one to 90 months). Of the eight patients who survived the immediate postoperative period, the average follow-up after surgery was 29 months (range 10 to 42 months). In this group are included four patients who are no longer living. These four patients had an average follow-up period of 25 months (range 10 to 42 months) from surgery to death.

This information regarding the longevity of patients in the postoperative period is similar to that reported in the literature. In the most extensive report, by Favaloro et al,[7] 80 patients who underwent aneurysmectomy were followed for a period of up to seven years. In this group, there were a total of 12 hospital deaths, and 19 late deaths during the follow-up period. The average time elapsing from surgery until death was 19 months. The average duration of the follow-up period from surgical intervention until the publication of the report was 14 months in the surviving patients. The most frequent cause of late death in these surgical patients was recurrent myocardial infarction.

Similarly, Cooley et al reported an early series of 37 patients in which aneurysmectomy was performed.[8] There were eight hospital deaths and five late deaths. The late deaths occurred after an average follow-up interval of 18 months from the time of surgery. Of the remaining 24 patients still alive, the average follow-up period was 31 months at the time the report was published. Likewise, Graber et al have reported on a series of 23 patients treated surgically for removal of a ventricular aneurysm.[14] In this group, there were five hospital deaths and seven patients who died after an average follow-up period of 26 months. Of the remaining 11 patients still alive, the average period of follow-up was 25 months.

Using the more liberal angiographic criteria for the diagnosis of ventricular aneurysm, Gorlin et al found that 24 out of a group of 100 patients sustaining an acute myocardial infarction developed some form of ventricular asynergy.[11] Only one of these patients died of intractable congestive heart failure. Deaths in the remaining seven patients occurred either suddenly or as a result of recurrent myocardial infarction. In a similar report, Mourdjinis et al concluded that approximately 16 percent of patients developed a ventricular aneurysm following an acute myocardial infarction.[39] Yet only a relatively small percentage of these patients exhibited signs and symptoms related solely to the presence of a ventricular aneurysm.

For this reason, medical treatment is initially recommended for patients with complications of myocardial infarction related to ventricular asynergy.[7] Frequently, patients have a satisfactory response to medical treatment and will not require surgical intervention. Under these circumstances, the long-term outlook appears to be relatively favorable and is dependent upon the adequacy of myocardial perfusion. If patients continue to experience refractory congestive heart failure, uncontrolled ventricular arrhythmias, or recurrent peripheral systemic emboli, then consideration must be given to surgical intervention, since as many as 75 percent of patients showing more extensive left ventricular dysfunction die as a result of congestive heart failure or recurrent myocardial infarction.[16]

In this study, aneurysmectomy was reserved for those patients who remained symptomatic in spite of optimal medical therapy. Ideally, a surgical candidate should have good basilar constrictor activity in conjunction with an anterior and/or apical aneurysm and a competent mitral valve apparatus. In addition, there should be good coronary vascular supply to the remaining contractile portion of the left ventricle. Under these circumstances, a favorable operative result may be expected.[10] In most instances, however, patients considered for surgery have less favorable ventricular function and more extensive occlusive coronary artery disease. Under these circumstances, correspondingly less favorable surgical results may be anticipated. When this approach for selecting a treatment program was used, the long-term result for both the medically and surgically treated group of patients was similar. In both instances, the degree of underlying coronary artery disease was the prime factor in determining the patient's long-term prognosis. Recent reports suggest that more favorable long-term surgical results may be obtained when a coronary artery bypass procedure is combined with an aneurysmectomy.[9,40] Additional studies of the type reported here will be required in order to assess the long-term results of such intervention.

ACKNOWLEDGMENTS

The authors wish to express their appreciation to Mrs. Patricia Frick and Miss Arlene Scarlatelli for their help in preparing this manuscript. Illustrations were prepared by Mr. William Brent.

References

1. Hunter J (1757): An account of the dissection of morbid bodies. A manuscript copy in the Library of the Royal College of Surgeons no. 32:30–32
2. Zeigler E: Uber myomalacia cordis. Virchows Arch [Pathol Anat] 90:211–12, 1882
3. Berk CS: Operation for aneurysm of the heart. Ann Surg 120:34–40, 1944
4. Likoff W, Bailey CP: Ventriculoplasty—excision of myocardial aneurysm. JAMA 158:915–20, 1955
5. Davis RW, Ebert PA: Ventricular aneurysm, a clinical-pathologic correlation. Am J Cardiol 29:1–6, 1972
6. Schlichter J, Hellerstein HK, Katz LN: Aneurysm of the heart: a correlative study of one hundred and two proved cases. Medicine 33:43–86, 1954
7. Favaloro RG, Effler DB, Groves LK, et al: Ventricular aneurysm—clinical experience. Ann Thorac Surg 6:227–42, 1968
8. Cooley DA, Hallman GL, Henley WS: Left ventricular aneurysm due to myocardial infarction. Arch Surg 88:114–21, 1964
9. Johnson WD, Flemma RJ, Lepley D Jr, Ellison EH: Extended treatment of severe coronary artery disease: a total surgical approach. Ann Surg 170:460–83, 1969
10. Key JA, Aldridge HE, MacGregor DC: The selection of patients for resection of left ventricular aneurysm. J Thorac Cardiovasc Surg 56:477–83, 1968
11. Gorlin R, Klein MD, Sullivan JM: Prospective correlative study of ventricular aneurysm. Am J Med 42:512–31, 1967
12. Edwards JE: An Atlas of Acquired Diseases of the Heart and Great Vessels, vol. 2. Philadelphia and London, WB Saunders, p 615, 1961
13. Criteria Committee, New York Heart Association, Inc: Diseases of the Heart and Blood Vessels: Nomenclature and Criteria for Diagnosis, 6th ed. Boston, Little, Brown, 1964, pp 112–13
14. Graber JD, Oakley CM, Pickering BN, et al: Ventricular aneurysm: an appraisal of diagnosis and surgical treatment. Br Heart J 34:830–38, 1972
15. Cheng TO: Incidence of ventricular aneurysm in coronary artery disease. Am J Med 50:340–55, 1971
16. Dubnow MH, Burchell HB, Titus JL: Postinfarction ventricular aneurysm. Am Heart J 70:753–60, 1965
17. Clark WH, Russell M: Recurrent ventricular tachycardia in association with ventricular aneurysm. Am J Cardiol 31:529–30, 1973
18. Bryson AL, Parisi AF, Schechter E, Wolfson S: Shortening ventricular arrhythmias by exercise. Am J Cardiol 32:995–99, 1973
19. Graham AF, Miller DC, Stinson EB, et al: Surgical treatment of refractory life-threatening ventricular tachycardia. Am J Cardiol 32:909–12, 1973
20. Lane FJ, Carroll JM, Levine HD, Gorlin R: The apex-cardiogram in myocardial asynergy. Circulation 37:890–99, 1968
21. Petersen JL, Johnston W, Hessel EA, Murray JA: Echo-cardiographic recognition of left ventricular aneurysm. Am Heart J 83:244–50, 1972
22. Cokkinos DV, Hallman GL, Cooley DA, Zamalloa O, Leachman RD: Left ventricular aneurysm: analysis of electrocardiographic features and post-resection changes. Am Heart J 82:149–57, 1971
23. Groden BM, James WB: Significance of persistent R-ST elevation after acute myocardial infarction. Br Heart J 31:34–36, 1969
24. Kittredge RD, Cameron A: Abnormalities of left ventricular wall motion and aneurysm formation. Am J Roentgenol Radium Ther Nucl Med 116:110–24, 1972
25. Dock S: The ventricular pulsation in myocardial infarction: a fluoroscopic and kymographic study. Diseases of Chest 27:282–97, 1955
26. Kurtzman RS, Lofstrom JE: Detection and evaluation of myocardial infarction by image amplification and cinefluoroscopy. Radiology 81:57–64, 1963
27. Herman MV, Gorlin R: Implications of left ventricular asynergy. Am J Cardiol 23:538–47, 1969
28. Baxley WA, Jones WB, Dodge HT: Left ventricular anatomical and functional abnormalities in chronic postinfarction heart failure. Ann Intern Med 74:499–508, 1971
29. Klein MD, Herman MV, Gorlin R: A hemodynamic study of left ventricular aneurysm. Circulation 35:614–30, 1967
30. Parmley WW, Chuck L, Kivowitz C, Matloff JM, Swan HJC: In vitro length-tension relations of human ventricular aneurysms. Am J Cardiol 32:891–94, 1973
31. Watson LE, Dickhaus DW, Martin RH: The residual contracting left ventricle in patients with left ventricular aneurysm. Circulation Suppl 45, 46:419, 1972

32. Arthur A, Basta L, Kioschos M: Factors influencing prognosis in left ventricular aneurysmectomy. Circulation Suppl 45, 46:502, 1972

33. Sanders CA, Buckley MJ, Leinbach RC, Mundth ED, Austen WG: Mechanical circulatory assistance. Circulation 45:1292–1313, 1972

34. Schattenberg TT, Giuliani ER, Campion BC, Danielson GK Jr: Postinfarction ventricular aneurysm. Mayo Clinic Proc 45:13–19, 1970

35. Groden BM, James WB, McDicken I: Cardiac aneurysm after myocardial infarction. Postgrad Med J 44:775–84, 1968

36. Bruschke VG, Proudfit WL, Sones FM Jr: Prognosis study of 590 consecutive nonsurgical cases of coronary disease followed 5–9 years. Circulation 47:1154–1163, 1973

37. Richards DW, Bland EF, White PD: A completed twenty-five-year follow-up study of patients with myocardial infarction. J Chronic Dis 4:415–22, 1956

38. Pell S, D'Alonzo CA: Immediate mortality and five-year survival of employed men with a first myocardial infarction. N Engl J Med 270:915–22, 1964

39. Mourdjinis A, Olsen E, Raphael MH, Mounsey JPD: Clinical diagnosis and prognosis of ventricular aneurysm. Br Heart J 30:497–513, 1968

40. Merin G, Schattenberg TT, Pluth JR, Wallace RB, Danielson GK: Surgery for postinfarction ventricular aneurysm. Ann Thorac Surg 15:588–91, 1973

98

INCREASED LIFE EXPECTANCY AFTER CORONARY VEIN GRAFTS COMPARED TO PEDICLES

William H. Sewell

INTRODUCTION

A statement that has been made many times in recent years in informal conferences, formal meetings, and medical literature, is that there is no evidence that coronary grafts prolong life. Information is available on survival rates after vein graft surgery, but until recently no acceptable control series have been reported.

Sheldon et al (1972) reported an operative mortality of 4 percent of 1,000 vein graft patients, an additional loss of 2.3 percent during the first postoperative year, and an average five-year attrition rate (including operative mortality) of 4.1 percent. In comparison, he reported an annual attrition rate of 6.8 percent among patients with arteriographically documented severe coronary sclerosis treated without surgery.

Most cardiologists seem to favor a prospective study with patients randomized into medical or surgical groups. However, a series of sham operations in some respects would be better because a patient's confidence that he is protected from a heart attack could conceivably affect survival rates. A sham operation series could be used if death caused by the operation can be eliminated, as there would be no operative mortality in a true medical control series.

A prospective study using a sham operation is not likely to be performed on a large scale, but retrospective studies are possible if vein graft patients are compared with a series of mammary

Aided by the Donald Guthrie Foundation for Medical Research.

artery implant patients. Such a comparison would seem valid if a patient surviving a mammary implant can be assumed to have an equal or better life expectancy than if he had not had surgery. Although such an assumption could be questioned, it seems within the realm of probability.

Previously published criteria (Sewell, 1974) have been established for the preoperative classification of vein graft patients into a low-risk group or a high-risk group. The low-risk patients in general are comparable to a previously published series of patients (Sewell, 1969) with internal mammary artery pedicle implants. Mammary artery implants were considered contraindicated in certain high-risk patients who would now be accepted for vein graft surgery.

PATIENT POPULATION

Vein graft operations without aortic clamping were done on 263 patients between April 1970 and January 1974. Of these, 215 were considered in the low-risk group. The operative mortality was 1.9 percent (four of 215). The other 48 were done in the high-risk group with a mortality of 25 percent (12 of 48).

Follow-up coronary and graft arteriography was done by the end of the third postoperative month on 98 percent of the vein graft survivors. Of these, 178 were done over one year ago. Follow-up for one year or until death was obtained on 164 patients (92 percent). Of these, 136 were found to have all grafts patent and functioning well; 28 were found to have one or more grafts occluded although some patients had one or more functioning grafts (Fig. 1). Follow-up of at least one year (or until death) was obtained on all of

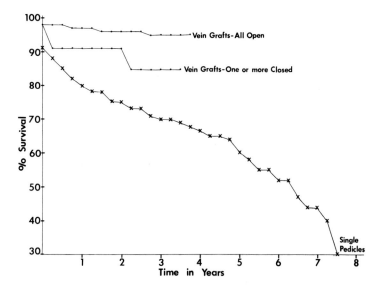

FIG. 1. Absolute survival. Life table presentation of 136 patients with all vein grafts open, 28 patients with one or more grafts closed, (plus 2 operative deaths), and 125 surviving pedicle patients (plus 12 operative deaths).

125 patients discharged alive after mammary pedicle implants between 1962 and 1966.

Age

The age range among the patients with all vein grafts patent was 24 to 69 years with an average of 51 years. Among those with one or more grafts occluded, the age range was 34 to 66 years with an average of 49 years. In the pedicle series, the age range was 34 to 59 years with an average of 45 years. Any bias introduced in the series because of age differences might be expected to favor the pedicle group.

Sex

In the group of patients in which all vein grafts were patent and functioning, 92 percent were male and 8 percent were female. Of the group with occluded vein grafts 80 percent were male and 20 percent were female. Of the males 87 percent had all grafts patent, whereas only 68 percent of the females retained function in all grafts.

Severity of Sclerosis

In the patent vein graft series of patients, 20 percent had one major coronary branch involved, 52 percent had two, and 28 percent had three. Comparable percentages among the occluded vein graft group were 20 percent, 53 percent, and 27 percent. Comparable percentages among the pedicle patients were 37 percent, 42 percent, and 21 percent. This indicates that more

of the pedicle patients had single lesions and more of the vein graft patients had triple lesions. Any bias introduced by this factor would be expected to favor survival in the pedicle series.

Congestive Failure

A patient was not accepted in the pedicle series if he had a left ventricular end-diastolic pressure of 15 mm Hg or higher if he also had triple coronary lesions. Patients were not accepted in the good-risk vein graft group if the ejection fraction was 0.30 or lower. Though not strictly comparable, this means that the vein graft patients in general had more ventricular damage than the pedicle patients.

RESULTS

Among the patients with all vein grafts patent, 135 survived the first postoperative year and one suffered a cardiac death during this period. Thirteen of the 125 pedicle patients suffered non-surgically related cardiac deaths during a comparable period. Three of the 28 patients in the occluded vein graft group died.

Comparison of the one postoperative death and 135 one-year survivors in the vein graft group with the 13 deaths and 112 survivors in the pedicle group was made. One-year survival rate was higher in the vein graft group (p < 0.001). If the two operative deaths during that period are included, then comparison of three deaths and 135 survivors with the same pedicle series is significant at $p < 0.01$. Comparison between the occluded vein graft group and the pedicle group demonstrates no difference.

Two-year follow-up information is available on 103 of the above patent vein graft patients. One of these died a noncardiac death during this period, but there were no cardiac deaths. Comparison with the three cardiac deaths among the 98 comparable pedicle patients does not indicate a significant difference. There were no deaths during the second postoperative year among the 16 eligible patients with occluded vein grafts.

There was one noncardiac death among the 46 eligible patients with patent vein grafts during the third postoperative year; there were no cardiac deaths. There was one noncardiac death among the 92 comparable pedicle patients. These differences are not of statistical significance.

Adding both vein graft series together gives two operative and four postoperative deaths among 166 patients. Comparing this with 13 deaths among 125 pedicle patients is significant at $p < 0.05$.

DISCUSSION

The implication of the study is that a patient can expect increased life expectancy if he can be offered vein graft surgery with a low mortality risk and a high chance of all grafts being patent. A recently published follow-up study (Sewell, 1974) showed a 97 percent patency rate with 79 side to side anastomoses between a vein graft and coronary artery, and patency of 87 percent of the 54 end to side anastomoses on 54 patients. Ninety-eight percent of the patients had one or more patent grafts with an average of 2.3 per patient.

SUMMARY AND CONCLUSIONS

A retrospective comparison was done between a series of 125 patients surviving mammary artery pedicle implantation and 164 comparable patients surviving vein graft operations. The cardiac death rate among patients with all vein grafts patent is significantly lower than the cardiac death rate among pedicle patients ($p < 0.001$). The death rate among the patients with one or more vein grafts occluded is not better than in the pedicle series, but the total (including operative mortality) of six deaths among 166 vein graft patients is significantly lower than the one-year mortality among the pedicle patients ($p < 0.05$).

Based on past experience, a patient meeting the criteria for the low-risk vein graft group can be offered surgery with a 2 percent operative risk, an 87 percent chance of all grafts remaining patent, and a 97 percent chance of surviving the first postoperative year. This represents an increased survival rate when compared to the pedicle group ($p < 0.05$), and compared to medical management alone if single pedicles are equal to or better than medical management alone.

References

Sewell, WH: Coronary Disease Management: Coronary Arteriography, Nitrates, and the Triple Pedicle Operation. St Louis, Warren H. Green, 1969

Sewell, WH: Improved coronary vein graft patency rates with side-to-side anastomoses. Ann Thorac Surg 17: 538, 1974

Sheldon WC, Rincon G, Effler DB, Proudfit WL, Sones FM Jr: Vein graft surgery for coronary artery disease: survival and angiographic results among the first one thousand patients. Circulation (Suppl 2) 46:2–110, 1972

99

MYOCARDIAL REVASCULARIZATION BY INTERNAL THORACIC ARTERY IMPLANTATION
Late Follow-up

Gulshan K. Sethi, Stewart M. Scott,
and Timothy Takaro

In 1946, Vineberg proposed the idea of implantation of the internal thoracic artery in the ischemic myocardium for its revascularization,[22] and the first clinical attempt was made by him in 1950.[23] Since then, and prior to introduction of direct coronary arterial surgery, internal thoracic arterial implantation was the commonest procedure for angina pectoris. It has been confirmed angiographically that the internal thoracic artery when implanted in the ischemic ventricular wall remains patent and establishes connection with the coronary arterial system. However, the degree of coronary arterial opacification at implant angiography has been found to be an unreliable index of the volume of blood flow through the implant, because the intensity of implant and coronary arterial opacification can be altered with the position of the tip of the catheter in relation to the internal thoracic arterial orifice and with the pressure of injection of the contrast material in the implant.[3,20] Among 40 angiographically patent implants, Ellestad reported nine of them to have no measurable blood flow and six of these patients, with no flow through the implant, had good clinical results.[5]

The relative physiologic significance of the contribution of blood through the implant to coronary arterial circulation and the degree of subjective and objective improvement following surgery remain controversial. There seem to be almost as many favorable clinical reports as those that are unfavorable or inconclusive.

CLINICAL EXPERIENCE

From 1962 to 1969, there were 198 patients with disabling angina pectoris and significant coronary occlusive disease of vessels supplying the anterolateral or a combination of anterolateral and posteroinferior left ventricular myocardial wall who underwent myocardial revascularization by using one or both internal thoracic arteries as pedicle implants. Prior to surgery these patients were subjected to selective coronary angiography, which demonstrated that all the patients had significant anterolateral ischemia, and 104 (51.5 percent) had concomitant significant posteroinferior disease as well. One hundred and eighty-five patients had implantation of the left internal thoracic artery, and 13 patients underwent implantation of both internal thoracic arteries. The implants consisted of a pedicle containing internal thoracic artery and vein, surrounding endothoracic fascia, pleura, and sternocostalis muscle.[19]

The operative mortality (death within 30 days following surgery) was 8.5 percent (17 patients) and another 17 patients (8.5 percent) died during the first year. The operative mortality was 15 percent among the 13 patients who underwent bilateral implantation. Late follow-up (up to 10.5 years) was obtained in all of the remaining 164 patients. In the majority of patients, routine examination was performed at six-month intervals following surgery. In the remainder, clinical information was obtained through other Veterans' Administration agencies, family physicians, a special questionnaire, or by telephone contact with the patient or his family, if the patient was dead. Specific information was obtained concerning physical activity level, myocardial infarction following surgery, congestive heart failure, reduction of use of coronary dilators, and change in severity and frequency of anginal attacks after operation in comparison to the preoperative status.

LATE FOLLOW-UP

Of 164 patients who survived more than one year, 146 (89 percent) had follow-up implant angiography at least once. Seventy of these had a second arteriogram two or more years following operation, and 25 had a third arteriogram three to six years after surgery. The arteriograms in 139 patients were of single implants and in seven of bilateral implants. On review of arteriograms of 139 single implants, 11 (eight percent) demonstrated occlusion. Sixty-five (61 percent) were patent with visualization of myocardial blush or fine coronary vessels. These were classified as "low-grade" arteriograms. Forty-three (31 percent) were patent with opacified large coronary arteries and usually veins as well. These were termed "high-grade" arteriograms (Table 1). The implant patency rate among seven patients with bilateral implants who underwent implant angiography was 78.5 percent (Table 2).

Late follow-up was complete in all 164 patients. An attempt was made to correlate coronary arterial opacification at implant arteriography with symptomatic relief of angina, incidence of postoperative myocardial infarction, congestive heart failure, physical activity level, and late cardiac death. No correlation was noted in any of these parameters. Symptomatic improvement in angina

TABLE 1. Classification of Implant Arteriograms According to Opacification of Coronary Vessels in 139 Single Implants

	NO.	%
Occluded[a]	11	8
Low-grade[b]	85	61
High-grade[c]	43	31

[a]*Implant occluded with no coronary vessels visible.*
[b]*Implant patent and producing a myocardial blush or opacifying small coronary vessels.*
[c]*Implant patent and opacifying large coronary vessels.*

TABLE 2. Correlation of Implant Opacification and Relief of Angina in Seven Patients with Bilateral Implants

PT. NO.	IMPLANT		ANGINA			FOLLOW-UP PERIOD, MOS	SURVIVAL STATUS
	Right	Left	B	S	W		
1	H	O	–	x	–	13	Dead
2	L	O	–	x	–	46	Alive
3	L	L	–	x	–	55	Alive
4	L	H	–	–	x	50	Alive
5	O	L	x	–	–	50	Alive
6	L	L	x	–	–	50	Alive
7	L	L	x	–	–	48	Dead

B: better; O: occluded implant; S: same; L: low-grade opacification; W: worse; H: high-grade opacification.
Reproduced from Sethi et al: Internal thoracic arterial implants: longterm followup. Chest 64:235, 1973.

TABLE 3. Degree of Angina Relief Correlated with Implant Arteriographic Grades in in 139 Patients with Single Implant

IMPLANT ANGIOGRAM	ANGINA				TOTAL
	Improved	Same	Worse	Undecided	
Occluded	5 (46%)	3 (27%)	2 (18%)	1 (9%)	11
Low-grade	31 (37%)	39 (46%)	6 (7%)	9 (10%)	85
High-grade	14 (33%)	21 (49%)	3 (7%)	5 (11%)	43

Reproduced from Sethi et al: Internal thoracic arterial implants: longterm follow-up. Chest 64:235, 1973.

was noted in 46 percent of the patients with occluded implants, in 37 percent of the patients with low-grade opacification, and in 33 percent with high-grade opacification (Table 3). Seven of 39 patients (18 percent) in the low-grade opacification group and six of 20 (30 percent) in the high-grade opacification group had initial improvement in their angina, which gradually became worse, and at last follow-up they claimed to have no change in the angina in comparison to the preoperative status.

There were 108 deaths among this group of 198 patients. Of these, 60 were cardiac in origin, and a death was defined as "cardiac" if the primary cause of death was due to some manifestation of arteriosclerotic heart disease, including myocardial infarction, cardiac arrhythmias, or congestive heart failure. A sudden death at home was also attributed to cardiac origin. Other causes of death are shown in Table 4. In 16 patients, the exact cause of death could not be determined. The terminal course was progressively increasing weakness, fatigue, and occasional signs of congestive heart failure. However, these were not grouped *under known "cardiac" deaths* but were due to *unknown causes.*

Thirteen patients who continued to have disabling angina underwent dorsal sympathectomy

TABLE 4. Causes of Death in 108 Patients

CAUSE OF DEATH	NO.	%
Operative deaths	17	15.7
Late cardiac deaths	60	55.6
Unknown causes	16	14.8
Various malignancies	5	4.6
Associated with other surgical procedures	5	4.6
Following implant or coronary angiography	3	2.8
Hepatic dysfunctions	2	1.9

for symptomatic relief. This opportunity was utilized to measure directly the blood flow through the internal thoracic arterial implant at surgery. Seven of these 13 patients had arteriograms showing "low-grade" opacification, and six had arteriograms showing "high-grade" opacification by the criteria mentioned previously. Implant flows by electromagnetic flow meter measurement averaged eight ml per minute with a range of four to 19 ml per minute. Approximately 6 ml was the average flow in the "low-grade" group as compared to 11 ml in the "high-grade" group. Temporary manual occlusion of the implant for five minutes did not change the electrocardiogram or cardiac function as observed at operation. However, in one patient we noticed significant ST segment depression in lead III on temporary occlusion of implant at the time of direct coronary arterial surgery (Fig. 1). This indicated to us that the myocardium was probably dependent upon the implant and led to the decision not to divide it.

Repeat coronary angiography, usually at the time of implant angiography, was performed in 91 patients one to five years following surgery. Fifty-four patients (59 percent) showed progression of coronary arterial disease, and 18 of these (33 percent) showed progressive increase of disease in the right coronary artery. The presence of a new occlusion, further stenosis of an already diseased vessel, or new stenosis in a previously uninvolved artery were considered as evidence of progression of the coronary arterial disease. No correlation between progression of coronary arterial disease and degree of coronary arterial opacification during implant angiography was noted. However, improvement in coronary arterial opacification was seen in seven patients who had serial implant angiograms, and five of these showed progression in coronary arterial disease.

Among 77 patients with single implants who are still alive and have been followed from four to

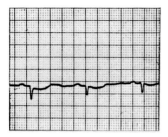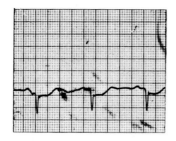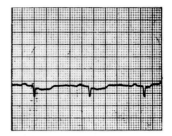

FIG. 1. Intraoperative electrocardiographic changes in a patient whose implant was clamped temporarily. Left: before clamping pedicle. Middle: pedicle clamped. Right: pedicle unclamped. (Reproduced from Sethi, et al: Internal thoracic arterial implants: longterm follow-up. Chest 64:235, 1973.)

10.5 years, there was no definite correlation between symptomatic relief and angiographic findings. Improvement in angina was noted in 50 percent of patients in whom the myocardial ischemia was limited to anterolateral left ventricle (in the area of the implant), as compared to 43 percent when the patient had both anterolateral and posteroinferior ischemic myocardium.

DISCUSSION

Internal thoracic arterial implantation represents one of the many techniques of indirect revascularization of the ischemic myocardium. Evaluation of the results of this procedure has usually been based on mortality rate, symptomatic improvement, and angiographic patency, and evidence that this operation is of benefit has rested largely upon the reduction or disappearance of angina pectoris. Unfortunately, previous experience with other medical and surgical methods of treatment of angina has amply demonstrated the unreliability of such uncontrolled observations.

One cannot deny the validity of the evidence of angiographic patency of internal thoracic arterial implants and of the formation of communicating vessels between the internal thoracic artery and coronary arterial system. However, the demonstration of implant patency and communication with the coronary arteries does not necessarily imply that a significant amount of blood is being delivered to the ischemic myocardium through these channels. It has been conclusively demonstrated, both clinically and experimentally, that the degree of coronary arterial opacification by way of implant arteriography is highly dependent upon the technical factors during angiography. The intensity and extent of coronary arterial visualization at implant angiography can be varied by altering the position of the tip of the catheter in relation to the internal thoracic arterial orifice or by altering the pressure of injection of contrast material. Even injection of contrast material in the subclavian artery may produce a major temporarily significant elevation in the internal thoracic arterial flow.

TABLE 5. Flow Measurements in Chronic Internal Thoracic Arterial Implants in Dogs

INVESTIGATOR	FLOW (ML/MT)	
	Range	Average
Vineberg	8–55	11
Provan	–	28
Criollos	13–47	29
Barner	2.2–7.6[a]	–
Mallette	–	14
Dart	3–22	12

[a]*2.2 to 7.6 ml per 100 gms of left ventricle.*

The available data, regarding volume of blood flow through the implant, is conflicting in experimental animals (Table 5) and scanty in human beings (Table 6). In patients, Taylor and Gorlin,[21] and Kay and associates [11] have utilized indirect techniques to measure the flow through the implant. These techniques are subject to inherent errors. The correlation of volume flows obtained by electromagnetic flow meter and indirect techniques have not been well established.

Most clinical and experimental results of internal thoracic arterial implantations cast serious doubt upon the value of this procedure for providing a significant extra cardiac blood supply to the ischemic myocardium. Kaiser and associates studied the metabolic and functional contribution of blood flow in five angiographically patent chronic implants in dogs that also had ameroid constrictors on their coronary arteries. Occlusion of the implants failed to alter myocardial extraction of oxygen, pyruvates, and lactate, or ventricular function; nor did these patent implants prevent significant changes in the above parameters during and following occlusion of the remaining patent left coronary artery.[9]

Kassenbaum and associates reported clinical improvements in 50 percent of their patients. However, only 15 percent of them had satisfactory collateralization. Electrographic evidence of myocardial ischemia induced by stress exercise or hypoxia remained present in most of the patients. Only three patients reverted from a positive stress test to a negative one, and only one showed development of corresponding excellent collaterals

TABLE 6. Flow Measurements in Chronic Internal Thoracic Arterial Implants in Humans

INVESTIGATOR	METHOD	RANGE	AVERAGE
Taylor	Isotope (Kr 85) Method	50–100 ml/ 100 gms of LV	–
Kay	Cineangiographic volume flow studies	25–40 ml	35 ml
Dart	Direct electromagnetic flow studies	4–19 ml	8 ml
Ellestad	Double contrast technique using CO_2 and hypaque	0–48 ml	16.2 ml

from the implant.[10] Langston and associates studied 18 patients who had had bilateral implants. Thirteen of these demonstrated deterioration of cardiac hemodynamics as indicated by low cardiac index, decreased stroke index, and increased pulmonary arterial wedge pressure. Six of these patients also had poorer left ventricular contractility on ventriculography.[13] McAllister and associates demonstrated improvement in left ventricular function in only eight percent of their patients who were evaluated one year after implant surgery.[15]

Balcon et al evaluated 20 patients postoperatively by stressing the heart with atrial pacing. Only three of them showed objective improvement associated with arteriographic evidence of intramyocardial anastomosis between implant and the coronary arterial system. However, clinical improvement was noted in 60 percent of the patients in this group, and there was no correlation between angiographic findings and clinical results. The authors concluded that in most of the subjectively improved patients some mechanism other than revascularization was responsible for clinical success.[1]

Greenberg and associates reported that the diagnosis of myocardial infarction was either confirmed (18 percent) or suspected (10 percent) among a group of 40 patients who underwent implant surgery. The incidence of confirmed postoperative myocardial infarction was much higher in the bilateral implant group (30 percent) as compared to patients undergoing single implant (5 percent).[8] It is conceivable that deterioration of cardiac function following surgery may be attributed to myocardial injury at surgery. This has been documented in animals following internal thoracic arterial implantation by McNamara and Urschel.[16]

Gorlin and Taylor reported 16 of 20 patients who produced lactate preoperatively reverted to normal lactate extraction one year after surgery.[7] Kemp and associates found a positive correlation between reversal of normal lactate metabolism, angiographic patency, and clinical improvement following internal thoracic arterial implantation.[12] However, the significance of these changes of myocardial metabolism have been seriously questioned. The metabolic studies do not reflect altered perfusion to a specific segment of the heart muscle since the biochemical analysis is performed on coronary sinus blood, which represents a pooled sample of total myocardial mass. Secondly, the metabolic changes have not been recorded consistently enough to claim them as a routine consequence of surgery.[14] The change in lactate metabolism may be explained by conversion of the ischemic area of myocardium to infarction, scar, or a metabolically inert area.[13]

We confirmed that there was no correlation between incidence of postoperative myocardial infarction, symptomatic improvement, or survival rate with degree of coronary arterial opacification during implant angiography, which others have also noted.[1,2,3,18] One may attribute this poor correlation to the fact that single implants were used in some patients with both anterolateral and posteroinferior myocardial ischemia. However, among the 77 patients who are still alive with single implant and in whom up-to-date reliable data are available, 40 had recognizable myocardial ischemia only in the anterolateral wall of the left ventricle, while the remaining patients had both anterolateral and posteroinferior disease. Statistically, there was no significant difference between implant opacification and symptomatic relief in either group. Razavi and associates at the Cleveland Clinic, on review of 500 patients with bilateral implants, also concluded that symptomatic improvement did not correlate with angiographic findings.[17]

A cumulative survival curve of these 198 patients who underwent internal thoracic arterial implants was constructed by using Life Table Methods (Fig. 2). It was compared with the survival curve, obtained from the Metropolitan Life Insurance Company, in a group of patients with ischemic ST segment depression after exercise. In these patients, the survival curve was constructed on the data obtained at stress electrocardiography and degree of ST segment depression criteria advocated by Robb (Grade 1, depression of 0.1 to 0.9 mm, Grade 2, depression of 1 to 1.9, Grade 3, depression of more than 2 mm).[4] The survival curve of our patients approximated the curve of a group of patients with severe ischemic changes (Grade 3) who were not treated surgically (Fig. 3).

A comparison of survival curves based on angiographic classification among surgically and nonsurgically treated patients with angina pectoris was also attempted. Our patients had an average angiographic score of about nine, but the survival curve was comparable with the group of patients with angiographic score of more than 10, representing severe ischemic disease, who were not treated surgically (Fig. 4).[6] Based on these studies, we have concluded that the cumulative survival curve has not been significantly altered by the surgical procedure.

A hypothesis that would explain the results in an occasional patient in whom the contribu-

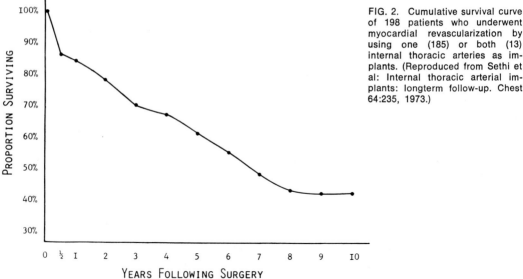

FIG. 2. Cumulative survival curve of 198 patients who underwent myocardial revascularization by using one (185) or both (13) internal thoracic arteries as implants. (Reproduced from Sethi et al: Internal thoracic arterial implants: longterm follow-up. Chest 64:235, 1973.)

tion of blood flow through the implant to the coronary arterial circulation seems to be of physiologic significance depends upon the following sequence of events. The implant is placed in an area that becomes progressively more ischemic weeks and months after implant surgery because of progression of coronary arterial disease proximal to the site of the implant. When this happens, the usually small and insignificant communications between the implant and myocardial vessels

in the granulation tissue, which form in the process of healing of the myocardial wound made at the time of implant surgery, become physiologically significant. This occurs because of the gradual development of a gradient between the implanted internal thoracic artery and the coronary artery distal to the progressing coronary arterial lesion. Under these circumstances, an arteriogram of an implant showing initially insignificant anastomoses with the coronary circulation, might at

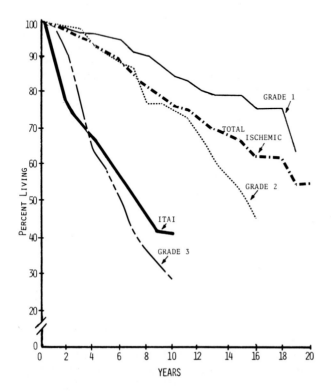

FIG. 3. Comparison of cumulative survival curve of patients undergoing internal thoracic arterial implant (ITAI) and nonoperated patients with various grades of ischemic changes on stress electrocardiography. (Adapted from "Detection and prognosis in coronary artery disease," Metropolitan Life Ins Co Stat Bull 53:3, 1972.)

FIG. 4. Comparison of survival curve of patients undergoing internal thoracic arterial implant (ITAI) and nonoperated patients with varying degrees of coronary arteriosclerosis as seen on coronary angiography. (Adapted from Friesinger, et al: Prognostic significance of coronary arteriography. Trans Assoc Am Physicians 83:78, 1970.)

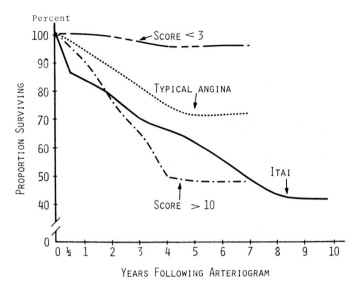

subsequent arteriography show significant improvement in coronary opacification, presumably indicative of improvement in collaterals and implant flow. This sequence of events apparently occurs uncommonly enough so that longevity in a large number of patients does not appear to be significantly affected. From this evidence and in view of the availability of direct coronary arterial surgery, it appears that implantation of the internal thoracic artery does not now seem to be a reasonable modality of surgical treatment to offer to the patient with angina pectoris.

References

1. Balcon R, Leaver D, Ross D, Ross K, Sowton E: Internal mammary artery implantation. Lancet 1: 440, 1970
2. Barner HB, Harada Y, Jellinek M, Mudd JG, Kaiser GC: Coronary flow and myocardial function after myocardial revascularization. Surg Forum 18:105, 1967
3. Dart CH Jr, Kato Y, Scott SM, et al: Internal thoracic (mammary) arteriography. A questionable index of myocardial revascularization. J Thorac Cardiovasc Surg 59:117, 1970
4. Detection and prognosis in coronary artery disease. Metropolitan Life Ins Co Stat Bull 53:3, 1972
5. Ellestad MH: Double-contrast angiography in human internal mammary implants. Ann Thorac Surg 12:428, 1971
6. Friesinger GC, Page EE, Ross RS: Prognostic significance of coronary arteriography. Trans Assoc Am Physicians 83:78, 1970
7. Gorlin R, Taylor WJ: Selective revascularization of the myocardium by internal mammary artery implant. N Engl J Med 275:283, 1966
8. Greenberg BH, McCallister, BD, Frye RL, Wallace RB: Serum glutamic oxaloacetic transaminase and electrocardiographic changes after myocardial revascularization procedure in patients with coronary artery lesion. Am J Cardiol 26:135, 1970
9. Kaiser GC, Barner HB, Jellinek M, Mudd JG, Hanlon CR: Metabolic assessment of internal mammary artery implantation in the dog. Circulation 41:Suppl 2, 49, 1970
10. Kassenbaum DG, Judkins MP, Griswold HE: Stress electrocardiography in the evaluation of surgical revascularization of the heart. Circulation 40:297, 1969
11. Kay EB, Suzuki A: Myocardial revascularization by bilateral internal mammary artery implantation. Experimental and clinical data. Am J Cardiol 22: 227, 1968
12. Kemp HG, Manchester JH, Amsterdam EA, Taylor WJ, Gorlin R: Internal mammary artery implantation: effect on myocardial lactate utilization. Circulation 41:Suppl 2, 55, 1970
13. Langston MF, Kerth WJ, Selzer A, Cohn, KE: Evaluation of internal mammary artery implantation. Am J Cardiol 29:788, 1972
14. Likoff W: Myocardial revascularization: A critique. NY J Med 70:1983, 1970
15. McAllister BD, Richmond DR, Saltups A, et al: Left ventricular hemodynamics before and one year after internal mammary artery implantation in patients with coronary artery disease and angina pectoris. Circulation 42:471, 1970
16. McNamara JJ, Urschel HC Jr: Acute influence of internal mammary artery implantation on ventricular function. Circulation 39:Suppl 1, 67, 1969
17. Razavi M, Heupler FA, Germanovich E, Effler DB, Sones M, Jr: Long-term clinical and angiographic results in bilateral internal mammary artery implants. Circulation 46:Suppl 2, 208, 1972
18. Sethi GK, Scott SM, Takaro T: Myocardial revascularization by internal thoracic arterial implants: longterm follow-up. Chest 64:235, 1973
19. Sewell WH: Surgery for acquired coronary disease. Springfield, Ill, CC Thomas, 1967
20. Suma K, Hammond GL, Buckley MJ, Austen WG: Hemodynamic studies of short-term and long-term internal mammary artery implants. Ann Thorac Surg 7:13, 1969
21. Taylor WJ, Gorlin R: Objective criteria for internal mammary artery implantation. Ann Thorac Surg 4:143, 1967
22. Vineberg AM, Miller GG: Internal mammary coronary anastomosis in surgical treatment of coronary artery insufficiency. Canad Med Assoc J 64:204, 1951
23. Vineberg AM: Development of anastomosis between coronary vessels and transplanted internal mammary artery. Canad Med Assoc J 55:117, 1946

100

AORTOCORONARY BYPASS SURGERY
Review of 2,711 Patients *

Robert J. Hall, Efrain Garcia, Mahdi S. Al-Bassam,
and John T. Dawson

Coronary artery disease, a major cause of disability and death, has currently become a topic of intense medical interest. Attention has turned in this direction largely because of expertise in the anatomic definition of the intravascular lesions by coronary cineangiography developed by Sones and associates,[26] and development of the first consistently successful surgical approach to the problem, aortocoronary saphenous vein bypass grafting, by Favaloro [11] and Johnson.[19] A review was made of the immediate and long-term results of coronary artery bypass surgery (CAB) performed at our institution since August 1969. Patients who had simultaneous valve, ventricular aneurysm, or aortic aneurysm surgery were not included in this report.

CORONARY BYPASS SURGERY

Composition of the Patient Population

Patients seen at the Texas Heart Institute originate from widespread areas of the United States and many foreign countries. While many undergo complete evaluation at our institution, others are referred for evaluation and surgical consideration after having undergone coronary angiogaphy elsewhere. Those who undergo CAB [18] are predominantly men (87 percent),

have a high incidence of previous myocardial infarction(s) (79 percent), or have experienced an acute infarction within one month before surgery (5.3 percent), have an average coronary artery score of 9.2 (graded on a scale of 0 to 15 according to the method of Friesinger and associates [12]), are symptomatic because of angina pectoris (98.6 percent), and are predominantly in functional classifications III (72 percent) or IV (24 percent) (New York Heart Association). Congestive heart failure, past or present, was noted in 22 percent and the preinfarction syndrome in 9.5 percent.

Early Mortality

Among all 2,711 patients who underwent CAB alone, with or without endarterectomy, at our institution through December 31, 1973, early mortality (within the first 30 days after operation) was 6.2 percent.[7] Of 1,030 patients who had CAB alone in 1973, forty-six (4.5 percent) early deaths occurred. There was one death (0.9 percent) in 112 single, 14 (3.8 percent) in 370 double, and 29 (5.3 percent) in 548 triple or more CAB procedures. The wide range of reported figures for surgical or early mortality is in large part the result of the variable extent of disease and type of patients accepted for CAB, by differing groups. We have carefully monitored early mortality in order to isolate as many determinants as possible. The direct cause of early deaths was predominantly cardiac in origin (88 percent),[18] over one-third of which were caused by immediate failure of myocardial pump function and another one-third by postoperative myocardial infarction. Analysis of the composition of the surviving and the nonsurviving groups has

* All coronary artery bypass operations reported in this review were performed by Drs. Denton A. Cooley, Grady L. Hallman, and their associates. Their permission to review these patients is gratefully acknowledged.

TABLE 1. Factors Adversely Influencing Survival Following Coronary Artery Bypass Surgery

Simultaneous endarterectomy
Age of patient
Female sex
Left ventricular failure
Moderate to severe left ventricular dysfunction
Recent prior acute infarction
Preinfarction angina
Coronary artery score
Involvement of main left coronary artery

delineated a number of determinants that adversely effect survival (Table 1).

FACTORS ADVERSELY INFLUENCING SURVIVAL

Simultaneous Endarterectomy

Endarterectomy was performed concomitantly with CAB in 32 percent of the first 1,105 patients who underwent the procedure from October 1969 to March 1972. These patients had a higher coronary artery score, and endarterectomy was accomplished by blunt dissection and traction without the use of special techniques such as gas dissection. The saphenous vein bypass was anastomosed to the site of endarterectomy. While simultaneous endarterectomy has extended the procedure to vessels that otherwise could not have been considered for bypass, it also has increased early mortality (9.3 percent with, in comparison to 5.3 percent without endarterectomy) and was accompanied by a higher rate of postoperative graft occlusion.[18]

Age of Patients

Early mortality was lowest in the fifth decade of life (4.2 percent) and highest in the seventh and eighth decades (9.6 percent).[18]

Female Sex

We previously documented an early mortality twice as great in women as in men [18] and have attempted to elicit those factors that lead to this increased surgical risk. Although women on the average were three years older than men, the age difference was not the sole cause of the higher early mortality since an increase in the risk for women who underwent CAB was seen in every decade except the fourth.[18] In a recent study involving the first 1,372 consecutive CAB

TABLE 2. Comparison of Risk and Other Factors in 1,221 Men and 151 Women Who Underwent Coronary Artery Bypass

FACTOR	NO. MEN	%	NO. WOMEN	%
Diabetes mellitus	110	9.0	32	21.2
Hypertension	71	5.8	47	31.1
Preinfarction angina	78	6.4	29	11.6
Recent infarction	90	7.4	20	13.2
Electrocardiogram				
ST injury	320	26.2	66	43.7
T injury	318	26.0	62	41.0
Average coronary artery score	9.24		7.95	
Autopsy cardiac weight	545 gm		453 gm	

patients,[1] major differences were noted between certain characteristics of the men and women patients (Table 2). Diabetes mellitus, hypertension, preinfarction angina, and recent myocardial infarction occurred nearly three times more frequently in women than in men, and ischemic T-wave and ST segmental changes of subendocardial injury were present nearly twice as often in women. In spite of these differences, the designated coronary artery score was slightly lower in the women. A general impression that women have smaller hearts was substantiated by studying the weight of hearts of women from autopsy specimens. It is our opinion that women more frequently have generalized vascular abnormalities, more diffuse and widespread coronary disease, poorly reflected in the gross coronary artery score, and from a technical standpoint, smaller hearts and coronary vessels—all of which contribute to an increased surgical risk.

Left Ventricular Failure and Dysfunction

Prior congestive heart failure, elevation of left ventricular end-diastolic pressure (above 25 mm Hg) and moderate or severe abnormalities of ventricular wall motion on left ventricular cineangiography were observed twice as often among those patients who did not survive surgery.[18]

Recent Myocardial Infarction

Early observations at our institution revealed that surgery performed within 30 days of a myocardial infarction adversely influenced early mortality.[18] A subsequent review of the role of recent infarction in the outcome of CAB revealed a 36 percent mortality when surgery was carried out within the first 24 hours, 40 percent when surgery occurred within the first week, and 16 percent when CAB was performed between eight to 30 days after a recent infarction. The majority of these patients underwent CAB because of serious consequences of a recent infarction including recurrent ventricular tachyarrhythmia, shock, congestive failure, recurrent cardiac arrest, and persistent severe chest pain. A number of survivors in this group represented retrieval from grave complications of a recent infarction. Patients who experienced infarction earlier than 30 days before CAB sustained no increased risk from CAB surgery. Those individuals who had not experienced a previous infarction demonstrated the lowest early mortality after CAB surgery (4.1 percent).[10] We believe CAB is contraindicated in the first 30 days following acute infarction unless it is performed to cope with grave and life-threatening complications in a patient who is not responding satisfactorily to aggressive medical therapy.

Preinfarction Angina

This syndrome is characterized by recurrent or continued coronary chest pain at rest, in the absence of Q-wave changes and enzyme elevation and usually accompanied by ST segment depression or subendocardial injury at least during the periods of pain. The increased mortality rate of patients who experienced preinfarction angina and who were managed medically has recently been detailed by Gazes.[14] Our observations show that these patients also have an increased surgical risk: 18 of 137 (13.1 percent) died in the first 30 days after CAB.[10] Whether some of these patients may have experienced a nondocumented acute myocardial infarction rather than the preinfarction angina syndrome was not always clear. The clinical judgment regarding the timing of surgical intervention in patients with prefarction angina is difficult.

Coronary Artery Score

The extent of coronary artery involvement, as reflected in the coronary artery score,[12] influenced the outcome of surgery. The coronary artery score was lower (9.1) in patients who survived in comparison to those who died (10.6).[6,18] This factor was even more pronounced in the group of patients who had concomitant ventricular aneurysm surgery (score of 8.9 in survivors versus 11.8 in nonsurvivors).[6]

Involvement of Main Left Coronary Artery

The increased risk involved in treating patients with main left coronary lesions—medically, at cardiac catheterization, during treadmill exercise testing, or with CAB—has recently been reported by others.[24,25] In our patients, main left arterial lesions were present in 5.1 percent of survivors and in 23 percent of the patients who died in the early period after CAB.[6]

Mortality in Low-Risk Patients

In our patients who were under the age 70, were of either sex, had a coronary artery score below 13, and had none of the other "high-risk" factors, early mortality following CAB was only 1.6 percent and late mortality was 1 percent.[6] Appreciation of the composition of different reported surgical series is essential for an understanding of varying data on early and late mortality.

SURGICAL SEQUELAE

Complications of Surgery

The predominant complications of CAB surgery[18] included arrhythmias, myocardial infarction, postpericardiotomy syndrome, and congestive heart failure (Table 3). Myocardial infarction

TABLE 3. Complications in 1,105 Patients Who Underwent Coronary Artery Bypass

COMPLICATIONS	NO. PTS.	%
Arrhythmia	232	21.0
Atrial	148	13.4
Ventricular	84	7.6
Myocardial infarction	156	14.1
Neurologic	59	5.3
Minor	33	3.0
Major	26	2.4
Postpericardiotomy syndrome	46	4.2
Congestive heart failure	43	3.9
Pulmonary	30	2.7
Urinary	30	2.7
Serous cavity hemorrhage and effusion	19	1.7
Thromboembolic and thrombophlebitis	13	1.2
Wound infection	10	0.9
Hepatitis	9	0.8
Renal failure	6	0.5
Other, miscellaneous	24	2.2

Many patients had multiple complications.

TABLE 4. Causes of Death in Patients Who Underwent Coronary Artery Bypass

CAUSE	NO. PTS.
Early (within 30 days postop)	
Could not come off pump	24
Acute myocardial infarction postop	24
Cardiac arrest, unresponsive[a]	12
Cardiac failure[a]	4
Neurologic	4
Miscellaneous	5
Total	73
Late (after 30 days postop)	
Acute myocardial infarction	6
Congestive heart failure	3
Cardiac arrest	2
Neurologic	1
Pulmonary embolism	1
Noncardiac in origin	1
Peripheral emboli	1
No cause ascertained	10
Total	25

[a]No autopsy performed or acute infarction observed at autopsy in these patients.

occurred in 14.1 percent of the first 1,105 patients. The causes of early and late deaths were predominantly cardiac in origin (Table 4).

Postoperative Myocardial Infarction

Postoperative myocardial infarction, indicated by new or substantially widened permanent Q-waves seen electrocardiographically, could be substantiated by serum enzyme increases above those seen in patients with uncomplicated CAB.[8] Postoperative infarction occurred more frequently in patients who had simultaneous endarterectomy[8,18] and resulted in more frequent postoperative congestive heart failure and decreased frequency of clinical improvement at long-term follow-up evaluation.[9]

FOLLOW-UP DATA OF SURVIVORS

Long-term Follow-up

Follow-up data have been compiled through June 1973 of 1,404 survivors of all CAB operations performed from August 1969 to September 1972, without other associated procedures other than endarterectomy.[17] Of the survivors (Table 5), 5.3 percent were lost to follow-up. Sixty-four late deaths (4.6 percent) were recorded. Angina was completely relieved in 65 percent, significantly improved in 20 percent, remained unchanged in 11 percent, and became worse in 4 percent of the survivors. Complete relief and improvement of angina occurred with greater frequency in patients who underwent multiple bypass procedures, apparently reflecting more complete and adequate revascularization. Since multiple bypass procedures were performed with increasing frequency during the progress of this series of patients, it is also possible that the higher frequency of improvement merely reflects a shorter period of follow-up study.

Of 943 patients with stable angina, 46 patients (4.9 percent) were lost to follow-up, and 33 (3.5 percent) died in the late period after surgery. Angina was relieved or improved in 87.5 percent of the survivors and remained the same or became worse in 12.5 percent of the survivors —results essentially identical to those in the total group (Table 6).

Follow-up for a period up to 46 months disclosed a late (after one month) attrition rate of

TABLE 5. Coronary Artery Bypass Alone: Follow-up through June 1973 of All Patients from Aug. 1969 through Sept. 1972

	NO. PTS.	%	BYPASS					
			Single	%	Double	%	Triple	%
Total series	1,404		304		822		278	
Late deaths	64	4.6	10	3.3	45	5.5	9	3.2
Unknown	75	5.3	15	4.9	43	5.2	17	6.1
Known survivors	1,265		279		734		252	
Angina								
Complete relief	823	65	149	53	470	64	204	81
Improved	251	20	65	23	153	21	33	13
Same	141	11	41	15	88	12	12	5
Worse	50	4	24	9	23	3	3	1

TABLE 6. Long-term Follow-up through September 1972 in 943 Patients with Stable Angina Who Underwent Coronary Bypass

	NO. PTS.	%	
Late deaths	33	3.5	
No follow-up	46	4.9	
Known survivors	864	91.6	
Angina relieved	558	64.6 }	87.5%
Angina improved	198	22.9 }	
Angina same	79	9.1 }	12.5%
Angina worse	29	3.4 }	

2.9 percent per annum for the total group; 3.2 percent per annum for patients with preinfarction angina; and 1.8 per annum for those with stable angina (Fig. 1).

The overall (early and late) survival rate of our total series at four years is 82.7 percent compared to the four-year survival rate of 70 percent in patients treated medically according to Sones (Fig. 2).[4]

Influence of Antithrombotic Therapy on Survivors

Of the 1,404 survivors of CAB, adequate follow-up drug data derived from an evaluation of the effects of postoperative antithrombotic therapy were available on 1,078 survivors.[3] The groups of patients receiving antithrombotic agents were similar in character to those not on such regimens. All groups of patients receiving long-term Coumadin, Persantine, and aspirin experienced higher survival rates than those not on drug therapy (Fig. 3). Evidence favored the group on aspirin, and it is our current practice to continue long-term aspirin alone or with Persantine in the postoperative period.

Survival Curve of Patients with Preinfarction Angina

The actuarial curve generated by patients with preinfarction angina in our series has been examined.[2] The cumulative three-year survival including the early mortality was 78.4 percent, slightly less than the 82.7 percent survival rate recorded in our patients as a whole. These results of surgical therapy appear to compare favorably with Gazes's data on medical treatment alone where the cumulative three-year survival was 69 percent in his total series and 37 percent in a subgroup whom he defined as presenting a high risk.[14]

Incidence of Postoperative Myocardial Infarction

The occurrence of postoperative myocardial infarction after the first month following surgery was reviewed in the total follow-up data of the

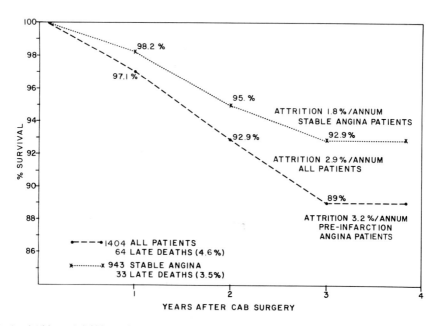

FIG. 1. Attrition of 1,404 survivors of coronary artery bypass (operated through September 1972) followed up to 46 months.

FIG. 2. Survival curve (actuarial method) for 1,510 patients who underwent coronary artery bypass at the Texas Heart Institute (St. Luke's Episcopal Hospital) from August 1969 through September 1972 (follow-up data through June 1973). The 4 percent, 6 percent, 10 percent, and 6.8 percent attrition curves are drawn from studies of Bruschke et al [4] describing the survival of medically treated patients with single-, double-, and triple-vessel disease and their whole group of 590 patients, followed 5 to 9 years after coronary arteriography.

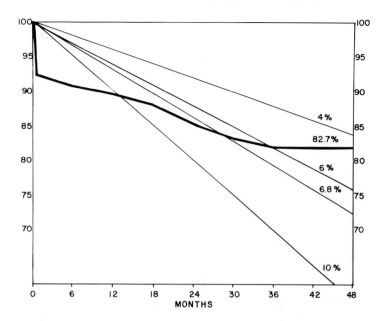

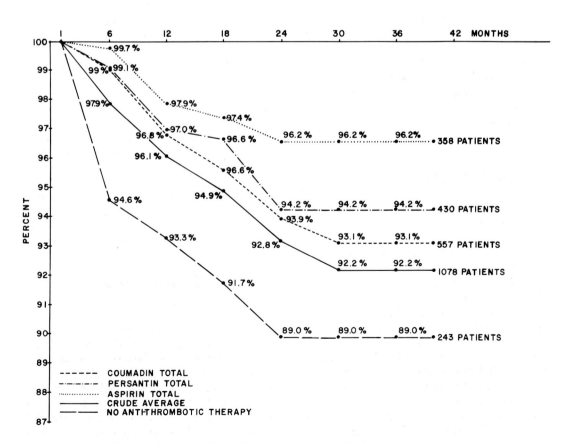

FIG. 3. Survival in patients receiving antithrombotic therapy following aortocoronary bypass.

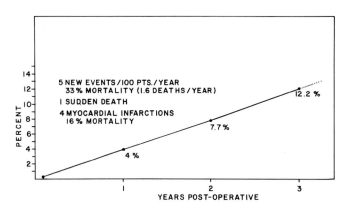

FIG. 4. Cumulative incidence of myocardial infarction after the first month following surgery in patients who underwent coronary artery bypass through September 1972.

series of patients who underwent operation through September, 1972. The cumulative incidence of infarction (Fig. 4) included four episodes per 100 patients per year with a fatality rate of 16 percent. If sudden deaths are included (approximately one per 100 patients per year), a total of five new cardiac events per 100 patients per annum occurred, with a fatality rate of 33 percent (attrition of 1.6 percent per annum). The similarity of fatality rates for all new events (33 percent) and for myocardial infarction (16 percent) in this postoperative series was strikingly similar to the fatality rates for new events in the natural history of coronary disease. Noncardiac events accounted for 25 percent of the deaths, and other cardiovascular causes for 42 percent of the deaths in this series of patients. Unfortunately, there is no acceptable yardstick for comparing the incidence of infarction and cause of death in a medically treated, comparable group of patients.

INVASIVE STUDIES

Graft Patency and Ventricular Function

The size and varying origins of our patient population have precluded angiographic restudy of all CAB patients on a routine basis. The restudy of one subgroup of patients from our institution has been accomplished by Leatherman and colleagues.[21-23] In this group of 200 patients, 60 percent were restudied on a random basis while 40 percent were restudied because of atypical or typical manifestations of their coronary artery disease, either continuing or recurrent after CAB. Men constituted 83 percent of this subgroup, slightly less than the composition of our total series.[18] Of 356 grafts, 267 (75 percent) were patent. All grafts were patent in 63 percent, at least

one in 89 percent, and none in 14 percent of these patients. Both the existence of diabetes mellitus and the performance of endarterectomy reduced the incidence of graft patency. Postoperative myocardial infarction occurred in 16 percent of these patients and occurred with greater frequency among those who underwent endarterectomy (24 percent) than in those who did not require endarterectomy (13 percent). Left ventriculography revealed an apparent improvement in myocardial function in 15 percent, no change in 66 percent, and decreased function in 19 percent of the 96 patients who had adequate pre- and postoperative evaluation. Graft patency in the groups of patients whose ventricular function was judged to be improved, unchanged, or worse was 78 percent, 69 percent, and 44 percent, respectively, revealing a correlation between graft occlusion and impaired ventricular dynamics.[22] These findings were similar to those reported by Ross and associates.[15] The incidence of graft patency of 80 percent in patients studied for atypical pain, in contrast to a range of 53 percent to 37 percent in those restudied for classical angina, congestive heart failure, or postoperative infarction also demonstrates a relationship between graft patency and long-term results of surgery.

Pathologic Changes in the Saphenous Vein Bypass Graft

Klima and Milam[42] from our institution have shown that saphenous vein graft occlusion is due primarily to intraluminal thrombosis. Although luminal narrowing caused by fibrous intimal proliferation in the vein graft was observed in many of the long-term survivors, the majority exhibited patency even at two to three years following surgery. This latter process is similar to that observed by others in saphenous vein grafts used in peripheral arterial reconstructive surgery and in experimental animals. Recent thrombosis was observed in some of the long-term survivors, and in only one case was saphenous vein obstruction due to fibrous intimal proliferation.

NONINVASIVE STUDIES

Objective Measures of Improvement Following CAB Surgery

While improvement or complete relief of angina has been noted in 85 percent of our survivors, it is argued by some that such improvement may be the consequence of either the natural course of the disease, infarction of ischemic areas, or a placebo effect from surgery. It is possible that each of these factors probably plays some role in a certain percentage of patients, and the total evaluation of the procedure cannot rest upon subjective data. In an earlier report on pre- and postoperative treadmill exercise testing of CAB patients, we noted a 75 percent conversion to a negative response.[13] An increase also occurred in the average maximal heart rate achieved and the average duration of the test in the postoperative period. Reversion to a negative response in those patients who underwent simultaneous endarterectomy was only 63.7 percent. In a smaller group subjected to exercise testing by Leatherman,[22] there was a lower percentage (50 percent) of reversion to a negative response postoperatively. Treadmill and other forms of exercise testing add some objective evidence to support the subjective improvement noted in patients after CAB. It should be recognized, however, that an occasional patient with angina treated medically can demonstrate a reversion from a positive to a negative exercise test response and that some patients will show reversion following recovery from a nonfatal myocardial infarction, without surgical intervention, presumably because of either enhanced collateralization or infarction of the ischemic area.

Serial Treadmill Testing

A more recent study of serial treadmill testing in patients up to 26 months after CAB[16] revealed an 18 percent late reversion to a positive response (greater than 1 mm ST segment depression) in 56 patients whose response was negative on the first postoperative treadmill testing procedure. In those patients whose first postoperative study was negative, subsequent conversion to a positive test occurred in only 5 percent of patients whose test was negative preoperatively, in 18 percent of those who were not tested preoperatively (most often because of the angina at rest or preinfarction angina syndrome), and in .26.9 percent of those whose preoperative test was positive. While complete angiographic restudy of these patients has not been accomplished, late conversion to a positive treadmill test appears to be associated, in equal frequency, with either progression of the disease in the native circulation or late bypass graft occlusion presumably due to occlusion from intimal fibrous proliferation. Late recurrence of symptoms after a period of absence of angina and normal exercise tolerance has been observed in some of these patients. These observations cast some shadow of concern upon the long-range efficacy of CAB surgery, both because of the incompletely defined potential for late graft occlusion at this time and the variable and presently unpredictable rate of progression of the disease in the native coronary circulation. Since these patients did not represent a group randomly selected for serial follow-up, and since some underwent exercise testing and restudy because of recurrence of symptoms, it is possible that the percentage of reversions to a positive test identified in this small group is greater than would be found in the series as a whole. Further observations are required to clarify these initial observations.

CURRENT ROLE OF CAB SURGERY

Coronary artery bypass must be evaluated from four aspects: (1) relief of symptoms, (2) improvement of myocardial function, (3) prevention of myocardial infarction, and (4) prolongation of life.

There is little doubt, from both our series and that of others, that *relief of symptomatic angina* is achieved with a high order of frequency and results in occupational rehabilitation and improvement in the quality of life. CAB can be recommended with confidence to patients whose response to medical therapy is inadequate and who are incapacitated by angina pectoris, if their angiographic anatomy permits surgical intervention. There is little evidence that symptoms of myocardial failure decrease after CAB and the presence of congestive heart failure and seriously impaired ventricular function significantly increase the surgical risk.

Improvement in myocardial function after CAB surgery, as assessed by left ventricular angiography, occurs infrequently except in cases of preinfarction angina [5] where the abnormalities of ventricular wall motion are presumably on an "ischemic" basis rather than the result of fibrotic scar replacement. Additional diagnostic tools are necessary to distinguish preoperatively reversible ischemic wall motion abnormalities from irreversible scar. Such maneuvers, currently under investigation, would greatly enhance selection of patients for CAB surgery.

Our own data relative to long-term *prevention of myocardial infarction* are preliminary and at present do not permit one to draw any decisive conclusions. While designed to prevent, CAB surgery actually causes myocardial infarction in the postoperative period in from 6 percent to 14 percent [18] of patients who undergo operation. While some of these infarctions terminate fatally or impair long-range improvement, others are clinically "benign" and do not appear to alter the recovery or long-range status of the patient. The occurrence of these "forced" infarctions in a controlled situation may play a role in the incidence and timing of subsequent postoperative infarctions, and more information is required to clarify this point. Data on the seriousness of the preinfarction syndrome suggest that surgical intervention may prevent myocardial infarction and carry a smaller risk than medical management. Even in this area, decisive information is lacking, but the cumulative actuarial data appear favorable.

On the assumption that *prolongation of life* is a proven fact, prophylactic CAB surgery remains highly controversial. While it is enticing to view with favor the actuarial data in surgical series, it is still hazardous to compare any non-randomized surgical series with a medically treated and *assumed comparable series* (frequently from another institution) and conclude that the data indicate life is prolonged. Results of preliminary serial treadmill exercise testing suggest, at least in some patients, that the atheromatous process is a progressive one and bypass surgery is palliative. Conclusive data will require longer follow-up and careful evaluation of randomly treated series.

If one could predict, in the clinical course of coronary artery disease, the likelihood of imminent sudden death or acute myocardial infarction with its potential for either a fatal outcome or serious destruction of heart muscle, then one could recommend CAB surgery with great confidence before such catastrophic sequelae. We currently view the syndrome of preinfarction an-

gina as one such warning. It is hoped that in the continued intensive study of coronary artery disease—its natural course, its clinical and exercise premonitory warnings, its angiographic and ventriculographic signs—we will gain the perceptiveness required to use properly timed surgical intervention with progressive effectiveness.

ACKNOWLEDGMENT

We gratefully acknowledge the assistance of Mary McReynolds, RRA, MPH, Research Assistant; Patrick Edwards, BS, Director of Computer Projects; and Joyce Staton, BS, Editorial Assistant, of the Texas Heart Institute.

References

1. Al-Bassam MS, Hall RJ, Dawson JT, et al: Increased risk factors in women undergoing coronary artery bypass. (Unpublished data)
2. Al-Bassam MS, Hall RJ, Garcia E, Hallman GL, Cooley DA: Early and late follow-up results of coronary artery bypass in patients with preinfarction angina. (Unpublished data)
3. Al-Bassam MS, Hall RJ, Garcia E, et al: Evaluation of the effects of antithrombotic therapy on survival following aortocoronary bypass surgery. Presented before the American College of Cardiology, Feb 14, 1974, New York
4. Bruschke AVG, Proudfit WL, Sones FM Jr: Progress study of 590 consecutive non-surgical cases of coronary disease followed 5–9 years; I: arteriographic correlations. Circulation 47:1147, 1973
5. Chatterjee K, Swan HJC, Parmley WW, Sustaita MHS, Matloff J: Influence of direct myocardial revascularization on left ventricular asynergy and function in patients with coronary heart disease. Circulation 47:276, 1973
6. Cooley DA, Dawson JT, Hallman GL, et al: Aortocoronary saphenous vein bypass: results in 1,492 patients, with particular reference to patients with complicating features. Ann Thorac Surg 16:380, 1973
7. Cooley DA, Hall RJ: Surgical and early mortality with CAB surgery at the Texas Heart Institute Oct 1969 to July 1973. (Unpublished data)
8. Dawson JT, Garcia E, Hall RJ, Cooley DA: Serum enzymes after coronary artery bypass (CAB) surgery [abstract]. Circulation 46 (Suppl 2):144, 1972
9. Dawson JT, Hall RJ, Garcia E, Cooley DA: Myocardial infarction after coronary artery bypass (CAB) surgery [abstract]. Circulation 46 (Suppl 2):144, 1972
10. Dawson JT, Hall RJ, Hallman GL, Cooley DA: Mortality of coronary artery bypass after myocardial infarction [abstract]. Am J Cardiol 31:128, 1973
11. Favaloro RG: Saphenous vein graft in the surgical treatment of coronary artery disease. J Thorac Cardiovasc Surg 58:178, 1969
12. Friesinger GC, Page EE, Ross RS: Prognostic significance of coronary arteriography. Trans Assoc Am Physicians 83:78, 1970
13. Garcia E, Treistman B, El-Said G, Cooley DA, Hall RJ: Treadmill evaluation of coronary artery bypass surgery [abstract]. Circulation 46 (Suppl 2):154, 1972

14. Gazes PC, Mobley EM Jr, Faris HM, Duncan RG, Humphries GB: Preinfarction (unstable) angina—a prospective study—ten year follow-up. Circulation 48:331, 1973

15. Griffith SC, Achuff SC, Conti CR, et al: Changes in intrinsic coronary circulation and segmental ventricular motion after saphenous-vein coronary bypass graft surgery. N Engl J Med 288:589, 1973

16. Guttin J, Garcia E, Hall RJ: Serial treadmill testing following CAB surgery. Am J Cardiol 35:142, 1975

17. Hall RJ, Al-Bassam MS, Garcia E, Hallman GL, Cooley DA: Coronary artery bypass: four years' follow-up. (Unpublished data Texas Heart Institute, Houston)

18. Hall RJ, Dawson JT, Cooley DA, et al: Coronary artery bypass. Circulation 48 (Suppl 3):146, 1973

19. Johnson WD, Flemma RJ, Lepley D Jr, Ellison EH: Extended treatment of severe coronary disease: a total surgical approach. Ann Surg 170:460, 1969

20. Klima T, Milam J: Pathology of aortocoronary artery autologous saphenous vein graft [abstract #37]. Coronary Artery Medicine and Surgery: Concepts and Controversies, Texas Heart Institute, February 21–23, 1974, Houston

21. Leatherman LL, Rochelle DG, Dawson JT, et al: Coronary arteriography after coronary artery bypass (CAB) surgery [abstract]. Circulation 46 (Suppl 2):181, 1972

22. Leatherman LL, Rochelle DG, Montgomery BR: Coronary artery bypass follow-up. (Unpublished data)

23. Leatherman LL, Rochelle DG, Montgomery BR, Hallman GL, Cooley DA: Coronary artery bypass surgery—graft patency [abstract]. Circulation 48 (Suppl 4):190, 1973

24. Pichard AD, Sheldon WC, Shinji K, Effler DB, Sones FM Jr: Severe arteriosclerotic obstruction of the left main coronary artery: follow up results in 176 patients [abstract]. Circulation 48 (Suppl 4):53, 1973

25. Sharma S, Khaja F, Heinle R, Goldstein S, Easly R: Left main coronary (LMC) artery lesions: risk of catheterization, exercise test and surgery [abstract]. Circulation 48 (Suppl 4):53, 1973

26. Sones FM Jr, Shirey ER: Cine coronary arteriography. Mod Concepts Cardiovasc Dis 31:735, 1962

101

CORONARY ARTERY SURGERY IN THE YOUNG ADULT

David A. Hughes, Lloyd A. Youngblood, John C. Norman,
and Denton A. Cooley

Aortocoronary bypass utilizing reversed saphenous vein segments is becoming accepted therapy in arteriosclerotic coronary artery disease.[7,11] The indications for, and the anticipated results of, this procedure in patients over the age of 40 are becoming established. There is very little information available, however, regarding coronary artery bypass surgery in the younger patient. The purpose of this report is to present a series of 73 patients below the age of 40 who have undergone aortocoronary bypass, commenting particularly on etiologic factors predisposing to the early development of arteriosclerotic coronary artery disease, the indications for surgery, and the postoperative results.

PATIENT POPULATION

Between October 1969 and March 1972, there were 1,275 patients who underwent aortocoronary bypass at our institutions. Of these, 73, or 5.7 percent, were below the age of 40 years; they ranged in age from 28 to 39 years. Their mean age was 35.9 years. Sixty-six were male and seven female.

Angina pectoris was present in 94.5 percent of these patients. Forty-eight percent had sustained a single previous myocardial infarction and 27 percent had a history of multiple previous infarctions. An additional 9 percent had electrocardiographic evidence of previous infarctions without any history of heart attack. Symptoms of congestive heart failure were present in 22 percent. Eighty-five percent of these patients were in the New York Heart Association functional classes III and IV.

Seventeen patients were operated upon urgently with a diagnosis of preinfarction angina, characterized by increasing anginal pain lasting longer than 30 minutes and showing poor response to rest and sublingual trinitroglycerin. Eleven of these 17 had a history of previous myocardial infarction.

Preoperative laboratory data showed significant elevations in serum cholesterol (> 270 mg percent) in 49 percent, and in serum triglycerides (> 150 mg percent) in 64 percent. Thirty percent had fasting blood glucose levels greater than 100 mg percent, but only three had significant glucosuria. No patient was being treated for diabetes mellitus at the time of surgery. Fifty-six percent of the patients were considered to be overweight in accordance with a standard height nomogram.[6] Twenty-seven percent were hypertensive with systolic pressures greater than 140 mm Hg and diastolic pressures greater than 90 mm Hg. Fifty-eight percent gave a significant family history of arteriosclerotic heart disease. Eighty-eight percent acknowledged smoking a package or more of cigarettes daily.

ANGIOGRAPHIC ANALYSES

All patients underwent preoperative selective coronary angiography and left ventriculography. Coronary arteriograms were scored using the method of Friesinger, Page, and Ross,[4] in which each of the three main coronary arteries (right, left anterior descending, and circumflex) is graded on a scale of 0 to 5 where 0 = no disease and 5 = complete obstruction. A total score of 0 to 3 is considered minimal disease, while one of 10 to 15 is severe disease. Using this method, 36 percent of the patients had mild disease, 33 percent moderate disease, and 30 percent were considered to have severe arteriosclerotic coronary artery disease.

One patient had no significant disease (although he was functionally Class IV and had a history of previous myocardial infarction). The left anterior descending coronary artery (LAD) was 50 percent or more occluded in 81 percent, the right coronary artery (RCA) in 73 percent, and the circumflex coronary artery (CX) in 51 percent. Fifty-eight percent had one or more vessels totally occluded. Single-vessel disease (greater than 50 percent occlusion) was present in 30 percent of the patients, double-vessel disease in 35 percent, and three vessels were involved in 34 percent.

Left ventricular end diastolic pressures were elevated (> 12 mm Hg) in 55 percent with 16 percent having marked elevations ranging from 25 to 42 mm Hg. Left ventriculography revealed some degree of ventricular dysfunction in 27 percent.

OPERATIVE PROCEDURES

One hundred and twenty bypass procedures were performed on these 73 patients. A single bypass graft was done in 44 percent, two bypass grafts in 48 percent, and three grafts in 8 percent. Coronary endarterectomy by blunt dissection was accomplished 22 times in 17 patients followed by saphenous vein bypass. These procedures were performed utilizing cardiopulmonary bypass under mild to moderate hypothermia and ischemic cardioplegia. The pump-oxygenator was primed with 5 percent dextrose in water. The period of cardiac ischemia ranged from 24 to 52 minutes.

The associated surgical procedures undertaken at the time of coronary artery bypass were resection of ventricular aneurysm (2), plication of ventricular aneurysm (1), resection of aneurysm of the ascending aorta (1), and resection of subaortic stenosis (1). None of these patients required valvular replacement.

POSTOPERATIVE COURSE

The most commonly occurring abnormality among these patients postoperatively was S-T and T-wave changes on electrocradiography. These changes were noted in 23 percent of all patients and 35 percent of those having an endarterectomy. In those having only coronary bypass, the frequency of occurrence paralleled the number of arteries bypassed. These electrocardiographic abnormalities did not appear to add to the operative mortality or affect the late results of the procedure,

and are of uncertain significance. Other postoperative complications and their frequency of occurrence are listed in Table 1.

TABLE 1. Frequency of Postoperative Complications

	NO.	%
Electrocardiographic abnormalities	17	23
Arrhythmias		19
Atrial	10	14
Ventricular	6	8
Congestive heart failure	6	8
Pulmonary edema	2	3
Pneumonia	1	1
Atelectasis	3	4
Postpericardiotomy syndrome	5	7
Anemia	4	6
Psychiatric disturbances	2	3
Postoperative infections	2	3

MORTALITY

Of these 73 patients undergoing aortocoronary bypass, one died during surgery and three died within the first 30 postoperative days, constituting a surgical mortality of 5.5 percent. The patient who died at surgery developed ventricular fibrillation at the induction of anesthesia and had a massive myocardial infarction intraoperatively. A second patient had early thrombosis of his bypass graft with infarction and when reexplored became dependent upon cardiopulmonary bypass and succumbed to low output cardiac failure. The third patient died of bronchopneumonia and pulmonary insufficiency, and the fourth of refractory congestive heart failure. These deaths are summarized in Table 2.

Factors that appeared to correlate statistically with surgical mortality in this series were increased

TABLE 2. Causes of Surgical and Late Mortality

CAUSE	NO.	DAYS POSTOP
Surgical Mortality (<30 days postoperatively)		
Ventricular fibrillation and myocardial infarction	1	0
Low output cardiac failure	1	14
Congestive heart failure	1	14
Pneumonia	1	11
Late Mortality (>30 days postoperatively)		
Excessive anticoagulation	1	50
Myocardial infarction	2	56 and 390
Congestive heart failure	1	240

preoperative left ventricular end diastolic pressure, a history of multiple preoperative myocardial infarctions, and endarterectomy (17.7 percent mortality vs 1.8 percent for patients who did not have endarterectomy). The presence of congestive heart failure preoperatively had no effect on surgical mortality. The duration of cardiopulmonary bypass and the number of coronary vessels bypassed did not affect mortality. No patient diagnosed as having preinfarction angina, regardless of other factors, expired.

Causes of late mortality are listed in Table 2. Factors affecting late mortality were (1) the presence preoperatively of congestive heart failure, elevated left ventricular end diastolic pressure, or ventricular dysfunction, and (2) history of multiple preoperative myocardial infarctions. There was no correlation of late deaths with preoperative functional classification or the number of vessels bypassed. There were no late deaths among those patients who had endarterectomies and survived the immediate postoperative period. There were no late deaths among patients undergoing resection or plication of dyskinetic areas of left ventricle. Two of three patients, however, with dysfunctional left ventricular segments that were not repaired, died. In retrospect, excision of these segments might have altered the outcome. Postoperative follow-up of 90 percent of this group of patients has ranged from two to 32 months (mean 10.2 months).

RESULTS

Of those patients who complained of angina preoperatively, 96 percent were improved and 69 percent obtained complete relief. Shortness of breath was considered improved in 82 percent of patients who had this symptom. Seventy percent of those patients who complained of easy fatigability or exercise intolerance were improved.

Eight patients with abnormal preoperative treadmill tests were retested postoperatively. Of these, six reverted to normal, showing no evidence of myocardial ischemia. Left ventricular end diastolic pressures were reevaluated postoperatively in 11 patients. In seven patients whose preoperative LVEDP was less than 25 mm Hg, no change was noted. All four patients whose preoperative left ventricular end diastolic pressures were greater than 25 mm Hg showed improvement with decreases of 15, 13, 7, and 6 mm Hg, respectively.

Postoperative coronary angiography was performed in 19 patients with 29 bypass grafts, three

in the second postoperative week because of suspected graft thrombosis, and 16 from five to 32 months (mean 13.0 months) after surgery. Of those restudied before discharge, three of six grafts were occluded. Of the remaining 23 grafts studied postoperatively, 87 percent were patent. The patency rate for all grafts studied (N: 29) was 79 percent. Grafts to the right coronary artery remained patent in 54 percent (7 of 13). All grafts to the left anterior descending and circumflex were patent (16 of 16).

In patients studied in whom endarterectomies had been performed, grafts to the vessels that had endarterectomy were patent in only 40 percent versus 88 percent for vessels on which endarterectomy was not required. No graft that was patent at discharge and that bypassed a vessel on which endarterectomy was not performed became occluded during the period of follow-up.

DISCUSSION

Coronary artery occlusive disease was considered rare among patients less than 40 years of age until the period following the second world war. Medical records and pathologic specimens from the large body of young men mobilized for World War II service were analyzed by Yater and his colleagues [12,13,14] at the Armed Forces Institute of Pathology. Their report, published in 1948, documented over 800 cases of myocardial infarction and correlated them with pathologic findings of over 400 autopsies. The median age of this series was 32.7 years. The comprehensiveness of Yater's study and the number of patients presented focused attention on the younger patient with coronary artery disease and led one authority [10] to conclude that coronary artery disease among military populations was a problem of major medical proportion.

Autopsies reported by Spain et al in 1953 [8] documented the presence of coronary arteriosclerosis in asymptomatic males less than 46 years of age who had died from violence. Final confirmation of the ubiquitous nature of the coronary atheromatous lesion came with the publication in the same year of the comprehensive study by Enos, Holmes, and Beyer [2] of autopsy findings in young men killed in battle during the Korean War. Coronary lesions at various stages were found in 77 percent of the patients studied, representing a continuum from the earliest observed lesion, fragmentation of the internal elastic lamina, to high-grade obstruction by atheromatous plaques.

The exact etiology of coronary atherogenesis remains unknown. Numerous theories regarding the "initial" lesion have been advanced; these include intramural hemorrhage, intramural accumulation of excess lipid substances, hypercholesterolemia, monocytic infiltration of the intima, thrombus and fibrin deposition, and fragmentation of the internal elastic lamina.[3] Whatever the precipitating factors, it is now widely accepted that some degree of coronary arteriosclerosis exists in essentially every male past puberty, and perhaps begins to occur coincident with extrauterine life.

Histologically, there is no difference between the coronary atheroma of young and elderly patients. The primary difference appears to be the rate of accumulation of the plaques. A number of factors correlate with early development. Hanashiro and associates[5] have identified certain "risk factors" among males sustaining myocardial infarctions prior to age 50, which predispose to coronary disease. They are as follows: abnormal intravenous glucose tolerance tests, elevations of serum cholesterol and triglycerides, history of cigarette smoking, hypertension, obesity, and positive family history of coronary artery disease. These findings parallel our observations.

A comparison of patients less than 40 years of age with the 1,202 patients of age 40 or greater undergoing coronary artery bypass during the same period at our institutions reveals the extent of coronary atherosclerosis to be somewhat greater among the older patients (mean coronary artery score of 9.2 versus 7.8 for younger patients). Multiple coronary bypass grafts were required more frequently in older patients (79 percent versus 56 percent in the younger age group). Endarterectomy was also performed somewhat more frequently in the patients 40 years of age or older. Associated surgical conditions were more frequently present in older patients (14 percent as opposed to the younger (7 percent). This is almost entirely due to the increased incidence of valvular disease in the older age group.

Overall surgical mortality was 8.5 percent for patients 40 years of age or older and 5.5 percent for younger patients. This increased operative risk is primarily due to the increased mortality associated with concomitant surgical procedures, particularly valve replacement, among older patients. Operative mortalities among older and younger patients undergoing only coronary artery bypass or endarterectomy and bypass were 6.7 and 5.9 percent, respectively.

Other investigators[1,9] have noted that patency rates for vein grafts are similar for right, left anterior descending, and circumflex coronary bypasses. Our series of patients below age 40 showed a marked tendency toward late occlusion of grafts to the right coronary artery.

SUMMARY

Of 1,275 patients undergoing aortocoronary artery vein bypass procedures for coronary artery occlusive disease at our institution between October 1969 and March 1972, seventy-three (6 percent) were between the ages of 28 and 39 (mean 35.9 years).

In this young adult group, the factors predisposing to early obstructive coronary artery disease were abnormalities in lipid and carbohydrate metabolism and cigarette smoking. Incapacitating or preinfarction angina were the presenting symptoms in 94.5 percent. Eighty-six percent of these young adults were classified as functional Class III or IV. Thirty-four percent had coronary artery scores of 10 or greater.

The surgical mortality was 5.5 percent. The factors affecting early and late mortality were multiple preoperative myocardial infarctions, congestive heart failure, and ventricular dysfunction. Endarterectomy associated with coronary bypass increased the risk of early and late graft thrombosis and adversely affected mortality in the immediate postoperative period. The coronary artery scores were lower and multiple bypasses and endarterectomy less frequently required in this young group of patients in comparison with those 40 or more years old. The operative mortality was comparable in both age groups.

Symptomatic improvement was obtained in 96 percent of this group of young patients. The overall graft patency in this group of patients as determined by postoperative angiography was 79 percent. Grafts to the right coronary artery demonstrated a greater propensity for thrombosis than those to the left anterior descending or circumflex coronary arteries.

Coronary artery occlusive disease is not uncommon in young adults. The accumulating results seem to justify operative intervention.

References

1. Effler DB, Favaloro RG, Groves LK, Loop FD: The simple approach to direct coronary artery surgery —Cleveland Clinic Experience. J Thorac Cardiovasc Surg 62:503, 1971
2. Enos WF, Holmes RH, Beyer J: Coronary disease among United States soldiers killed in action in Korea; preliminary report. JAMA 152:1090, 1953

3. Friedman M: Pathogenesis of Coronary Artery Disease. New York, McGraw Hill, 1969, pp 136–47

4. Friesinger GC, Page EE, Ross RS: Prognostic significance of coronary arteriography. Trans Assoc Am Physicians 83:78, 1970

5. Hanashiro PK, Sanmarco ME, Selvester RH, Blankenhorn D: Risk factors in males with premature atherosclerosis. *Abstracts* from Coronary Artery Medicine and Surgery, Houston, Feb 1974, p. 29

6. Metropolitan Life Insurance Company, 1959. From Thorn GW and Bondy PK in Principles of Internal Medicine, edited by T. R. Harrison, New York, McGraw Hill, 1962, p. 187

7. 1971 Reflection of 1970 Statistics. Report of the Subcommittee on Surgery for Coronary Disease, American College of Chest Physicians Chest 61: 475, 1972

8. Spain DM, Bradess VA, Huss G: Atherosclerosis in males less than 46 years of age. Ann Intern Med 38:254, 1953

9. Walker JA, Friedberg HD, Flemma RJ, Johnson WD: Determinants of angiographic patency of aortocoronary vein bypass grafts. Circulation 45 (Suppl I) 86, 1972

10. White PD: Coronary heart disease in mid-century with note concerning its military importance. US Armed Services Med J 2:357, 1951

11. Wilson WS: Aortocoronary saphenous vein bypass: a review of the literature. Heart Lung 2:290, 1973

12. Yater WM, Traum AH, Brown WG, et al: Coronary artery disease in men 18–39 years of age, Part I. Am Heart J 36:334, 1948

13. Yater WM, Traum AH, Brown WG, et al: Coronary artery disease in men 18–39 years of age, Part II. Am Heart J 36:481, 1948

14. Yater WM, Traum AH, Brown WG, et al: Coronary artery disease in men 18–39 years of age, Part III. Am Heart J 36:683, 1948

102

EARLY AND LATE FOLLOW-UP STUDIES OF EJECTION FRACTION AND GRAFT STATUS AFTER CORONARY ARTERY BYPASS SURGERY

Carl S. Apstein, Susan A. Kline, David C. Levin,
Harold A. Baltaxe, R. G. Carlson,
and Thomas Killip

INTRODUCTION

The effect of coronary bypass surgery on left ventricular function is uncertain (Manley and Johnson, 1972; Editorial in Lancet 1:137, 1973). In a selected group of patients with a recent acute increase in anginal symptomatology ("acute coronary insufficiency," "intermediate syndrome," or "impending myocardial infarction") successful surgery was associated with improved left ventricular function (Sustaita et al, 1972; Chatterjee et al, 1972). However, ventricular contractility has not generally improved after surgery in patients with chronic, stable angina (Spencer et al, 1971; Kouchoukos et al, 1972; Hammermeister et al, 1974).

The present study was performed in order to determine the effect of coronary bypass graft surgery on left ventricular function in patients with a stable level of angina pectoris. The influence of preoperative myocardial contractility on postoperative graft patency was also studied.

METHODOLOGY

The pre- and postoperative angiograms in patients who underwent coronary bypass graft surgery over a two-year period at the New York Hospital–Cornell Medical Center were reviewed. Twenty-six patients had technically adequate pre- and postoperative angiographic studies and are included in this report. The 26 patients represent one-fifth of the patients who underwent this operation during the two-year period.

All patients had significant coronary artery disease demonstrated by coronary angiography and angina pectoris of varying severity. However, no patient was judged to have "crescendo" or "preinfarction" angina or acute coronary insufficiency.

A total of 51 grafts were implanted in the 26 patients. Early follow-up studies of left ventricular and graft angiograms took place in 20 patients at an average postoperative interval of 14 days. Later follow-up studies were performed in 13 patients at an average of nine months after surgery.

Ventricular function was analyzed by calculating the ejection fraction (EF) (Sandler and Dodge, 1968; Kennedy et al, 1970; Chatterjee et al, 1971) and mean rate of circumferential fiber shortening ($\overline{V}_{CF}$) (Karliner et al, 1971). Postoperative graft status was assessed by hand injections of angiographic contrast solution into the venous bypass grafts.

All patients were requested to return for late follow-up angiographic reevaluation. The patients who returned for the late follow-up studies were a representative sample of all patients who were eligible for reevaluation (survival for at least six months after surgery); there was no significant difference in preoperative EF, $\overline{V}_{CF}$, or severity and extent of coronary atherosclerosis in the group who returned for late follow-up angiograms and those who did not. Thus, conclusions based on the patients restudied at late follow-up can reasonably be extrapolated to the group as a whole.

TABLE 1. Graft Patency at Early Follow-up in Relation to Preoperative Ejection Fraction

	PREOP EJECTION FRACTION		
	≥0.50	<0.50	Total
Number of Patients	11	9	20
Number of grafts	20	22	42
Patent grafts[a]			
Number	20	16	36
Percent	100	73	86
Occluded grafts[a]			
Number	0	6	6
Percent	0	27	27

[a] $\chi^1 = 4.33, p < 0.05.$

RESULTS

Early Follow-up Studies (Average of Two Weeks after Surgery)

GRAFT PATENCY. The relationship between preoperative ejection fraction and graft patency is shown in Table 1. The overall postoperative graft occlusion rate was 14 percent; however, all graft occlusions occurred in patients who had an abnormal preoperative ejection fraction (< 0.50). Thus the risk of graft occlusion in the early postoperative period was zero if the preoperative EF was normal, but patients with an abnormal preoperative EF had an early graft occlusion risk of 27 percent. The association between risk of graft occlusion and preoperative EF was significant at $p < 0.05$.

VENTRICULAR FUNCTION. Left ventricular function, as measured by ejection fraction and mean rate of circumferential fiber shortening, was not significantly changed for the total group of 20 patients in the early postoperative period. However, a subgroup of seven patients had moderate impairment of LV function preoperatively with a mean ejection fraction of 0.38 (range: 0.20 to 0.50). This group of patients demonstrated a moderate improvement in ejection fraction from 0.38 to 0.47 ($p < 0.05$) in the early follow-up period. Patients who had a normal preoperative EF continued to have normal LV function 14 days postoperatively (Fig. 1).

Thus, the early postoperative period was characterized by a 27 percent risk of graft occlusion for patients with subnormal preoperative ejection fractions, but no risk of graft occlusion with a normal preoperative ejection fraction. A modest increase in ejection fraction occurred in patients who had had moderately subnormal ejection fractions preoperatively.

Thus, there is a paradoxical increase in ejection fraction in the group of patients with the

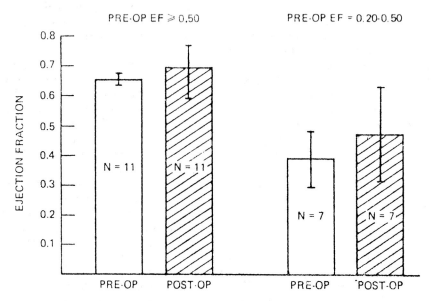

FIG. 1. Preoperative and Early Postoperative Ventricular Function. Patients are grouped on the basis of the preop EF. Those with a normal preop EF had no significant change after surgery. Patients with a moderately abnormal preop EF had a small but significant (p < 0.05) increase in the early postoperative period. (Each bar graph represents the mean value ± the 95 percent confidence limit.)

highest rate of graft occlusion, namely those with an abnormal preoperative EF. The increase in EF in the immediate postoperative period may not be entirely due to the bypass graft but may also be related to an optimal, enforced medical regimen and a period of bed rest. Furthermore, two of the seven patients who improved their postoperative EF had been digitalized between the pre- and postoperative studies.

Late Follow-up Studies (Average of Nine Months after Surgery)

GRAFT PATENCY. The late follow-up studies showed a further increase in graft occlusion. Eight grafts out of the 28 implanted in this group of 14 patients were occluded, representing a 29 percent risk of occlusion. In addition, the proximal segment of the grafted coronary artery became occluded in three cases as indicated by lack of bidirectional flow of radiopaque contrast solution from the vein graft into the anastamosed coronary artery.

The overall risk of graft occlusion during both the early and late follow-up periods is shown in Table 2. Graft occlusion is less likely (7 percent) in those patients who had a preoperative EF > 0.50 than in patients with a preoperative EF < 0.50 (37 percent risk of occlusion, p < 0.05).

VENTRICULAR FUNCTION. Both

TABLE 2. Graft Patency in Both Early and Late Follow-up Periods: Relation to Preoperative Ejection Fraction

| | PREOP EJECTION FRACTION | | |
	$\geqslant 0.50$	< 0.50	Total
Number of patients	16	10	26
Number of grafts	29	22	51
Patent grafts[a]			
Number	27	14	41
Percent	93	63	80
Occluded grafts[a]			
Number	2	8	10
Percent	7	37	20

$^{a}X^2 = 5.15, p < 0.05.$

ejection fraction and mean rate of circumferential fiber shortening were decreased in the late follow-up studies in the 13 patients so studied. Ejection fraction decreased from 0.57 to 0.49 and circumferential fiber shortening decreased from 1.35 to 1.18 circumferences/second. Both changes were statistically significant (p 0.05) (Fig. 2). However, a subgroup of patients could be culled who maintained their normal preoperative ejection fraction. The four patients who maintained their normal preoperative ejection fraction had all grafts patent and had maintained patency of the proximal segment of the grafted native coronary artery. The group of nine patients who had suffered graft occlusion or had occluded the proximal segment of

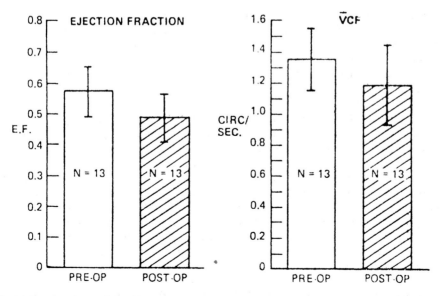

FIG. 2. Preoperative and Late Postoperative Ventricular Function (All Patients). The mean values for EF and $\bar{V}_{CF}$ showed a significant decrease (p < 0.05) nine months after surgery in the 13 patients studied. (Each bar represents the mean ± 95 percent confidence limit.)

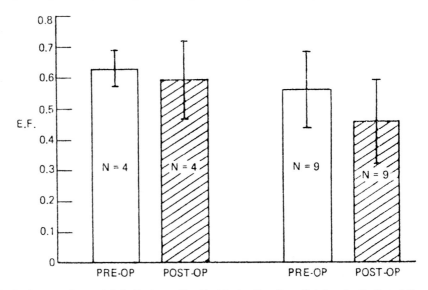

FIG. 3. Preoperative and Late Postoperative Ventricular Function: Relation to Graft and Coronary Artery Patency. The 13 patients reported in Figure 2 are grouped on the basis of venous graft and coronary artery patency. In the four patients who had all venous grafts patent and who had maintained patency of the grafted coronary artery, there was no decrease in ejection fraction (two bars on left). The nine patients whose venous grafts or proximal segments of the grafted coronary arteries had become occluded showed a significant decrease in ejection fraction; $p < 0.05$ (two bars on right). (Each bar represents the mean value ± 95 percent confidence limit.)

the grafted coronary artery had a significant decline in EF from 0.55 to 0.45 (Fig. 3).

DISCUSSION

The results of this study indicate that a subnormal preoperative EF is associated with a higher risk of venous graft occlusion postoperatively and that the majority of patients have poorer LV function nine months after surgery than they had preoperatively.

The correlation between risk of graft occlusion and a decreased preoperative EF may be related to a lesser velocity and volume of flow through the venous graft (Walker et al, 1972). Patients with abnormal LV function may have more myocardial fibrosis and a higher resistance to flow through the region of myocardium being perfused by the venous bypass graft.

Regardless of mechanism, the empirical correlation between an abnormal preoperative EF and a higher risk of graft occlusion indicates that a decreased preoperative EF decreases the chance for successful surgery.

Ventricular function in the early postoperative period increased slightly in patients who were abnormal preoperatively (Fig. 1). However, late follow-up studies showed a significant decline in both EF and $\overline{V}_{CF}$; only the minority of patients

with no graft occlusions and no new occlusions of the proximal segment of the coronary artery had no decrease in LV function.

Thus the long-term effect of bypass graft surgery upon left ventricular EF in patients with chronic stable angina and left ventricular dysfunction is not encouraging. All patients with an abnormal preoperative left ventricular EF eventually suffered graft occlusion and a further decline in ventricular function. Several patients with normal preoperative function became abnormal postoperatively. No patient, in the nine-month follow-up period, had a significant improvement in an abnormal preoperative ventriculogram.

Our results and conclusions complement previous studies following coronary bypass graft surgery. It would seem apparent that the mere presence of a new supply of oxygen could not convert scar tissue into functioning sarcomeres; however, depression of function due to oxygen lack could theoretically be reversed if the ischemia were corrected before myocardial necrosis occurred. Thus Chatterjee et al (Sustaita et al, 1972, and Chatterjee et al, 1972) have reported a significant early postoperative improvement in left ventricular contractility, in the immediate postoperative period in a selected group of patients with a recent acute increase in the severity of their anginal syndrome. In contrast Spencer et al (1971) failed to observe an improvement in left ventricular function in patients with chronic congestive heart failure secondary to ischemic heart disease. In this series (Spencer et al, 1971) the presence of both severe angina and congestive heart failure was associated with a better surgical prognosis than the presence of congestive heart failure alone, suggesting that the symptom of angina pectoris is a manifestation of the existence of ischemic but viable myocardial tissue. Manley and Johnson (1972) also note that improvement in cardiac failure with revascularization is uncertain and that patients with abnormal preoperative ventriculograms have a much less impressive improvement in ergometry studies than patients with normal preoperative ventriculograms.

A recent study (Hammermeister et al, 1974) employing serial ventriculography in patients who underwent this operation reached conclusions similar to ours. The postoperative study occurred at an average of four months postoperatively. Despite marked symptomatic relief of angina and improved objective exercise performance, there was no consistent improvement in postoperative left ventricular function in this series.

Blood flow provided by bypass grafts has been shown to influence contractility. Rees et al (1971) examined postoperative ventricular function in patients with 100 percent graft patency. All patients had normal left ventricular function preoperatively and were studied at an average of three months after surgery. Graft patency was associated with a slight increase in ejection fraction within the normal range; occlusion of the vein grafts was associated with a decrease in EF from 0.59 to 0.50, a change that was not statistically significant but that suggested that graft occlusion might prove deleterious. Bolooki et al (1971) demonstrated that graft occlusion for a two-minute period was associated with a decline in left ventricular contractility in five of nine patients during studies performed on the operating table immediately after bypass grafting. However, no correlation with preoperative left ventricular function was reported; hence neither of these studies (Rees et al, 1971 and Bolooki et al, 1971) provides evidence that bypass graft surgery can improve chronic left ventricular dysfunction.

Systolic time intervals after coronary artery bypass have shown sustained improvement in ventricular performance three months after surgery (Johnson et al, 1972). The PEP/LVET ratio (preejection period/left ventricular ejection time) decreased from a mean of 0.479 preoperatively to a mean of 0.409 at the time of three-month follow-up period. If one extrapolates these data to the study of Garrard et al (1970), these values

correspond to ejection fractions of 0.53 and 0.61 respectively. Thus, these patients were similar to our group of patients with slight-to-moderate impairment of preoperative function who showed early postoperative improvement.

The general conclusions that we draw from the above studies and our own are as follows:

1. The new blood supply provided by bypass graft surgery can improve LV function in patients with acute ischemia which has not progressed to necrosis.
2. There is a slight improvement in LV function in the early (14 day to three months) postoperative period in selected patients with slight-to-moderate preoperative abnormalities of LV contraction.
3. Late follow-up (nine months) is associated with a general decrease in LV function. Those patients with abnormal preoperative contractility had a higher risk of graft occlusion and a further decline in LV function. Some patients with normal LV function preoperatively became abnormal at the time of late postoperative follow-up.
4. Thus, subnormal LV function in the setting of a stable pattern of angina should not be an indication for surgery and should probably be considered a relative contraindication since the risk of operative mortality is greater, as is the risk of postoperative graft occlusion.

References

Bolooki H, Rubinson RM, Michie DD, et al: Assessment of myocardial contractility after coronary bypass grafts. J Thorac Cardiovasc Surg 62:543–53, 1971

Chatterjee K, Sacoor M, Suttin GC, et al: Assessment of left ventricular function by single plane cine angiographic volume analysis. Br Heart J 33:565–71, 1971

Chatterjee K, Swan HJC, Parmley WW, et al: Depression of left ventricular function due to acute myocardial ischemia and its reversal after aortocoronary saphenous-vein bypass. N Engl J Med 286:1117–22, 1972

Editorial: Coronary bypass surgery. Lancet 1:137, 1973

Garrard CL Jr, Weissler AM, Dodge HT: The relationship of alterations in systolic time intervals to ejection fraction in patients with cardiac disease. Circulaton 42:455–62, 1970

Hammermeister KE, Kennedy JW, Hamilton GW, et al: Aortocoronary saphenous vein bypass: failure of successful grafting to improve resting left ventricular function in chronic angina. N Engl J Med 290: 186–92, 1974

Johnson A, O'Rourke RA, Karliner JS: Effect of myocardial revascularization on systolic time intervals in patients with left ventricular dysfunction. Circulation 45 (Suppl 1):91–96, 1972

Karliner JS, Gault JH, Eckberg D, et al: Mean velocity

of fiber shortening. A simplified measure of left ventricular myocardial contractility. Circulation 44: 323–33, 1971

Kennedy JW, Treeholme SE, Kasser IS: Left ventricular volume and mass from a single plane cine angiocardiogram. A comparison of anteroposterior and right anterior oblique methods. Am Heart J 80:343–52, 1970

Kouchoukos N, Doty DB, Buettner LE, et al: Treatment of post-infarction cardiac failure by myocardial excision and revascularization. Circulation 45 (Suppl 1):72–78, 1972

Manley H, Johnson D: Effects of surgery on angina (pre- and post-infarction) and myocardial function (failure). Circulation 46:1208–21, 1972

Rees C, Bristow JD, Kremkau EL, et al: Influence of

aortocoronary bypass surgery on left ventricular performance. N Engl J Med 284:1116–20, 1971

Sandler H, Dodge HT: The use of single plane angiocardiograms for the calculation of left ventricular volume in man. Am Heart J 75:325–34, 1968

Spencer FC, Green GE, Tice DA, et al: Coronary artery bypass grafts for congestive heart failure: a report of experiences with 40 patients. J Thorac Cardiovasc Surg 62:529–42, 1971

Sustaita H, Chatterjee K, Matloff JM, et al: Emergency bypass surgery in impending and complicated acute myocardial infarction. Arch Surg 105:30–35, 1972

Walker SA, Freidberg HE, Flemma RJ, et al: Determinants of angiographic patency of aortocoronary vein bypass grafts. Circulation 45 (Suppl 1):86–90, 1972

103

THE EFFECT OF AORTOCORONARY SAPHENOUS VEIN BYPASS ON RESTING LEFT VENTRICULAR FUNCTION IN PATIENTS WITH CHRONIC ANGINA

K. E. Hammermeister and J. W. Kennedy

Resting ventricular performance measured by quantitative angiocardiographic determination of left ventricular volumes and ejection fraction was studied pre- and postoperatively in 55 patients undergoing saphenous vein bypass grafting for angina pectoris. The clinical success of the procedure was documented by symptomatic improvement in 82 percent (45 of 55), increase in treadmill maximal exercise capacity in 52 percent (22 of 42), normalization of ischemic ST segment in 76 percent (22 of 29) of those with preoperative exertional ST depression, and a graft patency rate of 83 percent (88 of 106). Sixteen percent had an intraoperative myocardial infarction. There were no significant changes in end-diastolic volume (EDV), end-systolic volume (ESV), or systolic ejection fraction for the group as a whole following saphenous vein bypass grafting. Analysis of patient subgroups showed that ejection fraction was unchanged postoperatively for the 40 patients with all patent grafts, for the 24 patients who had neither a preoperative nor intraoperative myocardial infarction, or for the 24 patients in whom all obstructed coronary vessels were successfully bypassed. Left ventricular contraction plots were unchanged postoperatively in 62 percent (34 of 55), improved in 20 percent (11 of 55), and worse in 18 percent (10 of 55).

We conclude that saphenous vein bypass grafting does not alter resting left ventricular performance and should not be offered to patients whose primary symptoms are those of left heart failure or who have markedly impaired ventricular performance (ejection fraction less than 33 percent).

INTRODUCTION

Myocardial revascularization using aortocoronary saphenous vein bypass grafts for patients with angina pectoris has been enthusiastically received because of a high incidence of symptomatic relief and low surgical mortality. The effect of this procedure on ventricular performance is still a matter of controversy and may be important in providing objective data in support of the efficacy of this operation. From animal studies, it is clear that hypoxia depresses myocardial contractility and that reoxygenation within a reasonable period of time restores myocardial function (Tyberg et al, 1970). This study was undertaken to examine the hypothesis that successful saphenous vein bypass grafting in patients with angina would result in improved resting ventricular performance as measured by quantitative angiography.

METHODS

Patient Population

Fifty-five adult patients (54 males and one female; age range 32 to 65, mean 46) who have undergone saphenous vein bypass grafting constitute the basis of this report. Fifty-four were operated on because of symptomatic disabling angina pectoris and one because of exertional ventricular tachycardia. Twenty-three had had one or more myocardial infarctions from one month to 13 years prior to surgery. Four patients had mitral regurgitation, one requiring valve replacement, and one valvuloplasty. Only two had symptoms of heart failure at rest. Aortocoronary saphenous vein bypass grafting was performed with hypothermic cardiopulmonary bypass on a fibrillating ventricle with the aorta cross-clamped, as necessary for hemostasis. Mean graft flow measured with an electromagnetic flowmeter in 32 grafts in 18 patients averaged 65 ml/min (range 11 to 250 ml/min). Postoperative studies were carried out as a part of routine evaluation of all patients operated upon. The only criterion for inclusion in this study was technically adequate quantitative left ventricular angiography before and after surgery.

Evaluation pre- and postoperatively included resting ECG and maximal treadmill exercise electrocardiogram (Bruce and Hornsten, 1969). A preoperative myocardial infarction was diagnosed if the patient had typical Q-waves on the ECG and/or typical history with diagnostic enzyme changes. An intraoperative myocardial infarction was diagnosed only if an early postoperative tracing showed new Q-waves, except for one patient who two days postoperatively developed marked ST depression and enzyme elevation not previously present. A positive ischemic response to maximal exertion was diagnosed in patients not on digitalis if the ST segment was flat or down-sloping and depressed greater than 1 mm, and if resting ST segment depression was not present. Maximal exercise performance was expressed as functional aerobic impairment (FAI), the percent decrement from age, sex, and activity predicted maximal oxygen intake (Bruce, 1971). A change of 10 percent or more between the pre- and postoperative study was considered significant.

Cardiac Catheterization

After informed patient consent cardiac catheterization was performed with the subject at rest, in the supine position, and with no or light (ie, diazepam 10 mg, IM) premedication. Preoperative catheterization included selective coronary angiography and left ventriculography performed with power injection of 60 to 70 ml sodium-meglumine diatrizoate through a 7 or 8F catheter over three to four seconds. In nine patients left ventricular angiocardiography was recorded on 35 mm cine film at 60 frames per second in the right anterior oblique (RAO) projection. The remaining 46 underwent biplane direct filming at 12 exposures per second in the anteroposterior and left lateral projections. In all cases the same filming technique and projection were used in the pre- and post-

operative studies. Postoperative evaluation was carried out an average of five months after surgery (range 1 to 14) and consisted of selective injection of the bypass graft(s) and a left ventricular angiogram.

Evaluation of the Data

The number of obstructive lesions per patient was taken as the number of the three major vessels (right, left anterior descending, and circumflex) with at least one point of 75 percent or greater reduction in cross-sectional area. The adequacy of revascularization was assessed by comparing the number of patent grafts with the total number of obstructed vessels.

Left ventricular volumes were calculated using the area-length method from biplane large films (Dodge et al, 1960) or from the single plane RAO cineangiograms (Kennedy et al, 1972). Overestimation of left ventricular volume by the latter technique was corrected by the use of regression equations relating the two techniques (Kennedy et al, 1970). All patients were in sinus rhythm. When premature beats occurred early

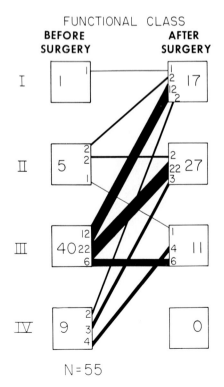

FIG. 1.   Changes in functional class following saphenous vein bypass surgery are shown.

in the injection, the beat following the post extrasystolic beat was used for analysis. Stroke volume (SV) was computed as end-diastolic volume (EDV) minus end-systolic volume (ESV), and ejection fraction was SV/EDV. Cardiac index (CI) was SV/M^2 times heart rate (HR).

Contraction plots were drawn and graded as previously described (Hamilton et al, 1970). Briefly, end-diastolic and end-systolic chambers were outlined, and the films superimposed according to the long axis of the chamber and the midpoint of the long axis. Contraction plots were graded on a scale of I to V where I is normal, II is borderline (contraction asymmetry involving less than 25 percent of the ventricular surface), III is localized akinesis or hypokinesis (25 to 75 percent of the ventricular surface involved), IV is localized dyskinesis (paradoxical motion), V is diffuse akinesis or hypokinesis (greater than 75 percent of ventricular surface involved).

The statistical significance of the difference between the means of the preoperative study versus the postoperative study was analyzed using Student's t-test for paired data.

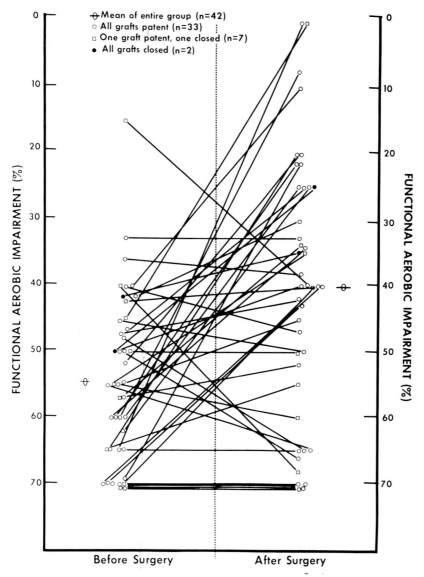

FIG. 2. Changes in functional aerobic impairment (percent decrement from age, sex, and activity status predicted maximal aerobic capacity) are shown following saphenous vein bypass surgery for the 42 patients with pre- and postoperative maximal treadmill exercise testing. The change in the mean FAI from 54 ± 12 percent to 40 ± 20 percent following surgery represents a statistically significant (p < 0.01) improvement in maximal aerobic capacity.

TABLE 1. Exercise, Hemodynamic, and Quantitative Angiographic Data before and Five Months after Saphenous Vein Bypass Grafting

	NO. PTS.	FAI	HR	EDV/M²	ESV/M²	SV/M²	EF (%)	LVEDP (mm Hg)	CI
All patent grafts	40								
Pre		55 ± 13[c]	76 ± 13	81 ± 22	39 ± 19	42 ± 12	52 ± 13	12 ± 6	3.1 ± 0.8
Post		41 ± 20[b]	86 ± 16[b]	77 ± 22	37 ± 20	40 ± 11	52 ± 13	10 ± 4	3.4 ± 1.0
No MI and all patent grafts	17								
Pre		53 ± 15[d]	71 ± 13	79 ± 15	36 ± 12	43 ± 7	55 ± 8	11 ± 5	2.9 ± 0.5
Post		43 ± 23	79 ± 15	73 ± 13	31 ± 7	43 ± 9	58 ± 7	10 ± 5	3.3 ± 0.8
No MI	24								
Pre		54 ± 14[e]	72 ± 14	81 ± 18	37 ± 14	44 ± 10	54 ± 9	12 ± 5	3.1 ± 0.7
Post		43 ± 20[a]	85 ± 16[b]	76 ± 21	36 ± 16	41 ± 10	54 ± 11	11 ± 5	3.5 ± 1.0
Total revascularization	24								
Pre		55 ± 11[b]	75 ± 13	81 ± 19	37 ± 15	44 ± 12	53 ± 12	11 ± 5	3.2 ± 0.9
Post		41 ± 21[b]	88 ± 17[b]	71 ± 18[b]	35 ± 17	38 ± 13	52 ± 15	9 ± 4	3.3 ± 1.1
One or more patent grafts	51								
Pre		54 ± 13[g]	76 ± 14	82 ± 22	41 ± 19	42 ± 11	51 ± 12	11 ± 5	3.2 ± 0.9
Post		41 ± 20[b]	86 ± 16[b]	80 ± 23	41 ± 21	40 ± 11	50 ± 13	11 ± 4	3.4 ± 0.9
Abnormal preop EF	25								
Pre		55 ± 12[h]	79 ± 14	94 ± 26	56 ± 20	38 ± 10	41 ± 7	11 ± 6	3.0 ± 1.0
Post		37 ± 16[b]	89 ± 17[b]	94 ± 27	54 ± 25	42 ± 13	45 ± 13	10 ± 4	3.6 ± 1.0[a]
All patients	55								
Pre		54 ± 12[i]	76 ± 14	85 ± 22	42 ± 19	42 ± 11	51 ± 12	11 ± 6	3.2 ± 0.9
Post		40 ± 19[b]	85 ± 16[b]	81 ± 25	42 ± 22	40 ± 11	50 ± 13	11 ± 4	3.4 ± 0.9

FAI: functional aerobic impairment; HR: heart rate; EDV: left ventricular end-diastolic volume; ESV: left ventricular end-systolic volume; SV: stroke volume; EF: ejection fraction; LVEDP: left ventricular end-diastolic pressure; CI: cardiac index; MI: myocardial infarction.
[a] *Statistically significant change from the preoperative mean ($p < 0.05$).*
[b] *Statistically significant change from the preoperative mean ($P < 0.01$).*
[c] to [i] *Exercise testing performed on 33, 15, 19, 20, 40, 17, and 42 patients, respectively.*

operatively despite the same or greater workloads and maximal heart rates in all except five (Fig. 3).

Angiographic Results

There were 110 major vessels with significant obstruction in the 55 patients for an average of 2.0 obstructed vessels per patient. Of a total of 106 grafts attempted, 88 were patent for a patency rate of 83 percent. Some revascularization (at least one patient graft) was accomplished in 51 of the 55 patients (93 percent), but in only 24 (44 percent) were all significantly obstructed major coronary arteries successfully bypassed.

Left ventricular end-diastolic pressure (LVEDP), EDV, ESV, and ejection fraction (Table 1, Figs. 4 to 6) showed no significant change following saphenous bypass grafting for the group as a whole. However, heart rate at the moment of left ventricular angiography increased significantly at the postoperative study from 76 ± 14 to 85 ± 16 beats per minute with a small decrease in stroke volume from 42 ± 11 to 40 ± 11 ml/m^2 such that cardiac index did not change significantly (Table 1). The ejection fraction improved more than 10 percent in only nine patients, but decreased more than 10 percent in 12 patients. In these 12 patients with significant decrements in ejection fraction, the graft patency rate (79 percent) and percent of significantly obstructed vessels successfully bypassed (64 percent) were not different from the group as a whole, but the rate of intraoperative infarction was somewhat greater ($4/12 = 33$ percent). Contraction plots showed little change following surgery with 37 remaining the same, nine showing improvement and nine showing a poorer contractile pattern (Fig. 7).

Since no improvement in ventricular function could be demonstrated for the group as a whole, those subgroups of patients most likely to have a favorable result were selected out and the data re-analyzed (Table 1). The 40 patients with all grafts patent again showed no change in ejection fraction. There was a small, statistically non-significant decrease in EDV. The 24 patients who never had a myocardial infarction either preoperatively or intraoperatively also showed no change in ejection fraction. Very similar results were obtained for the 24 patients in whom all significantly obstructed major coronary arteries were successfully bypassed. Finally, since those patients with normal left ventricular ejection fraction preoperatively might be expected to show little change in ventricular performance following successful re-

RESULTS

Clinical Evaluation

Following surgery, 45 of the 55 patients (82 percent) improved one or more functional classes, nine were unchanged, and one went from Class II to III (Fig. 1). Nine patients (16 percent) sustained intraoperative myocardial infarctions.

Pre- and postoperative exercise data were available in 42 patients. There was a statistically significant improvement in FAI in the group as a whole (Fig. 2, Table 1). Improvement in FAI of 10 percent or greater occurred in 22 of the 42 (52 percent) while worsening of FAI of 10 percent or greater occurred in five (12 percent). Failure to improve exercise performance was not related to graft closures, as four of 10 with one or more closed grafts improved their exercise performance. Preoperatively 33 of 42 patients were limited by chest pain at maximal exertion. Postoperatively only nine had pain on exercise testing, the remainder stopping with fatigue and dyspnea. Twenty-two of the 29 with an ischemic ST response preoperatively had a negative response post-

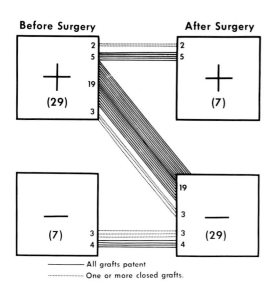

FIG. 3. The ST segment response to maximal exercise for 36 patients not on digitalis and without resting ST segment depression is shown before and after saphenous vein bypass surgery. A positive response consists of a flat or down-sloping ST segment depressed 1 mm or greater from the base-line PR segment. The change in ST response following surgery is highly significant statistically (p < 0. 01) using the Chi² test.

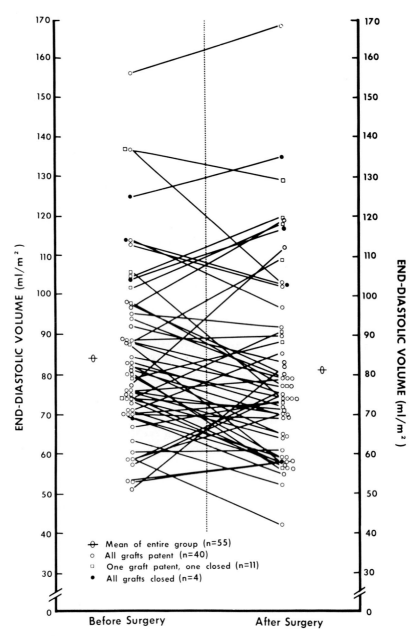

FIG. 4. Left ventricular end-diastolic volume is shown before and following saphenous vein bypass surgery. For the group of 55 patients, mean preoperative end-diastolic volume (85 ± 22 ml/M^2) did not differ significantly from the mean postoperative value (81 ± 25 ml/M^2).

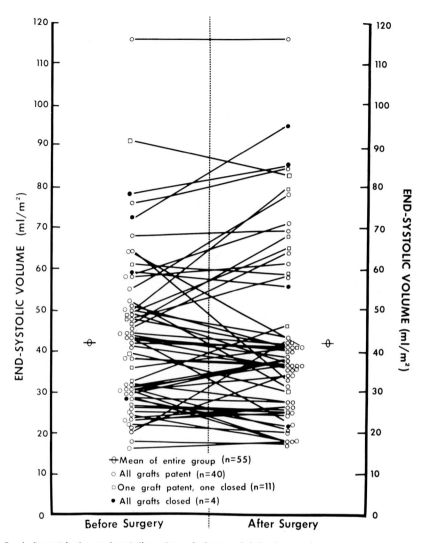

FIG. 5. Left ventricular end-systolic volume before and following saphenous vein bypass surgery is shown. For the group of 55 patients, mean preoperative end-systolic volume (42 ± 19 ml/M²) did not differ significantly from the postoperative value (42 ± 22 ml/M²).

vascularization, the patients whose preoperative ejection fraction was greater than two standard deviations below the normal mean (Kennedy et al, 1966) (ejection fraction ≤ 0.50) were analyzed separately. Again, there was no significant change in EDV, ESV, or ejection fraction following surgery (Table 1).

DISCUSSION

This study was initiated to test the hypothesis that adequate myocardial vascularization in patients with angina pectoris would result in improved ventricular performance. If patients with angina did have reversible, impaired contractility,

then improvement in ventricular function would be objective evidence supporting the adequacy of revascularization. This study has failed to demonstrate consistent improvement in resting ventricular performance as measured by ventricular volumes, ejection fraction, SV, CI, and LVEDP following saphenous vein bypass grafting. Even in selected subgroups of patients who might be expected to do well, ie, those with all grafts patent, those who have never had documented myocardial necrosis, and those in whom all significantly obstructed major vessels were successfully bypassed (Table 1), no improvement in resting left ventricular performance could be demonstrated.

There are four possible explanations for the failure of this study to document improvement in

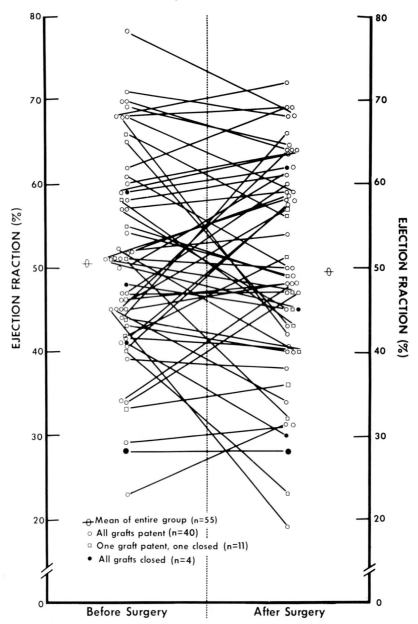

FIG. 6. Left ventricular ejection fraction before and following saphenous vein bypass surgery is shown. There is no statistically significant change from before (51 ± 12 percent) to after (50 ± 13 percent) surgery for the group of 55 patients.

ventricular performance following saphenous vein bypass grafting: (1) revascularization in this group was technically inadequate or incomplete in comparison with the general experience, (2) saphenous vein bypass grafting, like other surgical attempts at myocardial revascularization preceding it, does not improve blood delivery to ischemic muscle, (3) the techniques that we used to study ventricular performance were insensitive to changes that actually occurred, and (4) resting

ventricular dysfunction in patients with stable angina is not usually reversible.

Blood flow through the grafts in our patients at the time of surgery was similar to that obtained by other groups (Johnson et al, 1970a). Our graft patency rate (83 percent), rate of symptomatic improvement (82 percent), improvement in quantitated maximum exercise performance, and disappearance of electrocardiographic manifestations of ischemia at maximal exertion cer-

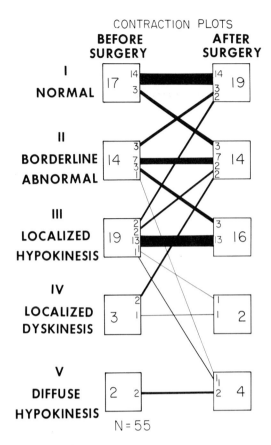

CONTRACTION PLOTS
BEFORE **AFTER**
SURGERY **SURGERY**

I
NORMAL

II
BORDERLINE
ABNORMAL

III
LOCALIZED
HYPOKINESIS

IV
LOCALIZED
DYSKINESIS

V
DIFFUSE
HYPOKINESIS

N = 55

FIG. 7. Left ventricular contraction plots before and following saphenous vein bypass surgery are shown. See text for descriptions of classification. Following surgery no change in contraction plot was seen in 37 patients, while 9 became worse and 9 improved.

tainly compare favorably with the general experience. The number of intraoperative myocardial infarctions (9/55 or 16 percent) is comparable to that previously reported (Hultgren et al, 1971; Achuff et al, 1972; Brewer et al, 1973).

While it has now become clear that older techniques of myocardial revascularization such as internal mammary artery implantation result in relatively little increase in myocardial blood flow (Dart et al, 1970), all evidence to date indicates that flows through the vein grafts are substantial in relation to total myocardial blood flow (Johnson et al, 1970a; Greene et al, 1972) and that the mass of myocardium perfused via the graft represents a significant proportion (ie, 25 to 50 percent) of total myocardial mass (Greene et al, 1972). In addition, the normalization of exertional ischemic ST changes following surgery as reported here and elsewhere (Lapin et al, 1973) indicates that previously ischemic myocardium is either adequately perfused or no longer viable. While intra-

operative myocardial necrosis undoubtedly accounts for ST normalization and pain relief postoperatively in some patients, reversal of exertional myocardial ischemia is likely the mechanism in most patients.

In this study, quantitative left ventricular volume measurements and qualitative analysis of the left ventricular contractile pattern were made from high quality biplane direct film angiograms exposed at 12/sec in 84 percent of the patients, with similar analyses being made from high quality single plane cineangiograms in the remainder. Using these techniques, abnormalities in resting ventricular performance were detected in a high proportion of the patients preoperatively—ie, ejection fraction greater than one standard deviation below the normal mean of 0.67 ≤ 0.08 (Kennedy, et al, 1966) in 40 of 55—and definitely abnormal contraction patterns were detected in 24 of 55. However, additional abnormalities of ventricular contraction or dysfunction in the previously normal resting ventricle can be brought out by stress such as atrial pacing (Dwyer, 1970). While our data fail to show improvement in resting ventricular performance, it is possible that stress-induced abnormalities may be corrected with revascularization concomitant with relief of stress-induced pain (angina). This subject is currently being investigated.

Heart rate was increased an average of 10 beats per minute at the postoperative study, compared with the preoperative study. Since all patients were studied after they were fully recovered from surgery (average of five months), the nonspecific stress of surgery, anemia, postoperative pain, or fever were not present. Nor was undue anxiety evident; degree of sedation, personnel, and catheterization technique were similar. Stroke volume was reduced slightly, such that cardiac output did not change significantly.

We conclude that the failure of apparently successful saphenous vein bypass grafting to improve resting ventricular performance or segmental contraction abnormalities indicates that resting ventricular dysfunction is due to myocardial fibrosis or scarring and is irreversible. Despite obvious angiographic evidence of obstructive coronary disease, sufficient blood is reaching the remaining viable myocardium to allow normal resting contractile function. With exercise or stress, coronary blood flow and myocardial oxygenation become inadequate, resulting in both pain and its physiologic correlate, abnormal contractile performance. Evidence for abnormal contractile performance during angina is abundant, ie, appearance of gallop rhythm, appearance of ischemic bulge, and transient elevation of LVEDP. We surmise that viable myocardium, which is sufficiently ischemic to have impaired contractility, will usually result in ischemic pain.

Several previous studies failed to demonstrate improved resting left ventricular performance following aortocoronary bypass surgery. Young et al (1971) (seven patients), Deal et al (1973) (16 patients), Itscoitz et al (1973) (10 patients), and Arbogast et al (1973) (23 patients) failed to show an improved EF in patients with patent grafts whereas the latter two studies showed deterioration in patients with occluded grafts. The 71 patients studied by Griffith et al (1973) failed to show improvement in contraction pattern. Kitamura et al (1972) reported improved EF following bypass surgery in nine patients, but each of these patients also had resection of a dyskinetic portion of left ventricular myocardium that would reduce EDV and thereby improve the EF if stroke volume changed little following surgery.

The studies by Johnson et al (1970b) and Rutherford et al (1972) showing improved ventricular performance following vein bypass grafting are also compatible with our data and conclusions, since these investigators studied a measure of ventricular function (LVEDP) during stress (exercise or atrial pacing).

Data that appear to disagree with our conclusion that resting ventricular dysfunction in the absence of pain is irreversible have been presented by Rees et al (1971) and Chatterjee et al (1973). In the former study, the group of eight patients showing improved ejection fraction following saphenous vein bypass grafting had normal mean preoperative ejection fractions, which increased to the high-normal range postoperatively, a change consistent with an unrecognized inotropic stimulus postoperatively. The patients in the latter study all underwent postoperative catheterization less than two weeks following surgery. This is a time when pain, anemia, fever, and the nonspecific "stress" of surgery may all result in sympathetic stimulation. Increased excretion of catecholamines during this period has been documented (Boudowas et al, 1973). In support of increased sympathetic stimulation at the postoperative study is the 21 percent increment in heart rate and 58 percent increment in calculated cardiac index in these 29 patients. The mean postoperative cardiac index was 6.5 L/min/M^2) in the eight patients with patent grafts who were said to have improved myocardial function by Rees et al, (1971). These data indicate that at least some of the improvement in ejection fraction seen in these patients was due to sympathetic stimulation and not to myocardial revascularization. In contrast, cardiac index was

in the normal range in our 55 patients and in all subgroups (3.0 to 3.5 L/min/M^2) with no change following surgery. Heart rate was somewhat higher at the postoperative study in our patients, but not as much as in the patients reported by Chatterjee et al (1973). The subgroup of Chatterjee et al (1973) showing the greatest increase in ejection fraction and wall motion were those with preinfarction angina. Such patients undergoing preoperative study during a period of active ischemia may have greater potential for reversible myocardial dysfunction. No patients in our group had their preoperative study during acute ischemic episodes.

Finally, two clinical trials corroborate these concepts. Spencer et al (1971) and Kouchoukos et al (1972) have reported a high mortality rate and little symptomatic improvement in patients who underwent myocardial revascularization primarily because of symptoms of left ventricular dysfunction.

The failure of saphenous vein bypass grafting to improve resting ventricular performance does not negate its value for the symptomatic relief of angina. However, those anginal patients with resting ventricular dysfunction who are limited by pain preoperatively may expect to continue to have impaired ventricular performance postoperatively, with exertional limitation from dyspnea and fatigue instead of angina pectoris. Patients whose primary symptoms are those of left ventricular failure or who have these symptoms at rest should not be offered myocardial revascularization, since left ventricular function is not likely to improve. In addition, patients with severe left ventricular dysfunction have an inordinately high operative mortality (mortality: 33 percent with ejection fraction less than 33 percent in our experience of nine patients).

The ultimate worth of this procedure for myocardial revascularization will only be known when prospective randomized studies demonstrate its effect on rate of myocardial infarction and mortality. Until these data become available, we feel this procedure should be primarily reserved for patients who are severely limited by angina, do not have left heart failure, have suitable coronary anatomy, and an ejection fraction greater than 33 percent.

References

Arbogast R, Solignac A, Bourassa MG: Influence of aorto-coronary saphenous vein bypass surgery on left ventricular volumes and ejection fraction. Am J Med 54:290, 1973

Achuff S, Griffith L, Humphries JON, et al: Myocardial damage after aorto-coronary vein bypass surgery. J Clin Invest 51 (no 6):1a, 1972 (abstract)

Boudowas H, Lewis RP, Karayannacos PE, Vasco JS: The effect of saphenous vein graft surgery upon left ventricular function. Paper presented to 22d Annual Scientific Session of American College of Cardiology, San Francisco, February 17, 1973

Brewer DL, Bilbro RH, Bartel AG: Myocardial infarction as a complication of coronary bypass surgery. Circulation 47:58, 1973

Bruce RA: Exercise testing of patients with coronary heart disease. Ann Clin Res 3:323, 1971

Bruce RA, Hornsten TR: Exercise stress testing in evaluation of patients with ischemic heart disease. Prog Cardiovasc Dis 11:371, 1969

Chatterjee K, Swan HJC, Parmley WW, et al: Influence of direct myocardial revascularization on left ventricular asynergy and function in patients with coronary heart disease. Circulation 47:276, 1973

Dart CH Jr, Scott S, Fish R, Takaro T: Direct blood flow studies of clinical internal thoracic (mammary) arterial implants. Circulation 41 (Suppl II):64, 1970

Deal P, Elliott LP, Bartley TD, Wheat MW Jr, Ramsey HW: Quantitative left ventriculography in the immediate postoperative period after aorto-coronary bypass. J Thorac Cardiovasc Surg 66:1, 1973

Dodge HT, Sandler H, Ballew DW, Lord JD: The use of biplane angiocardiography for the measurement of left ventricular volume in man. Am Heart J 60:762, 1960

Dwyer EM Jr: Left ventricular pressure-volume alterations and regional disorders of contraction during myocardial ischemia induced by atrial pacing. Circulation 42:1111, 1970

Greene DG, Klocke FJ, Schimert GL, et al: Evaluation of venous bypass grafts from aorta to coronary artery by inert gas desaturation and direct flowmeter techniques. J Clin Invest 51:191, 1972

Griffith LSC, Achuff SC, Conti CR, et al: Changes in intrinsic coronary circulation and segmental ventricular motion after saphenous-vein coronary bypass graft surgery. N Engl J Med 288:589, 1973

Hamilton GW, Murray JA, Kennedy JW: Quantitative angiocardiography in ischemic heart disease. Circulation 45:1065, 1972

Hultgren HN, Miyagawa M, Buck W, Angell WW: Is-
chemic myocardial injury during coronary artery surgery. Am Heart J 82:624, 1971

Itscoitz SB, Shepherd RL, Glancy DL, et al: Deterioration of myocardial function following aorto-coronary bypass operation. Clin Res 21:427, 1973 (abstract)

Johnson WD, Flemma RJ, Lepley D Jr: Determinants of blood flow in aortic-coronary saphenous vein bypass grafts. Arch Surg 101:806, 1970a

Johnson WD, Flemma RJ, Manley JC, Lepley D Jr: The physiologic parameters of ventricular function as affected by direct coronary surgery. J Thorac Cardiovasc Surg 60:483, 1970b

Kennedy JW, Trenholme SE, Kasser IS: Left ventricular volume and mass from single-plane cineangiocardiogram. Am Heart J 80:343, 1970

Kennedy JW, Baxley WA, Figley MM, Dodge HT, Blackmon JR: Quantitative angiocardiography: I: the normal left ventricle in man. Circulation 34:272, 1966

Kitamura S, Echevarria M, Kay JH, et al: Left ventricular performance before and after removal of the noncontractile area of the left ventricle and revascularization of the myocardium. Circulation 45:1005, 1972

Kouchoukos NT, Doty DB, Buettner LE, Kirklin JW: Treatment of postinfarction cardiac failure by myocardial excision and revascularization. Circulation 45 (Suppl I):72, 1972

Lapin ES, Murray JA, Bruce RA, Winterscheid L: Changes in maximal exercise performance in the evaluation of saphenous vein bypass surgery. Circulation 47:1164–73, 1973

Rees G, Bristow JD, Kremkau EL, et al: Influence of aorto-coronary bypass surgery on left ventricular performance. N Engl J Med 284:1116, 1971

Rutherford BD, Gau GT, Danielson GK, et al: Left ventricular hemodynamics before and soon after saphenous vein bypass graft operation for angina pectoris. Br Heart J 34:1156, 1972

Spencer FC, Green GE, Tice DA, et al: Coronary artery bypass grafts for congestive heart failure. J Thorac Cardiovasc Surg 62:529, 1971

Tyberg JV, Yeatman LA, Parmley WW, Urschel CW, Sonnenblick EH: Effects of hypoxia on mechanics of cardiac contraction. Am J Physiol 218:1780, 1970

Young WG Jr, Sabiston DC Jr, Ebert Pa, et al: Preoperative assessment of left ventricular function in patients selected for direct myocardial revascularization. Am Thorac Surg 11:395, 1971

104

HEMODYNAMIC ASSESSMENT AND PULMONARY BLOOD VOLUME ALTERATIONS FOLLOWING CORONARY ARTERY BYPASS SURGERY

Joseph D. Cohn, Meena M. Mehta, Rogelio Trespicio, Micki A. Rosenbloom, and Louis R. M. Del Guercio

The introduction of aortocoronary bypass has led to the widespread application of surgery for acquired coronary artery disease. Numerous reports have described preoperative selection criteria for this revascularization procedure, intraoperative management, postoperative graft function, and mortality. The efficacy of the technique of coronary artery bypass surgery is well established. Further measures, however, must be developed with a view toward reduction of intraoperative and postoperative morbidity and mortality.

Mortality from coronary artery bypass surgery has ranged from 1.5 to 10 percent (Alderman, Matloff, et al, 1973; Anderson, Hodam, et al, 1972; Effler, Favaloro, et al, 1970; Janke, 1973; Lea, Tector, et al, 1972; Morris, Reul, et al, 1972). The operative and early postoperative mortality and morbidity have been almost entirely limited to patients with congestive heart failure or intraoperative infarction (Lea, Tector, et al, 1972). In addition, postoperative pulmonary abnormalities and pulmonary embolism have also been described as common complications (Alderman, Matloff, et al, 1973; Gott, Brawley, et al, 1973), similar to the incidence of complications occurring following other major surgical procedures.

The introduction of continuous monitoring techniques and the availability of hemodynamic profile assessment have provided methods for the analysis of cardiovascular and pulmonary function in the immediate postoperative period. Early detection and assessment of altered hemodynamic function may be used as a guide to appropriate and timely therapeutic intervention. Optimal maintenance of cardiovascular and pulmonary function in the immediate and early postoperative period should then provide a framework for improved postoperative hemodynamics and metabolic response and lead to further reduction in the incidence of postoperative complications.

METHODS

Hemodynamic profile analysis was performed in 30 consecutive patients undergoing elective coronary artery bypass surgery. The mean age for all patients was 53.7 years, with a range of 33 to 69 years. The male-to-female ratio was 3.1:1. Patients were selected for coronary artery bypass surgery on the basis of incapacitating angina. Proximal segmental obstructive disease was demonstrated on cinecoronary angiography and ventricular ejection fraction was greater than 50 percent in all cases. Forty-four percent of the patients underwent single coronary artery bypass, and the remainder underwent multiple grafting procedures.

Hemodynamic assessment was performed following volume replacement and cardiovascular stabilization in the early postoperative period. Nonphysician personnel were trained in the procedures required for hemodynamic assessment, blood sampling techniques, and data reduction, and they routinely performed all studies. During the procedure all patients were maintained on assisted ventilation with 100 percent inspired oxygen. Blood samples were obtained from the indwelling central arterial and right atrial catheters for oxygen and carbon dioxide tension, pH, hemoglobin, hematocrit, lactate, and pyruvate determinations. Arterial and central venous pressures were recorded on a monitoring system,* and cardiac output studies were performed by the indocyanine green dye indicator-dilution method. Data reduction and derived data calculations were performed by use of an electronic digitizing unit † and programmable calculator.‡ Computer programs based upon previously described computation methods for analysis of dye dilution curves (Cohn and Del Guercio, 1966; Siegel, Greenspan, et al, 1968) and algorithms for blood acid-base and blood gas calculations (Thomas, 1972) provided rapid assessment of hemodynamic and pulmonary function. Primary and derived data were provided on a timely basis and in a format for ready interpretation by the attending physician. The capability of performing serial assessments of hemodynamic function allowed effective modification of therapy directed toward improved cardiovascular function.

Hemodynamic assessment included recording of pulse rate and arterial and venous pressures. Cardiac output was computed from the indicator dilution curve and derived data based upon these parameters included cardiac index, stroke volume, stroke index, left ventricular stroke work, mean ejection rate, and peripheral resistance. Data from blood gas analyses, pH, hemoglobin, and hematocrit determinations allowed calculation of oxygen saturation corrected to patient temperature, arteriovenous oxygen difference, oxygen consumption, and venoarterial admixture (Finley, Lenfant, et al, 1960). Serum lactate and serum pyruvate concentrations were determined by enzymatic methods § and are included in the hemodynamic assessment.

A complete hemodynamic profile analysis was performed by nonphysician personnel at two and 20 hours following surgery. In addition, at the 20-hour period pulmonary blood volume assessment was performed by a noninvasive indicator dilution method (Cohn, Ito, et al, 1974; Del Guercio, Cohn, et al, 1973). During this procedure a portable solid state X-ray detector array was positioned under the patient and aligned with a collimated X-ray generator source located

over the patient (Fig. 1). Rapid injection of nonradioactive, radio-opaque, contrast material into the right atrium during constant X-ray transmission allowed recording of multiple transthoracic contrast dilution curves reflecting indicator transit through the heart and lungs. Pulmonary transit time was estimated from the appearance of indicator in right and left heart chambers and allowed calculation of pulmonary blood volume. Detectors positioned over the peripheral lung field provided recording of pulmonary capillary arrival times, thus defining pulmonary arterial and pulmonary venous blood volume dimensions (Cohn and Holden, 1972).

Data were grouped to compare hemodynamic profiles at two and 20 hours following surgery by the Student's t-test (Randall, 1962). In addition, data analyses were performed to assess the relationship of single and multiple graft procedures on hemodynamic function in the postoperative period.

RESULTS

Hemodynamic profiles for all patients were compared at two hours and 20 hours following coronary artery bypass surgery, and pulmonary blood volume analysis was performed during the 20-hour study period. All patients in the study group survived the operative procedure and were subsequently discharged from the hospital.

During the initial study, at the two-hour period, mean values for central arterial pressure were 117/70, mean 87 mm Hg. Central venous pressure averaged 10 mm Hg and cardiac index was 2.72 L/min/M², within the normal range. Stroke index was slightly decreased at 32 ml/M² and the mean pulse rate was 88/min. Peripheral vascular resistance averaged 1378 dyne/sec/cm⁻⁵, demonstrating mild vasoconstriction. The mean hemoglobin level was 11.3 gm percent reflecting the effects of moderate hemodilution related to intraoperative management. Arterial oxygen tension during ventilation with 100 percent oxygen was somewhat depressed, reflecting intrapulmonary shunting, and a mean value of venoarterial admixture of 20.6 percent was obtained. Mild metabolic acidosis is demonstrated during the two-hour hemodynamic profile assessment: Arteriovenous oxygen difference averaged 5.14 vol percent, and oxygen consumption, based upon cardiac output and arteriovenous difference measurements, was 249 ml/min. Arterial lactate was elevated to 5.64 mM/l (normal: 0.3 − 0.8 mM/l) and arterial

* Datascope Physiological Monitor, Datascope Corporation, Paramus, NJ.
† Model GP-2 BCD Graf/Pen. Science Accessories Corporation, Southport, Conn.
‡ Wang Model 600 Programmable Calculator. Wang Laboratories, Inc, Tewksbury, Mass.
§ Rapid Lactate Stat-pack and Pyruvate Stat-pack. Calbiochem, La Jolla, Calif.

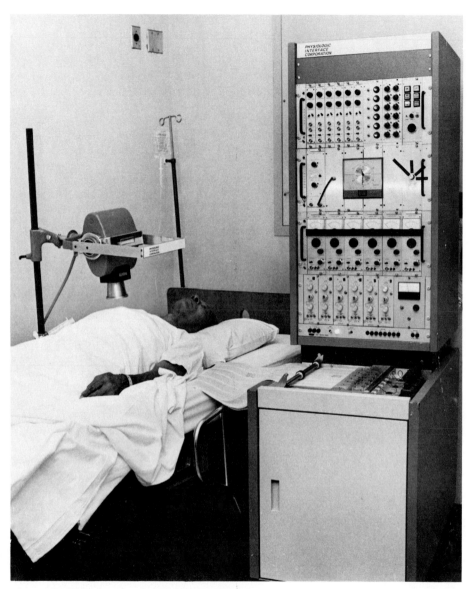

FIG. 1.   The portable contrast dilution analysis system (Contrast Dilution Analysis System, Physiologic Interface Corporation, Livingston, NJ) consists of a solid state X-ray detector array positioned under the subject and a collimated X-ray source. Multiple, simultaneous indicator dilution curves were recorded during continuous X-ray transmissions and following injection of nonradioactive, radio-opaque contrast material into the central circulation. Indicator dispersion allows computation of pulmonary transit times and provides data for calculation of pulmonary blood volume.

pyruvate was elevated to 0.31 mM/l (normal: 0.03 − 0.10 mM/l).

Data from the two-hour and 20-hour studies were analyzed by the Student's t-test for significant differences and are recorded in Table 1. Average values for central arterial pressures were unchanged. Cardiac index increased to 3.22 l/min/M², and the difference was significant at $P < 0.05$. The mean value for stroke index increased from 32 to 41 ml/M² and was associated

with a decrease in pulse rate to 80/min. Central venous pressure decreased from 10 to 7 mm Hg and was associated with a rise in left ventricular stroke work from 71 to 91 gm/M, reflecting improved myocardial function. Blood gas analyses demonstrated a slight decrease in oxygen tension during 100 percent oxygen ventilation, though this was not statistically significant. Mild respiratory alkalosis was demonstrated during the 20-hour study period, reflecting the effect of mild

TABLE 1. Hemodynamic Profile Analysis in 30 Patients Following Coronary Artery Bypass Surgery

	2 HRS. POST SURGERY ($\bar{x} \pm SD^a$)	20 HRS. POST SURGERY ($\bar{x} \pm SD^a$)	P
Blood pressure, systolic mm Hg	117 ± 20	117 ± 17	>0.9
Blood pressure, diastolic mm Hg	70 ± 15	66 ± 9	<0.3
Blood pressure, mean mm Hg	87 ± 17	83 ± 12	<0.4
Central venous pressure, mean mm Hg	10 ± 4	7 ± 2	<0.01
Cardiac output $1 \cdot min^{-1}$	5.04 ± 1.57	5.99 ± 2.07	<0.1
Cardiac index $1 \cdot min^{-1} \cdot M^{-2}$	2.72 ± 0.82	3.22 ± 0.94	<0.05
Stroke volume ml	59 ± 22	76 ± 27	<0.02
Stroke index $ml \cdot M^{-2}$	32 ± 11	41 ± 12	<0.01
Pulse min^{-1}	88 ± 16	80 ± 13	<0.05
Peripheral resistance $dyne \cdot sec \cdot cm^{-5}$	1378 ± 624	1138 ± 383	<0.1
Left ventricular stroke work $gm \cdot M$	71 ± 34	91 ± 40	<0.1
Mean ejection rate $ml \cdot sec^{-1} \cdot M^{-2}$	117 ± 34	152 ± 44	<0.8
Hemoglobin gm %	11.3 ± 1.4	11.0 ± 1.5	<0.6
$P_A O_2$ mm Hg	332 ± 99	295 ± 133	<0.2
$P_A CO_2$ mm Hg	39 ± 7	33 ± 6	<0.01
pH_A	7.34 ± 0.05	7.48 ± 0.05	<0.01
Base excess$_A$ $meq \cdot 1^{-1}$	-4 ± 2	2 ± 3	<0.01
$P_V O_2$ mm Hg	45 ± 10	38 ± 7	<0.01
$P_V CO_2$ mm Hg	46 ± 6	38 ± 6	<0.01
pH_V	7.29 ± 0.05	$7.45 \pm .04$	<0.01
Base excess$_V$ $meq \cdot 1^{-1}$	-4 ± 3	2 ± 2	<0.01
Arterial oxygen saturation %	99.7 ± 0.6	99.1 ± 2.0	<0.2
Venous oxygen saturation %	72.4 ± 9.8	72.2 ± 7.7	>0.9
Arteriovenous oxygen difference vol %	5.14 ± 1.62	4.71 ± 1.19	<0.4
Oxygen consumption $ml \cdot min^{-1}$	249 ± 93	280 ± 80	<0.3
Oxygen consumption $ml \cdot kg^{-1}$	3.41 ± 1.25	3.64 ± 0.86	<0.5
Venoarterial admixture %	20.6 ± 9.2	18.3 ± 6.3	<0.4
Serum lactate $mM \cdot 1^{-1}$	5.64 ± 3.12	3.40 ± 2.51	<0.1
Serum pyruvate $mM \cdot 1^{-1}$	0.31 ± 0.11	0.20 ± 0.09	<0.05

^{a}*Mean ± standard deviation.*

hyperventilation during assisted ventilation. In addition, the average value for base excess was recorded as 2 mEq/1 representing a significant increase compared to the immediate postoperative study. Arterial and mixed venous oxygen saturations were unchanged, and there was a slight decrease in arteriovenous oxygen difference, which was not statistically significant. Likewise, oxygen consumption and venoarterial admixture remained unchanged. Serum lactate and serum pyruvate decreased and these changes were of significance at $P < 0.1$ and $P < 0.05$, respectively.

Pulmonary vascular volumes were determined at the 20-hour study period by the non-invasive contrast dilution analysis method (Table 2). Pulmonary blood volume averaged 273 ml/M². Pulmonary arterial blood volume based upon the arrival time to the peripheral lung field was found to be 161 ml/M², and pulmonary venous blood volume was similarly computed to be 116 ml/M².

Hemodynamic data were further analyzed to assess cardiovascular and metabolic response following surgery for single and multiple coronary

artery grafting procedures. The average of the mean blood pressure values during the two-hour study period was increased in the multiple grafting group (93 mm Hg) compared to the patients undergoing single coronary artery bypass procedures (79 mm Hg), and this was statistically significant at $P < 0.05$. Significant differences also included diminished pulse rate and increased left ventricular stroke work in patients undergoing multiple grafting procedures. In addition, blood gas analyses demonstrated a slight but significant increase in arterial and mixed venous pH and

TABLE 2. Pulmonary Blood Volume

	20 HRS. POST SURGERY ($\bar{x} \pm SE^a$)	NORMAL SUBJECTS (Yu, 1969) ($\bar{x} \pm SE^a$)
PBV $ml \cdot M^{-2}$	273 ± 27	271 ± 8
PBV$_A$ $ml \cdot M^{-2}$	161 ± 17	
PBV$_V$ $ml \cdot M^{-2}$	116 ± 17	

^{a}*Mean ± standard error.*

diminished fixed base deficit in the group of patients undergoing multiple coronary artery grafting. The remaining hemodynamic parameters, including recorded and derived data, did not demonstrate statistically significant differences. Furthermore, analyses of all data at the 20-hour period demonstrated complete absence of statistically significant differences between the single and multiple grafting groups related to any of the recorded or derived variables including hemodynamic and blood gas parameters and pulmonary vascular volume determinations.

Cardiopulmonary bypass support during coronary artery bypass surgery was utilized in 25 of the 30 patients in this study. In five patients, coronary artery grafting was performed without circulatory assistance. Because of sample size, however, relevant comparison of hemodynamic function in these two groups of patients was not possible.

The duration of cardiopulmonary bypass in the 25 patients in whom circulatory support was utilized was 97 ± 44 (SD) minutes. The lowest intraoperative pH was 7.30 ± 0.04 (SD) and the intraoperative fixed base replacement was 68 ± 44 (SD) mEq sodium bicarbonate. Analysis of the hemodynamic profiles related to intraoperative acidosis and duration of cardiopulmonary bypass did not establish these variables to be of statistical significance in this study.

DISCUSSION

Physiologic assessment by analysis of the hemodynamic profile provides information related to hemodynamic function, pulmonary function, and metabolic responses. The physiologic alterations following coronary artery bypass surgery in patients with satisfactory preoperative ventricular function demonstrate stabilization of hemodynamic parameters and mild elevation in cardiac index. Progressive increase in ventricular performance over the first 20 hours following surgery is illustrated by improvement in ventricular function as reflected by a decrease in central venous pressure and an increase in left ventricular stroke work as well as an increase in stroke index. Mild metabolic acidosis, related to intraoperative cardiopulmonary bypass support, returned toward normal by the 20-hour study and was associated with postoperative diuresis. In addition, mild respiratory alkalosis related to mechanical assisted ventilation was also present. Though arteriovenous oxygen difference and oxygen consumption were within normal limits, moderate venoarterial admixture was evident from data analyzed during 100 percent oxygen ventilation. The intrapulmonary shunt was unchanged over the study period.

Pulmonary blood volume was determined to be within normal limits by the 20-hour study. The relationships between pulmonary artery and pulmonary venous blood volume calculations illustrate abnormal distributions of blood flow (Yu, 1969) confirming the presence of altered pulmonary function in the early postoperative period (Naimark, Dugard, et al, 1968).

Serum lactate and serum pyruvate were found to be considerably elevated in the early postoperative period, probably reflecting diminished tissue perfusion during cardiopulmonary bypass as well as other factors (Cady, Weil, et al, 1973; Moffitt, Tarhan, et al, 1973; Oliva, 1970; Weil and Afifi, 1970). Arterial lactate and pyruvate levels significantly decreased over the 20-hour period as previously demonstrated by Moffit and coworkers in patients undergoing open heart surgical procedures (Moffitt, Tarhan, et al, 1973).

The serial physiologic patterns demonstrated by hemodynamic profile assessments document the cardiovascular and metabolic response to coronary artery grafting procedures and associated intraoperative circulatory support measures. The significant and progressive improvement in hemodynamic function over the period of study implicates the presence of an initial phase of postoperative myocardial depression, which gradually improves. The etiology of the initial decrement in cardiac output and myocardial function is not defined by this investigation. Further evaluation of the hemodynamic function of patients undergoing coronary artery bypass procedures without the use of pump oxygenator support may provide an answer in this regard. These investigations are currently being performed.

Experimental and clinical studies of the evaluation of lactate concentration as an indicator of the severity of shock and as a predictor for survival have demonstrated significant correlation of mortality with elevated arterial lactate concentration (Cady, Weil, et al, 1973; Weil and Afifi, 1970). Limited correlation, however, has been documented in relation to values for excess lactate (Huckabee, 1958), arterial pyruvate concentration, and lactate/pyruvate ratios (Weil and Afifi, 1970). Moffitt and associates (Moffitt, Tarhan et al, 1973) have also demonstrated intraoperative and postoperative elevations in arterial and mixed venous lactate and pyruvate concentrations. Their findings were similar to those found in this study and suggested that glucose priming solution during cardiopulmonary bypass accounted for these abnormalities.

It is apparent, however, that the elevated lactate levels do not correlate with survival probability in the present investigations. Weil and Afifi (1970) and Cady and coworkers (1970) documented survival probability with plasma lactate concentration. For a plasma lactate concentration of 5.64 mM/1, the average lactate concentration at the two-hour study period, the predicted survival probability indicated by these authors was less than 30 percent. This predictive assessment is inconsistent with the results of our clinical investigation, which indicates return of arterial lactate and pyruvate concentrations toward normal following coronary artery bypass surgery, associated with 100 percent patient survival.

Comparison of data from patients undergoing single and multiple coronary artery grafting procedures demonstrated slight differences in hemodynamic function immediately following surgery. However, at the 20-hour study period these changes were no longer apparent and both groups demonstrated identical hemodynamic profiles. These findings demonstrate that similar cardiovascular function is present in both patient groups and implies that underlying myocardial disease, rather than the severity of coronary artery obstructive disease, is the determinant of hemodynamic and metabolic responses following coronary artery bypass surgery.

Evaluation of pulmonary function based upon blood gas parameters and noninvasive contrast dilution analysis demonstrates significant elevation in venoarterial admixture and alterations in pulmonary blood flow patterns in the postoperative period. These abnormalities persist past the 20-hour study period at which time hemodynamic and metabolic functions have stabilized and returned toward normal. These alterations in distribution of ventilation and perfusion have been demonstrated in response to shock, transfusion, and pump oxygenator support (Cook and Webb, 1968; Henry, 1968; Jouasset-Strieder, Cahill, et al, 1966; Veith, Hagstrom, et al, 1968). Though the etiology of these physiologic alterations may reside in a multitude of interactions, attempts to reduce further the magnitude of these hemodynamic abnormalities may provide a basis for early improvement in pulmonary function and reduction in the pulmonary complications particularly related to coronary artery bypass procedures.

References

Alderman EL, Matlof HJ, Wexler L, Shumway NE, Harrison DC: Results of direct coronary artery surgery for the treatment of angina pectoris. N Engl J Med 288:535, 1973

Anderson RP, Hodam R, Wood J, Starr A: Direct revascularization of the heart: Early clinical experience with 200 patients. J Thorac Cardiovasc Surg 63:353, 1972

Cady LD, Weil MH, Afifi AA, et al: Quantitation of severity of critical illness with special reference to blood lactate. Critical Care Medicine 1:75, 1973

Cohn JD, Del Guercio LRM: A nomogram for the rapid calculation of cardiac output at the bedside. Ann Surg 164:109, 1966

Cohn JD, Holden FM: Roentgen dilution curve analysis of pulmonary blood flow distribution during hemorrhage. Invest Radiol 7:67, 1972

Cohn JD, Ito K, Del Guercio LRM: Gamma-ray densitometry in the analysis of hemodynamic function. In Harmison LT (ed), Proceedings National Conference on Research Animals in Medicine, National Heart and Lung Institute, Washington, 1973, p 1085

Cook WA, Webb WR: Pulmonary changes in hemorrhagic shock. Surgery 64:85, 1968

Del Guercio LRM, Cohn JD, Ito K, Haas G, Huth GC: Clinical cardiovascular studies with solid state contrast dilution analysis. In Kaufman L, Price DC (eds), Proceedings Symposium on Semi-conductors in Medicine. University of California, San Francisco and US Atomic Energy Commission, Conf-730321, 1973

Effler DB, Favaloro RG, Groves LK: Coronary artery surgery utilizing saphenous vein graft techniques: clinical experience with 224 operations. J Thorac Cardiovasc Surg 59:147, 1970

Finley TN, Lenfant C, Haab P, Piper J, Rahn H: Venous admixture in the pulmonary circulation of anesthetized dogs. J Appl Physiol 15:418, 1960

Gott VL, Brawley RK, Donahoo JS, Griffith LSC: Current surgical approach to ischemic heart disease. Curr Probl Surg May 1973

Henry JN: The effect of shock on pulmonary alveolar surfactant. J Trauma 8:756, 1968

Huckabee WE: Relationships of pyruvate and lactate during anaerobic metabolism: II. Exercise and formation of O_2 debt. J Clin Invest 37:255, 1958

Janke WH: Restricted use of extra-corporeal circulation in coronary bypass surgery. Contemp Surg 3:75, 1973

Jouasset-Strieder D, Cahill JM, Byrne JJ: Pulmonary capillary blood volume in dogs during shock and after retransfusion. J Appl Physiol 21:365, 1966

Lea RE, Tector AJ, Flemma RJ, et al: Prognostic significance of a reduced left ventricular ejection fraction in coronary artery surgery. Circulation 46, Supplement 2:49, 1972

Moffitt EA, Tarhan S, McGoon DC: Whole-body metabolism during and after open-heart surgery. Canadian Anesthesiology Society Journal 20:607, 1973

Morris GC, Reul GJ, Howell JF, et al: Follow-up results of distal coronary artery bypass for ischemic heart disease. Am J Cardiol 29:180, 1972

Naimark A, Dugard A, Rangno RE: Regional pulmonary blood flow and gas exchange in hemorrhagic shock. J Appl Physiol 25:301, 1968

Oliva PB: Lactic acidosis. Am J Med 48:209, 1970

Randall JE: Elements of Biophysics, 2d ed. Chicago, Year Book Medical Publishers, 1962

Siegel JH, Greenspan M, Cohn JD, Del Guercio LRM: A

bedside computer and physiologic nomograms. Arch Surg 97:480, 1968

Thomas LJ: Algorithms for selected blood acid-base and blood gas calculations. J Appl Physiol 33:154, 1972

Veith FJ, Hagstrom JWC, Panossian A, Nehlsen SL, Wilson JW: Pulmonary microcirculatory response to shock, transfusion, and pump-oxygenator proce-

dures: a unified mechanism underlying pulmonary damage. Surgery 64:95, 1968

Weil MH, Afifi AA: Experimental and clinical studies on lactate and pyruvate as indicators of the severity of acute circulatory failure (shock). Circulation 41:989, 1970

Yu PN: Pulmonary blood volume in health and disease. Philadelphia, Lea and Feibiger, 1969

105

EFFECT OF MYOCARDIAL REVASCULARIZATION ON REDUCED LEFT VENTRICULAR COMPLIANCE IN ISCHEMIC HEART DISEASE

Richard R. Miller, Dean T. Mason, Albert E. Iben,
Edward J. Hurley, Arthur J. Lurie, Robert Zelis,
and Ezra A. Amsterdam

The effects of myocardial revascularization on altered left ventricular diastolic compliance in coronary heart disease are unknown. Although previous clinical observations have documented improvement in hemodynamic and contraction variables following restoration of myocardial perfusion in coronary disease (Chatterjee, Swan, et al, 1972; Chatterjee, Swan, et al, 1973; Rees, Bristow et al, 1971), data pertaining to the reversibility of abnormal left ventricular distensibility are lacking. Thus, amelioration of pulmonary congestive symptoms following coronary artery bypass surgery may be related to improved compliance of the ventricle with consequent favorable alterations of its diastolic pressure-volume relation, in addition to enhancement of cardiac contractile properties. This investigation was carried out to determine whether, and to what degree, abnormalities of left ventricular diastolic compliance in patients with ischemic heart disease are influenced by successful coronary artery bypass.

PATIENTS AND METHODS

Twenty-two patients undergoing left heart catheterization and selective coronary arteriography preoperatively and two to 70 weeks (mean 16 weeks) following coronary artery bypass surgery comprised this study. The 22 patients were selected to achieve maximum uniformity in one of

Supported by NIH Research Program Project Grant HL-14780.

two groups, so that only patients with all grafts patent or all grafts occluded were selected for evaluation. Accordingly, 14 patients with one to three patent aortocoronary saphenous bypass grafts or left internal mammary artery to left anterior descending coronary artery (LAD) anastomoses (Group I) were compared to eight patients with all grafts or anastomoses occluded (Group II). All patients were in normal sinus rhythm, and no patient had mitral regurgitation as assessed by left ventricular angiography. The average number of major coronary arteries with significant (> 75 percent) proximal stenoses was 2.2 in Group I with patent grafts and was 2.6 in Group II with occluded grafts. The mean number of saphenous bypass grafts and/or internal mammary to LAD anastomoses was 1.6 in patients with patent grafts and 1.7 in patients with occluded grafts. Four patients with patent grafts and three with occluded grafts had preoperative evidence of myocardial infarction. Three patients with patent grafts and two with occluded grafts had electrocardiographic evidence of intraoperative or postoperative myocardial infarction. Eight additional patients with normal coronary arteriography and left ventricular function served as normal controls.

Left ventricular total diastolic compliance (distensibility) is defined as $(\triangle V/\triangle P)$, where $\triangle V$ equals diastolic volume change obtained from stroke volume index determined from dye dilution cardiac output and corrected for body surface area and $\triangle P$ equals change in left ventricular diastolic pressure. The expression $(\triangle V/\triangle P)$ was further modified by normalizing with end systolic volume index (ESI): [$\Delta V/\Delta P(V_{ESI})$]. This ratio is termed ventricular diastolic specific compliance (Smith, Russell, et al, 1972).

The reciprocal of the expression for compliance ($\Delta P/\Delta V$) provides an index of total left ventricular diastolic stiffness. There is a linear relationship between mean ventricular diastolic pressure ($\overline{p}$) and total diastolic ($\Delta P/\Delta V$), and the slope of this linear plot has been termed the passive elastic modulus (Diamond, Forrester, 1972). Utilizing a constant volume and the same contrast agent for each patient during preoperative and postoperative left ventricular angiography, this procedure represents a uniform increment of stress upon the left ventricle consisting of a sudden osmotically related volume load and to a lesser extent a direct toxic effect. Accordingly, indices of total left ventricular diastolic compliance and stiffness were determined immediately prior to and 10 minutes following left ventricular angiography preoperatively and postoperatively.

RESULTS

The 14 patients in Group I with patent grafts at postoperative coronary arteriography had an increase in ejection fraction from a preoperative value of 57 percent to 66 percent following surgery ($p < 0.01$). In contrast the eight Group II patients with graft occlusion demonstrated no significant change in this parameter postoperatively: 64 percent to 61 percent ($p > 0.05$).

Utilizing the expression [$\Delta V/\Delta P(V_{ESI})$] as an index of left ventricular compliance, the eight normal patients had a mean specific left ventricular compliance of 0.180, while the patients with coronary stenoses had presurgical values of 0.100 ($p < 0.05$ compared to normals) and 0.109 ($p < 0.05$ in the groups with sub-

sequent patent and occluded grafts respectively. There was no significant difference ($p > 0.05$) in the reduced compliance in Groups I and II. Following surgery, patients with open grafts demonstrated an increase in this index of compliance to 0.149 ($p < 0.05$); patients with graft occlusion had no significant change: 0.102 ($p > 0.05$) (Fig. 1).

Graft patency was related to a decrease in the index of left ventricular stiffness [($\Delta P/\Delta V)/\overline{p}$]: 0.041 preoperatively to 0.034 ($p < 0.05$) postoperatively (Group I); patients with occluded grafts (Group II) exhibited no change in this index: 0.047 to 0.045 ($p > 0.05$).

The slopes of the plot obtained from ($\Delta P/\Delta V$) and $\overline{p}$ were linear and the same in both groups of coronary patients prior to operative intervention (Fig. 2, A and C). Following surgery, patients with open grafts had a reduction in this slope from a $= 0.033$ to a $= 0.019$ ($p < 0.05$) (Fig. 2, A and B), while patients with graft failure had no significant change: a $= 0.036$ to a $= 0.032$ ($p > 0.05$) (Fig. 2, C and D).

The stiffness response to a sudden increase in intravascular volume quantified by [($\Delta P/\Delta V)/\overline{p}$] 10 minutes following angiography returned toward normal following successful coronary artery bypass. The eight normal patients demonstrated a 9 percent increase in this index of stiffness following ventriculography, compared ($p < 0.05$) to preoperative increases of 31 percent and 39 percent in the patients with subsequent patent and occluded grafts respectively. After surgery this response was reduced to 17 percent ($p < 0.05$) in Group I patients with patent grafts and 36 percent ($p > 0.05$) in Group II patients with closed grafts. Thus, the left ventricle appears to withstand sudden volume loads with less alteration of its total pressure-

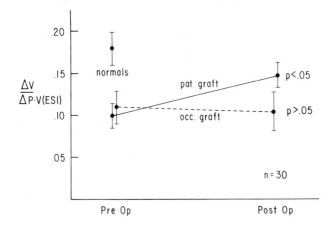

FIG. 1. Effects of coronary artery bypass on total left ventricular diastolic specific compliance in patients with patent (pat) grafts compared to patients with occluded (occ) grafts. Preop: preoperation; postop: postoperation. The index of compliance obtained from normal patients is shown.

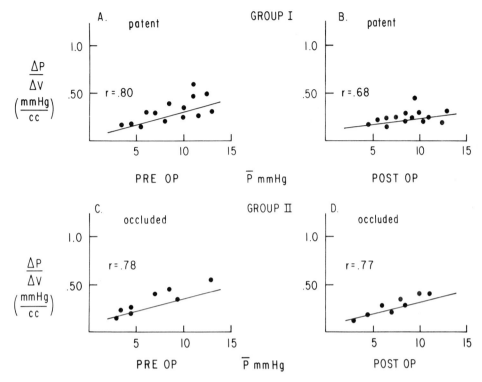

FIG. 2. Effects of coronary artery bypass on the relation between total left ventricular diastolic stiffness and mean left ventricular diastolic pressure in patients with patent grafts (Group I) compared to patients with occluded grafts (Group II). The slope of this linear regression relates directly to wall stiffness.

volume relationship following reestablishment of coronary blood flow.

DISCUSSION

This study demonstrates the reversible nature of depressed left ventricular diastolic compliance occurring consequent to myocardial ischemia by restoration of myocardial blood flow. Since diminished left ventricular distensibility may result in elevated pulmonary venous pressure, improvement in abnormal left ventricular pressure-volume relations may play an important role concomitant with enhanced contractile properties in the relief of congestive symptoms following myocardial revascularization (Bristow, Van Zee, et al, 1970; Covell, Ross, 1973; Levine, 1972).

Previous investigations have demonstrated a reduction in left ventricular compliance corresponding with the onset of myocardial ischemia (Dwyer, 1970; Forrester, Diamond, et al, 1972). Immediately following myocardial infarction compliance may increase, while in the healing stage following infarction, there is an abnormal decrease in compliance apparently related to scar formation

(Forrester, Diamond, et al, 1972; Hood, Bianco, et al, 1970). Patients with chronic stable symptomatic coronary disease have a significant reduction of left ventricular distensibility, and the extent of this abnormality is related to the severity of diseased coronary arteries, the presence of previous myocardial infarction, and the degree of abnormal left ventricular segmental contraction (Miller, Zelis, et al, 1973). Although changes in ventricular compliance related to ischemia have not previously been known to be correctable, alterations in compliance associated with chronic volume overload have been shown to be at least partially reversible in some patients as demonstrated in children following repair of ventricular septal defects (Jarmakani, Graham, et al, 1971) and following surgical correction of aortic insufficiency (Gault, Covell, et al, 1970). Further, experimental studies have shown a progressive return toward normal in parameters of left ventricular diastolic compliance following correction of large left-to-right shunts (McCullogh, Covell, et al, 1972).

In the present study patients selected for patency of all grafts or occlusion of all grafts demonstrated significant differences in several derived indices of total left ventricular diastolic compliance and stiffness. Chronically scarred left ventricular segments have been shown by *in vitro* studies of resected aneurysms from patients to have diminished compliance, and it is doubtful if the alterations exhibited by these fibrosed fibers are reversible (Parmley, Chuck, et al, 1973). In this regard, of the 14 of our patients with patent grafts, seven patients with no prior or intercurrent myocardial infarction had an increase in left ventricular specific compliance $[\Delta V/\Delta P/(V_{ESI})]$, which was greater than the seven patients with patent grafts and evidence of myocardial infarction with dyssynergy either prior to surgery or occurring following surgery. Thus, it appears that when these aneurysmal areas are extensive by angiographic assessment, the extent of improvement of total left ventricular diastolic compliance is limited even when coronary blood flow is restored to a potentially viable area of myocardium.

In summary, this investigation has demonstrated by several expressions of compliance, favorable alterations in left ventricular diastolic distensibility in coronary patients with patent aortocoronary bypass grafts or internal mammary to left anterior descending coronary artery anastomoses. Thus, evidence is provided for improvement in an additional abnormal parameter of left ventricular function following successful myocardial revascularization, which affords further support for the physiologic utility of coronary bypass procedures in properly selected patients.

References

Bristow JD, Van Zee BE, Judkins MP: Systolic and diastolic abnormalities of the left ventricle in coronary artery disease. Circulation 42:219–338, 1970

Chatterjee K, Swan HJC, Parmley WW, et al: Depression of left ventricular function due to acute myocardial ischemia and its reversal after aortocoronary saphenous-vein bypass. N Engl J Med 286:1117–22, 1972

Chatterjee K, Swan HJC, Parmley WW, et al: Influence of direct myocardial revascularization on left ventricular asynergy and function in patients with coronary heart disease. Circulation 47:276–86, 1973

Covell JW, Ross J: Nature and significance of alterations in myocardial compliance. Am J Cardiol 32:449–55, 1973

Diamond G, Forrester JS: Effect of coronary artery disease and acute myocardial infarction on left ventricular compliance in man. Circulation 45:11–19, 1972

Dwyer EM: Left ventricular pressure-volume alterations and regional disorders of contraction during myocardial ischemia induced by atrial pacing. Circulation 42:1111–22, 1970

Forrester JS, Diamond G, Parmley WW, Swan HJC: Early increase in left ventricular compliance after myocardial infarction. J Clin Invest 51:598–603, 1972

Gault JH, Covell JW, Braunwald E and Ross J: Left ventricular performance following correction of free aortic regurgitation. Circulation 42:773–80, 1970

Hood WB, Bianco JA, Kumar R, Whiting RB: Experimental myocardial infarction IV. Reduction of left ventricular compliance in the healing phase. J Clin Invest 49:1316–23, 1970

Jarmakani JMM, Graham TP, Conent RV, Capp MP: Effect of corrective surgery on left heart volume and mass in children with ventricular septal defect. Am J Cardiol 27:254–58, 1971

Levine HJ: Compliance of the left ventricle. Circulation 46:423–26, 1972

McCullogh WH, Covell JW, Ross J: Left ventricular dilatation and diastolic compliance changes during chronic volume overloading. Circulation 45:943–51, 1972

Miller RR, Zelis R, Massumi RA, et al: Left ventricular compliance: Relation to different patterns of left ventricular dyssynergy. Am J Cardiol 31:147, 1973

Parmley WW, Chuck L, Kivowityz C, et al: In vitro length-tension relations of human ventricular aneurysms. Am J Cardiol 32:889–94, 1973

Rees G, Bristow JD, Kremkau EL, et al: Influence of aortocoronary bypass surgery on left ventricular performance. N Engl J Med 284:1116–20, 1971

Smith M, Russell O, Field BJ, Rackley CE: Left ventricular compliance and abnormally contracting left ventricular segments following myocardial infarction. Clin Res 20:398, 1972

106

IMPROVED LEFT VENTRICULAR ASYNERGY AND PUMP FUNCTION AFTER SUCCESSFUL AND UNCOMPLICATED DIRECT MYOCARDIAL REVASCULARIZATION

Kanu Chatterjee, Jack M. Matloff, V. S. Kaushik,
Hector Sustaita, Harold S. Marcus, William W. Parmley,
and H. J. C. Swan

Myocardial ischemia denotes diminished oxygen supply in relation to its demand. In patients with obstructive coronary artery disease, its distribution and severity are, as a rule, nonuniform and diverse. Such regional myocardial ischemia produces not only angina pectoris but also important changes in contractile state and compliance characteristics of the myocardium involved and thus may depress overall left ventricular pump function. Furthermore, left ventricular asynergy—ie, abnormalities of left ventricular systolic wall motion—frequently occurs in patients with obstructive coronary artery disease, which may cause further depression of left ventricular function. Although left ventricular asynergy usually results from the presence of scar tissue due to previous myocardial infarction, quantitatively, and qualitatively similar abnormalities of segmental wall motion may also be of consequence in the presence of viable but ischemic myocardial segments (Chatterjee et al, 1972).

In experimental models, myocardial ischemia produced by temporary coronary artery occlusion is consistently associated with akinesis or hypokinesis of the affected wall segments. However, recovery of normal motion of the hypoxic myocardium occurs if the occlusion is promptly relieved (Hood et al, 1969; Tennant and Wiggers, 1935). Aortocoronary artery bypass surgery provides supplementary channels of blood supply and may restore blood flow to the ischemic myocardial segments. Therefore, following direct myocardial revascularization by aortocoronary bypass surgery,

partial, or complete recovery of normal wall motion might be expected. As a consequence of improved segmental wall motion, overall left ventricular pump function should also improve.

SEGMENTAL WALL MOTION

That striking improvement in abnormalities of segmental wall motion may occur in some patients following successful aortocoronary artery bypass surgery is illustrated in Figure 1. Marked hypokinesis involving large anteroapical areas seen in preoperative left ventriculograms was replaced by normal systolic motion following aorto-left-coronary artery bypass surgery. Improvement in abnormalities of segmental wall motion are commonly observed after successful and uncomplicated aortocoronary bypass surgery in patients without previous transmural myocardial infarction (Chatterjee et al, 1973). Postoperative changes in segmental wall motion in patients with preinfarction syndrome and also in patients with chronic ischemia without previous infarction are shown in Figures 2 and 3, respectively. An assessment of abnormalities of left ventricular systolic wall motion was determined from single plane (RAO) cineangiography (Greene et al, 1967). Seven of the eight patients with the preinfarction syndrome had reduced wall motion preoperatively involving one or more segments, which corresponded in general to the angiographically determined coronary artery lesions. In six patients with reduced

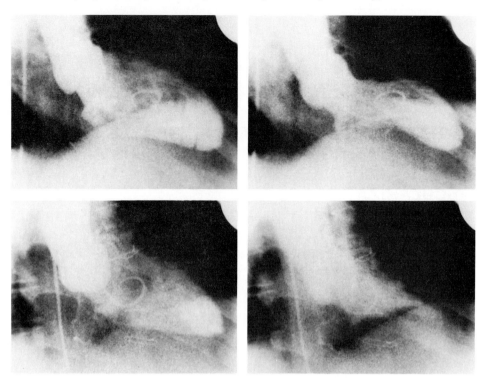

FIG. 1. Preoperative and postoperative left ventricular cineangiograms of a patient with "pre-infarction syndrome" who had aorto-left anterior descending coronary artery bypass surgery. In the upper panel the preoperative end-diastolic (left) and end-systolic (right) frames indicate marked hypokinesis involving large areas of anterior and apical segments. In the lower panel, postoperative end-diastolic (left) and end-systolic (right) frames reveal normalization of abnormalities of systolic wall motion. (Circulation 47:276, 1973)

anterior wall motion and in six of the seven patients with reduced apical motion preoperatively, significant improvement occurred following aorto-left-coronary artery bypass surgery. Inferior wall motion was reduced in three of these eight patients and improved postoperatively. Normal segmental wall motion, preoperatively, remained normal postoperatively.

In patients with chronic ischemia but without previous infarction similar improvements in abnormalities of segmental wall motion may occur following successful and appropriate bypass surgery (Fig. 3). In seven of 10 patients anterior wall motion improved postoperatively. Similarly, in three patients apical motion and in three patients inferior wall motion improved postoperatively. In patients with previous myocardial infarction, however, some abnormalities of wall motion persist in the area of infarction as determined by preoperative electrocardiograms. As compared to a patient without previous infarction (Fig. 4, left panel) in whom normalization of segmental wall motion occurred postoperatively, in a patient with previous anterior infarction (Fig. 4, middle panel)

abnormalities of anterior wall motion remained even after successful left coronary artery bypass. Similarly in patients with inferior wall infarction (Fig. 4, right panel) inferior wall motion abnormalities persisted although movements in other areas occurred postoperatively. In general, individuals with limited anterior wall infarction demonstrate improvement in inferior wall motion and apical motion, whereas patients with inferior infarction showed improved anterior wall motion and apical motion following appropriate bypass surgery. Individuals with normal systolic wall motion preoperatively demonstrate no significant change postoperatively.

RELATION BETWEEN SEGMENTAL WALL MOTION AND EJECTION FRACTION

Along with the improvement in segmental wall motion, overall left ventricular pump function tends to improve in such patients. This is

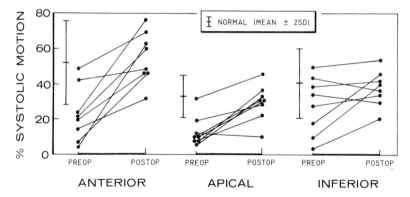

FIG. 2. Summary of postoperative changes in segmental wall motion in eight patients with the preinfarction syndrome. The normal range (mean ± SD) is indicated by the vertical bar to the left of each panel. Each patient is plotted individually (●). Quantitative assessment of left ventricular systolic wall motion both in normal controls as well as in patients having bypass surgery was performed according to the method described by Chatterjee et al: Circulation 47:276, 1973.

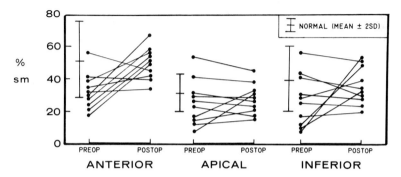

FIG. 3. Summary of postoperative changes in segmental wall motion in 10 patients with chronic ischemia and no previous infarct. The normal range is indicated as in Figure 2. (Circulation 47:276, 1973)

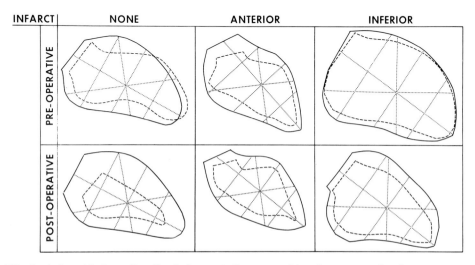

FIG. 4. Left ventricular wall motion before and after successful aortocoronary artery bypass surgery in three representative patients. The end-diastolic (solid line) and end-systolic (dashed line) frames together with the multiple hemiaxes (dotted lines) are superimposed for visual comparison. Left to right: A patient with the preinfarction syndrome and a high-grade LAD lesion, a patient with a previous anterior infarction, and a patient with a previous inferior infarction and anterior ischemia.

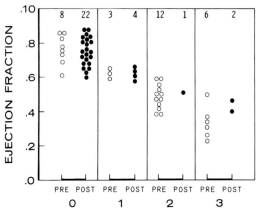

SEGMENTAL WALL MOTION ABNORMALITIES

FIG. 5. Relation between pre- and postoperative ejection fraction (vertical axis) and abnormalities of segmental wall motion (horizontal axis) in all patients. 0: no abnormality; 1, 2, 3: wall motion abnormalities involving one, two, or three segments. The number of patients in each group is designated at the top of each panel. The majority of patients had normal segmental wall motion and normal ejection fraction postoperatively.

illustrated in Figure 5. The majority of patients preoperatively had wall motion abnormalities involving one or more segments and in these patients ejection fraction—an index of left ventricular pump function—was also reduced. Only a few patients had normal segmental wall motion and ejection fraction preoperatively. Following appropriate and successful bypass surgery, however, the majority of patients had segmental wall motion in the normal range with normal ejection fraction. Only a few patients had significant wall motion abnormalities and reduced ejection fraction postoperatively.

CHANGES IN EJECTION FRACTION AND LEFT VENTRICULAR VOLUMES

After appropriate and successful aortocoronary artery bypass surgery, ejection fraction, determined angiographically, tends to improve in patients who have depressed ejection fraction preoperatively. Improved ejection fraction not only occurs in patients without previous infarction but also in patients with previous infarction (Fig. 6).

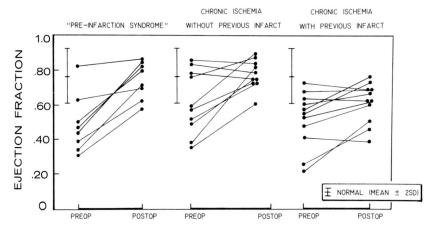

FIG. 6. Pre- and postoperative ejection fraction (vertical axis) in patients with the preinfarction syndrome (left), with chronic ischemia and no previous infarct (middle), and with a previous infarct (right). Ejection fraction was calculated from the left ventricular stroke volume (SV)/end-diastolic volume (EDV). SV was obtained by subtracting the angiographically determined end-systolic volume (ESV) from EDV. Left ventricular volumes were calculated from single plane (RAO) cineangiograms (Greene et al, 1967; Chatterjee et al, 1971) assuming the ventricle to approximate an ellipsoid of revolution. The long axis was determined directly, and the minor axis was determined by the area-length method of Dodge (1960). As calculated LV volumes from single plane cineangiograms in RAO projection over-estimate the actual volumes, correction was made for this overestimation using the regression equation of Herman et al (1969).

The vertical bar represents the normal range (mean ± SD) or ejection fraction.

TABLE 1. Pre- and Postoperative Hemodynamic Data and Derived Parameters of LV Function

PARAMETER	PATIENTS WITHOUT PREVIOUS INFARCT (N: 18)				PATIENTS WITH PREVIOUS INFARCT (N: 11)			
	Preop Reduced EF		Preop Normal EF		Preop Reduced EF		Preop Normal EF	
	Preop	Postop	Preop	Postop	Preop	Postop	Preop	Postop
Number	12	12	6	6	7	7	4	4
Ejection fraction	0.45 ± 0.03	0.74 ± 0.03[a]	0.78 ± 0.03	0.80 ± 0.03	0.44 ± 0.05	0.59 ± 0.05[a]	0.67 ± 0.03	0.66 ± 0.01[a]
Heart rate (beats/min)	76 ± 3	90 ± 3[a]	67 ± 4	86 ± 4[a]	85 ± 8	99 ± 5[a]	84 ± 5	104 ± 4[a]
Mean heart pressure (mm Hg)	93 ± 3	87 ± 4	86 ± 2	87 ± 7	101 ± 6	88 ± 5	96 ± 6	89 ± 12
LVEDP (mm Hg)	15 ± 1	10 ± 1[a]	8 ± 1	7 ± 1	17 ± 3	10 ± 2[a]	11 ± 3	7 ± 1
LVESP (mm Hg)	5.8 ± 0.8	2.6 ± 0.6	2.5 ± 0.8	2.0 ± 0.9	5.6 ± 1.1	3.0 ± 0.9	2.0 ± 0.3	0.9 ± 0.2
LV dP/dt (mm Hg/sec)	1271 ± 79	1602 ± 91[a]	1606 ± 277	1698 ± 389	1122 ± 84	1685 ± 226[a]	1512 ± 241	1662 ± 114
SWI (g-m/m²)	49 ± 6	78 ± 6[a]	78 ± 9	84 ± 16	59 ± 10	71 ± 10	85 ± 1	73 ± 1
EDV (ml/m²)	114 ± 12	97 ± 9[a]	85 ± 6	86 ± 13	106 ± 5	108 ± 8	100 ± 9	97 ± 3
ESV (ml/m²)	71 ± 12	23 ± 4[a]	16 ± 3	14 ± 3	57 ± 5	41 ± 6[a]	33 ± 3	31 ± 1
SV (ml/m²)	43 ± 3	73 ± 8[a]	70 ± 7	71 ± 10	49 ± 6	67 ± 9[a]	67 ± 7	64 ± 1
VCE at 5 mm Hg (ml/sec)	1.3 ± 0.1	1.8 ± 0.1[a]	1.6 ± 0.1	1.6 ± 0.3	1.3 ± 0.1	1.9 ± 0.2[a]	1.7 ± 0.3	1.9 ± 0.1

EF: ejection fraction; EDV: end-diastolic volume; ESV: end-systolic volume; SV: stroke volume; LVESP: left ventricular end-systolic pressure; LVEDP: left ventricular end-diastolic pressure; SWI: stroke work index; LV dP/dt: left ventricular peak dP/dt; VCE: contractile element velocity at 5 mm Hg.
[a] $P < 0.05$.

Thus, in six patients in the preinfarction group and in six with chronic ischemia, ejection fraction improved significantly following appropriate bypass surgery. Of seven patients with previous infarction who had decreased ejection fraction preoperatively, ejection fraction increased significantly in six following surgery. In patients with normal ejection fraction preoperatively, with or without previous infarction, no significant change occurs following surgery.

Changes in left ventricular volumes following surgery are shown in Table 1. Most patients had normal or near normal end-diastolic volume preoperatively, but in many there was an increase in end-systolic volume and a decrease in ejection fraction. Postoperatively, there was little or no change in end-diastolic volume in patients with normal ejection fraction; preoperatively, there was

no significant change either in end-systolic volume or stroke volume. In patients with depressed ejection fraction preoperatively, there was, however, significant decrease in end-systolic volume and increase in systolic volume and ejection fraction.

CHANGES IN CONTRACTILE STATE

Improved left ventricular pump function was also suggested by increase in stroke work index along with decrease in left ventricular end-diastolic pressure in those patients who demonstrated improved ejection fraction postoperatively (Table 1). Improved pump function was associated with increased contractile state. Increased ejection fraction postoperatively due to reduction

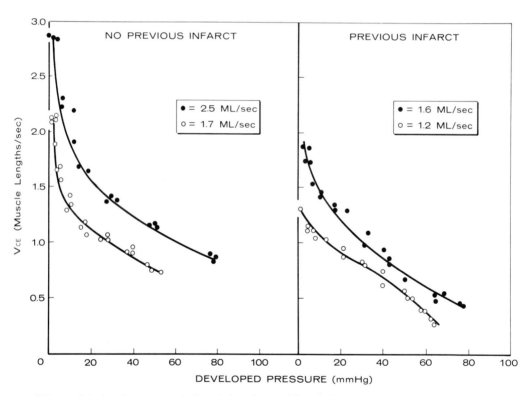

FIG. 7. Calculated pressure velocity relations before (o) and after surgery (●) in two patients, one without (left) and one with (right) previous infarction. Overall mean contractile element velocity (V_{CE}) was calculated from the simultaneously recorded LV pressure pulse and its first derivative (dP/dt), using the formula $V_{CE} = dP/dt/KP$, where P is the developed isometric pressure and K is the series elastic constant. This calculation is based on the three component Maxwell model of muscle mechanics (Parmley et al, 1972). A value of 32/muscle length was used for the series elastic constant K (Yeatman et al, 1969). Since the above formula for V_{CE} approaches infinity as developed pressure approaches zero, the value of V_{CE} at 5 mm Hg developed pressure was used as an approximation of Vmax. V_{CE} at 5 mm Hg was calculated from three consecutive beats and averaged. Definite postoperative improvement in myocardial contractility in both patients is evident by the shift of the pressure velocity curves upward and to the right. The inset values represent V_{CE} at 5 mm Hg developed pressure.

in end-systolic volume without any change in end-diastolic volume suggests more efficient left ventricular systolic emptying. As there was no significant reduction in afterload (systemic pressure) or increase in preload (end-diastolic pressure) following surgery, postoperative increase in stroke volume must be related to improved contractile state.

This assumption is supported by the fact that derived indices of contractility increased significantly in those patients who had increased ejection fraction postoperatively. Without any change in preload (end-diastolic pressure) or afterload (arterial pressure), LV maximum dP/dt increased significantly. Pressure velocity curves obtained from simultaneously recorded LV pressure pulse and its dP/dt showed a shift to the right and upward postoperatively (Fig. 7) and V_{CE} at 5 mm Hg (an approximation of Vmax) also increased significantly (Table 1). Higher heart rates observed postoperatively in most patients are unlikely to be the only cause for an increase in contractility indices because higher heart rates of similar magnitude were found postoperatively in patients who had normal ejection fractions both before and after surgery and who did not show any changes in contractile state.

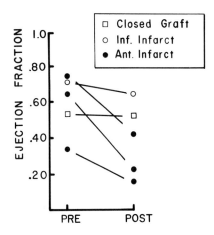

FIG. 8. Changes in ejection fraction in patients with closed grafts or with perioperative myocardial infarction. Ejection fraction either remained unchanged or deteriorated postoperatively in these patients.

ment was also seen in patients with isolated right coronary artery bypass in the presence of triple vessel disease. In the presence of previous myocardial infarcts or chronic congestive heart failure with considerable cardiomegaly, left ventricular function tends not to improve despite successful and uncomplicated aortocoronary bypass surgery (Fig. 9).

LEFT VENTRICULAR FUNCTION IN PATIENTS WITH UNSUCCESSFUL BYPASS OR WITH PERIOPERATIVE COMPLICATIONS

In patients with occluded grafts or who developed perioperative myocardial infarction, left ventricular function and segmental wall motion frequently deteriorated (Fig. 8). Lack of improve-

CHANGES IN CORONARY RESERVE FOLLOWING SUCCESSFUL AORTOCORONARY ARTERY BYPASS SURGERY

Uncontrolled angina of effort still remains the major indication for surgical therapy in patients with obstructive coronary artery disease. Therefore, it is important to assess the influence

FIG. 9. Changes in LV volumes and ejection fraction in a patient with preoperative chronic congestive heart failure and considerable cardiomegaly following successful aortocoronary artery bypass surgery. No improvement in left ventricular function was noted in this patient.

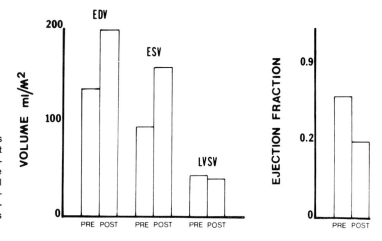

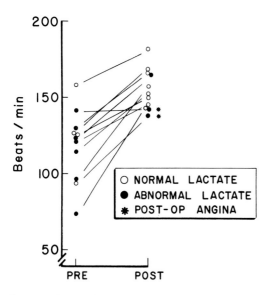

FIG. 10. Pre- and postoperative atrial pacing stress in 11 patients with coronary artery disease who had successful aortocoronary artery bypass surgery. All patients developed angina preoperatively and 7 patients had abnormal transmyocardial lactate extraction rate indicative of anaerobic metabolism at angina. Postoperatively, in all but one patient, heart rate could be increased to a much higher level, and only 2 patients developed angina. However, 3 patients had abnormal lactate extraction rates postoperatively.

of aortocoronary artery bypass surgery not only on left ventricular mechanical function but also on its metabolic function and coronary reserve. Subjective improvement in angina following surgery is common. Such subjective improvement, however, may be very deceptive when assessing the results of any therapeutic interventions in patients with obstructive coronary artery disease. Furthermore, improvement of angina in some patients may be due to perioperative myocardial infarction and hence may not indicate successful surgical therapy. Objective data are, therefore, necessary for evaluation of changes in metabolic function and coronary reserve following bypass surgery.

Improved effort tolerance with minimal or no electrocardiographic changes indicative of myocardial ischemia following successful bypass surgery has been reported. Data regarding changes in coronary reserve following such therapy are scarce. Preliminary studies, however, suggest that following successful aortocoronary artery bypass surgery, coronary reserve improves significantly in the vast majority of patients. Thus, during atrial pacing studies, the heart rate can be increased to a much higher level postoperatively without inducing angina in most patients (Fig. 10). Abnormal transmyocardial lactate extraction rate indicative of myocardial ischemia at the time of angina was observed preoperatively, in the majority of patients and tended to revert to normal extraction rate postoperatively, suggesting im-

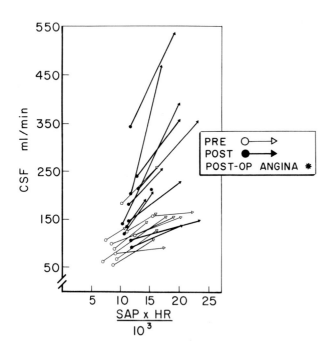

FIG. 11. Pre- and postoperative global myocardial blood flow at control (circle) and maximum stress (arrow) that could be achieved during atrial pacing study. Coronary blood flow (vertical axis) was determined by continuous infusion thermodilution technique, by inserting a pre-shaped "Ganz" catheter in the coronary sinus (Ganz et al, 1971). Myocardial stress (horizontal axis) was calculated from the product of peak systolic pressure (SAP) and heart rate (HR). Postoperatively (thick lines) global myocardial blood flow increased markedly and steeply at the maximum stress achieved compared to the preoperative values (thin lines).

FIG. 12. Changes in global myocardial oxygen supply following aortocoronary artery bypass surgery in patients with obstructive coronary artery disease. Oxygen supply, ml/min, was calculated from the product of coronary blood flow, ml/min, measured by thermodilution technique and arterial oxygen content in vol percentage. Symbols are the same as in Figure 11. In most patients, global myocardial oxygen supply increased significantly, postoperatively, at the maximum stress that could be achieved during atrial pacing study.

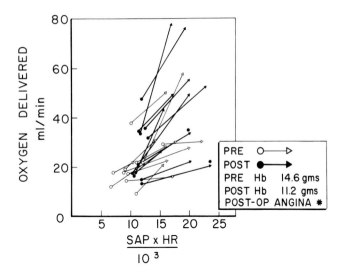

proved metabolic function. Furthermore, total myocardial flow and myocardial oxygen supply can markedly increase in the majority of patients during stress following surgery compared to preoperative values (Figs. 11 and 12).

Not all patients, however, show similar improvements in coronary reserve or cardiac metabolic function, nor is this expected. Improvement in metabolic function and coronary reserve not only depends on the presence of technically adequate grafts, but also on the number of coronary artery branches grafted, changes and progression of disease in the native coronary arteries, postoperative changes in the collateral circulation, and other factors that still are not apparent. Nevertheless, preliminary results suggest that, at least in selected patients, following successful and appropriate coronary bypass surgery, significant improvement in coronary reserve may occur. Marked improvement and even normalization of left ventricular function may occur in properly selected patients with the preinfarction syndrome or with chronic ischemia and no previous infarct. Although left ventricular asynergy tends to persist in areas of previous infarction, overall improvement in left ventricular pump function and contractile state may still occur following successful and appropriate bypass surgery.

ACKNOWLEDGMENT

We gratefully acknowledge the assistance of William Ganz, MD, DSc, FACC in the cardiac metabolic studies and the editorial assistance of Mrs. Sharman Jamison.

References

Chatterjee K, Saccoor M, Sutton GC, Miller GAH: Assessment of left ventricular function by single plane cineangiographic volume analysis. Br Heart J 33: 565, 1971

Chatterjee K, Swan HJC, Parmley WW, et al: Depression of left ventricular function due to acute myocardial ischemia and its reversal after aorto-coronary saphenous-vein bypass. N Engl J Med 286: 1117, 1972

Chatterjee K, Swan HJC, Parmley WW, et al: Influence of direct myocardial revascularization on left ventricular asynergy and function in patients with coronary heart disease: with and without previous myocardial infarction. Circulation 47:276, 1973

Dodge HT, Sandler H, Ballew DW, Lord JD: The use of biplane angiocardiography for measurements of left ventricular volume in man. Am Heart J 60:762, 1960

Ganz W, Tamura K, Marcus HS, et al: Measurement of coronary sinus blood flow by continuous thermodilution in man. Circulation 44:181, 1971

Greene D, Carlisle R, Grant C, Bunnell I: Estimation of left ventricular volume by one plane cineangiography. Circulation 35:61, 1967

Herman HJ, Singh R, Dammann JF: Evaluation of myocardial contractility in man. Am Heart J 77:755, 1969

Hood WB Jr, Covelli VH, Norman JC: Acute coronary occlusion in pigs: effects of acetyl strophanthidin. Cardiovasc Res 3:441, 1969

Parmley WW, Chuck L, Sonnenblick EH: Relation of Vmax to different models of cardiac muscle. Circ Res 30:34, 1972

Tennant R and Wiggers CJ: The effect of coronary occlusion on myocardial contraction. Am J Physiol 112:351, 1935

Yeatman LA Jr, Parmley WW, Sonnenblick EH: Effects of temperature on series elasticity and contractile element motion in heart muscle. Am J Physiol 217: 1030, 1969

107

DELINEATION OF IMPROVED VENTRICULAR WALL MOTION AFTER CORONARY REVASCULARIZATION

W. Peter Geis, Rostam G. Ardekani, Shahbudin H. Rahimtoola, and Constantine J. Tatooles

The usual rationale employed when recommending myocardial revascularization for ischemic heart disease is for the relief of angina pectoris and/or the improvement of blood flow to nutritionally deprived ventricular myocardium. The present discussion confines itself to the latter hypothesis, ie, that occlusive disease of major coronary arteries results in regional abnormalities in mechanics caused by deprivation of blood flow to the muscle mass distal to the occlusion. The ultimate fate of the myocardial region distal to a coronary lesion depends upon the severity of stenosis,[1,2,3] the abruptness of onset of the coronary hemodynamic deficit,[4] the presence or absence of effective collateral vessels from nearby regions that have adequate coronary blood flow,[5,6] and the presence or absence of pronounced small vessel arterial disease.[7-10] The nutritionally deprived segment of ventricular wall may become infarcted as has been demonstrated with acute coronary occlusion experimentally,[11] or it may retain its metabolic integrity in the absence of mechanical function.[12]

CORONARY OCCLUSION, REGIONAL BLOOD FLOW, AND ASYNERGY

Acute occlusion of a single coronary artery has been shown by Tennant and Wiggers[13] to result in regional loss of mechanical activity of the compromised muscle. Using myographic recordings, these investigators were the first to show

regional suppression of myocardial contractility during acute ischemia. Later, Prinzmetal et al[14] and Dack et al[15] reported similar regional abnormalities in ventricular wall motion after acute coronary occlusion using electrokymograms or roentgenkymograms. More recently, Tatooles and Randall[16] adopted use of the strain gauge arch to demonstrate regional ventricular wall "bulging" during acute coronary occlusion in dogs. These investigators showed suppression of contractility with short periods of occlusion and paradoxical lengthening of the involved region with longer periods of occlusion. Further, release of the occluding ligature most often resulted in restoration of shortening with ventricular systole, strongly suggesting the absence of irreversible ischemic damage during short periods of occlusion. In contrast, under similar circumstances, Wiggers[17] showed that restoration of normal contractile function would not occur after 60 minutes of sustained vessel occlusion. His data imply that long periods of acute coronary occlusion always result in irreversible damage to contratile components in the ischemic area.

Contrariwise, Tatooles and Randall[16] infrequently observed continued ventricular contractility after coronary occlusion. They surmised that occasionally collateral blood flow was adequate to maintain the nutritional integrity of the ischemic region. Cohen et al[18] corroborated these conclusions experimentally, using the strain gauge arch. They documented absence of regional ventricular contraction after acute coronary occlusion in dogs. However, when these investigators applied the strain gauge arch to an ischemic area two to four weeks after gradual occlusion of the anterior descending coronary artery, muscle shortening

Supported in part by USPHS Grant HE 08682 and the Chicago Heart and Lung Institute.

occurred concomitant with ventricular systole. They postulated that the small intercoronary collateral vessels in the dogs [19] grew, multiplied, and matured during the two-to-four week interval corroborating the already known histological evidence for growth of collateral vessels after acute coronary occlusion.[20] These directionally normal length changes recorded many weeks after experimental coronary occlusion suggest strongly that the "irreversible" changes observed by Wiggers [17] and by the latter investigators are at least, in part, due to profound local ischemia, but not infarction of muscle. It is hypothesized that the temporal improvement in regional blood flow occurred along with development of collateral vessels to viable myocardium. The gradual improvement in blood flow to the ischemic, viable region improved nutrition enough to effect a return of mechanical function.

Certainly, anginal attacks and acute myocardial infarction have been shown recently to result in ventricular asynergy.[21,22,23] Whether the ischemic region of myocardium progresses to infarction, maintains its metabolic integrity without mechanical function, or whether the local wall dysfunction is transient will in large part depend upon the extent to which collateral vessels are able to improve blood flow. Should an adjacent coronary artery and its vascular tributaries be free of occlusive disease, then collateralization will presumably improve regional blood flow enough to maintain metabolic integrity of the majority of the involved muscle. Further, as demonstrated experimentally, mechanical shortening of the ischemic segment may return within two weeks.[18] In contrast, if the flow to nearby vessels is also compromised, the ability of collateral vessels to improve mechanical events in the ischemic region may be dramatically reduced. These relations have been meticulously documented experimentally by Cohen et al [18] by altering circumflex coronary artery flow and pressure independent of anterior descending coronary artery flow. At intervals greater than two weeks after occlusion of the anterior descending vessel, contractility of the myocardial region distal to the occluded vessel was determined. Step-wise decline in circumflex artery flow resulted in dramatic suppression of contractility in the region distal to the anterior descending artery. Further, administration of nitroglycerin to dilate collateral vessels accomplished augmentation in regional contractility when circumflex artery flow was in the normal range, but not when circumflex artery flow was suppressed. Each of these observations delineate the necessity of hemodynamic integrity of circumflex artery flow in order to deliver adequate collateral blood flow to the region distal to the occluded anterior descending artery.

In the absence of collateral vessels and/or in the presence of occlusive disease in an adjacent vascular bed, acute regional myocardial ischemia will more than likely result in either acute infarction, permanent loss of mechanical activity without infarction, or a combination of the two. It is reasonable, therefore, to conclude that a noncontractile segment of ventricular myocardium may remain viable, but nonfunctional, solely due to poor blood supply to the region. Further, it is appropriate to assume that such a viable segment of ventricular wall will convert to active mechanical shortening with ventricular systole if revascularization is accomplished—whether it be by coronary artery bypass [24] or by myocardial implantation.[25] The dilemma is, of course, that neither ventriculographic analysis nor coronary angiography will define whether a dysfunctional region is viable noncontractile myocardium or infarcted, fibrotic ventricular wall.

VENTRICULOGRAPHIC DETERMINANTS OF ASYNERGY

Herman et al [26] described a spectrum of regional abnormalities in left ventricular wall motion in patients with ischemic heart disease. They delineated three types angiographically: regional hypokinetic motion (asynergesis), regional noncontractile wall (akinesis), and regional paradoxical expansion of ventricular wall (dyskinesis). These abnormalities in the pattern of ventricular muscle contraction were thought to be capable of adversely affecting ventricular chamber dynamics leading to clinical cardiac failure.

Hypothetically, hypokinetic wall motion represents a segment of myocardium that has the ability to develop tension to a lesser extent than the remainder of the muscle mass of the ventricular chamber and is probably the most subtle expression of asynergy. The akinetic wall segment develops tension enough to resist lengthening during systole, while the dyskinetic region of wall is not capable of developing enough tension to resist lengthening during ventricular systole. At the far end of the spectrum is ventricular aneurysm,[27] which not only reduces the muscle mass available for development of tension but also sequesters ventricular blood in the dilated area. Corroborating evidence for this hypothesis comes from Enright and coworkers, who have delineated the detrimental effect of regional left ventricular wall dysfunction upon ventricular chamber dynamics.[28] They determined ventricular stroke work at various left ventricular end-diastolic volumes before and after occlusion of the anterior descending coronary artery in dogs. The classic Starling preparation was used to keep heart rate and aortic outflow resistance constant. Ventricular function was uniformly suppressed after coronary occlusion. Function was, however, returned to control values after removal of the occluding ligature. The directional alterations in ventricular function with intermittent coronary occlusion provide corroboration of the reversibility of abnormalities in regional wall motion alluded to by Tatooles and Randall.[16] The latter investigators further provide directionally appropriate alterations in ventricular chamber dynamics associated with coronary occlusion and regional muscle dysfunction demonstrated by the strain gauge arch. The reversal of suppressed ventricular chamber function after removal of coronary occlusion suggests that the region of viable ischemic myocardium is unable to develop forces comparable to the active forces generated by the remainder of the chamber, thus effecting distention of the area. Both Wiggers[29] and Gregg[30] postulated this reversible phenomenon as the mechanistic cause of the decrement in ventricular chamber function observed during acute coronary occlusion. Later studies by Nishimura[23] and, independently, by Forman[24] have corroborated the value of the strain-gauge-arch method in evaluating regional ventricular wall dysfunction in ischemic heart disease. Further, the latter investigators, as well as Cohen et al,[16] have determined the strain gauge arch to be the most sensitive means of determining alterations in blood flow to ischemic viable ventricular myocardium.

OPERATIVE DETERMINATION OF MECHANICAL EVENTS IN HUMANS

Improvement in regional wall motion with resultant improved left ventricular chamber dynamics as a consequence of coronary artery bypass surgery appears to be an interesting hypothesis in the treatment of ischemic heart disease in humans. There are, however, a number of subtle pitfalls to this approach. When given a group of patients with occlusive disease to one or more major coronary arteries and—by definition—compromise of left ventricular chamber function, the following issues arise. First, must regional dysfunction or asynergy be demonstrated at ventriculographic analysis in order to conclude that revascularization will improve chamber mechanics? Empirically,

there are large groups of patients who have experienced clinical heart failure and occlusive coronary disease without ventriculographic evidence of asynergy. Many have subsequently received coronary bypass procedures. Most of these patients have experienced postoperative resolution of heart failure and improvement in ventricular performance at repeat cardiac catheterization.[24] By inference, these patients have had improvement in ventricular mechanics and probably have had some degree of asynergy whether or not it was demonstrable angiographically. Moreover, patients with three-vessel disease have a decline in blood flow to most, if not all, areas of left ventricular muscle. Since asynergy implies that a portion of myocardium develops less total tension when compared to the remainder of the chamber muscle due to a disparity in perfusion, the muscle with greater contractility will then stretch the compromised myocardium resulting in chamber asynergy. If all areas have diminished flow and equally suppressed contractility, as may often occur in three-vessel disease, then asynergy may not be apparent.

Second, if asynergy is demonstrated, does the dysfunctional zone represent viable muscle mass, rigid scar tissue with high elastic modulus, or fibroelastic tissue with a compliance equal to or greater than the remainder of ventricular muscle mass? Certainly, ventriculographic analysis cannot be used to answer this question. Moreover, the dysfunctional region may contain viable muscle mass that is unable to depolarize due to high impedance scarring or other pathologic factors interfering with conduction to muscle. If the latter circumstances are present, revascularization will not improve regional contractility nor will chamber dynamics be improved.

In an effort to evaluate the functional nature of myocardium distal to the occlusive disease, we determined regional left ventricular wall motion in the operating theatre during coronary artery bypass procedures in 13 patients. Since the studies already alluded to as well as those of Nishimura[31] and, independently, of Forman[32] have corroborated the value of the strain-gauge-arch method of determining regional ventricular wall dysfunction in ischemic heart disease, strain gauge arches were chosen as the most sensitive means of determining alterations in regional blood flow and regional ventricular mechanics. Each patient had preoperative ventriculography and coronary angiography. Results of the preoperative studies are shown in Table 1. Column-Disease delineates the sites of occlusive disease angiographically. Four patients had disease of three vessels, five had disease of the right coronary artery (RCA), and the anterior descending artery (LAD), while two had disease of the LAD and circumflex artery (CIRC), and two had disease confined to the LAD. Column-type indicates the directional abnormality in regional wall motion in each patient. Three patients had no asynergy at ventriculographic analysis, four had hypokinetic wall motion, two had a region of akinesia, while four had dyskinetic motion or paradoxical distension with ventricular systole. Note that two of the patients with three-vessel disease had no evidence of asynergy angiographically. Column-location indicates the region of left ventricle with abnormal motion.

Intraoperatively, a strain gauge arch was sutured to the region of ventricular wall that was dysfunctional or to the area distal to the LAD disease in the three without asynergy. In the two cases with three-vessel disease and no apparent asynergy, a gauge was placed on each of two areas of the chamber to search for asynergy. In all cases, a second arch was sutured either to "normal" myocardium adjacent to the bifurcation of the left coronary artery or to the myocardium of the right ventricle in cases with circumflex artery disease. Regional muscle motion was recorded prior to cardiopulmonary bypass and during total cardiopulmonary bypass with decompression of the left ventricle. By emptying the left ventricle it was possible to decrease external forces tending to stretch the diseased area and to decrease wall stress, thus accomplishing an increment in collateral blood flow. These data were recorded to determine whether the dyskinetic wall would convert to systolic shortening in the absence of load. After aortocoronary bypass, repeat measurements of wall motion were recorded.

Figure 1 delineates the type of recording obtained from one patient with LAD disease and hypokinetic wall motion angiographically at the apico-inferior left ventricle (LVA). Note the downward deflection of the tracing (arrow) occurring 80 msec after the QRS of the ECG, reflecting paradoxical lengthening during ventricular systole. The lengthening occurs concomitant with shortening of nonischemic myocardium at the base of the left ventricle (LBV), as indicated by upward deflection at the arrow. This area converted to directionally appropriate shortening with ventricular systole after performance of aortocoronary bypass. In contrast, Figure 2 delineates comparable recordings prior to aortocoronary bypass from a patient with three-vessel disease and no evidence of asynergy angiographically. Gauges were placed on the posterior left ventricle (LVP) and on the base of the left ventricle (LVB). In both areas, upward deflections (arrows) occur along with ventricular systole indicating muscle shortening in both areas. This patient demonstrates lack of asynergy in spite of severe ischemic heart disease suggesting that a global compromise of blood flow effects suppression of the inotropic state throughout the chamber. In this setting, there is little disparity in the development of active tension in the various areas resulting in lack of asynergy.

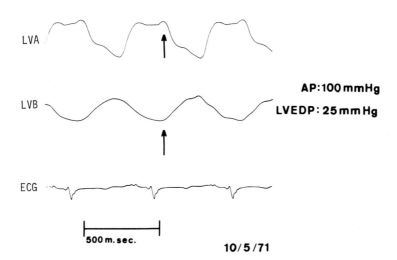

FIG. 1. Strain-gauge-arch recordings of regional left ventricular wall motion during 2 complete cardiac cycles from an apico-inferior segment (LVA) and from the base of the left ventricle (LVB) in a patient with occlusive disease of anterior descending coronary artery. Recordings taken prior to cardiopulmonary bypass and prior to aortocoronary bypass. ECG is surface electrocardiogram. Upward deflection is shortening and downward deflection is lengthening. AP: aortic pressure; LVEDP: left ventricular end-diastolic pressure.

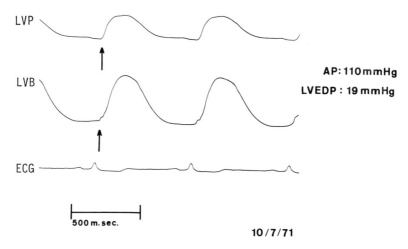

AP: 110 mmHg

LVEDP : 19 mmHg

500 m. sec.

10/7/71

FIG. 2. Strain-gauge-arch recordings of regional left ventricular wall motion during two complete cardiac cycles from the posterior wall (LVP) and from the base (LVB) near the circumflex artery origin in a patient with occlusive disease of the circumflex, anterior descending, and right coronary arteries. Recording taken prior to cardiopulmonary bypass. Upward deflection in each segment is shortening during ventricular contraction.

Table I depicts results obtained from all patients using the strain gauge method intraoperatively. None of the patients with no asynergy on cineangiogram had asynergy using the arch, nor did one patient with hypokinetic motion preoperatively have asynergy. Four patients exhibited conversion of systolic paradoxical motion to shortening with systole after unloading of the left ventricle, demonstrating conclusively the presence of muscle mass capable of tension development, but obviously of much less magnitude than the remainder of the myocardium. Note that these four patients ex-

TABLE 1. LV Asynergy: Cardiac Catheterization and Cineangiograms

PT.	DISEASE	TYPE	LOCATION
AB	LAD/RCA	None	–
FM	3-vessel	None	–
LW	3-vessel	None	–
KL	LAD/RCA	Hypokinesia	Inferolateral
ES	LAD/RCA	Hypokinesia	Inferior
HB	LAD/Circ	Hypokinesia	Apicoinferior
GG	LAD/RCA	Hypokinesia	Inferior
RM	LAD/Circ	Akinesia	Apical
RJ	3-vessel	Akinesia	Apicoinferior
AB	3-vessel	Dyskinesis	Apical
GC	LAD/RCA	Dyskinesis	Posteroinferior
FS	LAD	Dyskinesis	Apicoanterior
JB	LAD	Dyskinesis	Apicoanterior

Circ: circumflex coronary artery; LAD: left anterior descending coronary artery; and RCA: right coronary artery.

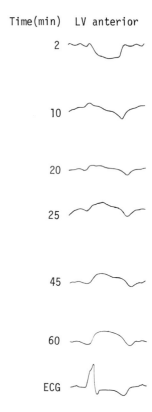

FIG. 3. Sequential recordings of regional left ventricular wall motion from anterior surface (LV anterior column) of chamber. Recordings taken 2 to 60 minutes after aortocoronary (AC) to anterior descending coronary artery (LAD). Downward reflection at 2 minutes is lengthening with systole, which gradually converts to upward deflection with systole after 60 minutes, representing shortening during systole.

hibited a wide spectrum of wall motion angiographically. After revascularization, two further patients exhibited conversion of paradoxical motion to shortening with systole. One patient continued to exhibit paradoxical muscle lengthening with systole until 60 minutes following revascularization. Recordings from this patient are in Figure 3. The obvious downward deflection during ventricular systole two minutes after revascularization represents lengthening of muscle during ventricular contraction. At 25 and 45 minutes after revascularization, the deflections appeared to be gradually converting to shortening with systole. At 60 minutes postrevascularization, the definite upward deflection documents improved wall function following enhancement of blood flow.

Two patients continued to exhibit paradoxical lengthening of the diseased segment 60 minutes after revascularization. In each of these, the region was considered to be nonfunctional, and, in each case, a ventriculotomy incision was performed in the dyskinetic area. In each, an endocardial thrombus—not observed at ventriculography—was noted and removed. The ventriculotomy incisions were then closed using an everting mattress suture technique to exclude the dysfunctional zone from the functioning chamber.

CINE-VENTRICULOGRAPHY VERSUS STRAIN GAUGE ARCH

The strain gauge arch appears to represent a more sensitive method for determining ventricular asynergy than ventriculography. Three aspects of this disparity are worth consideration. First, the strain gauge arch records linear displacement of ventricular muscle and thereby delineates either shortening or lengthening of muscle in a single plane. In contrast, regional wall motion determined at cine-ventriculography measures bulk wall motion toward or away from the center of a sphere (LV chamber). When a segment of ventricular wall moves less vigorously toward the center during systole, the region is considered hypokinetic. However, the region of ventricular muscle may lengthen during systole and the increment in length be undetectable angiographically as long as the radius of curvature of the segment does not change dramatically. In our series (Table 2), three of four patients who exhibited regional hypokinetic wall motion angiographically proved to show regional muscle lengthening during systole intraoperatively. Similarly, regional akinesia was demonstrated angiographically in two patients; in each of these the akinetic area exhibited paradoxical lengthening utilizing the strain gauge. In the latter circumstance, lack of regional wall motion demonstrable at ventriculography therefore represents systolic lengthening in a segment that resists "bulging." Further, ventriculographic demonstration of dyskinesis occurred in four patients, and, as expected, regional paradoxical lengthening occurred in each of these cases when recordings were determined at operation.

Second, ventriculograms tend to underestimate the margins of the ventricular chamber due to radiographic limits of resolution. Underestimation of volume would tend to lead to overestimation of wall motion. Thus, a region of ventricular

TABLE 2. Left Ventricular Asynergy

CINEANGIOGRAM	(SGA) INTACT VENOUS RETURN	CARDIOPULMONARY BYPASS		(SGA) INTACT VENOUS RETURN
		Before AC Bypass LVEDP = 0 (SGA)	After AC Bypass LVEDP = 0 (SGA)	
None	None	None	None	None
None	None	None	None	None
None	None	None	None	None
Hypokinesia	Shorten	Shorten	Shorten	Shorten
Hypokinesia	Distention	Shorten[a]	Shorten	Shorten
Hypokinesia	Distention	Shorten[a]	Shorten	Shorten
Hypokinesia	Distention	Distention	Shorten[a]	Shorten
Akinesia	Distention	Shorten[a]	Shorten	Shorten
Akinesia	Distention	Distention	Distention	Distention
Dyskinesis	Distention	Shorten[a]	Shorten	Shorten
Dyskinesis	Distention	Distention	Shorten[a]	Shorten
Dyskinesis	Distention	Distention	Distention	Distention
Dyskinesis	Distention	Distention	Equivocal	Shorten[a]

[a]Shortening with ventricular systole.
LVEDP: left ventricular end-diastolic pressure; AC: aortocoronary; SGA: strain gauge arch.

wall may be lengthening with systole, have a smooth mural thrombus on its endocardial surface, and have a paradoxical motion undemonstrable on cine ventriculograms. Last, the strain gauge arch is sutured to the ventricular muscle from its epicardial surface and more than likely does not record transmural wall motion. It is influenced most by the shells of muscle nearer the epicardial surface. It is highly probable that measurements of length change may be exaggerated when recorded from the surface of a sphere of larger diameter (epicardial) when compared to a sphere of smaller diameter (endocardial).

REGIONAL WALL MOTION AND MUSCLE MECHANICS

While it is valuable to determine intraoperatively the functional integrity of a zone of left ventricular asynergy as well as document its improvement after revascularization, a significant dilemma occurs prior to operative intervention. As alluded to earlier, the regional dysfunctional zone may represent nutritionally deprived muscle with compliance similar to that of the remainder of muscle mass. Enright has shown that acute occlusion of the anterior descending coronary artery does not alter the end-diastolic pressure (EDP)–end-diastolic volume (EDV) relation,[28] although it does suppress left ventricular function, ie, there is less ventricular work at any given EDP and circumference with outflow resistance held constant.[33] Since EDP has been shown to be a direct reflection of resting muscle segment length,[34] the initial muscle length (L_1) of the "normal" myocardium should be the same at any given EDP or EDV as it would have been in the absence of segmental ischemic disease. Enright's data delineate a more profound suppression of ventricular stroke work (VSW) at larger EDV (ie, longer L_1). He used the formula

$$VSW = \frac{SV \times (AoP - EDP)}{100}$$

where SV = stroke volume (ml), AoP = mean aortic pressure (cm H_2O), and EDP = end-diastolic pressure. The rather pronounced suppression of function at high loads must be due to decline in SV. Depressed SV implies a decline in peak chamber pressure developed due to a decline in dp/dt and a shift to the left in the net force-velocity and length-tension relations. These investigators calculated force-velocity relations following occlusion of the anterior descending coronary

artery and demonstrated a shift to the left of the curve especially at high loads. These results imply a suppression of active force generated by the chamber at any given contractile element velocity. These calculations, however, assume an evenly distributed force and wall stress of a thick-walled sphere.[35] This is obviously not the case when the ischemic portion of the wall is functioning partially as a series elastic (SE) component. Further, whether the stiffness of the ischemic zone will be greater than that of the true SE during chamber contraction will depend upon whether the ischemic segment generates tension during ventricular contraction. If the area generates enough tension to increase its stiffness, then less internal shortening of the healthy contractile mass will occur during isovolumic contraction.

Contractile element velocity V_{CE} is directly proportional to the rate of tension development (dT/dt), and inversely proportional to SE stiffness (dT/dl), ie:

$$V_{CE} = \frac{dT/dt}{dT/dl}.^{36}$$

By examination, the equation shows that the stiffer the diseased region the greater the dT/dt—ie, assuming the V_{CE} to be constant at any given load (although suppressed from normal due to the net decrease in muscle mass of the chamber available for development of tension). Contrariwise, if the diseased wall generates no tension, then the stiffness will be less (dT/dl), and the rate of tension developed by the chamber (dT/dt) will be less.

Moreover, as alluded to above, the less stiff the diseased region is during the contractile process, the greater the internal shortening of contractile elements. Exaggerated internal contractile element shortening—especially late in contraction—is akin to controlled release experiments in papillary muscle preparations, which results in uncoupling of contractile components and resultant suppression of peak active tension.[37] Thus, at least three potential mechanisms exist to suppress chamber function in the presence of an ischemic region of ventricular wall: (1) decrease in effective contractile mass, (2) the degree to which the ischemic segment either increases its stiffness or remains less stiff during the active contractile state, and (3) the resultant internal shortening and uncoupling of contractile elements due to the SE nature of the diseased segment.

A mechanistic approach to this theory has recently been demonstrated in the papillary muscle preparation by Tyberg, Parmley, and Sonnenblick.[38] They mounted two papillary muscles in

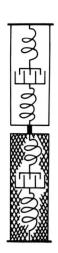
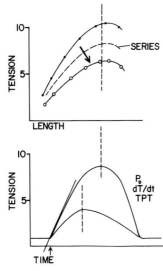

has a suppressed rate of development of tension (dT/dt), suppressed time to peak tension (TPT), and a suppressed peak tension developed (P_o). When the two muscles are in series, it appears obvious that during the entire duration of active contraction there is a disparity between the active tension in the nonischemic versus the ischemic muscle. In the isometric setting, therefore, the nonischemic muscle will shorten and stretch the ischemic muscle. These relations fully corroborate the theoretical hypothesis described earlier and are diagrammatically depicted in the lower portion of Figure 5. The rectangles on the left represent the two muscles during relaxation. During isometric contraction (right rectangles), the ischemic muscle (shaded) lengthens in response to the greater tension developed by the nonischemic muscle. The SE contribution of the ischemic muscle is analogous to the loss of developed tension described by Parmley and Sonnenblick [39] due to the inherent compliance in *in vitro* muscle preparations except that the ischemic muscle represents compliance of greater magnitude.

Three possibilities exist regarding the functional relation of a dysfunctional segment of ventricular wall to chamber dynamics. Figure 5 illustrates the alternatives. The shaded area of the ventricular chamber sketch represents the regional wall dysfunction. First, the shaded area may be composed of ischemic myocardium, which is viable but develops little tension due to inadequate blood flow. This relation has been discussed in

FIG. 4. Diagrammatic sketch on the left illustrates two muscles in series, a well-oxygenated, healthy muscle (nonshaded) and non-oxygenated, ischemic muscle (shaded). Upper graph at the right illustrates length–active tension relations for the oxygenated muscle alone (upper curve, solid circles), for the ischemic muscle alone (lower curve, open circles), and for the two muscles in series (center, interrupted line). Lower graph at the right illustrates the active tension curve during contraction from the oxygenated muscle (upper curve) and from the ischemic muscle (lower curve). Vertical interrupted lines indicate peak tension (P_o) and the time to peak tension (TPT) of each curve. dT/dt is rate of development of tension. See text for details.

series as schematically represented in Figure 4 (left side). The shaded lower rectangle represents ischemic muscle, while the upper muscle is not ischemic. Examination of the length-tension relations for the ischemic muscle, nonischemic muscle, and the two muscles in series were determined. The two curves on the right of Figure 4 illustrate schematically the pattern of results. Upper graph shows three length-tension curves. The upper curve is for nonischemic muscle, the lower curve the ischemic muscle, and the middle curve the length-tension relation for the muscles in series. Even cursory examination of the curves reveals a markedly greater development of active tension by the healthy muscle at any given L_1 when compared to that of the ischemic muscle. Moreover, the length-tension relation for the two muscles in series demonstrates less tension developed at any L_1 when compared to the healthy muscle alone, suggesting strongly that the normal muscle shortens, elongates the ischemic muscle, and dissipates energy by internal length alterations.

The lower graph illustrates the course of a single contraction for the ischemic and the nonischemic muscle. Note that the ischemic muscle

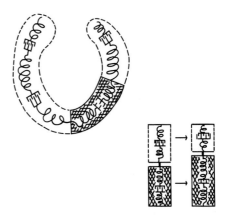

FIG. 5. Horseshoe sketch represents left ventricular chamber, and rectangular diagrams are myocardial muscle segments. Shaded areas represent segments that are either ischemic muscle, distensible noncontractile segment, or rigid nondistensible scar. Rectangular segments illustrate (from left to right) shortening of healthy muscle (nonshaded) and compensatory lengthening of diseased segment (shaded) without external shortening of the combined segments. See text for details.

detail above. Second, the diseased zone might represent distensible fibroelastic tissue with low stiffness and no contractile elements. If this is the case, then chamber dynamics are suppressed by the three aforementioned factors occurring during chamber contraction, ie, decreased total muscle mass, decreased development of tension by the chamber due to lengthening of the elastic segment during isovolumic contraction, and mechanical uncoupling due to internal shortening of the contractile components. In this situation, the latter two mechanisms will most likely present a more profound deterioration of chamber dynamics than would occur if the segment were ischemic muscle, because the elastic segment will exhibit a lower stiffness during ventricular systole than that of ischemic, poorly contracting viable myocardium. Further, an elastic-like segment imposes an alteration in the EDP-EDV relation during diastole. If the segment is less stiff than the remainder of the myocardium during diastole, then for any given increment in EDV, the increase in resting length of the elastic segment will be greater than the increment in resting length in the normal myocardium. As a result, at any given EDV, the L_1 of the healthy myocardium will be less, or alternately, a greater EDV will be required to attain a comparable L_1 for healthy myocardium when compared to the same ventricular chamber in the absence of a dysfunctional region. In this setting, therefore, the inotropic state will be suppressed at any fixed EDV, adding another detrimental mechanistic factor to adverse chamber dynamics.

The third possibility is rigid scar formation in the malfunctioning region. In this setting, the formation of fibrous scar with high stiffness will not lengthen during diastolic filling, and, therefore, the L_1 of the healthy myocardium will be longer for any specified EDV. The increment in L_1 at a given EDV actually benefits chamber dynamics due to the Frank-Starling mechanism. Further, during active contraction, little or no lengthening of the rigid area will occur nor will any internal shortening of contractile components during isovolumic contraction. The single major factor effecting a decline in chamber function in the presence of a zone of high stiffness is the decrease in contractile mass due to the presence of the fibrotic region.

Certainly, ischemic regions of left ventricular wall are composed of a combination of all of the above components in humans with ischemic heart disease. Whether the ischemic segment functions as poorly contracting muscle, rigid scar, or elastic-like tissue will depend upon the predominance of one of the three. It is, however, evident

that revascularization of vessels to an ischemic region of myocardium will plainly improve ventricular function. It is further apparent that a segment of distensible elastic-like region will have more profound detrimental effects upon chamber function than either rigid scar or ischemic muscle. For these reasons we presently feel that intraoperative determinations of regional wall motion should be made prior to and after aortocoronary bypass in all elective cases of occlusive coronary artery disease. Moreover, if a diseased region continues to lengthen after revascularization, the segment should be incised for two reasons. First, closure of the incision with eversion technique will effectively exclude the segment from the functional left ventricular chamber. Second, the likelihood of finding a mural endocardial thrombus is high. And, last, this mechanistic approach to the treatment of coronary artery disease raises an issue relevant to the management of patients with three-vessel disease. We believe that correction of flow to only a portion of the myocardium in the group of patients with three-vessel disease may actually increase the severity of asynergy and result in deterioration of ventricular function. We, therefore, recommend a concerted effort adequately to revascularize *all* major myocardial regions in patients with three or more vessel disease.

References

1. James TN: The coronary circulation and conduction system in acute myocardial infarction. Prog Cardiovasc Dis 10:410, 1968
2. Diethrich EB, Liddicoat JE, Kinard SA, et al: Surgical significance of angiographic patterns in coronary arterial disease. Circulation 35:1–155, 1967
3. Proudfit WL, Shirey EK, Sones FM: Distribution of arterial lesions demonstrated by selective cinecoronary arteriography. Circulation 36:54, 1967
4. Strong JP, McGill HC: The natural history of coronary atherosclerosis. Am J Pathol 40:37, 1962
5. Horwitz LD, Gorlin R, Taylor WJ, Kemp HG: Effects of nitroglycerin on regional myocardial blood flow in coronary artery disease. J Clin Invest 50:1578, 1971
6. Goldstein RE, Stinson EB, Epstein SE: Effects of nitroglycerin on coronary collateral function in patients with coronary occlusive disease. Am J Cardiol 31:135, 1973 (abstr)
7. Blumenthal HT, Alex M, Goldenberg S: A study of lesions of the intramural coronary artery branches in diabetes mellitus. Arch Pathol 70:13, 1960
8. Gross L, Kugel MA, Epstein EZ: Lesions of the coronary arteries and their branches in rheumatic fever. Am J Pathol 11:253, 1935
9. James TN, Brik RE: Pathology of the cardiac conduction system in polyarteritis nodosa. Arch Intern Med 117:561, 1966
10. Saphir O, Ohringer L, Wong R: Changes in the intramural coronary branches in coronary arteriosclerosis. Arch Pathol 62:159, 1956
11. Cohen MV, Eldh P: Experimental myocardial in-

farction in the closed-chest dog: controlled production of large or small areas of necrosis. Am Heart J 86:798, 1973

12. Gorlin R, Klein MD, Sullivan JM: Prospective correlative study of ventricular aneurysm. Am J Med 42:512, 1967

13. Tennant R, Wiggers CJ: Effect of coronary occlusion on myocardial contraction. Am J Physiol 112: 351, 1935

14. Prinzmetal ML, Schwartz LL, Corday E, et al: Studies of the coronary circulation: VI: loss of myocardial contractility after coronary artery occlusion. Ann Intern Med 31:429, 1949

15. Dack S, Paley DH, Sussman ML: A comparison of electrokymography and roentgenkymography in the study of myocardial infarction. Circulation 1:551, 1950

16. Tatooles CJ, Randall WC: Local ventricular bulging after acute coronary occlusion. Am J Physiol 201:451, 1961

17. Wiggers CJ: The problem of functional coronary collaterals. Exp Med Surg 8:402, 1950

18. Cohen MV, Downey JM, Sonnenblick EH, Kirk ES: The effects of nitroglycerin on coronary collaterals and myocardial contractility. J Clin Invest 52:2836, 1973

19. Blum RL, Alpern H, Jaffe H, Lang TW, Corday E: Determination of interarterial coronary anastomoses by radioactive spheres: effect of coronary occlusion and hypoemia. Am Heart J 79:244, 1970

20. Schaper W: The Collateral Circulation of the Heart. Amsterdam: North Holland Publishing Company, 1971

21. Harrison TR: Some unanswered questions concerning enlargement and failure of the heart. Am Heart J 69:100, 1965

22. Karliner JS, Ross J Jr: Left ventricular performance after acute myocardial infarction. Prog Cardiovasc Dis 13:374, 1971

23. Kazamias TM, Gander MP, Ross J Jr, Braunwald E: Detection of left ventricular wall motion disorders in coronary artery disease by radarkymography. N Engl J Med 285:63, 1971

24. Johnson WD, Lepley D: An aggressive surgical approach to coronary disease. J Thorac Cardiovasc Surg 59:128, 1970

25. Vineberg AM, Walter J: The surgical treatment of coronary artery heart disease by internal mammary artery implantation. Dis Chest 45:190, 1964

26. Herman MV, Heinle RA, Klein MC, Gorlin G: Localized disorders in myocardial contraction. N Engl J Med 277:222, 1967

27. Klein MD, Herman MV, Gorlin R: Hemodynamic study of left ventricular aneurysm. Circulation 35: 614, 1967

28. Enright LP, Hannah H, Reis RL: Effects of acute regional myocardial ischemia on left ventricular function in dogs. Circ Res 26:307, 1970

29. Wiggers CJ, Wegria R, Pinera B: The effects of myocardial ischemia on the fibrillation threshold: the method of spontaneous ventricular fibrillation following coronary occlusion. Am J Physiol 131: 309, 1940

30. Gregg DE: Coronary Circulation. Philadelphia: Lea and Febiger, 1950

31. Nishimura A, Giron F, Birtwell WC, Soroff HS: Evaluation of collateral blood supply by direct measurement of the performance of ischemic myocardial muscle. Trans Am Soc Artif Intern Organs 16:450, 1970

32. Forman R, Kirk ES, Downey JM, Sonnenblick EH: Nitroglycerin and heterogeneity of myocardial blood flow: reduced subendocardial blood flow and ventricular contractile force. J Clin Invest 52:905, 1973

33. Braunwald E, Frye RL, Ross J: Studies on Starling's law of the heart: determinants of the relationship between left ventricular end-diastolic pressure and circumference. Circ Res 8:1254, 1960

34. Mitchell JH, Linden RJ, Sarnoff SH: Influence of cardiac sympathetic and vagal nerve stimulation on the relation between left ventricular diastolic pressure and myocardial segment length. Circ Res 8:1100, 1960

35. Covell JW, Ross J Jr, Sonnenblick EH, Braunwald E: Comparison of the force-velocity relation and the ventricular function curve as measures of the contractile state of the intact heart. Circ Res 19: 364, 1966

36. Hill AV: The heat of shortening and the dynamic constants of muscle. Proc Roy Soc (London) Ser B 126:136, 1938

37. Brady AJ: Active state in cardiac muscle. Physiol Rev 48:570, 1968

38. Tyberg JV, Parmley WW, Sonnenblick EH: In-vitro studies of myocardial asynchrony and regional hypoxia. Circ Res 25:569, 1969

39. Parmley WW, Sonnenblick EH: Series elasticity in heart muscle: its relation to contractile element velocity and proposed muscle models. Circ Res 20:112, 1967

108

LATE HEMODYNAMIC EVALUATION OF PATIENTS WITH AORTOCORONARY BYPASS GRAFTS

Brian C. Morton, John E. Morch, Peter McLaughlin,
Harold Aldridge, Bernard Goldman,
and Alan S. Trimble

INTRODUCTION

The real impact of aortocoronary bypass graft operations on coronary artery disease will only be determined by the evaluation of long-term results. Early postoperative follow-up studies have reported marked relief of angina pectoris (Najmi et al, 1974). However, only long-term detailed reevaluation including angiography will determine graft patency, myocardial infarction incidence, and survival.

This study was performed as the initial phase of a longitudinal postoperative study. We set out to determine at late follow-up the symptomatic state of the patient (including employability), the incidence of myocardial infarction, and the graft patency rate. Estimation of any impact on survival will require a longer follow-up and will only be available at a later phase of the longitudinal study.

MATERIAL AND METHODS

From March 1969 to December 1972, a total of 314 patients had aortocoronary bypass graft surgery performed at the Toronto General Hospital, with a 2.5 percent in-hospital mortality. All patients had stable angina graded by the New York Heart Association Classification and were uncontrolled symptomatically with medical therapy including short- and long-acting nitrate preparations and high doses of beta blocking drugs. Smoking habits and work histories were recorded. Investigations included the following: a resting 12 lead electrocardiogram, fasting blood sugar, cho-

Supported by the Ontario Heart Foundation.

lesterol, triglyceride, and lipoprotein electrophoresis. Cardiac catheterization was performed including left ventricular angiogram and selective coronary arteriograms on 35 mm cine film with a Phillips image intensifier with multiple projections. Ejection fractions were calculated from the left ventricular angiograms and used as an indication of ventricular function. The single plane method (Covvey et al 1972) was used for calculating the ejection fraction. Grafts were only performed if narrowing of the vessel lumen was 75 percent or greater and the distal run-off 1.5 mm or greater in diameter. No patients had gross generalized left ventricular dysfunction.

Of the original group of 314 patients, 100 patients volunteered to return for follow-up investigation 12 to 24 months postoperatively (mean 19.7 months). There were 93 males and seven females ranging in age from 32 to 65 years (mean 52.2 years). Internal mammary implants were done in conjunction with aortocoronary bypass grafting in seven patients. The preoperative assessment indicated above was repeated at the time of follow-up. In addition, the vein grafts were selectively opacified in two views.

RESULTS

Clinical

All patients preoperatively were symptomatically classes II to IV (NYHA)* but postoperatively 74 percent were asymptomatic or mildly symptomatic in class I (see Fig. 1). The largest group of patients were class III preopera-

* All further gradation of symptoms by classes refers to the NYHA classification.

TABLE 1. Graft Patency According to Date of Surgery

	FIRST 50 PTS. (8/69–8/71)			SECOND 50 PTS. (9/71–7/72)			TOTAL
	LAD	RC	Circ	LAD	RC	Circ	
Number of grafts	40	29	1	37	32	3	142
Patent grafts	27	22	1	29	26	2	107
Percent patency	67	76	ns	78	81	ns	75

tively, but postoperatively 54 of 65 (83 percent) were asymptomatic or class I. By contrast, of 20 class IV patients preoperatively, only 12 (60 percent) were asymptomatic or class I postoperatively. There were 33 asymptomatic postoperative patients who originated primarily in class III (20 patients), but five were preoperatively class IV. Only seven patients in the total group failed to improve. Seven patients with internal mammary implants in addition to an aortocoronary bypass graft showed no significant difference from the group who had grafts alone.

Graft Patency

Seventy-five percent of 142 grafts in 100 patients were patent at late follow-up (Table 1). Patency rates for specific vessels were similar, but the patency of the second 50 patients (left anterior descending artery 78 percent, right coronary artery 81 percent) was significantly higher than the rates for the first 50 patients (left anterior descending 67 percent, right coronary artery 76 percent). In 107 patent grafts, narrowings were seen proximally in three, distally in eight, and diffusely in four.

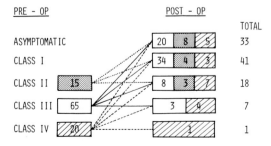

PRE - OP   POST - OP

		TOTAL
ASYMPTOMATIC	20 8 5	33
CLASS I	34 4 3	41
CLASS II	15 → 8 3 7	18
CLASS III	65 → 3 4	7
CLASS IV	20 → 1	1

FIG. 1. Comparisons of preoperative (left) and postoperative (right) symptomatology in 100 patients with stable angina pectoris uncontrolled by medical therapy. The NYHA classification of angina was used. Totals for the postoperative classes appear in far right column.

Graft Patency vs Clinical Result

The relationship between the clinical status and graft patency is shown in Table 2. The degree of symptomatic improvement by number of classes (eg, class III to class I would be improvement by two classes) is shown with the graft patency rates in column two. Improvement by three classes was associated with the highest patency rate of 84 percent in a large group of 23 patients. (Although an 88 percent patency rate was seen in some patients who improved four classes the numbers were small, ie seven/eight patients). Larger numbers of patent grafts were found in those patients showing greater improvement, ie 16 patients with 13 patent grafts (0.8 graft/pt) improved by one class compared to 23 patients with 31 patent grafts (1.3/pt) who improved by three classes.

PERIOPERATIVE MYOCARDIAL INFARCTION

Comparisons of pre- and immediate postoperative electrocardiograms showed a perioperative infarct in 15 patients as indicated by the appearance of new Q-waves. The relationship of perioperative infarction to graft patency is shown

TABLE 2. Relationship of Clinical Postoperative Improvement to Graft Patency

DEGREE OF IMPROVEMENT	NO. PTS.	GRAFT PATENCY RATE	PERIOP INFARCTION
No improvement	7	4/8 (50%)	0
1 class	16	13/18 (72%)	5
2 classes	49	49/71 (70%)	3
3 classes	23	31/37 (84%)	4
4 classes	5	7/8 (88%)	2

TABLE 3. Perioperative Infarction: LAD Grafts

	ANTEROSEPTAL	ANTERIOR	ANTEROLATERAL
Number of patients	3	6	1
Patency at follow-up	2	3	0
Clinical	2–1 classes	2–3 classes	1 class
Improvement	1–2	3–2 classes	–
(NYHA Classes)	–	1–1 classes	–

TABLE 4. Perioperative Infarction RCA Grafts

	INFERIOR	LATERAL
Number of patients	4	1
Patency at follow-up	2	1
Clinical	1–1 classes	–
Improvement	1–3 classes	2
(NYHA classes)	2–4 classes	–

in Tables 3 and 4 and summarized in the last column of Table 2.

Eight of the 15 patients with myocardial infarctions had patent grafts at follow-up examinations. All infarcts were in the distribution of the grafted vessel. In this group the clinical improvement was by only one class in four patients with all grafts occluded and by two or more classes in 11 patients with one or more grafts patent.

Ventricular Function

Twenty-eight patients had comparisons of the left ventricular ejection fraction before and after surgery (Table 5). Five patients increased and 13 decreased their ejection fractions after surgery. Of the 10 unchanged, seven were normal preoperatively and no improvement could be expected. The myocardial infarction rate was too low to permit any conclusions. Graft patency was less (55 percent) in patients with decreased ejection fractions than those with unchanged ejection fractions (70 percent), but the number of patients was small.

Risk Factors

Forty-three of 57 grafts (75 percent) performed in patients with normal triglyceride levels were open compared to 62 of 84 grafts (74 percent) in patients with elevated triglyceride levels. Similarly, no difference in graft patency was seen in patients with normal cholesterol levels compared to hypercholesterolemic patients.

Eighty-five percent of patients smoked more than one package of cigarettes a day. Forty-five percent continued smoking at follow-up. There was no difference in graft patency between pa-

tients who continued to smoke after surgery and patients who were nonsmokers or had stopped smoking before surgery.

Work History

Sixty-five percent returned to their former jobs although some had reduced requirements for physical exertion.

DISCUSSION

All patients in this study were markedly symptomatic before surgery in spite of vigorous medical therapy, including high doses of short- and long-acting nitrate preparations and beta blocking drugs. Postoperatively, 93 percent of the patients were improved symptomatically by one or more NYHA classes. Thirty-three asymptomatic patients, able to carry on heavy exertion without pain, were remarkable. Although preoperatively 18 of the patients in this asymptomatic group were in class II, 20 started in class III, and five in class IV. Improvement by numbers of classes as shown in Table 1 correlates with graft patency. For example, improvement by three classes was associated with an 84 percent patency in 23 patients. Those patients with a larger number of patent grafts per patient showed the most marked improvement.

The difficulties in evaluating symptomatic relief of angina are well recognized. Placebo responses of up to 35 percent following surgery (Beecher, 1961) have been documented, and spontaneous remissions of angina are well known. However, it is unlikely that either the placebo responses or spontaneous remissions would persist

TABLE 5. LV Ejection Fractions
(No. Patients: 28)

	NO. PTS.	GRAFT PATENCY	PERIOP INFARCTION
Increased	5	5/6	2
Unchanged	10	12/17	0
Decreased	13	11/20	1

in many patients for the long interval between surgery and follow-up study. Furthermore, it is recognized that distinguishing the improvement from one class to another, ie III to II, might be difficult in some patients. Improvement by two or more classes as seen in 77 of our patients is more readily detectable and reproducible by different examiners. Similar degrees of improvement have been reported by other authors (Cannom et al, 1974). Some bias may have been introduced because the more symptomatic patients volunteered to return for follow-up examination.

The high degree of late graft patency was encouraging. Better case selection and surgical techniques led to higher patency rates in the second 50 of the 100 patients. Although still of concern, only 11 showed segmental narrowing and 4 diffuse narrowing of the graft. Lespérance et al (1973) reported that only 5 percent of grafts open at one year occluded by the third year. No reduction in graft patency in patients with increased triglycerides, compared to normolipemic patients, was documented contrary to reports by Allard et al (1972).

Myocardial infarction in the perioperative period was of concern. Fifteen of our patients developed new Q-waves in the distribution of the grafted vessel. Subendocardial damage is obviously not estimated by the Q-wave criteria. Although four patients in this group with their sole graft occluded improved, it was only by one class. Of the remaining 11 patients with myocardial infarctions with at least one graft patent, only two improved by one class but nine improved by more than one class. Myocardial infarctions in the perioperative period do not necessarily mean that grafts have been occluded and significant symptomatic improvement is possible if at least one graft is patent. No definite contribution to left ventricular dysfunction because of transmural infarction could be detected in any of the patients (Table 5). Our data on ventricular function are in general agreement with Hammermeister et al (1974) and other reports and showed a varied response at rest, postoperatively.

The potential effectiveness of aortocoronary bypass surgery was evident as 65 percent of the patients returned to their former jobs. Although many patients were functionally capable of working they remained out of work because of attractive disability benefits or reluctance of employers to rehire them.

In summary, a high percentage of patients with medically uncontrolled angina with good ventricular function can be improved symptomatically with a low surgical mortality rate and a high long-term graft patency. Perioperative myocardial infarctions and failure to improve ventricular function consistently are disappointing. Further improvements in surgical techniques with reductions of perioperative infarctions and reductions in mortality will permit consideration of prophylactic vein grafts for patients with severe proximal stenosis of coronary arteries who are either mildly symptomatic or asymptomatic following myocardial infarctions.

ACKNOWLEDGMENT

We would like to thank Drs. Bigelow, Key, Heimbecker, Brown, Greenwood, Watt, Noble, Morrow, Adelman, Schwartz, MacMillan, and Wigle for permitting us to include their patients in this study.

References

Allard C, Ruscito O, Goulet C: The influence of serum triglycerides on the fate of aorto-coronary vein grafts. Can Med Assoc J 107:213, 1972

Beecher H: Surgery as placebo. A quantitative study of bias. JAMA 176:88, 1961

Cannom DS, Miller DC, Shumway NE, et al. The long term follow up of patients undergoing saphenous vein bypass surgery. Circulation 46, 1974, p 77

Covvey H, Adelman A, Felderhof C, Taylor K, Wigle E: Television/computer: dimensional analysis interface with special application to left ventricular cineangiograms. Comput Biol Med 2:221, 1972

Hammermeister KE, Kennedy JW, Hamilton GW, et al. Aortocoronary saphenous-vein bypass. Failure of successful grafting to improve resting left ventricular function in chronic angina. N Engl J Med 290:186, 1974

Lespérance J, Bourassa M, Saltiel J, Campeau L, Grondin C: Angiographic changes in aortocoronary vein grafts: lack of progression beyond the first year. Circulation 48, 1973, p 633

Najmi M, Ushiyama K, Blanco G, Adam A, Segal B: Results of aortocoronary artery saphenous vein bypass surgery for ischemic heart disease. Am J Cardiol 33:42, 1974

109

EVALUATION OF MYOCARDIAL PERFUSION BY DIRECT INJECTION OF RADIOACTIVE PARTICLES FOLLOWNG CORONARY BYPASS SURGERY

Glen W. Hamilton, John A. Murray, Eugene Lapin,
David Allen, Karl E. Hammermeister,
and James L. Ritchie

Postoperative coronary graft arteriography provides anatomic detail but does not provide definitive information about the volume or regional distribution of graft flow. We have studied the myocardial distribution of coronary graft flow by the direct injection of ^{99m}Tc or ^{113m}In MAA at the time of postoperative angiography in 40 vein bypass grafts, four internal mammary–LAD anastomoses, and a single anterior internal mammary implantation. Scintillation camera images following catheterization provided high-quality images of myocardial perfusion from which the size and uniformity of the primarily grafted area could be determined and the degree of collateral flow judged.

Compared to the assessment of flow by angiography the size of the area of myocardium perfused was not helpful in predicting graft flow. Collateral flow was more readily appreciated on the myocardial perfusion study (53 percent) than by angiography (18 percent) and was greater in degree in 42 percent. The presence of collateral flow on the perfusion study was uniformly associated with good graft flow angiographically. Adequate graft flow by angiography and documentation of the region supplied by perfusion study was not always associated with improved regional contraction.

Four studies of internal mammary–LAD anastomosis showed major perfusion of the mediastinum and intercostals in two cases and predominantly myocardial perfusion in two.

Overall, the qualitative assessment of regional perfusion by this technique was felt to aid in the evaluation of graft function in 35 percent.

INTRODUCTION

Delivery of an increased volume of coronary flow and distribution of that flow to previously underperfused areas of myocardium are the primary goals of coronary bypass surgery. Postoperative coronary and bypass graft arteriography demonstrate anatomic detail but do not provide definitive information regarding the volume or regional distribution of graft flow. Direct injection of hydrogen gas (Greene et al, 1972) or ^{133}Xe (Lichtlen et al, 1972) into a coronary graft allows determination of "average" myocardial blood flow; however, they do not delineate regional perfusion abnormalities. In fact, as pointed out by Greene et al (1972), failure to find a monoexponential washout curve with these techniques is evidence that flow is not evenly distributed throughout the revascularized segment.

Measurement of graft flow using videodensitometry as reported by Smith et al (1971) provides absolute volume flow in cc/min but is not well suited for study of regional distribution. Regional myocardial washout studies of ^{133}Xe with a scintillation camera (similar to those reported by Cannon et al [1972ab] in patients with coronary disease) would delineate regional flow changes following surgery but require a scintillation camera in the cardiac catheterization laboratory.

In contrast to ^{133}Xe or H$_2$ washout studies, the injection of radioactive macroaggregated albumin (MAA) particles directly into the coronary arteries at the time of angiography allows study of the distribution of flow after completion of the catheterization (Ashburn et al, 1971; Endo et al, 1970; and Weller et al, 1972). We have used this technique to study the regional distribution of coronary graft flow following the direct injection of ^{99m}Technetium and ^{113m}Indium labeled particles into coronary grafts at the time of angiography. Reported here are the results of regional perfusion studies using this technique and the relationships of the perfusion study to other parameters of graft function.

MATERIALS AND METHODS

Forty-five graft myocardial perfusion studies were performed in 34 patients undergoing routine postoperative catheterization to assess the results of coronary artery surgery. Clinical assessment included history, physical, chest X-ray, and EKG. Separate informed consent was obtained for the postoperative assessment and for the myocardial perfusion study. High specific activity ^{99m}Technetium macroaggregated albumin (Tc MAA) was prepared using stannous chloride (Allen et al, 1973). The resultant Tc MAA contained 1.5–3.0 millicuries of ^{99m}Tc on 30,000 to 60,000 particles of MAA. Ninety percent of the particles were from 20 to 40 microns in size with no particles exceeding 100 microns in diameter. In some studies, a similar preparation tagged with ^{113m}Indium was used to study two coronary grafts simultaneously. Standard graft angiography was performed by either the Sones or Judkins technique. Graft patency and adequacy of flow was assessed qualitatively as good, fair, or poor, by two independent observers. The presence or absence of collateral

flow and the area supplied were noted. Following angiography, 1.5 millicuries TcMAA or InMAA was injected directly into the graft or internal mammary artery, flushed in with saline, and the catheter position confirmed by contrast angiography. Care was taken to flush the catheter free of contrast material two minutes prior to the injection of the MAA to minimize the hemodynamic effects of radiographic contrast material (Kloster et al, 1972, and Gould et al, 1974). Biplane ventriculography was performed to assess ventricular volume, ejection fraction, and contraction pattern.

Following catheterization, the patients were taken to the nuclear medicine laboratory for myocardial imaging. We obtained 100,000-count scintiphotos using a Nuclear-Chicago HP scintillation camera in the right anterior oblique (RAO), anterior, left anterior oblique (LAO), left lateral, left posterior oblique (LPO), and posterior positions. For studies employing only ^{99m}Tc, a low-energy parallel 4,000-hole collimator was used. For studies of both ^{113m}In and ^{99m}Tc, a parallel 1,000-hole medium energy collimator was used.

Each myocardial perfusion study was evaluated by two observers without prior knowledge of the angiographic findings. The size of the primary graft area was graded as normal or decreased and assessed for uniformity of flow. Images demonstrating collateral flow were assessed regarding the region or regions of myocardium supplied.

RESULTS

Regional perfusion studies were performed in 40 saphenous vein bypass grafts (SVBG), four

TABLE 1. Regional Perfusion Studies

	SVBG			INT. MAM.		TOTAL	PERCENT
	RCA	LAD	Circ	LAD	Vineberg		
Number of grafts	14	16	10	4	1	45	
Angiographic flow							
Good	13	12	10	2	0	37	82
Fair	0	2	0	0	0	2	4
Poor	1	2	0	2	1	6	13
Myocardial perfusion size							
Normal	14	15	10	2	1	42	93
Decreased	0	1	0	2	0	3	7
Collateral flow present							
Angio	3	4	1	0	0	8	18
Perfusion	8	10	5	1	0	24	53
Collateral flow greater on perfusion than angio	6	7	5	1	0	19	42
Perfusion aided interpretation	5	4	4	3	0	16	35

SVBG: saphenous vein bypass graft; RCA: right coronary artery; LAD: left anterior descending coronary artery; Circ: circumflex coronary artery.

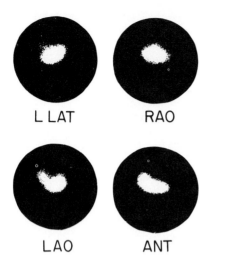

FIG. 1. Scintiphotos of a saphenous vein bypass graft (SVBG) to the distal right coronary artery (RCA). The "ball and tail" configuration is best appreciated in the LAO view. The tail represents flow to the right ventricular myocardium and the ball represents flow to the inferior myocardium supplied by the posterior descending coronary artery. LLAT: left lateral; LAO: left anterior oblique; RAO: right anterior oblique.

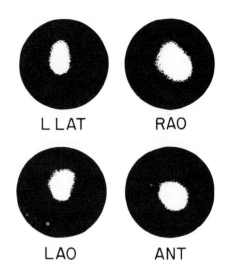

FIG. 2. Scintophotos of a saphenous vein bypass graft (SVBG) to the left anterior descending coronary artery (LAD). In the anterior (ANT) and right anterior oblique (RAO), the entire left ventricle appears to be visualized. The left anterior oblique (LAO) and the left lateral (LLAT) views clearly show the activity to be anterior representing the anterior, ceptal, and anterior-lateral portion of the left ventricular myocardium.

direct internal mammary-to-anterior descending anastomoses, and a single anterior wall Vineberg implant (Table 1). Injection of ^{99m}Tc or ^{113m}Indium MAA produced no symptoms or changes in either the ECG or aortic pressure. Scintiphotos of regional perfusion were of high quality in all but two early cases, in which there was inadequate labeling of the MAA particles. Imaging time per view was one to two minutes with ^{99m}Tc and two to four minutes with ^{113}In, resulting in a total study time of 30 to 45 minutes.

Normal images of patent saphenous vein bypass grafts (SVBG) judged to have good flow angiographically to the left anterior descending (LAD), circumflex, and right coronary artery (RCA) are shown in Figures 1 to 3. Overall, the RAO or anterior view combined with an LAO or left lateral view provided the most information. Right coronary grafts had a "ball and tail" configuration. The length of the "tail," which represents flow to the right ventricular myocardium, was variable, depending on the location of the SVBG anastomosis to the right coronary artery or posterior descending artery and the presence or absence of retrograde flow up the right coronary artery. Vein grafts to the left anterior descending or circumflex coronary arteries or their branches were not readily distinguishable in the anterior or RAO views; however, the LAO or left lateral clearly showed the perfused area to be anterior (LAD) or posterior (circumflex) (Figs. 2 and 3).

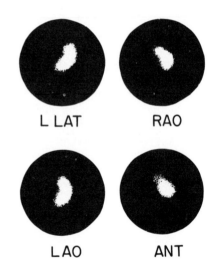

FIG. 3. Scintiphotos of a saphenous vein bypass graft (SVBG) to the circumflex coronary artery. The pattern of activity resembles a SVBG to the left anterior descending in the anterior and right anterior oblique (RAO) images. On the left lateral (LLAT) and left anterior oblique (LAO) views the area of activity is clearly seen to be posterior in the posterior and posterior-lateral part of the left ventricular myocardium. Circ: circumflex coronary artery.

Comparison of regional distribution following coronary artery injection preoperatively and graft injection postoperatively in the LAD and circumflex areas is presented in Figure 4. This patient had separate coronary ostia for the LAD and circumflex arteries, allowing selective injec-

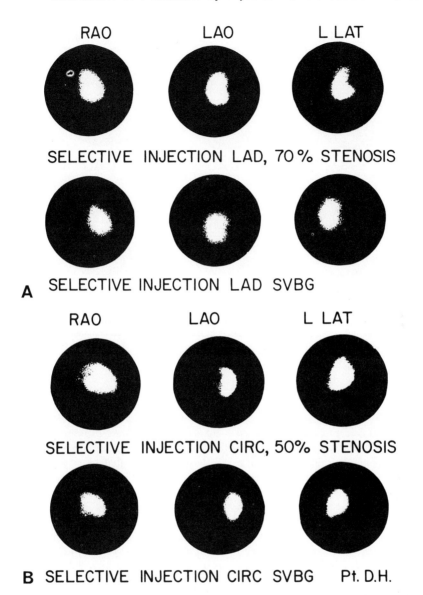

FIG. 4. Scintiphotos of a single patient with a 70 percent left anterior descending (LAD) stenosis, a 50 percent circumflex (Circ) stenosis, and a total occlusion of the right coronary artery. The upper images in A and B were made by selective injection of the LAD (A) and circumflex (B). Separate ostia for the LAD and circumflex made the selective injection possible. The lower images followed selective injection of saphenous vein bypass grafts (SVBG) to the LAD and circumflex respectively. The primary LAD and circumflex areas are the same in both studies. However, collateral flow to the inferior left ventricle normally supplied by the right coronary artery was more prominent on the preoperative study than on the SVBG study. The inferior collateral flow is best visualized on the right anterior oblique (RAO) and left lateral (LLAT) images in A and on the RAO and left anterior oblique (LAO) in B. Angiography demonstrated LAD to right coronary collateral on the preoperative study. No angiographic collateral was noted on the circumflex injection preoperatively or on the SVBG injections postoperatively.

tion of these vessels prior to surgery. In spite of a 70 percent stenosis in the LAD and a 50 percent stenosis in the circumflex vessels, regional distribution was normal in both primary areas preoperatively (Fig. 4). Flow to the inferior myocardium was seen with both injections and represents collateral to a totally occluded right coronary artery. Postoperatively these areas were perfused by SVBG's, which were separately injected with ^{99m}Tc and ^{113m}In MAA. The regional distribution

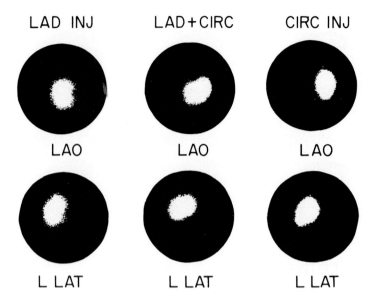

FIG. 5. Single and composite images of a patient with saphenous vein bypass grafts to the circumflex (Circ) and left anterior descending (LAD) coronary arteries. The composite (LAD + Circ) image was made by superimposing 50,000 counts of both the 99mTc window and the 113mIndium window on the same polaroid film. The relationship of the LAD and Circ areas is easily appreciated. LAO: left anterior oblique; LLAT: left lateral.

of flow through the SVBG to the LAD and circumflex areas is virtually identical to that noted on the preoperative injection of the native circulation. Collateral flow to the inferior left ventricle normally supplied by the RCA is much less prominent on the postoperative study. Angiography revealed collateral flow from only the LAD to RCA preoperatively and no collateral flow postoperatively.

Single and composite views of a patient with SVBGs to the circumflex and LAD are shown in Figure 5 to demonstrate the relationship of these two areas in the LAD and left lateral views. Although there is some overlap of areas, in both views it is possible to distinguish clearly the circumflex from the LAD area.

Collateral flow to areas other than the primarily grafted area was easily visualized. Figure 6 demonstrates a SVBG to the LAD with collateral flow to the circumflex and RCA areas. Since the distribution of tagged particles is dependent upon blood flow (Domenech et al, 1969, and Rhodes et al, 1971) the relative concentration of activity in the perfused areas depicts the relative distribution of blood flow from the graft. Collateral flow was more easily appreciated on the myocardial perfusion study than by angiography (Table 1, Fig. 7). Collateral flow was visualized on the myocardial

perfusion study in 24 cases (53 percent) and by angiography in eight (18 percent). The extent of collateral flow was greater on the myocardial perfusion study than that visualized by angiography in 42 percent (Table 1). In no case was angiographic collateral visualized in the absence of perfusion study evidence of collateral flow.

The size of the area of myocardium perfused was not directly related to the angiographic assessment of graft flow (Table 1, Fig. 7). Normal-sized perfusion areas were seen in all 37 grafts judged to have good flow angiographically, and in five of eight grafts judged to have fair or poor flow. A decreased perfusion area was noted in the remaining three grafts judged to have poor flow. The single Vineberg studied demonstrated a large area of anterior myocardial perfusion comparable to that usually seen with SVBG to the LAD coronary artery. However, angiographic flow was felt to be poor and subsequent measurement at surgery demonstrated flow rates of only 10 to 15cc/min. The size of the area of myocardium perfused was thus a measure of relative flow distribution, not absolute graft flow. It is notable, however, that in all 24 graft perfusion studies showing collateral flow to the areas other than the primary graft, graft flow was judged to be good angiographically. The recognition of collateral flow was therefore an

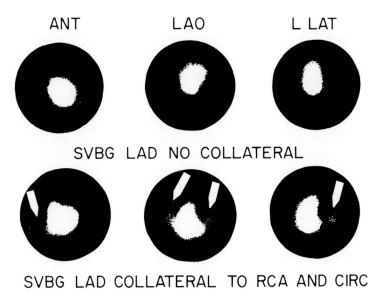

ANT   LAO   L LAT

SVBG LAD NO COLLATERAL

SVBG LAD COLLATERAL TO RCA AND CIRC

FIG. 6. Images of two normal saphenous vein bypass grafts (SVBG) to the left anterior descending (LAD) coronary artery. The upper images show no collateral flow, and the lower images demonstrate prominent collateral to both the right coronary area (anterior view; left arrow in the LAO view) and the circumflex coronary area (left lateral view; right arrow in the LAO view). Angiographic collateral flow was noted to the right coronary artery but not to the circumflex coronary artery. LAO: left anterior oblique; LLAT: left lateral, RCA: right coronary artery.

indicator of good flow through the graft. The area of the primary graft appeared uniform in all cases.

In five cases SVGB's to vessels supplying hypokinetic or akinetic areas of myocardium were studied. In an additional two cases, collateral flow to hypokinetic or akinetic areas was present on the perfusion study. In spite of adequate graft flow angiographically and documentation of adequate regional perfusion by imaging, improvement in regional contraction and ejection fraction was not uniformly seen. Only three of seven showed improvement in contraction pattern with an increased ejection fraction (increase > 10 percent).

In four studies of regional perfusion following direct internal mammary–to–left anterior descending anastomosis, a scintigraphic pattern similar to that seen with a SVBG to the left anterior descending was noted (Fig. 8). Flow to nonmyocardial areas via internal mammary branches was routinely visualized. In two cases the nonmyocardial flow was judged to be minimal or moderate (estimated to be less than 20 percent of total). In the other two studies, the majority of flow delivered by the internal mammary was to nonmyocardial areas—intercostal arteries and mediastinum.

Considering all 45 cases, the myocardial per-

FIG. 7. Comparison of graft flow judged angiographically with the size of the primary perfusion area on the myocardial images and the assessment of collateral flow by the two methods. Collateral flow was visualized more frequently on the perfusion study and was of greater magnitude in 42 percent. Angio: angiogram; myoc: myocardial; coll: collateral; norm: normal; decr: decreased.

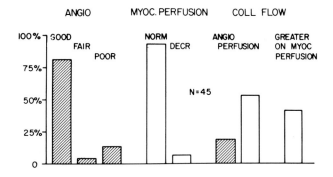

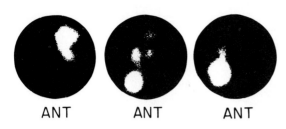

FIG. 8. Anterior-view images of 3 internal mammary-to-left anterior descending grafts. The image on the left shows virtually all flow in the mediastinum while the right image shows most flow to the myocardium. The center image demonstrates flow to both the mediastinum and the myocardium.

fusion study was judged to provide useful information in 35 percent (Table 1). Most often this was due to visualization of collateral flow not appreciated by angiography.

DISCUSSION

Our initial interest in the direct injection of ^{99m}TC or ^{113m}In MAA into coronary grafts was stimulated by the difficulty in judging the adequacy of flow in saphenous vein grafts by angiography. Since the coronary graft and the native circulation both supply the myocardium competitively, it was hypothesized that the size of the perfused area might correlate with absolute volume flow in the graft. This hypothesis was incorrect— grafts with low flow could have the same relative distribution as grafts with high flow rates. The perfusion study thus portrayed relative regional myocardial distribution of graft flow but provided relatively little information regarding the volume of flow. Although the size of the primarily grafted area perfused was not helpful in judging graft flow, the presence of myocardial perfusion to other areas via collaterals was always associated with good graft flow by angiography. It seems unlikely that this association will pertain in all cases; even if graft flow is minimal, collateral flow to less well perfused areas could be present. We currently consider the presence of collateral myocardial perfusion to be helpful in assessing the amount of graft flow. Nonuniformity of activity or maldistribution within the primary graft area was not seen by simple visual inspection. It is possible that more quantitative image analysis by computer could bring out subtle abnormalities in flow distribution.

The ability to appreciate collateral flow was much better on the perfusion study than on the angiogram. Not only was collateral flow more frequently visualized (53 percent vs 18 percent), but the extent of the collateral flow was greater on the perfusion study in 42 percent. This is likely due to the fact that the two techniques depend on different principles for visualization. While angiography depends on opacification of a sufficiently sized vessel, myocardial imaging with MAA depends on capillary blockage without regard to the caliber of the vessel delivering flow.

Failure to find uniform improvement in regional myocardial contraction with adequate graft flow by angiography and normal regional perfusion was of interest. Whether, in fact, this was due to inadequate flow misjudged as adequate on the angiogram or failure of local contraction in spite of adequate regional flow, is uncertain. It does not appear from this study that localized maldistribution was the cause of the failure to improve contractile performance.

The results reported here indicate that direct injection of coronary grafts with MAA, although useful in defining regional distribution of the flow delivered, is not a measure of the quantity of flow delivered. Combination of washout techniques (Greene et al, 1972; and Lichtlen et al, 1972), which measure flow in cc/min/gram of myocardium, with an estimate of the myocardial mass perfused from the myocardial perfusion study would allow a reasonable estimate of the absolute volume of graft flow. Measurement of both regional distribution and washout of ^{133}Xenon injected directly into the coronary graft would provide both a measure of flow and regional distribution. This would, however, require a scintillation camera in the catheterization laboratory.

Assessment of volume flow by videodensitometry (Smith et al, 1971) and regional distribution by the technique described here would provide a measure of both absolute volume flow and distribution. Alternatively, the transit time of the injected bolus could be quantitated using a scintillation camera. Based on the transit time and size of the graft, volume flow could be calculated directly.

At the present time, the described method of studying the regional distribution of graft flow is probably the most widely applicable technique and is available to any facility with a scintillation camera or scanner. The complete lack of toxicity noted here confirms the safety of this technique as reported by Weller et al (1972) and Ashburn et al (1971). The technique was easily performed and provided information useful in the evaluation of coronary graft function in about one-third of the patients studied.

References

Allen DR, Nelp WB, Cheney F, Harnett DE: Studies of acute cardiopulmonary toxicity of SN–MAA in the dog. Submitted (J Nuc Med, Oct 1973)

Ashburn WL, Braunwald E, Simon AL, et al: Myocardial perfusion imaging with radioactive-labelled particles injected directly into the coronary circulation of patients with coronary artery disease. Circulation 44:851–56, 1971

Cannon PJ, Dell RB, Dwyer EM Jr: Measurement of regional myocardial perfusion in man with ^{133}xenon and a scintillation camera. J Clin Invest 51:964–77, 1972a

Cannon PJ, Dell RB, Dwyer EM Jr: Regional myocardial perfusion rates in patients with coronary artery disease. J Clin Invest 51:978–94, 1972b

Domenech R, Hoffman J, Noble M, et al: Total and regional coronary blood flow measured by radioactive microspheres in conscious anesthetized dogs. Circ Res 25:581–96, 1969

Endo M, Yamazaki T, Konos, et al: The direct diagnosis of human myocardial ischemia using ^{131}I–MA via the selective coronary catheter. Am Heart J 80: 498–506, 1970

Gould KL, Lipscomb K, Hamilton GW: A physiologic basis for assessing critical coronary stenosis: instantaneous flow response and regional distribution during coronary hyperemia as measures of coronary flow reserve. Am J Card 33:87–94, 1974

Greene DG, Klocke FJ, Schimert GL, et al: Evaluation of venous bypass grafts from aorta to coronary artery by inert gas desaturation and direct flow meter techniques. J Clin Invest 51:191–96, 1972

Kloster FE, Friesen WG, Green GS, Judkins MP: Effects of coronary arteriography on myocardial blood flow. Circulation 46:438–44, 1972

Lichtlen P, Moccetti T, Halter J, Schonbeck M, Senning A: Postoperative evaluation of myocardial blood flow in aortocoronary artery vein bypass grafts using the xenon-residue detection technique. Circulation 46:445–55, 1972

Rhodes B, Stern H, Buchanan J, Zolle I, Wagner H: Lung scanning with ^{99m}Tc-microspheres. Radiology 99:613–21, 1971

Smith HC, Frye RL, Davis GD, et al: Measurement of flow in saphenous vein-coronary artery grafts by roentgen videodensitometry. Circulation suppl to vol 43 and 44:389, 1971

Weller DA, Adolph RJ, Wellman HN, et al: Myocardial perfusion scintigraphy after intracoronary injection of ^{99m}Tc-labelled human albumin microspheres. Circulation 46:963–75, 1972

110

TREADMILL EXERCISE TEST FOLLOWING CORONARY ARTERY SURGERY

W. Charles Helton, Frederick W. Johnson, John Hornung,
R. Bradford Pyle, Kurt Amplatz, Naip Tuna,
and Demetre M. Nicoloff

Aortocoronary bypass grafting has gained widespread use in the last five years for the symptomatic relief of angina pectoris (and, it is hoped, for the prevention of myocardial infarction). The popularity of this procedure has been enhanced by the recent reports of a low operative mortality with a high yield of symptomatic relief in elective procedures (Anderson et al, 1971; Cannom et al, 1974; Favaloro, 1971; Reul et al, 1972). Indeed, at present, the principal indication for this form of surgery is the subjective alleviation of the symptoms of chronic disabling angina (Johnson and Lepley, 1970; Spencer, 1970).

The current literature is replete with evaluations of the pre- and postoperative state based largely on subjective parameters. However, there is a relative paucity of objective assessments of the efficacy of direct aortocoronary revascularization. One method of approach to this problem is by the use of graded exercise during electrocardiography (treadmill testing) as a means of indirectly assessing myocardial oxygen demand and coronary blood flow.

If aortocoronary revascularization of the heart does improve myocardial oxygenation with a resultant relief in ischemic myocardial pain, then patients with a preoperative exercise limitation due to angina should demonstrate an improved exercise tolerance postoperatively if oxygen delivery is increased. Furthermore, enhanced postoperative exercise tolerance should correlate well with the disappearance of ischemic S-T changes in the postoperative exercise cardiogram and with graft patency (Lapin et al, 1973).

In an effort to study this hypothesis, we have evaluated the pre- and postoperative response to maximal graded work by the use of treadmill electrocardiography in 81 patients undergoing direct aortocoronary bypass grafting for ischemic heart disease in an effort to demonstrate objective changes attributable to surgery. Heart rate at the point when the target rate was reached or at the time of positivity of the test was used as a corollary to myocardial oxygen demand and coronary blood flow and has been related to graft patency and subjective improvement.*

METHODS

Patient Profile (Table 1)

TABLE 1. Age, Sex Distribution, and Preoperative Risk Factors of 81 Patients Included in Study

	MALE		FEMALE		TOTAL	
	No.	%	No.	%	No.	%
Sex	72	89	9	11	81	
Prev. MI	39	54	5	55	44	54
Angina at rest	24	33	3	33	27	33
Preinfarctional angina	6	8	2	22	8	10

Eighty-one normotensive or controlled hypertensive patients, both pre- and postoperatively, ranging from 28 to 73 years of age were studied

Supported by Minnesota Medical Foundation, Research Number 0697 5884.

* Target rate: 85 percent of age-adjusted maximal heart rate.

before and three months after coronary artery bypass by treadmill cardiography and cineangiography. Twenty-seven of these patients had ischemic changes on resting cardiograms and had angina at rest. These patients were considered too ill to undergo exercise evaluation and were considered by definition to have a positive preoperative treadmill test. However, all patients did undergo postoperative treadmill testing. All patients had chronic disabling angina preoperatively, with 54 percent having had at least one myocardial infarction prior to surgery.

These 81 patients constituted 87 percent of the survivors of 98 elective coronary artery bypass procedures without concomitant ventricular aneurysmectomy or valve replacement. The three month postoperative mortality for these patients was five percent. The only selection criterion for this study was that the patients agreed to a pre- and postoperative evaluation. However, pre- or postoperatively, patients who were unable to reach their age-related target rate due to generalized fatigue, but not ischemic changes on EKG or angina, were excluded from the study because they were felt to have an inconclusive test not reflecting maximal stress. None of the patients was too ill postoperatively to undergo exercise evaluation.

Angiographic Technique

Selective coronary arteriography and selective catheterization of the bypass graft was carried out with all patients at rest in the supine position following light sedation with Seconal. Angiographic catheters were introduced into the femoral artery percutaneously and passed in a retrograde fashion to the level of the coronary ostia and to the ostia of the bypass graft. Five to 10 cc of 60 percent Renografin was selectively injected into each coronary ostia and the bypass graft, while 60 frames/sec of 35 mm cine filming was being performed or cut films at 3 to 5/sec were being taken (Judkins, 1968; Sones and Shirey, 1962).

The coronary vessels were graded as normal, less than 50 percent occluded, 50 percent to 75 percent occluded, 75 percent to 95 percent occluded and totally occluded. The bypass graft was graded as either patent or occluded.

Surgical Technique

Reversed autologous saphenous veins were harvested from the medial thigh and were grafted from the ascending aorta to a point distal to the stenosis as determined by the preoperative angiogram and observations made at surgery. In 23 patients, an internal mammary-coronary artery anastomosis was done in lieu of or in addition to a saphenous vein graft. Aortic anastomoses were done with partial occlusion of the vessel. All coronary anastomoses were done under ischemic hypothermic arrest with extracorporeal oxygenation.

Exercise Testing

A complete clinical evaluation and a control resting standard 12 lead electrocardiogram were done prior to exercise evaluation both pre- and postoperatively. A multistage treadmill test of maximal exercise capacity was then done by having the patient exercise for three minutes at each stage on a variably inclined treadmill (Bruce and Horsten, 1969; Bruce, 1971). Treadmill speeds were progressively increased as follows: 1.7 mph at 10 percent grade, 2.5 mph at 12 percent grade, 3.4 mph at 14 percent grade, 4.2 mph at 16 percent grade, 4.9 mph at 18 percent grade, 5.5 mph at 20 percent grade, and 6.0 mph at 22 percent grade. During exercise, continuous cardiac monitoring was carried out by a V_5 precordial lead. After cessation of exercise, a standard simultaneous 12-lead electrocardiogram was done in the supine position and continued every 60 seconds for four minutes, then every two minutes for a full 10-minute recovery period or longer if indicated. The test was considered positive and terminated if during the exercise period prior to or after attaining the target rate, or during the recovery period, any electrocardiographic abnormalities not present on the resting cardiogram developed—namely, progressive horizontal elevation or depression of the S-T segment ≥ 1 mm (0.1 mv) in any lead.

The test was terminated and considered inconclusive if any of the following developed prior to attaining the target rate or before the test was judged as positive:

1. symptoms suggestive of cerebral vascular insufficiency or leg claudication;
2. excessive dyspnea, fatigue, cyanosis, pallor;
3. a fall in blood pressure or heart rate with increasing exercise;
4. chest pain with negative EKG findings;
5. development of arrhythmias such as multifocal or unifocal PVC's (two or three in close succession or in runs of two or more), heart block, or tachyarrhythmias;

6. development of incomplete or complete bundle branch block, either right or left.

Patients whose tests were terminated for any of the above reasons were not included in this study since they were felt to have an inconclusive test not reflecting maximal stress.

Data Analysis

The postoperative treadmill test was considered positive but improved if the test met the criteria for positivity as mentioned above but with a heart rate at the time of positivity 20 percent greater than the preoperative value. Values for pre- and postoperative maximal heart rate and functional class were tested by the Student's t-test for statistical signficance and found to have a P-value of < 0.005. Postoperatively the patients were categorized into one of three treadmill groups: Group I: improved (includes both patients who were positive preoperatively and negative postoperatively as well as those who were positive preoperatively and postoperatively but significantly improved postoperatively); Group II: unchanged over preoperative; and Group III: worse than preoperative.

RESULTS

Clinical Evaluation

Of the 81 patients studied, 69 (85 percent) related symptomatic improvement after surgery, whereas 12 (15 percent) did not. Of the 62 patients who were in an employable age group (up to 60 years old), 36 (58 percent) were unable to work preoperatively because of disabling

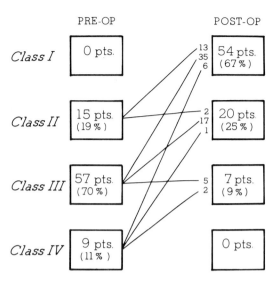

FIG. 1. Changes in preoperative NYHA Functional Class following aortocoronary bypass procedures in 81 patients.

angina. Of this disabled group, 19 (53 percent) returned to work prior to the three-month postoperative examination.

Preoperatively, of the 81 patients, there were none in the NYHA Functional Class I, there were 15 (19 percent) in Class II, 57 (70 percent) in Class III, and nine (11 percent in Class IV. Postoperatively there were 54 (67 percent) in Class I, 20 (25 percent) in Class II, seven (9 percent) in Class III, and 0 in Class IV (Fig. 1).

Exercise Test (Fig. 2)

Preoperatively four patients (5 percent) had a negative test and 77 patients (95 percent) had a positive test. Twenty-seven (27) patients

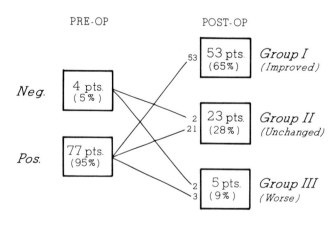

FIG. 2. Changes in preoperative exercise electrocardiograms after aortocoronary bypass procedures in 81 patients included in study.

FIG. 3. Composition of postop treadmill groups expressed as percent NYHA Functional Class.

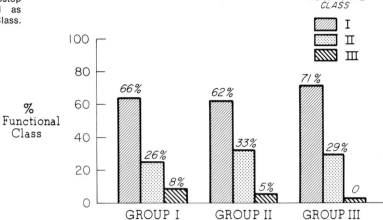

were not studied preoperatively because of angina at rest and were considered by definition to have a positive test. Postoperatively, the patients were divided into three groups: Group I: (improved) 53 patients (65 percent); Group II: (unchanged) 23 patients (28 percent); and Group III: (worse) five patients (6 percent). Group II included two patients who had negative tests pre- and postoperatively. Likewise, Group III included two patients who had negative tests preoperatively and positive tests postoperatively.

The relationship between postoperative treadmill status and NYHA Functional Class is summarized in Figure 3. Treadmill Group I (improved) had 66 percent in NYHA Functional Class I, 26 percent in Class II, and eight percent in Class III. Treadmill Group II (unchanged) had 62 percent in Functional Class I, 32 percent in Class II, and five percent in Class III. Group III (worse) had 71 percent in Class I, 26 percent in Class II, and 0 percent in Class III.

If one looks at the inverse of this relationship—namely, the number of patients within each functional class with respect to postoperative treadmill grouping—there is no significant difference in the distribution of the patients. Functional Class I had 65 percent in Treadmill Group I, 28 percent in Group II, and seven percent in Group III. Functional Class II had 65 percent in Treadmill Group I, 30 percent in Group II, and 5 percent in Group III. Functional Class III had 71 percent in Treadmill Group I, 29 percent in Group II, and none in Group III.

Graft Patency

In the 81 patients there were a total of 127 grafts, with overall patency rate of 75 percent.

There were 37 single grafts, 42 double grafts, and two triple grafts. Twenty-eight of the single grafts were patent at three months; 22 of the 42 double-graft patients had both vein segments patent at the time of study; 18 had one open and one occluded; and two had both occluded. In the group with triple grafts (two patients), one patient had all grafts patent and one had one graft occluded.

Graft Patency vs Exercise Test (Table 2)

SINGLE GRAFTS. Of the 28 grafts that were open, 21 (75 percent) were in the Treadmill Group I (improved), five (18 percent) were in the Group II (unchanged), and two (seven percent) were in Group III (worse). Of the nine occluded single grafts, six (67 percent) were in Group I, two (22 percent) in Group II, and one (11 percent) in Group III.

TABLE 2. Relation of Postoperative Graft Patency to Postoperative Treadmill Group

GRAFT STATUS	POSTOP TREADMILL GROUP		
	Group I	Group II	Group III
Single (37 pts.)			
Open	21	5	2
Closed	6	2	1
Double (42 pts.)			
2 open	14	7	1
1:1	11	6	1
2 closed	1	1	0
Triple (2 pts.)			
3 open	–	1	–
2:1	–	1	–
1:2	–	–	–
3 closed	–	–	–

DOUBLE GRAFTS. Of the 22 double grafts that had both bypass segments patent, 14 (64 percent) were in Treadmill Group I, seven (32 percent) in Group II, and one (5 percent) in Group III. In the group with one occluded (18 patients), 11 (61 percent) were in Group I, six (33 percent) in Group II, and two (11 percent) in Group III. In the two patients with both grafts occluded one patient was in Group I and one in Group II.

TRIPLE GRAFTS. Of the two patients with triple grafts, both were in Group II, one had all grafts patent and one had one graft occluded.

The relation between over-all graft patency within each Treadmill Group is demonstrated in Table 3. Group I had a patency rate of 76 percent, Group II of 73 percent, and Group III of 71 per cent. The inverse relationship is depicted in Table 4. In the group of patients with all grafts patent (51 patients), 35 patients (69 percent) were in Treadmill Group I, 13 (25 percent) in Group II, and three (6 percent) in Group III. In the group with all grafts closed at three months (12 patients) seven (59 percent) were in Group I, four (33 percent) in Group II, and one (8 percent) was in Group III.

TABLE 3. Overall Graft Patency within Each Postoperative Treadmill Group

	TOTAL	NO. PATENT	% PATENT
Group I	79	60	76
Group II	41	30	73
Group III	7	5	71

DISCUSSION

The use of coronary artery bypass procedures for the treatment of ischemic heart disease is widespread. To a large degree, the generalized acceptance of this procedure is based on its ability to relieve the pain of disabling angina at an acceptable operative risk to the patient. Early reports relevant to the efficacy of this procedure have dealt primarily with subjective parameters. Only recently has the major focus of investigators shifted to an objective evaluation of pre- and postoperative myocardial function in an effort to determine what, if any, changes are related to surgery.

One method of approach to the problem is

TABLE 4. Relation of Number of Patients with All Grafts Patent, One Open/One Closed and All Closed to Postop Treadmill Group

	ALL PATENT		1 OPEN/ 1 CLOSED		ALL CLOSED	
	No. Pts.	%	No. Pts.	%	No. Pts.	%
Group I	35	69	11	61	7	59
Group II	13	25	6	33	4	33
Group III	3	6	1	6	1	8
Total	51		18		12	

to assess, preoperatively and postoperatively, the changes in attainable myocardial oxygen consumption (MVO_2) and, therefore, coronary blood flow, at the time of appearance of ischemic changes on EKG during graded exercise. It has been previously shown that the heart rate times blood pressure product is an accurate index of myocardial oxygen demand (Katz and Feinberg, 1958; O'Brien et al, 1965). However, more recently it has been demonstrated by Kitamura et al that heart rate alone affords a reasonable approximation of myocardial oxygen consumption and coronary blood flow (Kitamura et al, 1972). If it is assumed that angina and/or ischemic changes on EKG are due to a relative insufficiency of myocardial blood flow to a segment of myocardium, then improving the coronary blood flow to that segment should relieve ischemic pain and reverse, at least to some degree, the EKG changes. Furthermore, the reversal of such EKG changes should correlate well with graft patency and subjective parameters of improvement, changes in NYHA functional class.

If one views the postoperative treadmill groups with respect to graft patency (Table 3), it is surprising to find that all three treadmill groups reflect similar patency rates indicating that there may be no relation of postoperative treadmill function to graft patency. This indication is further confirmed if the patients are categorized by graft patency (Table 4) and then evaluated as to postoperative treadmill grouping. When this is done, there appears to be no statistically significant difference in the distribution of patients throughout the groups comprised of differing degrees of graft patency with respect to postoperative treadmill performance. Furthermore, if one examines the postoperative treadmill groups with respect to postoperative NYHA functional class, there is no significant difference in the distribution of the NYHA functional categories within the three treadmill groups.

These findings suggest that there may be

no relationship between postoperative improvement or nonimprovement in treadmill performance and graft patency. These findings are consonant with those of Hammermeister, who reported significant improvement in functional aerobic impairment (FAI) as determined by exercise electrocardiography in patients with one or more grafts closed (Hammermeister et al, 1974).

There are several possible explanations for the failure of this study to document a consistently positive relationship between improvement in exercise tolerance (and supposedly coronary blood flow) and graft patency:

1. Demonstration of a patent graft by angiographic techniques is a qualitative assessment of graft patency and as such bears no relation to quantitative flow *in vivo*.

2. Neovascularization of the coronary macrocirculation may not uniformly be reflected in ischemic areas due to obstructions in the microcirculation of the affected areas that are not apparent on preoperative angiograms.

3. Frank infarction of the preoperatively borderline ischemic myocardium may frequently occur during surgery resulting in an unidentifiable postoperative scar that does not generate ischemic pain and EKG changes and as such may be responsible for the abolition of preoperative ischemic changes and pain.

4. Changes in exercise performance in ischemic myocardium may not accurately reflect changes in myocardial oxygen demand (MVO$_2$) and coronary blood flow in the same manner as it does in normal myocardium.

The lack of quantitative correlation between graft patency and changes in exercise performance is consonant with the lack of correlation between graft patency and changes in other parameters of ventricular function such as systolic ejection fraction, end diastolic pressure, and cardiac index reported by others and observed in our unpublished data.

SUMMARY

Eighty-one patients undergoing coronary artery bypass procedures for ischemic heart disease were studied preoperatively and three months postoperatively by treadmill electrocardiography. Sixty-five percent demonstated impovement in exercise tolerance postoperatively, 28 percent were unchanged, and seven percent were worse. There was no significant correlation between graft patency and postoperative treadmill performance.

References

Anderson RP, Hadom R, Wood J, Starr A: Direct revascularization of the heart: early clinical experience with 200 patients. J Thorac Cardiovasc Surg 63:353, 1971

Bruce RA: Exercise testing of patients with coronary heart disease. Ann Clin Res 3:323, 1971

Bruce RA, Hornsten TR: Exercise testing in evaluation of patients with ischemic heart disease. Prog Cardiovasc Dis II:371, 1969

Cannom DS, Miller DC, Shumway NE, et al: The long term follow-up of patients undergoing saphenous vein bypass surgery. Circulation 49:77 Jan 1974

Favaloro RG: Surgical treatment of coronary arteriosclerosis by saphenous vein graft technique. Am J Cardiol 28:493, 1971

Hammermeister E, Kennedy JW, Hamilton GW, et al: Aorto-coronary saphenous vein bypass: failure of successful grafting to improve resting left ventricular function in chronic angina. N Engl J Med 290 (4):186, Jan 24, 1974

Johnson WD, Lepley D: An Aggressive Surgical Approach to Coronary Artery Disease. J Thorac Cardiovasc Surg 59:128, 1970

Judkins MP: Percutaneous transfemoral selective coronary arteriography. Radiol Clin N Am 6:467, 1968

Katz LN, Feinberg H: The relation of cardiac effort to myocardial oxygen consumption and coronary flow. Circ Res 6:656–59, 1965

Kitamura K, Jorgensen CR, Gobel FL, Taylor HL, Wang Y: Hemodynamic correlates of myocardial oxygen consumption during upright exercise. J Appl Physiol 32(4):516–22, 1972

Lapin ES, Murray JA, Bruce RA, Wintersheid L: Changes in maximal exercise performance in the evaluation of saphenous vein bypass surgery. Circulation 47: 1164 June 1973

O'Brien KP, Higgs LM, Glancy DL, Epstein SE: Hemodynamic accompaniments of angina: a comparison during angina induced by exercise and atrial pacing. Circulation 39:735, 1965

Reul GJ, Morris GC, Howell JF, Crawford ES, Selter WJ: Current concepts in coronary artery surgery: a critical anaysis of 1,287 patients. Ann Thorac Surg 14:243, 1972

Spencer FC: Venous bypass grafts for occlusive disease of the coronary arteries. J Thorac Cardiovasc Surg 59:128, 1970

Sones FM, Shirey EK: Cine Coronary Arteriography. Mod Concepts Cardiovasc Dis 31:735, 1962

III

SYMPTOMATIC RESULTS OF AORTOCORONARY BYPASS COMPARED WITH POSTOPERATIVE EXERCISE PERFORMANCE

Robert E. Cline, Arthur J. Merrill, Charles N. Thomas, Raymond G. Armstrong, and William Stanford

INTRODUCTION

Aortocoronary bypass has now become a widely accepted surgical procedure for the treatment of angina pectoris. Symptomatic improvement can be obtained in the majority of patients with a low operative morbidity and mortality in properly selected cases (Cooley et al, 1973; Gott et al, 1973; Thomas et al, 1973). Although numerous clinical reports have documented the excellent subjective response to this procedure, there is a lack of objective information regarding the postoperative physiologic response with respect to cardiac performance or exercise capacity. The placebo effect of both surgical and medical methods of treatment of angina have been recognized for many years (Cobb et al, 1959; Dimond et al, 1960; Ross, 1972). If the current enthusiasm for coronary bypass surgery is to be maintained, additional objective evidence of benefit should be obtained in the postoperative period. This has stimulated us to perform these preoperative studies of exercise performance in a group of patients having coronary bypass surgery for a correlation with the angiographic and symptomatic results that followed operation.

METHOD

This study utilized 30 adult patients who were selected from a group of more than 150 individuals who had undergone aortocoronary bypass procedures at Wilford Hall USAF Medical Center. Patients were selected for this study on the basis of having had complete preoperative and postoperative angiographic evaluation and studies of treadmill exercise performance. Each patient had a detailed clinical evaluation including complete history and physical examination with careful assessment of his functional classification (NYHA). All of the patients had failed to respond to a strict trial of conservative medical therapy and were considered to be incapacitated by angina pectoris preoperatively. None of the patients had any other complicating factors such as ventricular aneurysm or valvular heart disease. Preoperative and postoperative selective coronary angiograms were performed using either the Sones or Judkins technique. Single-plane left ventricular angiograms were used for calculation of ejection fraction and assessment of abnormal patterns of ventricular contraction. The same angiographic studies were repeated six to eight weeks following surgery with the addition of selective angiography of the coronary bypass grafts.

Exercise testing was conducted using the graded Bruce multistage treadmill test protocol (Bruce and Hornsten, 1969) with exercise continued for three minutes at each stage (Stage I: 1.7 mph at 10 percent grade; Stage II: 2.5 mph, 12 percent grade; Stage III: 3.4 mph, 14 percent grade; and Stage IV: 4.2 mph, 16 percent grade). The exercise test was terminated with the onset of severe angina, fatigue, ischemic EKG changes, or significant fall in blood pressure or heart rate. Heart rate and systolic blood pressure were recorded prior to exercise, at the end of each stage of testing, and at the time the test was terminated. Treadmill testing was performed on all patients five to seven days preoperatively and six to eight weeks following surgery.

The operative procedures were carried out using standard techniques of cardiopulmonary bypass with mild hypothermia. Autogenous saphenous veins were employed for the bypass grafts in 26 patients. In four patients the left internal mammary artery was anastomosed directly to the left anterior descending coronary artery. Twenty-two of the patients had two or more coronary bypass grafts, while eight of the patients had a single graft procedure. None of the patients had Vineberg intramyocardial mammary artery implants.

RESULTS

Postoperative clinical evaluation of these 30 patients revealed that 28 (90 percent) had dramatic improvement in their anginal symptoms, and 26 (87 percent) were totally free of angina pectoris. Four of these patients who had relief of angina postoperatively developed new symptoms of congestive heart failure that responded to medical therapy.

Postoperative cardiac catheterization revealed patency of all bypass grafts in 14 patients and occlusion of one or more grafts in the remaining 16 patients, five of whom had occlusion of all their bypass grafts. In spite of closure of all grafts, four of these five patients were relieved of their angina but developed symptoms of congestive heart failure. Left ventricular angiograms suitable for postoperative analysis were obtained in 22 pa-

tients. Six with normal preoperative ejection fractions showed no postoperative changes. Improvement in the postoperative ejection fraction or ventricular wall motion was observed in seven patients. There were nine individuals (seven of whom had one or more occluded grafts) who demonstrated a postoperative reduction in their ejection fraction or impaired patterns of ventricular contraction.

The results of the postoperative exercise testing are included in Table 1, which summarizes all of the postoperative results. The maximum heart rate, duration of exercise and functional aerobic impairment are not included since they are less reliable indices of cardiac performance than the Rate Pressure Product (RPP) (Redwood et al, 1972). Although 20 of the 30 patients demonstrated an increased RPP postoperatively, the mean change for the entire group was not statistically significant ($P > 0.10$). However, if the five patients with all grafts occluded are eliminated from the analysis, a significant overall improvement in the maximum RPP was observed ($P < 0.05$). More importantly, there was noted to be a highly significant change in the postoperative RPP in the 14 patients with all grafts patent ($P < 0.001$). This is in contrast to the absence of any significant change in RPP in the 16 patients with one or more of their grafts occluded at the time of the postoperative study.

Figure 1 illustrates the individual preoperative and postoperative changes in maximum RPP and provides a comparison between patients with all bypass grafts patent and those with one or more occluded grafts.

TABLE 1. Postoperative Maximal RPP (Heart Rate Times Blood Pressure Product) Obtained during Bruce Multistaged Treadmill Exercise Testing

	ALL PATIENTS (30)	ALL GRAFTS PATENT (14)	ONE OR MORE GRAFTS OCCLUDED (16)
Angina			
No. pts. improved	28	14	14
No. pts. worse	2	0	2
Comments	90% improved	100% improved	88% improved
Exercise testing [HR X BP (RPP)]			
No. pts. improved	20	14	6
No. pts. worse	10	0	10
Comments	Mean Δ RPP + 4.5 X 10^3 (p: ns)	Mean Δ RPP + 13.5 X 10^3 (p $<$ 0.001)	Mean Δ RPP − 3.2 X 10^3 (p: ns)
Ventriculogram[a] (EF)			
No. pts. improved	7	4	3
No. pts. worse	9	2	7
Comments	No change in 6 pts.	No change in 4 pts.	No change in 2 pts.

[a]*Only 22 patients had ventriculograms that were adequate for measurement of ejection fraction.*

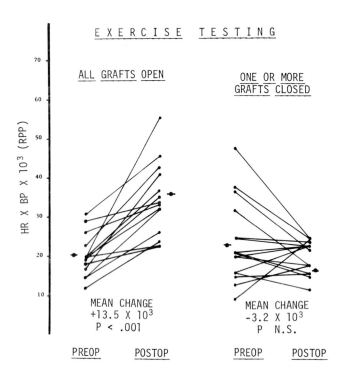

FIG. 1. Summary of postoperative symptomatic results, changes in maximal-exercise-induced RPP (heart rate times blood pressure product), and ventriculographic observations in the 30 patients studied.

The postoperative ventriculograms in eight patients were inadequate for study of patterns of contraction or ejection factors. Six of the remaining 22 patients had normal preoperative ventricular ejection fractions and wall motion that was unchanged postoperatively. In seven patients there was significant improvement in the postoperative ventriculogram. Nine individuals had postoperative reduction in ejection fraction and impairment of wall motion; seven of these had one or more occluded grafts.

A detailed analysis of each patient's ventricular angiograms demonstrated a good correlation between graft patency, increase of exercise performance, and improvement of wall motion abnormalities on the postoperative left ventricular angiograms. Three patients, however, were observed to have an increased postoperative exercise capacity but a reduction in the ventricular ejection fraction with appearance of new wall motion abnormalities.

DISCUSSION

The majority of these patients were relieved of their anginal symptoms by the surgical procedure. It should be noted, however, that four of the five patients with all their grafts occluded at the time of the postoperative angiography had improvement in their angina, which emphasizes the

problems encountered in defining surgical results on the basis of subjective clinical evaluation alone. Dramatic symptomatic improvement in these patients may either result from a placebo effect or be a result of a perioperative myocardial infarction, which has been observed to occur in a significant number of patients who undergo coronary bypass surgery (Brewer et al, 1973). The additional postoperative physiologic and angiographic assessment of these patients, therefore, provided the only reliable method of accurately defining the therapeutic benefits of these surgical procedures.

We limited our analysis of postoperative exercise performance to the measurement of the product of the systolic blood pressure and the heart rate (RPP), which has been observed to represent a reliable index of myocardial oxygen demand (Robinson, 1967). The change in the RPP reflects the capacity of the heart to increase its work in response to exercise. This response, of course, depends upon the availability of oxygen, which, in turn, is related to the coronary blood supply. Therefore, the ability to achieve an increased RPP postoperatively without symptoms demonstrates the capacity for greater cardiac work, which generally requires an enhanced myocardial blood supply, indicating a successful myocardial revascularization procedure. Other exercise parameters such as maximum duration of exercise are affected by overall physical conditioning and may not reflect alterations in cardiac performance (Redwood et al,

1972) and, therefore, are not included in this analysis. Although the maximum RPP for the total group of patients was not significantly improved following surgery, when the five patients with occluded bypass grafts were eliminated, there was an overall increase in the maximal RPP. This, of course, suggests a good correlation between functional improvement and objective anatomical evidence of revascularization—ie, graft patency.

The most important observation in this regard was the highly significant postoperative increase in the RPP of the 14 patients who had all grafts patent at the time of the postoperative study. This improvement in exercise performance directly contrasts with the lack of any overall increase in the postoperative RPP of the remaining 16 patients who had one or more of their bypass grafts occluded. Lapin et al (1973) in a similar study were unable to demonstrate significant improvements in the exercise performance of their group of patients with occluded grafts. Bartel et al (1973) have also reported a greater incidence of ischemic ECG change during treadmill testing in patients with "incomplete revascularization" (ie, one or more occluded grafts or stenotic coronary lesions that were not bypassed) as compared with patients who had "complete revascularization." Matloff et al (1973), in a recent postoperative study of 72 patients, have also observed a significant correlation between clinical improvement and graft patency. Our findings provide additional objective evidence to support the concept of these three previous reports (Lapin et al, 1973; Matloff et al, 1973; Redwood et al, 1972) that angiographic evidence of successful revascularization correlates well with the observed improvement in exercise capacity or anginal symptoms.

The analysis of the alterations in the ventricular angiograms of our patients provides useful additional information that can be correlated with the changes in exercise capacity to help define the functional benefit achieved by the coronary bypass procedures. More than half of our patients had either normal or improved postoperative ejection fractions, which correlated well with graft patency and the ability to increase the maximum postoperative rate times pressure product. Most of the remaining patients with reduced postoperative ejection fraction had one or more occluded grafts and reduced exercise performance. The most relevant ventriculographic observations relate to the isolated changes in segmental abnormalities of wall motion or contractile patterns of ischemic zones that were unique to each patient and were impossible to quantitate numerically. They did, however, permit an objective assessment of the physio-

logic benefit of the individual grafts. It was evident from a critical review of the ventricular angiograms that those individuals with regions of impaired ventricular contraction before surgery usually demonstrated improvement postoperatively if all of the grafts supplying these areas were patent. Conversely, little change or, more often, progression of ventricular asynergy was often observed in the patients with occluded grafts and was usually accompanied by a reduction in the calculated ejection fraction.

Although these abnormalities in wall motion are impossible to quantitate, they are easily recognized and, when correlated with the areas of coronary stenosis, graft patency, and changes in exercise performance, constitute a valuable part of the evaluation of surgical results. Chatterjee et al (1973), in a recent review of postoperative hemodynamic and angiographic results in 29 patients with patent bypass grafts, noted a similar improvement in segmental wall motion abnormalities following successful revascularization. They observed greatest improvement in eight patients with preinfarction syndrome and no previous infarction, which adds credence to the concept that normal function can be restored to ischemic, but viable myocardium by coronary bypass procedures. However, the occasional disparity that was observed in some of our patients, between enhanced exercise capacity and lack of ventriculographic improvement, emphasizes that failure to employ both exercise testing and angiography in the follow-up evaluation can lead to incorrect conclusions regarding the physiologic benefit that is obtained from coronary bypass procedures.

These observations of the postoperative improvement of clinical status, exercise performance, segmental wall motion, and graft patency help to confirm the hypothesis that successful anatomical myocardial revascularization usually produces physiologic benefit in addition to symptomatic relief of disabling angina pectoris. This study also illustrates the importance of objective physiologic testing for the proper assessment of surgical results since the relief of symptoms or the patency of some of the grafts does not always result in improved cardiac performance.

SUMMARY

Thirty adult patients who underwent coronary bypass surgery had complete preoperative and postoperative studies that included a careful clinical evaluation, cardiac catheterization, and standardized treadmill exercise testing. The majority of these patients had relief of their angina pectoris by the surgical procedure. Fourteen of these patients with all grafts patent were essentially asymptomatic and had a significant improvement in exercise performance. In contrast, although most of the remaining 16 patients with occlusion of one or more grafts had relief of their angina, there was no overall significant improvement in their exercise performance. Postoperative change of left ventricular ejection fraction or ventricular contraction patterns were in most instances similar in direction and magnitude to the results obtained with exercise testing. These follow-up data indicate that significant physiologic benefit is associated with anatomic evidence of "complete revascularization" as demonstrated by the postoperative angiographic studies. Although patients with one or more occluded grafts may have relief of angina, this does not ensure an improvement of exercise capacity or a correction of ventricular wall motion abnormalities. These observations emphasize the need for additional efforts to perform multiple postoperative physiologic studies in addition to angiographic confirmation of bypass graft patency. This will permit a more objective assessment of surgical results and help to define guidelines for the future clinical application of these revascularization procedures.

References

Bartel AG, Behar VS, Peter RH, Orgain ES, Kong Y: Exercise stress testing in evaluation of aortocoronary bypass surgery. Circulation 58:141, 1973

Brewer DL, Bilbro RH, Bartel AG: Myocardial infarction as a complication of coronary bypass surgery. Circulation 47:58, 1973

Bruce RA, Hornsten TR: Exercise stress testing in evaluation of patients with ischemic heart disease. Prog Cardiovasc Dis 11:5, 1969

Chatterjee MB, Swan JC, Parmley WW, et al: Influence of direct myocardial revascularization on left ventricular asynergy and function on patients with coronary heart disease. Circulation 57:276, 1973

Cobb LA, Thomas GI, Dillard DH, Merendino KA, Bruce RA: An evaluation of internal mammary ligation by a double-blind technic. N Engl J Med 260:22, 1959

Cooley DA, Dawson JT, Hallman GL, et al. Aorto-coronary saphenous vein bypass. Ann Thorac Surg 16, 1973

Dimond EG, Kittle CF, Crockett JE: Comparison of internal mammary artery ligation and sham operation for angina pectoris. Am J Cardiol 5:483, 1960

Gott VL, Brawley RK, Donahoo JS, Griffith LS: Current surgical approach to ischemic heart disease. Curr Probl Surg, May 1973

Lapin ES, Murray JA, Bruce RA, Winterscheid L: Changes in maximal exercise performance in the evaluation of saphenous vein bypass surgery. Circulation 57:1164, 1973

Matloff HJ, Alderman EL, Wexler L, Shumway NE, Harrison DC: What is the relationship between the response of angina to coronary surgery and anatomical success? Circulation supp 3, 57 and 58: 168, 1973

Redwood DR, Rosing DR, Epstein SE: Circulatory and symptomatic effects of physical training in patients with coronary artery disease and angina pectoris. N Engl J Med 286:18, 1972

Redwood DR, Rosing DR, Goldstein RE, Beiser GD, Epstein SE: Importance of the design of an exercise protocol in the evaluation of patients with angina pectoris. N E J Med 286:959, 1972

Robinson BF: Relation of heart rate and systolic blood pressure to the onset of pain in angina pectoris. Circulation 40:1073, 1967

Ross RS: Surgery in ischemic heart disease, angina pectoris and myocardial infarction. DM, July 1972

Thomas CS, Alford WC, Burrus GR, Stoney WS: Aorto-to-coronary artery bypass grafting. Ann Thorac Surg 16:2, 1973

112

PATHOLOGY OF AORTOCORONARY ARTERY AUTOLOGOUS SAPHENOUS VEIN GRAFTS

Tomas Klima and John D. Milam

INTRODUCTION

Aortocoronary bypass using autologous saphenous vein graft is now the principal myocardial revascularization procedure being done.[3,4,5,8,9,10]

Since 1969, over 5,000 aortocoronary artery autologous saphenous vein graft bypass procedures were performed in the Division of Cardiovascular Surgery of the Texas Heart Institute. Of those who died, 159 nonselective postmortem examinations were performed and are included in our studies.

Our objectives were to review systematically morphologic findings of the patients who died at various time intervals following aortocoronary homologous saphenous vein bypass graft procedures and to correlate the clinical results with our findings.

MATERIAL AND METHODS

Of the total number of 159 patients, 37 single, 74 double, and 48 triple bypasses were done. Thus, 329 saphenous vein grafts were implanted. In all the bypasses, single grafts to single peripheral arterial branches were used, except in one instance, when a reverse Y-shaped graft was anastomosed into two coronary artery branches of the left coronary artery.

In one patient, a second bypass procedure was performed after six months, when the patient's condition gradually became worse and the original bypasses were found by angiography to be occluded. Three new saphenous vein grafts were placed after excision of two occluded grafts. At the end of surgery, the patient developed a cardiac arrest and could not be resuscitated.

Morphologic evaluation of the heart specimens included grading the severity of the coronary artery disease and assessing the degree of myocardial fibrosis as well as of myocardial hypertrophy. The findings were correlated with the postoperative survival in Table 1 and Figure 1 and by patient's age in Table 2 and Figure 2. In both instances, the incidence of recent myocardial infarct was also included and evaluated.

Although any grading of morphologic change is arbitrary, evaluation of the coronary arteriosclerosis was made in terms of minimal, moderate, and severe. Minimal change comprised an occasional arteriosclerotic plaque without significant compromise of the lumen. Moderate change included occasional stenosis which did not compromise the lumen more than 30 percent; severe change indicated a greater degree of arteriosclerosis than moderate, eg multiple stenosis, compromising the lumen more than 30 percent, or a single stenosis of a high degree (over 70 percent).

Minimal myocardial fibrosis was consistent with focal microscopic interstitial fibrosis. Moderate fibrosis implied a few foci of interstitial fibrosis observed grossly; any greater degree of fibrosis was designated as severe. This included multiple foci of fibrosis and transmural scars, as well as ventricular aneurysms, even when these were resected as a single lesion.

For grading of myocardial hypertrophy, the following classification was used:

	Males	Females
None	up to 360 g	up to 320 g
Minimal	up to 400 g	up to 360 g
Moderate	up to 500 g	up to 460 g
Severe	more than 500 g	more than 460 g

TABLE 1. Relationship of Severity of Coronary Arteriosclerosis, Myocardial Fibrosis, and Myocardial Hypertrophy to Survival Time after Surgery and Incident of Recent Myocardial Infarcts

	SURVIVAL TIME AFTER SURGERY IN DAYS									
	0	1	3	7	14	30	90	180	730	1,095
No. Myocardial infarcts	24	11	13	7	9	3	3	1	1	0
Coronary Sclerosis										
None or minimal	3	1	1	2	–	–	–	–	–	–
Moderate	4	1	1	1	2	1	1	–	1	–
Severe	53	36	14	11	10	6	6	1	2	1
% Infarcts moderate and severe	(45)	(30)	(87)	(59)	(75)	(43)	(43)	(100)	(33)	(0)
Myocardial fibrosis										
None or minimal	8	5	3	1	3	1	1	–	–	–
Moderate	13	9	11	3	2	–	–	–	–	–
Severe	39	24	2	10	7	6	6	1	3	1
% Infarcts moderate and severe	(46)	(33)	(100)	(54)	(100)	(50)	(50)	(100)	(33)	(0)
Myocardial hypertrophy										
None or minimal	6	3	1	–	1	1	–	–	–	–
Moderate	19	11	4	4	3	–	1	–	1	–
Severe	35	26	11	10	8	6	6	1	2	1
% Infarcts moderate and severe	(45)	(30)	(87)	(50)	(82)	(50)	(43)	(100)	(33)	(0)
Total no. cases	60	38	16	14	12	7	7	1	3	1
% MI	(40)	(29)	(83)	(50)	(75)	(43)	(43)	(100)	(33)	(0)

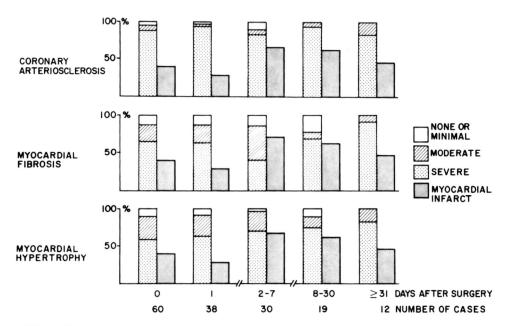

FIG. 1. Severity of coronary arteriosclerosis, myocardial fibrosis, and myocardial hypertrophy and the relationship to survival time after surgery; incidence of recent myocardial infarcts.

TABLE 2. Relationship of Severity of Coronary Arteriosclerosis, Myocardial Fibrosis, and Myocardial Hypertrophy to Patient's Age and Incidence of Recent Myocardial Infarcts

	AGE GROUP					
	20–29	30–39	40–49	50–59	60–69	70–79
No. Myocardial Infarcts	1	4	13	23	22	3
Coronary Sclerosis						
None or minimal	1	1	1	4	–	–
Moderate	–	1	1	6	3	1
Severe	1	5	28	51	47	8
% Infarcts moderate and severe	(100)	(67)	(45)	(40)	(44)	(33)
Myocardial Fibrosis						
None or minimal	1	1	4	13	4	–
Moderate	–	1	4	11	16	2
Severe	1	5	22	37	30	7
% Infarcts moderate and severe	(100)	(67)	(50)	(48)	(48)	(33)
Myocardial Hypertrophy						
None or minimal	–	2	4	6	1	–
Moderate	1	4	7	15	15	–
Severe	1	1	19	40	34	9
% Infarcts moderate and severe	(50)	(80)	(50)	(42)	(45)	(33)
Total no. cases	2	7	30	61	50	9
% MI	(50)	(57)	(43)	(38)	(44)	(33)

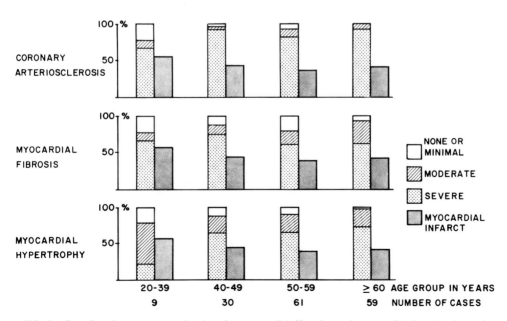

FIG. 2. Severity of coronary arteriosclerosis, myocardial fibrosis, and myocardial hypertrophy and the relationship to patient's age; incidence of recent myocardial infarcts.

TABLE 3. Other Cardiovascular Surgical Procedures in Addition to Aortocoronary Bypasses and Incidence of Recent Myocardial Infarcts

ADDITIONAL PROCEDURES	SURVIVAL TIME AFTER SURGERY IN DAYS								TOTAL
	0	1	3	7	14	30	90	180	
Aortic valve replacement[a]	10	3	5	2	1	1	2	1	25
Mitral valve replacement[a]	2	2	1	1	–	–	–	–	6
Resection of ventricular aneurysm	4	2	2	3	–	–	1	–	12
Resection of ascending aorta[b]	2	–	1	–	–	–	–	–	3
Total	18	7	9	6	1	1	3	1	46
Myocardial infarcts	3	1	4	3	1	0	2	1	15
Percent infarcts of total									(33)

[a]*In three patients both aortic and mitral valves have been replaced.*
[b]*Two patients with Marfan's Syndrome in addition to the repair of ascending aortic aneurysm by dacron graft; aortic valve replacement by prosthesis performed.*

Of the total of 159 patients in our series, 46 underwent coronary bypass procedures combined with other major cardiovascular corrective surgery; these are shown in Table 3, together with the incidence of recent myocardial infarctions.

The microscopic examination of the hearts included sections through the bypass graft at the takeoff point (inflow), from the middle segment, at the reentry point (outflow), and at any unusual or remarkable sites. Routine hemotoxylin-eosin stains were employed, and special stains (Verhoeff-Van Gieson, Masson's Trichrome, Movat's, Wilder's PAS, and Alcian Blue stains) were performed selectively.

In addition to routine autopsy techniques, postmortem coronary angiography was performed in 79 of the cases.

The first method employed was an aortic root injection, a combination of the methods of Baroldi, Scomazzoni, and Rissanen.[2,13] The aortic ostium is blocked by an inflated Foley catheter, and a 50 percent mixture of barium sulfate (Micropaque) in water (in some cases with 5 percent gelatin) is injected into the aortic root. The coronary arteries, as well as the aortocoronary bypasses, are perfused under a pressure of 120 mm Hg either simultaneously or in a two-step injection. In the later modification, the balloon of the Foley catheter was first overinflated in order to block the aortic ostium as well as the coronary artery ostia. The perfusion of the aortocoronary bypasses was started, the pressure maintained for three minutes, and the specimen X-rayed. The balloon was then partially deflated in order to open the coronary artery while maintaining occlusion of the aortic ostium. A second-step injection through the coronary arteries followed, again for a period of three minutes under a controlled pressure of 120 mm Hg.

The second method of injection was direct cannulation of the ostia of the bypasses as well as the coronary arteries. The barium-gelatin mass was injected, in some studies, into the bypasses first and then into the coronary arteries. In other cases, these steps were reversed. The modification of this technique allowed us to inject, separately, in some cases, the right coronary artery system and the corresponding bypasses; and, later, the left coronary system with its corresponding bypasses. Accurate pressure controls were not employed in the direct injections.

Flushing of the vascular system by saline was useful prior to injection of contrast material, since it prevented artifacts caused by air bubbles.

Following injection, X-ray films were exposed in different projections using mammography film by Kodak. Siemens and Faxitron X-ray machines were used. The first films included the pictures of the noninjected heart specimen in order to disclose any areas of calcification.

Following X-ray studies, the heart specimens were fixed in 10 percent formalin, and routine gross and microscopic examinations followed.

MORPHOLOGIC FINDINGS

Several studies on postoperative morphologic changes of saphenous vein grafts have been reported.[5,6,7,11,12,14,15] In general, our findings are in agreement with those previously published. The findings could be divided into two separate groups, depending on whether the graft remained patent or became occluded in the early postoperative period.

If the vein graft functions, it is exposed to a higher arterial pressure than the saphenous vein in its natural position. The intima undergoes fibrous proliferation, which becomes quite prominent with time, depending on the continued function of the graft (Fig. 3). Fibroblasts are seen somewhat circularly oriented within an intracellular substance, which is sometimes dense collagen but often initially has a myxoid character. Occasionally, smooth muscle cells appear (Fig. 4). The changes in the media are not striking and include mainly degeneration of elastic fibers. The adventitial tissue does not appear to be altered.

Similar changes have been observed in humans as well as in experimental animals (such as at venous sites of arteriovenous fistulas and venous grafts used in femoropopliteal and other bypasses), and the term "arterialization of the vein" has been frequently used. Since the resulting thickening of the graft wall does not correspond morphologically to an arterial wall, the term "intimal fibrous proliferation" has been proposed.[14,15]

The intimal proliferation at first builds up the mural strength of the graft as a response to the pressure; however, if the proliferation is excessive, it gradually reduces the lumen and eventually results in a fibrous obliteration. A transverse section through the graft generally has a circular configuration and rarely an elliptical shape.[1]

If the graft occludes in the early postoperative period, this is invariably caused by thrombosis (Fig. 5). There are several critical points where the thrombosis may start: (1) the proximal aorto-saphenous graft anastomosis (the so-called takeoff point of the graft), (2) the distal saphenous graft–coronary artery anastomosis (the reentry point of the graft), (3) sites of the venous valves of the graft, and (4) points of constriction of the graft, ie, at the ligature sites of the original venous branches. Complete thrombotic luminal occlusion of a segment at any level is then a starting point for a continuous and total thrombosis of the graft. A mural thrombus, for example, on a venous valve, might not result in a total occlusion of the graft.

The development of a thrombus within the graft follows the general alterations of a thrombus as seen at any place within the body: central liquefaction, peripheral organization, and recanalization develops into a strikingly rich system of newly formed capillaries and arterioles, not unlike the so-called cavernous transformation of a thrombus (Figs. 6, 7). In other cases of graft occlusion, a solid fibrous band is the result. In both instances, a transverse section through the obliterated graft discloses an elliptical and markedly flattened shape.

The intraluminal conditions causing thrombosis are stasis, turbulence, and/or reduced velocity of blood flow. The above-mentioned critical points are sites where one could certainly expect irregularities of blood flow. Therefore, different modifications of the anastomoses have been adapted to position them at suitable angles toward the aortic root, as well as toward the coronary arteries.

In rare instances, mechanical damage to the wall of the graft causes intramural hemorrhage or even necrosis. Thrombosis may often start in these parts of the graft.

Among the extramural causes of thrombotic occlusion, compression of the graft is naturally the most serious condition. This could be due to pericardial fibinous exudate (Fig. 8), and subsequent fibrous adhesions (Fig. 9), pericardial hemorrhage or effusion, another overlying and crossing graft at the takeoff site, or stretching of a short graft over the surface of the heart. Also kinking or angulation of the graft due to external traction by fibrinous or fibrous adhesions may compromise patency. In some instances, a combination of several different factors had to be considered, including the aforementioned causes as well as disorders of coagulation (Fig. 10).

EVALUATION OF POSTMORTEM ANGIOGRAPHY

The direct aortic root injection is preferable because the injection is performed under controlled pressure. Also no manipulation in the areas of the coronary artery and aortocoronary graft ostia is needed, and therefore any compromise of the lumen in these sites could be readily visualized by injection of the contrast mass. The method is technically more difficult, and some leaks through the aortic ostia occasionally occur that necessitate flushing of the cavity of the left ventricle to one of the many pulmonary veins via the left atrium prior to X-raying the specimen. If the contrast mass is not entirely removed from the left ventricle, the resulting films include artifacts.

The cannulation of the ostia of aortocoronary arteries is technically less difficult; however, insertion of any cannula can remove or dislocate intraluminal material causing a compromise of the lumen at the ostium. Perfusion of the peripheral cardiac circulation is usually better, and the different combinations mentioned above are very useful for evaluation of the collateral vasculature. The drawback of noncontrolled pressure should be borne in mind, since almost always the pressure exerted by a syringe greatly exceeds the physiologic arterial pressure of the coronary arteries *in vivo*. Therefore, visualization of the coronary artery system and the bypass grafts generally is more complete than might be expected *in vivo*.

Generally, angiography is a very valuable

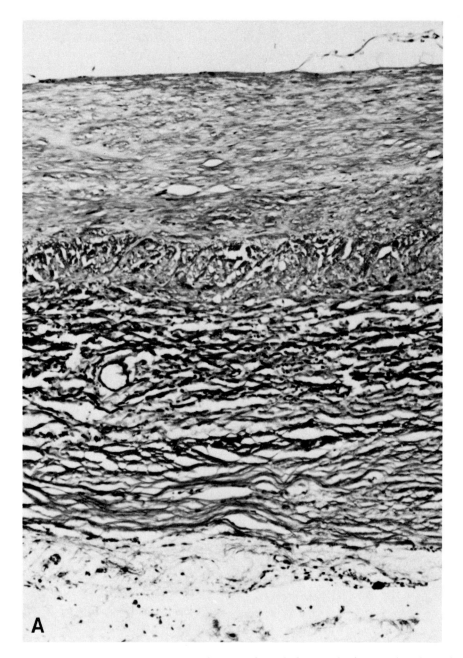

FIG. 3. A. Histologic section through a saphenous vein graft that remained patent for 14 months; 54-year-old man. Note intimal thickening by fibrous proliferation with collagenization of the thickened intima and media. Hematoxylin-eosin: ×109.

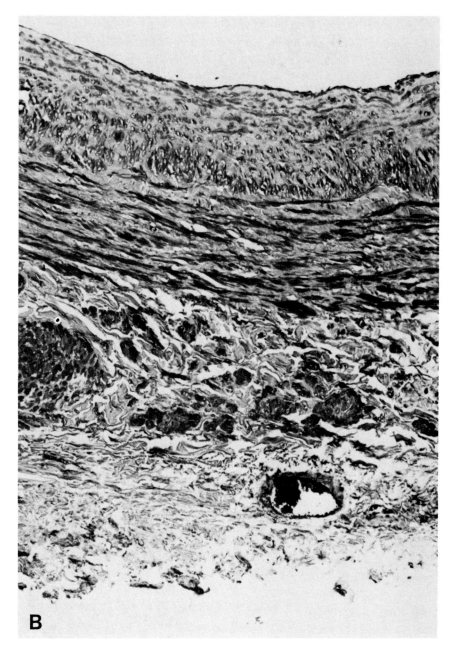

FIG. 3, B. Photomicrograph of a segment of a normal saphenous vein of 42-year-old man. Masson-Trichrome: ×106.

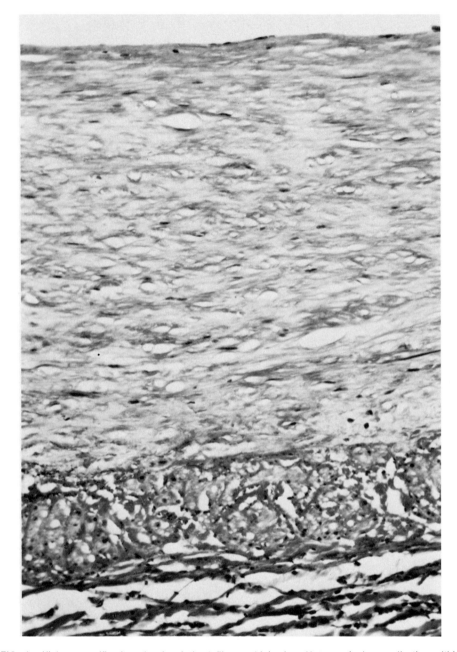

FIG. 4.   Higher magnification showing intimal fibrous thickening. Note marked vacuolization within the intimal fibrous proliferation. Elastic Verhoeff's-Van Gieson: ×280.

FIG. 5. Aortocoronary saphenous vein bypass, 6 days postoperative status; 44-year-old man. Patent bypass to the periphery of the left anterior descending coronary artery, thrombosed bypass to the left diagonal coronary artery branch. Anterior view. Plication of a recent myocardial infarct, lateral wall left ventricle, with attached Dacron strip.

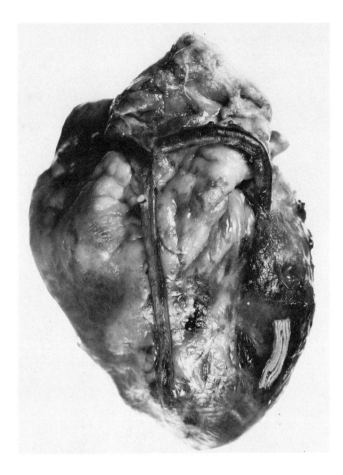

FIG. 6. Occluded bypass with multiple recanalized channels in the organized thrombus. Six months postoperative status. Note increase and irregular elastic fibers of the outer zone of tunica media and elastica. Elastic Verhoeff's-Van Gieson: ×54.

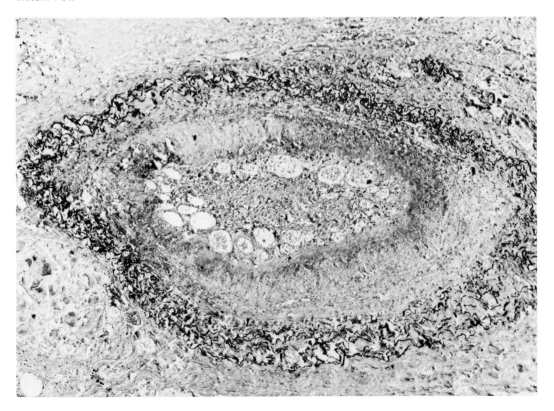

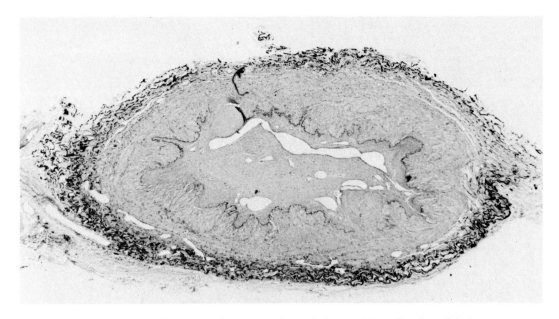

FIG. 7. Transverse section of an occluded saphenous vein bypass, 14 months after original surgery; 54-year old man. Note marked recanalization of the lumen otherwise occluded by organized thrombus. Elastic fibers are seen forming internal lamella, being increased and irregular in the outer zone, mostly in the adventitia. Elastic Verhoeff's-Van Gieson: ×44.

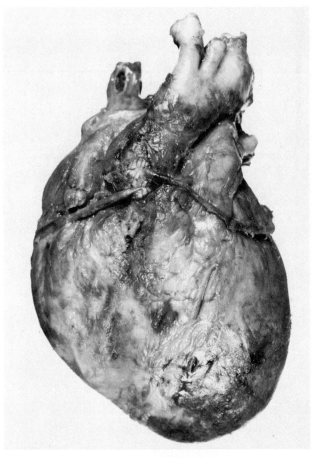

FIG. 8. Aortocoronary bypasses to right coronary artery and left obtuse marginal coronary artery. Three days postoperative obtuse status; 66-year-old female. Both venous grafts occluded by recent thrombosis. Anterior view.

FIG. 9. Aortocoronary artery bypasses, two years postoperative status; anterior view; 55-year-old male. Note extensive pericardial fibrous adhesions. Three grafts: the one to the right coronary artery is occluded; the grafts to the left anterior descending and left circumflex branches remained patent.

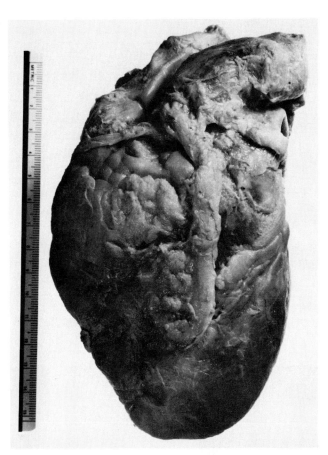

FIG. 10. High-power view of the occluded bypass to the left coronary artery, anterior descending branch, showing marked recanalization with one arteriole-like vascular channel, right lower portion of the picture. Note again elastic fibers forming internal lamella and increase in the adventitia. Elastic Verhoeff's-Van Gieson: ×77.

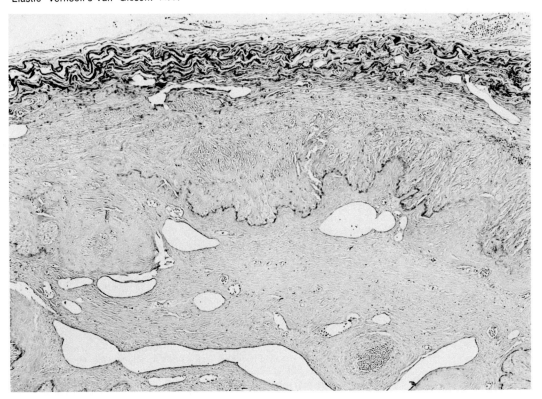

addition to the postmortem examination of the heart, regardless of the technique used. Combined with a proper gross and microscopic study, it invariably contributes to a better postmortem evaluation of the coronary circulation as well as of the grafts (Figs. 11 to 13).

DISCUSSION

Of a total of 159 patients who underwent postmortem examinations, 131 were males and 28 were females. The distribution year by year is shown in Table 4. The time of death following surgery varied from immediately postoperative to three years.

As seen in Table 5, the survival time for males and females does not significantly differ; therefore, further evaluation of our series is based

TABLE 4. Number of Autopsies in Persons Who Underwent Aortocoronary Saphenous Vein Bypass, 1969-73

	MALE	FEMALE	TOTAL
1969	–	1	1
1970	18	–	18
1971	29	7	36
1972	35	10	45
1973	49	10	59
Total	131	28	159

on the combined figures of both sexes. Also the data in Table 5 reveal that the majority of the fatalities survived one week or less following surgery; 71.7 percent survived three days or less, and 80.5 percent survived seven days or less. Only 11.9 percent of the patients in our series lived one

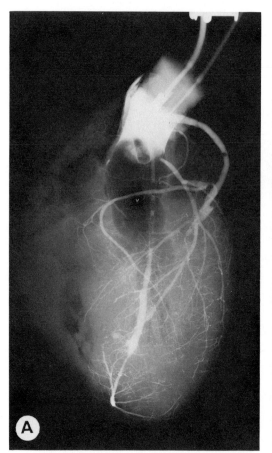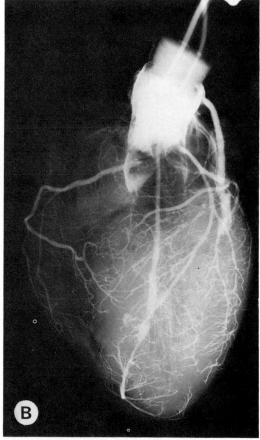

FIG. 11. Postmortem angiogram of a heart specimen with double aortocoronary bypass to the left anterior descending and left obtuse marginal coronary artery, 55-year-old man. Injection in two steps showing filling through the bypass only to the left coronary artery system (A); filling through both bypasses and coronary artery ostia showing the entire coronary system (B). Autopsy findings: minimal arteriosclerotic change of the main right coronary artery.

FIG. 12. Angiogram of a heart specimen showing filling through the bypass to the left anterior descending coronary artery. Fair filling of the periphery with retrograde extension to a point of occlusion of the left anterior coronary artery (arrow); 53-year-old female. Autopsy findings: single occlusion of the left anterior descending coronary artery by organized thrombus, otherwise minimal arteriosclerotic changes. Mitral valve replacement by prosthesis.

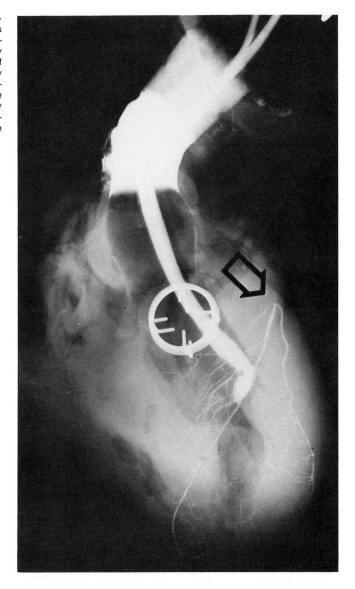

TABLE 5. Survival Time after Surgery in Days

DAYS AFTER SURGERY	MALE	FEMALE	TOTAL
0	47	13	60
1	32	6	38
3	14	2	16
7	14	–	14
14	9	3	12
30	6	1	7
90	5	2	7
180	–	1	1
365	–	–	–
730	3	–	3
1,095	1	–	1
Total	131	28	159

month or longer. The critical care time appears to be in the first few days postoperatively.

In Table 6, there is grouping of the cases according to length of survival and the incidence of occluded grafts. Of 126 grafts in patients dying immediately after surgery, none were occluded, and of 88 grafts in patients dying during the first 24 hours after surgery, four (5 percent) were occluded. The percentage of occluded grafts increases with survival time.

The majority of cases exhibited moderate or severe coronary artery atherosclerosis, moderate, or severe myocardial fibrosis and moderate to severe myocardial hypertrophy. Also the association of re-

TABLE 6. Total Number of Saphenous Vein Grafts and Percentage of Occluded Grafts

DAYS AFTER SURGERY	TOTAL NO. GRAFTS	NO. OCCLUDED GRAFTS	% OCCLUDED GRAFTS
0	126	0	(0)
1	88	4	(5)
3	26	7	(27)
7	27	8	(30)
14	25	6	(24)
30	16	5	(31)
90	11	8	(73)
180	1	0	–
365	–	–	–
730	7	3	(43)
1,095	1	1	(100)
Total	328	42	(13)

TABLE 7. Occurrence of Myocardial Infarcts

	DAYS AFTER SURGERY				
	0	1	2–7	8–30	⩾31
No. cases	60	38	30	19	12
Myocardial infarctions	24	11	20	12	5
Percent	(40)	(29)	(67)	(63)	(42)
Significance of differences between groups	⊢——$P<0.05$——⊣				
	⊢$P<0.01$⊣				
	⊢——$P<0.05$——⊣				

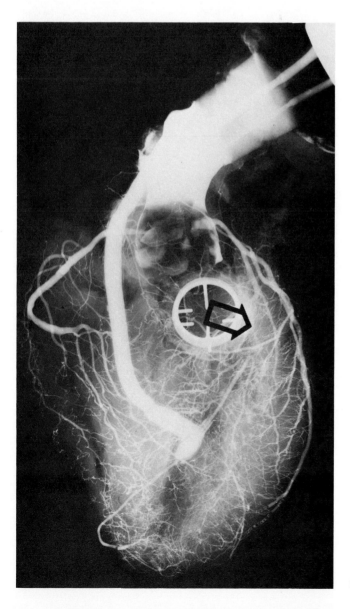

FIG. 13. Same case. Filling through both bypass and coronary ostia. Arrow indicates the site of occlusion of the left anterior descending coronary artery branch.

cent myocardial infarction is great in this group (Tables 1 and 2). Whereas the presence of moderate to severe coronary atherosclerosis may serve as an indication for the coronary artery bypass procedure, the coexistence of moderate to severe fibrosis or moderate to severe myocardial hypertrophy may predispose to an unfavorable outcome.

Frequently, other cardiovascular surgical procedures are performed simultaneously with coronary artery bypass. A listing of other procedures performed in cases of this series may be seen in Table 3. Twenty-five had aortic valve replacement with a prosthetic valve, and six had mitral valve replacement.

After a statistical analysis of the occurrence of myocardial infarcts (Table 7), the following conclusions may be drawn:

1. No direct relationship between myocardial infarcts and graft occlusion could be stated.
2. The incidence of coronary arteriosclerosis, myocardial fibrosis, and myocardial hypertrophy, and the coincidence of the myocardial infarcts in our series were not related to the patient's age.
3. The incidence of myocardial infarcts is not greater in those patients who underwent multiple cardiovascular surgical procedures.

SUMMARY

In 159 patients who died following aorto-coronary saphenous autologous bypass surgery, autopsy findings were analyzed. The morphologic findings of the saphenous vein grafts included mainly early occlusion by thrombosis, marked recanalization of the thrombosed grafts, as well as intimal fibrous thickening of the grafts, which remained patent for varying periods of time. It was found that the overall incidence of graft occlusion did not exceed 13 percent and that the incidence of recent myocardial infarct was not related to graft occlusion. The cause of myocardial failure appeared to be related to the severity of coronary arteriosclerosis, myocardial fibrosis, and myocardial hypertrophy.

References

1. Alonso DR, Carlson RG, Roters FA, Killip T, Lillehei CW: The patency and luminal diameter of distal coronary arteries in fatal, acute myocardial infarction. Arch Surg 104:826–30, 1972
2. Baroldi G, Scomazzoni G: Coronary circulation in the normal and pathologic heart. Armed Forces Institute of Pathology, Washington, DC, 1967
3. Effler DB, Favaloro RG, Groves LK: Coronary artery surgery utilizing saphenous vein graft techniques. J Thorac Cardiovasc Surg 59:147–54, 1970
4. Favaloro RG: Saphenous vein graft in the surgical treatment of coronary artery disease. J Thorac Cardiovasc Surg 58:178–85, 1969
5. Flemma RJ, Johnson WD, Lepley D, et al. Late results of saphenous vein bypass grafting for myocardial revascularization. Ann Thorac Surg 14:232–42, 1972
6. Grondin CM, Meere C, Castonguay Y, Lepage G, Grondin P: Progressive and late obstruction of an aorto-coronary venous bypass graft. Circulation 43:698–702, 1971
7. Grondin CM, Castonguay Y, Lesperance J, et al: Attrition rate of aorta-to-coronary artery saphenous vein grafts after one year. A study in a consecutive series of 96 patients. Ann Thorac Surg 14:223–31, 1972
8. Hall RJ, Dawson JT, Cooley DA, et al: Coronary artery bypass. Circulation, 47 and 48, suppl III: 146–50, 1973
9. Johnson WD, Flemma RJ, Lepley D: Direct coronary surgery utilizing multiple-vein bypass grafts. Ann Thorac Surg 9:436–44, 1970
10. Lesperance J, Bourassa MG, Biron P, Campeau L, Saltiel J: Aorta to coronary artery saphenous vein grafts: preoperative angiographic criteria for successful surgery. Am J Cardiol 30:459–65, 1972
11. Lesperance J, Bourassa MG, Saltiel J, Campeau L, Grondin CM: Angiographic changes in aorto-coronary vein grafts: lack of progression beyond the first year. Circulation 48:633–43, 1973
12. Marti MC, Bouchardy B, Cox JN: Aorto-coronary by-pass with autogenous saphenous vein grafts: histopathological aspects. Virchows Arch (Pathol Anat) 352:255–66, 1971
13. Rissanen VT: Double contrast technique for postmortem coronary angiography. Laboratory Investigation 23:517–23, 1970
14. Vlodaver Z, Edwards JE: Pathologic changes in aortic-coronary arterial saphenous vein grafts. Circulation 44:719–29, 1971
15. Vlodaver Z, Edwards JE: The pathologist approaches clinical coronary disease. Human Pathology 3:3–9, 1972

113

HISTOPATHOLOGIC CHANGES OCCURRING IN AORTOCORONARY ARTERY SAPHENOUS VEIN GRAFTS

Richard I. Staiman and Graeme L. Hammond

INTRODUCTION

During the past nine years there has been increasingly widespread use of autogenous saphenous vein aortocoronary bypass grafts for the treatment of occlusive coronary artery disease. The initial results have appeared very favorable,[2,6] but there have been isolated case reports [4,5] and several larger studies [6,7,10] that describe an obstructive process in the grafts called intimal proliferation. This process results in narrowing of the graft lumen and may result directly or indirectly in graft failure. The frequency, extent, and pathogenesis of this lesion are not understood and are essential questions that must be answered in the overall evaluation of this therapeutic modality.[3] It was with these goals in mind that this study was undertaken.

METHODS AND MATERIALS

Since May 1969, over 600 patients at the Yale–New Haven Medical Center have undergone aortocoronary bypass grafting using autogenous saphenous veins. Forty-five of these patients have expired, with subsequent postmortem graft examination. The survival range of this group of patients is from less than one hour to 45 months. One patient, who later succumbed, and two additional patients have had surgical graft revisions at three, 20, and 42 months, respectively. The grafts from these 48 patients form the basis of this study.

In 30 of the 43 autopsies, the grafts were removed intact, then flushed with and fixed in 10 percent formalin. After adequate fixation all grafts were serially cross-sectioned with suspicious and representative sections submitted for microscopic examination. The same procedure was followed for the surgical specimens. In the remaining 13 autopsies, the reports and all available slides were reviewed. No histologic sections were available on two autopsies.

All specimens were embedded in paraffin, sectioned at 5 microns, and stained with Hematoxylin and Eosin, Masson's trichrome, and Verhoeff's elastic tissue stains. Many sections were stained with Periodic-Acid-Schiff (PAS), Alcian Green, and Prussian Blue stains. Selected specimens were prepared by frozen section and stained for lipids with Oil-Red-O.

Whenever possible, sections of the original saphenous vein used at surgery or the contralateral saphenous vein removed at autopsy were obtained as controls. An additional 25 saphenous vein specimens were examined from autopsies performed on patients in the same age (36 to 69 years) but who had no history of vascular surgery.

For purposes of discussion, the patients will be divided into groups based on the postoperative age of the graft at the time it was examined.

Group I consists of 30 patients who died during the first 14 postoperative days. Twenty-one patients died during the first 24 hours, and this group includes all the operative deaths. Group II consists of seven patients who survived between 15 and 59 days. Group III consists of five patients (five autopsies and one surgical specimen) whose graft age was from 60 to 180 days.* Group IV was composed of two surgical specimens aged 20

* One patient had a surgical revision of his grafts with a complicated reanastomosis using new vein grafts, and he is included in groups II and III with graft specimens aged 40, 89, and 129 days.

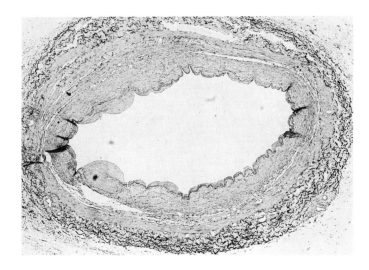

and 42 months and the grafts from one autopsy performed 45 months postoperatively.

RESULTS

Prior to discussing the histologic changes seen in saphenous veins used as grafts, it is worthwhile to review briefly the histology of the normal saphenous vein (Fig. 1).

The intima consists of the lining layer of endothelial cells and a thin subendothelial layer of fine connective tissue composed of a few scattered round or stellate cells and elastic fibers. This layer also contains longitudinally arranged smooth muscle fibers in the region of the valves.

The media is composed of circular smooth muscle fibers with varying amounts of interspersed collagen and fibroblasts. The adventitia is the thickest of the three layers and is composed of

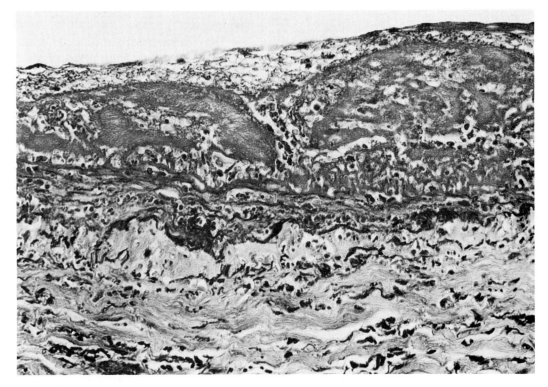

FIG. 2. Intima of a 24-hour-old bypass graft with thick fibrin meshwork on the surface. (Verhoeff's elastic tissue stain ×212.5.)

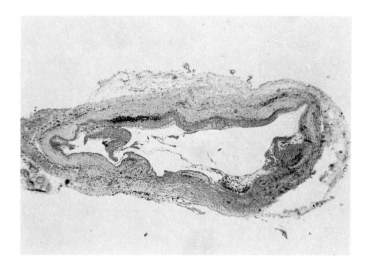

FIG. 3. Photomicrograph of saphenous vein graft in place for 24 hours. Fibrin deposits on the intima vary in size, shape, and distribution. (Verhoeff's elastic tissue stain ×40.)

loose collections of collagen and coarse elastic fibers.

Group I

In most patients surviving several hours and in all patients surviving over 24 hours, there is deposition of granular and fibrillary material on the endothelial surface (Fig. 2). This deposition of fibrin and platelets forms a meshwork that appears as a ribbon, as a loose lattice, or as pedunculated projections from the intimal surface (Fig. 3). Red blood cells may be trapped in the interstices, but red cells are not a major component of this material. These deposits vary from less than 10 microns to greater than 500 microns in thickness. Fibrin deposition is seen in all grafts at the aortic insertions with the fibrin being continuous over the aortic and venous surfaces (Fig. 4). In-

dentations in the venous lining appear particularly prone to fibrin deposition. Suture material, if it protrudes into the vascular lumen, is generally covered with fibrin. These deposits are usually present on the anastomotic sites, particularly the proximal, but they can and do occur either focally or diffusely throughout the length of the graft. Venous valves do not show increased fibrin deposits and are often uninvolved (Fig. 5). The presence of an acute inflammatory infiltrate on the endothelial surface is usually accompanied by increased deposition of fibrin. Grafts with an intact endothelium and good preservation of the media usually exhibit lesser amounts of fibrin deposition. Concomitant with fibrin deposition in many vessels is loss of endothelium, polymorphonuclear leukocytic infiltrates in the wall, edema of the media, and smooth muscle nuclear pyknosis and karyolysis. Several grafts have been seen at 24 to 48 hours

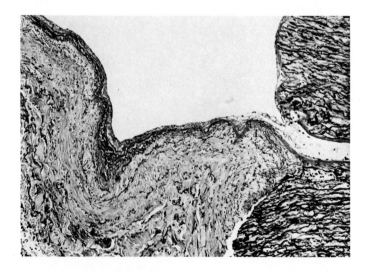

FIG. 4. Fibrin deposition on vein graft and aortic intimal surfaces after 24 hours. (Verhoeff's elastic tissue stain ×100.)

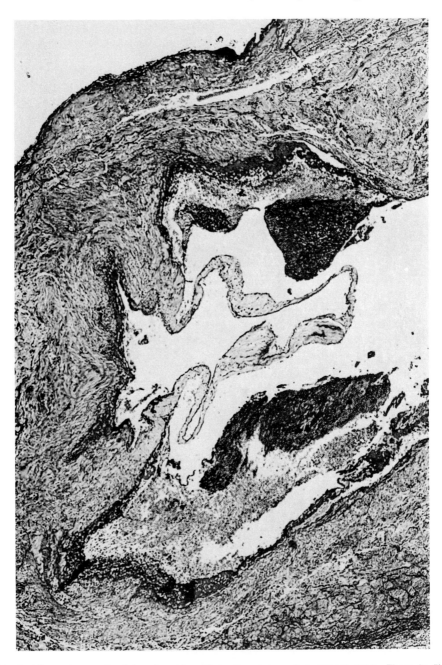

FIG. 5. Photomicrograph of two-day-old graft in the region of a venous valve. There is fibrin deposition on the adjacent intima, but the valve is uninvolved. (Verhoeff's elastic tissue stain ×40.)

postoperative in which no nuclear detail was visible in the intima or media and a dense inflammatory infiltrate was present at the endothelial surface (Fig. 6). These ischemic or degenerative changes are most prominent near the anastomotic sites, but the entire graft may be involved. Fibrin can be seen on the aortic endothelium as far as several centimeters from graft attachments and in coronary arteries at and distal to graft insertions. Grafts examined at 10 and 13 days were similar in appearance but with a markedly reduced inflammatory response. The media of the graft may appear slightly edematous or may exhibit the degenerative changes described above. The adventitia is usually

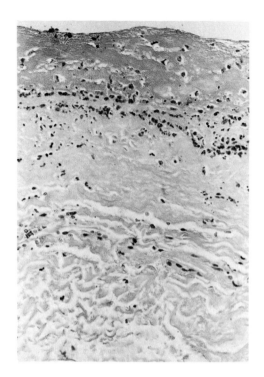

FIG. 6. Graft in place for 24 hours showing intimal fibrin deposits, acute inflammatory infiltrate, and medial muscle karyolysis. (Hematoxylin and eosin ×250.)

edematous and covered with a thick layer of organizing fibrin. Similar changes have not been seen in control grafts removed from these patients at surgery or at autopsy, or in the autopsy specimens of the nonvascular surgery group.

Group II

The seven patients in this group had grafts whose age was from 23 to 44 days. At the aortic origin, all grafts showed a markedly thickened intima. This layer covered most of the venous surface and extended onto the aortic surface for a distance of greater than one centimeter. As with the cases in Group I, this layer was especially pronounced on sutures extending into the vascular lumen (Fig. 7). The thickened intima appeared as a loose-fibrillary lattice that tended to be denser at the base than at the luminal edge. The cellularity of this thickened intima varied from patient to patient but tended to be consistent within the grafts of a given case. Most of the intimal cells were stellate or spindle-shaped cells, many of which stained as young myocytes. The cells in the deeper more compact region tended to be more round or oval, while in the loose superficial regions the cells exhibited more pleomorphism (Fig. 8). Polymorphonuclear leukocytes and red blood cells were uncommon. Many cells appear to sit in clear spaces or lacunae. Stains for mucin, polysaccharides, and lipids failed to demonstrate any of these materials in the clear spaces. A few mononuclear cells, some of which resemble macrophages, were seen. These cells did not contain hemosiderin pigment. Variable amounts of weakly staining, fine collagen fibers were seen between the cells, with the collagen being more prominent in the deeper layer. In all seven cases, the intimal layer measured up to several hundred microns in thickness at the aortic insertion. Within one centimeter from the graft origin, the intima tapered to a layer measuring 10 to 50 microns with focal regions of increased thickness. At the coronary artery insertions the thickness of the intimal layer was increased over the midgraft regions (Fig. 9). In one graft at 38 days, the insertion of the graft to the right coronary artery was occluded by recent thrombus. All other grafts were seen to be fully patent. In several cases venous valves were identified, and they exhibited minimal fibrin-coating and little if any

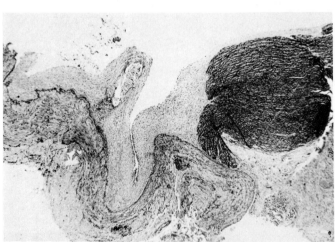

FIG. 7. Proximal anastomosis with organizing intimal layer extending over the graft and aortic surfaces after 38 days. A suture protruding into the vessel lumen is associated with a focal increase in intimal thickening. (Verhoeff's elastic tissue stain ×25.)

FIG. 8. Pleomorphic stellate and spindle-shaped young myocytes in the intima of a 33-day-old graft. (Masson's trichrome stain ×250.)

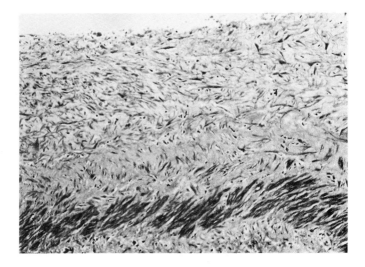

coating with thickened intima. In several sections, fresh deposition of fibrin was seen on the thickened intima (Fig. 10).

In the 23-day-old grafts, the smooth muscle fibers of the media appeared hyalinized with loss of nuclei. The media in all other cases was intact and appeared somewhat thickened. The smooth muscle fibers were well preserved but were often separated by bundles of collagen (Fig. 11). The amount of collagen appeared to be increased over that seen in controls and over that present in grafts of younger age.

The adventitia was thickened and covered with organizing granulation tissue.

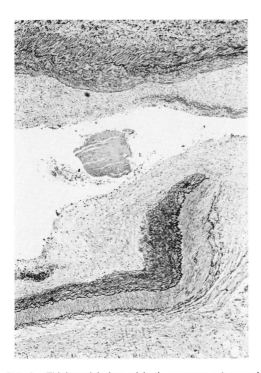

FIG. 9. Thickened intima of both coronary artery and venous graft at a distal anastomosis. There are fresh fibrin deposits present in the superficial intima of this 38-day-old graft. (Verhoeff's elastic tissue stain ×40.)

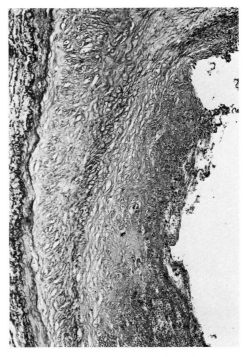

FIG. 10. Section of a 140-day-old graft showing organization of the deeper intima with fresh fibrin deposits at the luminal surface. (Verhoeff's elastic tissue stain ×100.)

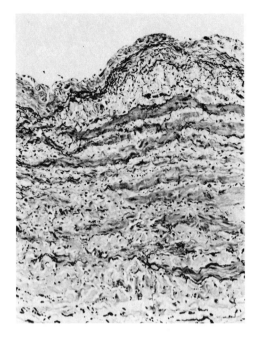

FIG. 11. Thirty-eight-day-old graft with medial muscle fibers separated by newly formed collagen. The intima in this midgraft section is only mildly thickened. (Verhoeff's elastic tissue stain ×100.)

Group III

The five patients in this group had a total of 11 vein grafts. Two grafts from different patients were occluded by old, organized, and recanalized thrombi. The walls of these grafts were extensively collagenized with an increase in fine and coarse elastic tissue. The intima in both cases did not appear thickened, suggesting early graft thrombosis. Smooth muscle cells were absent from the thrombi, but large numbers of hemosiderin-laden macrophages were present. The other graft present in each of these patients showed moderate (30 percent) and severe (90 percent) narrowing due to intimal thickening with superimposed recent thrombi. The 89-day-old surgical specimen was thrombosed and had an appearance similar to that of the thrombosed grafts.

The remaining three patients had a total of eight patent grafts. All eight grafts showed diffuse intimal thickening with 25 to 60 percent luminal narrowing (Fig. 12). The thickened intima was composed of loose fibrous tissue of varying degrees

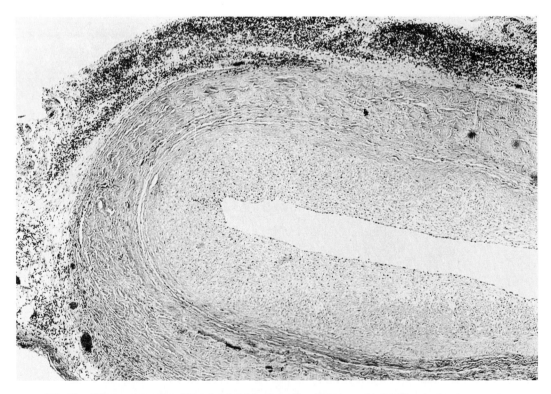

FIG. 12. Diffuse, circumferential intimal thickening after 164 days. (Verhoeff's elastic tissue stain ×34.)

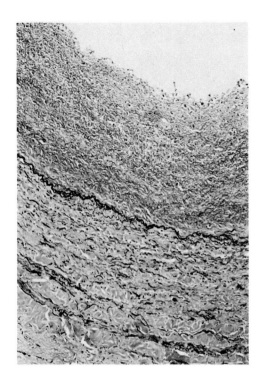

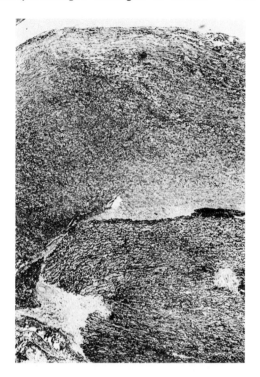

FIG. 13. Intima after 90 days with increased fibrosis toward the base of the layer. (Verhoeff's elastic tissue stain ×100.)

FIG. 14. Thick intimal layer (top) on the aortic surface adjacent to the graft insertion. (Verhoeff's elastic tissue stain ×40.)

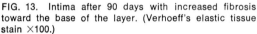

of cellularity. The fibrous tissue contained fine collagen and elastic fibers with increased amounts of collagen in the deeper portions of this layer (Fig. 13). Many of the cells present in the intima were smooth muscle cells. Hemosiderin-laden macrophages were absent. The intima was thicker at the aortic region than at the insertion (Fig. 14). The midportions of the grafts showed a uniformly

thickened intima which was thinner than at the anastomoses. There were no focal midgraft stenotic regions. Proliferating intima was seen on the aortic surface and in the coronary arteries at the anastomotic sites (Fig. 15). The intimal thickening tended to vary in amount from patient to patient but was generally uniform throughout each patient's grafts. The media in these grafts was also

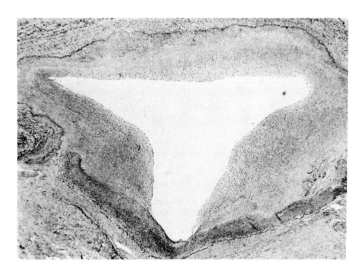

FIG. 15. Distal anastomotic site after 90 days. (Verhoeff's elastic tissue stain ×25.)

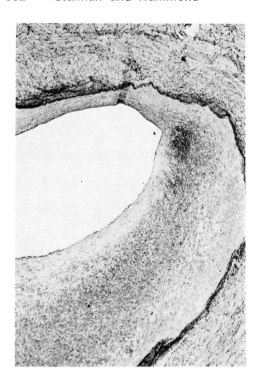

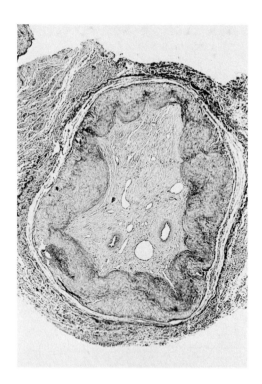

FIG. 16. Eccentric intimal thickening in a surgically excised specimen 20 months postinsertion. (Verhoeff's elastic tissue stain ×40.)

FIG. 17. Organized thrombus in portion of a vein graft surgically excised 42 months after insertion. (Verhoeff's elastic tissue stain ×40.)

thickened, with most of the increase due to additional collagen between the muscle layers. The adventitia showed extensive thickening secondary to fibrosis. All grafts had thickened walls and narrowed lumens with most of the narrowing due to the thickened intima.

Group IV

The surgical specimen removed at 20 months was patent but showed eccentric intimal thickening with 50 to 75 percent luminal narrowing (Fig. 16). The intima contained smooth muscle cells, fine elastic fibers, and coarser collagen fibers. The media was thickened with an increase in elastic and collagenous components. The adventitia was fibrosed. This vessel had a wall thickness of approximately two times that of the contralateral saphenous vein control removed at surgery for repair of the stenotic vessel. Most of the increase in thickness was secondary to the intimal proliferation. The 42-month-old surgical specimen exhibited phlebosclerosis and very minimal intimal proliferation. Superimposed was an old, organized thrombus (Fig. 17). It is noteworthy that both reoperated patients are alive and doing well 11 months after their surgical revisions.

The grafts from one patient were observed at autopsy 45 months postoperatively. The graft to the right coronary artery had a fibrotic wall, had no identifiable intimal thickening, and was occluded by organized thrombus. The graft to the left coronary artery showed a moderate amount of intimal thickening at the origin with a superimposed organizing thrombus. The intima showed extensive fibrosis with fewer cellular components as compared to younger grafts. The distal portions and graft insertions were similar in appearance to the previously described right coronary artery graft. The media of both vessels was densely fibrotic as was the adventitia.

DISCUSSION

In histopathologic studies of autogenous saphenous veins used for aortocoronary artery bypass, there has been little comment about alterations in grafts in place for less than one month. Vlodaver and Edwards (1971) report that no significant changes were seen in grafts present for less than seven days; and Kern, Dermer, and Lindesmith (1972) report only "minimal" intimal changes as being present in grafts in place for less than 30 days. The grafts from the 30 patients in this study who survived less than 14 days showed many significant changes. These findings include disruption of the endothelium with focal or diffuse fibrin deposition, acute inflammatory infiltrate within the swollen intima, and anoxic changes in the muscle of the media. Fibrin deposits were most pronounced at the insertions of the grafts and were continuous over the arterial and venous surfaces. Sutures when present in the lumen of the vessel serve as a nidus for fibrin precipitation. These observations are particularly significant when viewed in terms of the alterations observed in older grafts.

Among the theories on the etiology of the intimal lesion, the one generally favored is graft response to injury, especially to increased intraluminal pressure.[5,7,10] The circumferential distribution of the thickened intima, lack of early lesions, and absence of hemosiderin have caused most authors to doubt that this lesion represents organized mural thrombi. While the distribution has been variable, the general histologic features of reported vein graft lesions [4,5,7,8,10] have been relatively constant.

In view of the features described in Group I, it appears that the late intimal lesion may represent the response of the vein graft to focal and/or diffuse injury with subsequent epithelial damage, fibrin deposition, and subsequent organization. Since few red blood cells are trapped in the precipitated fibrin, the absence of hemosiderin-laden macrophages is not surprising.

Vlodaver and Edwards (1972) suggest that the lesion seen in coronary arteries distal to the graft insertion may represent a jet lesion.[11] Marti, Bouchardy, and Cox (1971), in their case number 6, show particular involvement of the proximal insertion in a graft that was 34 days old. This type of alteration was typical of our Group II patients. While it may not be the only factor involved, an etiology based on local trauma is consistent with the increased lesions found at the sites of insertion, especially those associated with intrusive suture material. Graft injury may also produce focal lesions elsewhere in the graft and the fibrocellular proliferation seen on the aortic surface and coronary arteries in the region of anastomosis. A generalized injury might result in the diffuse intimal lesions seen in Groups II and III. The loss of muscle from the media as seen in older grafts may represent a generalized early insult to the graft or late intimal and adventitial fibrosis with devascularization and anoxia.

Flemma et al (1973) report angiographic evidence that in patients with multiple bypasses

"one of many may be involved without any evidence of the process in other veins." This has not been observed in the patients in this study. When one graft is occluded and the others are grossly or microscopically patent, particularly if the occlusion is focal, then the etiology is most often thrombotic and not intimal thickening.

An important question raised with regard to the etiology of local lesions is the role of the venous valves. Thrombi in saphenous veins used as femoral-popliteal bypass grafts, as well as those used for aortocoronary bypass grafts, have been attributed to the presence of valves.[1,5,8,9] Valves have been identified microscopically in grafts from Groups I, II, and III. One patient in Group III had an organized thrombus involving a valve located less than 0.3 centimeters from the distal insertion. In all other cases, the amount of fibrin deposition or intimal thickening associated with the valve was no greater than, or even less than, the adjacent portions of the graft. These findings strongly suggest that with the use of reversed veins, the valves do not promote intimal proliferative lesions and when not at an anastomotic site do not promote thrombosis.

None of the patients studied exhibited occlusion of a graft on the basis of intimal thickening alone. All graft closures have been based on thrombus formation. This has been observed in grafts showing intimal thickening, but the majority of thrombosed grafts appear to occur early prior to the intimal response and probably within the first 30 postoperative days. In a large angiographic follow-up study, Flemma et al (1973) found no graft closures occurring after the 18th postoperative month. Garrett et al (1973) studied a patient seven years postgrafting and found his graft to be patent. Although the extent of the intimal thickening appears to increase for the first six to 12 months, we have not found that graft occlusion is inevitable. The large number of asymptomatic, angiographically patent, long-term survivors corroborates this observation.

The removal, preparation, latent periods, and anastomotic procedure are all potential sources of injury to the vessels involved in the grafting. The evidence of vessel injury, the type and distribution of the response, and the progressive organization that appears to follow suggest that early injury may be the basis of, or at least contribute to, the process called intimal proliferation. It would also appear that early and/or late thrombosis may be sequelae of these injuries. These findings suggest that the ultimate fate of a vein graft may to a great extent be determined at the time of its placement, and any measures that minimize injury to the vessels involved also maximize the chances of a successful outcome.

References

1. Barner HB, Judd DR, Kaiser GC, Willman, VL, Hanlon CR: Late failure of arterialized in situ saphenous vein. Arch Surg 99:781–86, 1969

2. Flemma RJ, Walker JA, Gale H, et al: Is vein bypass here to stay: early and long-term observations. Adv Cardiol 9:124–33, 1973

3. Garrett HE, Dennis EW, Debakey ME: Aortocoronary bypass with saphenous vein graft: seven-year follow up. JAMA 227:792–94, 1973

4. Grondin CM, Meere C, Castonguay Y, Lepage G, Grondin P: Progressive and late obstruction of an aorto-coronary venous bypass graft. Circulation 43:698–702, 1971

5. Hamaker WR, Doyle WF, O'Connell TJ, Gomez AC: Subintimal obliterative proliferation in saphenous vein grafts: a cause of early failure of aorto-to-coronary artery bypass graft. Ann Thorac Surg 13:488–93, 1972

6. Hammond GL, Poirier RA: Early and late results of direct coronary reconstructive surgery for angina. Thorac Cardiovasc Surg 65:127–33, 1973

7. Kern WH, Dermer GB, Lindesmith GC: The intimal proliferation in aortic-coronary saphenous vein grafts: light and electron microscopic studies. Am Heart J 84:771–77, 1972

8. Marti MC, Bouchardy B, Cox JN: Aorto-coronary bypass with autogenous saphenous vein grafts: histopathological aspects. Virchows Arch Abt A Path Anat 352:255–66, 1971

9. McCabe M, Cunningham GJ, Wyatt AP, Rothnie NG, Taylor GW: A histological and histochemical examination of autogenous venous grafts. Br J Surg 54:147–55, 1967

10. Vlodaver F, Edwards JE: Pathologic changes in aortic-coronary arterial saphenous vein grafts. Circulation 44:719–28, 1971

11. Vlodaver F, Edwards JE: The pathologist approaches clinical coronary disease. Hum Pathol 3:3–9, 1972

114

SIMULATION OF ATHEROGENESIS BY COMPUTER DISPLAY TECHNIQUES

HARVEY GREENFIELD

INTRODUCTION

Most investigators concerned with the pathogenesis of atherosclerosis assume that its occurrence, progression, and possible regression largely depend upon dietary factors. Indeed, clinical programs for the prevention and treatment of atherosclerosis are directed toward the manipulation of serum lipids. There is a considerable body of medical evidence that points toward the importance of blood cholesterol content and, in turn, the linking of such content to the nutrient composition of the diet. One cannot ignore studies that compared coronary vessels of Americans killed in the Korean conflict with Japanese control subjects and found equal resultant damage to the coronary elastica (Enos et al, 1955) but that also showed that the control group's lesions evolved into simple scars while the American group's lesions developed into continually growing atheromatous processes. In turn, others (Friedman and Byers, 1962) concluded that relative absence of cholesterol in the Japanese diet apparently caused the control group's resulting lesions not to develop further, whereas the presence of cholesterol aggravated the healing process that is normal to the initial elastica injury in the American cases.

Genetic history and types of stress have also been recognized as etiologic factors in atherosclerosis; however, they have been emphasized by re-

searchers to a lesser extent. In turn, the relative roles of the vascular wall and the blood flow in vascular degeneration have been debated since the atherosclerotic process was first described. These concepts have been studied to even a lesser degree. It is this investigator's contention that localization of the atherosclerotic process is determined to no mean extent by rheologic factors, including the geometrics of arterial branching, intraluminal pressure and pulse contour, properties of the blood and blood-intima interface, and the physical properties of the vessel wall. Amplifying this contention, we should regard the vascular wall as having a large role in the initiation of vascular degeneration as well as in the later manifestations of such localization, seen clinically (Reemtsma et al, 1970). Others (Mustard et al, 1964; Downie et al, 1963) recognize a multitude of interactive mechanisms that include hydraulic factors and arterial wall changes. Fluid mechanics may play a part in the localization of lesions (Texon, 1957, 1960a, b) since the role of hydrodynamic laws has been emphasized and is evidenced by an irregular distribution of atherosclerotic lesions upon vascular walls (Wesolowski et al, 1965). Experimentally, some investigators (Lynn et al, 1970) have sought to obtain a vorticity map of the aortic bifurcation region while others (Spurlock, Homa, Durfee, 1968) studied dye streamlines in pulsating flow. Recently, hemodynamic theories of atherogenesis have been reviewed (Gessner, 1973), and the relative merits of pressure-related, wall shear stress, turbulence-related, and flow separation hypotheses have been examined.

The study of flow-related hypotheses has been extended by the present investigator in an attempt to develop simulations of desired medical

Supported by National Institutes of Health grant number HL-12202, and by Program Project grant number H3-PO1-HL-13738-02S1.

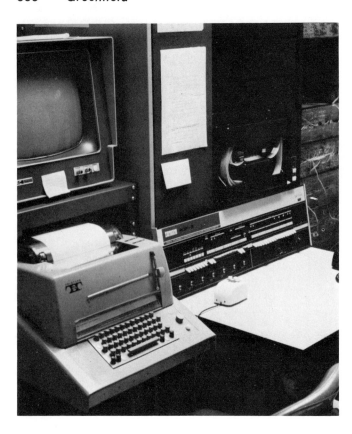

FIG. 1. Computer graphics display equipment. From Greenfield: Trans Am Soc Artif Int Organs 18:607, 1972

phenomena. Such simulations are the end products of mathematical analyses of the blood flow field and are desired in order to avoid amounts of unwieldy data that emanate from equations that are intractable except in particular, well-chosen situations. The resultant representations are made available through the employment of computer graphics, a tool that allows the computer to depict a physical system on a television-type screen and permits the viewer to interact with the natural-appearing representation. This chapter will present a feasibility study in the attempt to examine the development of a coronary atheromatous lesion and subsequent blood flow changes. Eventually, this new investigative effort should allow the investigator, with the aid of a computer, to walk into a simulated artery and watch the lesion grow with time.

COMPUTER GRAPHICS: ITS ROLES IN THE PROJECT

A small computer acting as a satellite to a larger computer some distance away is employed in the investigation (Fig. 1). The smaller computer processes data from a cathode-ray-tube (CRT) screen, gathers data to present to the larger computer, which has greater capability, and acts as a multiplex system for display information coming from the other computer. (A multiplex system transmits several signals simultaneously on the same circuit or channel.) Therefore, several satellite computers can be attached to the "mother" computer, allowing many investigators at teletypes to work at individual problems simultaneously.

A teletype allows the investigator to type in his computer program to the storage banks of the computer and then issue commands to the computer such as input of data and output of desired information. A small white box, called a "mouse," is a graphic input device that consists of a plastic unit in whose base two potentiometers are mounted. The mouse rests on two metal wheels, whose axes are at right angles to each other. As the mouse is rolled on a flat surface, its movements in the orthogonal directions are recorded by the rotation of the potentiometers and a phosphorus spot moves accordingly on the display screen. Pressing a button on the mouse allows contact at the dot between the computer's memory bank and the teletype. The computer interprets commands from the teletype concerning the dot position and constructs a drawing or deletes a geometric section as required or outputs numerical data upon the screen. Once a representation of an object is upon the screen, clever subroutines within the computer program can, by the use of matrix algebra concepts, cause the object (in perspective view) to rotate or translate its position, continually or by single frame, so as to allow complete scrutinization. Shading and even coloring of the object is possible. As in most fluid flow analyses, contour maps are used to present the data in pictorial form. The contour-mapping routine designed for this interactive graphics simulation program is more efficient as compared with other contour mapping routines available. The contour program is designed to plot an unlimited number of contour levels.

The use of contour maps to represent data on a two-dimensional grid, however, is rather insufficient. Ambiguities arise when the contour levels are not labeled with their associated values, for computer graphics displays have limited-view area. In addition, depending on the contour levels used, detailed information may be concealed between contours. To utilize the computer graphics resources fully, an isometric display program was designed to supplement the contour maps. The isometric plot maintains the spatial relationship of each data point on a plane and uses the third axis in the three-dimensional space to represent the functional values. The data array is represented by a family of curves, each representing a set of data points along one dimension in the data array. Each curve is plotted where it is not hidden by any of the curves previously plotted. The sequence of curves thus closely approximates a surface that represents the data array. In order to provide spacings between successive curve profiles, only every other curve profile is displayed in all isometric plots.

The combination of contour map and iso-metric view provides a detailed description of the solution. These displays, however, do not indicate the numerical values of the data at any point. In order to facilitate detailed examination of the solution, an interactive curve plotting program was developed. It allows the operator to examine the data values along a selected cross-section in the solution space. To select a particular cross-section, the mouse, used as an input device, is brought to the desired position on the contour plot. When one of the three buttons on the mouse is depressed, the current location of the electron beam is transmitted to the program. The data along that cross-section are plotted on a grid, and a dotted line is drawn on the contour map to indicate the location being examined. The grid is scaled appropriately by the program to ensure inclusion of all possible values. The operator has the option of displaying a particular curve or a family of curves for comparison. Results of such a methodology are seen in subsequent sections of this chapter.

THE SIMULATION PROCEDURE

In the attempt to analyze the movement and consequential change of the blood flow field about a lesion, an idealized projection of such an isolated protuberance was placed on a boundary wall, as shown in Figure 2. The obstacle and its surrounding flow field were then covered by a cellular network, which can be described as a computational mesh, the coordinate values of each cell node having been described to the computer and then stored in its memory. The Navier-Stokes equations that prescribe the two-dimensional flow (Greenfield, 1972a) about the obstacle on the wall were simplified by the use of the finite-difference method

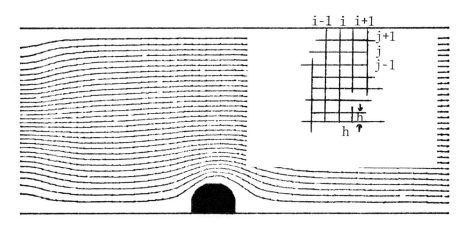

FIG. 2 Idealized lesion on an arterial wall, overlayed by a computational mesh. Streamlines have been formed.

(Fromm, 1963; Fromm and Harlow, 1963; Pearson, 1965). Such action allowed the extremely difficult, nonlinear equations to be simplified, resulting in a set of algebraic equations that were compatible with the computer. These approximations related the value of the dependent variable at a point in the computing mesh to the values at a number of symmetrically arranged neighboring mesh points, at one instant of time and then at succeeding time intervals. The solution becomes quite accelerated if the method of relaxation is used (Lawrensen, 1966). The approach made use of stream function and vorticity function values at each cell node after proper manipulation of the equations. The procedure was first attempted for obstacles that were parallel to the mesh boundaries (Greenfield and Brauer, 1969) since crossing the mesh lines was somewhat of an additional mathematical problem. A later and improved procedure allowed nonparallel results. This latter development was extremely important, for it allowed the positioning of side channels that emanate from the boundary wall. Blood flowing through a large channel such as the aorta could then have its path simulated as it moved into any smaller channel of the arterial tree. Although not discussed in this paper, the methodology has also been employed for analyzing the motion of occluders in prosthetic heart valves and the resulting sequel of events (Greenfield, 1972a, b; Greenfield and Hampton, 1973).

The computer program that allowed the above results contained subroutines that formed a horizontal velocity plot, a vertical velocity plot, a total velocity plot, a stream function depicture, the velocity vector form, and a vorticity function display. The computer program also included a subroutine, so that a hard copy of a single time frame of any plot could be drawn upon an automatic plotter.

The first group of flow studies that evolved proved the feasibility of the concept. As the investigation continued, specially employed numerical techniques permitted the fitting of curved boundaries into the desired two-dimensional flow problem. Again it was felt, however, that the methodology should be improved upon in order to bring the analysis technique closer to *in vivo* knowledge. At this point, the technique for forming the desired displays used vorticity and stream function values, as noted, for the primary dependent variables. Some disadvantages of this technique were its poor eventual extension to three-dimensional studies and the difficulty encountered in satisfying free-surface boundary conditions.

Also, true channel flow remained to be described, and pulsating motion and viscoelastic properties of the arterial wall were missing in the final solution. To overcome partially the difficulties, the Marker and Cell method (Harlow et al, 1966; Amsden and Harlow, 1970) has been studied and simplified for usage. This method used pressure and velocity as primary dependent variables and permits free surfaces, the latter useful for a pulsing, viscoelastic wall. The method also maintains accuracy with a minimum of computer time through the employment of a corrective procedure in the computer program. Stress equations were also programed so as to enlarge the simulation capabilities.

The next section includes some of the results and explanatory comments, of concern to parametric studies of an idealized lesion. These reviewed accomplishments will then be fitted into the larger study that involves processes for investigating the coronary arterial section that encloses the lesion.

LESION-PLAQUE SIMULATION STUDIES

Atherosclerotic lesions may be classified into three types: fatty streaks, fibrous plaques, and complicated lesions. In the following simulations, the terms lesion and plaque may be arbitrarily interchanged since the obstacle studied is an idealized one, in no particular stage of development. No detailed meaning is, therefore, given to the obstacle at this point.

For the sake of simplicity the first attempt to simulate an idealized lesion (or a plaque) was computer processed as if it were the hemisphere noted in Figure 2. The numerical technique that employs the vorticity and stream function as prime parameters permitted results such as exemplified in Figure 3. Figure 3 shows the vorticity plot (Greenfield, Brauer, Reemtsma, 1971) at one particular time frame and for a particular Reynolds number in their respective continuums of motion. (The Reynolds number being a dimensionless number, indicative of the ratio of flow inertial forces to viscous forces and which includes the flow velocity as a parameter.) The reader will note that emphasis is placed throughout such studies on the vorticity function. If vortices are assumed to be the forerunners of turbulence and they denote the positioning of eventual turbulent flow areas and turbulence can possibly denote shear stresses and the development of mural thromboses (Sako, 1962;

FIG. 3. Various computer-devised flow functions for an idealized atherosclerotic lesion. From Greenfield, Brauer, Reemtsma: In Parslow, Green (eds): Computer Graphics in Medical Research and Hospital Administration, 1971. Courtesy of Plenum Publishing Corp.

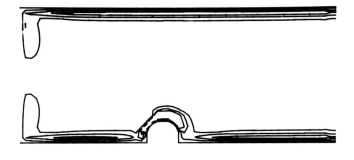

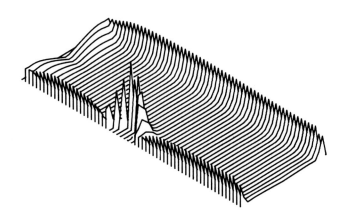

Scharfstein et al, 1963), such theoretical studies are of interest. Bruns et al (1959) discussed the possibility of turbulence inducing high-frequency vibrations, which may, in turn, induce a destructive effect upon the arterial wall. Subsequent healing at the turbulent position might be viewed as the processor to a lesion. If one views Figure 3 as an interim step in the formation of an idealized lesion, the isometric view shows the sharp peaks of turbulence and at what points an involved vibratory motion should be amplified.

If one also evaluates the velocity component pictorially along the y axis, it shows increased lateral value for the incremental time frame chosen. If one then compares computer-formed isometric plots of the horizontal and total velocities, it is seen that they appear equivalent. This would lead one to believe that since the total velocity is the vector sum of its horizontal and vertical components, the vertical velocity is quite small.

In an attempt to vary the shape of an idealized plaque radically, a square form was drawn upon the graphics display screen, rather than the previously seen hemisphere. This action presumes

that the investigator can draw any interim shape between the two extremes and then employ either numerical procedure. To exemplify this, the second numerical procedure was initiated in order that the blood flow be represented about the square plaque by particles. In this procedure, regions were opened to allow inflow and outflow in the flow regime. At a particular time in the sequence, the observer can see a vortex forming downstream and proximal to the obstacle tip. Subsequently, as the blood flow velocity increased, the flow became disoriented and randomly turbulent. (The obstacle shape was enlarged in the y coordinate direction to study also flow about a disc-type occluder tip in a prosthetic heart valve in other studies.) The procedure was then varied so as to view the flow about a hypothetical idealized square plaque in a half-filled channel. Figure 4 depicts a group of one-time-frame examples of the resulting continuum (Greenfield, 1973; Greenfield and DeBry, 1972). Such particle motion in a partially filled channel permits a free surface boundary to be duplicated, rather than the previously noted rigid wall boundary. Space does not allow the dis-

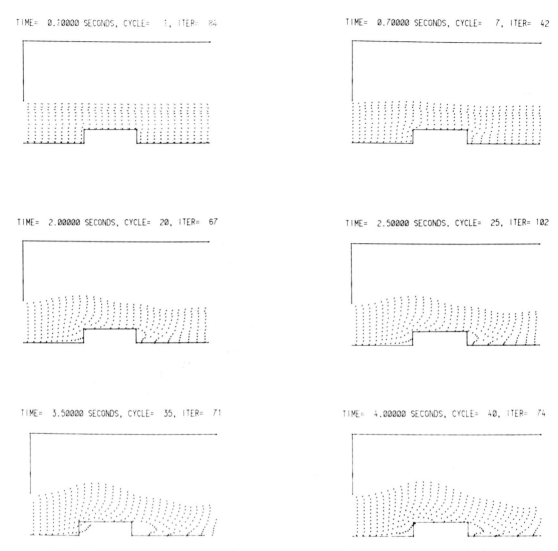

FIG. 4. Successive views of blood flow simulated by particles, employing a free surface boundary. From Greenfield: In Haga (ed): Computer Techniques in Biomedicine and Medicine, 1972. Courtesy of Mason and Lipscomb, Publishers, Inc.

play of various shapes that were studied and bracketed by the hemisphere and square advanced lesion models.

A particular study chosen to follow the above one was a shear stress simulation. It has been suggested that a localized change in pressure or shearing stress (Rodbard, 1958) may trigger certain biologic mechanisms that allow proliferation of the endothelial and subendothelial cells of the arterial wall. Fry (1968, 1969) has examined the influence of local wall shear levels on the erosion of the endothelium and has attempted to correlate high wall shear stress with common sites of lesion development. Although at least one investigator (Caro, 1971) has opted for lesion development

in regions of low wall shear, in part because of a shear-dependent diffusional efflux theory, the important point is that this investigator felt that shear stress studies should be simulated. To this end, an atherosclerotic ring or "plug," as portrayed in Figure 5, was assumed. Later, an asymmetric "plug" was studied.

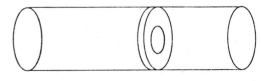

FIG. 5. A simplified arterial "plug."

Employment was made of a finite element approach (Ray and Davids, 1970) to analyze and then simulate blood flow in the inlet region of a tube when a "plug" was present (Cannon and Greenfield, 1972). Interest was aroused since the analysis could be extended to the viewing of blood flow velocity profiles and stress distributions about symmetric and asymmetric atherosclerotic plaques. Accuracy tests performed by Ray and Davids and the author indicated that the methodology allowed results that were within 3 to 5 percent of previously accepted solutions.

The applications of the finite element method permitted the arterial section to be divided into contiguous planes, each of which were then divided into cells. Any amount of cells were allowed (in cross-section) to be part of the plaque; however, no blood was allowed to flow "mathematically" through the plaque section. One assumed a rigid, constant diameter tube where there was no plaque or lesion. Other assumptions were laminar flow, a Newtonian fluid, and insignificant radial velocity.

The above approach permitted the investigator to command the computer to display the fluid velocity at each "cell" in the vascular vessel. In turn, this evaluation allowed the simulation of the velocity patterns (based upon chosen Reynolds numbers) and the shear stress distribution resulting from the blood flowing past an asymmetric

plaque or through a symmetric plaque, the latter constituting a plugged arterial section. Associated with each velocity profile was a value of the shear stress between the fluid of that particular plane and the vessel wall. These were assembled into a second display file and arranged to appear as a graph above the velocity profiles. The pressure gradient appeared at the bottom of the picture.

Figure 6 shows the simulation of the blood flow's velocity profiles, by particles, when no lesion is present. Notice that the shear stress and pressure gradients appear as one might assume such functional shapes to be for the inlet flow region position. Figure 7 shows the blood velocity profiles when a symmetric plaque was present at a particular vascular channel position and with a chosen plaque length. The user of the display system is able to position the plaque and change its length at will, with the aid of the light pen or mouse at his disposal. Not only can the investigator, via the teletype, specify the position, size, and shape of the plugged region, but is also able to create it one layer at a time, and subsequently view flow parameter changes as the plaque builds up.

It soon became obvious that the observer, looking at the screen, might confuse velocity profiles as the dots became irregular, particularly where the profiles changed shape in the plugged section. In order to ease the situation the particles that made up each velocity profile were con-

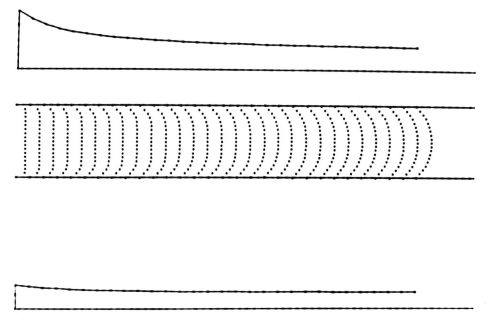

FIG. 6.   Arbitrary velocity profiles of simulated blood moving in an arterial channel with no atherosclerosis plaques present. (Shear stress gradient and pressure gradient are also shown.) From Greenfield: Int J Biomed Comput 4:31, 1973

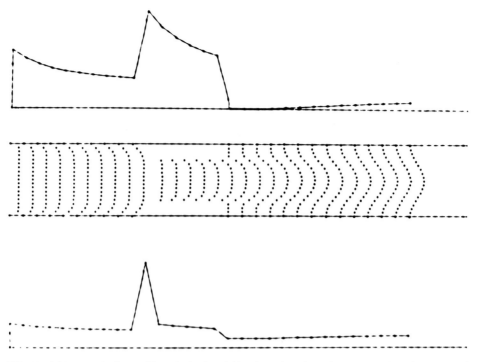

FIG. 7. Arbitrary velocity profiles of simulated blood moving through a symmetric atherosclerotic plaque in an arterial channel. Top view in the computer-formed display is the shear stress gradient, center view is the velocity profile group and the bottom view is the pressure gradient. Values change as plaque is lengthened and flow velocity is changed. From Greenfield, 1973: Int J Biomed Comput 4:31, 1973

nected via cubic splines (Ting and Greenfield, 1972; Greenfield, 1973), third-degree polynomials that are fitted to a set of data points. Such a procedure caused each velocity profile to have 11 times as many data points, which, when connected, formed pleasantly smoothed curves.

As was noticed, such blood velocity profiles were symmetric curves, for no atherosclerotic plaque was deemed to be present. Figure 8 depicts the result of placing a relatively thick, square-edged, axially symmetric obstruction in the flow field. Since that section of the flow field that is displayed may not contain the stenosis, that obstruction shape in cross-section was made to appear at the upper right boundary of the artery. It is realized, however, that for analytic purposes the computer reads the plaque position as being in the inlet flow region. Viewing the plaque as a cross-sectional shape allows interaction by light pen to change the shape. Shown on the screen is the maximum shear value on the plaque, along with its shear percent increase at that position compared to shear stress at the inlet. With the shape change to a triangle, the shear stress values changed, as seen in Figure 9.

The observer is also presented with numer-ical values of erythrocyte damage upon the dis-play screen. Such values were seen to change with the reshaping of the plaque at the inlet region of the flow regime. The red blood cell damage cal-culations were based upon the empirical studies (Nevaril et al, 1968) of others. Nevaril subjected thin layers of blood to varying degrees of shear stress and tabulated the resulting cell damage. In the present analysis, the outermost layer of fluid was assumed to correspond to the thin layer pos-tulated by Nevaril. At the point of maximum shear upon this layer, the corresponding damage was calculated according to Nevaril's results. This yielded the percent of blood cells damaged in that layer of fluid. This quantity was then multiplied by the percent of total vessel volume occupied by the outermost layer of fluid and stored in a dis-play file. Although the total area causing the shear stress is not nearly as great as that used by Nevaril, it is believed that results are approximately cor-rect, for Nevaril stated that findings were essen-tially independent of the duration of the shearing stress.

Figure 10 resulted when the case of an asym-metric lesion was programed as being present at the inlet region and on the left wall. It is obvious

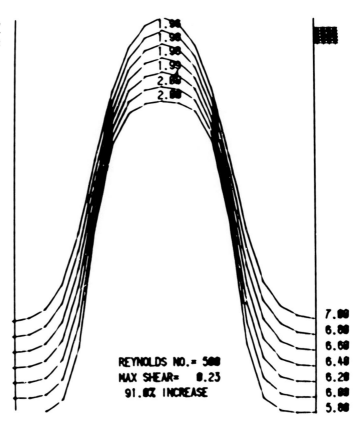

FIG. 8 Blood flow velocity profiles, downstream of a square-shaped annular obstruction. From Greenfield: J Assoc Adv Med Inst 6:254, 1972

REYNOLDS NO.= 500
MAX SHEAR=   0.23
91.0% INCREASE

7.00
6.80
6.60
6.40
6.20
6.00
5.80

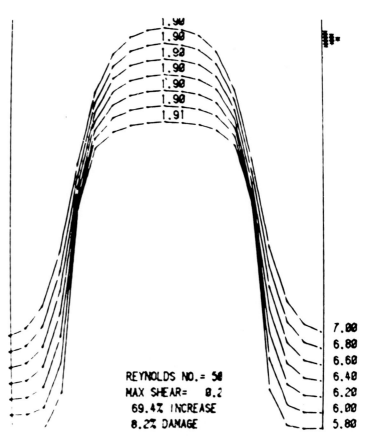

FIG. 9 Blood flow velocity profiles, downstream of a triangular, cross-sectioned-shaped annular obstruction.

REYNOLDS NO.= 50
MAX SHEAR=   0.2
69.4% INCREASE
8.2% DAMAGE

7.00
6.80
6.60
6.40
6.20
6.00
5.80

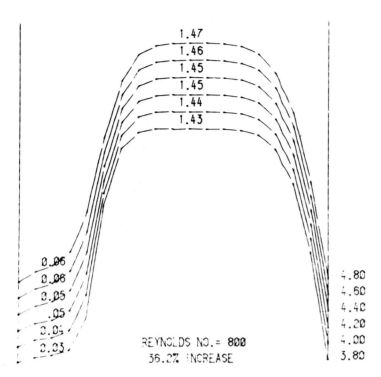

FIG. 10. Computer-simulated blood flow velocity profiles, downstream of the inlet region of a vascular channel, with a square-shaped asymmetric plaque present. From Greenfield: Int J Biomed Comput 4:31, 1973.

that with no lesion component present on the opposite wall the velocity profiles will be unaffected at that position.

Up to this point the reader has been presented with simulation capabilities that, by computer programing, permitted the analysis of various parameters about an ideal lesion or plaque, but only at a particular point in the growth cycle. It will now be seen that the simulation procedure can also be performed with the idealized lesion placed in a larger flow regime—a particular length of the arterial tree. As seen below in Figures 11 and 12, the advanced lesion was viewed as being present in a renal artery as well as in the abdominal aortic bifurcation (Greenfield and Brauer, 1971). Again, space requirements preclude the display of all the computer results except the vorticity function plots. The renal section and the aortic bifurcation were also joined for simulation of that connected regime (Greenfield and Kolff, 1972).

The renal artery simulation was programed so that the side channels angled at any desired inclination. The upper artery was seen to face upstream slightly to conform to displacements seen in angiograms. The capability of arbitrary angling allows the input of angiogram-formed patient data that show the amount of turbulence and possible resulting thrombi, compared to the amount of angle variance from the main blood flow.

Although not shown, the plotted stream

function for the renal arteries bore out physical concepts in that the streamlines were shown closer in proximity upstream of the side arteries, therefore permitting a lessening of flow energy downstream as flow is drained off in the side channels. A horizontal velocity plot showed the typical parabolic-type front for laminar flow, which then changed to a typical turbulent front in the main flow region between the side arteries. A total velocity plot again showed a proper physical amalgamation of the horizontal and vertical velocity components. The vorticity function, seen in Figure 11, became the subject of detailed sequential study within the particular portion of the backward facing side artery region. Figure 11's isometric plot in particular shows the extremely high vortex peaks in the upper channel, which was to be expected as the blood flow radically changed direction. Realizing this, the Reynolds number was continually changed in a montage of the components of Figure 11 to allow a transition from a slow initial rate of flow to slightly above an average blood flow velocity value in that particular area. One then notes the formation of a vortex in such a velocity regime, and if the observer views the small triangular-shaped vortex on the anterior wall, the breakup and re-formation of stream function lines in amplifying this vortex are clearly noticed.

In turn, comparison of Figure 12 with the arterial tree and its usually seen lesion sites shows

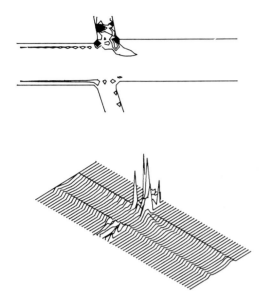

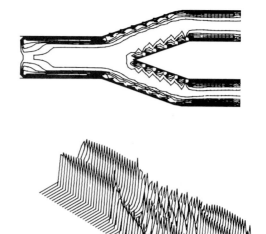

FIG. 11. Computer-simulated vorticity function plot for angled renal arteries. Isometric view shows variances in vorticity peaks at different positions. From Greenfield, Am J Surg 119:548–52, 1970

FIG. 12. Computer-simulated vorticity function plot for the abdominal aortic bifurcation. From Greenfield, Am J Surg 119:548–52, 1970

that the theoretical vorticity function plot appears equivalent for site-positioning with observed atherosclerosis sites.

INTERNAL VIEWING OF THE ARTERIAL TREE

With the study of the single advanced lesion amplified to where it is viewed *in situ* within an arterial tree section, a desirable second amplification would be the viewing of the affected area as if the viewer were transported inside the artery. Since the investigation at hand is a simulation procedure, it is obvious that such internal viewing would also be simulated. Such three-dimensional kinematic behavior has been duplicated by the employment of a head-mounted display helmet, which includes two miniature (0.5 inch square) cathode-ray-tubes (Sutherland, 1968). The computer-developed information, previously seen on the normal-size display screen, is now displayed upon the two miniature screens that are placed in tubes centered before the observer's eyes (Fig. 13). An incorporated optical system presents a stereoscopic image of the simulated data so that computer-projected objects enter and leave the observer's field of view in a natural manner. The helmet-wearing subject can move in a volumetric space of specified size, and as he moves toward the object, its apparent size and perspective ap-

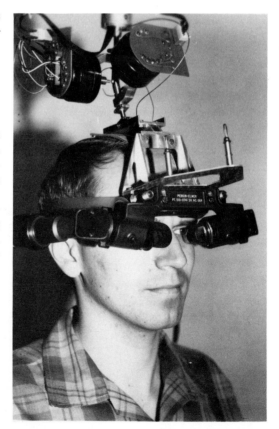

FIG. 13. An observer wearing the head-mounted display equipment. From Greenfield: Trans Am Soc Artif Int Organs 18:607, 1972

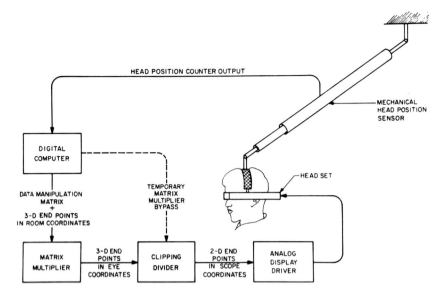

FIG. 14. Information flow components within the head-mounted display terminal. From Greenfield: Trans Am Soc Artif Int Organs 18:607, 1972

pearance change. Initially, there had appeared to be no particular application for this computer tool; therefore, its use was directed toward our attempt to walk into a simulated artery. A film was the outcome of this investigation. In the film the observer walked into an aortic section, turned into a renal artery, and then retraced his steps (Greenfield, Vickers, et al, 1971).

As shown in Figure 14, the head-mounted display consists of a head position sensor, the digital computer, a matrix multiplier, a clipping divider, and the head set. The head position sensor includes concentric moving shafts between the head set and the ceiling. By their movement, a certain volume of head motion is allowed. As the wearer moves, high resolution counters measure rotation at the shaft end and the head set while translation is measured along the shaft. These counters send signals to the computer for the defining of the observer's head position with respect to fixed room coordinates, in matrix form. Such data plus the data that define the coordinate values in matrix form for each point of the displayed object are combined by the matrix multiplier equipment. The computer can then manipulate all coordinate values to allow the illusion that the object rotates, translates, or changes size. As the observer walks toward and into an object, the clipping divider computes new end points for those object points that move out of the observer's peri-

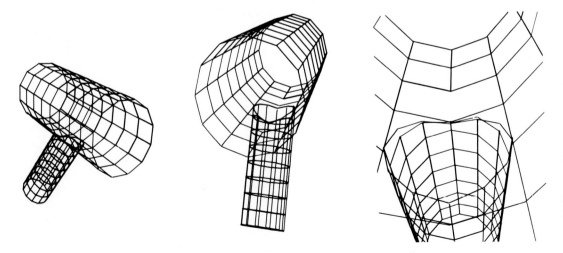

FIG. 15. Some views of the vascular configuration as simulated by the head-mounted display system. One notes the positioning of the observer within the artery, in certain frames of the film.

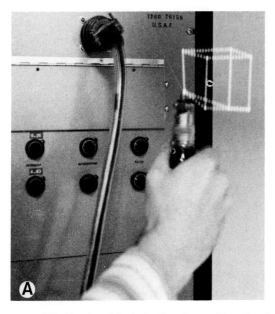 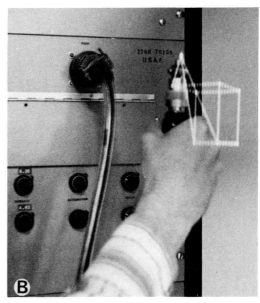

FIG. 16. A and B. A simple cube, positioned and varied in shape by use of the wand.

pheral vision, thus presenting the illusion that one has moved into the object. The head set presents the observer with synthetic objects defined by the computer's data file. Figure 15 exhibits some frames from the finished film. In another film, the observer also walked into a simulated prosthetic heart valve (not shown here).

Also to be mentioned is the wand (Vickers, 1973): This unit is a hand-held rod ancillary to the head-mounted display equipment. It permits the user to interact with the synthetic object that is suspended in space. One points to a point in the suspended image and forms contact with that point by pressing a button on the wand. A series of such buttons acts as the communication input to the computer. The observer can then move the wand to a different position in space with the immediate result that the object is elongated, fused, or added upon, as shown in Figure 16. The user can also "zoom in" for detailed study of a particular component or surface of the object.

DISCUSSION

The most ambitious phase of the overall investigation is presently being contemplated. It is one that employs all the simulation concepts seen to this point. It will be an attempt to duplicate a detailed history of a continually forming, atherosclerotic advanced lesion, with a proportionate interest in the coronary artery regime. The ration-

ale is twofold; not only is present knowledge of the complete growth cycle of a lesion a nondetailed but gross view gained from nonhuman experiments or mortalities, but also the importance of such coronary knowledge is obvious.

Assume that the investigator, using the head-mounted display system, positions himself in a simulated coronary artery. He then travels to a site of predilection for the initiation of a lesion, based upon the geometrics of the chosen channel and the fluid dynamics involved. It would certainly appear that a typical portion of the coronary arterial tree is a many-time amplification of the renal and/or aortic bifurcation geometry that has been previously simulated. In turn, although not specifically discussed, certain algorithms within our present capabilities, permit the wire form arteries of Figure 15 to be shaded, smoothed, and colored (Greenfield, 1972c) for a more natural appearance. As the observer hovers over the point of interest, having used the rotation feature to turn internally within the natural-appearing artery to face the wall, the initiation of the lesion's growth would be formed upon the usage of memory-stored equations describing the results of platelet diffusion theory, in conjunction with red cell augmented diffusion, via a transport mechanism (Monsler et al, 1970). The initial lesion might then appear as computer simulated in Figure 17. The observer by command to the computer can rotate and zoom in to view the eventual growth at a particular surface point (Fig. 18).

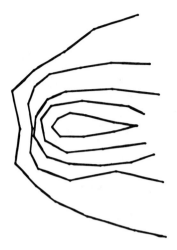

FIG. 17   Idealized plaque growth, computer simulated.

The asymptotic structure of the platelet aggregates will be described mathematically to allow subsequent computer algorithms to be defined. A detailed, growing surface section will then be formed in conjunction with a surface shading, via spline function theory. As the surface is changing shape, blood flow, represented by particles, would form streamlines, and turbulent eddies and stasis regions would appear. Attendant stress values at various positions would appear numerically upon the graphics display screen, in conjunction with visual results and typical red blood cell damage evaluation (all such capabilities have been exemplified in this chapter).

If the observer were able to touch the center fold of the simulated surface and then move it in an upward fashion to represent stress, the pulling action at one surface position would change the constraint values at the other surface position. Such action would denote steps in the growth cycle of a lesion. The pulling action, with its resulting stress analysis values plotted on the display, could well be performed by the "wand," in conjunction with the head-mounted display system. The new shape is then displayed in space or upon the display screen.

As the observer hovers over an area of interest, such man-machine interaction would allow continuous changes in equations for the theory to evolve and come closer to any available data. If,

in turn, a plaque, for example, does not correctly build up piecewise according to data, one can immediately erase a portion of the simulation. By computer command the flow can be initiated again about the reshaped plaque section. If the plaque, in its formative details, is seen to be approximate to some known part of the growth cycle, it is then assumed that the mathematical equations in the theory are correct. The sum of the interim steps that result will be compared to viewed lesions seen in animal experimentations or cadaver results. At present, we are performing experimental stress studies in a fluid about a model lesion so as to attempt verification of the computer simulations. If the procedure is successful, parts or eventually the whole of the formation of an atherosclerotic lesion would be displayed in minutes—equivalent to natural atheroma buildup that takes years to develop. Varying conditions and assumptions could be quickly interchanged and evaluated.

This investigator is convinced that fluid dynamic concepts and numerical analysis techniques have important roles in the studies of hemodynamic phenomena. The use of computer graphics allows information by man-machine interaction not previously available. It is realized that the task of forming results is still arduous and that continuous development of this interdisciplinary technique is required.

References

Amsden A, Harlow F: The SMAC method. Los Alamos Science Report LA-4370, 1970

Bruns D, Connolly J, Holman E, Stafer R: Experimental observations on post-stenotic dilatation. J Thorac Cardiovasc Surg 38:662, 1959

Cannon T, Greenfield H: Adaptability of computer graphics to studies of atherosclerosis pathogenesis. J Assoc Adv Med Instrum 6:250, 1972

Caro C, Fitz-Gerald J, Schroter R: Atheroma and arterial wall shear: observation, correlation, and proposal for a shear dependent mass transfer mechanism for atherogenesis. Proc R Soc London (Biol) 117: 109, 1971

Downie H, Mustard J, Rowsell H: Swine atherosclerosis: the relationship of lipids and blood coagulation to its development. Ann NY Acad Sci 104:539, 1963

Enos W, Beyer J, Holmes R: Pathogenesis of coronary disease in American soldiers killed in Korea. JAMA 158:914, 1955

Friedman M, Byers S: Excess lipid leakage: property of very young vascular endothelium. Br J Exp Pathol 43:363, 1962

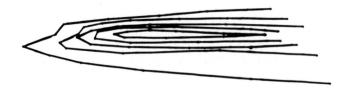

FIG. 18.   Computer rotation of a simulated plaque to a degree that would allow cross-sectional viewing before the growth cycle was varied.

Fromm J: A method for computing nonsteady incompressible viscous fluid flows. Los Alamos Science Report LA-2910, 1963

Fromm J, Harlow F: Numerical solution of the problem of the vortex street development. Phys Fluids 6:975, 1963

Fry D: Acute vascular endothelial changes associated with increased blood velocity gradients. Circ Res 22:165, 1968

Fry D: Certain chemorheologic considerations regarding the blood vascular interface with particular reference to coronary artery disease. Circulation suppl IV 40:38, 1969

Gessner F: Hemodynamic theories of atherogenesis. Circ Res 33:259, 1973

Greenfield H: Use of graphic terminal device for distributed system simulation studies in hemodynamics. In Haga E (ed): Computer Techniques in Biomedicine and Medicine New York, Auerbach, 1972a, p 149

Greenfield H: Large-scale numerical problems in biomedical studies. In Computer Graphics in Medicine, New York, ACM Press, 1972b, p 27

Greenfield H: Special address: studies of medical phenomena by computer graphics. Trans Am Soc Artif Int Organs 18:607, 1972c

Greenfield H: Investigations into particular human circulatory system phenomena by true computer-man interaction. Int J Biomed Comput 4:31, 1973

Greenfield H, Brauer C: Hemodynamic studies involving a computer simulation technique. Br Inst Elec Eng publ 51, 1969, pp 21–30

Greenfield H, Brauer C, Reemtsma K: Preliminary analysis of blood flow characteristics in the abdominal aorta by computer interpretation. In Parslow RD, Green RE (eds): Computer Graphics in Medical Research and Hospital Administration. London, Plenum, 1971, p 35

Greenfield H, DeBry R: Interactive graphic representation of hemodynamic phenomena. In Parslow RD, Green RE (eds): Proceedings International Conference on Line Interactive Computers, Middlesex, Brunel, 1972, p 573

Greenfield H, Hampton T, Gascoigne H, Kolff W: Photoelastic stress analysis of silastic poppet degeneration in prosthetic heart valves. Circ Res 23:54, 1973

Greenfield H, Kolff W: The prosthetic heart valve and computer graphics. JAMA 219:69, 1972

Greenfield H, Vickers D, Sutherland I, Kolff W, Reemtsma K: Moving computer graphics images seen from inside the vascular system. Trans Am Soc Artif Int Organs 17:381, 1971

Harlow F, Welch J, Shannon J, Daly B: The MAC method. Los Alamos Science Report LA-4325, 1966

Lawrensen D: Numerical methods. In Vitkovitch D (ed): Field Analysis. New York, Van Nostrand, 1966, p 102

Lynn N, Fox V, Ross L: Flow patterns at arterial bifurcations presented at 63d annual meeting, AIChE, Chicago, 29 Nov 1970

Monsler M, Morton W, Weiss R: The fluid mechanics of thrombus formation, presented at AIAA 3d fluid and plasma dynamics conf (AIAA paper no 70-787) Los Angeles, 29 June, 1970

Mustard J, Murphy E, Rowsell H, Downie H: Platelets and atherosclerosis. J Athero Res 4:1, 1964

Nevaril C, Lynch C, Alfrey C, Hellums J: Erythrocyte damage and destruction induced by shearing stress. J Lab Clin Med 71:784, 1968

Pearson C: A computational method for viscous flow problems. J Fl Mech 21:611, 1965

Ray G, Davids N: Shear stress analysis of blood-endothelial surface in inlet section of artery with plugging. J Biomech 3:99, 1970

Reemtsma K, Sandberg L, Greenfield H: Some theoretic aspects of vascular degeneration. Am J Surg 119: 548, 1970

Rodbard S: Physical factors in the progression of vascular lesions. Circulation 17:410, 1958

Sako Y: Effects of turbulent blood flow and hypertension on experimental atherosclerosis. JAMA 179:36, 1962

Scharfstein H, Gutstein W, Lewis L: Changes of boundary layer flow in model systems: implication for initiation of endothelial injury. Circ Res 13:580, 1963

Spurlock J, Homa M, Durfee R: Atherosclerosis etiology: further evidence of the role of hemodynamic effects. Res Mono, Atl Res Corp, Alexandria, Va, 1968

Sutherland I: A head-mounted three-dimensional display. Proc Fall Joint Comp Conf AFIPS Press, Montvale NJ, 33:757, 1968

Texon M: The hemodynamic concept of atherosclerosis with particular reference to coronary occlusion. Arch Int Med 99:418, 1957

Texon M: The hemodynamic concept of atherosclerosis. Am J Cardiol 5:291, 1960a

Texon M, Imparato A, Lord J: The hemodynamic concept of atherosclerosis: the experimental production of hemodynamic arterial disease. Arch Surg 80:47, 1960b

Ting D, Greenfield H: Spline function interpolation in interactive hemodynamic simulation. Int J Man-Mach Studies 4:256, 1972

Vickers D: Sorcerer's apprentice: head-mounted display and wand. Unpublished PhD thesis, Univ of Utah, Salt Lake City, 1973

Wesolowski S, Fries C, Sabin A, Sawyer P: Turbulence, intimal injury and atherosclerosis. In Sawyer PN (ed): Biophysical Mechanisms in Vascular Homeostasis and Intravascular Thrombosis. New York, Appleton-Century-Crofts, 1965, p 147

115

NEW APPROACHES TO THE UNDERSTANDING AND CHEMOTHERAPY OF ATHEROSCLEROSIS AND INTRAVASCULAR THROMBOSIS

P. N. Sawyer, B. Stanczewski, N. Ramasamy, and J. S. Keates

INTRODUCTION

Progressive insights into the causal mechanisms of arteriosclerotic peripheral vascular disease, the areas of the vascular tree and blood vessel wall involved with the progress of the disease, and techniques for their investigation have been provided by studies from many laboratories over the past several years (Sawyer et al, 1973). Atherosclerotic and thrombotic phenomena have been studied at different levels—biologic, biochemical, and physicochemical. The blood vascular interface is the site of a series of interactions that finally result in thrombus deposition. The morphology of normal and injured blood vessels and vessels with different degrees of atherosclerosis have been investigated using scanning electron microscopy (Stoner et al, 1973). The biochemical interactions leading to platelet plug formation and the factors that affect this process constitute a second mode of studying the problem, ie, the physical biochemistry at the interface (Wilner et al, 1968; Spaet and Al-Mondhiry, 1970; Mustard and Packham, 1971; Massini and Lucher, 1972; Jamieson et al, 1971; Barber and Jamieson, 1971). One of the most important and potentially rewarding approaches is a study of the interface at the physicochemical level (Sawyer, 1965a). Since thrombosis is mainly an interface phenomenon and many of the biochemical and metabolic processes are reflected in an alteration of charge, study of the charge distribution at the interface is quite useful. Thus a study of the electrical double layer at the blood-vascular interface and the interface potential of blood vessels and blood cellular elements yields valuable information on the effects of drugs, injury, and atherosclerosis on the vascular system. In this review, it is planned to describe briefly the methods that are used to study the interface both *in vivo* and *in vitro,* and the techniques used to study their effect in patients. We will discuss the recent results obtained for three classes—antithrombotic drugs, thrombolytic drugs, and drugs used for unrelated purposes (ie, oral contraceptives). The correlation between the clinical effects of drugs and the physicochemical phenomena at the blood vascular interface will be described. We will also describe a drug that was first studied at the interface level and based on these results was then used in clinical trials in our laboratories.

EXPERIMENTAL TECHNIQUES

The experimental techniques adopted for the study of reactions occurring at the blood vascular interface and the effect of drugs at the interface can be broadly divided into two classes, *in vitro* and *in vivo.* The clinical trials and the techniques used to assess the effects of drugs in the human body comprise the second group (Table 1).

In Vitro and *In Vivo* Physicochemical Methods

It is quite well known that when a solid comes into contact with a solution, an electric double layer is set up at the solid solution interface. This is a very general physicochemical interaction that is true of any solid-solution system

TABLE 1. Summary of Methods Used for Screening of Drugs

EXPERIMENTS		CLINICAL	
Technique	Area	Technique	Area
Electrophoresis (*in vitro*)	RBC Platelets Leukocytes	Plethysmography	Venous and arterial flow
Electroosmosis (*in vitro*)	Artery Vein	Ultrasonic Doppler	Arterial pressure
		Venogram	Venous patency
Streaming potential (*in vitro* and *in vivo*)	Artery Vein	Aortogram	Arterial condition
		Coagulation studies	
Rat mesentery (*in vivo*)	Arterioles and venules	Blood chemistry	
Precipitation potential (*in vitro*)	RBC Platelets WBC	Blood picture	
		EKG	
SEM (*in vitro*)	Artery Vein		
Coagulation			

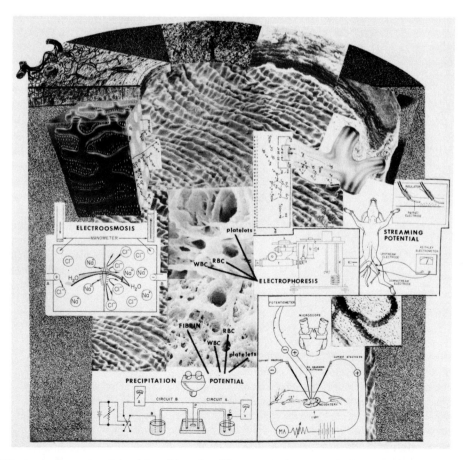

FIG. 1. A composite picture describing the different experimental techniques employed for the physicochemical evaluation of the blood vessel wall and cellular elements in blood.

(Kruyt, 1952; Davies and Rideal, 1963). Blood vessels and cells are normally negatively charged (Sawyer, 1965a). The electric double layer is about 10 to 15 Å thick; a voltage drop of 10^7 to 10^6 V/cm is associated with the double layer. A part of the potential drop of the double layer is called the zeta potential, and this parameter is a fairly good measure of the net charge of the interface. Three well-characterized electrokinetic phenomena are associated with the zeta potential; the streaming potential, electrophoresis, and electroosmosis. These are used to study the charge characteristics of the blood vessel wall and blood cells.

STREAMING POTENTIAL (*IN VITRO* AND *IN VIVO*). Streaming potential measures the potential developed across a pipe through which solution is flowing under a pressure difference (Sawyer, 1965a, 1966). This reflects the magnitude of the surface potential (zeta potential) and any change introduced by the adsorption of drugs. Figure 1 shows the arrangement for *in vivo* streaming potential measurements.

ELECTROPHORESIS (*IN VITRO*). Electrophoresis is the movement of charged particles under the influence of an external electric field (Kruyt, 1952). The surface charge characteristics of cellular elements of blood are measured using this technique (Fig. 1). This method is used to evaluate the effect of drugs administered *in vivo* on the surface charge of platelets, red and white cells.

ELECTROOSMOSIS (*IN VITRO*). This measures the flow of water across a membrane under the influence of an electric current (Kruyt, 1952). The effect of drugs on the modification of surface charge of blood vessels is ascertained using this technique. An animal is given a drug for a period of time, and at sacrifice the aorta and vena cava are removed and their electroosmotic characteristics measured immediately (Fig. 1).

PRECIPITATION POTENTIAL (*IN VITRO*). In this method the effect of drugs on blood cells is ascertained (Sawyer et al, 1964a, 1965b, 1965c). The adhesion of cells onto a bright platinum electrode at a set potential vs NHE is measured semiquantitatively by microscopically counting the cells. The number of cells adhering is plotted as a function of the applied potential. Antithrombotic drugs and drugs that affect platelet reactions alter the shape of the curve (number of cells adhered vs. the potential curve). The experimental setup is shown in Figure 1.

RAT MESENTERY COAGULATION TIMES (*IN VIVO*). This is a direct method that determines the effect of different pharmacologic agents on an intact vascular system (Sawyer, 1960). A drug is injected into rats, and the mesenteric vessels are observed under a microscope (Fig. 1). A small direct current is passed across the mesentery and the time taken for occlusion of vessels is measured. This current-induced occlusion time gives a clear indication of the thrombotic or antithrombotic nature of a pharmacologic agent.

SCANNING ELECTRON MICROSCOPY. Scanning electron micrographs of the blood vessel wall and the vascular system give a picture of the vessel surface and the cellular deposition. On sacrifice the vessels are fixed *in situ* within glutaraldehyde under pressure and examined using the SEM.

Clinical Trials

Pharmacologic agents that have passed through the different stages of development (eg, controlled tests on toxicity, *in vitro* and *in vivo* physicochemical evaluation, etc) and are suitable for an Investigational New Drug (IND) application from the Food and Drug Administration (FDA) are given patients. The following methods are employed to assess their effects in the body and these methods constitute an *in vivo* screen.

Patients on antiatherosclerotic or anticoagulant therapy proven to have arterial or venous disease as diagnosed by a combination of procedures, ie, arteriography and/or venography, blood flow determinations, EKG etc, are asked to return at one to two weekly intervals (where appropriate) for clinical examination and tests. At each subsequent visit a follow-up history and physical examination are done, measurements of "arterial blood flow volume" and venous function are made using mercury-in-rubber strain gauge plethysmography (Whitney, 1953; Egan, 1961; Dahn et al, 1967). The strain gauge is placed about the affected area and the change in limb volume due to venous filling rate following occlusion by a pressure cuff above the gauge, is recorded (Fig. 2). This record gives an indirect index of arterial blood flow volume expressed in ml/100ml tissue/min. Both resting and postischemic blood flow volumes are measured. Venous distensibility and emptying (Hällbröök and Göthlin, 1971) are measured with the patients' legs elevated 20 cm above the heart level. Here the venous occlusion cuff is applied until there is no further swelling of the limb (ie, the venous pressure becomes equal to,

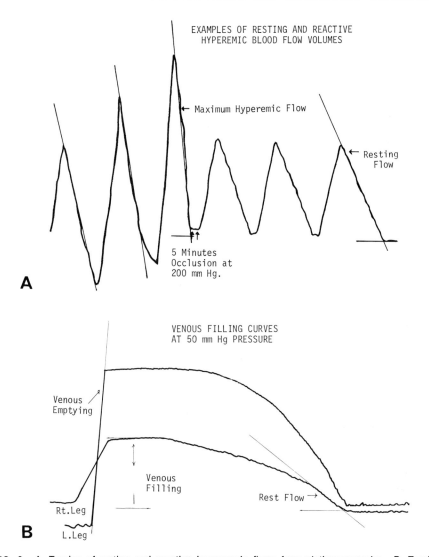

FIG. 2. A. Tracing of resting and reactive hyperaemic flows from plethysmography. B. Tracing of venous emptying and filling. Right—leg abnormal results as seen in phlebitic patients. Left—leg normal results.

or greater than, the occlusion cuff pressure). The amount of increase in volume is an index of venous distensibility (measured in ml/100 ml tissue). On release of the venous occlusion cuff, venous emptying is measured and expressed in ml/100ml tissue/min. Walking distances are recorded. Peripheral pulse pressures are measured by the ultrasonic Doppler technique (Kirby et al, 1969).

At each visit, routine blood samples are taken for fasting cholesterol levels, glucose levels, haematology, and coagulation studies. The coagulation studies include Lee White clotting, Thrombin (TRT), Activated Partial Thromboplastin, (APTT), and Recalcification Times (RTC).

RESULTS

The drugs evaluated on the physicochemical screen (electroosmosis, streaming potential, electrophoresis, rat mesentery, and precipitation potentials) and their specific clinical effects are discussed based on their employment (ie, antithrombotic, thrombolytic, and those used for unrelated purposes) (Table 2).

Table 3 compares the experimentally evaluated physicochemical effects with the clinical effects of a few of the pharmacologic agents studied.

TABLE 2. Classification of Some Pharmacologic Agents

ANTI-THROMBOTIC	THROMBOLYTIC	UNRELATED AGENTS
Heparin	Thrombolysin	Oral contra-ceptives
Protamine (heparin antagonist)	Arvin	–
Dextran 40 (plasma expander)	Reptilase	Aspirin
Aspirin	–	–
0-β-Hydrox-ethylrutoside (HR)	–	–

It is tabulated by the general degree of antithrombogenicity found experimentally, against the clinical results. It is seen that in general the drugs that increase the negative surface charge of the cells and vessel wall prolong the mesenteric occlusion time and have antithrombotic clinical effects.

DISCUSSION

One of the more interesting aspects of the use of the screening procedures described in this communication, for any chemical *in vitro,* is the obvious utility in terms of evaluating the effects of material on the surface chemistry of the various components that comprise the blood vascular system. Thus, one can determine the effect of any water-soluble compound on the surface charge characteristics and ultimately the antithrombogenic characteristics of virtually any chemical that is not totally destructive to the biologic interface. Our experience has been that significant modification of the vascular interface charge in the more negative direction tends to yield resistance to intervascular thrombosis. Loss or decrease in the negative surface charge of the various components of the vascular tree and more positive charge or loss of vascular interface potential are invariably indicative of a prothrombogenic characteristic for the materials in question. This provides a highly useful measurement of the thrombogenic side effects of many chemicals that are known to have other powerful biologic influences.

Antithrombogenic Drugs

HEPARIN.   Heparin, a sulfonated mucopolysaccharide, has powerful antithrombotic and anticoagulant effects in the vasculature. *In vitro* and *in vivo* studies show that it increases the negative surface charge of the blood cells and to a lesser extent of the arterial wall. Heparin inhibits the adhesion of platelets and blood cells to bright platinum electrodes maintained at a wide range of potentials (Fig. 3). It also significantly prolongs the electrically induced rat mesentery thrombosis time. In the injured blood vessel, heparin causes a reversal of the positive injury potential toward the normal negative value. SEM micrographs indicate that it modified thrombus formation and de-

TABLE 3. Physiochemical and Clinical Effects of Some Pharmacologic Agents Studied

PHYSIOCHEMICAL EFFECTS					DRUG	CLINICAL EFFECTS (BLOOD COAGULATION)			
Blood Cells		Blood Vessel		Mesentery		TRT	APTT	RCT	Bleeding
RBC	Platelets	Artery	Vein						
+++	+++	++	++	+++	Heparin	+	0	0	++
–	–	–	–	–	Protamine (heparin antagonist	N.D.			0
0	–	+	+	N.D.	Dextran 40	0	0	0	+
+	+	+	N.D.	+	Aspirin	+	0	0	+
0	0	++	++	++	0-β-Hydroxyethylrutoside	+	N.D.	++	+
0	0	+	+	++	Thrombolysin	+	+	+	N.D.
+	–	+	+	N.D.	Reptilase (1.8U/Kg)	+++	+++	+++	N.D.
Clotted		Clotted			(0.12U/Kg)			Clotted	
–	–	–	+	N.D.	Arvin (5U/Kg)	+++	+++	+++	N.D.
Clotted		Clotted			(0.5U/Kg)			Clotted	
		–	–	–	Mestranol	0	+	–	0
N.D.	0	–	N.D.	–	Norethindrone	0	+	+	N.D.
–	–	0	0	–	Mixed	0	0	–	N.D.

+, ++, +++: degree of antithrombogenicity.–:thrombogenic. 0: no effect. N.D.: not done

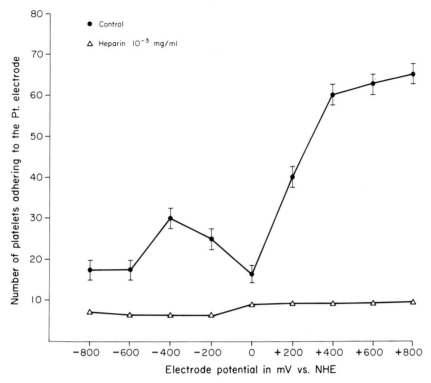

FIG. 3. Platelet adhesion on platinum electrodes as a function of potential. It is seen that in the presence of heparin thrombocytes do not adhere even at positive potentials.

position on the injured blood vessel wall (Fig. 4). Clinically it prolongs the bleeding time and demonstrates powerful anticoagulant effects, acting on Factor Xa, the conversion of prothrombin to thrombin and inhibiting the formation of fibrin in the presence of thrombin (Biggs and Denson, 1972).

PROTAMINE. Clinically, protamine is used as a neutralizing agent for heparin (Jorpes, 1971). When studied alone it demonstrates prothrombogenic effects on the vasculature causing the surface charge of the blood cells and vasculature to become less negative. The electrically induced rat mesentery thrombosis time is shortened to half the control time in the presence of protamine; thus the physicochemical effects are opposite to those induced by heparin.

DEXTRAN 40. Low Molecular Weight Dextran causes a minimal increase in the negative surface charge of blood cells but has a marked effect on blood vessels (Srinivasan et al, 1968). It is not as effective as heparin in reversing the positive injury potential to normal. The change in morphology of blood vessel wall injury due to perfusion of dextran before injury, is shown in Figure 5. Dextran has a dramatic masking effect

on red cell, white cell, and platelet "recognition," physically attaching to the surface of the cells, preventing or markedly reducing tendency for rouleaux formation (Kung-mien and Chien, 1973; Chien and Kung-mien, 1973) and preventing cell-cell and cell-wall interaction. The marginal effect on electrophoretic mobility of blood cells is suspected to be due to a change in viscosity of the medium. Clinically, dextran 40 has been used as a plasma expander and for improvement of blood flow (Pharmacia 1968). The bleeding time may be prolonged. The coagulation times are not greatly affected by dextran perfusion although the anti-thrombotic effect is ascribed to its effect on platelet aggregation (Nilsson and Eiken, 1964; Moncrief et al, 1963).

ASPIRIN. The antiinflammatory agent aspirin significantly increases the negative surface charge of both the blood vessel wall and of platelets and red blood cells. It also prolongs the electrically induced rat mesentery occlusion time. Clinically, aspirin administration causes a prolongation of bleeding time (Atac et al, 1970) and an increase in heparin sensitivity (FitzGerald and Butterfield, 1969). It inhibits platelet functions and

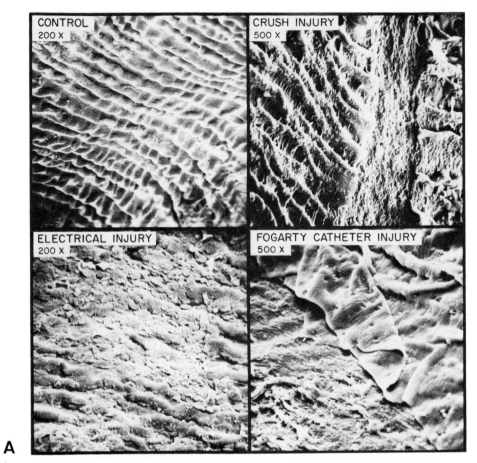

A

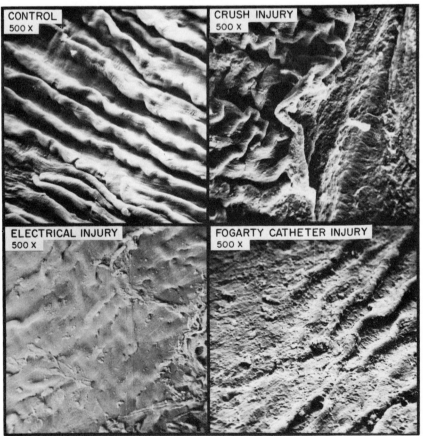

B

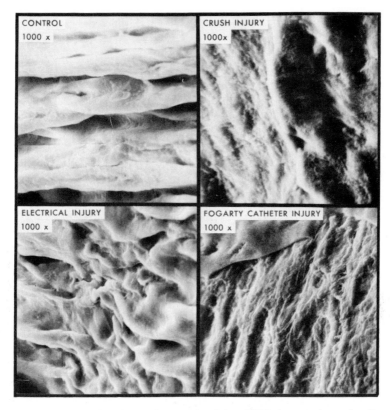

FIG. 5. The effect of administration of dextran after injury (SEM photographs at the site of injury).

prostaglandin formation (Somova, 1973). The aspirin effect can last for from two to 10 days after a single dose. Aspirin is used for secondary treatment of phlebitis (O'Brien, 1972).

Thrombolytic Agents

THROMBOLYSIN. Thrombolysin (human plasmin and fibrinolysin) is a proteolytic enzyme. Physicochemical studies show very little effect on the surface charge of blood cells, while the negative charge of blood vessel wall is enhanced. Rat mesentery occlusion times are markedly increased following large dosages (Lustrin et al, 1965). The effect of the drug in preventing thrombosis on the injured wall and the morphology of thrombus at site of injury is being studied. Clinically it has been used in thrombolytic therapy (Sawyer et al, 1964b). The blood coagulation times (TRT, APTT, RCT) are enhanced (Table 3).

ARVIN (ANCROD) AND REPTILASE. These snake (pit viper) venoms are proteolytic thrombinlike enzymes of low molecular weight. They function as defibrinating as well as defibrinogenating enzymes. They release fibrinopeptide-A from human fibrinogen. A high degree of hypocoagulability is observed without serious bleeding tendencies (Turpie et al, 1972; Blombäck 1972; Stocker and Egberg, 1972; Pizzo et al, 1972; Kwaan, 1972). Our findings show that there is very little effect on the surface charge of blood cells while there is limited increase in surface negativity of blood vessels. Coagulation studies show an extraordinary increase in TRT, APTT, and RCT times. This is expected as the enzymes function as defibrinogenating agents having a thrombinlike action. At low concentrations, plasma clots very rapidly making determinations impossible. Thrombus formation at the site of injury with administration of these enzymes is shown in Figures 6 and 7.

FIG. 4. Facing page: A. Scanning Electron Microscopic (SEM) photographs of injured blood vessel (control). B. The effect of administration of heparin after injury (SEM photographs at the site of injury).

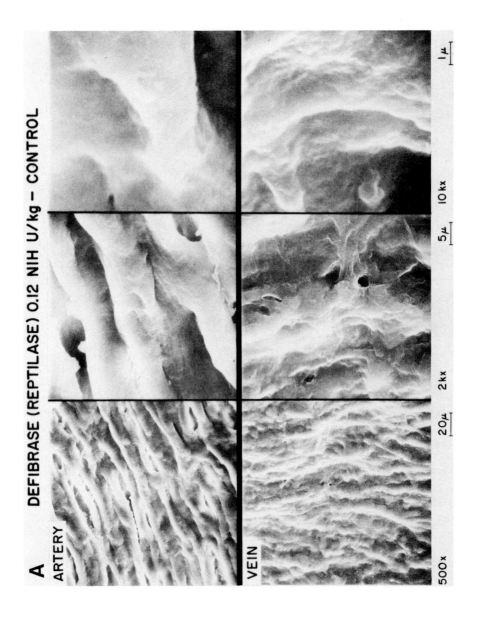

A   DEFIBRASE (REPTILASE) 0.12 NIH U/kg – CONTROL

ARTERY

VEIN

500x   20μ   2kx   5μ   10kx   1μ

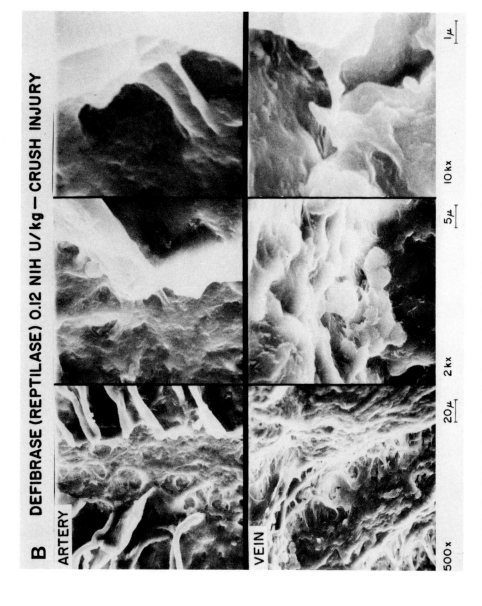

FIG. 6. SEM photographs of artery and vein (at different magnifications) of dogs administered reptilase (0.12 NIH U/Kg) and the effect of injury to the vessel. A. Control. B. Crush injury.

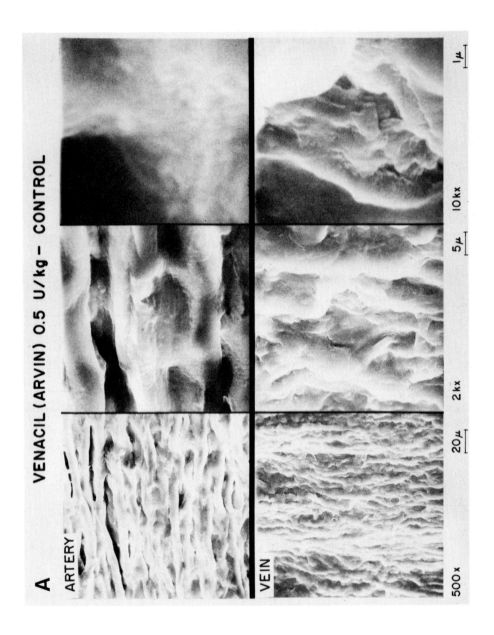

VENACIL (ARVIN) 0.5 U/kg – CONTROL

A

ARTERY

VEIN

1 µ

10 kx

5 µ

2 kx

20 µ

500 x

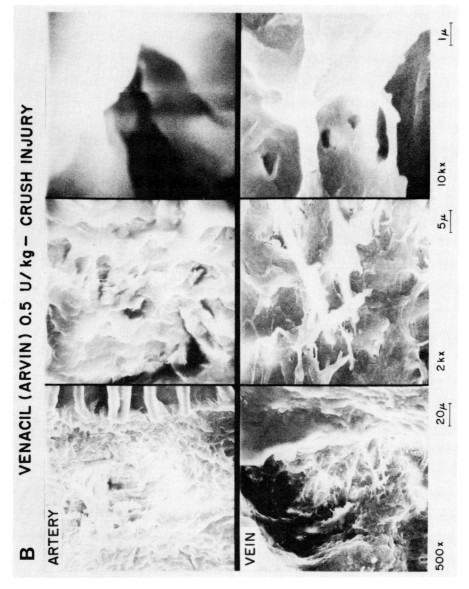

B VENACIL (ARVIN) 0.5 U/kg – CRUSH INJURY

ARTERY

VEIN

500 x 20 μ 2 kx 5 μ 10 kx 1 μ

FIG. 7. SEM photographs of artery and vein (at different magnifications) of dogs administered arvin (0.5U/Kg) and of the effect on injury. A. Control. B. Crush injury.

Drugs for Unrelated Uses

ORAL CONTRACEPTIVES. The steroid hormones used as oral contraceptives have been blamed for a number of thrombotic diseases in women (thrombophlebitis, embolism, and cerebrovascular accidents) (Vessey and Doll, 1969; Group Study, 1973; Sartwell et al, 1969; Alkjaersig et al, 1971). The effect of these hormones has been evaluated in our laboratories both in animal experiments and human subjects. These hormones have a marginal effect on the surface charge of platelets and red cells while the negative surface charge of blood vessels (artery and vein) dramatically decreases. This decrease is more pronounced with estrogenic compounds. Combined estrogen-progesterone administration markedly reduces the rat mesenteric occlusion time (less than half of the control) (Table 3). This may explain the prothrombotic effect of oral contraceptives on women. Coagulation times are affected differently, ie, thrombin times are unaffected while the APTT increases and RCT decreases for norethindrone. The data agree with other published results. It has been suggested that combined contraceptive therapy stimulates some and inhibits other coagulation proteins, the net effect being no change in the fibrinogen to fibrin conversion time (as demonstrated by the unchanged thrombin times) (Dugdale and Masi 1971; Asback et al, 1972).

0-β-HYDROXYETHYLRUTOSIDE (HR). *In vivo* studies of this drug (a flavonoid) have shown that while it significantly enhances the negative surface charge density of the blood vessel wall, it does not alter the surface charge of the blood cells. It also exhibits anticoagulant effects as demonstrated by a marked prolongation of rat mesentery occlusion times and increased thrombin and recalcification times. In experimental animals these effects become more apparent on long-term administration (one week to two months) (Comel and Laszt, 1972).

0-β-Hydroxyethylrutoside has been used clinically for the treatment of venous insufficiency and phlebitis in Europe for more than 15 years. More recently it has also been found to be effective in patients with atherosclerosis. Evidence from these clinical studies indicate that this drug has very low toxicity and that its beneficial effects become more apparent following long-term administration (FitzGerald et al, 1969; Sawyer, 1975). Because our experimental evidence also suggested that HR may have antiatherosclerotic effects in humans,

we proceeded to clinical trial (Srinivasan et al, 1971).

At present we are carrying out a controlled double blind trial study in patients with peripheral atherosclerosis. Surgery is not considered expedient in these subjects (1) because the disease is in its early stages; (2) because of heart or respiratory problems; or (3) because they have previously undergone surgery and require continued medication. Two grams a day of the drug is administered orally. Clinical effects are assessed every two weeks for three months (methods of testing were described in the previous section). Although this trial is not complete, the clinical and experimental evidence from European groups indicate that HR is effective in the relief of both venous and arterial diseases (FitzGerald et al, 1967, 1969, 1971; McEwan and McAndle, 1971).

CONCLUSIONS

A better understanding of the physical chemistry of intravascular thrombosis and the effects of various pharmacologic agents in modifying the processes at the vascular interface provides a new approach to the development of better antiatherosclerotic and antithrombotic agents. The effects of newer drugs for use in the cardiovascular system can be analyzed by the methods discussed. In the case of the drugs like oral contraceptive agents, we may be able, by this type of drug screening procedure, to predict any unexpected or undesirable side effects on the vasculature even at the animal experimentation stage.

ACKNOWLEDGMENTS

The authors thank the contributions by Drs. S. Srinivasan, J. Solash, D. Farhangian, G. E. Pasupathy, and G. E. Stoner, Messers. T. Boyd, T. R. Lucas, E. Ateyeh, Jr., R. Kron, G. W. Kammlott, and Mrs. L. Lucas, Miss J. Beeman, and Miss A. Redner to different aspects of the investigation reported in this review.

The work was made possible by financial support from (1) National Institute of Health (Grant No. HL 15123-02); (2) Zyma Nyon, Switzerland; and (3) Sawyer Foundation.

References

Alkjaersig N, Fletcher AP, Burstein R: Thromboembolism and oral contraceptive medication. Thromb Diath Haemor (Suppl.) 49: 125, 1971

Asbeck F, Bolter A, Henning, HD, et al: The mechanism of intravascular activation of the fibrinolytic system during hormonal contraception: a three month follow-up study. Haemostasis 1:108, 1972

Atac A, Spagnvol M, Zucker MB: Long term inhibition of platelet functions by aspirin. Proc Soc Exp Biol Med 133:1331, 1970

Barber AJ, Jamieson GA: Platelet collagen adhesion characterization of collagen glucosyl transferase on plasma membranes of human blood platelets. Biochim Biophysics Acta 252:533, 1971

Biggs R, Denson KWE: Natural and pathological inhibitors of blood coagulation. Chap 7 in Human Blood Coagulation Haemostasis and Thrombosis. Oxford, Blackwell Scientific Publications, 1972

Blombäck B: Mode of action of defibrinating enzymes with special reference to reptilase and arvin. Int Soc Thromb, Haemostasis. 3d Cong, Washington, DC Abstracts 46, 1972

Chien S, Kung-mien J. Ultrastructural basis of the mechanism of rouleaux formation. Microvasc Res 5:155, 1973

Comel M, Laszt PL (eds): Clinical Pharmacology: Flavonoids and Vascular Wall. Symposium Angiologica Santoriana, 4th International Symposium, S Karger, Basel, 1972

Dahn I, Lassen NA, Westling H: On the mechanism of delayed hyperaemia in the calf muscles in obliterative arterial disease. Cardiovascular Research I, 145–49:1967

Davies JT, Rideal EK: Interfacial phenomena, 2nd ed. New York, London, Academic Press, 1963

Dugdale M, Masi AP: Hormonal contraception and thromboembolic disease: effect of oral contraceptives on hemostatic mechanisms: a review of the literature. J Chron Dis 23:775, 1971

Egan CJ: The mercury strain gauge method of digital plethysmography, Alaskan Air Command Artic Aeromedical Lab. Technical Note AAL-TN 60, 14-17, 1960–61

FitzGerald DE: A clinical trial of troxerutin in venous insufficiency of the lower limb. Practitioner 198:406, 1967

FitzGerald DE, Butterfield WJH: A case of increased platelet antiheparin factor in a patient with Raynauds phenomenon and gangrene treated by aspirin. Angiology 20:317, 1969

FitzGerald DE, Butterfield WJ, Keates JS, Hodges M: The effect of hydroxyethylrutoside (HR) on peripheral blood flow: a preliminary report, 5th European Conference on Microcirculation Gothenburg Bibl Anat No. 10, 600–605 Karger, Basel, 1969

FitzGerald DE, Keates JS, MacMillan D: Chronic occlusive arterial disease: the results of blood flow studies in three groups of patients treated by exercise training; (O-β-hydroxyethyl)-Rutoside and Observation. In Bollinger A, Brunner U (eds): Aktuelle Problems in Der Angiologie, vol 13, Hans Huber, 1971

Group Study: Group for the study of stroke, oral contraception and increased risk of cerebral ischemia or thrombosis. N Engl J Med 288:871, 1973

Hällböök T, Göthlin J: Strain gauge plethysmography and phlebography in diagnosis of deep venous thrombosis. Acta Chir Scand 137:37, 1971

Jamieson GA, Urban LC, Barber AJ: Enzymatic basis for platelets collagen adhesion as the primary step in haemostasis. Nature [New Biol] 234:5, 1971

Jorpes JE: Heparin assays in blood. In Bang NU, Beller FK, Deutsch E, Mammen EF (eds): Thrombosis and Bleeding disorders. New York, London, Academic Press, 1971, p 277

Kirby RB, Kemmerer WT, Morgan JL: Transcutaneous Doppler measurements of blood pressure. Anesthesiology 31:86, 1969

Kruyt HR: Colloid Science, vol I. Irreversible Systems. Amsterdam, Elsevier Publishing Co, 1952

Kung-mien J, Chien S: Role of surface electric charge in red blood cell interactions. J Gen Physiol 61: 638, 1973

Kwaan HC: Current status of ancod and reptilase. Int Soc Thromb, Hemostasis, 3d Cong, Washington DC, Abstracts, p 50, 1972

Lustrin I, Breen H, Reardon D, Wesolowski SA, Sawyer PN: Comparative anticoagulant effects of coumadin, heparin and fibrinolysin on direct current thrombosis of rat mesoappendix vessels. Surgery 58:857, 1965

Massini P, Lucher EF: On mechanisms by which cell contact hinders the release reactions of blood platelets: the effects of cationic polymers. Thromb Diath Haemor 27, 120:1972

McEwan AJ, McArdle CS: Effect of hydroxyethylrutosides on blood oxygen levels and venous insufficiency symptoms in varicose veins. BMJ 2:138, 1971

Moncrief JA, Darin JC, Canizaro TC, Sawyer RB: Use of dextran to prevent arterial and venous thrombosis. Ann Surg 158:553, 1963

Mustard JF, Packham MA: Platelet reactions. Semin Hematol 8:37, 1971

Nilsson IM, Eiken O: Further studies on the effect of dextran of various molecular weights on the coagulation mechanism. Thromb Diath Haemor 11:38, 1964

O'Brien JR: A trial of aspirin in post-operative venous thrombosis. Int Soc Thromb Hemostasis 3d Cong. Washington, DC, Abstracts, 1972, p 42

Pharmacia (Pub): Blood flow improvement clinical and experimental data on Rheomacrodex. Pharmacia AB, 1968

Pizzo SV, Schwartz ML, Hill RL, McKee PA: The effects of ancrod and reptilase on fibrin formation and fibrin digestion. Int Soc Thromb Hemostasis, 3d Cong, Washington, DC, Abstracts 1972, p 48

Sartwell PE, Masi AT, Arhes FG: Thromboembolism and oral contraceptives an epidemiologic case control study. Am J Epidemiol 90:365, 1969

Sawyer PN (ed): Biophysical Mechanisms in Vascular Hemostasis and Intravascular Thrombosis. New York, Appleton-Century-Crofts, 1965a

Sawyer PN, Brattain WH, Boddy PJ: Electrochemical precipitation of human blood cells and its possible relation to intravascular thrombosis. Proc Natl Acad Sci 51:428, 1964a

Sawyer PN, Himmelfarb E, Lustrin I, Zuskind H, et al: Measurement of streaming potentials of mammalian blood vessels; aorta and vena cava in vivo. Biophys J 6:641, 1966

Sawyer PN, Reardon JH, Ogoniak JC: Irreversible electrochemical precipitation of mammalian platelets and intravascular thrombosis. Proc Natl Acad Sci 53:200, 1965b

Sawyer PN, Schaefer HC, Domingo RT, Wesolowski SA: Comparative therapy of thrombophlebitis. Surgery 55:113, 1964b

Sawyer PN, Srinivasan S, Redner A, et al: In vitro and in vivo effects of 0-β-hydroxyethylrutoside on the vascular system. To be published, 1975

Sawyer PN, Stanczewski B, Ramsey WR, et al: Electrochemical interactions at the endothelial surface. Journal of Supramolecular Structure, 417–36. New York, Alan R Liss Inc, 1973

Sawyer PN, Suckling EE, Wesolowski SA: Effect of small electric currents on intravascular thrombosis in the visualized rat mesentery. Am J Physiol 198: 1006, 1960

Sawyer PN, Wu KT, Wesolowski SA, Brattain WH, Boddy PJ: Electrochemical precipitation of blood cells on metal electrodes: an aid in the selection of vascular prosthesis. Proc Natl Acad Sci 53:294, 1965c

Somova L: Inhibition of prostaglandin synthesis in the kidney by aspirin-like drugs. Adv BioSci 9:335, 1973

Spaet T, Al-Mondhiry H: Inhibition of platelet adhesion to collagen by sulfhydryl inhibitors. Proc Soc Exp Biol Med 135: 878, 1970

Srinivasan S, Aaron R, Chopra PS, Lucas T, Sawyer PN: Effect of thrombotic and antithrombotic drugs on the surface charge characteristics of canine blood vessels: in vivo and in vitro studies. Surgery 64: 827, 1968

Srinivasan S, Lucas T, Burrowes CB, et al: Effects of some flavonoids of the surface charge characteristics of the vascular system and their antithrombogenic characteristics. Proceedings 6th European Conference on Microcirculation: Basel, Karger, 1971, p. 394

Stocker K, Egberg N: Reptilase as a defibrinogenating enzyme. Int Soc Thromb Hemostasis, 3d Cong, Washington, DC, Abstracts, 1972, p 46

Stoner GE, Chisholm GM, Lucas T, Srinivasan S, Sawyer PN: Vascular injury and thrombosis: a scanning electron microscopic study. Thrombosis Research 5:699, 1974

Turpie AGG, McNicol GP, Douglas AS: Ancrod (Arvin) a new anticoagulant. In Biggs R (ed): Human Blood Coagulation, Haemostasis and Thrombosis, ch 16. Oxford, Blackwell Scientific Publications, 1972

Vessey MP, Doll R: Investigation of relation between use of oral contraceptives and thromboembolic disease: a further report BMJ 2:651, 1969

Whitney RJ: The measurement of volume changes in human limbs. J Physiol 121:1–27, 1953

Wilner GD, Nossel HL, LeRoy EC: Aggregation of platelets by collagen. J Clin Invest 47:2616, 1968

116

CURRENT STATUS OF NONATHEROSCLEROTIC AND ATHEROSCLEROTIC MODELS OF MYOCARDIAL INFARCTION IN ANIMALS

WILLIAM B. HOOD, JR., RAJ KUMAR, WALTER H. ABLEMANN,
and JOHN C. NORMAN

The past decade has witnessed a burgeoning of experimental studies directed toward investigating the effects of myocardial ischemia and infarction in animals (Hood and Norman, 1972). This research emphasis has resulted from growing concern on the part of investigators over the epidemic proportions of coronary artery disease in our country. The two major causes of death from coronary artery disease—ie, cardiac arrhythmias and ischemic left ventricular failure—have both been reproduced in animal models. Although no currently available animal model successfully mimics all of the various facets of acute and chronic coronary artery disease in patients, much information of subsequent clinical value has been gained from the study of these models.

The purpose of this review will be to outline some of the methods that have been used to produce acute coronary occlusion in animals. Considerable detail will be given concerning nonatherosclerotic methods employed for most studies of arrhythmias and congestive heart failure. Some information is also included regarding currently available atherosclerotic models that may offer potential for the future in terms of accurately reproducing clinical syndromes.

Supported by USPHS Grants HL 14646, Contract 71-2498, HE 07299, PH 43-68-684, HE 5244, HE 10539, HE 14294, SF-57-111, Grant No. 71-1016 from the American Heart Association, the John and Mary Markle Foundation, and the Charles E. Merrill Trust.

NONATHEROSCLEROTIC MODELS

Methods of Producing Occlusion

Most studies of hemodynamics and arrhythmias have been carried out in animal preparations in which occlusion of a coronary vessel could be carefully controlled by the investigator. In general, these methods have employed thoracotomy with direct manipulation of a coronary vessel, or insertion of a catheter device within the vessel lumen to produce occlusion. Table 1 outlines a number of methods employed with the various characteristics, advantages, and disadvantages of each. *Direct ligation of a single large vessel* (Harris, 1950) has been commonly used. This method requires anesthesia and thoracotomy. Focal ischemia is induced, and discrete infarction of a portion of the left ventricular myocardium is produced. It is possible to define exactly the onset of ischemia and infarction, a characteristic that may be important when timed studies are being carried out. The incidence of ventricular fibrillation appears to vary according to the investigator. It is difficult to induce cardiogenic shock by this method, since ligation of a vessel large enough to produce shock invariably results in ventricular fibrillation. Because of the thoracotomy, serum enzymes are not valid in this model, unless isoenzymes are measured. The method is suitable for chronic studies in animals that are allowed to recover. *Ameroid constrictors,* metallic rings with inner coatings of

TABLE 1. Controlled Production of Coronary Vessel Occlusion

METHOD	THORACOTOMY REQUIRED	UNANESTHETIZED PREPARATION	FOCAL ISCHEMIA	EXACT TIMING OF INFARCTION	"TRIAL" OCCLUSIONS POSSIBLE	INCIDENCE VENTRICULAR FIBRILLATION	SHOCK MODEL	VALID SERUM ENZYMES	SUITABLE FOR CHRONIC STUDIES
Direct ligation of a single large vessel (Harris, 1950)	+	0	+	+	0	Variable	0	0	+
Aneroid constrictor (Vineberg et al, 1960)	+	+	+	0	0	?Low	0	Possibly	+
Microemboli (Agress et al, 1952)	0	0[a]	0	+	0	Variable	+	+	?
Coronary "plug" (Hammer and Pisa, 1962)	0	0[a]	+	+	0	?High	0	+	?
Multiple ligation of small vessels (Goldfarb and Gott, 1968)	+	0	+	+	0	?Low	+	0	0
Electrothrombosis (Weisse et al, 1969)	0	0[a]	+	+	0	?High	0	+	+
Mercury embolization (Lluch et al, 1969)	0	0[a]	±	+	0	Low	+	+	0
Metallic wire thrombosis (Kezdi et al, 1967)	0	+	+	0	0	?	0	+	+
Balloon cuff	+	+	+	+	+	Low	0	+	+

[a]Anesthesia generally employed, but probably not mandatory.
Reprinted from Hood and Norman, 1972.

hygroscopic material, may be placed around a coronary vessel; subsequently, the hygroscopic material swells and slowly occludes the vessel (Vineberg et al, 1960). The chief advantage of this method is that incidence of ventricular fibrillation is low, and the chief disadvantage is that exact timing of onset of infarction is not usually possible, unless elaborate monitoring procedures are employed. *Microembolization* of the coronary arteries by injecting small plastic spheres through a catheter (Agress et al, 1952) is a relatively simple method for producing infarction, but focal infarction of the type usually encountered clinically is not present. Shock commonly occurs in this model and subsequent serum enzyme rises accurately reflect the presence of infarction, since no surgery is required. Another noninvasive method is *"plugging"* *of a coronary artery* with a detachable catheter tip (Hammer and Piša, 1962). A variant of this technique is the insertion and subsequent inflation of a Fogarty catheter within a coronary lumen. *Multiple ligation of small coronary vessels* (Goldfarb and Gott, 1968) has been used chiefly to produce a controlled degree of cardiogenic shock. *Electrothrombosis* using a direct current passed through an electrode catheter inserted in a coronary lumen (Weisse et al, 1969) is another intraluminal method of producing coronary thrombosis, as is *mercury embolization* (Lluch et al, 1969), and insertion of *metallic alloy wires*, which subsequently thrombose (Kezdi et al, 1967).

The method that our laboratories have primarily employed to produce coronary occlusion is the insertion of a *balloon cuff coronary occluder* about a coronary artery, exteriorization of the inflation tubing, and subsequent controlled production of coronary occlusion when the animal has recovered from thoracotomy, as previously described by others (Chimoskey et al, 1967; Khouri et al, 1968). This method may be employed in unanesthetized animals, yields a relatively low incidence of ventricular fibrillation, allows "trial" occlusions that do not irrevocably commit the investigator to producing permanent infarction and is eminently suitable for studies requiring evaluation of enzyme elevations and other chronic changes resulting from myocardial infarction.

Studies carried out in unanesthetized animals appear to offer a distinct advantage in terms of simulating clinical syndromes. It can be shown that use of anesthesia produces different responses to coronary occlusion than those obtained in unanesthetized preparations (Kumar et al, 1971a). Most of the comments in the remainder of this discussion will be directed towards studies carried out in awake animals.

Hemodynamic Studies

PRESSURES, FLOW, AND HEART RATE. Studies carried out in our laboratories using dogs, pigs, calves, and baboons have revealed a reasonably consistent hemodynamic pattern following occlusion of a major coronary vessel. Tables 2 and 3 present results obtained from studies in a series of 15 intact conscious dogs and seven intact conscious calves before and after occlusion of the left anterior descending coronary artery. In both species the left ventricular end-diastolic pressure rises to abnormal levels, and there is a modest reduction in cardiac output. Heart rate increases substantially in the dog, but insignificantly in the calf. Aortic pressure is well-maintained in both species. In dogs these results have been reproduced in a much larger series of animals (Hood et al, 1970a; Hood et al, 1970b; Kumar et al, 1970a; Kumar et al, 1970b; Kumar et al, 1971b). With more severe left ventricular failure due to com-

TABLE 2. Left Anterior Descending Coronary Artery Occlusion in 15 Intact Conscious Dogs (Mean ± SEM)

	CONTROL	OCCLUSION
Left ventricular peak systolic pressure (mm Hg)	156 ± 6	142 ± 7[a]
Heart rate (beats/min)	82 ± 5	132 ± 9[a]
Left ventricular end-diastolic pressure (mm Hg)	6.8 ± 0.8	19.2 ± 1.8[a]
Cardiac output (L/min)	3.5 ± 0.3	2.8 ± 0.3[a]

[a]$p < 0.05$, paired differences.
Reprinted from Joison et al: *Trans Am Soc Artif Organs* 15: 417, 1969.

TABLE 3. Left Anterior Descending Coronary Artery Occlusion in Seven Intact Conscious Calves (Mean ± SEM)

	CONTROL	OCCLUSION
Aortic mean pressure (mm Hg)	129 ± 8	131 ± 10
Heart rate (beats/min)	103 ± 10	112 ± 8
Left ventricular end-diastolic pressure (mm Hg)	7.6 ± 1.6	15.7 ± 4.4[a]
Cardiac output (L/min)	5.2 ± 0.7	4.4 ± 0.6[a]

[a]$p < 0.05$, paired differences.
Reprinted from Molokhia et al: *Ann Thorac Surg* 10: 503, 1970.

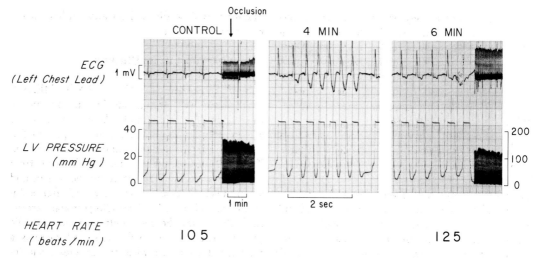

FIG. 1. Electrocardiographic and left ventricular (LV) pressure tracings made before and at 4 and 6 minutes after left anterior descending coronary artery occlusion in a baboon. LV pressure was measured at both high gain (rapid tracings) and low gain (slow tracings).

promise of flow in two major coronary vessels, systemic blood pressure, and cardiac output continue to be well-maintained, whereas heart rate may rise to levels as high as 160 to 180 beats a minute and left ventricular end-diastolic pressure to levels greater than 30 mm Hg (Hood et al, 1970b).

An example of tracings obtained illustrating these points from an experiment in a baboon is shown in Figure 1. Prior to coronary occlusion heart rate was 105 beats a minute and left ventricular end-diastolic pressure was in the range of 5 to 10 mm Hg. Four minutes after coronary occlusion a brief period of ventricular tachycardia was noted, but during a stable rhythm at six minutes the left ventricular end-diastolic pressure had risen to the range of 10 to 15 mm Hg, and heart rate had increased to 125 beats a minute. In this particular animal, the electrocardiogram failed to demonstrate the typical electrocardiographic changes of infarction at this time; however, analysis of serial electrocardiograms revealed that this was due to the transient occurrence of left anterior hemiblock (Fig. 2). Subsequent tracings, taken after disappearance of the hemiblock, showed characteristic ST segment elevation and eventual development of Q-waves over the affected area (Fig. 2). Subsequently, this same animal was studied during transient occlusion of the circumflex coronary artery, and at this time left ventricular end-diastolic pressure rose from the range of 10 mm Hg to greater than 20 mm Hg with an increase in heart rate from 116 to 128 beats a minute. There was a slight depression of left ventricular dp/dt, but aortic pressure was well maintained (Fig. 3).

Thus a relatively consistent array of hemodynamic abnormalities has been observed following occlusion of a major coronary vessel in several species of animals. More severe degrees of failure have also been produced by compromise of flow in two major coronary vessels in the dog (Hood et al, 1970b) and calf (Molokhia et al, 1970; Bernhard et al, 1970). Recent technologic developments have also made it possible to study chronically instrumented animals not subject to acute catheterization or sedation, and these techniques offer considerable promise for the future (Higgins et al, 1972).

STUDIES OF VENTRICULAR FUNCTION. We have also had some success in measuring ventricular function curves before and after acute myocardial infarction in unanesthetized animals. These methods have employed "pressure-loading" of the left ventricle, using transient aortic occlusion to cause a rise in both left ventricular systolic and diastolic pressures (Goodyer et al, 1962; Kumar et al, 1970a). To facilitate transient aortic occlusion in unanesthetized animals, we applied a loosely constricting band around the ascending aorta, placed so as to produce a gradient of approximately 3 mm Hg across the band (Fig. 4). This lightly constricting band was implanted at the time of thoracotomy for placement of the coronary occlusion balloon cuffs. Subsequently, a balloon catheter could be inserted for simultaneous transient aortic obstruction and measurement of left ventricular pressure (Fig. 4). Banding was necessary to prevent the balloon and catheter from being expelled into the descending aorta. Balloon inflation was performed under fluoroscopic control

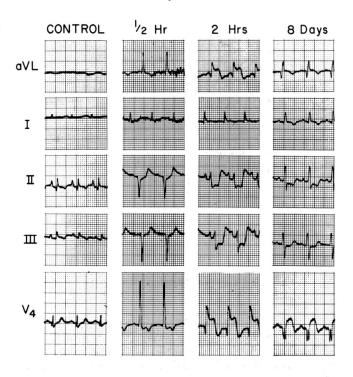

FIG. 2. Serial electrocardiograms made before (control) and at one-half hour, 2 hours, and 8 days after left anterior descending coronary artery occlusion in a baboon.

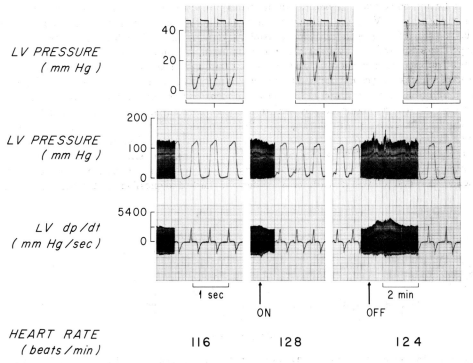

FIG. 3. Effects of transient circumflex coronary artery occlusion carried out following permanent occlusion of the left anterior descending coronary artery in a baboon. Nonsimultaneous high-gain (top) and low-gain (middle) left ventricular pressure tracings are shown, as well as the first derivative of left ventricular pressure (bottom).

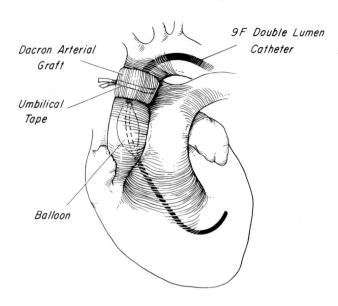

Dacron Arterial Graft

9F Double Lumen Catheter

Umbilical Tape

Balloon

FIG. 4. Diagrammatic representation of anterior view of canine heart, with banding of the aortic root just below origin of great vessels, using umbilical tape passed through protective cuff of dacron arterial graft. Also depicted is the double lumen catheter passed retrogradely into the left ventricle with the balloon used for aortic obstruction (shown partially inflated) in position just beneath the aortic band.

by injecting 10 to 50 ml of CO_2 into the obstructing balloon, which was left inflated for periods up to 12 seconds. In a total of 400 inflations, balloon rupture occurred eight times with no observable ill effects.

Characteristic ventricular pressure tracings during such a transient aortic occlusion are shown in Figure 5. There is a steady rise in left ventricular systolic and end-diastolic pressures during the period of obstruction. Ventricular function curves may be constructed by plotting individual systolic developed pressure and end-diastolic pressure for each beat during the period of obstruction (Fig. 6). Although sinus tachycardia occurs during such aortic obstruction, controlling the heart rate at a higher level by atrial pacing during obstruction did not influence the curves obtained (Fig. 7). We also noted that such ventricular function curves were reproducible with serial occlusions in the same animal (Fig. 8). Analysis of five or more ventricular function curves in each of six dogs

showed that the coefficient of variation for developed pressure at increments of 5 mm Hg end-diastolic pressure between 10 to 50 mm Hg did not exceed 4 percent. The small variability between five ventricular function curves obtained from one dog is illustrated in Figure 8. This observation is at variance with a previous report suggesting that ventricular function measured during pressure-loading produced by angiotensin is not reproducible with successive testing (O'Rourke et al, 1972), although these authors utilized stroke work determinations rather than developed pressure as a measure of ventricular function.

The methodology employed here permits construction of composite ventricular function curves by analyzing left ventricular developed pressure at 5 mm Hg increments of rise in left ventricular end-diastolic pressure, shown in Figure 9 for the entire series of 15 animals studied. When acute myocardial infarction is produced, there is a marked depression in the ventricular function

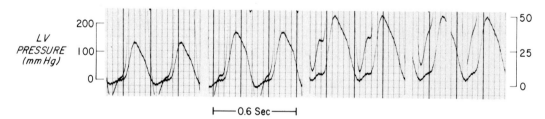

LV PRESSURE (mm Hg)

200

100

0

50

25

0

├── 0.6 Sec ──┤

FIG. 5. Left ventricular pressure tracings during pressure-loading of the left ventricle. Four pairs of beats obtained at intervals following aortic obstruction are shown. Simultaneous low-gain (left-hand scale) and high-gain (right-hand scale) tracings are displayed. Left-hand panel shows ventricular pressure tracings prior to obstruction, and next three panels show increasing elevations of both systolic and end-diastolic pressures during aortic obstruction.

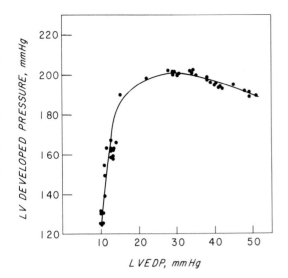

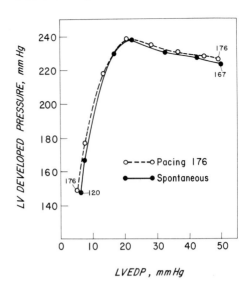

FIG. 6. Plot of a single left ventricular function curve obtained during aortic obstruction. Each point represents a single ventricular pressure pulse. LV developed pressure = LV peak systolic pressure − LV end-diastolic pressure. LVEDP: left ventricular end-diastolic pressure.

FIG. 7. Ventricular function curves obtained in one animal with and without controlled heart rate. In this example the animal's basal heart rate was 120 beats/min and rose to 167 beats/min with aortic obstruction. When atrial pacing at 176 beats/min was in effect, a virtually identical curve was inscribed. LVEDP: left ventricular end-diastolic pressure. Similar results were obtained in five other experiments.

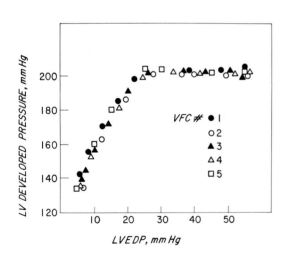

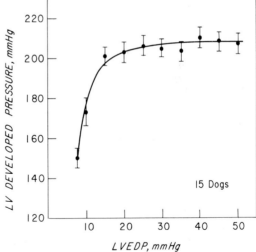

FIG. 8. Points obtained from five ventricular function curves in the same intact conscious dog. The points plotted were chosen at random along each curve and not all points are plotted. VFC: ventricular function curve; LVEDP: left ventricular end-diastolic pressure.

FIG. 9. Composite ventricular function curve in 15 intact conscious animals (mean ± SEM). LVEDP: left ventricular end-diastolic pressure.

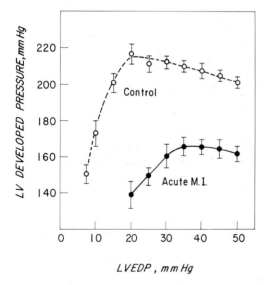

FIG. 10. Ventricular function curves in 12 animals before (control) and one hour after induction of acute myocardial infarction (MI). Points plotted as mean ± SEM. Ventricular function was depressed, as shown by a shift of the curve downward and to the right. The curves differ significantly from one another at every point (P < 0.01).

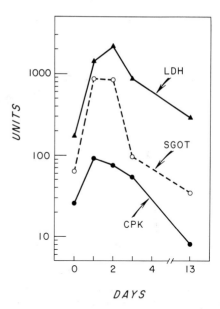

FIG. 11. Serum enzymes measured before, and 1, 2, 3, and 13 days after anterior descending coronary artery occlusion in a baboon. LDH: lactic dehydrogenase; SGOT: serum glutamic oxaloacetic transaminase; CPK: creatine phosphokinase.

curve analyzed in this manner. This was shown in a series of 12 animals in which acute anterior wall myocardial infarction was produced by balloon occlusion of the left anterior descending coronary artery (Fig. 10). This technique has been useful in assessing the long-term effect of myocardial infarction on left ventricular function (Kumar et al, 1970a) and also for studying the effects of inotropic agents on left ventricular function in acute myocardial infarction (Hood et al, 1969). The latter studies were carried out in anesthetized animals.

OTHER OBSERVATIONS. As noted in Table 1, the methods described here are useful for studies in which the effects upon serum enzymes are being observed (Hood et al, 1970a). Serial blood samples taken from a baboon following occlusion of the left anterior descending coronary artery, showing a rise in LDH, SGOT, and CPK, are illustrated in Figure 11.

Curiously, none of the species examined displayed agitation or other behavior suggesting that pain was present during coronary occlusion (Hood et al, 1970a; Norman et al, 1972). Whether this was due to the vessel dissection used for the implantation of balloons that might have injured the periarterial neural plexus remains unknown. Although caution has been taken in our studies to avoid vessel wall injury during dissection, this possibility cannot be excluded. It is also note-

worthy that some cases of clinical myocardial infarction are painless, and this is common in diabetics, suggesting that pain may be abated by the presence of neuropathy (Bradley and Schonfeld, 1962).

Studies of Arrhythmias

Animal models have also been useful for investigating the effects of coronary occlusion in causing cardiac arrhythmias (Harris, 1950), and for evaluating the effects of antiarrhythmic drugs (Stephenson et al, 1960). The majority of studies have been carried out in dogs, although pigs (Hurst et al, 1967) and other species have also been employed. In dogs, the arrhythmias that occur following coronary occlusion are characteristically of two types (Harris, 1950). Within the first 30 minutes after coronary occlusion, repetitive ventricular tachyarrhythmias, often resulting in ventricular fibrillation, may occur. Such a ventricular tachyarrhythmia is noted in Figure 2 following coronary occlusion in a baboon. We have noted that these "early" arrhythmias also occur in calves but may be delayed for up to one hour following occlusion (Molokhia et al, 1970). In dogs, a quiescent period free of ventricular arrhythmias follows this initial period of ventricular irritability; then, beginning four to eight hours after occlusion and lasting as long as two to three days, a period of rapid, sometimes intermittent, multifocal ventricular tachyarrhythmia occurs. Some animals may also die of ventricular fibrillation during this "late" period (Joison et al, 1969). Presumably the "early" arrhythmias correspond to those often occurring in patients at the onset of myocardial infarction that may result in sudden death. The "late" arrhythmias, which occur hours to days after infarction in dogs, do not closely correspond to any commonly observed clinical syndrome, although occasionally we have observed patients with sustained or recurrent ventricular arrhythmias lasting days or weeks after myocardial infarction. The reason for this difference between arrhythmia manifestations in experimental and clinical myocardial infarction remains unknown at the present time.

The occurrence of ventricular arryhthmias in animal experiments appears to correlate with the degree of ventricular damage. Although the clinical concept has been widely promulgated that ventricular fibrillation may readily occur in hearts with only minimal ischemic damage, and, indeed, often in hearts in which no coronary thrombosis is observed at postmortem, our experiments in animals suggest that the incidence of ventricular fibrillation is directly related to the mass of ventricular muscle subject to ischemic injury. Although some previous workers have suggested that there is a poor correlation between hemodynamic abnormalities and the occurrence of ventricular fibrillation in anesthetized dogs with coronary occlusion (Berglund et al, 1969), others have shown that decompression of the distended ischemic left ventricle lowers the incidence of ventricular fibrillation (Chardack et al, 1967). Furthermore, it is known that animals with large hearts maintain ventricular fibrillation more readily than animals with small hearts (Lown et al, 1963). This suggests that there may be a critical mass of myocardium that must be made ischemic for fibrillation to occur.

We analyzed the incidence of ventricular fibrillation in a series of 34 dogs subjected to coronary occlusion in relation to indices that indicated the severity of ischemia. Of the 34 animals, seven developed fatal ventricular fibrillation within the first half-hour after occlusion. Heart rate in this group rose from 103 ± 10 to 170 ± 9 beats a minute, and left ventricular end-diastolic pressure from 6.1 ± 1.1 to 18.2 ± 2.1 mm Hg (Fig. 12). All animals that developed a heart rate of 160 beats a minute or greater fibrillated, and in every animal that fibrillated the heart rate exceeded 130 beats a minute. Six additional animals died during the first 24 hours after onset of infarction. In these animals, heart rate rose during the first hour after coronary

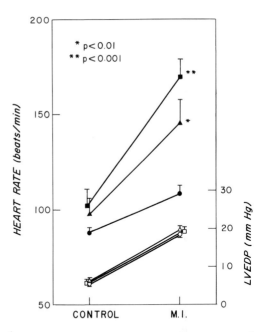

FIG. 12. Heart rate (closed symbols) and left ventricular end-diastolic pressure (open symbols) before (control) and after (MI) left anterior descending coronary occlusion in dogs. Squares indicate animals surviving less than one hour after occlusion, triangles animals surviving less than 24 hours, and circles represent long-term survivors.

occlusion fom 99 ± 8 to 146 ± 13 beats a minute, and left ventricular end-diastolic pressure from 7.4 ± 1.8 to 19.1 ± 2.7 mm Hg (Fig. 12). Twenty-one animals survived for at least one week after infarction, and in these animals heart rate rose from 88 ± 4 to 108 ± 5 beats a minute and left ventricular end-diastolic pressure rose from 6.4 ± 0.7 to 17.1 ± 1.1 mm Hg during the first hour after infarction (Fig. 12). A comparison of changes in heart rate in these three groups showed that animals dying in the first half-hour and in the first 24 hours after infarction had higher heart rates than surviving animals. The values for animals dying within 24 hours were intermediate between those dying within one-half hour and the long-term survivors (Fig. 12).

In contrast to the changes in heart rate, left ventricular end-diastolic pressure, while elevated after infarction, did not differ significantly in the three groups. Although degree of elevation of left ventricular end-diastolic pressure may give some indication of the severity of left ventricular failure, this is not necessarily true when effects of heart rate are accounted for. In this same preparation, it has also been shown that increasing the heart rate by rapid atrial pacing will lower the elevated left ventricular end-diastolic pressure after acute infarction (Kumar et al, 1971b). Thus the more rapid spontaneous heart rates in dogs surviving less than one-half hour and less than 24 hours may have prevented left ventricular end-diastolic pressures from rising to higher levels. Observations in calves vary somewhat from the above findings. In this species, sinus tachycardia is not a prominent finding after experimental infarction, whereas the height of elevation of left ventricular end-diastolic pressure does appear to be related to the rapidity with which subsequent ventricular fibrillation occurs (Molokhia et al 1970).

These studies suggest that the degree of ischemic injury, as manifested by rapid heart rates, was related to the occurrence of ventricular fibrillation and, indeed, may have been a major factor predisposing to the occurrence of this fatal arrhythmia. The study may have certain implications regarding myocardial infarction as it occurs in a clinical setting. The occurrence of ventricular fibrillation in patients following myocardial infarction is sometimes considered to be an "electrical accident," unrelated to the extent of underlying myocardial damage (Lawrie et al, 1967). The results of our studies of experimental canine myocardial infarction show that ventricular fibrillation is associated with extensive ischemic damage to the left ventricular myocardium. It may be that, in sudden death victims, the extent of myocardial injury is not appreciated because patients do not survive long enough for hemodynamic measurements to be made or for pathologic changes in the heart to become well-defined. Since sudden death is a major unresolved health problem, identified as requiring urgent attention (Lown and Ruberman, 1970), it is important to learn whether hemodynamic factors are as paramount in patients as they appear to be in experimental animals.

ATHEROSCLEROTIC MODELS

There is no evidence presently available to suggest that atherosclerotic models are intrinsically superior to the nonatherosclerotic ones for studying experimental myocardial infarction. If one takes the view that hemodynamic function and generation of arrhythmias are both critically related to the degree of left ventricular ischemic damage, then it may make little difference whether this is produced by ligating a coronary vessel or by slow occlusion of that vessel by natural processes. Furthermore, atherosclerotic models suffer from many of the disadvantages listed for certain types of

preparations in Table 1. Thus, for example, exact timing of the onset of infarction, and prediction of the locus of focal ischemia would be difficult for most atherosclerotic models. However, since gradual occlusion of multiple coronary vessels is the usual case in clinical coronary artery disease, it seems appropriate to investigate these models and to attempt to define their relevance to the clinical situation. The multiplicity of coronary lesions in most patients and the possibility that effects related to restriction of collateral flow from adjacent lesions may influence the progression of events in focal myocardial infarction may lend particular pertinence to atherosclerotic animal models.

Some progress has been made to date in producing animal models in which myocardial infarction occurs, sometimes accompanied by arrhythmias. These models in general depend upon altering dietary fat and cholesterol intake. A model of acute myocardial infarction in pigs has been produced by high-fat–high-cholesterol feeding combined with irradiation of the heart (Lee et al, 1971). These animals developed acute myocardial infarction, often with sudden death due to documented arrhythmias less than six months after inception of the atherogenic diet plus irradiation (Lee et al, 1973). More recently this rather unselective approach, which produces diffuse involvement of both large and small coronary vessels, has been improved upon by balloon denudation (Nam et al, 1973) of proximal coronary vessels using a balloon-tipped catheter, followed by high-fat–high-cholesterol feeding (Lee and Lee, 1974). Another model suitable for study of coronary atherosclerosis has been developed in the primate Macaca fascicularis (irus) by feeding butter fat and cholesterol (Kramsch and Hollander, 1968). This species develops severe proximal stenosing coronary lesions after approximately one to 1.5 years on the diet. Some of these animals have been observed to die suddenly, either during exercise or isoproterenol infusion, and the latter is accompanied by ischemic electrocardiographic changes (Kramsch et al, 1970). To date, no detailed hemodynamic studies for measuring pressure or volume in the affected left ventricle have been carried out in either of these preparations.

The ultimate utility of these atherosclerotic models for studying acute or chronic myocardial infarction remains to be determined. However, because these preparations simulate very closely the clinical occurrence of coronary artery disease in patients, it seems appropriate to carry on in these models the same kinds of studies that have previously been used only in nonatherosclerotic models.

SUMMARY

In recent years much information regarding the occurrence of both cardiac failure and arrhythmias has been gained from studies of nonatherosclerotic animal models of acute and chronic myocardial ischemia and infarction. Studies of unanesthetized preparations in multiple-animal species suggest a relatively consistent hemodynamic pattern of failure resulting from major-vessel coronary occlusion, characterized by sinus tachycardia, elevated left ventricular end-diastolic pressure, modest reduction in cardiac output, and maintenance of systemic arterial pressure. Ventricular function may be clearly demonstrated to be depressed in these preparations by pressure-loading of the left ventricle. Ventricular fibrillation is a common occurrence and appears to be related primarily to the mass of involved myocardium.

Such preparations have proven eminently suitable for studying the effects of the natural course of left ventricular failure following infarction, the effects of interventions upon left ventricular failure, and the effects of antiarrhythmic drugs upon ventricular arrhythmias. However, further advantages may accrue from studies of preparations with myocardial ischemia and infarction due to atheroma formation. Models developed in the pig and monkey are currently available for study.

ACKNOWLEDGMENT

We wish to thank Hynson, Westcott, and Dunning, Baltimore, Md., for the generous supplies of indocyanine green used in these experiments to measure cardiac output.

References

Agress CM, Rosenberg MJ, Jacobs, HI et al: Protracted shock in the closed-chest dog following coronary embolization with graded microspheres. Am J Physiol 170:536, 1952

Berglund E, Resnekov L, William-Olsson G, Ohrlund A: Hemodynamic measurements prior to ventricular fibrillation or asystole following experimental coronary occlusion. Thorax 24:626, 1969

Bernhard WF, LaFarge CG, Husain M, Yamamura N, Robinson TC: Physiological observations during partial and total left heart bypass. J Thorac Cardiovasc Surg 60:807, 1970

Bradley RF, Schonfeld A: Diminished pain in diabetic patients with acute myocardial infarction. Geriatrics 17:322, 1962

Chardack, WM, McRonald RE, Souther S, Gage AA: Comparison of the incidence of ventricular fibrillation from coronary artery ligation in the decompressed and loaded heart. J Cardiovasc Surg 8:446, 1967

Chimoskey JE, Szentivanyi M, Zakheim R, Barger AC: Temporary coronary occlusion in conscious dogs: collateral flow and electrocardiogram. Am J Physiol 212:1025, 1967

Goldfarb D, Gott VL: Cardiovascular alterations during declining and steady-state low cardiac output secondary to coronary insufficiency in the dog. J Thorac Cardiovasc Surg 56:578, 1968

Goodyer AVN, Goodkind MJ, Landry AB: Ventricular response to a pressure load: left ventricular function curves in intact animals. Circ Res 10:885, 1962

Hammer J, Pisa Z: A method of isolated, gradual occlusion of a main branch of a coronary artery in closed-chest dogs. Am Heart J 64:67, 1962

Harris AS: Delayed development of ventricular ectopic rhythms following experimental coronary occlusion. Circulation 1:1318, 1950

Higgins CB, Vatner SF, Franklin D, Braunwald E: Effects of experimentally produced heart failure on the peripheral vascular response to severe exercise in conscious dogs. Circ Res 31:186, 1972

Hood WB Jr, McCarthy B, Lown B: Aortic pressure loading in dogs with myocardial infarction. Am Heart J 77:55, 1969

Hood WB Jr, Joison R, Kumar R, et al: Experimental myocardial infarction: I: production of left ventricular failure by gradual coronary occlusion in intact conscious dogs. Cardiovasc Res 4:73, 1970a

Hood WB Jr, Kumar R, Joison J, Norman JC: Experimental myocardial infarction. V: reaction to impaired circumflex flow in the presence of established anterior myocardial infarction in intact conscious dogs. Am J Cardiol 26:355, 1970b

Hood WB Jr, Norman JC: Animal models of myocardial infarction: current limitations and future promise. In Harmison LT (ed): Research Animals in Medicine, Publ No (NIH) 72-333, Washington, DC, 1973, p. 41

Hurst VW III, Morris JJ, Zeft HJ, Hackel DB, McIntosh HD: Increased survival with prophylactic quinidine after experimental myocardial infarction. Circulation 36:294, 1967

Joison J, Kumar R, Hood WB Jr, Norman JC: An implantable system for producing left ventricular failure for circulatory assist device evaluation. Trans Am Soc Artif Int Organs 15:417, 1969

Kezdi P, Marshall WJ Jr, Stanley EL: Hemodynamic and biochemical measurements in experimental myocardial infarction. Am J Cardiol 19:135, 1967

Khouri EM, Gregg DE, Lowensohn HS: Flow in the major branches of the left coronary artery during experimental coronary insufficiency in the unanesthetized dog. Circ Res 23:99, 1968

Kramsch DM, Hollander W: Occlusive atherosclerotic disease of the coronary arteries in monkey (Macaca irus) induced by diet. Exp Molec Pathol 9:1, 1968

Kramsch DM, Huvos A, Hollander W: A primate model for the study of coronary (atherosclerotic) heart disease. Circulation 42: (Suppl III) 9, 1970

Kumar R, Hood WB Jr, Joison J, Norman JC, Abelmann WH: Experimental myocardial infarction. II: acute depression and subsequent recovery of left ventricular function: Serial measurements in intact conscious dogs. J Clin Invest 49:55, 1970a

Kumar R, Hood WB Jr, Joison J, et al: Experimental myocardial infarction. VI: efficacy and toxicity of digitalis in acute and healing phase in intact conscious dogs. J Clin Invest 49:358, 1970b

Kumar R, Hood WB Jr, Abelmann WH: Hemodynamic spectrum of left ventricular failure in experimental myocardial infarction. Am Heart J 82:713, 1971a

Kumar R, Joison J, Gilmour DP, et al: Experimental myocardial infarction. VIII: chronotropic augmentation of cardiac function in left ventricular failure of acute and healing stages in intact conscious dogs. J Clin Invest 50:217, 1971b

Lawrie DM, Greenwood TW, Goddard M, et al: Coronary-care unit in the routine management of acute myocardial infarction. Lancet 2:109, 1967

Lee KT, Jarmolych J, Kim DN, et al: Production of advanced atherosclerosis, myocardial infarction and "sudden death" in swine. Exp Molec Pathol 15:170, 1971

Lee KT, Lee WM, Han J, et al: Experimental model of study of "sudden death" from ventricular fibrillation or asystole. Am J Cardiol 32:62, 1973

Lee WM, Lee KT: Experimental model for study of advanced atherosclerosis and myocardial infarction in swine. Fed Proc 33:623, 1974

Lluch S, Moguilevsky HC, Pietra G, et al: A reproducible model of cardiogenic shock in the dog. Circulation 39:205, 1969

Lown B, Kaid Bey S, Perlroth M, Abe T: Comparative studies of ventricular vulnerability to fibrillation. J Clin Invest 42:953, 1963

Lown B, Ruberman W: The concept of precoronary care. Mod Concepts Cardiovasc Dis 39: no. 5, 1970

Molokhia FA, Asimacopoulos PJ, Kumar R, Hood WB Jr, Norman JC: Controlled production of left ventricular failure in intact calves using implanted coronary occluders. Ann Thorac Surg 10:503, 1970

Nam SC, Lee WM, Jarmolych J, Lee KT, Thomas WA: Rapid production of advanced atherosclerosis in swine by a combination of endothelial injury and cholesterol feeding. Exp Molec Pathol 18:369, 1973

Norman JC, Molokhia FA, Hood WB Jr: Primate models of ischemic left ventricular failure: absence of pain reaction with transient coronary occlusion. Fed Proc 31:628, 1972

O'Rourke RA, Pegram B, Bishop VS: Variable effect of angiotensin infusion on left ventricular function. Cardiovasc Res 6:240, 1972

Stephenson SE Jr, Cole RK, Parrish TF, et al: Ventricular fibrillation during and after coronary artery occlusion: incidence and protection afforded by various drugs. Am J Cardiol 4:77, 1960

Vineberg A, Mahanti B, Litvak J: Experimental gradual coronary artery constriction by ameroid constrictors. Surgery 47:765, 1960

Weisse AB, Lehan PH, Ettinger PO, Moschos CB, Regan TJ: The fate of experimentally induced coronary artery thrombosis. Am J Cardiol 23:229, 1969

117

MYOCARDIAL REVASCULARIZATION IN DIFFUSE CORONARY ARTERIOSCLEROSIS
Recent Experimental Progress

RAY C. J. CHIU

INTRODUCTION

Aortocoronary artery bypass graft, using either a saphenous vein or an internal mammary artery, has been performed in a large number of patients with considerable success. The anatomic studies of coronary occlusion by Schlesinger et al (1941) and more recently by Berger et al (1971) indicate that approximately two-thirds of the coronary lesions are localized and segmental, thus potentially amenable to the bypass operation. Other patients with either segmental or diffuse coronary arteriosclerosis suffer irreversible myocardial damage. For some patients, left ventricular aneurysmectomy is beneficial, while in others total organ replacement, either with an allograft or with a mechanical device, offers the only hope for survival.

Thus experimental studies aimed at revascularizing patients suffering from diffuse coronary arteriosclerosis and yet with viable myocardium are both timely and important. A small distal coronary artery may be a cause of precarious anastomoses during the constructon of an aortocoronary artery bypass graft, predisposing it to early occlusion. These patients are also candidates for an alternate surgical operation. Procedures currently employed or investigated with the objective of achieving myocardial revascularization in patients suffering from diffuse coronary arteriosclerosis include:

Supported by grants from the Medical Research Council of Canada and the Quebec Heart Foundation.

1. gas (carbon dioxide) and mechanical coronary endarterectomy;
2. myocardial arterial implantation; and
3. arterialization of the coronary veins.

The value of other adjunct procedures, such as omentopexy and epicardiectomy, is not well defined at present.

The clinical appraisal of coronary endarterectomy is discussed elsewhere. Myocardial arterial implantation has been widely applied in patients, but controversies remain on results obtained and there has been a major reappraisal of the rationale proposed for this procedure in the past several years. Another approach is the selective arterialization of coronary veins, because coronary veins are not involved in the arteriosclerotic process and because of the potential for immediate delivery of oxygenated blood to the ischemic myocardium. These developments will be discussed in perspective.

MYOCARDIAL ARTERIAL IMPLANT: RECENT EXPERIMENTAL REAPPRAISALS

Correlation of Patency, Blood Flow, and Ventricular Function Following Myocardial Arterial Implantation

The pioneering work of Vineberg (1946) to revascularize the ischemic heart with an intramyocardial arterial implant remained dormant for almost two decades. It was only after development of cinecoronary arteriography (Sones, Shirey, 1962)

947

that prolonged patency of such arterial implants was verified, which development was then followed by a surge of interest in this procedure. The number of patients receiving this procedure has declined in recent years with the advent of direct coronary arterial surgery, but this operation is still believed to be of value in selected patients (Effler, 1971). Although many patients report marked clinical improvement after such an operation, attempts to obtain objective evidence of benefit from this operation, such as with hemodynamic studies and stress tests, have met with controversial results (Langston, 1972). Thus a number of experimental studies have been conducted to elucidate the objective effects of myocardial arterial implants.

The success or failure of myocardial arterial implants have often been determined with postoperative angiography. In these arteries, however, the radiographic evidence of patency does not necessarily guarantee a significant blood flow. Yokoyama et al (1972) reported on dogs studied two to five months after myocardial arterial implantation. In spite of the high patency rate of the implants, blood flow through such arteries was virtually nil. Thus internal mammary arteriography appears to be a questionable index of myocardial revascularization and may not correlate either with the actual blood flow or with the clinical improvement (Dart et al, 1970). Wanibuchi et al (1972) studied left ventricular function three to seven months following arterial implant and ameroid constriction of the left anterior descending coronary artery. In these dogs, implant blood flow in the working heart was less than 10 ml/min, and no measurable change in left ventricular function was noted upon occlusion of the implant. Interestingly, however, left ventricular function in the implanted animals was significantly better than in those not receiving implants. It was thus thought to indicate that the implant procedure improved the intercoronary circulation and the redistribution of myocardial blood flow in the ischemic heart. A similar suggestion was made by Anabtawi et al (1969) that myocardial tunneling with or without the added increment of blood flow through the implanted artery may be beneficial to the ischemic heart. Postoperative angiography in many patients however has established the direct connection of the implanted artery with the distal portion of the occluded artery, with retrograde perfusion of the coronary artery. It appears clear that delayed implant-to-coronary anastomoses do occur, presumably as a result of the dual blood supply of granulation tissue in the myocardial tunnel (Baird et al, 1970). The initial small capillary connections from implant to coronary arteries may enlarge and become direct arteriolar channels if exposed to a significant pressure gradient.

The Nature of Early Runoff of Myocardial Arterial Implants

The rationale for myocardial arterial implants and the reason why such implants remain patent have been reappraised. The original hypothesis of Vineberg, which met with considerable skepticism for decades, was suddenly accepted and widely quoted in textbooks and literature in the mid-1960s, together with sudden acceptance of this procedure (Effler, 1971; Urschel, 1967). This hypothesis was based on the earlier anatomic studies of Grant (1926), Wearn et al (1933), and others, who used the techniques of serial histological sections and corrosion casts to describe the so-called myocardial sinusoids in the heart. These structures were thought to be very thin-walled irregular vascular spaces, measuring 100 to 250μ in diameter and composed of an endothelial layer with or without minimal supportive tissues. Vineberg surmised that this "sponge-like network of endothelial lined myocardial sinusoidal system" would provide a unique runoff for the bleeding artery, thus avoiding the formation of hematoma and maintaining its patency. Although this concept of myocardial arterial implant runoff is convenient and of historical value, its validity has been challenged in a number of recent studies. At present, the existence of so-called arterioluminal and arteriosinusoidal vessels is debatable (Netter, 1969), and the evidence for their existence is considered inconclusive. Direct flow studies of myocardial arterial implants, such as those conducted by Baird et al (1971), indicate that the initial forward flow, contrary to earlier reports, is near zero. Their attempts to infuse more than 0.25 ml/min of blood through the arterial implants led to the development of suprasystolic pressure and the formation of myocardial hematomas. Cheanvechai et al (1972) reported on patients with ruptured myocardial hematomas following myocardial arterial implantation. It was suggested that such hematoma and rupture may occur when the artery is implanted into an area of myocardial dyskinesia, as the decreased intramyocardial pressure allows the initial blood flow through the implanted artery in contrast to a normal myocardium in which high intramyocardial pressure produces enough resistance to prevent hematoma formation (Chiu et al, 1973).

The nature of the early runoff of the myocardial arterial implant was also elucidated morphologically. Chiu et al (1973) used nucleated chicken erythrocytes as markers to trace the intramyocardial distribution of blood coming from the implanted artery. As shown in Figure 1, light and electron microscopic studies reveal that the blood introduced into the myocardial tunnel escapes into the interstitial space, which is not bound by endothelium. Thus the interstitial space that exists as a continuum, intermeshing with the "syncytium-like myocardium," provides minimum initial runoff for the arterial implant. The correlation of such findings with those obtained from corrosion cast studies indicate that any initial communications that may exist between the implant and the coronary vessels are produced by traumatic disruption of the vascular bed in the process of creating a myocardial tunnel. Thus neither the patency of the implanted vessel nor the later development of implant-to-coronary vascular anastomosis depends on the existence of so-called sinusoidal spaces in the myocardium. Such a conclusion appears justified in view of the findings of Carlson et al (1969) who demonstrated that blind venous segments with no blood flow at all tunneled into the myocardium remain open, while similar segments lying in the pleural cavity occlude rapidly. They postulated that phasic to-and-fro blood flow within the venous segment compressed by the contracting myocardium produces mechanical defibrination, leading to implant patency in spite of total absence of distal runoff. Yet that such a theory may not fully explain implant patency is illustrated by the work of O'Grady et al (1972) and others in which a splenic artery was implanted into the parenchyma of the kidney. These renal implants were found to remain patent for a prolonged period of time and alleviated hypertension associated with renal ischemia. No "sinusoidal system" has been described in the kidney, and since the kidney is not a contractile organ, one would not expect to-and-fro movement of blood contained in the implanted splenic artery.

It is apparent that the final story for a myocardial arterial implant procedure has not been told. The crucial question remains the amount of blood actually delivered through an implanted artery and not merely the radiographic evidence of patency and the subjective responses of the patient. Further experimental clarification of the mechanisms for patency and effectiveness may not only enhance our knowledge of the scientific basis of this procedure but also extend its possible application to other organs.

SELECTIVE ARTERIALIZATION OF THE CORONARY VEIN

Historical Background: Arterialization of the Coronary Sinus

The concept of arterializing the coronary venous system for treatment of myocardial ischemia is not new. Pratt (1898) reported his experimental studies on nourishing the heart through the vessels of Thebesius and coronary veins. Claude Beck (1948) carried out extensive experimental studies to arterialize the coronary sinus and determined its effects on myocardial ischemia. They found reduced mortality following ligation of the three main coronary arterial branches with this procedure. Histologically, the myocardium distal to an occluded artery had many patent vascular channels. The arterialized coronary sinus and its tributaries showed hyperplasia of the intima, but none of the veins became occluded. A number of human patients were operated upon with this so-called "Beck II" operation, with some encouraging results. Although Beck's procedure failed to receive wide acceptance (Favaloro, 1970), the concept of perfusing the coronary sinus with arterialized blood to maintain myocardial viability persisted. Blanco et al (1956), Lillehei et al (1956), Gott et al (1957), Hammond et al (1967), and Spann et al (1969) used the retrograde coronary sinus perfusion as a method of myocardial protection in coronary occlusion and during aortic valve surgery, both in experimental and in clinical conditions. They studied myocardial contractility, along with hemodynamic and biochemical parameters, and reported that such perfusion afforded a measure of protection to the myocardium during ischemia. Eckstein et al (1953) studied the acute physiological effects of arterialization of the coronary sinus. The retrograde flow that was established supplied from 14 to 25 percent of the normal myocardial oxygen requirement. They suggested that this is insufficient to maintain normal myocardial contraction, but probably enough to prevent ventricular fibrillation. That the retrograde flow was limited and the myocardial hypoxia persisted was thought to be due to the restriction in capillary outflow with expansion of the coronary vascular bed. Recently, we have further studied in dogs the coronary hemodynamics associated with retrograde perfusion of the coronary sinus using a calibrated roller pump. When the heart was excised and retrograde perfu-

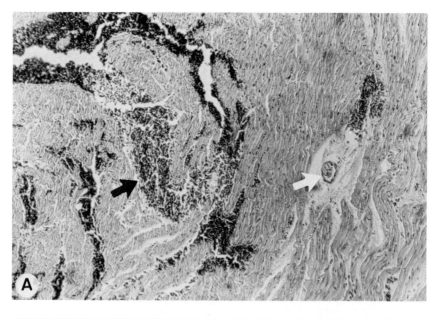

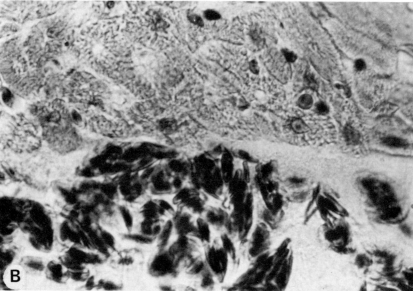

FIG. 1. Early runoff of the canine myocardial arterial implants traced with the infusion of nucleated chicken erthyrocytes. Light and electron microscopic studies show that the chicken RBCs are in the interstitial space not bound by endothelium (A, black arrow), and in juxtaposition with the sarcolemma of the muscle fibers (C), and thus are not in the so-called sinusoidal spaces. In contrast, the nonnucleated canine RBCs are found within the endothelium-lined coronary vessels (A, white arrow, and D). From Chiu and Scott: J Thorac Cardiovasc Surg 65:772, 1973

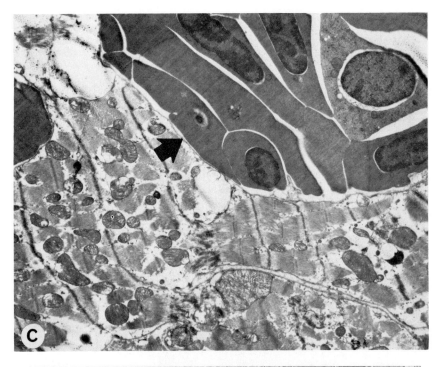

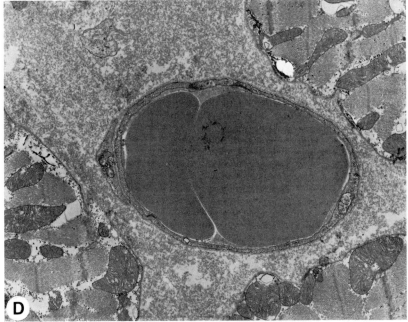

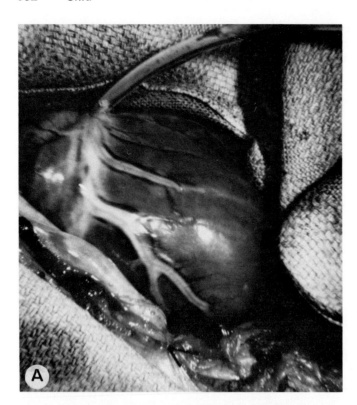

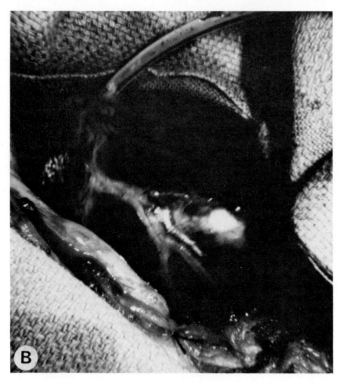

FIG. 2.   Before (A) and after (B) the retrograde infusion of India ink via the great cardiac vein, delineating the area of myocardium perfused.

sion was carried out *ex vivo*, blood pumped into the coronary sinus traversed the myocardial capillaries and exited via the coronary arteries, pouring out the coronary ostia at the root of the aorta. The resistance encountered in retrograde and antegrade perfusion of coronary vessels was found to be approximately the same under such *ex vivo* conditions. At a mean perfusion pressure of 100 mm Hg, blood flow was about 100 to 150 ml/min. When similar perfusion was performed *in vivo* in the beating heart, retrograde perfusion through the coronary sinus encountered a very high resistance, with or without ligation of the main coronary arteries. When a pump flow rate of over 100 ml/min was maintained, perfusion pressure often rose to as high as 200 mm Hg with subsequent myocardial hemorrhage and edema.

Another source of difficulty for arterializing the coronary sinus may be related to the anatomy of coronary veins in humans. The largest veins that enter the coronary sinus are the "great," "middle cardiac veins," and the "posterior left ventricular vein" (Netter, 1969). The orifices of these veins may be girded by unicuspid or bicuspid valves that are fairly well developed. Only the oblique vein of the left atrium (Marshall) never has a valve. These valves, if not rendered incompetent by dilatation of the veins, may provide resistance during retrograde perfusion.

THE RATIONALE

Selective Arterialization of the Coronary Vein Draining an Ischemic Area of the Myocardium

1. Perfusion of the myocardium with a preexisting vascular channel, such as the coronary artery distal to an obstruction or a coronary vein accompanying an obstructed artery, is the most reliable way to deliver blood to an ischemic area promptly.
2. The coronary venous system is never involved in the arteriosclerotic process, even though the accompanying coronary artery may be diffusely occluded.
3. Major coronary veins may possess valves at their orifices. Selective aortocoronary vein grafts with anastomoses beyond (upstream) the valves allows unobstructed retrograde blood flow.
4. In contrast to arterialization of the coronary sinus, the selectively arterialized coronary vein is provided with an adequate immediate runoff due to the interconnection of the coronary veins, and thus obviates the development of myocardial edema, congestion, and hemorrhage (Figs. 2 and 3).

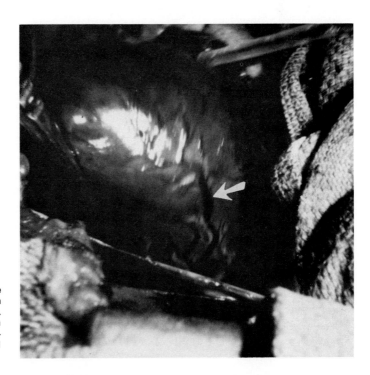

FIG. 3. Immediate runoff available for the arterialized great cardiac vein demonstrated with India ink injection. The collateral connections between the great cardiac vein with the posterior vein of the left ventricle and middle cardiac vein are shown.

5. With the present-day mechanical cardiac support during operation and the technique of microvascular anastomosis, such a procedure should be feasible with acceptable mortality.

FEASIBILITY OF IMMEDIATELY PROTECTING THE MYOCARDIUM FROM ISCHEMIA WITH SELECTIVE CORONARY VEIN ARTERIALIZATION

Kolff's group (Arealis et al, 1973; Sallam et al, 1973; and Bhayana et al, 1974) described their experience in arterializing the great cardiac veins in dogs and sheep, connecting the internal mammary artery to the coronary vein with either a cannula or by direct anastomosis. Using the epicardial electrocardiogram, these authors demonstrated that ischemia following occlusion of the anterior descending coronary artery can be reversed with retrograde perfusion of the accompanying vein.

EARLY RUNOFF FROM THE ARTERIALIZED CORONARY VEIN

Figure 2 demonstrates an area of canine myocardium perfused by the retrograde infusion of India ink into the great cardiac vein. We found that the area corresponded well with the ischemic zone produced by the ligation of the anterior descending coronary artery. Figure 3 illustrates the collateral connections between the great cardiac vein and the posterior vein of the left ventricle and middle cardiac vein. These connections apparently provided enough immediate runoff even when the accompanying artery was "diffusely" occluded by injecting polyvinyl acetate plastic (Fig. 4) or large microspheres.

TECHNIQUE OF SELECTIVE ARTERIALIZATION OF THE CORONARY VEIN IN SHEEP

Our technique (Chiu, Mulder, and Mercer) involves anaesthetizing sheep with intravenous (external jugular vein) injection of pentobarbital, followed with nitrous oxide and halothane anaesthesia. The sheep are intubated, and positive pressure ventilation is provided with a respirator. An orogastric tube is inserted to avoid aspiration. The chest is entered through a sternal splitting incision, and the left internal mammary artery is dissected out with ligation of its branches. Initially, the operation was performed with cardiopulmonary bypass and induced ventricular fibrillation, but later we found that it was technically feasible to accomplish such anastomoses without cardiopul-

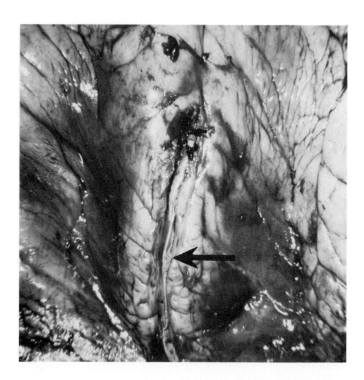

FIG. 4. An experimental model of "diffuse coronary arteriosclerosis" produced by the injection of polyvinyl acetate plastic into the anterior descending coronary artery. The plastic occluding "core" is shown.

FIG. 5. Internal mammary artery (arrow) to great cardiac vein anastomosis in sheep (A and B).

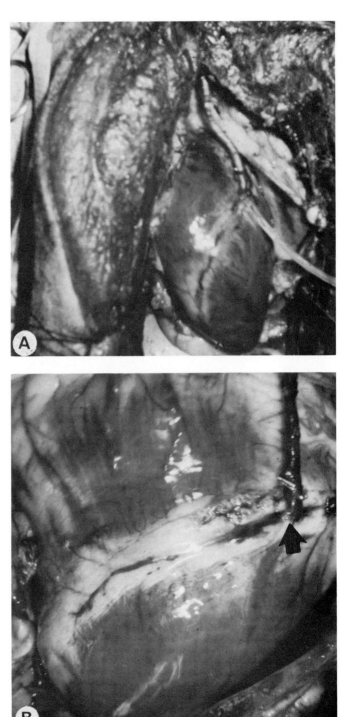

monary bypass support. One hundred and fifty units/Kg of heparin are injected intravenously, and two 3-0 silk sutures are looped around the vein above and below the selected site of anastomosis as snares to control bleeding. The advantage of this procedure, in comparison with the coronary artery bypass graft, is that in the former the anastomosis can be made at any site of the vein most accessible during the operation, whereas in the coronary artery bypass graft, the site of anastomosis has to be distal to the obstructing lesion and therefore is determined by the location of the arteriosclerotic plaque. A longitudinal incision is made through the epicardium and the superficial wall of the vein, and the anastomosis is accomplished with 6-0 polyethylene sutures, in a manner similar to coronary artery bypass grafts (Fig. 5). The coronary vein proximal to the site of anastomosis and the anterior descending coronary artery are occluded. The sheep tolerate such procedures well, recover from anaesthesia, and are often on their feet within two hours of operation.

RESULTS

Although more than 15 sheep have been operated upon to date, the experiment is still in progress and the results are preliminary. The blood flow through the internal mammary artery is measured with a square wave electromagnetic flow probe immediately upon the establishment of the anastomosis. As shown in Figure 6A, flow up to 90 cc/min was recorded, and the flow pattern appeared to be similar to that of the coronary artery bypass graft. The color of a coronary vein became pink immediately upon arterialization, and

the animal tolerated well the diffuse occlusion (Fig. 4) of the anterior descending coronary artery, without developing myocardial cyanosis. Such cyanosis can be clearly recognized within several minutes in control sheep in which the anterior descending coronary artery was ligated without the revascularization procedure. Figure 6B illustrates the flow through the internal mammary artery 10 days following the establishment of the internal mammary artery to great cardiac vein anastomosis, with simultaneous ligation of the anterior descending coronary artery. The myocardium appears viable, and histologic studies reveal patent coronary vessels and capillaries filled with blood and healthy myocardial fibers but also focal areas of fibrosis (Fig. 7). The corrosion cast (Fig. 8) demonstrates the arterialized great cardiac vein and the patent anastomosis. The left ventricular systolic and end-diastolic pressures remained normal.

Comments

More experiments and longer periods of observation are needed to establish the value and limitations of this particular procedure. Ten days following arterialization of the great cardiac vein, no significant dilatation of the venous collaterals is noted. However, it is possible that such intervenous connections may enlarge in time, resulting in shunting away the arterialized blood from the capillary bed and the tissue. The arterialized vein may also develop intimal proliferation. Longer periods of observation on patency, nutritional rather than total blood flow through the arterialized vein, as well as further objective evidence of myocardial protection are needed. Such studies are in progress.

Flow ml / min.   **Flow ml / min.**

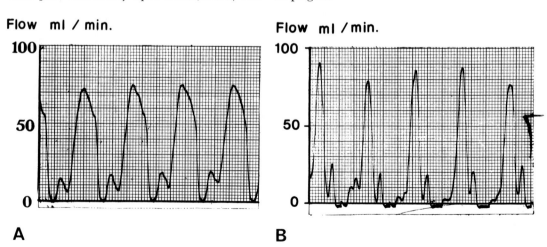

A   B

FIG. 6. Blood flow through the internal mammary artery immediately after (A) and 10 days after (B) the construction of the internal mammary artery to great cardiac vein anastomosis in sheep.

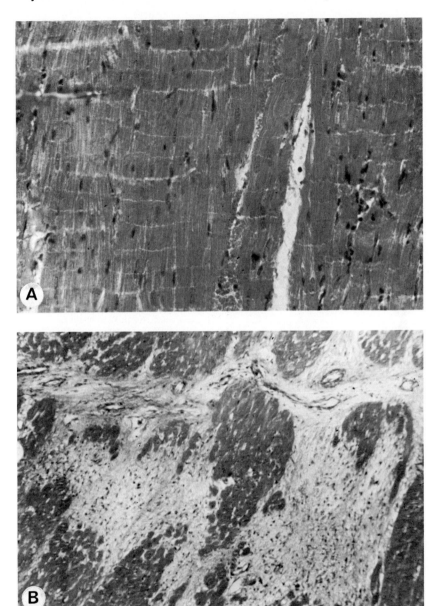

FIG. 7. Myocardial biopsy from area perfused by the arterialized great cardiac vein, obtained 10 days after the occlusion of the anterior descending coronary artery. (A) normal myocardial fibers, and (B) areas of focal necrosis and fibrosis.

SUMMARY AND CONCLUSIONS

Several surgical procedures are being investigated in order to revascularize the myocardium of patients suffering from diffuse coronary arteriosclerosis that are not amenable to the aortocoronary artery bypass graft. Experimental reappraisal of the rationale for the widely performed myocardial arterial implant procedure has been reviewed, and the newer concept of selective arterialization of coronary vein is discussed in perspective. Preliminary studies carried out in several centers and in our own laboratory indicate that this procedure can deliver oxygenated blood promptly to the ischemic myocardium in patients suffering from diffuse occlusion of the coronary artery. Further investigations are in progress in order to determine long-term potentials of the procedure, as well as possible limitations.

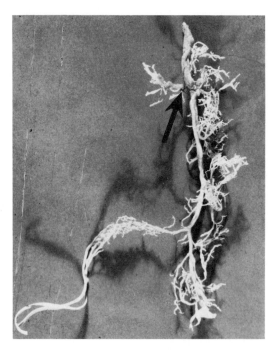

FIG. 8. Corrosion cast demonstrating the arterialized great cardiac vein, and the patent anastomosis (arrow) 10 days after operation.

References

Anabtawi IN, Reigler HF, Ellison RG: Experimental evaluation of myocardial tunnelization as a method of myocardial revascularization. J Thorac Cardiovasc Surg 58:638, 1969

Arealis EG, Volder JGR, Kolff WJ: Arterialization of the coronary vein coming from an ischemic area. Chest 63:462, 1973

Baird RJ, Ameli FM: The reasons why an internal mammary implant stays patent and why it forms anastomoses. J Cardiovasc Surg 2:195, 1970

Baird RJ, Shah PA, Ameli FM: The initial flow through an internal mammary artery implanted into the myocardium. J Thorac Cardiovasc Surg 61:456, 1971

Beck CS, Stanton E, Batinchok W, Leiter E: Revascularization of the heart by graft of systemic artery into the coronary sinus. JAMA 137:436, 1948

Berger RL, Stary HC: Assessment of operability by the saphenous vein bypass operation. N Engl J Med 285:248, 1971

Bhayana JN, Olsen DB, Byrne JP, Kolff WJ: Reversal of myocardial ischemia by arterialization of the coronary vein. J Thorac Cardiovasc Surg 67:125, 1974

Blanco G, Adam A, Fernandez A: Direct experimental approach to the aortic valve; acute retroperfusion of the coronary sinus. J Thorac Surg 32:171, 1956

Carlson RG, Edlich RF, Laude AJ, Bonnabeau RC, Gans H, Lillehei CW: A new concept for the rationale of the Vineberg operation for myocardial revascularization. Surgery 65:141, 1969

Cheanvechai C, Effler DB: Postoperative myocardial rupture. Ann Thorac Surg 13:458, 1972

Chiu CJ, Scott HG: The nature of early run-off in myocardial arterial implants. J Thorac Cardiovasc Surg 65:768, 1973

Dart CH Jr, Kato Y, Scott SM, Fish RG, Nelson WM, Takaro T: Internal thoracic (mammary) arteriography: a questionable index of myocardial revascularization. J Thorac Cardiovasc Surg 59:117, 1970

Eckstein RW, Hornberger JC, Sano T: Acute effects of elevation of coronary sinus pressure. Circulation 7:422, 1953

Effler DB: Myocardial revascularization: direct or indirect? (Editorial) J Thorac Cardiovasc Surg 61:498, 1971

Favaloro RG: Surgical treatment of coronary arteriosclerosis. Baltimore, Williams and Wilkins Co, 1970

Gott VL, Gonzalez JL, Zuhdi MN, Varco RL, Lillehei CW: Retrograde perfusion of the coronary sinus for direct vision aortic surgery. Surg Gynecol Obstet 104:319, 1957

Grant RT, Reguir M: The comparative anatomy of the cardiac coronary vessels. Heart 13:285, 1926

Hammond GL, Davies AL, Austen WG: Retrograde coronary sinus perfusion: a method of myocardial protection in the dog during left coronary artery occlusion. Ann Surg 166:39, 1967

Langston MF, Kerth WJ, Selzer A, Cohen KE: Evaluation of internal mammary artery implantation. Am J Cardiol 29:788–92, 1972

Lillehei CW: Direct vision correction of calcific aortic stenosis by means of a pump-oxygenator and retrograde coronary sinus perfusion. Diseases of the Chest 30:123, 1956

Netter FH, Yonkman FF: "Heart" Ciba 1969, p 17

O'Grady JF, Bonakdarpour A, Reichle RM, Reichle RA: Effect of renal revascularization by splenic artery implantation on experimental renovascular hypertension. J Surg Res 13:67, 1972

Pratt FH: The nutrition of the heart through the vessels of Thebesius and the coronary veins. Am J Physiol 1:86, 1898

Sallam IA, Kolff WJ: A new surgical approach to myocardial revascularization—internal mammary artery to coronary vein anastomosis. Thorax 28:613, 1973

Schlesinger MJ, Zoll PM: Incidence and localization of coronary occlusions. Arch Pathol 32:178, 1941

Sones FM Jr, Shirey EK: Cine coronary arteriography. Mod Concepts Cardiovasc Dis 31:735, 1962

Spann JF Jr, Mason DT, Zelis R: Retrograde perfusion of the coronary sinus with oxygenated blood at systemic pressure in experimental coronary occlusion: A new therapeutic concept for the treatment of pump failure. Circulation suppl 3:190, 1966

Urschel HC Jr: Surgery for coronary artery disease. In Norman JC (ed): Cardiac Surgery. New York, Appleton-Century-Crofts, 1972, p 447

Vineberg AM: Development of anastomosis between coronary vessels and transplanted internal mammary artery. Can M Assoc J 55:117, 1946

Wanibuchi Y, Mundth ED, Wright JEC, Austen WG: The effect of indirect myocardial revascularization on left ventricular function. Ann Thorac Surg 12:93–98, 1972

Wearn JT, Mettier SR, Klompp TC, Zchiesche LJ: The nature of vascular communications between the coronary arteries and the chamber of the heart. Am Heart J 9:143–64, 1933

Yokoyama M, Sakakibara S: Blood flow measurements in internal mammary artery implanted into the myocardium. Ann Thorac Surg 13:154, 1972

118

RETROVENOUS ARTERIALIZATION OF ISCHEMIC MYOCARDIUM

Don B. Olsen, J. M. Bhayana,
and J. P. Byrne

INTRODUCTION

Six hundred thousand people die each year from coronary artery disease in the United States. The problem is further emphasized by the fact that one-third of all male deaths in the Western world among men between the ages of 45 and 54 years are attributed to coronary artery disease, as well as 25 percent of all male deaths between the ages of 35 and 44. If we add the debilitation of young adults to those ending in death, the magnitude of the problem becomes even clearer. Therefore, until the biochemist, nutritionist, and cell biologist discover breakthroughs into the basic etiology of this condition, we must either endure the disease or attempt to cure the afflicted. Measures in the control and/or abatement of coronary artery disease can be categorized as (1) reduction of ventricular work by therapeutic agents such as nitroglycerin, beta adrenergic blocking agents, or severe constraint on physiologic function or (2) the delivery of more oxygen into the ischemic myocardium by O_2 inhalation or surgical intervention in arterial occlusion. Surgical intervention by coronary artery bypass procedures is the only procedure today that shows any real possibility of returning the patient to a productive life. This is reflected in the literature ie Effler, 1969; Favaloro, Effler and Grove, 1970; Johnson and Lepley, 1970. The literature is replete with articles discussing

Supported by the Development Fund of the Division of Artificial Organs to which contributions have been made by Maurice Warshaw, Mrs. Mary Hercik, Ethicon, Tom Hartford, and many others, including St. Marks Hospital SLC, Utah 84112.

one-year survival (Johnson, Auer and Tector, 1970; Grodin et al, 1972) and five years' survival (DeWeese, 1971) in revascularization of the myocardium. Further articles describe the outcome (Lawrence et al, 1973; Grodin et al, 1973; Schoonmaker et al, 1973).

REVIEW OF THE LITERATURE

Early Findings

Three hundred years ago the anatomic basis for revascularization of the myocardium was initiated. In 1669, Lower dissected the coronary arteries and demonstrated the presence of intercoronary anastomosis; his dissection was facilitated by injection techniques. Vieussens, in 1706 and 1715, injected the coronary arteries and the veins with mercury and saffron dye and reported that this injection material passed into the heart cavities through small openings in the endocardium.

These communications were further described by Thebesius in 1708. Grant and Viko in 1929 reconfirmed Thebesius's work wherein the veins that bear his name communicate directly from the coronary veins to the ventricular cavities. The number and position of these foramina are variable but are most constant on the right ventricular side of the septa and on the papillary muscles of the left ventricle. In a study of the metabolism of the heart and lungs, Evans and Starling in 1913 found that only 60 percent of the coronary blood returned via the coronary sinus. This early work was later confirmed and reported by Gregg in 1953. Sixty-four to 83 percent of the coronary blood drains through the coronary sinus. Thus, luminal anastomoses account for 20 to 40 percent of the coronary artery blood perfusion in the normal heart. There is evidence that greater percentages can pass these luminal anastomoses (Beck et al, 1948; Smith, 1962) in disease states.

It is now well recognized that coronary arterial flow into the myocardium is intermittent and predominantly occurs during diastole. This is consistent with the first investigations and descriptions of coronary circulation in the horse studied by Radatel in 1872 and reconfirmed by Wood in 1968 who stated, "During systole, ventricular contraction prevents blood flow through the coronary vessels which penetrate the left ventricular muscle. The large arteries on the surface dilate to form an elastic reservoir which in diastole acts as an accessory pump forcing the blood into the myocardium."

The early work by Beck and associates (1948 through 1954) predated cineangiography and extracorporeal circulation techniques, which had led in part to nonacceptance of their pioneering efforts. In a two-step procedure they ligated the coronary sinus then two weeks later arterialized it with an arterial graft from the aorta. Gregg and Dewald in 1938 reported that pressures in the ligated coronary sinus equaled the aortic pressure, but at the time of the subsequent anastomosis the pressure had returned to the preligation level, as reported by Thornton and Gregg in 1939. The experimental animals could not tolerate cessation of the total coronary artery supply but were able to survive major branch ligation, ie, left anterior descending artery. However, present-day investigators are reevaluating Beck's earlier work, and their procedure was recently used clinically by Moll et al, 1973.

Dr. Kwan-Gett in 1969 and 1970, in this laboratory, first experimented with the possibility of retrograde perfusion into the myocardium by way of a specific coronary vein. He placed a small silastic cannula from the internal mammary artery into the anterior interventricular vein (parallels the left anterior descending artery, LAD, hereafter referred to as the LAD vein). When the LAD was ligated there were no electrocardiographic (EKG) changes manifested if the LAD vein was perfused. When the internal mammary artery was clamped, ischemia of the myocardium was evidenced by elevated S-T segments on the EKG. These changes could be reversed by perfusing the vein with oxygenated blood. Subsequently, Arealis, Volder, and Kolff (1973) published preliminary results of this technique. Anterolateral ischemic changes were evident in leads 1, AVL, and epicardial in the form of elevation of the S-T segment with inversion of the T-wave. Perfusion of the coronary vein from the internal mammary artery was followed by a gradual improvement in these electrocardio-

graphic changes. If at this point the internal mammary artery was clamped, the electrocardiographic changes reappeared. This process could be reversed several times. The hemodynamic changes were variable. The induction of myocardial ischemia in the sheep produced a variable drop in the blood pressure shortly after the ischemic changes were evident in the electrocardiograms. The left atrial pressure was elevated in some of the animals studied by Sallam and Kolff in 1973.

Bhayana, Olsen, et al (1974) reported on the reversibility of the electrocardiographic changes in ischemic myocardium by perfusing the vein that drains the area with oxygenated blood. The electrocardiographic changes were most easily observed in the epicardial leads. The standard leads do not depict the early ischemic condition of the myocardium in the sheep or the calf. The epicardial leads did not demonstrate appreciable S-T segment changes up to 60-minute post LAD ligation when the LAD vein was perfused. Flow studies were done on seven sheep where a small plastic cannula was used to connect the internal mammary artery to the coronary vein with the coronary vein and LAD ligated. The flows ranged from a low of 22 cc a minute to a high of 96 cc per minute with a mean of 44 cc per minute.

Recent and Previously Unreported Research Findings

In three animals where only the LAD vein was ligated between the first and second primary diagonal branches of the LAD, the venous blood pressure was measured with a strain gauge and recorded on a Sanborn recorder. It was found that during ventricular systole the intravenous pressure peaked at 38 mm Hg with an electronic mean of 22 mm Hg and the diastolic pressure was 6 mm Hg. These pressures are unusually high; however, one must be aware that the coronary artery supplying the myocardium in this area is still intact and that all of the collecting venules were channeled into the coronary vein draining this area and runoff channels of this venous system had been occluded.

POSTMORTEM ANGIOGRAPHY AND VENOGRAPHY

Initially, Angioconray (Malinkrodt) was injected into the LAD vein of the excised calf and sheep hearts. All injections were made at 100 mm Hg with a constant air pressure system. These hearts were subsequently fixed in formalin and

FIG. 1. Photographs of radiographs of 1 cm slices of arteriogram (A) and venogram (B) of calf hearts. Angioconray (Malinkrodt) was injected at 100 mm Hg pressure. Note the extent of infiltration of the contrast media into the septum in both the arteriogram (A) and venogram (B).

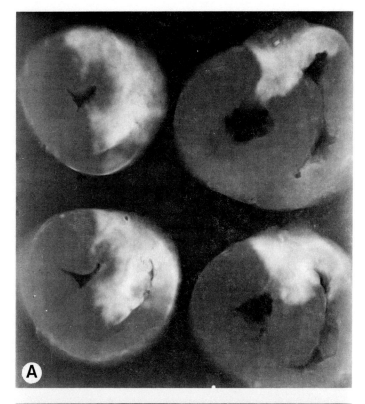

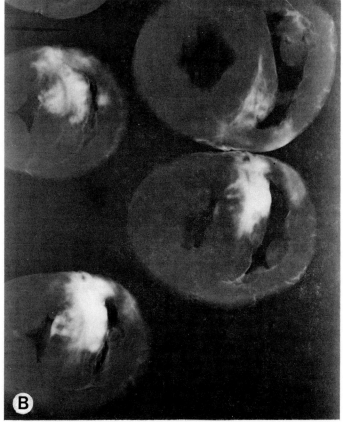

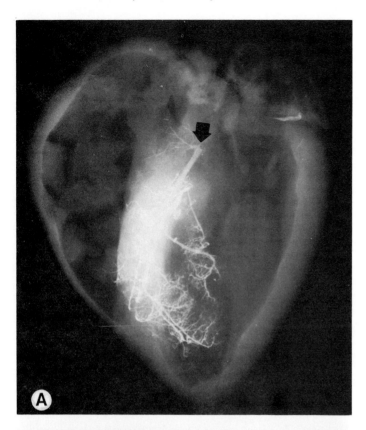

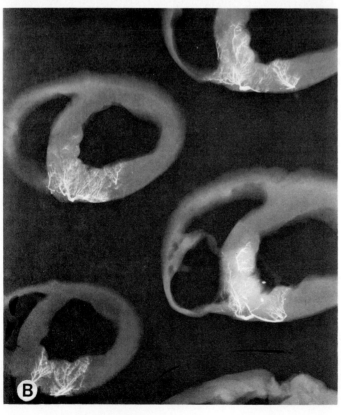

FIG. 2. Photograph of a radiograph made of the sheep heart. The modified Schlesinger mass (no formalin was added to the media) was injected into the LAD vein (interventricular vein) of a beating sheep heart and was later fixed in formalin and radiographed. A. The intact heart and the arrow is the point of injection into the LAD vein. B. The same heart as A radiographed in 1 cm thick slices.

then radiographed in two dimensions; they were then sliced in about 1 cc sections and laid out on a radiographic plate and again radiographed (Fig. 1).

In the excised postmortem heart the angioconray did leave the intravascular spaces and infiltrate the intramyocardial tissues. Subsequent studies were then done using Schlesinger mass (Schlesinger, 1938) and modified Schlesinger mass (Rodriguez and Reiner, 1957). These masses were injected into both the coronary artery and the left anterior descending coronary artery and also into an adjoining vein in both excised sheep and calf hearts and radiographs were then taken. These contrast media stayed in the vascular beds of the tissue injected and passed down to vessels approximately 20 microns in diameter. The ramifications and distribution of the LAD vein injections (Fig. 2) paralleled very closely with that of the LAD artery injections. It is of particular interest to visualize the degree of arborization and the distribution of very minute channels into the septa and papillary muscle area of the left and right ventricles (Fig. 3).

After radiographing some of the LAD vein

injected specimens, sections of the septa were taken for routine histopathology. Figures 4 and 5 are photo micrographs of the septa from the vein injected hearts. The injected mass is demonstrable in the venous system and vessels at the intramyocardial fiber level. The muscular arteries are devoid of any injection mass. Many of the small venules come in close proximity to the endocardium of both the right and left ventricular surfaces.

On gross observation the majority of the injected mass, leaving the intravascular venous system, appeared in the right ventricle, coronary sinus, and left ventricle in that order (Fig. 6).

LEFT INTERNAL MAMMARY ARTERY: CORONARY VEIN ANASTOMOSIS

Ligation of the left anterior descending coronary artery in the six sheep, described in the article by Bhayana, Olsen, et al, 1974, resulted in marked S-T segment changes in epicardial electrograms and subsequently ended in ventricular fibrillation and death. More recently death occurred in

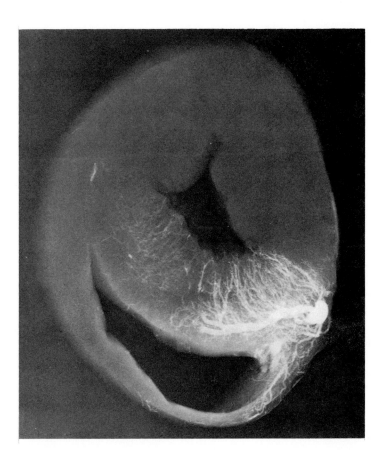

FIG. 3. Photograph of a radiograph of an LAD venogram of a calf heart. The slice is 1 cm thick and shows the arborization of the coronary vein with minute branches deep into the septum. Note the contrast media within the small veins in close proximity to the endocardial surfaces of the ventricles.

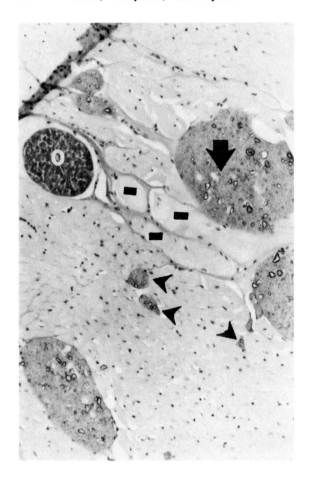

FIG. 4. Photomicrograph (approximately 300 magnification) of the left ventricular septum from the radiographed section of Figure 3. The LAD vein was injected with Schlesinger's mass and the heart fixed in formalin and prepared for standard histopathological evaluation. The Schlesinger's mass fills the larger veins, as well as the smaller intramyocardial venules (arrows). The capillaries are devoid of the injected mass (bar). In the upper left of the photograph (O) is a sarcosporidial cyst, an unrelated entity but a very commonly found innocuous myocardial inclusion of adult sheep and cattle.

five sheep and three calves when the LAD artery and vein were ligated between the first and second diagonal branches. Death occurred in all the ligated animals in as little as 20 minutes or as long as 90 minutes. We have thus established that the sheep and calf cannot tolerate ligation of the LAD artery or the LAD artery and vein.

DISCUSSION

There has been very little new or additional study on the coronary arterial or venous vascular system since Smith's work in 1962. His well-documented review article coupled with his own investigations established the relationships between the coronary artery system and the capillaries and venous systems with their various communicating anastomoses. These observations constitute a strong basis for the retrovenous perfusion of the myocardium.

Smith (1962) and Parsonnet (1953) point out a somewhat consistent veno-veno-anastomosis

in man between the interventricular vein (LAD vein) and either the posterior vein (Smith) or the middle cardiac vein (Parsonnet). The authors have not encountered this as a consistent finding in the sheep or calf heart. If and when it is encountered, it can be readily ligated to prevent an arteriovenous shunt.

Silver et al, in 1973 reported on a sequential study delineating the pathogenesis of these observed alterations in venous grafts. In a series of grafts studied from 12 hours to seven months the characteristic changes were as follows: (1) an acute inflammatory reaction with loss of endothelium and extensive medial necrosis within seven days was observed; (2) at one month he observed, first, subintimal proliferation, and, second, fibrous tissue replacement of the tunica media, and, third, evidence of graft revascularization; (3) at seven months the subintimal proliferation condensed and matured, and there were definite arterial channels in the graft wall. They suggested that graft ischemia was the mechanism responsible for these observed changes and that the medial fibrosis and intimal hyperplasia was a reparative process. The question immediately arose, would this vein graft ischemia occur in the coronary veins? We suggest that these changes will not occur in the coronary veins for the following reasons: First, the saphenous vein grafts are removed from their environment and from all surrounding tissues including their arterial blood supply; second, the pressures that they are submitted to are unusually high and are prolonged over a period of time without any supportive tissues surrounding the vein wall; third, a stretching of the endothelium and vein walls will allow for the ischemic condition described by Silver et al (1973), but the inherent coronary veins remain undisturbed in their surrounding environment. Their vasa vasorum remains intact. The surrounding structure, including the very adherent epicardium, lends support to the vein, thus limiting its overall distention. We further suggest that the arterial systolic diastolic pulse waves described by Radatel (1872) and Wood (1968) are somewhat similar to the venous pressures in the ligated vein we report here. The very adherent

epicardium and the underlying contracting myocardium create a dynamic situation in the coronary vein similar to muscular arteries in the peripheral vasculature. We, therefore, suspect no intimal or medial changes in the natural coronary veins paralleling those in venous bypass grafts.

Moll et al (1973) report empirically that blood delivered via the coronary sinus goes back into the arteries. When the arteries are ligated, this blood eventually goes by way of small fetal veins that are dormant in the adult and is channeled into the four cavities of the heart. Using this as a rationale, Moll et al have used a saphenous vein bypass from the descending aorta, through the wall of the right atrium and into the coronary sinus with ligation or closure of the coronary ostium in five patients. They reported that the SGOT and CPK values were normal on the first postoperative day and that cineangiograms demonstrated patency and flow from the saphenous vein grafts. This work was on five patients who had undergone previous coronary artery bypass procedures without success. They further report cessation of angina in

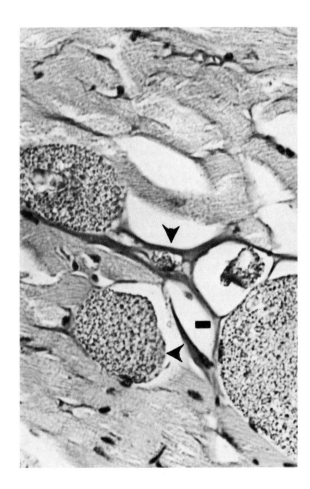

FIG. 5. Photomicrograph of higher power (approximately 800 magnification) of the same specimen as Figure 4. See Figure 4 for legend.

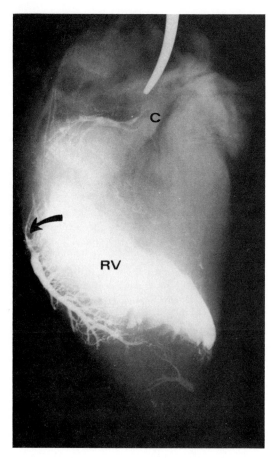

FIG. 6. Photograph of a radiograph of an LAD venogram of a sheep heart. The point of injection is at the arrow. The large mass of contrast media is in the right ventricle (RV) and the coronary ostium (C) in the right atrium.

all patients. This investigation took the same approach described by Beck and associates in the late 1940's. The revascularization of the entire myocardium is an extension of our work reported here. Nevertheless, at this time, Beck's unique approach deserves further evaluation and consideration in light of new surgical techniques, as well as equipment and instrumentation. Magovern (1974) describes six patients where the internal mammary artery was anastomosed directly to the left anterior descending vein. Follow-up studies included higher O_2 saturation of coronary sinus blood and postoperatively cineangiographic studies indicate perfusion in all but one patient. All six of his patients tolerated the procedure well, and the results are promising and merit further investigation.

There yet remain several pertinent, but still unanswered, questions. First, where does the blood go? To what extent are arteriovenous shunts created? What alterations occur in the coronary vein and myocardium in long-term studies? Will collaterals develop from the venous system to other veins and/or the heart cavities since the heart has been shown to have that propensity? Concentrated efforts by competent research teams with present-day sophisticated equipment and techniques will answer these and other less obvious questions.

CONCLUSIONS

Over the last 300 years evidence has accumulated and elucidated the anatomic and physiologic basis for revascularizing the ischemic myocardium. This evidence has not indicated that only the arterial vasculature be utilized for this procedure. There has been adequate evidence that would suggest that the always healthy myocardial venous system might offer a new and yet untapped conduit system for effective introduction of additional oxygenated blood into the ischemic myocardium. The authors have presented the facts, as available in the literature, and made available the observations from their own investigations. The evidence thus presented would support the retrovenous arterialization of the ischemic myocardium in patients, while conceding that further research in some areas is needed.

ACKNOWLEDGMENTS

To Dr. W. J. Kolff for his enthusiastic, investigative leadership, and motivation into new areas of research, Mr. Jeff Monroe for the postmortem arteriograms and venograms of the sheep and calf hearts, and the entire staff for supporting these investigations.

References

Arealis EG, Volder JGR, Kolff WJ: Heart revascularization by internal mammary coronary vein anastomosis. Diseases of the Chest 63:462, 1973

Beck CS, Stanton E, Batiuchok W, Leiter E: Revascularization of heart by graft of systemic artery into coronary sinus. JAMA May:436, 1948

Beck CS, Leighninger DS: Operations for coronary artery disease. JAMA November:1226, 1954

Bhayana JN, Olsen DB, Byrne JP, Kolff WJ: Reversal of myocardial ischemia by arterialization of the coronary vein. J Thorac Cardiovasc Surg 67:125, 1974

DeWeese JA, Rob CG: Autogenous venous bypass grafts five years later. Ann Surg 174:346, 1971

Effler DB: The role of surgery in the treatment of coronary artery disease. Ann Thorac Surg 8:376, 1969

Evans CL, Starling EH: The part played by the lungs in the oxidative processes of the body. J Physiol 46: 413, 1913

Favaloro RG, Effler DB, Grove LK: Direct myocardial revascularization by saphenous vein graft. Ann Thorac Surg 10:97, 1970

Grant RT, Viko LE: Observations on the anatomy of the thebesian vessels of the heart. Heart London 15: 103, 1929

Gregg DE: Coronary circulation in health and disease. Philadelphia, Lea and Febiger, 1953, p 11

Gregg D, Dewald D: Immediate effects of the occlusion of the coronary veins on the collateral blood flow in the coronary arteries. Am J Physiol 124:435, 1938

Grondin C, LePage G, Castonguay Y, et al. Aorto-coronary vein graft: technical modifications that may improve short and long-term results. Can J Surg 16:4, 1973

Hahn RS, Beck CS: Revascularization of the heart. Circulation 5:801–9, 1952

Johnson WD, Lepley D Jr: An aggressive surgical approach to coronary disease. J Thorac Cardiovasc Surg 59:128, 1970

Johnson WD, Auer JE, Tector AJ: Late changes in coronary vein grafts. Am J Cardiol 26:640, 1970

Kwan-Gett CS: Surgeon at the Division of Artificial Organs. Data in laboratory records and in-house reports, 1969–70

Lower R: Tractatus de Corde, London, 1669

Magovern G: Personal communications. Pittsburgh

Moll J, Dziatkowiak A, Rybinski K, Edelman M, Ratajczak-Pakalska E: Arterialisierung des sinus coronarius. Indikationen, Technik, Ergebnisse, Thoraxchirurgie 21:295–301, 1973

Parsonnet V: The anatomy of the veins of the human heart with special reference to normal anastomotic channels. J Med Soc NJ 50:446, 1953

Radatel F: Recherches experimentales sur la circulation dans les arteres coronaires. Paris, A Delahaye, 1872

Rodriguez FL, Reiner L: A new method of dissection of the heart. Am J Pathol 63:160, 1957

Sallam IA, Kolff WJ: Arterialization of the specific vein that drains an acutely ischemic area of the myocardium: an experimental study. Thorax 28:613, 1973

Schlesinger MJ: An injection plus dissection study of coronary artery occlusions and anastomoses. Am Heart J 15:528, 1938

Schoonmaker F, Grow J, Prevedel A, Hopeman A, Demong C: Direct coronary arterial revascularization. Rocky Mt Med J December 1973

Silver J, MacGregor D, Agarwal V, Lixfield W: Aorto-coronary bypass graft: early histological changes in dogs. Can J Surg 16:4, 1973

Smith GT: The anatomy of the coronary circulation. Am J Cardiol 9: 327–42, 1962

Thebesius AC: Dissertatio medica de circulo sanguinis in corde. Lugduni Batavorum, 1708. Elsevier

Thonton JJ and Gregg DE: Effect of chronic cardiac venous occlusion on coronary arterial and cardiac venous hemodynamics. Am J Physiol 128:179, 1939

Vieussens R: Nouvelles decouvertes sur le coeur. Paris, 1706.

Wood PH: Disease of the heart and circulation. 3d ed, Philadelphia, Lippincott, 1968

119

FACTORS INFLUENCING THROMBUS GENERATION IN ARTIFICIAL HEARTS

Peter B. Mansfield, Lester R. Sauvage,
and James C. Smith

INTRODUCTION

Throughout the course of surgical therapy for cardiovascular disease, the problem of thrombus accumulation is ever present. Vascular prosthetic grafts, artificial valves, artificial hearts, and even veins and arteries used for bypass procedures are constantly threatened with thrombus accumulation. There are at least three major factors that play a determining role in the generation of thrombus. These include (1) the blood-conduit interface, (2) the artificial conduit material and construction, and (3) the blood coagulation status of the host. Table 1 gives a more detailed breakdown of specific factors within each category.

This chapter, which evaluates potential solutions to thrombus generation in calves, includes experiments involving each of the three factors. These experiments were designed to find a successful technique for preventing significant thrombus buildup in artificial conduits and left ventricular assist devices.

MATERIALS AND METHODS

Preoperative Care

Holstein and Jersey calves weighing from 60 to 100 kg were used in these experiments. They were admitted for a one-week observation period before entering the appropriate protocol sequence.

Research supported by National Institutes of Health contracts nos. NIH-NHLI-71-2060-01, -02, and -03.

Surgical Procedure

Following the administration of atropine, anesthesia was induced with nose cone ether. The calf was then intubated and maintained on Fluothane and room air. All surgery was performed via a left thoracotomy.

Aortic Tubular Graft

A tubular, nonporous graft (Table 2) 20 mm in diameter and 50 mm long was used to replace an excised segment of the descending

TABLE 1. Major Factors in Thrombus

I. Blood conduit interface
  A. Blood flow
    1. Velocity
    2. Wall movement
  B. Surface lining material
    1. Raw
    2. Cell linings
    3. Thrombus covering
II. Conduit construction and mechanical requirements
  A. Wall
    1. Porous
    2. Nonporous
  B. Conduit contour
    1. Crimping
    2. Smooth
III. Blood coagulation status
  A. Clotting factors
  B. Platelets (CPA, PA, CA, CP)
  C. Fibrinolysis
  D. Hemodilution
  E. Anticoagulants
    1. Heparin
    2. Coumadin

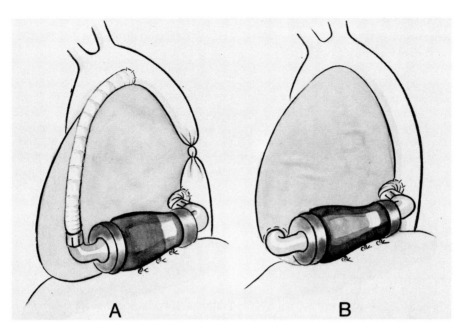

FIG. 1. Left Ventricular Assist Device Configuration. A. Nonpumping aorta-to-aorta configuration. Woven Teflon grafts attach the inlet and the outlet portions of the pump to the aorta. The aorta is tied off completely between these limbs. In this configuration the device is acting as a passive conduit. This configuration tends to increase thrombus deposition since the device is handling less than total cardiac output and there is no movement of the pump bladder wall. B. Left-ventricular-to-descending-aorta configuration. The left ventricular assist device is designed for use in this configuration. An inlet tube at the left ventricular apex brings blood to the device, which then pumps it into the aorta. In these experiments the bladders were continuously pumped and a near total cardiac output passed through the device.

TABLE 2. Aortic Tubular Nonporous Materials

SURFACE MATERIAL	CORONA DISCHARGE	STERILIZATION IRRADIATION	PARYLENE C COATING	TUBE DIMENSIONS	
				I.D.	Length
Polypropylene microfiber–B (Union Carbide)[a]	Yes	5 mr	0.5 micron	20 mm	50 mm
Nonwoven nylon (Abcor)[b]	Yes	2.5 mr	1.0 micron	20 mm	50 mm

[a]Union Carbide Corporation (Plastics Division); River Road; Bound Brook, New Jersey 08805.
[b]Abcor Corporation; 341 Vassar St., Cambridge, Mass. 02139.

aorta. Everting, end-to-end anastomoses were performed, using 3-0 Tycron suture material. Aortic cross-clamp time for the resection and both anastomoses averaged 12 minutes. Heparin, 100 units per kg of body weight, was administered three minutes prior to aortic cross-clamping and was reversed with 0.5 mg of protamine per 100 units of heparin, 15 minutes after releasing the clamps. Postoperative serial blood studies included hematocrits, platelet counts, white blood cell counts, and fibrinogen levels. Detailed postmortem studies of the aorta, graft, lungs, kidneys, spleen, and liver were carried out at the specified intervals. All animals were kept in the laboratory under direct supervision during the entire course of the experiment.

Pump Systems

Left ventricular assist devices were implanted in calves either in the left-ventricular-to-descending-aorta position, or the aorta-to-aorta position (Fig. 1). The assist pumps were Model 6, manufactured by TECO.* These devices had a maxi-

* Thermo Electron Corporation, 85 First Ave. Waltham, Mass. 02154.

mum stroke volume of 60cc and contained pumping bladders made from Nichols Polyurethane (Bernhard, Bankole, et al, 1971). The bladder surfaces were flocked Dacron attached to the polyurethane backing and were also manufactured by TECO. Pumping was accomplished via a transcutaneous air pressure line connected to the space between the pump housing and the pump bladder. Pumping was asynchronous and required pressure pulses of approximately 3 psi to activate the device properly.

The assist pumps were attached as shown in Figure 1. In the aorta-to-aorta position, the aorta was ligated between the two points of attachment. However, while the influence of reduced flow through the device was studied, this tie was left partially open. Woven Teflon grafts were sewn to the aorta and attached to the ends of the pump with a push-on connector.

In the left-ventricular-to-descending-aorta position, an inlet tube was inserted into the left ventricle via the apex. A Teflon graft was sewn end-to-side to the descending aorta and attached to the distal pump end by means of a clip connector. The pump housing was then secured to the diaphragm.

Tissue Culture

Fibroblasts and endothelial cells were obtained from calves using techniques previously described (Mansfield and Wechezak, 1968; Wechezak and Mansfield, 1973) (Figs. 2 and 3). The cells were grown on glass cover slips for *in vitro* studies of platelet activation. Aortic tubular grafts had cells seeded onto their surfaces in two stages in the course of one week and were maintained in culture until the graft was inserted in the aorta. The insertion technique and the administration of heparin and protamine were identical to the procedures used with unlined grafts.

Anticoagulant Protocols

HEPARIN. At the time of surgery, three minutes prior to excision of the aortic segment, 100 units of heparin per kg of body weight was administered intravenously. No protamine was administered following completion of the insertion of the aortic tubular graft. Four hours following the initial intravenous heparin dose, 400 units of Bio-Heprin (sodium heparin, 10,000 units per

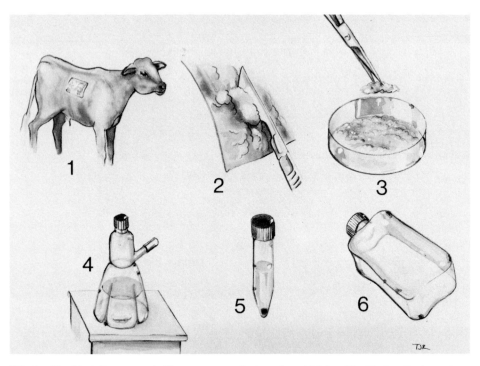

FIG. 2. Fibroblast Procurement. The sequence of steps for obtaining fibroblast cells for culture is shown. A skin flap is elevated on the side of the animal, and granulation tissue allowed to build up. Granulation tissue is then excised, minced, and digested with Trypsin (4) to separate the individual cells. The cells are then centrifuged into a pellet, which is seeded into a prescription bottle for growth in tissue culture. The entire sequence takes approximately one week.

ml) per kg of body weight was given subcutaneously. This dose of Bio-Heprin was repeated 12 hours later. Every 12 hours for the remainder of the study, 800 units of Bio-Heprin per kg of body weight was given subcutaneously. Monitoring of the effectiveness of the heparin was accomplished by following coagulation times, prothrombin times, and partial thromboplastin times from blood drawn just prior to each heparin administration. The heparin dose was adjusted to maintain the animal at full therapeutic levels.

COUMADIN. The calf was started on oral coumadin, 10 mg per day, four days prior to surgery. When the therapeutic level was reached, the dosage was lowered to approximately 5 mg per day as needed to maintain therapeutic levels as judged by daily prothrombin times. Coumadin was not administered either the day before surgery or the day of surgery. At the time of surgery, 100 units of heparin per kg of body weight was administered intravenously three minutes prior to excision of the aortic segment. Fifteen minutes after completion of the tubular implant, 0.5 mg of protamine was given per 100 units of heparin administered. The animals were maintained on coumadin throughout the remainder of the experiment, with dosages regulated by daily prothrombin times.

COUMADIN-PERSANTINE-ASPIRIN. The calf was started on oral doses of all three drugs, four days prior to surgery. Initial dosage of coumadin was 10 mg per day; when the therapeutic level was reached, the dosage was lowered to approximately 5 mg per day as needed to maintain the therapeutic level. Persantine was given as a single oral dose of 400 mg once daily, and aspirin, 1.2 gm, was also given daily as a single oral dose. Coumadin was not administered the day before surgery, nor the day of surgery, but persantine and aspirin were continued daily throughout the experiment, including the day of surgery. Heparin, 100 units per kg of body weight, and protamine, 0.5 mg per 100 units of heparin, were given during surgery as described above. Coumadin was restarted on the day following surgery, at initial doses of 5 mg per day, and was continued throughout the remainder of the experiment, with dosages regulated by daily prothrombin times.

COUMADIN-ASPIRIN. The calf was started on oral coumadin, 10 mg per day, four days prior to surgery. When the therapeutic level was reached, the dosage was lowered to approximately

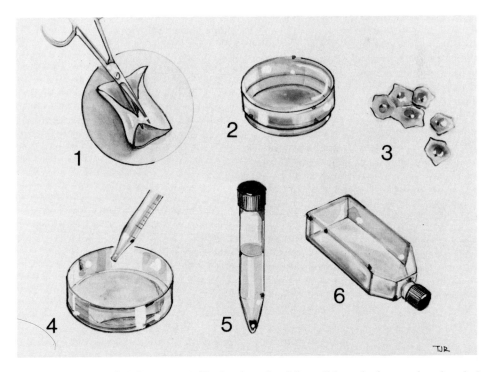

FIG. 3. Endothelial Cell Procurement. The jugular vein of the calf is excised, opened, and soaked in chelating solution to separate the endothelial cells as shown in (3). Pipette washing of the surface removes more cells. The supernatant is then centrifuged, and the cells obtained are seeded in prescription flasks of Falcon plastic.

5 mg per day as needed to maintain therapeutic levels. Coumadin was not administered the day before surgery, nor on the day of surgery. The calf was also started on a single daily dose of oral aspirin, 1.2 gm per day, four days prior to surgery. The aspirin was continued throughout the experiment, including the day of surgery. The standard heparin-protamine routine was used during implantation. Coumadin was restarted on the day following surgery, at initial doses of 5 mg per day, regulated by daily prothrombin times, and continued throughout the remainder of the experiment.

COUMADIN-PERSANTINE. The calf was started on oral coumadin, 10 mg per day, four days prior to surgery. When the therapeutic level was reached, the dosage was lowered to approximately 5 mg per day as needed to maintain therapeutic levels. Coumadin was not administered the day before surgery nor on the day of surgery. Persantine was administered orally as a single dose of 400 mg per day beginning four days preoperatively and continuing throughout the remainder of the experiment, including the day of surgery. The standard heparin-protamine routine was used during implantation. Coumadin was restarted on the day following surgery, at initial doses of 5 mg per day, and was continued throughout the remainder of the experiment, with dosages regulated by daily prothrombin times.

PERSANTINE-ASPIRIN. The calf was started on single oral doses of persantine, 400 mg per day, and aspirin, 1.2 gm per day, four days prior to surgery, and was continued at these levels throughout the remainder of the experiment, including the day of surgery. The standard heparin-protamine routine was used during implantation.

DEXTRAN. Approximately one hour prior to aortic graft implant, 100 cc of Dextran 70 was administered IV push and followed with a continuous 20 cc/hour IV infusion for the duration of the experiment. The standard heparin-protamine routine was used during implantation.

LOW-DOSAGE COUMADIN-PERSANTINE-ASPIRIN. The calf was started on single oral doses of each of the three drugs, four days prior to surgery. The dosages were maintained at the same levels throughout the experiment, including the day of surgery. Coumadin: 1 mg per day. Persantine: 400 mg per day. Aspirin: 1.2 gm per day. The standard heparin-protamine routine was used during implantation.

HEMODILUTION. During the thoracotomy, 1 unit (500 cc) of blood was withdrawn from the calf and replaced with 1,500 cc of lactated ringer's solution. A hematocrit was then done to determine the dilution level. The process was repeated until the hematocrit reached 20 percent. The aortic resection and tubular implant were then carried out. Heparin, 100 units per kg of body weight, was given three minutes before aortic resection, and protamine, 0.5 mg per 100 units of heparin, was given 15 minutes after completion of the implant. No drugs were administered during the remainder of the experiment. The blood was not reinfused.

RESULTS

Bare Surface Aortic Tubular Graft Studies

EARLY THROMBUS DEPOSITION. In determining the characteristics of early *in vivo* thrombus deposition, three variables have been considered. The first is graft material, the second is influence of heparin before and after reversal by protamine, and the third is the length of implantation. All tubular grafts were inserted as described under "Materials and Methods" above.

The first control study evaluated the influence of time on thrombus accumulation and resolution. Both Abcor and Union Carbide surfaces, without cell linings, were used in this study. Figure 4, shows the average maximum and average minimum thrombus depth over the surface of each tubular aortic graft after removal at the indicated time following insertion. The grafts showed significant thrombus deposition within seconds to minutes after the aortic clamps were opened. Despite complete haparinization (infinite clotting times), thrombus in the form of platelets, fibrin, and entrapped red blood cells was seen on the surface of both types of material. This layering was thinner on the Union Carbide material than on the Abcor material during the period of time before the heparin was reversed with protamine. Following reversal of heparin with protamine, the progression of thrombus buildup was similar on both materials. A rapid buildup occurred during the first 12 to 24 hours, in which the thrombus obtained a maximum depth of approximately 1.5 mm. The thrombus layer then began to thin in random areas, suggesting humoral fibrinolytic activity. With both materials, thrombus depth decreased over the subsequent three to five days, with a maximum average depth of approximately 0.8 mm at 10 days.

Figure 5 demonstrates the changes in surface configuration of the thrombus on these grafts and shows the constituents of the thrombus

FIG. 4. A. Average maximum and average minimum thrombus depth on aortic tubular grafts of nonwoven nylon (Abcor). Note the separation of time frames in the left and right halves of the graft. Heparin administered during the graft insertion was reversed with protamine at 15 minutes. Peak levels of thrombus were found from 12 to 24 hours. Humoral fibrolytic activity removed thrombus more rapidly than it was deposited after the first 24 hours of insertion. B. Average maximum and average minimum thrombus depth found on polypropylene microfiber aortic tubular grafts (Union Carbide). The time course of thrombus deposition was similar to that seen in the Abcor implant, with the exception that almost no thrombus deposition occurred during the first 15 minutes prior to Heparin reversal with protamine. The evidence of humoral fibrolytic activity was again seen.

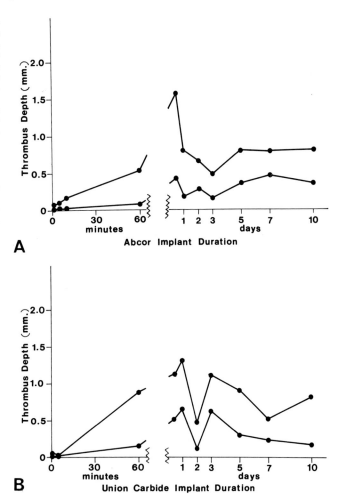

formed as seen microscopically. As can be appreciated from the drawings, the thrombus that formed while heparinization was in effect consisted initially of platelets and fibrin and, by 10 minutes, included red blood cell entrapment in the meshwork. Following reversal of the heparin with protamine, a marked increase in the depth of thrombus occurred, with more prominent red blood cell entrapment within the fibrin-platelet network and, in particular, a sharp increase in the number of white blood cells included within the superficial part of the thrombus. White ridges or spots were seen on the surface of the thrombus (very similar to the white caps on the sea in a high wind) and consisted mainly of white blood cells, fibrin, and platelets without red blood cell entrapment. The rapid increase in thrombus occurred between 12 and 24 hours and was associated with marked white cap activity. Vast islands of white blood cells were present at the thrombus surface.

By two days the number of white caps had begun to diminish. During the same interval, there had been significant fibrinolysis of previously deposited thrombus. The average depth had decreased from 1.5 mm to approximately 0.9 mm, and by five days the first organizational activity at the anastomotic line had begun. This organizational activity consisted of the migration of macrophages across the anastomotic junction into the thrombus. These cells appeared to thin and organize thrombus locally at the suture lines, and endothelial cells from the surface of the adjacent aorta began to move over the thrombus shortly thereafter. This process is called pannus ingrowth. At 10 days, the average maximum thrombus depth was near 0.8 mm, and pannus ingrowth had progressed aproximately 1 mm onto the graft.

The dynamic sequence of thrombus formation is thus an immediate deposition of platelets and fibrin, literally within seconds of the time blood passes through the graft, and a rapid increase in thrombus depth following return of coagulation capability to normal (reversal of heparin by protamine). The thrombus depth appears

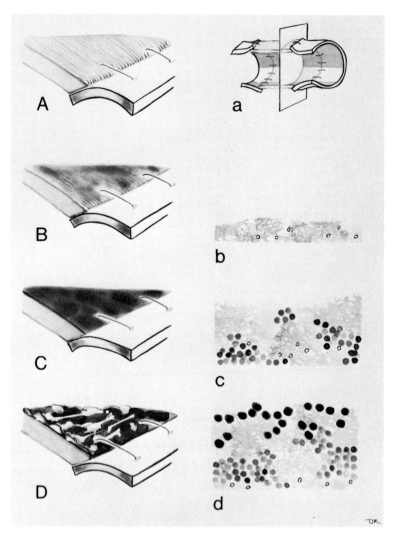

FIG. 5.   Time Course of Early Thrombus Deposition in Aortic Tubular Grafts. (Drawings are from ×600 magnification.)   A. Aortic graft anastomosis prior to blood flow. Drawing depicting section plane for microscopic study.   B. One minute following institution of blood flow, heparin not reversed. Thrombus deposited is a complex of platelets and fibrin with minimal red cell entrapment. The deposit surrounds fibers of the surface material of the graft.   C. Graft surface 10 minutes after institution of flow, heparin not reversed with protamine. The thrombus color has changed from pale to deep red and has increased in depth to approximately 0.1 mm. c. Microscopically, red blood cell entrapment has become more marked: a platelet fibrin complex continues to add thrombus at the surface.   D. Sixty minutes following institution of flow. Heparin has now been reversed with protamine. There is very rapid accumulation of thrombus and multiple ridges and isolated spots of white debris on the surface of the thrombus (whitecaps). d. Microscopically, white blood cells have now appeared in significant numbers. They are concentrated at the surface of the thrombus, associated with the platelet fibrin complex there. Red blood cell entrapment continues to account for a significant portion of the thrombus depth.

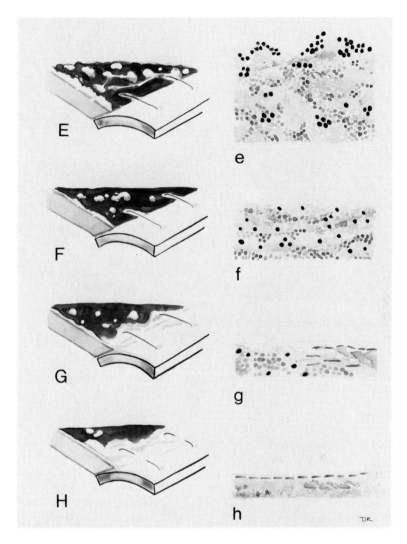

FIG. 5. E. Twenty-four hours following institution of flow. Thrombus is now reaching its maximum depth and is more uniform over the entire surface of the graft. White caps remain in evidence but are somewhat fewer in number. Early evidence of humoral fibrolytic activity thinning the thrombus is seen. e. Microscopically, the white blood cells remain prominent at the platelet-fibrin-complex surface of the thrombus. Red blood cell boundaries are becoming slightly less distinct, but entrapment continues, particularly between white caps. F. Three days following implantation. Thrombus depth has been reduced through humoral fibrolytic activity. White caps are significantly less abundant. f. Microscopically, white blood cell numbers at the surface are reduced, there is thinning of the platelet-fibrin red blood cell entrapment thrombus, and occasional white blood cells are seen throughout the thrombus as well as on the surface.   G. Five days following implantation. Grossly the thrombus has thinned even further from humoral fibrolytic activity, and now at the suture lines there is evidence of pannus ingrowth starting. White caps are occasionally seen. g. Microscopically, entrapped red blood cells have become more indistinct, white blood cells are less frequently seen, and at the anastomotic margin, macrophages have begun to enter the thrombus. These are followed closely by endothelial migration from the aortic wall on the surface of the thrombus. H. Ten days following implantation. Thrombus depth is essentially unchanged from five days, except at the suture lines where pannus ingrowth has thinned the thrombus significantly. Collagen, demonstrated by stains, is only seen in association with the ingrowing pannus.

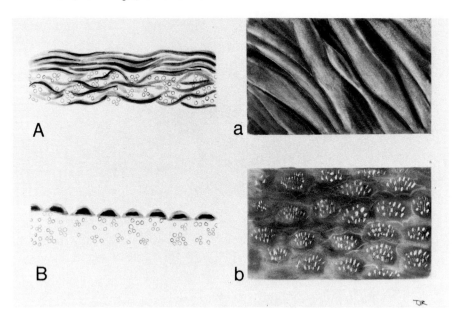

FIG. 6. Fibroblast and Endothelial Cell Growth on Microfabrics. (Drawings of fibroblasts are from ×454 magnification. Drawings of endothelial cells are from ×573 magnification.) A. Conceptual drawing of fibroblast growing on microfabric surface. The cells penetrate into the fiber web as well as covering it on the surface with multiple layers of cells. a. Grossly, fibroblasts form a type of syncytium, show no evidence of contact inhibition, and grow in multiple layers. B. Endothelial cells grow only on the surface of the fiber web and do not penetrate between individual fibers. b. The endothelial cells show contact inhibition and form monolayers.

to reach a maximum between 12 and 24 hours after implantation. Fibrinolytic activity appears to exceed the rate of thrombus deposition over the subsequent few days and by 10 days the thrombus depth has been reduced to approximately 60 percent of its previous maximum. Additional thinning of the thrombus occurs by pannus ingrowth initiated at the suture lines. This organization is apparently accomplished by invasion of the thrombus with macrophages, with subsequent reduction in thrombus depth, and eventual covering by migrating endothelial cells from the adjacent aorta. Collagen stains have demonstrated that collagen present on the surface of the tubular grafts occurs only in association with these invading macrophages.

In these nonporous tubular grafts, any graft material that became covered with thrombus appeared to be of little importance in the subsequent addition and resolution of thrombus.

LATE THROMBUS DEPOSITION. Another series of calves was studied at longer implant times, using both Abcor and Union Carbide aortic tubular grafts (Fig. 5). The animals were sacrificed at four weeks, six weeks, four months, and six months. The results demonstrated a slow but continuous decrease in the maximum thickness of thrombus (with a single exception at four months), and a continuing ingrowth and reduction of thrombus by pannus organization from the suture line. At four weeks, the average maximum depth was approximately 0.6 mm, at six weeks it was 0.5 mm, at four months it was 0.4 mm, and at six months it was approximately 0.4 mm. The minimum depth seen was the result of a combination of initial fibrinolytic activity and subsequent pannus ingrowth from the anastomotic lines. At six months, this had reduced the thrombus near the suture lines, where pannus ingrowth and organization was completed, to approximately 0.1 mm.

Tissue Cultured Cell-Lined Aortic Tubular Graft Studies

IN VITRO STUDIES. Fibroblast and endothelial-like cells were obtained from calves, maintained in culture, and grown on the surface of tubular grafts using tissue culture techniques (Figs. 2 and 3). As shown later in Figure 6, fibroblasts covered the artificial surface by growing within the fiber network as well as covering the surface. The endothelial-like cells attached themselves only to the surface of the artificial material and did not grow down into the fiber network. *In vitro* testing of platelet adherence to cell surfaces was accomplished by obtaining platelet concentrates from autologous calf blood, layering them over fibroblast or endothelial-like cells grown on glass, and studying the resultant reaction with scanning electron microscopy. Figure 7 shows that the smooth fibroblast surface activated platelet metamorphosis, resulting in attachments of the platelets to the surface of the fibroblast. In contrast, the platelets were activated minimally, if at all, when in contact with endothelial-like cell surfaces.

IN VIVO FIBROBLAST-LINED AORTIC GRAFTS. Once seeded with autologous fibroblasts in tissue culture, both Abcor and Union Carbide aortic tubular grafts were implanted in the descending aorta and subsequently evaluated at two days, two weeks, four weeks, six weeks, four months, and six months. A similar control group of unlined grafts was done concurrently. The fibroblast cell-lined tubes developed significantly deeper thrombus, usually by a factor of two or more, than the unlined control grafts. Table 3 presents the average thrombus depth as a function of implant duration for the controls and the fibroblast-lined tubes. The incidence of renal infarcts was low in both series (Mansfield, 1972).

A similar series of fibroblast-lined tubes, using allogenic fibroblasts, showed even greater thrombus development than that developed on the autologous cells. A study of endothelial-like cell-lined aortic tubular grafts is in progress.

Anticoagulation Studies

The investigation of the time course of thrombus generation suggested that the first few seconds of blood flow through artificial conduits is very significant in determining the final outcome of the surface thrombus deposition. Therefore, our anticoagulant protocols for drugs that do not act immediately upon injection are protocols involved in establishing therapeutic levels prior to surgery and to continue these levels immediately following surgery. All animals were carefully monitored by appropriate anticoagulation tests and were maintained in therapeutic ranges just prior to and continuously following surgery until sacrifice. Animals were sacrificed at one, two, and four weeks following implantation. Each anticoagulation protocol had three animals with Abcor grafts and three animals with Union Carbide grafts.

HEPARIN ANTICOAGULATION. Despite documented therapeutic level of heparin anticoagulation from the time of surgery to the time of sacrifice, specimens at one week showed thin pebbly red blood cell and fibrin surface thrombus. White caps were prominent on the lining surface. The average maximum thrombus depth was 1.0 mm (Fig. 8). At two weeks, obvious pannus organization with covering endothelial ingrowth had occurred from each suture line, and the thrombus was thinned centrally by humoral fibrinolytic activity. By four weeks, the endothelial ingrowth had reached approximately 10 mm from each suture line. Central thinning had progressed and the maximum average depth of thrombus was 0.5 mm. No renal infarcts were found in any animals on heparin anticoagulation.

COUMADIN ANTICOAGULATION. One week following implantation, animals maintained on therapeutic levels of coumadin anticoagulation demonstrated thrombus and fibrin buildup of a significant depth, averaging 1.4 mm. White caps were rare and the surface was that of soft, friable clot with a lacy fibrin network (Fig. 8A). By two weeks there was spectacular resorption of the thrombus. Endothelial pannus ingrowth had occurred for a few millimeters from each anastomosis. At four weeks, there was a generous ingrowth of pannus (10 mm), with lysis of all but the central portions of the original thrombus. It appears significant that there were renal infarcts in some animals on the coumadin anticoagulation.

COUMADIN, PERSANTINE, AND ASPIRIN ANTICOAGULATION. In marked contrast to the one-week specimens on heparin and

TABLE 3. Average Maximum Thrombus Depth in mm

IMPLANT DURATION	UNLINED CONTROL GRAFTS		FIBROBLAST-LINED GRAFTS	
	Abcor	Union Carbide	Abcor	Union Carbide
4 wks	0.5	0.6	1.4	1.6
6 wks	0.6	0.4	2.4	1.3
4 mos	1.1	0.4	1.4	1.9
6 mos	0.4	0.4	1.7	1.5

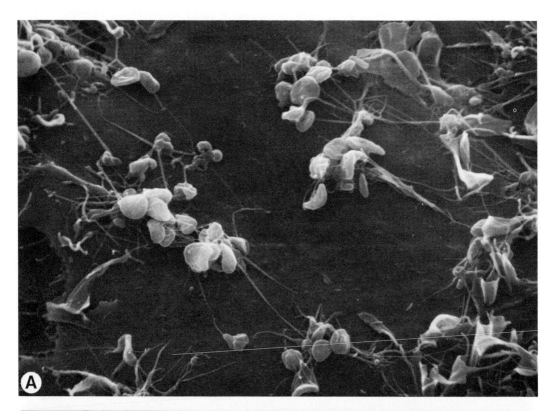

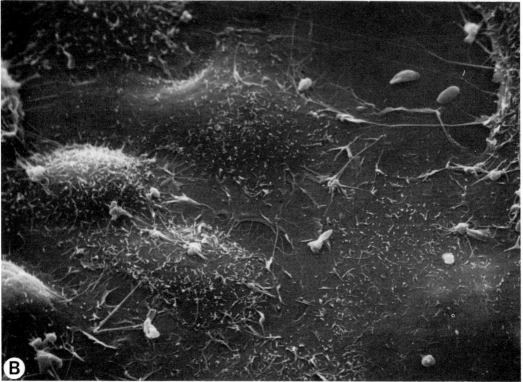

FIG. 7. Platelet Activation by Cellular Surfaces. A. Scanning electron photomicrograph of activated platelets on the surface of a smooth fibroblast cell. Activation is evidenced by clumping and strandlike cytoplasmotic projections and attachment to the fibroblast surface. B. Scanning electron photomicrograph of endothelial cells grown in culture and exposed to the same concentration of platelets as in A. Significant activation of platelets is not seen, and most platelets are found between cell bodies. The majority of platelets were found at the margin of the specimen, unactivated.

FIG. 8. Average maximum thrombus depth found on aortic tubular grafts (Abcor, Union Carbide) under varying anticoagulation protocols. Depth at any time greater than 0.5 mm is considered unsatisfactory. Note that some protocols allow initial rapid thrombus buildup but, subsequently, very significant humoral fibrinolytic activity reduces the thrombus to minimal level (eg, coumadin). In contrast, other protocols have thin thrombus depths initially, but thrombus continues to deposit with time (eg, persantine and aspirin). Most favorable are those protocols that maintain thrombus at low levels (eg, coumadin, persantine, and aspirin).

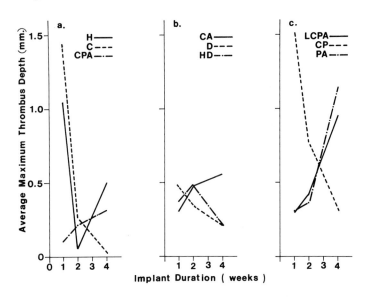

coumadin anticoagulation, which showed significant platelet, fibrin, and red blood cell thrombus formation, animals maintained on a combination of coumadin, persantine, and aspirin showed almost no deposition on the graft surface, and an average maximum depth of approximately 0.1 mm. Significant pannus ingrowth was present at the anastomotic margins. No white caps were seen on any of the coumadin-persantine-aspirin specimens. White blood cells, a prominent component of thrombus, which had been seen with the heparin, coumadin, and control studies, were seen in this protocol only occasionally in the one-week specimen and rarely in specimens later than that. At two weeks, there was some loss of red blood cell entrapment in the thrombus, the white blood cells were rare, and there were no white caps and only a minimal increase in total average thrombus depth (0.2 mm). At four weeks, marked pannus ingrowth had occurred to over 15 mm from each suture line. Average maximum thrombus depth had reached 0.3 mm (Fig. 8A). White blood cells were rarely seen. No renal infarcts were seen in any animals on this anticoagulation protocol.

COUMADIN-ASPIRIN ANTICOAGULATION. Grafts in animals maintained on coumadin and aspirin showed uniform thrombus covering at one week, which averaged 0.3 mm. White caps were present. Pannus ingrowth had begun. At two weeks, lysis activity was significant, and no white caps were seen, although the thrombus depth had increased to an average of 0.5 mm. Pannus ingrowth from the suture lines had covered 5 mm from each end. At four weeks, the average depth had increased to 0.6 mm and pannus in-

growth had extended to 10 mm (Fig. 8B). Renal infarcts were seen in the four-week specimens.

DEXTRAN ANTICOAGULATION. Animals maintained on Dextran 70 (20 cc/hour) infusions showed average maximum thrombus depths of 0.5 mm at one week. Evidence of humoral fibrinolytic activity was present and white caps were seen. At two weeks, the average thrombus depth had diminished to approximately 0.4 mm, white caps were still present, and pannus ingrowth was approximately 3 mm from each suture line. At four weeks the average thrombus depth had diminished to 0.2 mm (Fig. 8B), white caps were occasionally seen and pannus ingrowth extended approximately 10 mm from each suture line. Two to four renal infarcts were seen in each of the animals in this series.

HEMODILUTION ANTICOAGULATION. Animals who had blood removed and replaced with Ringer's lactate until they reached a hematocrit of approximately 20 showed, at one week, thrombus that was pale (less red blood cell entrapment) and had reached a maximum depth of approximately 0.4 mm. Rare white caps were seen. By two weeks, the depth had increased to approximately 0.5 mm, white caps were still present, and pannus ingrowth averaged 3 mm from each suture line. At four weeks, further fibrinolytic activity was evident; the average maximum thrombus depth was 0.2 mm and pannus ingrowth had reached approximately 10 mm from each suture line (Fig. 8B). No white caps were seen. Multiple renal infarcts were seen in all animals on this anticoagulant protocol.

LOW-LEVEL   COUMADIN-PERSAN-

TINE-ASPIRIN ANTICOAGULATION. At one week, these animals showed an average thrombus depth of 0.3 mm. White caps were absent and thrombus covering was uniform. At two weeks, the average thickness had increased to 0.4 mm, white caps were present, and there were irregular areas of pannus ingrowth up to 3 mm from the suture line. There was evidence of rather marked humoral fibrinolytic activity scattered randomly throughout the remainder of the thrombus. At four weeks, maximum thrombus depth had increased on the average to 0.9 mm, white caps were present, and pannus ingrowth from the anastomotic margins had reached approximately 5 mm from the suture line (Fig. 8C). Renal infarcts were seen in all animals with grafts implanted two weeks or longer.

COUMADIN-PERSANTINE ANTICOAGULATION. At one week, the thrombus on the graft surface was irregular, shaggy, and with multiple areas of white cap formation. The initial depth averaged 1.5 mm. Surface contour and configuration was very similar to the pure coumadin anticoagulant series. At two weeks, the average thrombus depth had diminished to 0.8 mm, there were a few residual white caps, and evidence of fibrinolytic activity was marked but randomly scattered throughout the graft surface. Pannus ingrowth had reached 3 mm. At four weeks, the average thrombus depth had further diminished to 0.3 mm (Fig. 8C). White caps were not seen, and

pannus ingrowth had extended to approximately 10 mm from the suture lines. Large numbers of renal infarcts were seen in most animals in this group.

PERSANTINE-ASPIRIN ANTICOAGULATION. At one week, thrombus covering was uniform over the surface, and the average depth was 0.3 mm. White caps were not seen. At two weeks, thrombus depth averaged 0.4 mm, white caps were present in small numbers, greater red blood cell entrapment was evident, and pannus ingrowth was approximately 3 mm in from the suture line (Fig. 8C). At four weeks, despite obvious proteolytic activity in random areas, the thrombus depth had increased to an average of 1.1 mm, multiple white caps were now in evidence, and pannus ingrowth had reached approximately 10 mm from the suture line margins. Renal infarcts were seen in all animals on this anticoagulant protocol.

Influence of Local Turbulence, Blood Velocity, and Artificial Wall Movement

LOCAL TURBULENCE. The influence upon thrombus generation of an uneven anastomosis, which generates local turbulent flow, may be seen in Figure 9. Thrombus, which normally overlies the artificial surface, is washed away by the turbulent eddy current created by the inexact approximation of graft and aorta. In our series, the

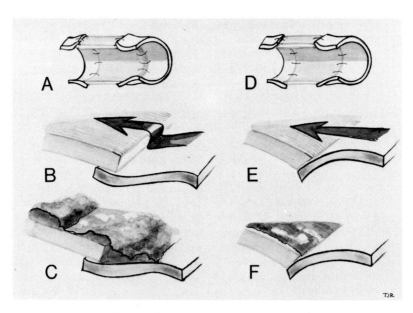

FIG. 9.   Influence of Turbulence on Thrombus Generation. A, B, C. When anastomotic irregularities occur, turbulent flow is generated (B), and irregular thrombus deposition occurs (C). This is in marked contrast to thrombus deposition when the aorta-graft anastomosis is even, and flow is nonturbulent (D, E, F).

FIG. 10. Influence of Flow on Thrombus Deposition. A. Left ventricular assist device as passive conduit in aorta-to-aorta position. With the aorta completely obstructed between inlet and outlet grafts from the pump, all flow is directed through the device. This is approximately 5 liters per minute, and flow velocities are approximately 26 cm/sec in the pump chamber. B. When the aorta is left partially open, blood flow is divided between the device and the aorta. This reduces velocities to approximately 10 cm/sec in the pump chamber. Thrombus depth is three times greater when only half the flow is through the pump.

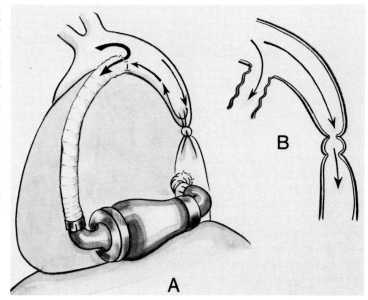

major thrombus erosion occurred an average of 1.2 cm distal to the proximal anastomosis. This phenomenon was not seen at the distal anastomosis. The aortic endothelium distal to the graft, as judged by silver nitrate staining, appeared intact.

BLOOD VELOCITY. These tubes had internal diameters of 18 to 20 mm. With an average blood flow in the descending aorta of approximately 5 liters per minute in these animals, the approximate velocity of flow was 26 cm per second. During the course of these experiments, TECO Model 6 left ventricular assist pumps were inserted in the aorta-to-aorta position with the descending aorta ligated between the two attachments (Figs. 1 and 10). When the aortic tie was not completely occlusive, the flow was divided approximately equally between the descending aorta and the nonpumping assist device (Fig. 10). In these cases,

thrombus deposition was two to four times as deep as in those cases in which flow through the graft was greater because the aorta was completely occluded (Fig. 10).

ARTIFICIAL WALL MOVEMENT. TECO Model 6 pumps, lined with a flocked Dacron surface bladder, and placed in the left-ventricular-to-descending-aorta position (Fig. 1), showed significant differences in thrombus depth depending on whether or not the bladder walls were moving. With activation of the device, bladder wall movement was significant, and thrombus depth was significantly less than on those bladders without wall movement. This finding suggests that not only velocity of flow but also movement and flexibility at the blood conduit interface can play a significant role in thrombus deposition (Fig. 11) (Bernhard, Bankole, et al, 1971).

FIG. 11. The Influence of Wall Movement on Thrombus Deposition. A. Assist device in aorta-to-aorta position, no bladder wall movement. a. Significant thrombus deposition is seen at one week (3 mm). B. assist device in aorta-to-aorta position, bladder pumping continuously. b. Thrombus deposition is much less than when device is used as a passive conduit (1 mm thrombus depth).

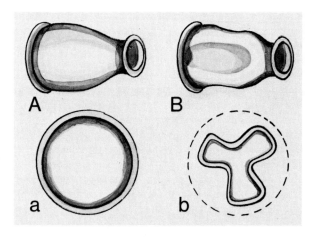

DISCUSSION

There are several considerations unique to assist-pump devices that determine acceptable levels of thrombus generation within the device. First, the pump must work in a satisfactory manner, continuously, from the moment of implantation. A technique for preventing thrombus deposition that produces satisfactory thrombus levels at two months is unacceptable if in the interim thrombus depths are sufficiently deep that they make the system malfunction. Second, since left ventricular assist devices not only pump blood down the aorta, but retrograde up the aorta to the cerebral circulation, embolic phenomena occurring at any time following implantation are unacceptable if strokes are to be avoided.

Third, the assist-pump system is nonporous, so that interstices ingrowth from surrounding tissues cannot aid in organizing the thrombus on the inner surface. Fourth, there are wide variations in blood-conduit interface movement, in velocity of flow, and in transient periods of blood stagnation present between beats of the pump. In addition, when the device is in clinical use, it is likely that there will be periods of time during which the unit may be nonfunctional. These may be intervals of a few minutes, or periods of days to months during which the device may not be needed to support the patient, but is left in place. Fifth, the mechanical requirements for the bladder itself are a severe test of industry's manufacturing capabilities. These requirements must be combined with a surface material that is satisfactory as a blood-conduit interface.

The ultimate technique for the prevention of thrombus buildup in left ventricular assist devices will depend in part upon the specific clinical situation. A patient who will not come off cardiopulmonary bypass following open heart surgery is certainly not a candidate for an autologous cell-lined pump system. On the other hand, an individual with severe chronic failure, who needs intervals of support to get over intercurrent illness such as viral pneumonitis, is a good candidate because his condition may allow the necessary time to preline a pump with his own cells. Thus, it may be necessary to tailor the technique of thrombus prevention to the individual patient. The advantages and disadvantages of each of the three surfaces (with and without anticoagulation) evaluated in this study are presented below.

Bare Lining Surface without Anticoagulation

Bare blood-conduit surface pump systems have the advantage of immediate availability. They can be stored in a sterile condition. As with all surfaces, they require a highly reliable bladder backing material. They also require surface characteristics that minimize thrombus generation and do not tend to cause peripheral embolization. To date, manufacturing techniques have usually necessitated a bladder constructed of two separate layers: a backing material and a bonded overlay of a special surface material. Separation of these two components during use has been a significant problem. The Abcor nonwoven nylon is a system made out of a single material, removing the necessity for bonding.

In the present study, thrombus deposition on the bare grafts (without anticoagulation) at 24 hours was between 1 and 1.6 mm maximum average depth (Figs. 4A and 4B). These data were obtained in aortic tubular grafts, where the environment is far *less* conducive to thrombus generation than that in assist device pumping systems. In the assist-pump, 1.5 mm thrombus depth in the area of the inlet or outlet valves could cause serious malfunction. Embolic phenomena were seen with both the Union Carbide and Abcor grafts within 10 days of insertion, though they were less frequent with the Abcor grafts.

Unfortunately, surfaces that tend to prevent thrombus formation because of their nonwettability also tend to have a higher incidence of peripheral embolization. Fibrin and thrombus do not attach well, and this causes embolization when moving blood shear forces exceed attachment forces. Successful utilization of bare lining surfaces depends on a modest initial thrombus deposition and an effective humoral fibrinolytic system to reduce the thrombus to acceptable depth levels quickly. Thrombus attachment forces must exceed the shear forces present in the device. In addition, if the device is to be used without anticoagulants during long-term implantations, surface irregularities should be minimal to avoid late embolic phenomena generated at these sites.

Cell-Covered Linings

Since autologous cell linings require several weeks to prepare, the cell-lined system has no application for emergency situations. The cells must be autologous in origin to avoid unwanted immune responses after implantation of the device. Once collected from the patient and cultured, the cells are seeded onto the graft material using tissue culture techniques. With current methods, these linings have a finite storage time.

Although a cell-lined system would require the same mechanical characteristics for the pump bladder system, the surface characteristics of the bladder need only be able to support cellular growth. Depending on cell type, this may be difficult or relatively easy to accomplish (Wechezak and Mansfield, 1973). Cell-lined systems will be of value only if they remove the need for anticoagulants. They are capable of self-regeneration, and endothelial-like cells used in recent experiments appear to control the depth of underlying thrombus and cellular activity. To be clinically useful, cell-lined bladders must reduce embolic risks to the patient. Potentially, they can accomplish this by (1) repairing surface irregularities through cellular regeneration, and (2) retarding, and possibly preventing, platelet activation and thrombus generation.

Persons experienced in tissue culture techniques are needed to establish cell lines in culture and to attach the lining to the bladder. The system cannot be sterilized after cellular growth has been initiated. Infection must be prevented by excellence of technique. Viral contamination could be a significant deterrent to effective utilization of cell linings.

Autologous fibroblasts are not satisfactory as lining cells even though they are hardy, grow rapidly, and cover the bladder surface well. As seen in Table 3, fibroblast-lined grafts at four weeks to six months had significantly greater depth of thrombus than did the unlined control graft systems. The incidence of peripheral embolization as determined by renal infarction was similar to the unlined control grafts. Recent developments in the growth of endothelial cells in culture and the *in vitro* demonstration of reduced platelet adherence to these cell surfaces suggest that further evaluation of endothelial cell linings should be undertaken.

Bare Lining Surfaces with Anticoagulation

The addition of anticoagulants to the bare lining surfaces provides certain advantages. Sterile units would be available for emergency use. Although the mechanical function of the bladders would have to be as strictly reliable as for the bare surfaces without anticoagulation, the standards for surface characteristics would not need to be as strict. Certain practical problems associated with surgery, however, might be encountered. The data presented from this study, as seen in Figure 8, demonstrate that not all anticoagulation protocols are effective when used with these assist devices. In addition, the risk of significant intraoperative and postoperative bleeding at the time of surgical insertion and the possibility that such insertion may follow open heart surgery (extracorporeal circulation) may compound the problem of bleeding. In addition, the postoperative anticoagulation protocols are not without continuing risk to the patient of hemorrhage in vital areas or of excessive blood loss.

One factor, not thoroughly evaluated as yet, is whether the anticoagulation protocol must be instituted before surgery or whether equally satisfactory results can be obtained by institution of the protocols at the time of, and subsequent to, surgical implantation. Since thrombus is laid down, despite complete heparinization, within seconds of blood flow through artificial devices (Figs. 4A and B), it seems likely that anticoagulant protocols should be instituted at the time the device is implanted and continued thereafter. (We have not found that this approach has led to excessive blood loss at, or following, surgery in these animals.) Thus, if certain anticoagulants reduce the amount of thrombus forming prior to enhancement of humoral fibrinolytic activity, average thrombus depth should be minimized.

Thrombus

The composition and depth of thrombus deposited on the surfaces in our studies was a very dynamic balance. As seen in Figure 5, initially, platelets and fibrin were deposited in thin layers, while heparin was in effect.

Within this framework, which was perhaps 60 microns thick, red blood cells began to be trapped. Very shortly thereafter, and particularly upon the reversal of heparin with protamine, white blood cells attached to platelet fibrin complexes, particularly at the surface of the thrombus. Grossly pale elevations on the surface of the thrombus (white caps) developed, leading to continuing red cell entrapment. Although one suspects that lysis activity was going on simultaneously, at this stage the rate of thrombus deposition far exceeded any humoral fibrinolytic activity. At 12 to

24 hours following initiation of blood flow through the grafts, evidence was found that lysis may be more rapid than thrombus generation. In the period of two to 14 days, continuing fibrolytic activity usually reduced the total thickness of thrombus. Additional help in reducing thrombus was generated from the suture line. Pannus ingrowth with macrophage activity and subsequent endothelial ingrowth reduced thrombus depth significantly. (Figs. 4A, 4B, and 5). This pannus ingrowth, however, was not available to areas remote from the suture line, such as the left ventricular assist device pump bladder. In such areas, cellular activity to remove and organize thrombus had to come from fallout seeding. Characteristic morphology of early thrombus generation is seen in Figure 5.

Attention must be called to the role of the white blood cell in thrombus deposition within vascular conduits (Petschek and Madras, 1969). The phase of rapid increase in thrombus depth was always associated with marked white blood cell attachment at the surface. Many white blood cells were found, far exceeding what could be expected from any conceivable skimming or eddy effects. Once entrapped in the thrombus, they disappeared rapidly and were replaced at the surface of the deepening thrombus by other white blood cells. It appears significant that this reaction could be influenced by certain anticoagulant protocols. The most successful protocol, a combination of coumadin, persantine, and aspirin, at no time showed any white cap formation, and the reduced number of white blood cells at the surface was conspicuous. This suggests that the influence of persantine and aspirin on clot formation may extend beyond an influence on the platelet. Whether these drugs alter the white blood cell or the white blood cell-platelet-fibrin complex is unknown. Intensive research is needed in this area. Possibly, antimetabolite drugs (nitrogen mustard) or immunosuppressives (Immuran) might influence thrombus generation in vascular conduits.

Embolic Phenomena

The ultimate aim is to avoid all embolic phenomena originating in association with assist devices. Nonwettable surfaces tend to accumulate loosely held thrombus, and subsequent shear forces within the vascular system lead to high incidence of peripheral embolization. In these studies, peripheral (renal) emboli were frequently seen. They were seen in all cases of bare surface without anticoagulants, all cases of fibroblast cell linings, and

in many of the anticoagulant protocol experiments. Most significant, perhaps, is the finding that when white caps were absent, peripheral emboli were rarely seen. A complete absence of emboli occurred with the use of coumadin-persantine-aspirin anticoagulation protocol. Rare white caps and very rare emboli were seen with the heparin protocol. With the coumadin protocol, emboli were seen early, but once marked proteolytic activity was seen, further emboli were rare. There did not appear to be any correlation between depth of thrombus and peripheral embolization.

Clinical Implications of Left Ventricular Assist Device

The results of these experiments have focused our attention on certain critical aspects of thrombus generation in left ventricular assist devices. First, thrombus is initiated immediately upon starting blood flow through the device. In the calf, peak levels of thrombus deposition occur between 12 and 48 hours, and the resolution is dependent upon fibrinolytic activity of humoral origin. Interpreting these results for use in other species must be done with caution.

Second, leukocytes appear to play a significant role in thrombus generation within vascular conduits actively carrying blood. Third, the demonstrated effectiveness of certain anticoagulation protocols makes it possible that their combination with other protocols (eg, hemodilution) at the time of surgery may reduce the stringent requirements for lining surface characteristics.

Fourth, anticipating the need for emergency use of these systems, the availability of aspirin and persantine in parenteral forms would be of particular benefit. Fifth, the antithrombogenic techniques used in association with left ventricular assist devices must be capable of preventing thrombus generation and embolic phenomena under all hemodynamic conditions associated with the use of the device, including deactivation for prolonged periods.

Applications to Current Clinical Practice

Arterial vascular prostheses and artificial heart valves currently in clinical use generate thrombus on their surfaces. The incidence of embolic phenomena associated with their use, particularly with artificial valves in low-flow areas (eg, mitral valve), is high. Since thrombus forms very rapidly following surgery, well ahead of the time most clinical programs initiate long-term anti-coagulation, reconsideration of current postoperative anticoagulation protocols seems warranted.

The patency rate of coronary artery bypass grafts associated with distal endarterectomy is lower than the patency rate of bypass grafts without endarterectomy (Urschel et al, 1974). After endarterectomy, the exposed surface is very conducive to platelet adherence, and progressive thrombus accumulation may account for the increased closure rates seen clinically. We now utilize hemodilution prime, Dextran 70 started before heparin reversal with protamine and continued until the chest tubes are out and the coumadin-persantine-aspirin therapy has reached therapeutic levels. The endarterectomized patients are kept on this protocol for six months followed by coumadin for one year.

Retrieval of artificial conduits and valves at postmortem provides a unique opportunity to study thrombus generation in the human. Careful documentation including photographs, clinical history, and microscopic examination, particularly of specimens retrieved early following surgery, may give us insight to human responses to artificial surfaces. Such information would be invaluable in evaluating potential problems relative to thrombus generation when these assist devices are ultimately applied to man.

Hemodilution

The influence on thrombus deposition of hemodilution with Ringer's lactate was an unexpected finding. Two animals bled from their anastomotic suture lines intraoperatively and their volume loss was replaced with Ringer's lactate. At sacrifice, their grafts were remarkably free of thrombus compared to other animals with similar surgery but without hemodilution. These two animals were removed from the study and a separate protocol for elective hemodilution was included. The results (Fig. 8) indicate that the protocol can be very effective in reducing thrombus.

This protocol warrants further study, since it could be an extremely practical approach for reducing thrombus in all areas of vascular surgery. We have no evidence that hemodilution increases bleeding in the clinical situation, and thus it may be applicable with very little risk of undesired hemorrhage.

References

Bernhard WF, Bankole MA, LaFarge CG, Bornhorst W, et al: Development of an experimental model for functional cardiac replacement. Surgery 70:205 1971

Mansfield PB: Tissue cultured endothelium for vascular prosthetic devices. Report to Medical Devices Applications Program. NIH-NHLI-71-2060-1. National Heart and Lung Inst. US Dept of Health, Education, and Welfare, Public Health Service, 1972

Mansfield PB, Wechezak A: Tissue cultured cells as an endothelial lining of prosthetic materials. In Organ Perfusion and Preservation, Norman JC (ed), Appleton-Century-Crofts, 1968, pp 189–202

Petschek HE, Madras PN: Thrombus formation on artificial surfaces. In Artificial Heart Program, National Heart Institute: Artificial Heart Program Conference, 1969, p 271

Urschel HC Jr, Razzuk MA, Wood RE: Long-term follow-up of coronary vein bypass grafts: appraisal of factors influencing patency. In Coronary Artery Medicine and Surgery, Norman JC (ed), Appleton-Century-Crofts, 1975, pp 619–34

Wechezak A, Mansfield PB: Isolation and growth characteristics of cell lines from bovine venous endothelium. In Vitro 9:39 1973

120

OVERCOMING PRESENT OBSTACLES TO THE ARTIFICIAL HEART

Jeffrey L. Peters, J. Volder, E. J. Hershgold,
Don B. Olsen, S. R. Greenhalgh,
John H. Lawson, and W. J. Kolff

Experience in over 200 total heart replacements in calves has indicated specific problem areas that have to be overcome before the artificial heart can be used in man. *In vivo* and *in vitro* studies indicated that biocompatibility of the pumping ventricles is one problem. This includes blood component damage, coagulation abnormalities, and formation of microemboli. Silicone rubber covered with dacron fibrils has been used as the intima of the artificial heart. Progressive deposition of blood proteins occurs on the fibrils with diminishing blood damage. The next major problem has been hemodynamic function of the artificial ventricles. Comparative mock circulation studies of nine different artificial hearts showed cardiac output curves with slopes of 0.04 to 0.88 L/min/0 to 5 mm Hg at 100 mm Hg outflow pressure. The artificial hearts have been diaphragm driven (usually pneumatic) and have been operated at a fixed rate, driving pressure, and duty cycle. Aortic pressures have been in the normal range (125 to 175 systolic and 60 to 100 mm Hg diastolic pressure), but in almost all experiments there has been pulmonary hypertension (systolic pressure above 50 mm Hg) and calves have required intermittent respiratory support. Calves have been able to stand,. eat, and function normally up to 94 days. The maximum cardiac output is 12 L/min, which may be enough for human candidates. Inflow obstruction of both the right and left ventricles at the level of the natural right and left remnant atria has resulted in atrial pressures greater than 20 mm Hg (particularly in the right atrium) and pulsatile atrial pressures of 10 to 20 mm Hg, which have been shown to be due in part to improper fit, regurgitation of valves, asynchronous atrial-ventricular contractions, and the use of high diastolic ventricular contractions, and the use of high diastolic ventricular vacuum. The progressive rise of right ventricular filling pressure with the time of pumping has been reduced with the use of a better fitting artificial ventricle. High-pulsatile atrial pressures have been reduced with the use of a large-volume compliant artificial atrium. Another problem has been the use of two driving lines and numerous pressure recording lines coming out of the thorax, which have led to lethal infections. New percutaneous leads, implantable power sources, and indirect measurement of hemodynamic events should minimize this problem. Prolonged survivals of calves with total artificial hearts both in our laboratory and other laboratories in the United States have stimulated innovative advances in artificial heart technology and brought us closer to application in man.

Supported in part by the National Institutes of Health via the National Heart and Lung Institute, Grant 5-PO1-HL-13738-03 and by Contract NO1-HT4-2905 and by the John A. Hartford Foundation, the Christina Foundation, the Lad L. and Mary Hercik Fund, and Mr. Maurice Warshaw.

INTRODUCTION

During the last two decades government and private industry have placed emphasis on the development of cardiac assist devices and total artificial hearts (Hastings, Harmison, 1969; Cooper,

TABLE 1. Long-Surviving Calves with Total Circulatory Support

LABORATORY	INVESTIGATORS	SURVIVAL TIME (days)	TYPE OF HEART	COMMENTS
Salt Lake City	Kolff et al	94	Air-driven, diaphragm-type silicone rubber with dacron fibril intima; Bjork-Shiley valves	Calf reoperated after 23 days to remove adhesions over the atria; terminal event—excessive fibrin buildup on intima and valves resulting in decreased cardiac output; evidence of embolization; infection
Jackson, Miss.	Akutsu et al	25	Air-driven, sack-type silicone rubber with dispersion coating intima; fabricated flap and bicuspid silastic valves	Progressive increases of inflow pressures with time of pumping; anemia and evidence of embolization infection; terminal event—cerebral thromboembolism
Boston	Bernhard, Lafarge et al	17	Air-driven diaphragm ventricles, polyurethane with dacron fibril intima; attached to natural heart, which was in ventricular fibrillation; modified Bjork-Shiley valves	Mean cardiac output—6.9 L/min, normal pulmonary and systemic pressures; anemia; right-sided pneumonia; calf sacrificed
Cleveland	Nosé et al	17	Air-driven diaphragm type heart of "biolized" pericardium, natural (tricuspid) bovine valves	Gradual increase of venous pressures and atrial pulsatility during first two weeks; infection; infarction of kidneys; terminal event—rupture of the left ventricle

Harmison, 1971; and Nosé, 1970). A recent artificial heart assessment panel of the National Heart and Lung Institute was presented with an estimate of approximately 16,000 to 50,000 potential yearly candidates for heart replacement (Totally Implantable Artificial Heart, NHLI Artificial Heart Assessment Panel, 1973). Most of these candidates would have coronary heart disease, rheumatic heart disease, or ischemic heart disease with hypertension. The implications of total heart replacement on our society are not fully defined; however, the continued research efforts in the United States and in some foreign countries suggest that the time of human heart replacement with a prosthetic device is not far away.* The greatest advances in total heart replacement have occurred in the last three years. This has been mainly mani-

* Workshop on Left Ventricular Assist Pumps. Washington, DC, NIH, October 28, 1973.

fested in the prolonged survival of calves by total circulatory maintenance with prosthetic ventricles for periods of more than three months (Table 1). The problems that plagued short-term survival in the early years (Nosé, 1970), such as fit of the prosthetic device in the chest, minimal perfusion capabilities, and surgical implantation, have in part been circumvented by new technology contributed by disciplines in both the medical and physical sciences. The following report surveys the experiences of three years in problem-oriented artificial heart research at the University of Utah. The general research approach to the development of an artificial heart suitable for implantation in man has been to use a device of minimal complexity, which fits in the chest and provides a basal cardiac output. Design criteria based on both *in vitro* and *in vivo* evaluation are continually upgraded. As new technology occurs in allied fields, it is incorporated into the heart design (eg, new biomaterials, better-performing prosthetic valves).

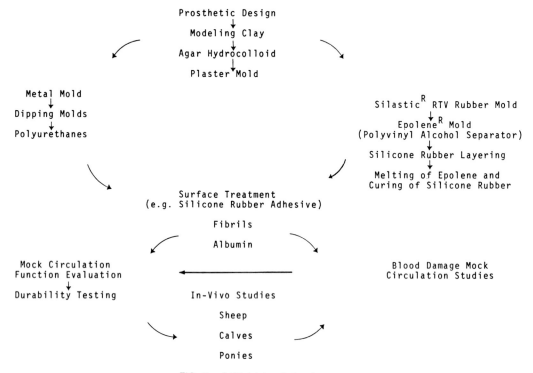

FIG. 1. Artificial heart development.

METHODS AND MATERIALS

Prosthetic Fabrication

All fabrication of artificial hearts can be performed in house from the design concept to a finished product ready for implantation. This capability is a tremendous advantage, particularly in minimizing delay time and cost of fabrication of new devices and for modification of currently used prostheses. Procedures for construction have been previously described (Kessler, Foote, et al, 1971), and Figure 1 illustrates the flow diagram of the steps to a finished product, including the evaluation of function and durability testing.

Presently raw, Silastic 372® medical grade sheeting, 372 medical grade tubing and Dow Corning 92-009® dispersion coating or polyurethane is used. The thickness of raw sheeting or polyurethane with and without dacron reinforcing ranges from 0.03 to 0.06 inches. Pressure monitoring taps consist of $\frac{3}{16}$ inch (ID) by $\frac{5}{16}$ inch (OD) tubing bonded to connector dacron grafts. All metal components, such as valve housing and connecting ring supports, are coated with 0.005 inch Silicone rubber dispersion or polyurethane. Application of uncured Silastic® sheeting or polyurethane is similar for most of the prostheses. The electrostatic nature of the nonwettable surface requires a dust-free atmosphere and the use of sterile gloves to prevent contamination. Silastic® sheeting is handled only by the surplus edges, except when molding intricate forms for which stainless steel dental plastic instruments are employed. Mold surfaces are nonporous and highly polished to provide a smooth surface for molded materials, such as housings and diaphragms, which will eventually be blood-interface materials.

In Vitro Evaluation

Short-term and long-term testing is performed on all heart models prior to utilization in implantation experiments. This ranges from pumping of the single diaphragm with compressed air to detailed function curves of an entire heart in a mock circulation. A rating system for all hearts has been developed in order to increase quality control and prevent costly errors (Foote, Greenhalgh, Peters, 1973). Essentially, two types of mock circulations have been developed to evaluate pumping performance and blood damage by prosthetic ventricles. One mock circulation consists of two chambers (venous and arterial) filled with

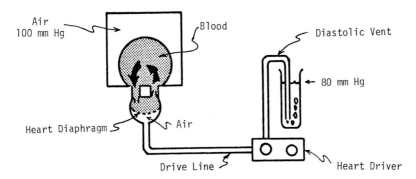

FIG. 2. *In vitro* blood damage evaluation system (5 liter) with air-driven diaphragm ventricle. Pressure on box is 100 mm Hg simulating outflow pressure. The difference in box pressure, height of the blood column, and positive pressure on the diaphragm during diastole simulate effective diastolic pressure. There are two identical systems for comparison of a single variable with fresh blood from a single source.

water or saline solution and separated by a resistance valve. Compliances are 1 and 25 ml/mm Hg for the arterial and venous chambers, respectively. Flow is read out directly from an electromagnetic flowmeter with a flow probe built into the outflow tract of the mock circulation (Donovan, 1972). Function curves (filling pressure versus cardiac output) are determined by varying the inflow pressures (utilizing a vacuum to regulate the venous chamber). Any driving parameters to be used *in vivo* are evaluated *in vitro*. A second electromagnetic flowmeter has been placed on the inflow side to determine valve regurgitation (Backman et al, 1974). Traces of the flow waveform are recorded on a strip chart recorder and graphically integrated to determine the forward and back flow through the valve over several cycles of pumping. A ventricle is usually pumped from two to six hours to ensure proper valve functions and to further ensure that the dacron fibril intima is firmly attached and that there are no leaks in the diaphragm or housing. Function curves for nine

different artificial ventricles have been evaluated. It is to be noted that the mock circulation does not duplicate *in vivo* characteristics completely (such as effects of respiration on cardiac output and effects of asynchronously beating atria on ventricular filling); however, information from specific ventricular characteristics can be used to determine hemodynamic parameters indirectly after implantation (Foote, 1973). A second mock circulation consisting of a silicone rubber sphere encased in a plexiglass chamber is used to evaluate relative blood damage by prosthetic ventricles (Peters et al, 1973a, 1974a; Carter et al, 1974. Three models of this system consisting of a 5-liter, 2-liter, and 1-liter volume sphere have been developed (Fig. 2). Each system is studied in duplicate with fresh, anticoagulated bovine blood such that one parameter (eg, intima or driving parameters or entire heart design) can be compared with respect to relative blood damage. Outflow pressure can be regulated by applying an air pressure to the box and inflow pressure (effective diastolic pressure) can be reg-

FIG. 3. *In vitro* blood damage evaluation system (2 liter). Outflow and inflow pressure in each system is 40 mm Hg. One system (left) is a standard reference system; the other (right) serves as the test system. Hemolysis index ratio may be determined between the standard ventricle and a test ventricle.

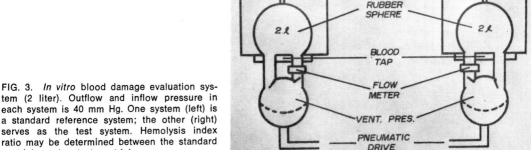

ulated in a diaphragm heart by venting the diaphragm to a positive pressure during diastole (Fig. 3). In most studies outflow and inflow pressures are identical at 40 mm Hg. An initial study was performed with the 5 liter system, utilizing an 8 cm Kwan-Gett ventricle with a smooth silicone rubber surface as a standard and dacron cloth, dacron fibril (before and after being pumped in a calf) intimas in an 8 cm Kwan-Gett test ventricle. Both ventricles had Bjork-Shiley inflow and outflow valves and were pumped at identical driving, outflow, and inflow parameters. Free plasma hemoglobin is determined by scanning spectrophotometry of sequential blood samples.

Hemolysis index (HI) is determined from the relationship:

$$\text{HI (gms/100 L)} =$$

$$\cfrac{\cfrac{Slope}{(\text{mg \% free plasma}} \cdot \cfrac{Syst.\,Vol.}{\text{hgb/min)} \,(\text{L})} \cdot \cfrac{\%\,Plasma}{(100\text{-Hct})}}{\cfrac{(\text{L/min})}{Cardiac\ Output} \cdot 100}$$

Carter et al (1974) have recently used the 2-liter system to study the difference in platelet function between a fibril and smooth-surface prosthetic ventricle. Platelet adhesiveness was measured by a modified method (Hellem, 1970). Durability studies are carried out by prolonged pumping on a mock circulation filled with water (Kwan-Gett et al, 1969). This allows fatigue studies to be performed on the valves, diaphragm, and housing and to evaluate the pneumatic driving system.

In Vivo Studies

The three-month-old bovine weighing approximately 80 kg has been used mainly for implantation studies. However the bovine and the adult pony have been used for acute studies (Peters, Donovan, et al, 1972a) evaluating artificial hearts. Preoperative conditioning of Holstein-Frisian calves (Peters, Donovan, et al, 1972b; Peters, Imlay, et al, 1972c) and normal values for blood chemistry and respiratory function have been previously described (Peters, Hess, et al, 1973b).

Artificial Heart Implantation Procedures

A variety of surgical implantation procedures have been utilized with the artificial heart. In order to minimize surgical trauma and to evaluate the effects of blood damage of the artificial heart, independent of cardiopulmonary bypass, two im-

plantation methods, deep hypothermia, and double bypass of the natural heart, have been employed. Dr. Jun Kawai introduced deep hypothermia in our laboratory as a method of implanting the artificial heart (Kawai et al, 1971, 1972). The fasted, preconditioned calf is induced with scopolamine (0.015 mg/kg) and brevane (5 mg/kg), intubated and placed on a Bird respirator (Mark 14), with halothane gaseous anesthesia. The calf is then instrumented with ECG electrodes, femoral arterial blood pressure catheter, external jugular vein catheter (for Ringer's lactate solution infusion), and a rectal temperature probe. The calf is placed in an ice bath and the rectal temperature is brought to 24C (range 22.5 to 25C). On the operating table, cooling is maintained by ice bags on the head, neck, and groin. The chest is open by a midsternal split and the great vessels are dissected and ligated after heparin (1 mg/kg) is given. Once the rectal temperature has decreased to 21C, blood is expelled from the natural heart and, with hyperventilation, from the pulmonary circulation. Both circulatory and respiratory arrest are maintained during the implantation of the artificial heart, which usually takes 45 minutes. The artificial heart is pumped slowly at first and at low pressures in order to detect and repair blood leaks and to prevent the pulmonary and systemic circulation from being exposed to sudden high pressures and flows. Protamine sulfate is administered (1.5 mg/kg), four chest drainage tubes are inserted and the chest is closed. The calf is then placed in a warm water bath (40 C) until the rectal temperature reaches approximately 34 C. Afterwards the calf is placed in a specially designed restraint cart. This method has been slightly modified for use with the adult pony (weight 100 kg). One modification includes an isoproterenol drip administered during surface cooling to prevent cardiac arrest above 23 C. Four ponies have been studied with this method of deep hypothermia as animal models for artificial heart implantation.

A second technique of implantation of the artificial heart (double bypass) without cardiopulmonary bypass was developed by Dr. Clifford Kwan-Gett (Kwan-Gett et al, 1971). In this method the calf, after anesthesia, is positioned midway between the dorsal and right lateral position for a fourth intercostal thoracotomy. The aortic graft is anastomosed to the descending aorta and the pulmonary graft is anastomosed to the pulmonary artery. The calf is then positioned on the dorsal surface and a transverse thoracotomy completed. A left atrial connector is anastomosed and the left ventricle is attached and primed for pumping. In a like manner, the right ventricle is attached to the right atrial connector. After ventricular fibrillation is induced and both artificial ventricles are maintaining the circulation, pulmonary artery and aortic roots are clamped, divided, and sutured. The ventricles are then clamped and removed. The two artificial ventricles are then fitted into the middle of the thorax and attached to each other. Chest tubes are inserted, and the chest is closed.

The standard method for open-heart surgery, cardiopulmonary bypass, is used routinely in our laboratory along with our other procedures (Peters et al, 1972b). It is particularly useful for initial evaluation of a new artificial heart for which fit in the thorax and vessel connections are not standardized. It allows for direct end-to-end anastomosis of the great vessels as compared to the double bypass technique which utilizes end-to-side anastomoses. It allows more time for implantation compared to the deep hypothermia method (limit of circulatory and respiratory arrest of one hour), which utilizes direct end-to-end anastomosis quick connects.

A Bentley oxygenator is used with a prime of 2,000 ml Ringer's lactate solution and 1,000 ml of Dextran 40. Blood drainage is from the inferior vena cava by way of the right atrium and the superior vena cava by way of the right jugular vein. Blood is returned to the right femoral artery. The duration of total bypass varies from one to three hours with an average of approximately one and one-half hour.

Surgical implantation is performed by both midsternal or right thoracotomy with the use of cardiopulmonary bypass. Implantation of the larger atomic energy heart (both right and left ventricles connected) requires a midsternal approach while individual ventricles may be inserted via a right thoracotomy. The use of right thoracotomy seems to minimize the postoperative complications of a midsternal thoracotomy, including the increased risk of infection, bleeding, and the difficulty of having the calf lying upright on the incision area.

Prosthetic Ventricles

Three models of artificial hearts have been investigated. The 7 cm hemispherical (Kwan-Gett et al, 1970) and the 8 cm hemispherical (Kwan-Gett et al, 1971) air-driven diaphragm ventricles with stroke volumes of 100 and 150 cc, respectively. Valves used in these ventricles include silicone rubber flap inflow and outflow valves, tricuspid outflow valves, and Bjork-Shiley disc valves. A second pneumatic ventricle, elliptical in shape with a stroke volume of approximately 160

cc, was developed in 1973 (Jarvik, 1973; Oster et al, 1973). Bjork-Shiley valves are employed in both the outflow and inflow positions. The third model developed and tested in the last two years is a mechanically driven diaphragm heart with Bjork-Shiley valves designed for implantation with an atomic energy power source (Backman et al, 1973; Smith et al, 1974). This device is currently driven by an electric motor, which is implanted in the abdomen. The driving mode is alternate, allowing one ventricle to fill while the other ventricle is ejecting blood at 120 b/min. The outer housing is collapsible to provide intrinsic regulation of cardiac output and to prevent collapse of the atria and inflow vessels when filling pressure is decreased.

In conjunction with the hemispherical ventricle, an artificial right atrium and left atrium (Fig. 4) has been developed. The right atrium has a volume of 120 cc and a compliant inner diaphragm vented to atmosphere (Peters et al,

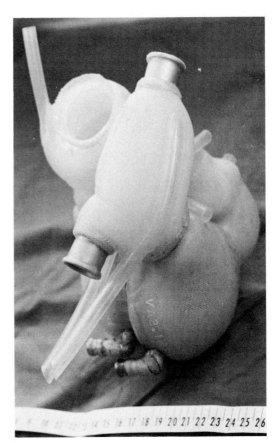

FIG. 4. Hemispherical ventricles with artificial right atrium (rings for attachment of superior and inferior vena cava) with two air vents to a compliant inner diaphragm; spherical artificial left atrium with diaphragm vent line.

1973d). Surfaces of all devices have included smooth silicone rubber adhesive or dacron fibrils attached to silicone rubber.

Standard intensive care procedures and physiological monitoring are employed after implantation (Peters et al, 1972b; Lawson et al, 1974). This includes blood chemistry analysis, pulmonary, hemodynamic, and renal function studies. Twenty-four-hour care is provided by two trained personnel (four- to eight-hour shifts). Special coagulation studies are performed by the hematology division utilizing standard methodology and modified tests for the bovine (platelet function, coagulation factors, fibrinogen, and platelet survival time) (Hershgold et al, 1972). Recent studies in an extracorporeal loop with the artificial heart pumping part of the blood volume of calves (Kwan-Gett et al, 1971; Volder et al, 1973) have been performed on radioactive labeled platelets by surface scanning procedures and by counting radioactive labels found in body parts at autopsy.

Postmortem examination includes gross and microscopic pathologic studies utilizing both light and electron microscopy of selected tissues (Johnson et al, 1973; Olsen et al, 1973).

RESULTS

Implantation of the Artificial Heart

Deep hypothermia provides an interesting alternative to cardiopulmonary bypass, particularly in the bovine. Without the use of an oxygenator, free plasma hemoglobin cannot be detected with surface cooling to 20 C, and platelets are minimally affected. The lungs are deflated during the average 45-minute circulatory and respiratory arrest period, and there is minimal blood loss. Figure 5 illustrates the changes in blood pressure and temperature in the adult pony during surface cooling, which responds similarly to the bovine except that isoproterenol is required to prevent cardiac arrest at rectal temperatures above 20 to 23 C. In the four experiments with implantation of the artificial heart in the pony with deep hypothermia, clinical evidence of minimal brain damage occurred, including involuntary muscle tremors and shaking of the neck in two ponies. The pony, unlike the calf, is much stronger and difficult to control, particularly during rewarming, and requires anesthesia. Careful attention to blood gases and pH during rewarming has resulted in a 10-day survival of the bovine without neurologic impairment (Kawai et al, 1972). The long period of rewarming, ap-

proximating four hours, allows for suspension of the animal in a water bath immediately postoperatively, preventing body-weight pressure on a midsternal thoracotomy incision site. The lowered metabolic rate and gradual increase during rewarming allows correction of fluid balance over a prolonged period without adverse metabolic consequences as may occur at normothermia. The decreased heparin requirement, one-third to one-fifth the concentration used in cardiopulmonary bypass, improves hemostasis postoperatively.

Cardiopulmonary bypass has been the current method of choice for implantation. Figure 6 illustrates blood gases, pH, and base excess in the pony during cardiopulmonary bypass. Postoperative blood loss from the chest in both the pony and the bovine averages from 1,500 to 2,500 cc. Free plasma hemoglobin has ranged from 6 mg percent to 132 mg percent after cardiopulmonary bypass (Peters et al, 1973b). Increases in free plasma hemoglobin have been correlated with the increased time of bypass.

Hemodynamic Consequences of the Artificial Heart

MOCK CIRCULATION STUDIES.   Performance of nine different ventricles (Greenhalgh et al, 1974; Peters et al, 1974b) pumped as left ventricles are indicated in Table 2. Cardiac output curve slopes of five diaphragm-type ventricles, three sack-type, and one mechanical ventricle ranges from 0.04–0.88 L/min/0–5 mm Hg. Maximum cardiac output ranges from 3.8–11.9 L/min. These ventricles vary in design and driving parameters and have been used for total circulatory support and/or partial bypass of the natural heart. Figure 7 illustrates the comparison of the function curves of the nine artificial ventricles. The current artificial hearts in Utah have a maximum cardiac output of 11.9 L/min. The Bjork-Shiley valve in the artificial heart regurgitates. Figure 8 illustrates

TABLE 2. *In Vitro* **Function Tests
(at 100 mm Hg Output Pressure)**

ΔCO/ΔFP (0 to 5 mm Hg)	CO (L/min) (at 5 mm Hg FP)	MAXIMUM CO (L/min)
0.04	3.6	3.8
0.12	5.8	6.0
—	4.6	6.2
0.34	6.8	11.0
0.32	6.6	9.6
0.12	8.4	8.4
0.32	8.2	11.8
0.86	8.0	11.9
0.88	10.0	11.9

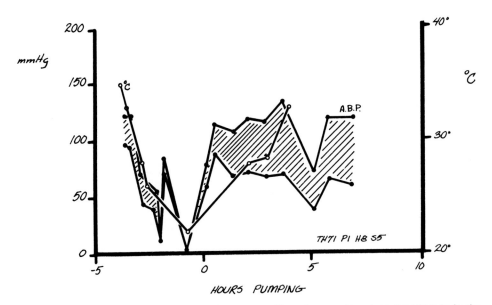

FIG. 5. Changes in temperature and blood pressure with surface cooling deep hypothermia in the adult pony. At 0 time the artificial heart begins pumping; a short time later the pony is placed in a warm water bath (40 C).

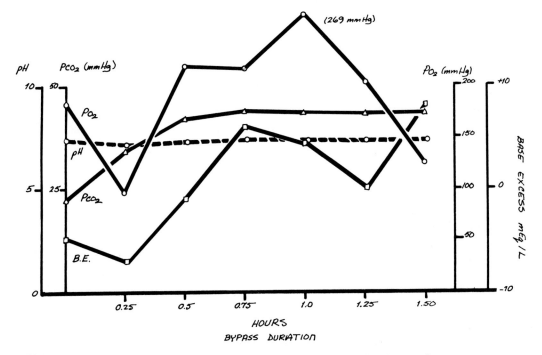

FIG. 6. Blood gases, pH, and base excess in the pony during cardiopulmonary bypass.

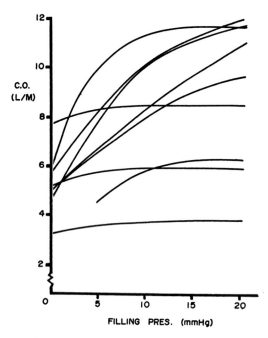

FIG. 7. Cardiac function curves performed on nine different ventricles in the USA, utilizing a mock circulation. Outflow pressure is maintained constant at 100 mm Hg.

sure in a noncompliant artificial right atrium attached to a hemispherical ventricle. Mean atrial pressure is 0 mm Hg, however, the pulse pressure fluctuates 20 mm Hg. When a compliant artificial right atrial diaphragm is vented to atmosphere with each beat, the C- and V-waves are damped (Fig. 12). Comparison of central venous pressure and mean artificial right atrial pressure in a calf during infusion of fluids and the turning off of ventricular diastolic vacuum illustrates that a large volume artificial atrium can prevent inflow obstruction and maintain mean inflow pressures

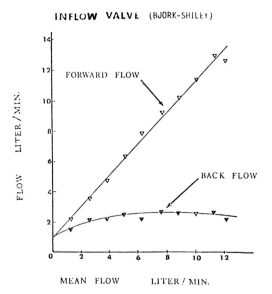

backflow of approximately 2 liters/min in the atomic energy heart at 120 b/min.

IN VIVO STUDIES.   Results of the 7 cm hemispherical ventricle indicated aortic pressures in the range of 125 to 175 mm Hg systolic pressure and 60 to 100 mm Hg diastolic pressure. Right ventricular pressures (above 100 mm Hg peak systolic) and pulmonary artery pressure (above 50 mm Hg peak systolic) were elevated from the normal. Figure 9 illustrates fluctuations in aortic and venous pressures in the pony with this ventricle. The pulse pressure gradually widened in this preparation over 24 hours of pumping. Implementation of the elliptical ventricles at lower ventricular driving pressures and larger stroke volume have produced aortic pressures in the range of 160/75 mm Hg (140/70 to 200/125 mm Hg). Mean pulmonary artery pressure has been reduced ranging from 15 to 45 mm Hg (usually around 25 mm Hg). Peak pulmonary systolic pressure has been 40 mm Hg and at times greater than 50 mm Hg. Comparison of central venous pressures between the hemispherical and elliptical heart show approximate normal values for the calf with the elliptical heart (Fig. 10). Both types of ventricles demonstrate elevated pulsatile atrial pressures many times in excess of 20 mm Hg. Figure 11 illustrates pulsatile atrial pres-

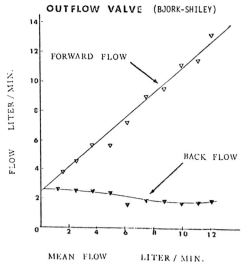

FIG. 8. Evaluation of regurgitation of the Bjork-Shiley inflow and outflow valves in the atomic energy heart on the mock circulation.

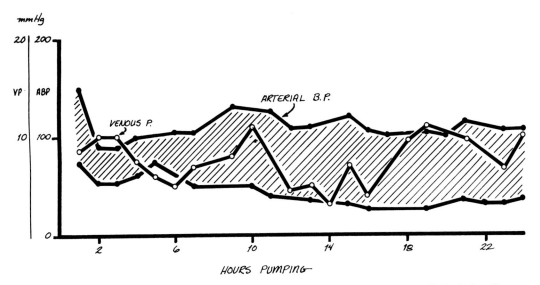

FIG. 9. Venous and aortic pressures in the adult pony after implantation of a hemispherical artificial heart. Cardiopulmonary bypass was utilized to implant the artificial heart.

close to 0 mm Hg (Fig. 13). Application of large diastolic ventricular vacuums can produce large cyclic atrial pressures below intrathoracic pressures, causing collapse of the venous inflow structures (Peters et al, 1974b) and reduce cardiac output.

BLOOD DAMAGE

IN VITRO STUDIES. Comparison of different surfaces in the 5-liter *in vitro* test system (Fig. 14) shows that a smooth surface causes the lowest hemolysis. After pumping in a calf, the

fibril surface, covered by a fibrin layer, produces approximately two times the damage of the standard; the fibril intima, and finally the dacron cloth intima produce the highest hemolysis when pumped at identical conditions for six hours. Hemolysis index (gms of free plasma hemoglobin/100 L blood pumped) is illustrated in Table 3 for the 8-cm hemispherical ventricle, the elliptical ventricle with a smooth surface, fibril surface, fibril surface after being pumped in a calf, and the atomic energy ventricle (mechanical driving waveform). The smooth surface atomic energy ventricle produces the lowest hemolysis index, followed

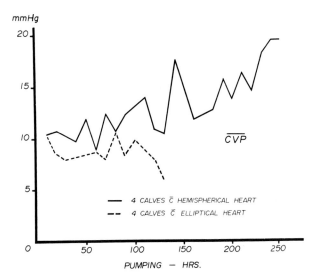

FIG. 10. Mean central venous pressure in 4 calves with an elliptical ventricle and 4 calves with a hemispherical ventricle.

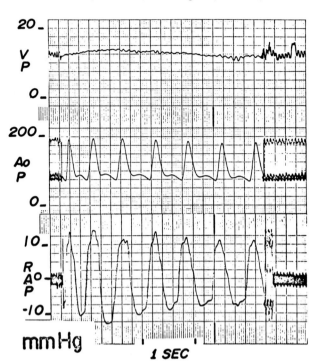

FIG. 11. Pulsatile atrial pressures in a noncompliant artificial right atrium connected to a hemispherical ventricle.

TABLE 3. *In Vitro* Blood Damage Evaluation

HEART DESCRIPTION	HEMOLYSIS INDEX	CONDITIONS OF TEST
8 cm Kwan-Gett Ventricle with Bjork-Shiley valves and smooth silicone rubber surface	0.024 ± .005 N = 12	Bovine blood at room temperature; outflow and inflow pressure = 40 mm Hg; duration of pumping = 2 hrs; 100 B/min; driving pressure = 6 psi
Jarvik elliptical ventricle with Bjork-Shiley valves and smooth silicone rubber surface	0.034 ± .01 N = 5	Bovine blood at room temperature; outflow and inflow pressure = 40 mm Hg; duration of pumping = 1 hr; 100 B/min; driving pressure = 2 psi
Jarvik elliptical ventricle with Bjork-Shiley valves and rough dacron fibril surface	0.072 ± .02 N = 5	Bovine blood at room temperature; outflow and inflow pressure = 40 mm Hg; duration of pumping = 1 hr; 100 B/min; driving pressure = 2 psi
Atomic energy ventricle with Bjork-Shiley valves and smooth silicone rubber surface	0.008 ± .003 N = 6	Bovine blood at room temperature; outflow and inflow pressure = 40 mm Hg; duration of pumping = 1 hr; 120 B/min
Jarvik elliptical ventricle with Bjork-Shiley valves and rough dacron fibril surface after having been pumped in a calf	0.009, 0.024	Bovine blood at room temperature; outflow and inflow pressure = 40 mm Hg; duration of pumping = 1 hr; driving pressure = 2 psi; 90 B/min (.009). 100 B/min (.024) after having been pumped 90 hrs in a calf

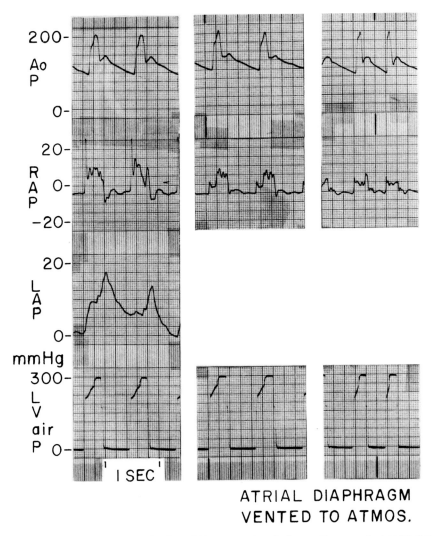

FIG. 12.   Right artificial atrium with C- and V-waves reduced after venting compliant atrial diaphragm to atmosphere with each ventricular cycle.

closely by the elliptical fibril surface ventricle after being pumped 90 hours in a calf (with a developed fibrin layer over the dacron fibrils). Figures 15 and 16 illustrate a fibril coat in a hemispherical ventricle that was pumped in a calf for 19 hours and then pumped for 24 hours on a mock circulation. Figure 15 is the 1,050 times magnification scanning photomicrograph illustrating a single fibril with loosened and fractured fibrin on the shaft. Figure 16 is a 220 times magnification scanning photomicrograph of the pumping dome in the same ventricle, illustrating the presence of many fibrils incompletely covered by fibrin.

Carter et al (1974) has demonstrated that a fibril and smooth-surfaced elliptical heart when compared to an unpumped control sack causes marked reduction in platelet retention (platelet adhesiveness). After one hour of pumping, values (for five identical experiments) included a 76.3 ± 3.6 (± standard error of the mean) platelet retention for the control sack, 42.5 ± 6.3 for the smooth ventricle and 15.0 ± 3.9 for the fibril ventricle.

IN VIVO STUDIES.   Effects of smooth and fibril surfaced hemispherical hearts on hemolysis have been previously described (Kawai et al, 1972). Figure 17 illustrates these values for free plasma hemoglobin for dacron fibril ventricles in five calves and smooth silicone rubber ventricles in four calves. These ventricles were implanted with deep hypothermia so there is no free plasma hemoglobin prior to pumping as might be measured

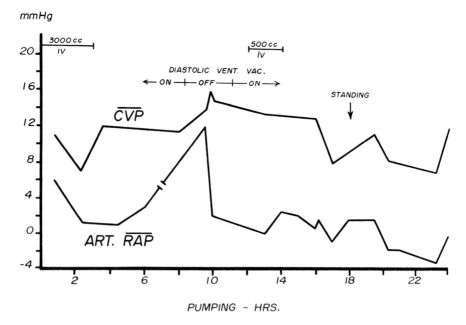

FIG. 13. Mean central venous pressure and right artificial atrial pressure in a calf with hemispherical ventricles. When the diastolic vacuum on the right ventricle is turned off, mean atrial and central venous pressure increases.

with the use of cardiopulmonary bypass. Lactic dehydrogenase (LDH) values in these experiments (control value of 612 mU/ml) range up to 828 mU/ml for the silicone rubber surface as compared to 5,470 mU/ml for the fibril surface. Present studies with the elliptical ventricles with shorter dacron fibrils demonstrate free plasma hemoglobin in the range of 10 to 25 mg percent and LDH values around 2,000 mU/ml.

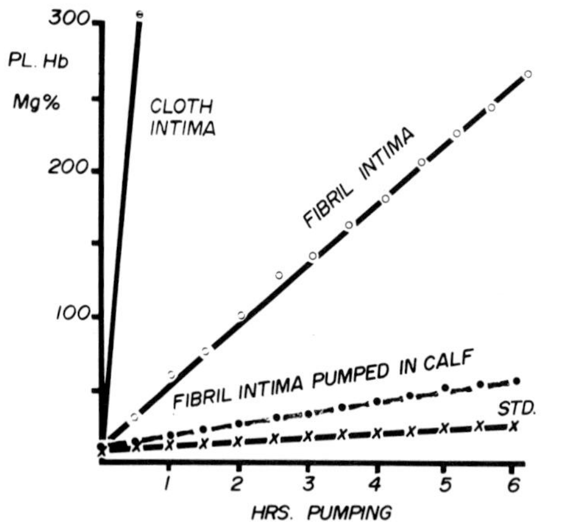

COAGULATION STUDIES. For the first five or six days of total heart pumping, a disseminated intravascular coagulation occurs. Fibrinogen levels diminish; the platelet count falls; the prothrombin time, partial thromboplastin time, and thrombin time are prolonged and the protamine sulfate paracoagulation test is positive. The platelet half-life is one-third of normal. These effects are related to the volume of blood pumped by the artificial heart and diminish as this volume is decreased from 100 to 50 to 10 percent of the total (Hershgold et al, 1972). After about six days of pumping, the intravascular coagulation becomes compensated with respect to the coagulation factors. The coagulation factors rise to normal or even supernormal levels, but fibrinogen survival measured at a time when fibrinogen levels are normal or high, is about one-third normal. The protamine-sulfate test, postive in the presence of fibrin monomer, remains positive. The rise of the coagulation parameters measured—the PT and the PTT—are within normal limits. Depending on the blood volume fraction, platelet attrition continues and is greater than compensatory platelet formation. The platelet count, in animals with total artificial hearts, first falls abruptly (both during cardiopulmonary bypass and initial pumping of the ventricles) and then continues to slowly diminish

FIG. 14. Comparison of different intima surfaces on mock circulation, utilizing a hemispherical ventricle with a smooth surface as a standard reference ventricle (see text). (8 cm Kg–BS VALVES; DR PRES = 6 psi; RATE = 100 b/min; percent systole = 35; DIAPHRAGM PRES [DIAST] = 80 mm Hg.)

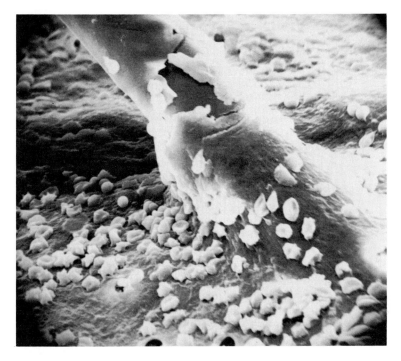

FIG. 15. Scanning photomicrograph of single fibril shaft with loosened fibrin layer. Intima had been pumped 19 hours in a calf and then 24 hours on a mock circulation. ×1500.

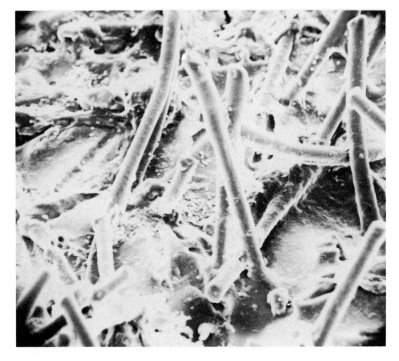

FIG. 16. Scanning photomicrograph of fibril surface of pumping dome after being pumped 19 hours in a calf and then 24 hours on a mock circulation. Protruding dacron fibrils can cause marked increase in hemolysis compared to a smooth silicone rubber surface. ×220.

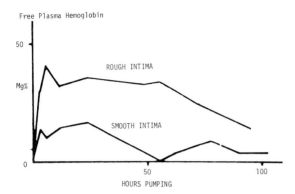

FIG. 17. Mean values of free plasma hemoglobin in 5 calves with a fibril ventricle and in 4 calves with a smooth silicone rubber surface ventricle (*in vivo* studies).

sometimes to counts one-sixth of normal. Platelet adhesiveness drastically drops and may become 0 throughout the course of an experiment. Sheetlike fibrin deposition occurs over the prosthetic surface and on valve connections (Fig. 18). The ^{51}Cr label derived from labeled autologous platelets is found at autopsy to have concentrated in the lung, liver, and spleen of the calves with artificial hearts. Compared to control calves, greater fractions of label are found in the lungs and liver (Hershgold EJ, 1974, personal communication).

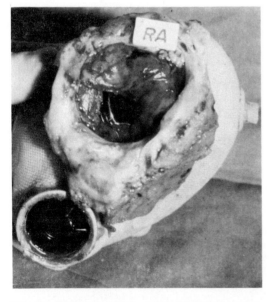

FIG. 18. Fibrin deposition almost completely occluding the inflow valve of the right ventricle (elliptical type) in a calf that survived 452 hours.

Quality of Life in Long-Surviving Calves

Calves with artificial hearts demonstrate normal alertness and respond to their surroundings. They seem to become accustomed to the intensive care environment and adapt to the noise of the pneumatic driving system, recording devices, and the many investigators entering and leaving the laboratory. At night an attempt is made to dim lighting and minimize external noise. Despite the abrupt change in life-style of a 90-day-old calf with implantation of the artificial heart and its sequellae, it has prolonged periods of unsupported respiration, alimentation, and spontaneous standing and lying in a specially designed cart. To date the physiologic effects of induced exercise have not been evaluated. Some calves, however, have succeeded in jumping out of the holding cart with great vigor and removing their ventricular drive lines.

Pathologic Effects of the Artificial Heart

A consistent finding in all calves is hepatomegaly either by physical examination after five days of pumping (Olsen D, 1974, personal communications) or at autopsy, for liver weight may exceed 3.5 times prepumping weight (normal liver weight is approximately 1.65 percent body weight) (Olsen et al, 1973). Central lobular necrosis is a common finding (Fig. 19) and has been related to the amount and time of exposure to high venous pressure. Edema of the root of the anterior mesenteric vessels and tail of the pancreas occurs and is frequently associated with ascites. Peripheral embolization occurs commonly in the lungs, kidneys, and brain. Polarized light on microscopic sections of tissues has revealed dacron fibrils that have broken away from the ventricular intima. Figure 20 illustrates one of these fibril emboli in the lung.

Mode of Termination

A review of 22 recent total heart experiments shows survivals ranging from 9 hours to 2,256 hours. Eight calves were terminated because of hemothorax, seven due to sepsis (Fig. 21 illustrates complete infection of the intimal surface of the elliptical ventricle), four because of pulmonary edema, three due to accidents, and two because of almost complete obstruction of the valves with fibrin deposition.

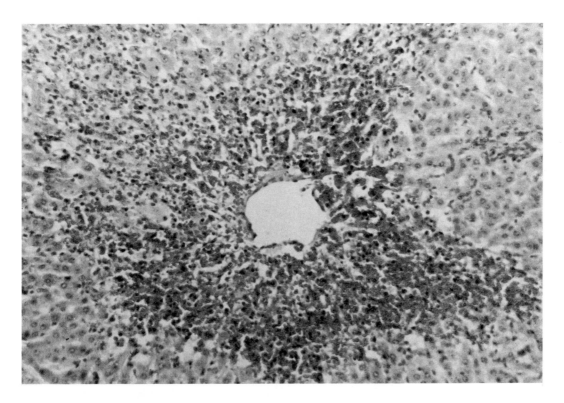

FIG. 19. Light microscopic section of liver tissue illustrating central lobular necrosis (area of central vein). This is a common finding in calves with artificial hearts.

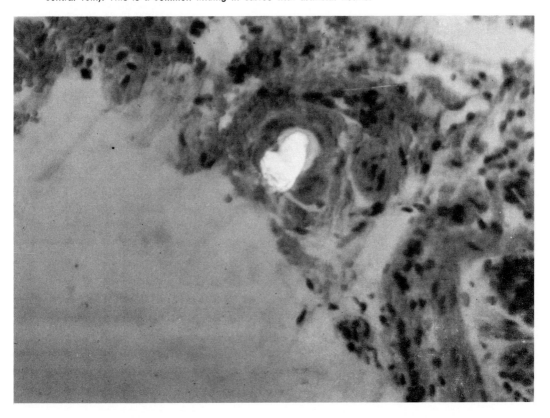

FIG. 20. Section of lung of calf pumped by a ventricle with a dacron fibril intima. Opacity in center of picture is a dacron fibril embolus. These fibrils are easily visualized with polarized light.

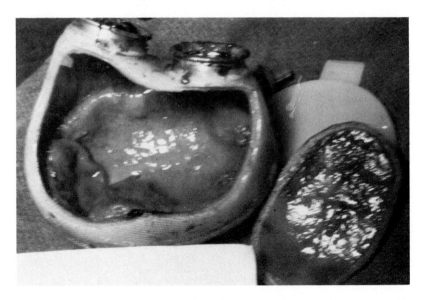

FIG. 21. Cutaway view of elliptical left ventricle after removal from a calf at autopsy. The entire fibrin-fibril intima is infected. The calf died from sepsis.

DISCUSSION

The results of artificial heart technology and implantation experiments are encouraging and provide incentive for continued research for a device that can maintain the circulation in man when failure of the natural heart occurs. Of particular interest is the prolonged survival of calves in the United States with at least four different models of artificial hearts, including one device connected to the fibrillating natural heart. Common problems to all of these devices include biocompatibility and durability. This has been manifested in continued red cell damage, evidence of embolization, or mechanical failure (tear or rupture of diaphragm). Anemia due to prosthetic valves is well documented, particularly with aortic valves (Santinga et al, 1973; Myhre, Rasmussen, 1969). Of necessity the current artificial hearts contain four prosthetic valves (except the biolized heart, which utilizes natural tricuspid valves). This may be a large factor in decreasing red cell survival and causing anemia or requiring blood transfusions in calves survivng 94 days. Since the introduction of Dacron fibril intimas with and without seeding by fetal fibroblasts (Bernhard et al 1969, 1972), there has been less evidence of embolization (Bernhard et al, 1969; Peters et al, 1973b). If surfaces are nontouching, a thin-fibrin membrane develops. Not all laboratories have been successful, however,

in preventing excessive fibrin buildup on the intima of the ventricles despite some form of anticoagulation. Fibrin deposition has been attributed mainly to the amount of flow through the device— higher flow causing less protein deposition (La-Farge et al, 1969, 1972; Bernhard et al, 1972)— and to the design of the ventricle, which may contain stasis areas (Phillips et al, 1972). The fibrin that deposits on the fibril surface converts a rough intima to a smooth surface, after which hemolysis becomes much less (Peters et al, 1973c, 1974a). The character of this surface has not been delineated for extensive periods and for cardiac outputs greater than 7 L/min. Evidence has been presented that fibrils can break off and embolize to major organs. The strength of attachment of the protein coat has not been quantified nor have the effects of changing pumping parameters (dp/dt, heart rate, percent systole) on surface integrity been reported. Smooth-surface artificial hearts ("biolized" artificial heart, silicone rubber adhesive), although demonstrating significantly less hemolysis initially (Peters et al, 1973c, 1974a), have greater evidence of embolization in the kidneys, brain, and lung (Henson et al, 1973; Peters et al, 1973b; Stanley, Kolff, 1973).

It is of great interest that hemorrhagic episodes other than early postoperative bleeding have not been a problem in long-surviving calves with artificial hearts. The main detrimental effects have been related to thromboembolic phenomena, with emboli being found in the lung, kidney, and brain at autopsy. In spite of a hypocoagulable state indicated by laboratory values, a state of compensation of coagulation exists (Hershgold et al, 1972). The preliminary evidence of an increased fraction of ^{51}Cr label in calves with artificial hearts (from autologous labeled platelets) in the lung and liver suggests that there may be reticuloendothelial system trapping of damaged platelets and also trapping of microemboli in the lungs (E. J. Hershgold, 1974, personal communication). The possible influence of hemolysis on coagulation factors and platelet function has been suggested in patients with prosthetic valves (Egeberg, 1972; Hellem, 1960, Myhre et al, 1971). Continuing hemolysis by the artificial heart and prosthetic valves could account for enhanced consumption of platelets and decrease in platelet adhesiveness.

Hemodynamically progressive increases in filling pressures have been reported (Peters et al, 1973d; Akutsu, 1973, personal communication) with the artificial heart. This has not been a problem with bypass of the natural heart—the natural atria and ventricles, providing both a reservoir and booster pumps (atria and/or ventricles) for filling of the prosthetic ventricle (Bernhard, 1972; C. G. LaFarge, 1973, personal communication). Part of the picture of increasing filling pressures on the right side of the heart and symptoms of artificial right heart failure have been ascribed to asynchronous atrial-ventricular contractions (remnant natural atria continue to contract, despite removal of coronary blood supply) (Peters et al, 1971, 1973d), inflow obstruction from compression of atria and great veins (Nosé et al, 1966; Peters et al, 1973d) increased fibrin deposition of the inflow valves (Jarvik et al, 1974), small atrial to ventricular stroke volume ratio (Brighton et al, 1973; Urzua, 1974, personal communication), and valvular regurgitation (Peters et al, 1972d, 1973c, 1974).

Implementation of better valves with less regurgitation (possibility of active valves), active artificial atria, or larger atrial ventricular stroke volume ratio may overcome these problems. A better-fitting ventricle or prosthetic atrium, which does not compress the inflow area, has demonstrated significant reduction of mean ventricular inflow pressures. Reduction of pulsatile atrial waves (C- and V-waves) may further improve inflow characteristics and increase cardiac output at lower inflow pressures. The slopes of the cardiac output curves of all prosthetic ventricles are less than the natural heart. However, this may not be an important factor for total circulatory maintenance. The interaction of the prosthetic pumping

parameters and their long-term effects on the physiologic system are still a matter for continued basic research (Kennedy et al, 1973). Most prosthetic ventricles are operated at fixed driving parameters (pressures, rate, percent systole). The effects of changing rates and/or stroke volume as a function of servo-feedback inputs other than filling pressure and intrinsic regulation of cardiac output, which is limited by the design (ie, diaphragm stiffness and maximum filling position) have not been investigated. One of the authors (JP, 1971) has suggested that an active ventricular function residual volume may be a useful addition to prosthetic ventricular function (Moulopoulos et al, 1973). This could be easily evaluated with a large-volume, sack-type artificial ventricle and hydraulic driving system.

The incidence of pulmonary arterial hypertension has been reduced by the better-fitting elliptical ventricle. However, this problem still occurs and needs to be studied in terms of optimum right ventricular driving pressure and dp/dt with an adequate cardiac output (Henson et al, 1973). The lung is known to be sensitive to numerous vasoactive substances, particularly serotonin, which could be continually released from damaged platelets. The lung is also sensitive to hemolyzed red cells and adenosine diphosphate, which has been demonstrated in the calf to cause increases in pulmonary artery pressure (Silove, 1971).

The quality of life in calves with total artificial hearts, despite the problems discussed, is surprisingly good. This is especially significant since these calves are approximately 90 days old and can be susceptible to pulmonary complications and viral and bacterial infections. If the use of the pony for artificial heart research can be improved in terms of implantation and postoperative management, the results may better approximate those of man. The pony is an adult animal and will not outgrow the artificial heart. The pony also has lungs similar to man (McLaughlin et al, 1961; Garner et al, 1971). Development of better percutaneous lead systems and implantable power sources (Backman et al, 1973) should decrease infectious complications that are now seen with air drive lines and pressure lines that exist from the thorax. The application of indirect methods to determine hemodynamic events by prosthetic hearts will also decrease the complications due to infection. It is still very important to know ventricular output under a variety of physiologic conditions. Until new flow-measurement devices are developed, conventional methods such as dye dilution (mean flow), electromagnetic, and ultrasonic flowmeters should be employed routinely, particularly for fixed driving parameter devices. Right and left ventricular cycle by cycle stroke output can ensure pulmonary and systemic circulatory matching and provide valuable physiologic information when cardiovascular changes occur.

The advances and innovative approach to total circulatory support in the last three years is encouraging. Survivals of calves approximating one month suggest that this technology could be applied in certain cases in man for short-term assist of the natural heart. A patient unable to be taken off cardiopulmonary bypass may, with enough time (eg, to overcome effects of anesthesia, myocardial ischemia), by prosthetic cardiac assist regain natural heart function. History has demonstrated the effectiveness of the artificial kidney for a variety of chronic and acute renal diseases. The artificial lung is now being used for reversible pulmonary (trauma, pneumonia) insufficiency (Hill et al, 1973). Perhaps the time has come to apply circulatory support devices in man with greater vigor.

References

Backman DK, Sandquist GM, Kolff WJ: Biomedical Engineering Support. Annual Report AT(11-1)–2155, July 15, 1972 to August 14, 1973

Bernhard WF, Husain M, George JB, Curtis GW: Fetal fibroblasts as a substratum for pseudoendothelial development on prosthetic surfaces. Surgery 66:284, 1969

Bernhard WF, LaFarge CG, Bornhorst WJ: Development of a bilateral circulatory support system. Annual Technological Progress Report, Contract No. 69-2182, Medical Devices Applications Program, National Heart and Lung Institute, June 1970–June 1972

Brighton JA, Wade CA, Pierce WS, Phillips WM, O'Bannon W: Effects of atrial volume on the performance of a sack-type artificial heart. Trans Am Soc Artif Intern Organs 19:567–72, 1973

Carter C, Peters J, Federer D, Hershgold EJ: Artificial heart effect on platelet function—a comparative in vitro study. Clin Res 22:177A, 1974

Cooper T, Harmison LT: Cardiopulmonary Support Systems: problems in clinical application. Transplantation Proceedings 3:1497–1501, 1971

Donovan FM: Thermodynamic studies of the artificial heart using a volume sensing mock circulation. Biomedical Engineering Society Proceedings, April 1972

Foote JL: Non-invasive measurement of inflow and outflow pressures in the artificial heart. 26 Annual Conf on Engineering in Medicine and Biology, Proceedings 15:22, 1973

Foote JL, Greenhalgh SR, Peters JL: In vitro artificial heart evaluation. 26 Annual Conf on Engineering in Medicine and Biology 15:27, 1973

Garner HE, Rosborough J, Amend J, Hoff HE: The grade pony as a new laboratory model in cardiopulmonary physiology. Cardiovascular Research Center Bulletin 9:91–103, 1971

Greenhalgh SR, Peters JL, Foote JL: Cooperative, comparative function testing of artificial hearts. To be presented, Association for Advancement of Medical Instrumentation, 9th Annual Meeting, April 1974

Hastings FW, Harmison LT: Artificial Heart Program Conference, Proceedings, 1,129 pages, June 1969

Hellem AJ: Platelet adhesiveness in Von Willebrand's disease. A study with a new modification of the glass bead filter method. Scand J Haematol 7:374, 1970

Henson E, Takano H, Takagi H, et al: Alterations in the lungs of sheep after implantation of the Akutsu total artificial heart, J Thorac Cardiovasc Surg 65:629–34, 1973

Henson E, Takagi H, Takano H, et al: Structural alterations in calves implanted with the Akutsu total artificial heart. J Thorac Cardiovasc Surg 66:99–104, 1973

Hershgold EJ, Kwan-Gett CS, Kawai J, Rowley K: Hemostasis, coagulation and the total artificial heart. Trans Am Soc Artif Intern Organs 18:181–84, 1972

Hill JD, et al: Post-graduate symposium, "Mechanical cardiorespiratory support/artificial heart." American Heart Association 27th Annual Meeting, November 1973

Jarvik R: Discussion on manuscript #90. Trans Am Soc Artif Intern Organs 19:588, 1973

Jarvik R, Oster H, Olsen D, Volder J, Stanley T: Design of an elliptical ventricle and results of 26 implantations in calves. Am Soc Artif Intern Organs Abstracts Vol 3, 20th Annual Meeting, 1974

Johnson SC, Kawai J, Kolff WJ: The significance of proper positioning of the artificial heart as revealed by a new method of autopsy. Submitted for publication

Kawai J, Peters J. Donovan F, et al: Implantation of a total artificial heart in calves under hypothermia with ten-day survival. J Thorac Cardiovasc Surg 64:45–60, 1972

Kawai J, Peters JL, Donovan FM, et al: Successful use of deep hypothermia for implantation of the artificial heart in calves. Circ Suppl II, vols 42 and 44, no 695, 184, 1971

Kennedy JH, DeBakey ME, Akers WW, et al: Progress toward an orthotopic cardiac prosthesis. Biomat Med Dev Art Org, 1:3–56, 1973

Kessler TR, Foote JL, Andrade JD, Kolff WJ: Methods to construct artificial organs. Trans Am Soc Artif Intern Organs 17:36–40, 1971

Kwan-Gett CS, Backman DK, Donovan FM, et al: Artificial heart with hemispherical ventricles II and disseminated intravascular coagulation. Trans Am Soc Artif Intern Organs 17:474–80, 1971

Kwan-Gett CS, Wu Y, Collan R, Jacobsen S, Kolff WJ: Total replacement artificial heart and driving system with inherent regulation of cardiac output. Trans Am Soc Artif Intern Organs 15:245–50, 1969

Kwan-Gett CS, Zwart HHJ, Kralios AC, et al: A prosthetic heart with hemispherical ventricles designed for lower hemolytic action. Trans Am Soc Artif Intern Organs 16:409–15, 1970

LaFarge CG, Bernhard WF, Robinson TC: A physiologic evaluation of the Baylor left ventricular bypass. Artificial Heart Program Conf Proceedings, 619–35, June 1969

LaFarge CG, Carr JC, Coleman SJ, Bernhard WF: Hemodynamic Studies during prolonged mechanical circulatory support. Trans Am Soc Artif Intern Organs 18:186–93, 1972

Lawson JH, Olsen DB: Postoperative care of calves with total artificial hearts. Am Soc Artif Intern Organs Abstracts vol 3, 20th Annual Meeting, 1974

McLaughlin RF, Tyler WS, Canada RO: A study of the subgross pulmonary anatomy of various mammals. Am J Anat 108:149, 1961

Moulopoulos S, Jarvik R, Kolff WJ: Stage II problems on the project of the artificial heart: J Thorac Cardiovasc Surg 66:662, 1973

Myhre E, Hellem AJ, Storkmorken H: Intravascular hemolysis, platelet consumption and platelet adhesiveness in patients with prosthetic heart valves. Scand J Thorac Cardiovasc Surg 5:13–15, 1971

Myhre E, Rasmussen K: Mechanical hemolysis in aortic valvular disease and aortic ball-valve prosthesis. Acta Med Scand 186:543–47, 1969

Nosé Y: Advances in biomedical engineering and medical physics. Cardiac Engineering, vol 3, New York, Interscience Publisher, John Wiley and Sons, 1970, 384 pages

Nosé Y, Sarin BL, Klain M, et al: Elimination of some problems encountered in total replacement of the heart with an intrathoracic mechanical pump: venous return. Trans Am Soc Artif Intern Organs 12:301–11, 1966

Olsen D, Van Kampen K, Volder J, Kolff WJ: Pulmonary hepatic and renal pathology associated with an artificial heart. Trans Am Soc Artif Intern Organs 19:578–82, 1973

Oster H, Olsen DB, Jarvik R, et al: Eighteen days survival with a Jarvik type of artificial heart. Surgery 77:113, 1975

Peters JL, Donovan FM, Backman DK, Kessler TR, Kolff WJ: Effects of the atria on the function of the artificial heart. 24th Annual Conference on Engineering in Medicine and Biology, Proceedings 13:234, 1971

Peters JL, Donovan F, Kawai J, Kolff WJ: An adult animal model for artificial heart research. Chest 62:374, 1972a

Peters JL, Donovan FM, Kawai J, et al: Preconditioning, implantation, and postoperative care of the artificial heart research calf. National Conference on Research Animals in Medicine, Proceedings, 1972b, pp 399–416

Peters JL, Imlay TF, Hess TO: The preconditioned Holstein calf for cardiovascular research. 23d Annual Session, American Association for Laboratory Animal Science, 1972c

Peters JL, Sandquist GM, Donovan FM, Kolff WJ: Effect of an active valve on the artificial heart. 3d Annual Meeting Biomedical Engineering Society, Abstract #43, 1972d

Peters JL, Donovan FM, Kawai J: Consequences of the diaphragm driven artificial heart—animal implantation and mock circulation studies. Chest 63:589–97, 1973a

Peters JL, Hess TO, Leach CS, et al: Hemic and spirometric profiles in calves used for cardiovascular research. Am J Vet Res 34: 1595–97, 1973b

Peters JL, Volder J, Kessler TR, et al: Use of the artificial heart for basic cardiovascular research. Chest 67:199–206, 1973c

Peters JL, Wood J, Kawai J, et al: Elimination of inflow obstruction to the artificial heart with artificial atria. Biomedical Engineering Society Proceedings 3:10, 1973d

Peters JL, Greenhalgh SR, Carter C, et al: In vitro and in vivo studies of blood damage by prosthetic ventricles. Presented—Engineering Studies of Blood Trauma, 77th National American Institute of Chemical Engineers, June 1974a

Peters JL, Greenhalgh SR, Foote JL, et al: Function, blood damage and dimensions of artificial hearts in the USA. Am Soc Artif Intern Organs Abstracts, vol 3, 20th Annual Meeting, 1974b

Phillips WM, Brighton JA, Pierce WS: Artificial heart evaluation using flow visualization techniques. Trans Am Soc Artif Intern Organs 18:194–201, 1972

Santinga JT, Kirsh MM, Batsakis JT: Hemolysis in different series of the Starr-Edwards aortic-valve prostheses. Chest 63:905–8, 1973

Silove ED: Effects of haemolysed blood and adenosine diphosphate on the pulmonary vascular resistance in calves. Cardiovasc Res 5:313–18, 1971

Smith L, Backman DK, Sandquist G, Kolff WJ: Development on the Implantation of a total nuclear-powered artificial heart system. Am Soc Artif Intern Organs 20:732–36, 1974

Stanley TH, Kolff WJ: The effects of smooth and Dacron lined Silastic artificial hearts on survival, blood cell destruction, serum bilirubin and embolization. Am Soc Artif Intern Organs Abstracts vol 2, 1973

The Totally Implantable Artificial Heart—Economic, Ethical, Legal, Medical, Psychiatric and Social Implications. Report by Artificial Heart Assessment Panel, Nat'l Heart and Lung Inst, June 1973

Volder J, Kwan-Gett C, Nielsen M, Kolff WJ, Hershgold EJ: In vivo testing of thrombogenesis of materials. Trans Am Soc Artif Intern Organs 29:210–12, 1973

121

AN ABDOMINAL LEFT VENTRICULAR ASSIST DEVICE (ALVAD): ACUTE AND CHRONIC EFFECTS ON LEFT VENTRICULAR MECHANICS

Stephen R. Igo, David A. Hughes, Joseph J. Migliore, Benedict D. T. Daly, and John C. Norman

Mechanical ventricular assistance has been proposed as a method of supporting the failing heart.[9] Our laboratories have concentrated on the design, development, and *in vivo* testing of an implantable, intraabdominal device (ALVAD) capable of temporarily supporting the left ventricle for periods of hours to days with subsequent transabdominal removal.[29]

Two major areas of experimental investigation have been undertaken. In acute canine experiments we have evaluated the hemodynamic effectiveness of the ALVAD in maintaining the circulation while decreasing left ventricular work. These experiments also serve to delineate the interaction of various biologic and mechanical variables for optimal device performance. Chronic experiments in calves have demonstrated the mechanical reliability and long-term effects of ALVAD assistance.

METHODS

Device Description and Implantation

The assist device (Fig. 1) is a single-chambered, pneumatically driven pump with a stroke volume of 65 ml (canine experiments) or 100 ml (bovine experiments). Blood is accepted from the apex of the left ventricle and ejected into the abdominal aorta.[26] Inlet and outlet caged

Silastic disc valves impart unidirectional flow. All blood-contacting surfaces of the pump, with the exception of the valve discs and dacron outlet graft, are flocked with a layer of polyester fibrils, 1 mil in diameter and approximately 10 mils in length. The main housing of the pump is implanted abdominally with the inlet tube tranversing the diaphragm to reach the left ventricular apex. The control system [7] is designed to accept an R-wave trigger from the electrocardiogram for synchronous operation, or operate at a fixed rate asynchronously. The drive pressure, systolic duration, vacuum level, synchronized ECG delay, and asynchronous rate are adjustable.

Implantation of the ALVAD for the acute canine experiments was done via a median sternotomy with a midline abdominal extension. Chronic experiments were performed on three- to six-month-old Hereford calves. For these animals, a left thoracotomy and left transverse celiotomy was utilized.

The woven dacron outflow graft is sutured end-to-side to the abdominal aorta below the renal arteries. The pumping chamber, filled with saline, is placed in the abdomen with the inflow tube transversing the diaphragm. For the chronic calf experiments, the pneumatic drive line is brought out of the abdomen through a separate small incision.

A Silastic attachment ring with an incorporated Teflon felt sewing ring is sutured to the apex of the left ventricle. A small incision is made in the center of the left ventricular apex, and a Foley retention catheter is passed into the ventricle, using a central stylet. After inflating the catheter balloon, a circular knife is passed over

Supported in part by USPHS Grant HL-14294-03 and Contract NO1-HL-73-2946.

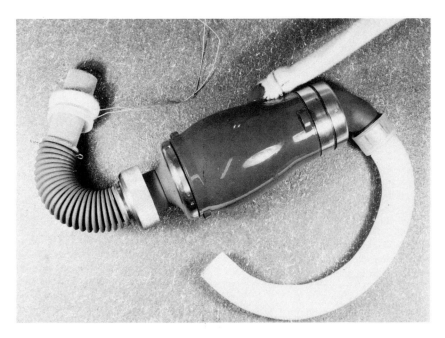

FIG. 1. View of abdominal left ventricular assist device (ALVAD).

the catheter and a full thickness cylindrical core of apical myocardium is excised. Under a carbon dioxide atmosphere, the catheter balloon is quickly deflated and the inlet tube of the pump is rapidly passed through the sewing ring into the left ventricle. A purse-string suture around the Silastic cuff of the sewing ring provides a tight seal and anchor for the inlet tube.

Data Acquisition (Acute Canine Experiments)

The acute effects of ALVAD pumping on ventricular function have been studied in both the nonischemic canine heart and during periods of induced myocardial ischemic injury.

In the group of animals with nonischemic hearts measurements of myocardial blood flow and oxygen consumption [23,24] were obtained by placing a short cannula in the coronary sinus. Coronary venous effluent was collected in a graduated cylinder over measured periods of time and returned to the systemic circulation. Simultaneous blood gas determinations were performed on coronary sinus and systemic arterial samples. Aortic pressure was measured via a polyethylene catheter passed into the thoracic aorta from the right carotid artery. Left ventricular pressures were measured via a short polyethylene catheter inserted through the anterior wall of the left ventricle. Pump driveline

pressure was measured from a side arm on the pneumatic drive line. Cardiac output [11] was measured by the indicator dilution method. For these measurements, 0.625 mg of indocyanine green dye was injected into the right atrium and blood was withdrawn from the main pulmonary artery through a Gilson densitometer.

In the group of animals with induced myocardial ischemic injury [17] the left anterior descending coronary artery was dissected distal to the first main branch. Umbilical tape was passed around the vessel to allow intermittent occlusion. Cardiac output was measured by means of a sine wave electromagnetic flow probe placed around the main pulmonary artery. The probe was calibrated in vivo by measuring simultaneously cardiac outputs by the indicator dilution method. A mercury-in-Silastic segment length gauge was sutured transversely onto the anterior surface of the left ventricle in the area to be rendered ischemic. The first derivatives of left ventricular pressure (dP/dt) and segment length (dL/dt) were obtained by means of electronic differentiators.

At the conclusion of each experiment, the heart was rapidly removed and a passive pressure-volume curve [32] of the left ventricle was determined with the pump inlet tube capped. End-diastolic volumes throughout each experiment were determined from the left ventricular end-diastolic pressure and postmortem pressure-volume curve.

Internal ventricular radius (r_1) was obtained from the left ventricular volume, assuming a spherical ventricular cavity, by the formula:

$$V = 4/3 \, \pi \, r_1^3$$

Mean myocardial wall tension was calculated from the formula:

$$T = \frac{Pr_1}{2h}$$

where P = left ventricular pressure, r_1 = internal ventricular radius, and h = instantaneous ventricular wall thickness.[32] Internal radius was calculated by subtracting the ejected volume from the end-diastolic volume. Wall thickness was calculated from r_1 and the instantaneous changes in external radius were derived from muscle segment length recordings.

The Maxwell-Hill two-component model of muscular contraction [16,36] was used to derive contractile element velocity (Vce) with the formula:

$$Vce = dl/dt + dc/dt$$

where dl/dt = the rate of lengthening of the series elastic component and dc/dt = the directly measured velocity of muscle shortening. In these experiments, Vce was expressed as a mean midwall velocity [17] with the formula:

$$Vce = \frac{dP/dt}{17.7(P) + 0.4718 \, dc/dt}$$

where dP/dt = the first derivative of left ventricular pressure, P = left ventricular pressure, and dc/dt = the directly measured first derivative of segment length divided by instantaneous segment length. Tension and velocity, during periods of ischemia, were calculated by a modification of the method of Hood.[16,17]

The pressure-time product was calculated from the mean ventricular pressure during contraction multiplied by the duration of systolic ejection. Stroke work was measured as mean ventricular pressure multiplied by the stroke volume. The ejection fraction was calculated as stroke volume divided by the end-diastolic volume.

Data Acquisition (Chronic Bovine Experiments)

The chronic hemodynamic effects of ALVAD pumping have been evaluated with cardiac catheterization and cineangiographic techniques two to four weeks following implantation. Left ventricular, central aortic, central venous, right ventricular, pulmonary artery, and pulmonary artery wedge pressures were measured via woven dacron cardiac catheters passed from the left carotid artery and external jugular vein. Left ventricular dP/dt, stroke work, ejection fraction, and pressure time product were calculated. The left ventricular end-diastolic, end-systolic, and stroke volumes were calculated from cineangiographic frames.

RESULTS

Acute Canine Experiments

Hemodynamic measurements obtained before and during left ventricular assist pumping in nonischemic canine hearts were compared (Table 1). When ALVAD pumping was instituted, the

TABLE 1. Effects of Abdominal Left Ventricular Assist Device Pumping on the Nonischemic Heart (N: 8)

	CONTROL	P VALUE	ALVAD ASSIST
Systolic aortic pressure (mm Hg)	93 ± 14.2	<0.01	69 ± 10.1
Diastolic aortic pressure (mm Hg)	70 ± 11.7	<0.01	104 ± 14.2
Peak left ventricular pressure (mm Hg)	93 ± 15.1	<0.01	16 ± 10.6
LV End Diastolic Pressure (mm Hg)	3.0 ± 0.7	<0.01	1.6 ± 0.3
Cardiac Output (L/min)	2.2 ± 1.2	NS	2.2 ± 1.1
Coronary blood flow (ml/min/100 gm)	26.8 ± 7.0	NS	21.0 ± 6.2
ΔA-V O_2 (ml%)	11.2 ± 2.5	<0.05	8.3 ± 3.0
Myocardial oxygen consumption (ml/min/100 gm)	2.83 ± 0.44	<0.01	1.61 ± 0.25
Max dP/dt (mm Hg/sec)	1491 ± 453	<0.01	804 ± 292
Pressure time product (mm Hg sec/B)	17.1 ± 3.2	<0.01	2.8 ± 1.0

Note: Mean values (± SD of mean) for control versus ALVAD assist states. Statistical significance was calculated by Student's t-test for paired differences.

aortic systolic pressure was phase shifted into diastole and increased an average of 12 percent (P < 0.01). Peak left ventricular pressure, pressure-time product, left ventricular end-diastolic pressure, and maximum left ventricular dP/dt showed measured reductions of 83, 84, 47, and 46 percent (P < 0.01), respectively, during ALVAD assist. Myocardial oxygen consumption was reduced 43 percent (P < 0.01). The diastolic aortic pressure increased 49 percent (P < 0.01). Myocardial oxygen extraction was reduced 26 percent (P < 0.05). Coronary blood flow and cardiac output were not significantly changed during ALVAD assist.

Hemodynamic measurements obtained before (control), during coronary occlusion and during occlusion with left ventricular assist were compared (Table 2).

Acute occlusion of the left anterior descending coronary artery resulted in the appearance of a cyanotic, dyskinetic area of muscle over the anteroapical surface of the left ventricle. This response was reflected by an increased degree of systolic expansion recorded by the muscle segment length gauge during isovolumic ventricular contraction (Fig. 2).

With the onset of induced segmental myocardial ischemia, the left ventricular end-diastolic pressure, end-systolic volume, and end-diastolic volume increased 57, 51, and 21 percent, respectively, (P < 0.01). Maximum left ventricular dP/dt, ejection fraction, and stroke work showed measured reductions of 20, 26, and 27 percent (P < 0.01), respectively. Diastolic aortic pressure and stroke volume decreased four and 16 percent (P < 0.05), respectively. The heart rate increased

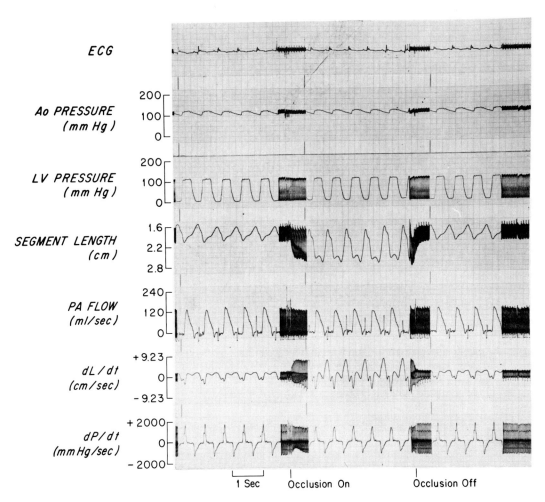

FIG. 2. Occlusion of left anterior descending coronary artery in a dog. Note fall in left ventricular dP/dt. Segment length gauge shows increased systolic expansion. Following release of occlusion, all values rapidly return to normal.

TABLE 2. Effects of Abdominal Left Ventricular Assist Device Pumping during Induced Myocardial Ischemia (N: 10)

	CONTROL	P-VALUE	OCCLUSION	P-VALUE	OCCLUSION + ALVAD
Heart rate (B/min)	119 ± 3.3	<0.05	122 ± 3.8	NS	121 ± 3.9
LV end-diastolic pressure (mm Hg)	6.18 ± 1.47	<0.01	9.71 ± 1.98	<0.01	4.05 ± 1.51
Stroke volume (ml/B)	24.1 ± 4.5	<0.05	20.2 ± 2.1	<0.01	24.9 ± 4.6
End-diastolic volume (ml)	50.5 ± 4.1	<0.01	61.0 ± 2.7	<0.01	37.0 ± 6.2
End-systolic volume (ml)	26.5 ± 3.0	<0.01	40.0 ± 2.2	<0.01	12.5 ± 3.0
Ejection fraction	0.47 ± 0.04	<0.01	0.35 ± 0.03	<0.01	0.62 ± 0.08
Cardiac output (L/min)	2.81 ± 0.55	NS	2.48 ± 0.33	<0.05	3.01 ± 0.59
Mean aortic pressure (mm Hg)	112 ± 5.6	NS	108 ± 5.0	NS	107 ± 6.8
Diastolic aortic pressure (mm Hg)	106 ± 4.3	<0.05	102 ± 4.6	<0.01	140 ± 5.2
Max dP/dt (mm Hg/sec)	1,750 ± 193	<0.01	1,400 ± 214	<0.01	300 ± 60
Peak tension (gm/cm²)	181 ± 4.9	NS	179 ± 5.8	<0.01	36 ± 4.1
Stroke work (gm m/B)	31.5 ± 2.7	<0.01	23.0 ± 1.6	<0.01	5.04 ± 0.6
Pressure-time product (mm Hg sec/B)	19.8 ± 0.8	NS	19.5 ± 0.9	<0.01	3.2 ± 0.8

Note: Mean values (±SD of mean) for control versus occlusion and occlusion versus occlusion + ALVAD states. Statistical significance was calculated by Student's t-test for paired differences.

3 percent ($P < 0.05$) during acute occlusion. Cardiac output, mean aortic pressure, pressure-time product, and peak developed ventricular tension were not significantly changed during the period following acute occlusion.

With the institution of left ventricular assist device pumping following induced segmental ischemia (Fig. 3), left ventricular end-diastolic pressure, end-diastolic volume, end-systolic volume, maximum left ventricular dP/dt, and stroke work were significantly reduced ($P < 0.01$). The pressure-time product and peak developed tension decreased 84 and 80 percent ($P < 0.01$), respectively. Stroke volume, diastolic aortic pressure, and ejection fraction increased 23, 37, and 77 percent ($P < 0.01$), respectively. Cardiac output increased 21 percent ($P < 0.05$). Heart rate and mean aortic pressure were not significantly altered from the acute occlusion state.

The instantaneous relations between segmental contractile element velocity (Vce) and developed ventricular tension were compared (Fig. 4). During the control state, Vce reached its peak approximately 40 msec after the onset of contraction. With occlusion, the Vce curve rose less sharply, the peak was lower and the entire curve was depressed below control determinations. This depression was reflected by a lower dP/dt/17.7 (P) ratio and larger negative dc/dt (Fig. 2). With ALVAD pumping during occlusion, the Vce curve rose sharply, and the peak increased toward control levels. This resulted in a 46 percent increase in peak Vce above the occlusion state. Systolic expansion of recorded muscle segment length was also reduced during ALVAD pumping (Fig. 3).

Chronic Bovine Experiments

In a recent series of 15 calves undergoing ALVAD implantation, the mean survival time was 41 days; the longest survival was 65 days. Increased survival time is attributed to refinements in anesthetic, operative, and postoperative management.[27,31]

The hemodynamic effects of ALVAD pumping in calves two to four weeks following implantation were compared (Table 3). With the initiation of ALVAD pumping, the mean aortic pressure was increased an average of 9 percent ($P < 0.01$). Left ventricular stroke work, maximum left ventricular dP/dt, and peak left ventricular pressure showed reductions of 69, 54, and 49 percent ($P < 0.01$), respectively. Left ventricular ejection fraction was increased 20 percent ($P < 0.01$); end-systolic volume was reduced 54 percent ($P < 0.05$). Left ventricular end-diastolic pressure, end-diastolic volume, stroke volume, and cardiac output were not significantly changed during ALVAD assist.

Cineangiographic analysis demonstrated that the cardiac output could be totally delivered by the ALVAD with retrograde filling of the ascending aorta and antegrade filling of the abdominal aorta (Fig. 5 to 7).

A representative tracing during ALVAD pumping is illustrated in Figure 8. During ALVAD pumping aortic pressure is phase-shifted into diastole and increased 30 percent. Heart rate, maximum left ventricular dP/dt, and peak left ventricular pressure are reduced 14, 65, and 84

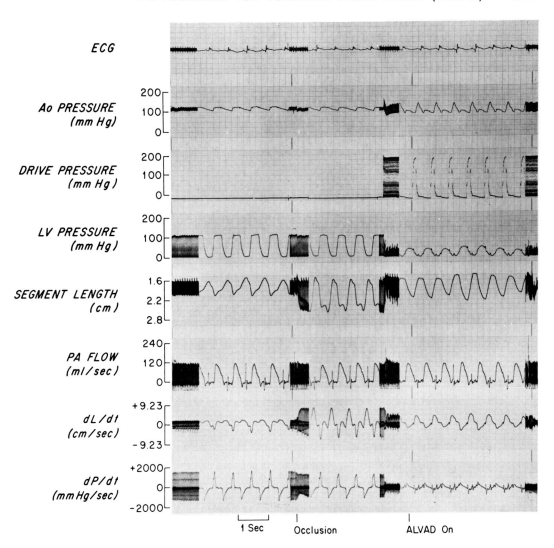

FIG. 3. Effects of ALVAD pumping during acute coronary occlusion. With ALVAD pumping, left ventricular pressure and dP/dt are reduced while peak systolic aortic pressure is phase-shifted into diastole and increased. Paradoxical systolic expansion of the ischemic muscle segment is also reduced during ALVAD assist.

TABLE 3. Chronic Effects of Abdominal Left Ventricular Assist Device Pumping in Calves

	CONTROL	P-VALUE	ALVAD ASSIST
Peak left ventricular pressure (mm Hg)	155 ± 7	<0.01	79 ± 2
LV end-diastolic pressure (mm Hg)	12.5 ± 3.5	NS	7.5 ± 3.5
Mean arterial pressure (mm Hg)	125 ± 2	<0.01	136 ± 1
Max dP/dt (mm Hg/sec)	1,950 ± 71	<0.01	900 ± 73
Stroke work (gm m/B)	208 ± 8	<0.01	65 ± 7
End-diastolic volume (ml)	150 ± 24	NS	135 ± 30
End-systolic volume (ml)	46 ± 8	<0.05	21 ± 3
Stroke volume (ml/B)	104 ± 23	NS	114 ± 38
Cardiac output (L/min)	6.72 ± 2.1	NS	6.74 ± 1.0
Ejection fraction	0.70 ± 0.01	<0.01	0.84 ± 0.01

Mean values (± SD of mean) for control versus ALVAD assist states. Statistical significance was calculated by Student's t-test for paired differences.

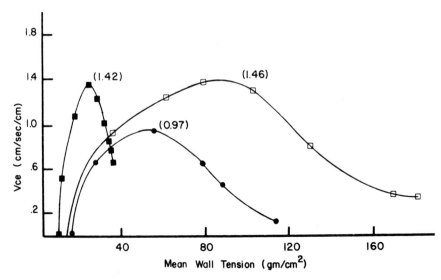

FIG. 4. Tension-velocity relationships. Following occlusion, peak V_{ce} was significantly depressed from control. With ALVAD pumping, the V_{ce} curve rises sharply with the peak velocity, increasing to control levels. Numbers in parentheses show peak V_{ce} values. Control ($\square$); ischemia ($\bullet$); ischemia and ALVAD ($\blacksquare$).

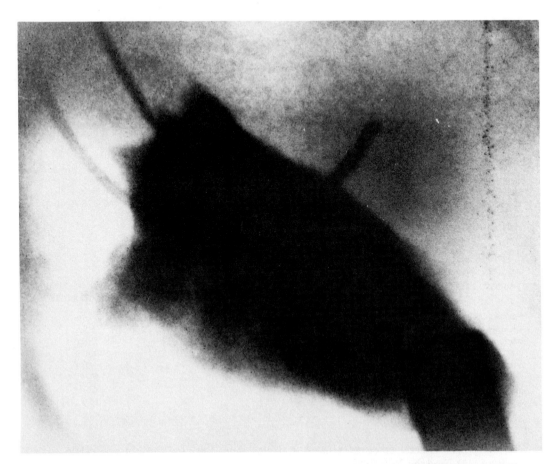

FIG. 5.   Bovine cineangiography; ventriculogram of end-diastole (ALVAD on).

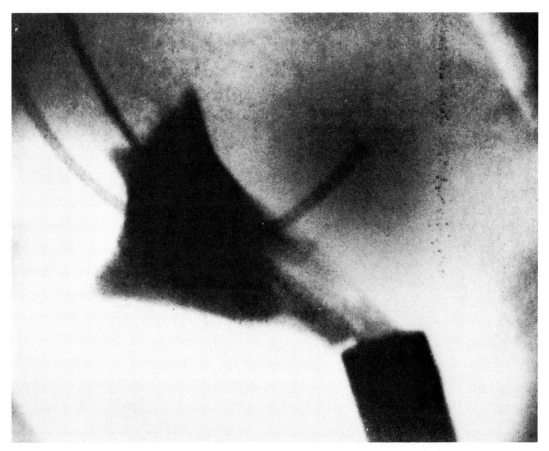

FIG. 6.   Bovine cineangiography: ventriculogram of end-systole. Aortic valve is closed; all flow is ejected into the ALVAD (ALVAD on).

percent, respectively. Right ventricular stroke volume and cardiac output are increased 21 and 4 percent, respectively.

ALVAD Removal and Effects of Retained Inflow Tubes

The abdominal configuration of the ALVAD facilitates its surgical removal; the thoracic incision need not be reopened. Studies were designed to document the safety of ALVAD removal and evaluate the effects of ALVAD inlet tube retention on hemodynamic function.

Two experimental groups were used. In the first group of three calves undergoing capped inlet tube implantation, two were sacrificed at two and 280 days postoperatively. The third died 49 days postoperatively during cardiac catheterization. In the second group of two animals, an ALVAD was implanted. Following seven and six days of ALVAD pumping, these calves were returned to the operating room, and the ALVAD was removed

through the previously made celiotomy incision. The inlet tubes were capped, and the outflow grafts were divided and oversewn. These calves have undergone cardiac catheterization 77 and 32 days post-ALVAD removal (Table 4). Both calves are alive and well at 213 and 123 days.

At the time of cardiac catheterization, the ejection fractions and cardiac outputs were within

TABLE 4. Chronic Hemodynamic Effects of Retained ALVAD Inflow Tubes

Peak left ventricular pressure (mm Hg)	163 ± 18
LV end-diastolic pressure (mm Hg)	13 ± 3.5
Mean arterial pressure (mm Hg)	133 ± 22
Max dP/dt (mm Hg/sec)	1,150 ± 71
Stroke work (gm m/B)	256 ± 16
End-diastolic volume (ml)	194 ± 33
End-systolic volume (ml)	62 ± 6
Stroke volume (ml/B)	132 ± 28
Cardiac output (L/min)	8.96 ± 0.14
Ejection Fraction	0.68 ± 0.03

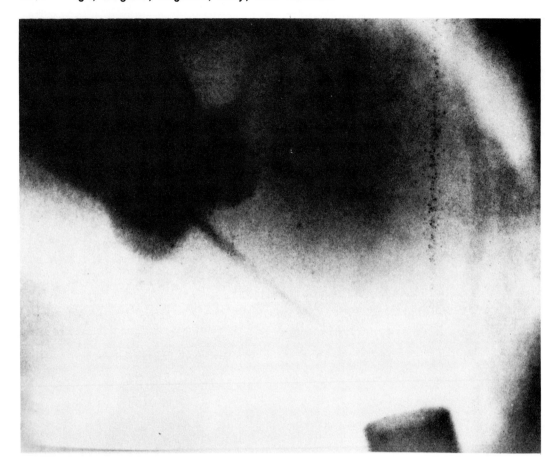

FIG. 7. Bovine cineangiography: retrograde filling of the aortic root and coronary arteries from the abdominal aorta (ALVAD on).

normal limits (Table 4); the end-diastolic pressures and volumes were minimally elevated.

On the basis of these findings further cineangiographic studies were undertaken. The cineangiographic films of the two calves with retained inflow tubes and three calves with implanted functioning ALVADs were analyzed. The equation describing the relation between ventricular axis ratio (AR) and internal radius (r_1) (Fig. 9) was found to be $AR = 0.65\ r_1 + 3.5$. The equation for the volume of a prolate ellipsoid [$V = 0.445\ (2r_1)^3$ (AR)] was used to calculate left ventricular volume (Fig. 10).*

The results of these studies show that in

* Cothran et al[8] have reported that a linear relationship exists between the internal left ventricular diameter and stroke volume during ventricular internal ejection. Similarly, a linear relation was found when left ventricular internal radius was plotted against the major-to-minor axis ratio. The equation describing this relationship was $AR = -0.6\ r_1 + 3$.

calves with inflow tubes implanted in the left ventricular apex, the degree of major axis shortening during ventricular ejection is reduced and that for any given internal radius the internal ventricular volume is increased. These findings are attributed to the fixed position of the ventricular apex to the inflow tube and diaphragm.

DISCUSSION

From an historical point of view, it is of interest that Carrel,[3] in 1910, and Jeger,[18] prior to 1923, reported experiments in which bypasses were established in experimental animals, from the left ventricle to the thoracic aorta, by means of vein grafts. Moreover, the subsequent work of Sarnoff, Donovan, and Case,[34] prior to 1953, is of particular interest. By means of a Lucite tube with a modified Hufnagel valve, the cardiac output was shunted from the left ventricular apex to the

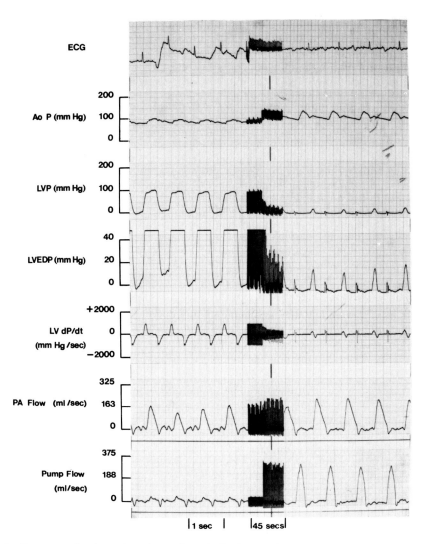

FIG. 8. Representative hemodynamic tracing obtained four days postoperatively during ALVAD pumping in the awake calf. Left ventricular pressure and dP/dt are reduced. Heart rate is reduced from 79 to 68 b/min during assist. Stroke volume and cardiac output are increased from 67 to 81 ml/b and 5.3 to 5.5 L/min, respectively, during ALVAD pumping.

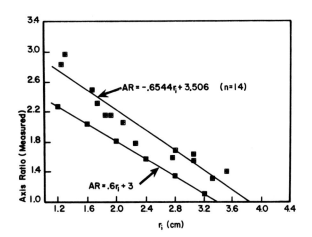

FIG. 9. Relationship of internal ventricular radius and left ventricular major-to-minor axis ratio for normal calves and those with retained ALVAD inlet tubes.

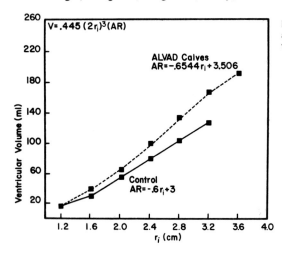

FIG. 10. Relationship of internal ventricular radius and left ventricular volume for normal calves and those with implanted inlet tubes.

descending aorta. In dogs so treated, the ascending aorta could be totally and permanently occluded without any apparent impairment of the circulation. Postoperatively, these animals ran, jumped, and swam and were not readily distinguishable from normal dogs. Detmer, Johnson, and Braunwald[10] have recently reported a similar method of bypassing the left ventricular outflow tract utilizing fresh aortic allografts.

Burch and DePasquale have noted that mechanical work performed by the heart is derived from the contractile tension of the ventricular wall and may be expressed as the integral of intraventricular pressure with respect to volume ($\int PdV$).[2] During the isovolumic phase of ventricular contraction, potential energy is imparted to the blood in the ventricular cavity. When the ventricular outflow valve opens, this potential energy is converted to kinetic energy. Very little additional work is performed by the ventricle during the ejection phase of systole.

The ALVAD is capable of maintaining or increasing cardiac output and systemic blood pressure while decreasing left ventricular pressure to a very low level (Tables 1 to 3). The left ventricle is thus transformed into a low-pressure chamber, which ejects into the mechanical "ventricle." As a result, there is a marked reduction in left ventricular work.

Tension development and the contractile state have been defined as being the two major determinants of myocardial oxygen consumption,[15] with coronary blood flow being regulated principally by myocardial oxygen demands.[4,28] If myocardial tension development increases, oxygen utilization increases and the myocardium becomes relatively hypoxic. This hypoxia is a stimulus for coronary vasodilation and increased coronary flow. Conversely, a significant decrease in myocardial wall tension, eg, during ALVAD assist,[24] causes the myocardium to become relatively hyperoxic. This causes increased coronary resistance and diminished blood flow.

A stable level of oxygen saturation is maintained in the coronary sinus under normal circumstances.[22] Case and Roven have demonstrated that there are limits to the degree of dilation and constriction possible for coronary vasculature.[4] If the myocardial oxygen demand is decreased, as during ALVAD pumping, the coronary vessels initially constrict to diminish oxygen transport. When the limit of constriction is reached, excess oxygen is returned to the coronary sinus. The coronary arteriovenous oxygen difference then diminishes (Table 1).

Following experimental coronary occlusion, blood flow and myocardial oxygen supply are reduced in the area supplied by the occluded vessel. The eventual size of the ischemic zone is dependent upon the degree of occlusion, distribution of collateral vessels, and other intrinsic factors such as stresses within the ventricular wall.[12,25] Regional noncontractile areas of myocardium result in a depression of effective ventricular performance. Such depressions in function may result in enlargement of the ventricular chamber, which leads to an increase in ventricular wall tension.

In the acute canine experiments with coronary occlusion the end-diastolic pressure, end-diastolic volume, and end-systolic volume increased significantly ($P < 0.01$) following occlusion, while cardiac output remained relatively unchanged.

With these changes, the ejection fraction decreased 26 percent (P < 0.01) from control values (Table 2). This reduction is mainly attributable to the loss of functional contractile muscle mass produced by the focal ischemic injury.[19]

During periods of induced myocardial ischemia, ALVAD assistance decreased peak wall tension 80 percent and increased the ejection fraction 77 percent. During assistance, the peak contractile element velocity increased 46 percent from acute occlusion levels. These findings suggest that ALVAD assistance increases the oxygen supply–demand ratio in acutely ischemic myocardium by reducing the oxygen demands of tension development. This reduction in ventricular wall tension and oxygen demand allowed the contractile function of the ischemic segment to increase.

Under normal conditions, myocardial blood flow is relatively evenly distributed across the left ventricular wall with approximately 80 percent of the flow occurring during diastole.[1] The subendocardium has been shown to be the most susceptible layer of the heart to changes in oxygen supply.[33] During left ventricular assist device pumping, peak tension development was significantly reduced. Phasic peak systolic pressure is phase-shifted into diastole (counterpulsation) and increased during ALVAD pumping. Coronary perfusion pressure (diastolic aortic pressure) was, therefore, increased (Table 2) during the assist state.

Urschel et al,[38] studying the effects of intra-aortic balloon counterpulsation, have shown increases in external ventricular performance (stroke volume) with no change in the contractile state of intact normal canine hearts. Balloon pumping effects on external performance during periods of myocardial ischemia were also examined; however, no comment was made on the contractile state during ischemia.

Shelbert et al[35] reported a significant reduction in active myocardial wall force in ischemic zones following experimental coronary occlusion. Counterpulsation was shown to produce a significant improvement in function in the ischemic zone, while reducing the area of ischemic injury. Spotnitz et al[37] reported the effects of arterial counterpulsation on left ventricular mechanics and oxygen consumption. Counterpulsation reduced peak wall stress, contractile element work, and fiber shortening work, while the extent of fiber shortening increased. Myocardial oxygen consumption was reduced during counterpulsation commensurate with the fall in wall stress.

LaFarge et al[20] have reported on the long-term physiologic effects of a similar but intrathoracic device. Studies were undertaken during periods of acute or chronic left ventricular failure. A normal or near normal physiologic state was maintained by left ventricular bypass, in calves with left ventricular failure, during periods of varying physiologic demand.

Recent investigations have stressed the importance of ejection impedance as a major determinant of external ventricular performance (stroke volume).[39,40] During periods when ventricular preload (end-diastolic volume) and contractility are constant, the stroke volume varies inversely as a function of the average impedance to ejection. Thus, a decrease in impedance will cause an increase in stroke volume, and increasing impedances have the opposite effect. It has also been noted that depressed hearts have a lower source impedance than normal hearts and have a greater flow sensitivity to changes in ejection impedance.

The rationale of lowering ejection impedance has recently been applied to patients in cardiogenic shock.[5,6,13,14,21] Chatterjee et al have reported on the use of vasodilator therapy (phentolamine or nitroprusside) in such patients.[5] Vasodilator therapy improved cardiac performance and affected the initial mortality of patients with severe pump failure. Of 15 patients with severe hemodynamic depression, nine (60 percent) survived. Improvement of left ventricular performance was accompanied by a decrease in coronary blood flow, myocardial oxygen consumption, and transmyocardial oxygen extraction (Table 1).

Improved ventricular performance, therefore, need not be accompanied by an increase in myocardial oxygen requirements. This effect is produced by reducing the resistance to ventricular ejection rather than altering the contractile state. Similar results have been obtained during ALVAD pumping in both normal and ischemic hearts (Table 5). The profound reduction of ejection impedance offered by the ALVAD results in a marked increase in ejection fraction (Tables 2 and 3). Since stroke volume is increased, forward flows to the central and peripheral circulations are

TABLE 5. Effects of ALVAD Pumping on Cardiac Performance

Ejection impedance (afterload)	↓
End-diastolic pressure and volume (preload)	↓
Wall tension	↓
Ejection fraction	↑
Cardiac output	↑
Coronary perfusion pressure	↑

increased (Table 2). Improved cardiac emptying results in a decrease in left ventricular end-diastolic volume, with a concomitant reduction in left ventricular end-diastolic pressure (Table 2). This primary reduction in afterload and secondary reduction in preload probably results in reduced oxygen requirements of focally ischemic areas of myocardium, leading to recruitment of previously ischemic noncontractile myocardial fibers (Fig. 4).

SUMMARY

Recent studies have demonstrated that left ventricular to aortic bypass decreases left ventricular work.[9,20,30] Our laboratories have extended these studies in the development and evaluation of an abdominal left ventricular assist device. This externally driven pneumatic pump is implanted subdiaphragmatically and actuated synchronously or asynchronously with the biologic heart. Blood is accepted from the left ventricular apex and ejected into the infrarenal abdominal aorta.

The results of the acute canine experiments demonstrate that the ALVAD is capable of markedly unloading the left ventricle while maintaining systemic perfusion. Under nonischemic conditions the ALVAD significantly reduces the oxygen demands of the left ventricle.

The findings in the animals with induced myocardial ischemia suggest that ALVAD assistance increases the oxygen supply–demand ratio in acutely ischemic myocardium by reducing the oxygen demands of tension development. This reduction in ventricular wall tension and oxygen demand allows the contractile function of the ischemic segment to increase.

The results of the chronic bovine experiments corroborated the acute canine studies and demonstrated the chronic hemodynamic effectiveness of ALVAD pumping for periods up to 65 days.

References

1. Becker L, Pitt B: Regional myocardial blood flow, ischemia and anti-anginal drugs. Ann Clin Res 3:353–61, 1971
2. Burch GE, DePasquale NP; Editorial: on resting the human heart. Am Med 44:165, 1968
3. Carrell A: On the experimental surgery of the thoracic aorta and the heart. Ann Surg 52:83–95, 1910
4. Case RB and Roven RB: Some considerations of coronary flow. Prog Cardiovasc Dis 6:45, 1963
5. Chatterjee K, Parmley WW, Ganz W, et al: Hemodynamic and metabolic responses to vasodilator therapy in acute myocardial infarction. Circulation 48:1183–93, 1973
6. Chatterjee K, Parmley WW, Swan HJC, et al: Beneficial effects of vasodilator agents in severe mitral regurgitation due to dysfunction of subvalvar apparatus. Circulation 48:684–90, 1973
7. Coleman S, Whalen R, Robinson W, Huffman F, Norman J: A preclinical drive console for a pneumatically-powered left ventricular assist device. Alin Res 20:854, 1972
8. Cothran LN, Hawthorne EW, Sandler H: An analysis of left ventricular dimensional changes in conscious animals. National Conference on Research Animals in Medicine (NIH Publ No 72-181, 1972 p 94
9. DeBakey ME: Mechanical circulatory support: current status. Am J Cardiol 27:1–2, 1971
10. Detmer DE, Johnson EH, Braunwald NS: Left ventricular apex-to-thoracic aortic shunts using aortic valve allografts in calves. Ann Thor Surg 11:417–22, 1971
11. Dove GB, Migliore JJ, Fuqua JM, Edmonds, CH, Robinson WJ, Huffman FN, Norman JC: An abdominal left ventricular assist device (ALVAD): experimental physiologic analyses III, cardiac output. Proceedings of 26th ACEMB, 15: 148, 1973
12. Eliot RS, Holsinger JW: A unified concept of the pathophysiology of myocardial infarction and sudden death. Chest 62:469–74, 1972
13. Franciosa JA, Guiha NH, Limas CJ, et al: Improved left ventricular function during nitroprusside infusion in acute infarction. Lancet 1:650, 1972
14. Gould L, Zahir M, Ettinger S: Phentolamine and cardiovascular performance. Br Heart J 31:154, 1969
15. Graham TP, Covell JW, Sonnenblick EH: Control of myocardial oxygen consumption: relative influence of contractile state and tension development. J Clin Invest 47:375–85, 1968
16. Hood WB, Covelli VH, Abelmann WH: Persistence of contractile behaviour in acutely ischaemic myocardium. Cardiovasc Res 3:249–60, 1969
17. Igo SR, Migliore JJ, Fuqua JM, Daly BDT, Norman JC: Effects of abdominal left ventricular assist device (ALVAD) on myocardial contractility during acute coronary occlusion. J Surg Res 1973 17:177–85, 1974
18. Jeger, Cited by Kuttner H: Chirurgische operationslehre. Ed 5, Leipsig, Barth, vol 2, 1923
19. Kitamura S, Kay JH, Krohn BG: Geometric and functional abnormalities of the left ventricle with a chronic localized noncontractile area. Am J Cardiol 31:701–7, 1973
20. LaFarge CG, Carr JG, Bernhard WF: Hemodynamic studies during prolonged mechanical circulatory support. Trans Am Soc Artif Int Organs 18:186–97, 1972
21. Majid PA, Sharma B, Taylor SH: Phentolamine for vasodilator treatment of severe heart failure. Lancet 2:719, 1971
22. Messer JV, Wagman RJ, Levine HJ: Patterns of human myocardial oxygen extraction during rest and exercise. J Clin Invest 41:725, 1962
23. Migliore J, Arthur J, Fuqua J, Dove G, Norman J: Myocardial arteriovenous oxygen content and derived consumption (qO_2) during abdominal left ventricular assist device (ALVAD) pumping. Clin Res 21:438, 1973
24. Migliore JJ, Dove GB, Fuqua JM, Edmonds, CH, Robinson WJ, Huffman FN, Norman JC: An abdominal left ventricular assist device (ALVAD): experimental physiologic analyses IV, myocardial blood flow. Proceedings, of 26th ACEMB, 15:149, 1973
25. Moir TW: Subendocardial distribution of coronary blood flow and the effects of antianginal drugs. Circ Res 30:621–27, 1972

26. Molokhia FA, Asimacopoulos PJ, Daly BDT, Huffman FN, Norman JC: An antiarrhythmic regimen for left ventricular assist device (LVAD) implantation in the calf. Clin Res 19:711, 1971

27. Molokhia FA, Asimacopoulos PJ, Daly BDT, Huffman FN, Norman JC: A simplified technique for left ventricular-to-aorta device (LVAD) implantation in the calf. Clin Res 19:711, 1971

28. Nasser MG, in Cardiovascular Dynamics by R. F. Rushmer. Philadelphia, WB Saunders, 1970, pp 276–77

29. Norman JC, Whalen RL; Daly BDT, Migliore J, Huffman FN: An implantable abdominal left ventricular assist device (ALVAD). Clin Res 20:855, 1972

30. Pierce WS, Aaronson AE, Prophet GA, Williams DR, Waldhausen JA: Hemodynamic and metabolic studies during two types of left ventricular bypass surgery. Surg Forum 23:176, 1972

31. Robinson WJ, Molokhia FA, Asimacopoulos PJ, Norman JC: Anesthesia for left ventricular assist device (LVAD) implantation in the calf. Clin Res 19:713, 1971

32. Ross J, Covell JW, Sonnenblick EH: Contractile state of the heart characterized by force-velocity relations in variably afterloaded and isovolumic beats. Circ Res 18:149–63, 1966

33. Ross RS: Pathophysiology of coronary circulation. Br Heart J 33: 173–84, 1971

34. Sarnoff SJ, Donovan TJ, Case RB: The surgical relief of aortic stenosis by means of apical-aortic valvular anastomosis. Circulation 11:564–75, 1955

35. Schelbert HR, Covell JW, Burns JW: Observations on factors affecting local forces in the left ventricular wall during acute myocardial ischemia. Circ Res 29:306–16, 1971

36. Sonnenblick EH: Implications of muscle mechanics in the heart. Fed Proc 21:975–90, 1962

37. Spotnitz HM, Covell JW, Ross J: Left ventricular mechanics and oxygen consumption during arterial counterpulsation. Am J Physiol 217:1352–58, 1969

38. Urschel CW, Eber L, Forrester J: Alterations of mechanical performance of the ventricle by intra-aortic balloon counterpulsation. Am J Cardiol 25: 546–51, 1970

39. Urschel CW, Sonnenblick EH: Determinants of cardiac performance. In YC Fung, N Perrone, M Anliker (eds): Biomechanics: Its Foundations and Objectives. Englewood Cliffs, NJ, Prentice-Hall, 1972, pp 303–16

40. Walker WE: Implications of studies of vascular impedance for assessment of left ventricular function. Cardiovascular Disease, Bulletin of the Texas Heart Institute 1:127–36, 1974

122

THE SMALL-CALIBER KNITTED ARTERIAL PROSTHESIS

S. Adam Wesolowski, Yoshiaki Komoto,
and Hatsuzo Uchida

Until recently, there had been only sporadic interest in the development of a small-caliber arterial prosthesis (less than 6 to 8 millimeters in diameter) because clinical demand had been minor and adequately enough fulfilled by the use of autologous vein. However, the recent widespread performance of aortocoronary bypass and increasing reports of late failure of autovein aortocoronary bypass grafts, the result of intimal hyperplasia [1,2] and other factors,[3,4] have been substantial enough to stimulate interest in the search for new bypass materials. Autologous internal mammary-coronary anastomosis [5] is being practiced more widely than before, but in the atherosclerotic patient, this artery is not always free of disease, especially about the orifice. Autologous radial arterial aortocoronary bypass has proven successful [6] but leaves something to be desired as a routine surgical procedure. Experimentally, small-caliber arterial homografts demonstrate a 50 percent occlusion rate three months after implantation.[7] For these reasons, a suitable long-term 4-mm-diameter class of flexible, porous arterial prosthesis would represent a significant tool for the practicing cardiac surgeon.

The lower diameter limit for continued patency of arterial prostheses for clinical bypass or interpolation has been 8 mm.[8] Although short-length prostheses of smaller caliber have been used successfully for arteriopulmonary shunts,[9] Harrison observed that a number of synthetic prostheses studied were not satisfactory for replacement of blood vessels less than 5 mm in diameter.[10] Jacobson noted that interpolated porous arterial grafts of 4 mm in diameter exhibited a 90 percent occlusion rate within 24 hours of implantation in spite of the use of microsurgical suture techniques.[11,12]

Small-diameter, solid-wall, elastic arterial prostheses have limited success even when the wall bears a negative electrical charge, but continued negative current application has a beneficial effect on implanted prostheses.[13] Sharp and associates [14] have also tested electrolour (dacron-velour fabric tubes sprayed with several coats of Bioelectric Polyurethane) and noted an 85 percent patency rate with 4-mm-diameter prostheses in the canine carotid artery 21 days after implantation. Recent reports of 3-mm-diameter expanded porous polytetrafluoroethylene prostheses are very encouraging with high patency rates for periods as long as 11 months after implantation.[15]

The present study is a report of a five-year experimental investigation of implantations of 113 small-caliber blood vessel prostheses, of which 93 were 4 mm diameter implanted into the adult dog and 20 were 6 mm tested in the adult dog and growing pig preparations.

MATERIALS, METHODS, AND RESULTS

The present studies were prompted as a result of observations in connection with the development and testing of finely knitted arterial prostheses.[16] It was noted that this class of "gossamer"

Supported in part by grants-in-aid from the National Heart Institute, National Institutes of Health, U.S. Public Health Service, Department of Health, Education, and Welfare, National Heart and Lung Institute.

materials handled and healed in such a fashion as to approach the assumed ideal specifications for a successful, porous, small arterial prosthesis.[17]

I. Technical characteristics
   A. Physical properties
      1. Finely knit, very thin wall
      2. Very flexible
      3. Very pliable
      4. Very conformable at anastomoses
   B. Accurate anastomotic technique

II. Healing properties
   A. Early healing
      1. Very porous
      2. Thin inner layer
   B. Late healing
      1. Stable inner capsule
      2. Thin inner capsule (less than 500 microns)
      3. Persistent flexibility
      4. Persistent elasticity (elastomechanical layer)

Six-millimeter-diameter prostheses had already been clinically tested in human application of these finely knitted materials.[18] The identification of a suitable experimental preparation was performed by the screening of three standard commercial 6-mm-diameter prostheses in the abdominal aortae of two adult dogs and 18 growing pigs. Standard anesthesia and operative techniques were used.[19] This preparation screening test demonstrated that the growing pig is not suitable for the screening of small-caliber arterial prostheses with our present knowledge but that the adult dog appears to be adequate for this purpose (Table 1, Fig. 1).

TABLE 1. Results of 6-mm ID Implants into Abdominal Aorta

DAYS OF IMPLANT	ADULT DOG (patent/total)	GROWING PIG (patent/total)
Milliknit (6 grafts)		
140-180		0/5
1,690	1/1	
Microknit (7 grafts)		
140-180		1/6 (septum)
942	1/1	
1967 Weavenit[a] (7 grafts)		
140-180		0/7
All materials, totals (20 grafts)		
	2/2	1/18

[a]*This Jersey knitted fabrication has been replaced by Meadox Medicals, Inc., with a different warp knit fabrication with different healing properties*

A series of 28 four-mm-diameter 40-needle-per-inch (npi) polyester prostheses of seven different water porosities * were implanted into both the femoral and carotid arteries of seven adult dogs under general pentobarbital anesthesia, varying the animal, left and right sides, neck and groin sites, and normal or loose tension with prostheses of each porosity. Normal tension was attained when the length of implanted prostheses was equal to the length of resected artery, and loose tension when the implanted prosthesis was longer. There was no correlation of patency of implant with different animals, or side, site, or tension of implant. A relationship was noted between the percentage of patent arterial implants at three days after implantation and the water porosity (Fig. 2). Patency was determined by palpation, arteriography, and removal after 72 hours. Recipient arteries varied from 2.0 to 3.5 millimeters outside diameter. Two of the seven materials demonstrated statistical patency (seven out of eight) at 72 hours, to be compared to Jacobson's control rate of less than 10 percent patency at the end of 24 hours after implantation.[12] One of these two prostheses was selected for further study.

Sixty-five selected (optimal porosity) 4-mm-diameter 40 npi polyester prostheses were further tested in adult dogs to gain insight into patency rates with time as follows: nineteen 5-cm-long interpolated grafts into carotid or femoral arteries; nine 5-cm-long interpolated grafts into the infra-renal abdominal aorta; twelve 10-cm long arteriovenous shunts, either carotid-jugular or femoro-femoral; and two 5-cm-long interpolated grafts into the external jugular vein. Control implants of 5-cm lengths were tested as follows: USCI-1963 4-mm DeBakey knitted polyester prostheses, two in carotid arteries; USCI ultralight-weight knitted prostheses of 4.5 millimeter diameter, 10 in carotid or femoral artery and 4 in abdominal aorta; 4-mm internal diameter polyester-reinforced Hydron implants, one in carotid artery and one in abdominal aorta; and 4 to 4.5 mm human saphenous venous heterografts, five in abdominal aorta. The gross patency rates are summarized in Table 2.

The gross patency rates demonstrate that the human heterograft vein, Hydron, and 1963-DeBakey prostheses and venous implants are undesirable at this time for further study. The ultra-lightweight USCI prosthesis demonstrates only partial

* Kindly supplied by Golaski Laboratories, Philadelphia.

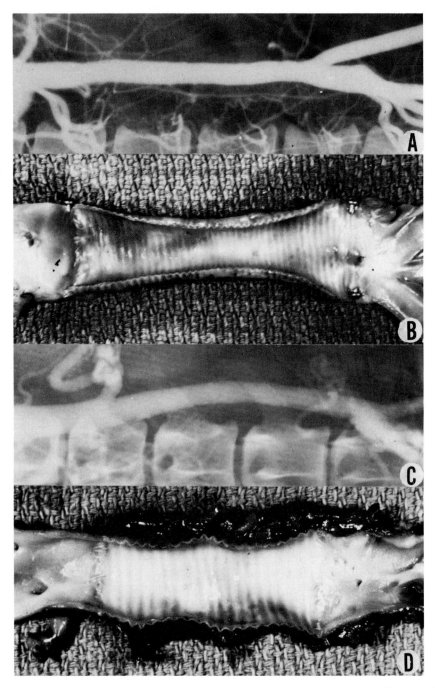

FIG. 1. Examples of screening of various 6-mm diameter finely knitted arterial prostheses in the abdominal aorta. A and B. Arteriogram and photograph, respectively, of 50-npi (Microknit) polyester prosthesis 942 days after implantation into mature dog. C and D. Arteriogram and photograph, respectively, of 40-npi (Milliknit) polyester prosthesis 1,690 days after implantation into mature dog.

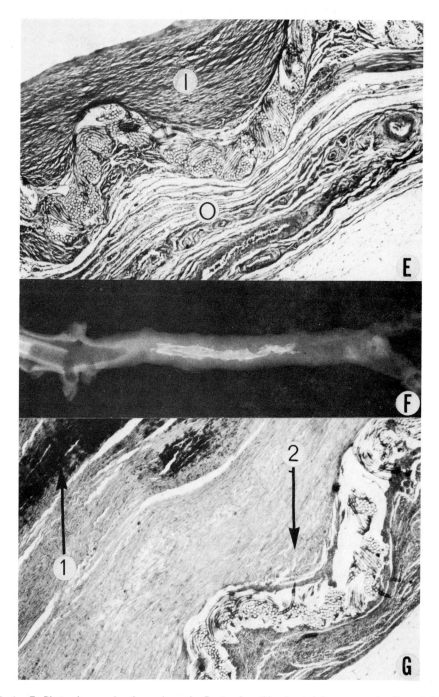

FIG. 1. E. Photomicrograph of specimen in B showing thin, healed inner capsule (I) and thin, healed outer capsule (O). ×25 Trichrome stain. F. Roentgenogram of Microknit prosthesis 146 days after implantation into growing pig. The calcification is within the thrombus and not in the inner capsule. G. Photomicrograph of specimen in F. Calcification is in the thrombus (arrow 1) and not in the usual calcification site in the inner capsule (arrow 2). ×25, H and E.

TABLE 2. Results Patency of 4-mm ID Implants

DAYS OF IMPLANT	CAROTID OR FEMORAL A. (patent/total 5-cm length)	ABDOMINAL AORTA (patent/total 5-cm length)	A/V SHUNT CAROT. OR FEM. (patent/total 10-cm length)	JUGULAR VEIN (patent/total 5-cm length)
Selected 40 npi knitted polyester (42 implants)				
2 hr		0/1		
2		1/1		
4	4/4	0/1		
5	2/2		2/2	
6		0/1		
7	2/2			
8		1/1		
15		0/1		
18	1/2		1/2	0/2
32			0/1	
40	1/1			
47	0/2		0/2	
62	1/2		0/2	
83		0/1		
104	2/2		0/1	
128			0/2	
1,085	1/2			
1,613		1/1		
1,690		1/1		
Total	14/19 (74%)	4/9 (44%)	3/12 (25%)	0/2
1963 USCI DeBakey knitted polyester (2 implants)				
7	0/2			
USCI ultraweight knitted polyester (14 implants)				
1		0/1		
2	1/1	0/1		
5	0/1			
7	0/4			
15	2/2			
110	0/2	0/1		
827		1/1 (septum)		
Total	4/10 (40%)	1/4 (25%)		
Reinforced hydron (2 implants)				
	0/1	0/1		
Human saphenous (5 implants)				
1		0/1		
6		0/1		
18		1/1		
32		0/2		
Total		1/5		

All materials, total implants: 65

success in terms of patency; it is possible that this prosthesis has never been optimized in construction with respect to healing and patency (cf Discussion). The selected 40 npi polyester fabrication shows the best gross, although less than statistical, patency (Figs. 3, 4).

Patency was determined by palpation of pulses and serial arteriography. Those grafts that were patent were recovered from animals sacrificed for serial healing studies; occluded impants were removed at discovery of nonpatency on the basis of loss of pulse and were verified by arteriography.

The gross patency results include all of the implants performed, including "technical errors" of implantation, because technique is an inherent determinant of patency of small-caliber arterial grafting, more so than in large-caliber implantation. In the case of the selected 40-npi prosthesis, patency-modifying factors include multiple implants in a single animal, experience with intraoperative heparinization, which leads to periprosthetic hematoma in the dog, and frequently repeated multiple-area arteriography. The ultra-lightweight implants were either one or two per animal with no femoral

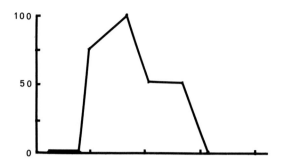

FIG. 2. Relationship between percentage of patent 4-mm diameter 40-npi arterial prostheses after three days' implantation in peripheral arteries of adult dog (ordinate) and the porosity of seven different porosities of the 40-npi polyester prosthesis (abscissa). Porosity is expressed in relative units. It would appear that the 40-npi prosthesis has an optimal porosity for patency of small-caliber arterial replacement.

implants in animals with an abdominal aortic implant. Correction for these modifying factors would tend to increase the patency rate lead of the 40-npi over the ultra-lightweight prosthesis.

The most important observations from the results of this study would appear to be:

1. The selected 4-mm-diameter 40-npi polyester prosthesis is
   a. promising for small-caliber peripheral arterial implantation (the blood flow through abdominal implants varied between 150 and 350 cc/min as measured by the square-wave electromagnetic flow meter at implantation or at sacrifice; patency without stenosis or septum formation and with persistently thin inner capsules has been observed for as long as four years, seven months [Figs. 3, 4, 5];
   b. of limited application for small-caliber peripheral arteriovenous shunts, none remaining patent for longer than three months (it should be noted that loop end-to-end shunts [Fig. 4D] are more successful than in-line end-to-side shunts. Side-to-side shunts were not tested. Occlusions appeared to be related to progressive stenosis of the vein just distal to the prosthetic-venous suture line in loop shunts);
   c. not promising for small-caliber peripheral venous implantation.
2. The USCI ultra-lightweight knitted polyester prosthesis as presently developed would not appear to be promising as a long-term small-caliber arterial prosthesis because no complication-free, long-term implant of this material has been observed (Fig. 6).
3. Reinforced Hydron prostheses have not been successfully developed for small- or large-caliber arterial implantations because of disruption of the material at suture lines (one 4-mm carotid, one 4-mm abdominal aorta, and five 10-mm thoracic aortic implants) within 15 days.
4. Human heterograft saphenous vein is not suitable for small-caliber canine arterial replacement.

DISCUSSION

It should be emphasized that in the assessment and comparison of various types of small-caliber prostheses, all implants—technical failures or not—should be included in the gross patency comparisons because the physical properties of the prosthesis *per se* can directly influence the suture technique and anastomotic quality and, therefore, patency.

Accuracy of suture technique is no doubt a determinant of the patency of small-caliber blood vessel surgery. The variables in technique accuracy can be summarized as follows:

1. Even circumferential spacing of sutures prevents offsetting of the anastomotic or closure lines and prevents pocket and pucker formation as well as delayed hemorrhage at suture lines. Even spacing of suture bites also allows smooth hemodynamic adaptation of diameter discrepancies and is probably the single most important determinant of accuracy in suture technique. Probably the most valuable aspect of the use of optical loupes or microsurgical techniques is the ease in obtaining evenness of suture placement. It has long been appreciated that a simple end-on coaptation ("over and over") suture produces less immediate stenosis in small vessel anastomoses and is indistinguishable from the everting mattress suture at six weeks in terms of patency, stenosis, and amount of internally visible suture material.[20]
2. Selection of size and type of suture material constitutes a presentday surgical mystique. It is true that the finest suture material for a given mechanical job is theoretically the most preferable, but in practice the concept of fine enough would appear to be valid. During this

FIG. 3. 4-mm 40-npi polyester prosthesis in canine carotid artery. A. Arteriogram of bilateral 5-cm length interpolated grafts three days after implantation. *Facing page*: B. Photomicrograph at three days showing fibrinous capsules (upper-inner, lower-outer). ×25, H and E. C. Photomicrograph at 105 days showing thin, healed stable inner capsule (upper) and thin, healed stable outer capsule (lower). ×25 Trichrome stain.

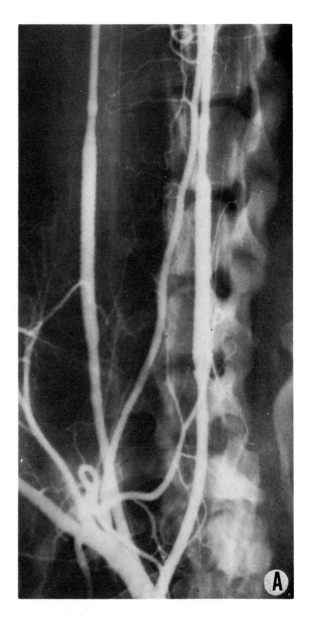

work it was determined that 5-0 dacron suture material is fine enough for 4-mm prosthetic implantation, but there could be no objection to the use of 6-0, 7-0, or 8-0 if so desired. The type of suture material can be of critical importance, since silk can fracture and lead to delayed suture line leaks with large-caliber prostheses.[21] Permanent synthetic sutures are, therefore, preferable in this application. It could prove, however, that silk may be an acceptable suture material for small-caliber prostheses because of the lessened wall tension of the smaller diameter according to Laplace's Law. The

rule of thumb, which appears to be axiomatic, is to use a fine enough suture material of the same formulation as the yarn of the prosthesis; eg, "dacron sutures for dacron prostheses."

3. Minimization of trauma, hypotension, dead space, and fluid collections are important to small-caliber blood vessel work as in all other types of clean surgical endeavors.

The most thought-provoking observation of the present study is the relationship between early small-caliber prosthetic implant patency and porosity. It should be stressed that the seven pros-

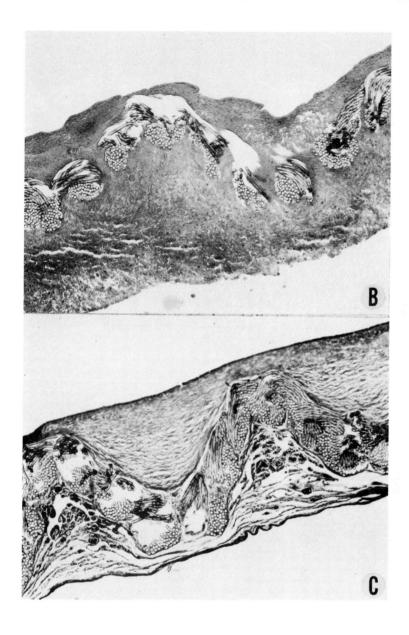

theses of different porosity initially screened were all of the same 40-npi knitted construction, the different porosities having been produced over a twofold range by varying the degree of compaction or shrinkage during the processing of otherwise identical material. It has been previously demonstrated that the 40-npi material has an optimum porosity for efficiency of preclotting and of late healing in connection with large caliber arterial prostheses.[16] It should be noted, parenthetically, that the optimum porosity of the 40-npi polyester prosthesis would appear to be different for large- and small-caliber sizes, perhaps as a result of dif-

ferent knitting techniques for the large- and small-caliber tubes. A major question raised by this observation is whether each particular prosthetic arterial construction has an optimum porosity for optimum overall results—eg, would the USCI ultra-lightweight 4.5-mm arterial prosthesis give a better result at a different porosity value, and has any arterial prosthesis really been optimized?

To the knowledge of the authors, no other prosthesis except the 40-npi knitted polyester has been optimized for porosity. Others have simply been biologically tested for adequacy upon delivery of the manufacturer's attempt, or of serial

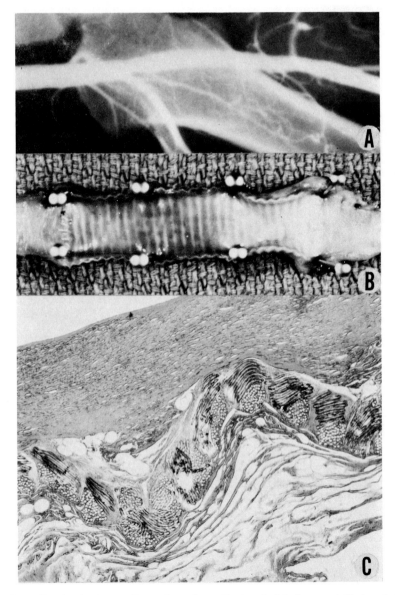

FIG. 4.   4-mm 40-npi polyester prostheses in canine subjects.   A. Arteriogram at 62 days in femoral artery.   B. Gross photograph at 1,085 days in femoral artery.   C. Photomicrograph at 1,085 days of specimen in B.

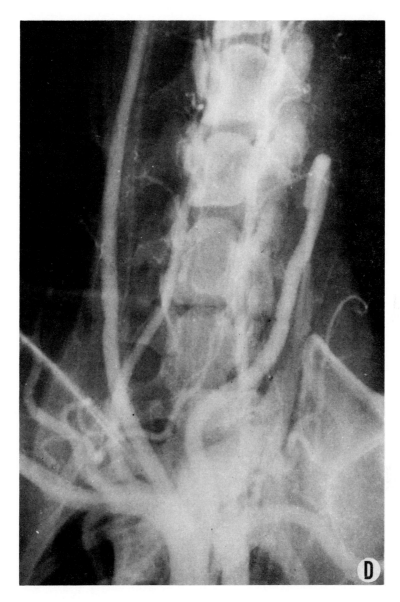

FIG. 4. D. Arteriogram at 37 days of 5-cm long right carotid prosthesis and 10-cm long left end-to-end loop carotid-jugular arteriovenous shunt.

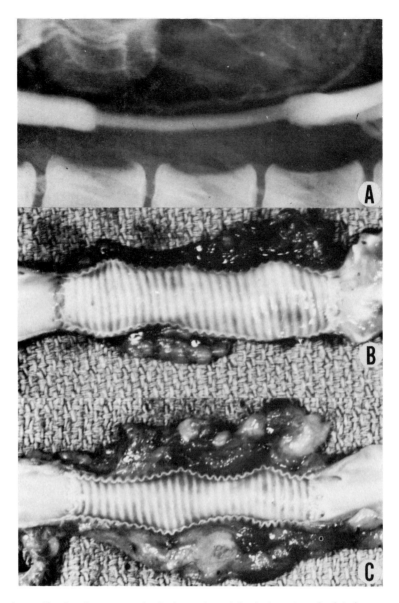

FIG. 5. 4-mm 40-npi polyester prosthesis in canine abdominal aorta. A. Arteriogram at 1,613 days. B. Photograph of specimen in A at 1,613 days. C. Photograph at 1,690 days.

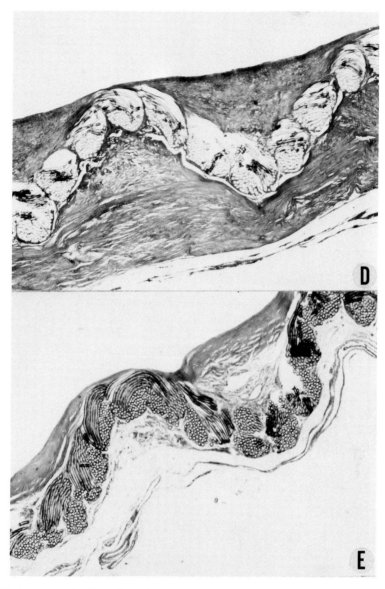

FIG. 5. Photomicrograph of specimen in B showing thin, stable capsules. ×25 Trichrome stain. E. Photomicrograph of specimen in C showing thin capsules. These recovered prostheses have ten percent residual linear elasticity related to the formation of an elastomechanical layer (surgical dissection plane) adjacent to the thin outer capsule.

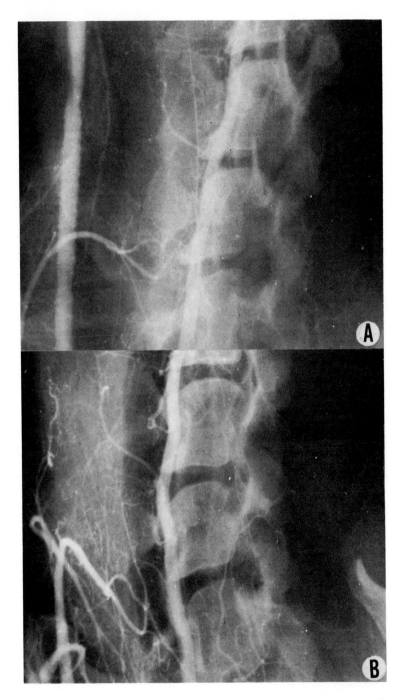

FIG. 6.   4.5-mm USCI ultra-lightweight polyester prostheses in canine subject. A. Arteriogram one day after implantation of 5-cm lengths into both carotid arteries. The right is patent; the left has occluded.   B. Repeat arteriogram of same area at three days showing bilateral thrombosis of carotid prostheses.

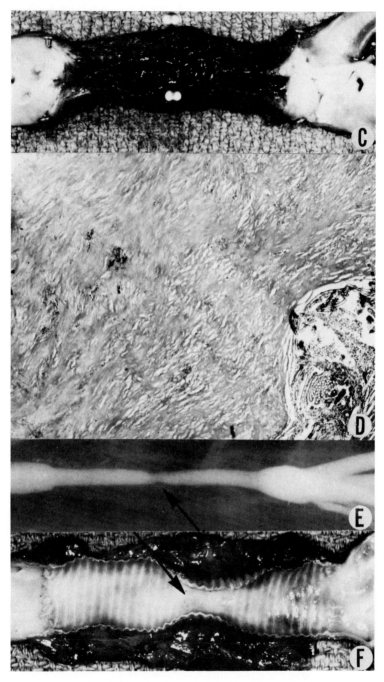

FIG. 6. C. 5-cm long abdominal prosthesis with recent thrombus 110 days after implantation. D. Photomicrograph of thick inner capsule of specimen in C with thrombus stripped away. ×25 Trichrome stain.   E. and F. Arteriogram and photograph, respectively, of USCI ultra-lightweight polyester implant with longest patency, 827 days, in abdominal aorta. Note secondary septum, a serious complication of healing (arrows), reducing effective lumen to 1.5 mm.

modifications as determined by the manufacturer. Porosity optimization of the 40-npi polyester prosthesis has, on the one hand, been a logical and necessary step in its development because its manufacture includes a shrinkage process unique, to our knowledge, to this class of arterial prostheses. These comments are not to be interpreted as praising the 40-npi prosthesis, or condemning any other, but should provide progressive insight into the development of the more critical arterial prosthesis—the small caliber. Finally, what other variables, in addition to porosity, can and should be optimized to produce the statistically ideal and permanently patent small-caliber arterial prosthesis for use in the aortocoronary and other body sites?

CONCLUSIONS

1. In the light of our present knowledge, the adult dog is preferable to the growing-pig preparation for the screening of small-caliber blood vessel prostheses. The challenge: to develop a small-caliber prosthesis that will also work in the growing pig.
2. Early and continued patency of the 4-mm diameter 40-npi knitted polyester arterial prosthesis is related to an optimal porosity.
3. The optimal porosity 4-mm diameter 40-npi arterial prosthesis has promise of statistical long-term patency up to observation periods of four years, seven months in the dog.
4. This same prosthesis would appear to be useful for only three-month periods as end-to-end loop arteriovenous shunts, which apparently fail as the result of continued changes leading to stenotic obstruction on the venous side adjacent to the prosthesis.
5. The relatively poor results of the 4.5-mm diameter USCI ultra-lightweight polyester prosthesis, and perhaps other prostheses as well, may be improved by optimization of porosity.
6. Finally, the study raises a basic question, What are the variables that determine statistical and permanent patency of small-caliber blood vessel prostheses?

References

1. Johnson WD, Auer JE, Tector AJ: Late changes in coronary vein graft. Am J Cardiol 26:640, 1970
2. Vlodaver C and Edwards JE: Pathologic changes in aortico-coronary arterial saphenous vein grafts. Circulation 44:719, 1971
3. Szilagyi DE, Elliott JP, Hageman JH, Smith RF, Dall'Olmo CA: Biologic fate of autogenous vein implants as arterial substitutes: clinical, angiographic and histo-pathologic observations in femoro-popliteal operations for atherosclerosis. Ann Surg 178:232, 1973
4. Jones M, Conkle DM, Ferrans VJ, Roberts WC, et al: Lesions observed in arterial autogenous vein grafts: light and electronmicroscopic evaluation. Circulation (Suppl III):198, 1973
5. Green GE, Stertzer SH, Reppert EH: Coronary arterial bypass grafts. Ann Thorac Surg 5:443, 1968
6. Carpentier A, Guermonprez JL, DePoche A, Frechette C, DuBost C: The aorta-to-coronary radial artery bypass graft. Ann Thorac Surg 16:111, 1973
7. Wesolowski SA, Sauvage LR, Golaski WM, Komoto Y: Rationale for the development of the gossamer small arterial prosthesis. AMA Arch Surg 97:864, 1968
8. Crawford ES, DeBakey ME, Cooley DA, Morris GC: Use of crimped knitted Dacron grafts in patients with occlusive disease of the aorta and of the iliac, femoral and popliteal arteries. In Wesolowski SA, Dennis C (eds): Fundamentals of Vascular Grafting. New York, McGraw Hill, 1963, pp 356–66, 372
9. Jones EL. Personal communication
10. Harrison JH: Synthetic materials as vascular prostheses. A comparative study in small vessels of nylon, Dacron, Ivalon, Sponge and Teflon. Am J Surg 95:3, 1958
11. Jacobson JH, Rosalio ES, Katsumura T: Influence of prosthesis diameter in small arterial replacement. Circulation 28:742, 1963
12. Jacobson JH: Personal communication
13. Sharp WV, Gardner DL, Andresen GJ: Adaptation of elastic materials for small vessel replacement. Trans Am Soc Artif Intern Organs 11:336, 1965
14. Sharp WV, Gardner DL, Andresen GJ, Wright J: Electrolour: a new vascular interface. Trans Am Soc Artif Intern Organs 14:73, 1968
15. Matsumoto H, Hasegawa T, Fuse K, Yamamoto M, Saigusa M: A new vascular prosthesis for a small caliber artery. Surgery 74:519, 1973
16. Wesolowski SA, Fries CC, McMahon JD, Martinez A: Evaluation of a new vascular prosthesis with optimal specifications. Surgery 59:40, 1966
17. Wesolowski SA, Golaski WM, Sauvage LR, McMahon JD, Komoto Y: Considerations in the development of small artery prostheses. Trans Am Soc Artif Intern Organs 14:431, 1968
18. Wesolowski SA, Sauvage LR, Komoto Y, McMahon JD: The long-term behavior of tissue and prosthetic arterial and cardiac valve implants. Proceedings of 17th Congress of the European Society of Cardiovascular Surgery, London, 1969, pp 41–55
19. Wesolowski SA: Evaluation of Tissue and Prosthetic Vascular Grafts. Springfield, Ill, Charles C Thomas Co, 1962
20. Sauvage LR, Wesolowski SA: The influence of suture method upon the incidence of thrombosis in artery-artery, vein-vein and artery-vein anastomoses. Surgery 36:227, 1954
21. Sawyers JL, Jacobs JK, Sutton JP: Peripheral anastomotic aneurysms. Arch Surg 95:802, 1967

123

THE EFFECTS OF ISOLATED CHANGES IN RIGHT VENTRICULAR CONTRACTILITY ON INTRAPULMONARY SHUNTING IN CALVES WITH ARTIFICIAL HEARTS

Theodore H. Stanley, Jay Volder, Hartmut Oster,
John Lawson, Willem J. Kolff,
and Don B. Olsen

INTRODUCTION

Although a number of therapies exist for treatment of the low-cardiac-output syndrome following myocardial infarction or open-heart surgery, most employ one or another of the vasoactive amines or some other cardiotonic agent (Kones, 1973). The majority of these pharmacologic interventions attempt to increase cardiac output by increasing myocardial contractility. While this may be desirable with respect to left ventricular (LV) function, it may also lead to very high rates of intraventricular pressure development in the right ventricle (RV), which could alter intrapulmonary perfusion pathways. Until recently there existed no experimental animal model that could be used to study the effects of isolated changes in the contractility of a single ventricle. The recent development of artificial hearts that can sustain animals in a relatively normal condition for periods longer than two weeks (Oster et al, 1975) presents us with a unique experimental animal model to study the effects of changes in function of a single ventricle. The object of this study was to quantitate the influence of contractility changes in the right ventricle on the pulmonary shunt (PS) fraction of

Supported in part by The National Institutes of Health via the National Heart and Lung Institute, Grant No. 3-POL-HL-13738-02-SL and by Contract No. HT4-2905 and by the John A. Hartford Foundation, The Christina Foundation, the Lad L. and Mary Hercik Fund, and Mr. Maurice Warshaw.

calves with artificial hearts whose left ventricular contractility was maintained constant.

METHODS

Ten 90–105-kg calves served as the experimental subjects. Each was anesthetized (with sodium brevital and then halothane) intubated, and placed in the supine position. After placement of femoral arterial and venous catheters the animals underwent cardiopulmonary bypass and had their natural hearts replaced with a Silastic ovoid (Jarvik) type of dacron fibril-lined artificial heart (Fig. 1). This artificial heart has been previously described (Oster et al, 1975). It is driven by compressed air and equipped with Bjork-Shiley Delrin disk valves. An artificial pulmonary artery made of woven dacron was attached proximally to the artificial heart and distally to the natural pulmonary artery. The artificial pulmonary artery and artificial left atrium contained taps to which pieces of high-pressure intravenous tubing were connected and brought out of the chest for mixed venous and left atrial blood sampling, pressure monitoring, and fluid administration.

All animals were mechanically ventilated with oxygen at concentrations of 40 to 100 percent and volumes of 10 to 20 ml/kg/breath for the first 24 hours postimplantation. Subsequently they were mechanically ventilated or allowed to breathe spontaneously known concentrations (21 to 70 percent) and volumes (4 to 12 ml/kg/breath) of oxygen or room air in order to maintain arterial oxygen tensions between 70 and 100 torr. During

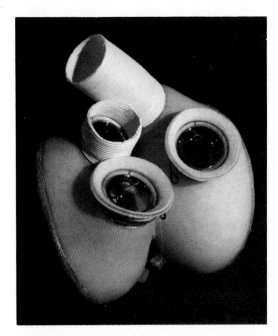

FIG. 1. Silastic ovoid (Jarvik) type of artificial heart used in these experiments.

the study periods the calves received 100 percent oxygen to breathe. Whole blood was given to maintain hematocrits above 30 percent, and lactated Ringer's solution in dextrose 5 percent water (10 to 30 ml/kg) was used daily to augment their natural diet of hay and water. No anticoagulants were used postoperatively.

The Artificial Heart Driving System

An intrinsic system of atrial pressure control, which has been previously described (Kwan-Gett et al, 1968; Kwan-Gett et al, 1969), was used in all the experiments. Basically the control system consists of two direct-acting three-way solenoid valves that apply compressed air through two air

drive lines during systole and exhaust air to atmosphere during diastole. With this system, the rate and therefore the volume of blood entering each ventricle during the diastolic period increases with an increase in atrial pressure. This volume is expelled during the next ventricular systole. As filling of the ventricle diminishes so does stroke volume. There is thus an inherent balance between the pulmonic and systemic circulatory systems, and extremes of high and low atrial and venous pressures are avoided.

The control system is capable of independent frequency and percent systole regulation by two dials on the control module (Figs. 2 and 3). During this study the artificial hearts were operated at a frequency of 90 to 100 beats/minute and a percent systole, which ranged from 30 to 40 percent of the cardiac cycle. The control module also has independent right and left air drive line pressure dials that change the rate of rise of ventricular air pressures. Compressed air is brought from an air compressor to the control module standing next to the calf's pen. From the control module, compressed air is conveyed through the chest wall of the artificial heart recipient to the artificial ventricles by two ⅜-inch tygon tube air drive lines. This air is introduced between the rigid outer housing of the artificial heart and the softer, pliable inner blood containing chamber at pressures that can be adjusted by one of two (one for RV and one for LV) air pressure drive line dials on the module. Air pressures used to drive the heart are usually between one to three lbs/sq inch (PSI) in the right ventricle and three to six PSI in the left.

Study Procedures

In these experiments calves were studied two to 15 days after receiving their artificial hearts when cardiovascular dynamics were stable. Each animal's RV maximum (max) rate of pressure de-

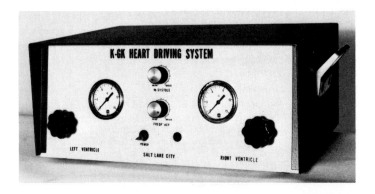

FIG. 2. Artificial heart control module.

FIG. 3. Artificial heart control module and compressed gas tank in cabinet below, which is used to power the artificial ventricles.

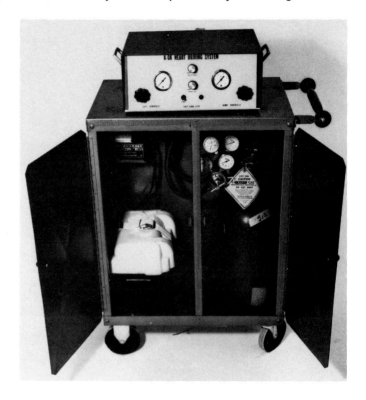

FIG. 3. Artificial heart control module and compressed gas tank in cabinet below, which is used to power the artificial ventricles.

velopment (dp/dt) was increased in increments of 100 to 250 mm Hg/sec from 300 to 6,100 mm Hg/sec by raising RV air drive line pressures in 0.1 to 0.3 PSI increments from 0.4 to 3.0 PSI. LV air driving pressures and max dp/dt's were maintained constant at 4.7 PSI and 2,800 to 3,200 mm Hg/sec respectively. Air driving pressures were sampled at the output portals of the control module and recorded along with pulmonary arterial and left atrial pressures on a Hewlett-Packard eight-channel recorder. Air drive line max dp/dt's were subsequently calculated by measuring the maximum slope of intraventricular pressure development during the isovolemic period of ventricular systole. Fifteen minutes after each change in RV max dp/dt samples of pulmonary arterial and left atrial blood were obtained for oxygen content analysis. Oxygen saturation was determined on an American Optical Company oximeter and pH and oxygen tension on a Radiometer digital acid-base analyzer. Rectal temperature was monitored with a Yellow Springs temperature probe and serum hemoglobin obtained from a Fisher Hemophotometer. Blood oxygen content was calculated from the hemoglobin concentration, pH, PO_2, and body temperature with a modified Sever-

inghaus slide rule and the pulmonary shunt obtained from the shunt equation as given below:

$$\frac{Q_S}{Q_T} = \frac{C_{AO_2} - C_{aO_2}}{C_{AO_2} - C_{VO_2}}$$

where Q_S = shunt blood flow
Q_T = total blood flow
C_{aO_2} = content of oxygen in 100 cc of arterial blood
C_{VO_2} = content of oxygen in 100 cc of mixed venous blood
C_{AO_2} = content of oxygen in 100 cc of end capillary blood (determined by subtracting alveolar pH_2O + PCO_2 + PN_2 from total atmospheric pressure)

RESULTS

Increases in RV max dp/dt resulted in progressive elevations in systolic, diastolic, and mean pulmonary artery pressures throughout the range of max dp/dt's studied (Fig. 4). The pulmonary shunt fraction was unaffected by RV max dp/dt

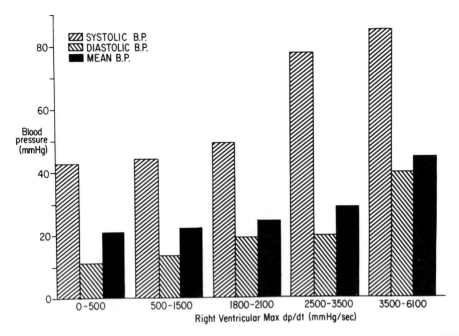

FIG. 4. Right ventricular max dp/dt vs pulmonary artery pressure in 10 calves with an artificial heart.

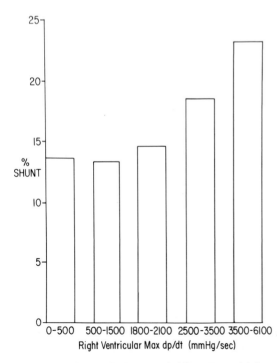

FIG. 5. Right ventricular max dp/dt vs percent intrapulmonary shunt in 10 calves.

changes between 300 to 1,800 mm Hg/sec, slightly increased by rises to 2,100 mm Hg/sec and significantly increased at all values > 2,100 mm Hg/sec (Fig. 5). With RV max dp/dt's between 2,500 and 3,500 mm Hg/sec the shunt fraction averaged 19.8 percent of the cardiac output, or 50 percent more than it did at dp/dt's between 1,400 and 1,800. With max dp/dt's between 3,500 to 6,100 mm Hg/sec the shunt fraction averaged 25.4 percent.

DISCUSSION

Although there are many reports of the effects of changes in ventilatory mechanics and patterns on the performance of the heart (Colgan et al, 1971; Colgan and Marocco, 1972; Cheney, 1973; Lysons and Cheney, 1972), the converse—that is, the effects of the heart on pulmonary function—has not been extensively investigated. One of the most important reasons for this is that, with the exception of cardiac rate, nonpharmacologic control of cardiac function is virtually impossible in the intact unanesthetized, close chest animal.

Furthermore, anesthesia, surgery, and cardiac dynamic changing pharmacologic agents all have direct effects on the pulmonary vascular system or tracheobronchial tree, which obscure their myocardial effects on pulmonary function (Nunn, 1964; Hillary et al, 1972; Marshall, 1964; Stone and Sullivan, 1972; Hickey et al, 1973; Colgan and Mahoney, 1969; Aviado, 1959; Muneyuki et al, 1971).

It is not surprising, therefore, that while some have found that increases or decreases in cardiac output, for example, result in corresponding changes in intrapulmonary shunting (Khambatta and Sullivan, 1973; Prys-Roberts et al, 1967; Lysons and Cheney, 1972; Cheney, 1973; Colgan et al, 1971), others have found the opposite (Modell and Milhorn, 1972; Stone and Sullivan, 1972; Marshall, 1966). Studies on the effects of positive inotropic agents on the pulmonary shunt fraction have been equally difficult to interpret (Fordham and Resnekov, 1968; Kreuzer, 1961; Tai and Read, 1967; Muneyuki et al, 1971; Silove et al, 1968). The obvious problem with all of the previous investigations is the inability to maintain stable control cardiopulmonary conditions while a change is made in a single cardiac parameter, ie, right ventricular contractility, left ventricular contractility, or cardiac output.

Recent progress in the design and development of an implantable, total artificial heart at the University of Utah may present a stable model to study some of the above problems (Stanley et al, 1973; Oster et al, 1975). Calves with their natural hearts removed and replaced with air-driven, pulsatile artificial hearts made of Silastic rubber now routinely survive between one and three weeks with normal body functions. These animals eat, drink, urinate, and defecate normally. They breathe room air, rarely require mechanical respiratory assistance, and with few exceptions have normal or close to normal cardiac outputs, arterial and venous blood gases, and spirometrically measured pulmonary function tests. They usually remain physiologically intact until a pulmonary or systemic embolus or massive infection overwhelms and kills them. Thus, they are very stable preparations for many days after their artificial heart is implanted. They are also very unique experimental animals because they are awake and functioning normally with artificial hearts, the dynamics of which can be selectively changed with the turn of a dial on the console standing next to the animal's pen. The artificial heart of course has no direct central nervous system connections and is unresponsive to drugs, hormones, and enzymes.

The results of this study, using our calf with

artificial heart model, indicate that in hearts with a fixed LV contractility or an inability to increase LV contractility, increases in RV contractility can significantly increase the intrapulmonary shunt fraction. This will increase the venous admixture of arterial blood, secondarily decrease coronary arterial oxygen content, and lead to myocardial hypoxia. A number of investigators have documented increases in the pulmonary shunt fraction after isoproterenol and other beta adrenergic agents (Kreuzer, 1961; Tai and Read, 1967; Muneyuki et al, 1971). Most have attributed this increase to a drug-induced alteration of ventilation-perfusion matching in the lung secondary to the drugs' effect on the pulmonary vasculature or bronchial smooth muscle. Our findings, while not denying this as a possible action, suggest that at least some component of the increase in shunt may be attributed to a comparable increase in right ventricular contractility. They also suggest that the artificial-heart-implanted animal model may be extremely important for further study and understanding of the complex interactions of the heart and lungs.

References

Aviado DM: Cardiovascular effects of some commonly used pressor amines. Anesthesiology 20:71, 1959

Cheney FW: The effects of tidal-volume change with positive end-expiratory pressure in pulmonary edema. Anesthesiology 37:600, 1973

Colgan FJ, Barrow RE, Fanning FL: Constant positive-pressure breathing and cardiorespiratory function. Anesthesiology 34:145, 1971

Colgan FJ, Mahoney EB: The effects of major surgery on cardiac output and shunting. Anesthesiology 31:213, 1969

Colgan FJ, Marocco PP: The cardiorespiratory effects of constant and intermittent positive-pressure breathing. Anesthesiology 36:444, 1972

Fordham RMM, Resnekov L: Arterial hypoxaemia. Thorax 23:19, 1968

Hickey RF, Visick WD, Fairley HB, Fourcade HE: The effects of Halothane anesthesia on functional residual capacity and alveolar-arterial oxygen tension difference. Anesthesiology 38:20, 1973

Hillary FD, Wahba WM, Craig DB: Airway closure, gas trapping and functional capacity during anesthesia. Anesthesiology 36:533, 1972

Khambatta HJ, Sullivan SF: Effects of respiratory alkalosis on oxygen consumption and oxygenation. Anesthesiology 38:53, 1973

Kreuzer F: Influence of catecholamines on arterial oxygen tension in anesthetized dogs. J Appl Physiol 16:1043, 1961

Kwan-Gett CS, Crosby MJ, Shoenberg A, Jacobsen SC, Kolff WJ: Control systems for artificial hearts. Trans Am Soc Artif Intern Organs 14:284, 1968

Kwan-Gett CS, Wu Y, Collan R, Jacobsen S, Kolff WJ: Total replacement artificial heart and driving system with inherent regulation of cardiac output. Trans Am Soc Artif Intern Organs 15:245, 1969

Lysons DF, Cheney FW: End-expiratory pressure in dogs with pulmonary edema breathing spontaneously. Anesthesiology 37:518, 1972

Marshall BE: Physiological shunting and deadspace during spontaneous respiration with Halothane-oxygen anesthesia and the influence of intubation on the physiological deadspace. Br J Anaesth 36: 327, 1964

Modell H, Milhorn H: Quantitation of factors affecting the alveolar-arterial PO_2 difference in thoracotomy. Anesthesiology 37:592, 1972

Muneyuki M, Urabe N, Kato H, et al: The effects of catecholamines on arterial oxygen tension and pulmonary shunting during the postoperative period in man. Anesthesiology 34:356, 1971

Nunn JF: Factors influencing the arterial oxygen tension during Halothane anesthesia wth spontaneous respiration. Br J Anaesth 36:327, 1964

Oster H, Olsen DB, Stanley TH, Volder J, Kolff WJ: Eighteen Days Survival with a Jarvic Type of Artificial Heart. Surgery 77:113, 1975

Prys-Roberts C, Kelman CR, Greenbaum RV: The influence of circulatory factors on arterial oxygenation during anesthesia in man. Anaesthesia 22:257, 1967

Silove ED, Inque T, Grove RF: Comparison of hypoxia, pH and sympathomimetic drugs on bovine pulmonary vasculature. J Appl Physiol 24:355, 1968

Stanley TH, Volder J, Kolff WJ: Extrinsic artificial heart control via mixed venous blood gas tension analysis. Trans Am Soc Artif Intern Organs 19:258, 1973

Stone JG, Sullivan SF: Halothane anesthesia and pulmonary shunting. Anesthesiology 37:258, 1972

Tai E, Read J: Response of blood gas tensions in aminophylline and isoprenaline in patients with asthma. Thorax 22:543, 1967

124

NUCLEAR-FUELED CIRCULATORY SUPPORT SYSTEMS
State of the Art

Fred N. Huffman, Kenneth G. Hagen, Benedict D. T. Daly,
Joseph J. Migliore, and John C. Norman

A totally implantable assist or total artificial heart should prove beneficial to a significant group of patients. For example, in the seven-year period between 1961 and 1968 at least 250,000 heart valves were implanted in patients in the United States alone.[24] These procedures were accompanied by operative and early mortalities between one and 10 percent. Implantable short, intermediate, and long-term assist or total cardiac prostheses could have lowered these mortalities appreciably.

A variety of energy sources such as biologic,[22,25] pneumatic,[6,20,31,45] electromagnetic,[1,8,29] and nuclear [37,46] are currently under evaluation. At the present, biologic fuel cell technology is not sufficiently advanced to permit its extrapolation to the power levels required for implantable circulatory support systems. Electromagnetic systems [4] have the disadvantage of requiring batteries of considerable bulk needing frequent recharging.[10,27,42] In comparison, radioisotope-fueled thermal engine systems [3,15,17,26,43,44,48] have the potential of ultimately providing prospective patients with untethered ranges of freedom not possible with pneumatic or rechargeable units. Radioisotope circulatory support systems will, however, subject their recipients to prolonged, low-level intracorporeal heat and radiation, minimally add to environmental background radiation, and constitute a small but finite hazard due to possible violation of fuel containment.[14] Our laboratories have been engaged for nearly a decade in the design, development and *in vivo* evaluations of nuclear-fueled circulatory support systems,[50] along with continued considerations of environmental, legal, social, and ethical aspects of their clinical use. This chapter summarizes some of the salient aspects of these studies and thoughts.

The development of a nuclear-fueled artificial heart requires the simultaneous resolution of a series of complex biomedical engineering, surgical, and cardiovascular physiologic problems within severe constraints of size and weight. The blood pump must provide adequate flow with antithrombogenicity and without hematologic damage. The power source to drive the blood pump must couple the radioisotope fuel capsule with a thermal engine and must be compact, reliable, and efficient. Heat rejected from the system must be dissipated by the body. The adjacent tissues must not be subjected to excessive temperature elevations or radiation. Moreover, the mechanical system must respond to physiologic demands.

The basic components of nuclear-fueled circulatory support systems [30] are a radioisotope heat source, a means of thermal insulation, a means of storing thermal energy, a thermal-to-mechanical converter (engine), a control unit, an actuator, and a blood pump. A genealogy of nuclear-fueled circulatory support systems is shown in Figure 1.

RADIOISOTOPE HEAT SOURCE [12,32,34,35,36,38,47]

Plutonium-238 (Pu-238) is the radioisotope of choice in all of the systems under development. It has a long half-life (89 years), an adequate power density (3.5 watt/cm^3), a low radiation output, an established containment technology, and a reasonable cost. The preferable fuel form is plutonium oxide, which has a high melting point (4,050° F) and is chemically and biologically inert. To minimize the probability of particulate inhalation if the encapsulation is compromised, the

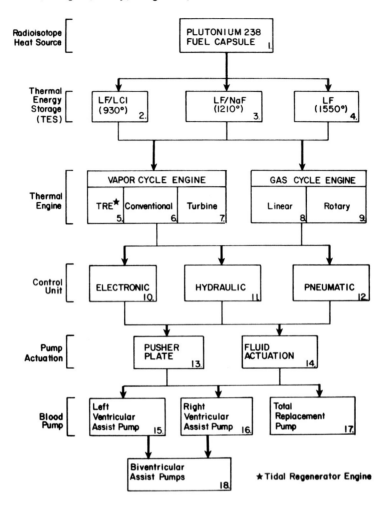

FIG. 1. Genealogy of nuclear-fueled circulatory support systems.

pellet is pressed and sintered. Enriching the plutonium oxide with Oxygen-16 diminishes generation of neutrons resulting from alpha bombardment of 0-17 and 0-18. The neutron dose rate can then be substantially reduced. Because Pu-238 is primarily an alpha emitter, its decay builds up a helium pressure inside a sealed capsule. The cumulative pressure and heat represents a containment problem. Consequently, to relieve the pressure, helium-vented fuel capsules that do not leak radioactivity are being developed.

MEANS OF THERMAL INSULATION (VACUUM FOIL) [40]

Most nuclear-fueled circulatory support systems employ heat source temperatures of approximately 1,000° F. Effective thermal insulation is required to minimize thermal losses and to protect the adjacent biologic tissues. Vacuum foil insulation is being utilized in all of the thermal engines currently under development. Such an insulation module consists of multiple metallic foils spaced in a vacuum canister. The foil layers (eg, titanium, copper, nickel, etc) are effective thermal radiation shields. The spacers are chosen as low thermal conductivity materials—eg, zirconia, silica, thoria, etc, in particle or fiber form. The vacuum environment eliminates gas conduction and convection. In effect, the vacuum foil insulation module functions as an 80-fold series of "Thermos" bottles, one within the other. Typically, the insulation heat loss with the engines at operating temperatures varies between five to 10 watts. Prototype units utilizing a variety of "getters," ie, materials that absorb and/or react with gases to maintain a high vacuum (as in electronic tubes), have not significantly degraded over test periods of two years.

MEANS OF THERMAL ENERGY STORAGE [4]

Thermal energy storage (TES) allows the fuel capsules to be structured for mean, rather than peak, power inputs. This results in decreased intracorporeal heat loads, radiation exposure, and cost. The TES material stores heat at high temperatures in the latent heat of fusion when the nuclear source thermal output exceeds the system consumption. Conversely, during periods of high activity, the molten TES material solidifies to provide the increased heat requirements of the engines.

Eutectic compositions of alkali-halide mixtures have been used because of high volumetric and gravimetric heat storage as well as melting points compatible with thermal engine design parameters. The temperature differentials required to melt the TES material or transfer heat from the TES material are usually less than 50 F. Compatibility tests of molten lithium halide salts in 304 stainless steel over two years have demonstrated the feasibility of storing heat by this technique.

THERMAL-MECHANICAL CONVERTERS (ENGINES) [15,30]

The thermal engines convert a fraction of the radioisotope decay heat into mechanical power (1.5 to 8 watts) to drive the blood pump. These miniature engines have volumes less than 500 ml and are either vapor or gas cyclical. In a vapor cycle engine (eg, a steam engine), the working fluid is alternately vaporized to provide high pressure (and work output) and condensed to give low pressure so that the components can be returned to their initial configurations. In a gas cycle engine (eg, a Stirling engine), the gas is periodically heated to give a high pressure and cooled to provide a low pressure.

Reversible gas cycle engines usually have higher theoretical efficiencies than vapor cycle engines. However, the vapor cycle engines have characteristics that allow comparable system efficiencies. The practical advantages of vapor cycle engines (high pressure differential, low compression work, and moderate operating temperatures) have resulted in wide application.

The developmental problems of the miniature engines used in artificial hearts have centered on minimizing pressure drops and void volumes

(empty spaces that are not necessary for engine function) while providing high heat fluxes. The small engine sizes require careful attention to restrict extraneous heat losses.

CONTROL UNITS [41]

The thermal engines can be coupled to the blood pump via hydraulic, pneumatic, or mechanical linkages. Most control units are interposed in this coupling circuit. Although assist and total heart systems differ in signal requirements and processing functions, the control logic of both types of systems are structured to pump all of the return flow over a wide range of physiologic demands. The assist control units are designed to counterpulse (ie, the mechanical pump ejects blood into the high pressure systemic circuit while the biologic heart fills). The biologic heart in systole ejects into the assist pump at low pressure, rather than through the aortic valve, regardless of heart rate or stroke volume. Logic units have been designed around electronic, hydraulic, and pneumatic components. Prototypes of all three of these types of logic systems have been tested *in vivo*. The fundamental control signal in all of the circulatory assist systems is the rate of change of blood filling the booster pump.

ACTUATORS

The blood pumps are usually actuated by either fluid pressure (pneumatic or hydraulic) or mechanically by pusher plates to collapse the pump chambers. Most pumps driven by an external console are actuated pneumatically. However, implantable pneumatic systems are hampered by problems of gas permeation, compressibility, lubrication, and heat transfer. These problems are eliminated or rendered more tractable with hydraulic actuation. One system under development (AEC/Westinghouse)[2,5,28] mechanically couples, via a flexible cable and Scotch yoke, the nuclear power source to the pusher plates of a total replacement pump.

BLOOD PUMPS

The blood pump can be an assist device (left ventricular [16,20] or right ventricular [21]) as well as a total replacement.[2] Because the left ventricle performs approximately 80 percent of the total work

TABLE 1. System Identification: Nuclear Artificial Hearts

AGENCY	FACILITY	SUBSYSTEM OPTIONS						STATUS
		Heat Source	TES	Engine	Controls	Actuator	Pump	
United States								
NHLI	Thermo-Electron	1	2	5	10	13	15	*In vivo* evaluations
NHLI	McDonnell-Douglas	1	3	8	11	13	15	*In vivo* evaluations
NHLI	Aerojet	1	3	8	12	13	15	*In vivo* evaluations
NHLI	ARCO	1	4	6	10	13	17	*In vitro* tests
NHLI	TRW	1	–	7	10	13	15	*In vitro* tests
AEC	Westinghouse	1	–	9	–	13	17	*In vitro* tests
West Germany								
–	Messerschmitt	1	–	8	–	–	–	

of the heart, major efforts have been focused on implantable left ventricular assist pumps. Biventricular systems utilizing a combination of left ventricular and right ventricular assist pumps can functionally replace the biologic heart. Blood compatibility (antithrombogenicity without denaturing or damaging protein and cellular elements) of prosthetic materials represents a fundamental and difficult set of incompletely understood problems. It involves a combination of fluid flow patterns, material properties, surface finishes, electrophysical factors, and blood chemistry. Thus far, the most successful pumps have used textured surfaces (flock or velour) upon which a biologic lining forms. A viable neointima can subsequently develop on the predominantly fibrin substrate.

It is evident that many combinations of the components of totally implantable assist or replacement options are possible. The subsystem identifications of the major efforts are summarized in Table 1.

Tidal Regenerator Engine Circulatory Assist System [9,15]

As an example of totally implantable nuclear-fueled systems, the tidal regenerator engine (TRE) circulatory assist system can be described in detail. Basically this implantable nuclear-fueled system converts a fraction of the decay heat from a 50-watt Pu-238 heat source into hydraulic power for driving a blood pump by means of a miniature steam engine (TRE). This system was the first to undergo *in vivo* testing. It has subsequently operated for a period of four-and-a-half days *in vivo*.

An idealized diagram of the TRE circulatory assist system is illustrated in Figure 2. The function of this system is to assume a large fraction of the work of the biologic heart by means of an assist pump connected between the apex of the left ventricle and the thoracic aorta. This assist pump removes the entire cardiac output from the left ventricle at low pressure ($\sim$30 mm Hg) and elevates it in pressure to perfuse the systemic circulation, ejecting during left ventricular diastole.

Pusher-Plate Left Ventricular Assist Pump

This left ventricular assist pump is designed for coupling to nuclear-fueled power sources and functions as a blood-cooled heat exchanger, a sensor for the control logic, and an integral pressure-volume transformer. An illustration of the pump used with the current nuclear power sources is shown in Figure 3. The entire surface of the pump, that comes in contact with the blood is flocked with polyester fibrils to promote the formation of a blood-compatible biologic lining. The pumping chamber is pancake-shaped. The upper surface of the bladder rolls under the action of the pusher-plate, attached to the integral pressure-volume transformer to propel the blood through the outlet tricuspid valve to the descending thoracic aorta. The bladder is designed to minimize stress and compliance as it is collapsed by the pusher-plate. It is fabricated from 1-mm-thick dacron-reinforced Silastic.

The nonflexing common wall between the blood and the plenum (filled with hydraulic fluid) is used for transferring heat, rejected from the nuclear energy system, from the hydraulic drive fluid into the blood. In this manner, the bladder is not subjected to significant temperature rises, and the parallel thermal path transfers most of the heat through a metal wall to the blood instead of through the elastomer bladder. Polyurethane foam is used to insulate thermally the heat exchanger plenum from the biologic left hemidiaphragm. A pressure-volume transformer is contained within the pump in such a manner that the volume swept by the transformer is the same as

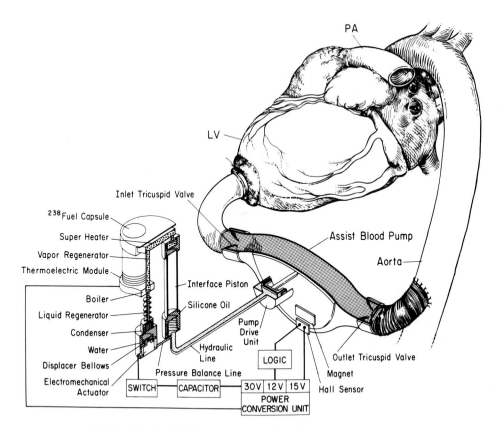

FIG. 2.   Idealized tidal regenerator engine circulatory assist system.

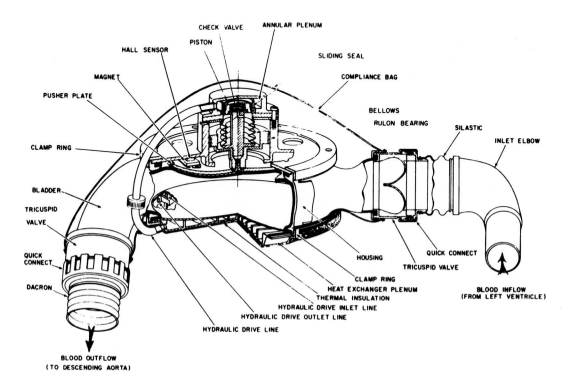

FIG. 3.   Cutaway drawing of the pusher-plate left ventricular assist pump.

that displaced by the collapsing bladder of the blood pump.

In addition, a Hall effect sensor, which provides a signal proportional to the magnetic field from a small permanent magnet attached to the pusher-plate, is mounted on the drive unit. Position as a function of time constitutes adequate information for counterpulsation control.

Tidal Regenerator Engine (TRE) [17]

This mechanically simple thermal engine does not contain valves or sliding seals. It is a vapor cycle analog of the regenerative gas cycle engine, which has characteristics in common with the Rankine and Stirling engines (eg, a boiler, condenser, and superheater similar to the Rankine engine and a displacer, vapor regenerator, and power piston similar to the Stirling engine). In addition, it has unique components, such as a liquid regenerator and an interface piston. As in the Stirling engine, there are only small differential pressures throughout regardless of wide pressure fluctuations. Unlike the Stirling engine, the tidal regenerator engine utilizes a liquid-to-vapor phase change that enables a small volume of working fluid to provide a high-pressure differential output with a moderate heat source temperature. As in the Rankine engine, the pressure work is low. Reliability is enhanced by the low speed (biologic heart rate) and moderate temperature operation. The engine supplies power at nearly constant pressure as needed for driving the blood pump without an intermediate hydraulic accumulator. This engine is also insensitive to spatial orientation.

Other than the liquid regenerator and condenser, all of the engine components that contact the vapor are maintained above the saturation temperature corresponding to the maximum engine pressure. The pressure throughout the engine corresponds to the temperature at the coldest point in the engine, which is always at the interface between the liquid and vapor phases (ie, pressure in the engine follows the temperature of the liquid vapor interface, which equilibrates to the temperature of the adjacent structures). Otherwise stated, this means that the engine can be controlled with the small energy required to displace a single drop of water from the condenser to the boiler. Because the engine utilizes a phase transition, less than 0.02 ml of water need be vaporized and condensed to vary the system pressure between 5 and 150 PSIA. Inasmuch as the engine is pressure balanced, only modest energy expenditure is required to displace the working fluid. This

makes the engine particularly suitable for electromechanical actuation. The tidal regenerator engine has achieved a cycle efficiency of 10 percent at a hydraulic output of 7 watts. Continued development of the single fluid, non-expanding engine is expected to yield cycle efficiencies up to 14 percent.

A binary version of the engine using both Dowtherm A and water working fluids is under development. The binary TRE has the potential to attain cycle efficiencies in the range of 20 to 30 percent. The binary TRE consists of two coupled engines so that the heat rejected from the high temperature engine (using Dowtherm A as the working fluid) is reused at a lower temperature by the lower temperature steam engine. Fundamentally, the binary efficiency is improved by elevating the effective temperature at which heat is added.

ELECTRONIC LOGIC

Electronic actuation gives this system the capability of synchronizing with the biologic heart in a counterpulsation mode regardless of biologic left ventricular rate and stroke volume. The Hall effect sensor mounted inside the pusher-plate left ventricular assist device provides an electric signal that is a function of pumping chamber position. To identify the times of pump filling and ejection, the Hall signal is interrogated by complementary metal oxide semiconductor (MOS) logic, which functions at very low power levels. Binary integrated circuits (flip-flops) whose output potentials are reversed by a pulse, are used for logic and memory. In addition to counterpulsing the engine from a normal input from the Hall effect sensor, the electronic logic circuitry has the capability of maintaining engine function when these signals may be lost. In this event, an interval timer triggers the pulsing circuit if the position sensor does not provide the expected signal within an arbitrary time span. As a result, the system will operate at a nearly fixed beat rate if no signals are received from the position sensor. A capacitor discharge energizes the electromechanical actuator, which may be either a binary solenoid or a miniature electric motor. Both have been used in *in vivo* and *in vitro* testing. The polarity of the current is reversed with each pulse by a solid-state reversing switch.

THERMOELECTRIC MODULE

The electrical power for the Hall sensor,

electronic logic and electromechanical actuator is provided by a thermoelectric module placed in thermal series with the superheater (900 F) and boiler (380 F) of the engine. The boiler heat, which is several times the magnitude of that of the superheater would normally be in a conventional steam engine degraded in temperature and in availability to perform work by the engine structure. In this system, however, the boiler heat is degraded through the thermoelectric module producing electricity to power the control logic virtually free from additional thermal input, ie, since the heat rejected from the cold junctions in the modules is reused in the boiler, the additional heat needed for the electrical requirements is less than 1 watt. On this basis, the control logic efficiency is higher than 95 percent. The electrical output from 39 bismuth telluride thermocouples in the thermoelectric unit is approximately 300 milliwatts at design temperature.

The Hall effect sensor requires approximately 50 milliwatts at 1.5 volts; the MOS logic consumes approximately 10 milliwatts at 12 volts. The logic power consumption, independent of the electromechanical actuation, is approximately 25 milliwatts. The actuator power consumption is proportional to biologic left ventricular rate. The total electrical power requirements vary from approximately 125 milliwatts at 60 beats per minute to 225 milliwatts at 120 beats per minute. The thermoelectric module delivers approximately 300 milliwatts (electrical) and 25 watts (thermal) to the boiler. Since the load potential of the thermoelectric module is 0.8 volts, a power conditioner unit must provide an output of 1.5 volts to the Hall effect sensor and a 12-volt output to the MOS logic and torque motor. The required pulse polarity reversal is achieved by a solid-state switch.

Binary pulse solenoids producing linear displacement and torque motors producing rotary displacement have been utilized as electromechanical actuators for displacing the water droplet for pressurization of the engine. In both instances, energy is utilized only during armature displacement. The direction of movement of the solenoid or the torque motor is dependent on polarity.

FUEL CAPSULE

The 50-watt Pu-238 fuel capsule is 1.28 inches in diameter, is 2.0 inches in length, and has a mass of 472 grams. The capsule temperature is approximately 1,000 F during typical engine operation. The 124 grams of substoichiometric ($PuO_{1.8}$) plutonium oxide fuel is pressed and sintered to 77 percent of theoretical density. A low neutron emission rate of 2.9×10^5 neutron/sec (corresponding to 2,720 neutrons/sec-gm Pu) is achieved by enriching the plutonia with Oxygen-16. The fuel pellet is triply encapsulated in tantalum, T-111, and Platinum-20 percent Rhodium. This heat source is designed to survive a maximum credible accident (2,400 F temperature) within five years after encapsulation.

Capsule qualification tests included (1) internal pressure (up to 6,000 psi at 2,300 F), (2) external pressure (3,000 psi for 15 min) (3) crush (20,000 lb for one hour), (4) impact (120 ft-lb), (5) puncture (44 fps onto ⅛ inch diameter pin), and (6) shear (10,000 lb for 1 hour), as well as (7) fire/corrosion, (8) thermal shock, (9) free drop, (10) water immersion, and (11) thermal exposure.

IN VIVO EVALUATIONS [7,13,49]

A representative TRE circulatory support system, prior to implantation, is shown in Figure 4. Polyurethane foam encases the power source. The metal tube and valve shown are used to evacuate and refill the system with xenon after the fuel capsule has been inserted and the unit sealed. The tube is subsequently occluded and covered with rapid-setting silicone rubber. The coiled umbilical cable is utilized to monitor the parameters of the system and is maintained transcutaneously for the duration of the experiment. The left ventricular assist pump is coupled to the TRE power source by hydraulic lines and a signal cable to the control logic. Initially, the pump is connected to a miniloop circuit that acts as a load and heat dissipater because the system must operate after insertion of the fuel capsule until the pump is operating in the calf.

The implantation procedure requires three incisions. The heart and descending thoracic aorta are exposed through a left thoracotomy. A left flank incision is extended toward the left upper quadrant for placement of the power source in the left retroperitoneal space and a small diaphragmatic incision allows insertion of the mini-loop and pump through the abdominal incision into the left hemithorax while the system is operating. Following implantation of the total system, the left hemidiaphragmatic leaf is repaired, the energy system is securely suspended from the left psoas tendon and the left ventricular assist pump is positioned on the left hemidiaphragm within the

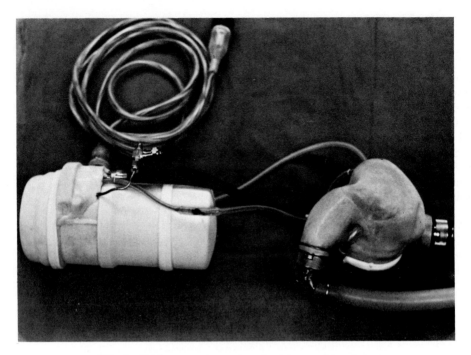

FIG. 4. Tidal regenerator engine circulatory assist system.

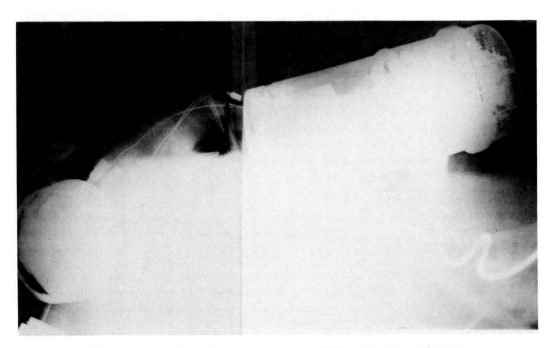

FIG. 5. X-ray of calf showing the position of the TRE power source and pump.

thoracic cavity. The TRE is then briefly stopped, the mini-loop is removed, and the pump is re-charged with saline.

The outflow tube from the pump is attached by means of a quick-connect coupling to a dacron graft sutured to the descending thoracic aorta. The inflow tube of the pump is inserted into the left ventricular apex and secured with a previously sutured dacron cuff. After the pump is connected, the engine is restarted and assist pumping ini-tiated. A X-ray of a calf standing postoperatively is shown in Figure 5. The printed circuit board of this control logic inside the TRE power source is evident.

Aside from programed interruptions to evalu-ate effectiveness, the system has synchronized with the biologic heart throughout the experiments. All temperatures have remained in an acceptable range and the rectal temperatures of the calves have re-mained within normal limits. Over the course of a 4.5 day study, there was no evidence of system malfunction until the pump drive bellows failed.

A representative data tracing obtained dur-ing an operative procedure following implantation is shown in Figure 6. This demonstrates lowering of peak systolic left ventricular pressure with the TRE system operating in a counterpulse mode. Synchronization of the system with the biologic heart without the use of EKG signals is evident by comparing the EKG with the engine pressure and pump displacement traces. The stroke volume of this nuclear-fueled circulatory support system during these studies was approximately 65 ml. At a biologic heart rate of 83 bpm, the pump output was approximately 5.4 liters per minute. Following transfer to the intensive care unit, this calf rapidly recovered, and its stroke volume exceeded that of the pump.

Blood gas measurements, pulmonary arterio-venous admixture, and compliance were serially measured.[13] Supportive respiratory therapy was varied and modified according to these results. A

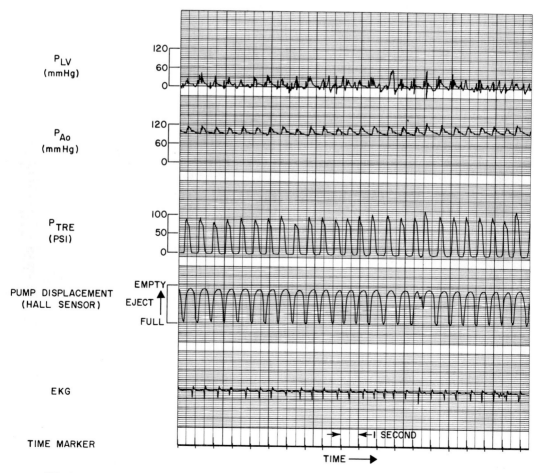

FIG. 6. TRE circulatory assist system performance. Note reduction of left ventricular pressure.

tracheostomy was performed. Weaning from the respirator was initiated on the first postoperative day by allowing the animal to breathe spontaneously with humidified oxygen for 15 minutes each hour. The length of this interval was increased to 30 minutes each hour on the third postoperative day. Supplemental volumes of fluid replacement (400 ml/hr) have been required to offset dehydration and hypovolemia, particularly during implantation and early postoperative periods. Decreasing fluid requirements on the third and fourth postoperative days have reflected stabilization and fluid mobilization from third spaces. Antibiotics have been administered in the immediate postoperative period and stopped on the third day because of possible adverse effects on gastrointestinal flora. Heparin has not been used as an anticoagulant. Rather, 1,000 ml of low molecular weight dextran is administered in daily aliquots. There has been no leukocytosis, and blood cultures obtained daily have been negative for significant growth. Approximately 50 watts of additional heat have been dissipated intracorporeally, and the plasma hemoglobin levels have remained below 10 milligrams percent. During the entire observation periods, the rectal temperatures have remained within normal limits. The most recent experiment was terminated when the bellows in the pump driver failed. This failure occurred in the bellows diaphragm rather than in the peripheral weld area. An improved design is being developed to increase the margin of safety in order to meet an "infinite" life criteria.

There was no evidence of thrombus within the pump at sacrifice. This observation is particularly significant in view of the avoidance of heparin and the utilization of dextran as an anticoagulant. A neointima developed within the pump over the four day observation period (Fig. 7). The thickness varied from approximately 200 microns to 500 microns. Elongated, fibroblast-like cells with lymphocyte-like nuclei suggested the origin of the neointima that developed in the presence of heat to be from circulating white blood cell types.

An unexpected finding associated with this most recent *in vivo* experiment was the discovery of a black powder on the fuel capsule when the TRE power source was opened to remove the Pu-238 heat source. Post-test investigations revealed that the material resulted from the catalytic carburization of ethylene oxide and/or its decomposition products. The ethylene oxide gas was absorbed from fiber thermal insulation during sterilization and was incompletely removed during subsequent vacuum cycles. The catalyst was the platinum-rhodium outer cladding of the heat source. Although this phenomenon does not represent a radiologic hazard, methods are under evaluation to eliminate the powder formation. A summary of NHLI nuclear-fueled circulatory assist system *in vivo* evaluations in our laboratories is given in Table 2. This tabulation indicates the increased system longevities with experience. There has been an attendant improvement in system-pumping capability.

INTRACORPOREAL HEAT

The feasibility of implantable nuclear-fueled circulatory support systems depends on the ability

TABLE 2. NHLI Nuclear-Fueled Circulatory Assist System Implantations[a]

IMPLANT DATE	CALF	CONTRACTOR	IMPLANT PERIOD (hrs)	SYSTEM FAILURE	ANIMAL CONDITION
14 Feb 72	28	Thermo-Electron	8	Kinked inflow tube	Good
17 Mar 72	30	McDonnell-Douglas	1	Overflow valve	Good
17 May 72	3	Thermo-Electron	7	Thermal instability	Good
31 May 72	31	McDonnell-Douglas	7	Overflow valve	Good
21 Feb 73	H-117	McDonnell-Douglas	12	Entrained gas in hydraulic system	Good
1 Mar 73	H-118	Aerojet	9	Thermal management induce fibrillation	Thermal injury
7 Mar 73	H-122	Thermo-Electron	112	Pump drive bellows leak	Good
16 Apr 73	H-125	Aerojet	73[b]	Foil insulation vacuum seal broken	Good
30 Apr 73	H-119	McDonnell-Douglas	29	Animal sacrificed	Pneumonitis
4 May 73	H-128	McDonnell-Douglas	5	Animal failure	Tachycardia
4 Dec 73	H-186	Aerojet	74[b]	Actuator bellows leak	Good
11 Dec 73	H-185	Aerojet	175[b]	Actuator bellows leak	Pulmonary edema

[a]*Cardiovascular Surgical Research Laboratories, THI.*
[b]*Externally cooled.*

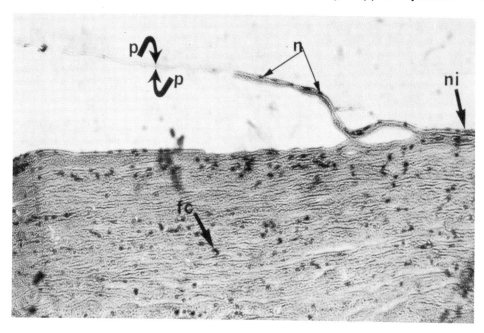

FIG. 7. Light photomicrograph (original magnification ×500) of the neointima (ni) and underlying tissue. The nuclei (n) of endothelial-like cells are seen on the neointima surface. Beneath this layer of cells are the densely staining, pyknotic nuclei of fibrocytes (fc) enmeshed in a fibrin mass. Part of the epithelial surface has torn away from the neointima proper during tissue preparation. This fortuitous artefact allows for the clear demonstration of the elongated, fibroblast-like cytoplasm (p), which extends laterally between adjacent neointimal nuclei.

of the body to dissipate the reject heat from the power source driving the blood pump.[39] In parallel experiments, we are studying the effects of intracorporeal nuclear radiation and additional thermal loads in experimental animals. These studies are a continuation of initial canine investigations using electrical heat exchangers[11,40] and subsequent efforts utilizing heat exchangers energized by 16- and 24-watt Pu-238 capsules.[18,23,33] The effects of RES (radiation equivalent source) -24 capsules that simulate the neutron and gamma radiation environments from 24-watt Pu-238 heat sources have been evaluated in dogs. The neutron source is Americium-241/Beryllium and the photon (gamma) course is the bremsstrahlung from Strontium-90 beta emission. More recently, RES-50 capsules that simulate the radiation dose rates from 50-watt Pu-238 heat sources have been implanted in primates. The RES-50 capsules also simulate the shape and density of a half-scale power source for driving a blood pump. They have been implanted retroperitoneally in the left lower quadrant and suspended from the psoas tendon.

A summary of the radioisotope-bearing animals is given in Table 3. Because of the limited number of animals and the restricted test periods,

TABLE 3. Dose Rates from Prototype Nuclear-Fueled Circulatory Assist System[a]

DISTANCE IN AIR FROM SURFACE OF POWER SOURCE (cm)	GAMMA PLUS NEUTRON DOSE RATES (through midplane of fuel capsule)	
	Maximum (mrem/hr)	Maximum (mrem/hr)
0	175	50
10	40	13
30	10	4
50	3.9	1.7
100	0.6	0.4

[a]The fuel capsule is not axially symmetric with the power source.

the conclusions thus far drawn from these studies are tentative. However, the long-term survivals in good condition of both Pu-238- and RES-implanted dogs and primates is encouraging. It appears that these experimental animals adjust their temperature regulation mechanisms to dissipate up to 0.5 watt/kilogram of additional heat without significant elevations in temperatures.

RADIOLOGIC CONSIDERATIONS [14,19]

Radiation exposure guidelines involve philosophy as well as physics and biology. As with other aspects of nuclear energy application, it is unreasonable to insist on no risk in the development and application of nuclear-fueled artificial internal organs that may have the potential for significant benefits. A search for totally riskless solutions usually leads to immobility. Therefore, decisions to proceed with the development of totally implantable nuclear-fueled circulatory support systems involve evaluations of the benefits in comparison with the risks. It is assumed that these judgments will be made on the bases comparable to those that have established the present permissible ionizing radiation levels in national security, occupational, general population, medical, educational, and television-viewing exposures.

The measured dose rates * (neutron plus gamma) from these circulatory assist systems are given in Table 3. These measurements were taken through the midplane of the 50-watt Pu-238 fuel capsule.

The radioisotope-bearing animals listed in Table 4 were exposed to dose rates higher than the dose rates listed in Table 3. Serial hematologic and metabolic data have ranged within normal values. In no instance was the demise of an animal attributable to radiation exposure. Postmortem examination has revealed possible radiation effects

---

* The basic unit of absorbed dose for ionizing radiation is the rad (Radiation Absorbed Dose). A dose of one rad indicates the absorption of 100 ergs of radiation per gram of absorbing material (1 millirad equals 1 mrad equals 0.001 in the space rad). A roentgen, or r, is defined only for x or gamma rays, which will deposit almost one rad in tissue (1 milliroentgen = 1 mr − 0.001 r). Some types of radiation, such as neutrons, induce a much more pronounced biologic response than x or gamma radiation for the same rad dose. The unit that accounts for the biologic response difference is the rem (Radiation Equivalent Man) (1 millirem equals 1 mrem equals 0.001 rem).

within a few centimeters of the sources. No evidence of radiation-induced neoplasms has been found. These results are in agreement with a related study sponsored by the United States Atomic Energy Commission. All recent lymphocyte cultures have indicated normal chromosomal morphology.

As previously indicated, radioisotope circulatory support systems have the potential for providing their projected recipients with degrees of freedom that cannot be achieved with pneumatically driven or electrically rechargeable units. Society allows and accepts options of statistically shortened life spans associated with hazardous occupations. It is reasonable and possible that it would also allow individuals bearing nuclear-fueled artificial internal organs the option of leading possibly statistically shorter but more meaningful lives, assuming that the risks are comparable to others accepted daily (eg, those associated with the use of automobiles, airplanes, electricity, pharmaceuticals, etc). It is probable that the possible genetic consequences would be acceptable provided that the radiation dose to the reproductive organs in the general population would be only a small fraction (eg, 1/100) of that due to natural background radiation.

The following tentative conclusions are supported by the available radiobiologic data, dose rate projections, ambient environmental radiation analyses, current radiation exposure guidelines, and fuel capsule containment studies:

1. The potential benefits of radioisotope-fueled circulatory support systems seem to outweigh the somatic radiation hazards.

2. The age distribution of the patient group should be such that the question of genetic effects to progeny will be, for the most part, rhetorical. For those individuals within the usual ages for fostering and child-bearing, the genetic risk may be appreciable enough that it would not be socially responsible to consider parenthood.

3. The somatic and genetic effects from the radiation of an encapsulated nuclear-fueled source to a patient's family, associates, and the general population do not appear to be a deterrent.

4. The primary problem of large-scale deployment of radioisotope-powered circulatory support systems is that of assuring fuel containment under all credible conditions. This will entail a great deal more analysis, design, and testing.

TABLE 4. Summary of Radioisotope-Bearing Animals

SPECIES	IDENTIFI-CATION	RADIO-ISOTOPE CAPSULE	IMPLANT SITE	SEX	IMPLANT DURATION (mos)[a]	STATUS
Dog	Plutina	16-W-Pu-238	Chest	F	25	Died (pulmonary embolus)
Dog	Wolf	24-W-Pu-238	Chest	M	26	Sacrificed
Dog	3403	RES-24	Chest	M	66	Alive and well
Dog	3308	RES-24	Chest	F	59	Died (infection-clostridium)
Dog	4172	RES-24	Abdomen	M	38	Died (pneumonia)
Dog	5932	RES-24	Abdomen	F	7	Died (sepsis)
Baboon	761-70	RES-50	Abdomen	M	31	Alive and well
Baboon	143-71	RES-50	Abdomen	M	18	Died (peritonitis)
Chimpanzee	191-71	RES-50	Abdomen	M	20	Died (sigmoid diverticulitis)
Baboon	1560	RES-50	Abdomen	M	11	Alive and well
Baboon	1190	RES-50	Abdomen	M	9	Alive and well
Baboon	H-159	RES-50	Abdomen	M	8	Alive and well
Baboon	H-160	RES-50	Abdomen	M	8	Alive and well

[a]Reference December 1973.

SUMMARY

Nuclear-fueled artificial hearts have reached the stage of *in vivo* evaluations. From the perspective of what remains to be accomplished before a nuclear-powered circulatory support system can be utilized clinically, it is clear that a great deal more work will be required. However, considered from the perspective of where these efforts were only a few years ago, substantial progress has been made. The current technology permits critical problems to be studied *in vitro* and *in vivo* in the context of complete systems.

GLOSSARY

Binary solenoid: A linear electromagnetic actuator whose armature is held in either of two positions by a permanent magnet after its translations.

Boiler: A heat exchanger for vaporizing the working fluid.

Cold junction: The junction between the dissimilar legs of a thermocouple, which is maintained at a low temperature relative to the hot junction.

Compression work: The work that must be supplied to the engine at the end of stroke to return it to the beginning-of-stroke configuration.

Displacer: Device that transfers the position of a fluid volume.

Dowtherm A: A fluorocarbon liquid with thermodynamic properties that are suitable for the second stage of a binary tidal regenerator engine.

Electromechanical actuator: Unit that converts electrical energy to mechanical energy (eg, solenoid or torque motor).

Eutectic: The composition of a mixture that has the lowest melting point.

Flip flops: Binary integrated circuits whose output potentials are reversed by a pulse.

Flock: A matted surface formed by attaching fibers with an adhesive.

Gas cycle: A thermodynamic engine in which power is extracted from a gas that is alternately heated and cooled.

Hall sensor: A sensor that provides a signal output proportional to the magnetic field.

Hydraulic accumulator: A compliant structure for reversibly storing and supplying hydraulic power.

Interface piston: High-thermal impedance piston that isolates the hot vapor from the cold liquid.

Liquid regenerator: Structure for improving thermodynamic cycle efficiency by storing heat from the liquid during depressurization for reuse during pressurization.

MOS logic: Metal-Oxide-Semiconductor electronics that function at very low power levels.

Phase transition: A change of physical state (eg, liquid-to-vapor).

Power piston: Piston for extracting the power output of the engine to a mechanical load.

Pressure balanced: A pneumatic/hydraulic configuration such that the pressure throughout the system is uniform.

Pressure-volume-transformer: A mechanism of converting a high pressure, small displacement into a low-pressure, large displacement.

Saturation temperature: The temperature at which a pure liquid in equilibrium with its vapor will have a given pressure.

Scotch yoke: A cam-driven mechanical linkage that translates circular motion into alternate right and left motions.

Stirling: A gas cycle engine invented by Robert Stirling in 1817.

Substoichiometric ($PuO_{1.8}$): Found to be a more chemically inert substance than true stoichiometric (PuO_2) plutonium dioxide.

Superheater: A heat exchanger for heating a vapor above its saturation temperature.

T-111: A high-strength, high-temperature alloy of tungsten, tantalum, and niobium.

Thermoelectric module: Converter of thermal-to-electrical energy using series connected thermocouples.

Thermal series: Sequential heat flow (as opposed to parallel flow) through stated components.

Vapor cycle: A thermodynamic engine in which power is extracted from a working fluid that is alternately vaporized and condensed.

Vapor regenerator: Structure for improving thermodynamic cycle efficiency by storing heat from the vapor during depressurization for reuse during pressurization.

Working fluid: The fluid in the engine that undergoes cyclic vaporization and condensation.

References

1. Altieri FD, Kudrick JA: Implantable electrical power source for an artificial heart system. Trans Am Nuclear Soc 13:505, 1970
2. Backman DK, Donovan FM, Sandquist G, Kessler T, Kolff WJ: The design and evaluation of ventricles for the AEC artificial heart nuclear power source. Trans Am Soc Artif Intern Organs, 1973, pp 542–52
3. Blair MG, Purdy DL: Preliminary developments of an implanted Rankine steam conversion system for circulatory support. Sixth Intersociety Energy Conversion Engineering Conference Proceedings: 299–309, 1971
4. Bluestein M, Huffman F: Development of a heat source for an implantable circulatory support power supply. Proceedings of the Artificial Heart Program Conference, RJ Hegyeli, ed. Washington, DC, US Government Printing Office, 1969, p 1037
5. Cole DW, Holman WS, Mott WE: Status of the USAEC's nuclear-powered artificial heart. Trans Am Soc Artif Intern Organs, 1973, pp 537–41
6. Coleman S, Whalen R, Robinson W, Huffman F, Norman J: A preclinical drive console for a pneumatically-powered left ventricular assist device. Clin Res 20(5):854, 1972
7. Daly BDT, Robinson WJ, Migliore JJ, Dove GB, Edmonds CH, Fuqua JM, Huffman FN, Norman JC: Implantable nuclear-fueled circulatory support systems VI: respiratory management and avoidance of bovine respiratory distress syndrome. Proc 26th ACEMB, Minneapolis, 1973, p 357
8. Fraim FW, Huffman FN: Performance of a tuned ferrite core transcutaneous transformer. IEEE Trans Biomed Eng 18:352–59, 1971
9. Hagen KG, Ruggles AE, Huffman FN, Daly BDT, Migliore JJ, Norman JC: Nuclear fueled circulatory support systems VIII: status of the tidal regenerator engine system. Proc of the Intersociety Engine Conversion Engineering Conference, Philadelphia, 1973
10. Hamlen RP, Siwek EG, Rampel G, Wechsler LD: Internal energy storage for circulatory assist devices. Chapter 86 in RJ Hegyeli (ed): Artificial Heart Program Conference Proceedings. Washington, DC, US Government Printing Office, 1969
11. Harvey RJ, Robinson TC, McCandless W, Bernhard WF, Bankole MA, Norman JC: Studies related to heat transfer and flow in an aortic prosthesis. Digest of the Seventh International Conference on Medicine and Biological Engineering, 1967, p 389
12. Harvey RJ, Robinson TC, Bernhard WF, Norman JC, van Someren L, LaFarge CG: Evaluation of the Rankine steam cycle as a power source for a portable artificial heart. Proceedings of Biomedical Engineering Symposium Progress in Biomedical Engineering. Ed, LJ Fogel, FW George Washington, DC, Spartan Books, 1967, pp 259–69
13. Huffman FN, Daly BDT, Hagen KG, Migliore JJ, Robinson WJ, Ruggles AE, Norman JC: An implantable nuclear-fueled circulatory support system. V: acute physiologic analyses. International Cardiovascular Society Proceedings, Barcelona, 1973
14. Huffman FN, Norman JC: Nuclear-fueled cardiac pacemakers. Chest 65:667–72, 1974
15. Huffman FN, Hagen KG, Ruggles AE, Harmison LT: Performance of a nuclear-fueled circulatory assist system utilizing a tidal regenerator engine. Seventh Intersociety Energy Conversion Engineering Conference Proceedings. 771–77, 1972
16. Huffman FN, Harmison LT, Whalen RL, Bornhorst WJ, Molokhia FA, Norman JC: A direct actuation left ventricular assist device (LVAD) suitable for integrating into a totally implantable system. Clin Res 19:710, 1971
17. Huffman FN, Coleman SJ, Bornhorst WJ, Harmison LT: A nuclear powered vapor cycle heart assist System. Sixth Intersociety Energy Conversion Engineering Conference Proceedings, 277–87, 1971
18. Huffman FN, Covelli VH, Sandberg G, Lee R, Norman JC: Studies of reject heat and radiation from implanted radioisotope sources. ASME 68-WA/ENER-11, 1968
19. Hughes DA, Edmonds CH, Huffman FN, Norman JC: Nuclear-fueled circulatory support systems:

9: histopathologic effects of chronic intracorporeal heat and radiation. Proceedings of 6th Congress of the Organ Transplantation Society, Varese, 1974 (in press)

20. Hughes DA, Edmonds CH, Igo SR, Daly BDT, Norman JC: An abdominal left ventricular assist device: experimental physiologic analyses. J Surg Res 17:255, 1974

21. LaFarge CG, Bankole M, Bernhard WF: Physiological evaluation of chronic right ventricular bypass. Circ (Suppl I) 43 and 44, 1971

22. Lahoda J, Liu CC, Wingard LB: Electrochemical evaluation of the activity of glucose oxidase immobilized by various methods. Seventh Intersociety Energy Conversion Engineering Conference Proceedings. 740–44, 1972

23. Liss RH, Huffman FN, Warren S, Norman JC: Electron microscopy and thermal analysis of neointima heated and irradiated in vivo for two years. Ann Thorac Surg 12:251, 1971

24. Magovern GJ: Letters. Science, vol 183:4121:149, 1974

25. Malachesky P, Holleck G, McGovern F, Devarakonda R: Parametric studies of the implantable fuel cell. Seventh Intersociety Energy Conversion Engineering Conference Proceedings. 727–32, 1972

26. Martini WR, Riggle P, Harmison LT: A radioisotope fueled Stirling engine artificial heart power system. McDonnell Douglas Astronautics Company (MDAC) Paper WD 1421, Richland, Washington 1971

27. Miller RA, Glanfield EJ: Development of an electrical energy storage system for use with a circulatory assist device. Chapter 87 in RJ Hegyeli (ed): Artificial Heart Program Conference Proceedings, Washington, DC, US Government Printing Office, 1969

28. Mott WE, Cole DW, Jr: Development of a nuclear-powered artificial heart. Trans Am Soc Artif Intern Organs, 1972, pp 152–57

29. Newgard PM, Eilers GJ: Skin transformer and power conditioning components. Chapter 78 in RJ Hegyeli (ed): Artificial Heart Program Conference Proceedings. Washington, DC, US Government Printing Office, 1969

30. Norman JC, Molokhia FA, Harmison LT, Whalen RL, Huffman FN: An implantable nuclear-fueled circulatory support system I: systems analysis of conception, design, fabrication and initial in vivo testing. Ann Surg 176 (4):492, 1972

31. Norman JC, Whalen RL, Daly BDT, Migliore J, Huffman FN: An implantable abdominal left ventricular assist device (ALVAD). Clin Res 20(5):855, 1972

32. Norman JC, Huffman FN, Molokhia FA, Asimacopoulos PJ, Warren S: Implantable nuclear power sources for artificial hearts: progress report, two years after implantation in the dog. Abstracts X International Cong of the International Cardiovascular Soc in conjunction with the XXIV Congrès de la Société Internationale de Chirurgie, Moscow, August 12–28, 1971

33. Norman JC, Pegg G, Sandberg GW, Lee R, Huffman FN: Effects of intracorporeal heat and radiation on dogs. Proceedings of the Artificial Heart Program Conference, RJ Hegyeli (ed): Washington, DC, US Government Printing Office, 1969, p 901

34. Norman JC, Covelli VH, Bernhard WF, Spira J: Implantable nuclear fuel capsules for artificial hearts: in vivo dosimetry. Surg Forum 10:140–41, 1968

35. Norman JC, Covelli VH, Bernhard WF, Spira J: An implantable nuclear fuel capsule for artificial hearts. Am Soc Artif Intern Organs 14:204–8, 1968

36. Norman JC, Covelli VH, Bernhard WF, Spira J: In vivo nuclear power 16 and 25 watt Pu 238 sources for artificial hearts. Circulation (suppl VI) 38(4):49, 1968

37. Norman JC, Harvey RJ, Covelli VH, McCandless WJC, Bernhard WF: Implantable power sources: continuing studies. Proceedings of 20th Annual Conference on Engineering in Medicine and Biology 9:3, Boston, 1967

38. Norman JC, Covelli VH, McCandless WJC, Bernhard WF: Feasibility of implantable Pu-238 power sources for circulatory assist devices. Circulation suppl 36:200, 1967

39. Norman JC, LaFarge CG, Harvey RJ, Robinson TC, van Someren L, Bernhard WF: Heat dissipation: a common denominator of implantable power sources for cardiac prostheses. Surg Forum 17: 162, 1966

40. Paquin ML: The multi-foil thermal insulation development program—a status report. Proceedings Intersociety Energy Conversion Engineering Conference, 1969, p 408

41. Peterson GH, Kessler AG, Thorne GH, Clark RR, Wood OL: All fluid control system to couple a Stirling engine gas compressor to a left ventricular assist device. Chapter 92 in RJ Hegyeli (ed): Artificial Heart Program Conference Proceedings. Washington, DC, US Government Printing Office, 1969

42. Powell RS: Electric energy systems for artificial hearts. Third National Conference on Electronics in Medicine, April 13–15, 1971, Boston

43. Riggle P, Noble JE, Emigh SG, Martini WR, Harmison LT: Development of a Stirling engine power source for artificial heart applications: a program review. Sixth Intersociety Energy Conversion Engineering Conference Proceedings: 288–98, 1971

44. Riggle P, Noble J, Emigh SG, Martini WR: Development of a Stirling engine power source for artificial heart applications: a program review. McDonnell Douglas Astronautics Company (MDAC) Paper WD 1610, 1971

45. Robinson WJ, Migliore JJ, Arthur J, Fuqua J, Dove G: An abdominal left ventricular assist device (ALVAD): experimental physiologic analyses II. Trans Am Soc Artif Intern Organs 19:229, 1973

46. Sandberg GW: Implantable nuclear power for an artificial heart: studies of the effects of intracorporeal heat and radiation. Thesis, Harvard Medical School, 1970

47. Sandberg GW, Jr., Huffman FN, Norman JC: Implantable nuclear power sources for artificial organs: physiologic monitoring and pathologic effects I. Trans Am Soc Artif Intern Organs 17:172, 1970

48. Watrous JD, Smith TH, Greenborg J, Andelin RL: A radioisotope heat source for artificial heart heat engines. McDonnell Douglas Astronautics Company (MDAC) WD 1883, 1971

49. Whalen RL, Molokhia FA, Jeffery DL, Huffman FN: Implantable nuclear-fueled LVAD: progress report. European Surgical Research 4:370, 1972 (abstract #171)

50. Hughes DA, Faeser RJ, Daly BDT, et al: Nuclear-fueled circulatory support systems XII: current status. Trans Am Soc Artif Intern Organs 20-B:737, 1974

INDEX